Autism and Child Psychopathology Series

Series Editor

Johnny L. Matson
Department of Psychology, Louisiana State University, Baton Rouge, LA, USA

For further volumes:
http://www.springer.com/series/8665

Johnny L. Matson · Peter Sturmey

Editors

International Handbook of Autism and Pervasive Developmental Disorders

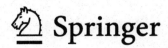 Springer

Editors
Johnny L. Matson
Department of Psychology
Louisiana State University
Baton Rouge
LA 70803, USA
johnmatson@aol.com

Peter Sturmey
Department of Psychology
Queens College
City University of New York
Flushing, NY 11367, USA
peter.sturmey@qc.cuny.edu

ISBN 978-1-4419-8064-9   e-ISBN 978-1-4419-8065-6
DOI 10.1007/978-1-4419-8065-6
Springer New York Dordrecht Heidelberg London

Library of Congress Control Number: 2011929778

Printed on acid-free paper

Springer is part of Springer Science+Business Media (www.springer.com)

Acknowledgements

We should like to thank Julie A. Worley and Alison M. Kozlowski for assistance in preparation of this manuscript.

Contents

Contributors

Trine Lise Bakken Psychiatric Department, Oslo University Hospital, Oslo, Norway, trinelise.bakken@ulleval.no

Bradley Bezilla The Hesley Group, Doncaster DN11 9HH, UK, brad.bezilla@hesleygroup.co.uk

Somer Bishop Kelly O'Leary Center for Autism Spectrum Disorders, Cincinnati Children's Hospital Medical Center, Cincinnati, OH 45229, USA, somer.bishop@cchmc.org

Asit B. Biswas Leicester Frith Hospital, Leicestershire Partnership NHS Trust, Leicester LE3 9QF, UK, asitbiswas@yahoo.co.uk

Sara Bobak Department of Psychiatry, The University of Michigan, Ann Arbor, MI 48109, USA, sbobak@med.umich.edu

Colin Andrew Campbell Department of Educational and Counselling Psychology, McGill University, Montreal, QC, Canada H3A 1B1, colin.campbell2@mail.mcgill.ca

Ira L. Cohen Department of Psychology, New York State Institute for Basic Research in Developmental Disabilities, Staten Island, NY 10314, USA, ira.cohen@opwdd.ny.gov

Susan Crawford Department of Education, University College Cork, Cork, Ireland, sc.miltown@gmail.com

Allison B. Cunningham Department of Psychology, University of California, San Diego, CA 92093-0109, USA, abcunning@ucsd.edu

Anthony J. Cuvo Center for Autism Spectrum Disorders, Southern Illinois University, Carbondale, IL 62901, USA, acuvo@siu.edu

Sahar Davarya Department of Psychology, Loyola College in Maryland, Baltimore, MD 21210, USA, sarah.davarya@gmail.com

James M. Day Center for Psychology of Religion, Catholic University of Louvain, 1348 Louvain-la-Neuve, Belgium, james.day@uclouvain.be

Dennis R. Dixon The Center for Autism and Related Disorders, Tarzana, CA 91356, USA, d.dixon@centerforautism.com

Sarah Dufek Department of Psychology, University of California, San Diego, CA 92093-0109, USA, sdufek@ucsd.edu

Svein Eikeseth Faculty of Behavioral Science, Akershus University College, N-2001 Lillestrøm, Norway, svein.eikeseth@hiak.no

Mayada Elsabbagh Centre for Brain and Cognitive Development, Birkbeck, University of London, London WC1E 7HX, UK, m.elsabbagh@bbk.ac.uk

Wendy H. Fitch Cleveland County Schools, Shelby, NC, USA, wfitch@clevelandcountyschools.org

Eric Fombonne Department of Psychiatry, Montreal Children's Hospital, Montreal, QC, Canada H3Z 1P2, eric.fombonne@mcgill.ca

Frederick Furniss School of Psychology, University of Leicester, Leicester LE1 7LT, UK, fred.furniss@hesleygroup.co.uk

Eynat Gal Department of Occupational Therapy, University of Haifa, Haifa 31905, Israel, egal@univ.haifa.ac.il

Mohammad Ghaziuddin Department of Psychiatry, The University of Michigan, Ann Arbor, MI 48109, USA, mghaziud@umich.edu

Daniel Gih Department of Psychiatry, The University of Michigan, Ann Arbor, MI 48109, USA, dgih@med.umich.edu

Christopher L. Gillberg Gillberg Neuropsychiatry Centre, Gothenburg University, Gothenburg, Sweden, christopher.gillberg@pediat.gu.se

Matthew S. Goodwin Massachusetts Institute of Technology, Program in Media Arts and Sciences, Cambridge, MA 02139-4307, USA, mgoodwin@media.mit.edu

Doreen Granpeesheh The Center for Autism and Related Disorders, Tarzana, CA 91356, USA, d.granpeesheh@centerforautism.com

Olive Healy School of Psychology, National University of Ireland, Galway, Ireland, olive.healy@nuigalway.ie

Sissel Berge Helverschou The National Autism Unit, Rikshospitalet, Oslo University Hospital, 0027 Oslo, Norway, s.b.helverschou@rikshospitalet.no

Thomas S. Higbee Department of Special Education and Rehabilitation, Utah State University, Logan, UT 84322-2865, USA, tom.higbee@usu.edu

Claudia List Hilton Department of Psychiatry, Washington University School of Medicine, St. Louis, MO 63110, USA, hiltonc@psychiatry.wustl.edu

Steve Holburn Institute for Basic Research in Developmental Disabilities, Staten Island, NY 10314, USA, holbursc@infionline.net

Julie K. Irwin Department of Psychology, University of Victoria, Victoria, BC, Canada V8W3P5, jkirwin@uvic.ca

Aaron A. Jones Quality Behavioral Solutions, Inc., Holliston, Massachusetts 01746, USA, djones@qbscompanies.com

Kimberly A. Kerns Department of Psychology, University of Victoria, Victoria, BC, Canada V8W3P5, kkerns@uvic.ca

Alison M. Kozlowski Department of Psychology, Louisiana State University, Baton Rouge, LA 70803, USA, alikoz@gmail.com

Debomoy K. Lahiri Department of Psychiatry, Psychiatry Research Institute, Indiana University School of Medicine, Indianapolis, IN 46202, USA, dlahiri@iupui.edu

Giulio E. Lancioni Department of Psychology, University of Bari, Bari, Italy, g.lancioni@psico.uniba.it

Geraldine Leader School of Psychology, National University of Ireland, Galway, Ireland, geraldine.leader@nuigalway.ie

Luc Lecavalier Ohio State University, Columbus, OH 43210, USA, luc.lecavalier@osumc.edu

Sophie E. Lind Department of Psychology, Durham University, Science Site, South Road, Durham, DH1 3LE, UK, sophie.lind@durham.ac.uk

Jennifer MacSween Department of Psychology, University of Victoria, Victoria, BC, Canada V8W3P5, macsween@uvic.ca

Lisa Madden Department of Educational and Counselling Psychology, McGill University, Montreal, QC, Canada H3A 1B1, lisa.madden@mail.mcgill.ca

Sara Mahan Department of Psychology, Louisiana State University, Baton Rouge, LA 70803, USA, srm101010@gmail.com

Garry L. Martin Department of Psychology, Rm. 129, St. Paul's College, University of Manitoba, Winnipeg, MB, Canada, gmartin@cc.umanitoba.ca

Harald Martinsen Institute of Special Needs Education, University of Oslo, Oslo, Norway, harald.martinsen@isp.uio.no

Johnny L. Matson Department of Psychology, Louisiana State University, Baton Rouge, LA 70803, USA, johnmatson@aol.com

Jane McCarthy Institute of Psychiatry, King's College London, London, UK, jane.m.mccarthy@kcl.ac.uk

Sarah Mohiuddin Department of Psychiatry, The University of Michigan, Ann Arbor, MI 48109, USA, smohiudd@umich.edu

Lauren Moskowitz Department of Psychology, Stony Brook University, Stony Brook, NY, USA, ljmoskowitz@gmail.com

Nathalie Nader-Grosbois Faculty of Psychology, Catholic University of Louvain, 1348 Louvain-la-Neuve, Belgium, nathalie.nader@uclouvain.be

Nozomi Naoi Okanoya Emotional Information Project, Japan Science Technology Agency, ERATO, and Graduate School of Education, Kinki District Invention Center, 14 Yoshida-Kawara-cho, Sakyo-ku, Kyoto 606-8305, Japan, nnaoi@educ.kyoto-u.ac.jp

Megan Norris University of Rochester Medical Center, Rochester, NY 14642, USA, megan.norris@osumc.edu

Kyle Pushkarenko Department of Kinesiology, Division of Science, Medicine Hat College, Medicine Hat, AB, Canada, kpushkarenko@mhc.ab.ca

Greg Reid Department of Kinesiology and Physical Education, McGill University, Montreal, QC, Canada H2W 1S4, greg.reid@mcgill.ca

Dennis H. Reid Carolina Behavior Analysis and Support Center, Morganton, NC 28680, USA, drhmc@vistatech.net

Joel E. Ringdahl Psychology Division, Department of Pediatrics, University of Iowa Children's Hosptial, Iowa City, IA 52242, USA, joel-ringdahl@uiowa.edu

Laura Schreibman Department of Psychology, University of California, San Diego, CA 92093-0109, USA, lschreibman@ucsd.edu

Laura J. Seiverling Department of Psychology, Queens College and The Graduate Center, City University of New York, Flushing, NY 11367, USA, ljs1284@gmail.com

Tyra P. Sellers Department of Special Education and Rehabilitation, Utah State University, Logan, UT 84322-2865, USA, tyrasellers@mac.com

Stacy Shumway Pediatrics and Development Neuroscience Branch, National Institute of Mental Health, Bethesda, MD 20892-1255, USA, shumways@mail.nih.gov

Nirbhay N. Singh American Health and Wellness Institute, Verona, VA 24484, USA, nirbsingh52@aol.com

Judy Singh American Health, Wellness Institute, Verona, VA 24484, USA, jsingh@ahwinstitute.com

Marlena N. Smith The Center for Autism and Related Disorders, Tarzana, CA 91356, USA, m.smith@centerforautism.com

Anne V. Snow Child Study Center, Yale University, New Haven, CT 06520, USA, annesnow@gmail.com

Deborah K. Sokol Department of Neurology, Riley Hospital for Children, Indiana University School of Medicine, Indianapolis, IN 46202, USA, dksokol@iupui.edu

Kerri L. Staples Faculty of Kinesiology and Health Studies, University of Regina, Regina, SK, Canada S4S 0A2, kerri.staples@uregina.ca

Peter Sturmey Department of Psychology, Queens College and The Graduate Center, City University of New York, Flushing, NY 11367, USA, psturmey@gmail.com

Jonathan Tarbox The Center for Autism and Related Disorders, Tarzana, CA 91356, USA, j.tarbox@centerforautism.com

Kendra Thomson Department of Psychology, St.Amant Research Centre, University of Manitoba, Winnipeg, MB (Manitoba), Canada, kthomson@stamant.mb.ca

Audrey Thurm Pediatrics and Development Neuroscience Branch, National Institute of Mental Health, Bethesda, MD 20892-1255, USA, athurm@mail.nih.gov

Elias Tsakanikos Department of Psychology, Roehampton University, London, UK, elias.tsakanikos@kcl.ac.uk

Jenny E. Tuzikow Institute for Basic Research in Developmental Disabilities, Staten Island, NY 10314, USA, jtuzikow@gmail.com

Lisa Underwood Institute of Psychiatry, King's College London, London, UK, lisa.underwood@kcl.ac.uk

Kerri Walters Department of Psychology, St.Amant Research Centre, University of Manitoba, Winnipeg, MB, Canada, kwalters@stamant.mb.ca

John Ward-Horner Department of Psychology, Queens College and The Graduate Center, City University of New York, Flushing, NY 11367, USA, wardhornerj@yahoo.com

David M. Williams Department of Psychology, Durham University, Science Site, South Road, Durham, DH1 3LE, UK, david.williams@durham.ac.uk

Keith E. Williams Feeding Program, Penn State Hershey Medical Center, Hershey, PA 17036, USA, feedingprogram@hmc.psu.edu

Alan S.W. Winton School of Psychology, Massey University, Palmerston North, New Zealand, a.winton@massey.ac.nz

Julie A. Worley Louisiana State University, Baton Rouge, LA 70803, USA, jules31h@hotmail.com

J. Helen Yoo Applied Behavior Analysis Laboratory, Department of Psychology, New York State Institute for Basic Research in Developmental Disabilities, Staten Island, NY 10314, USA, jhelen.yoo@opwdd.ny.gov

C.T. Yu Department of Psychology, St.Amant Research Centre, University of Manitoba, Winnipeg, MB, Canada, yu@stamant.mb.ca

About the Contributors

Trine Lise Bakken is educated as a psychiatric nurse and is employed as a researcher in the psychiatric department for people with intellectual disabilities and autism spectrum disorders at Oslo University Hospital, Norway. She has extensive experience in general psychiatry and for approximately 15 years has worked with mental health problems in individuals with intellectual disabilities. Her main area of research is schizophrenia and other psychoses in individuals with intellectual disabilities and autism spectrum disorders.

Brad Bezilla is a board certified behavior analyst and currently the head of Applied Behavior Analysis services with the Hesley Group in South Yorkshire, UK. He is also a member of the advisory panel for the UK ABA Competencies Project. Prior to moving to the United Kingdom, Brad worked for the May Institute in the United States for 18 years in a variety of roles. He was also a senior staff member with the National Autism Center, a continuing education instructor in applied behavior analysis through Fitchburg State College in Massachusetts, and a certified special education teacher.

Somer Bishop is a clinical psychologist and an assistant professor in the Division of Developmental and Behavioral Pediatrics at Cincinnati Children's Hospital Medical Center. Her research has focused mainly on assessment and diagnosis of autism spectrum disorders with a particular emphasis on differentiating symptom profiles in ASD from other developmental disorders. Dr. Bishop's current projects are funded by National Institute for Mental Health and National Institute for Child Health and Development and involve the development of improved screening tools for use in research studies of autism spectrum disorders.

Asit B. Biswas is a consultant psychiatrist with the Leicestershire Partnership National Health Service Trust and is training program director for higher specialist training in Psychiatry of Learning Disability at the East Midlands Deanery, Leicester, UK. Other appointments held include academic secretary to the Faculty of the Psychiatry of Learning Disability of the Royal College of Psychiatrists, London. His clinical and research interests include autism, mental illness, and challenging behavior in people with intellectual disability and the behavioral phenotype of velocardiofacial syndrome.

Sara Bobak is a research fellow in child and adolescent psychiatry at the University of Michigan, Ann Arbor.

Colin Andrew Campbell is currently completing his Ph.D. in school/applied child psychology at McGill University. His research there focuses on executive function. He has worked as a research assistant under Dr. Fombonne on a number of autism research projects at the Montreal Children's Hospital.

Ira L. Cohen is the chair of the Psychology Department at the New York State Institute for Basic Research where he also serves as head of the Behavioral Assessment and Research Laboratory. He received his doctorate in psychobiology from Rutgers University and his postdoctoral training at New York University Medical Center in experimental psychopathology and behavior therapy. He has performed research in autism since 1978 and his interests here include assessment and diagnosis, genotype–phenotype associations, early detection and intervention, assessing treatment outcome, and neural network models.

Susan Crawford is lecturer in the Physical Education and Sports Studies Department at University College Cork in the areas of health, motor development, adapted physical activity, and sports medicine. Her research interests lie in the areas of both motor learning and adapted physical activity.

Allison B. Cunningham is a graduate student in the University of California at San Diego Autism Intervention Research Program where she is pursuing a Ph.D. in experimental psychology. Her current research focuses on investigating methods of treatment individualization for children with autism, methods of matching child and family variables to appropriate treatments and on combining interventions into comprehensive child treatment programs.

Anthony J. Cuvo is emeritus professor of behavior analysis and therapy and emeritus founding director of the Center for Autism Spectrum Disorders at Southern Illinois University, a former distinguished research fellow of the National Institute of Handicapped Research, and fellow of the American Psychological Association, the American Psychological Society, and American Association of Mental Retardation. Dr. Cuvo has edited 2 books and authored 14 book chapters, over 100 journal articles, and other professional publications.

Sahar Davarya is currently a clinical psychology thesis track M.S. student at Loyola University in Maryland. She received her B.S. from the University of Maryland, Baltimore County, in developmental psychology. Her interest is studying emerging adults with a diagnosis of high-functioning autism who are transitioning out of school and trying to navigate the challenges of adult life.

James Meredith Day is professor in Catholic University of Louvain, Louvain-la-Neuve, Belgium, Institute for Psychological Science, Health and Psychological Development and Psychology of Religion Research Centers. He serves on the editorial and review boards of many journals. His scholarly publications include five books of which he is co-editor. He co-directs, with Michael Commons, at Harvard University, the project in cognitive complexity, religious cognition, and moral decision making.

Dennis R. Dixon is the director of analytics at the Center for Autism and Related Disorders. He received his Ph.D. in clinical psychology from Louisiana State University with a focus in developmental disabilities. He completed a postdoctoral fellowship at the Johns Hopkins University School of Medicine and specialized in the treatment of severe challenging behaviors. He currently serves on the editorial board of *Research in Developmental Disabilities* and *Research in Autism Spectrum Disorders*.

Sarah Dufek is a graduate student in the University of California, San Diego, Autism Intervention Research Program where she is pursuing a Ph.D. in experimental psychology. Sarah's current research is focused on examining practitioner utilization of evidence-based practice in community settings for diagnostic and intervention purposes.

Svein Eikeseth is a professor of psychology at the Department of Behavioral Science at Akershus University College, Norway. He is the founder and the director of the NOVA Institute for Children with Developmental Disorders, clinical and research director of UK Young Autism Project, and clinical and research director of Banyan Center, Stockholm, Sweden. Dr. Eikeseth has published a number of articles and book chapters on behavior analysis, conducted several outcome studies evaluating behavioral interventions for children with developmental disabilities, and authored and co-authored several papers on meta-analysis and effect evaluations of interventions for children with autism.

Mayada Elsabbagh completed her graduate training in the United Kingdom, Canada, and the United States. Her research in the areas of early infancy and developmental disorders is focused on understanding the brain basis of behavioral genetic disorders. This is achieved through converging methods to study brain development including EEG and eye tracking with behavioral and clinical assessment tools. Mayada is also active in public engagement with science, particularly in low- and middle-income countries.

Wendy H. Fitch   is the senior behavior analyst and lead school psychologist for Cleveland County Schools in North Carolina. She is a board certified behavior analyst and assists with educational programming for students with autism throughout the school system. Her duties include system-wide training of classroom and support staff in behavior analysis applications and directs parent-training and home-based intervention programs for young children with autism.

Eric Fombonne   trained in child psychiatry in France and was senior lecturer and reader at the Institute of Psychiatry, London, UK. He was then appointed as tenured professor of psychiatry at McGill University, head of the Division of Child Psychiatry at McGill University, and director of the Department of Psychiatry at Montreal Children's Hospital and holds the Canada Research Chair in Child Psychiatry. At Montreal Children's Hospital, he directs the autism spectrum disorder program, the largest clinical program in Quebec. His research activities encompass genetic, longitudinal, and epidemiological studies and clinical trials. He has published over 220 articles in peer-reviewed journals, 40 chapters in books, and is on the editorial board of several journals in the field of autism and child psychiatry.

Frederick Furniss   is a clinical psychologist with the Hesley Group, Doncaster, UK, and honorary lecturer with the School of Psychology, University of Leicester, UK. His main clinical and research interests are in assessment and intervention with severely challenging behavior in people with intellectual disabilities and/or autism spectrum disorders.

Eynat Gal   is an occupational therapist, specializing in the area of developmental disabilities and pervasive developmental disabilities and a faculty member of the Department of Occupational Therapy, University of Haifa. Her research focuses on investigation of underlying mechanisms that stand at the base of autistic behaviors such as sensory and social deficits, as well as functional aspects of autism and other developmental disabilities.

Mohammad Ghaziuddin   is professor of psychiatry at the University of Michigan, Ann Arbor, and director of child and adolescent psychiatry training. His main areas of clinical and research interest are the classification and comorbidity of autism spectrum disorders.

Daniel Gih   is a clinical fellow in child and adolescent psychiatry at the University of Michigan, Ann Arbor.

Christopher L. Gillberg   is professor of child and adolescent psychiatry at Gothenburg University, Sweden, visiting professor at Glasgow University, and honorary professor at the Institute of Child Health, London. He is consultant at Yorkhill Hospital, Glasgow, and the National Centre for Young People with Epilepsy, Lingfield. Professor Gillberg is the founding editor of *European Child & Adolescent Psychiatry* and is or has been editor of the *Journal of Autism and Developmental Disorders, Autism, Journal of Attention Disorders*, and the *Journal of Child Psychology and Psychiatry*. He is the recipient of The Swedish King's Medal for his contributions to child and adolescent psychiatry.

Matthew S. Goodwin   is the director of clinical research at the Massachusetts Institute of Technology, Media Laboratory, associate director of research at the Groden Center, Rhode Island, and co-chair of the Autism Speaks–Innovative Technology for Autism Initiative. He has an adjunct associate research scientist appointment in the Department of Psychiatry and Human Behavior at Brown University and is an adjunct assistant professor in the Department of Psychology at the University of Rhode Island. His research interests include developing innovative technologies for behavioral assessment, especially for use with developmentally disabled populations.

Doreen Granpeesheh   is the founder and executive director of the Center for Autism and Related Disorders and the founder and president of the Board of Autism Care and Treatment Today. She is a board certified behavior analyst with over 30 years of experience providing behavioral therapy to children with autism spectrum disorders. She currently serves on the US Autism and Asperger's Association Scientific Advisory Board and the Autism Society of America National Board.

Olive Healy   is lecturer in psychology in the National University of Ireland, Galway, and a certified behavior analyst with the Behaviour Analyst Certification Board®. She was responsible for opening and directing the first government-funded applied behavior analysis school for autism spectrum disorder in Ireland and has been involved in the establishment of four other treatment centers.

Sissel Berge Helverschou   is licensed as psychologist and specialist in clinical psychology within the field of psychological habilitation. She is an experienced psychologist in the field of autism and has for the last 10 years worked as researcher at the National Autism Unit, Oslo University Hospital, Norway. Her research has addressed psychiatric comorbidity in autism.

Thomas S. Higbee   is associate professor in the Department of Special Education and Rehabilitation at Utah State University and director of the Autism Support Services: Education, Research, and Training (ASSERT) program, an early intensive behavioral intervention training and research center for children with autism which he founded in 2003. He is a doctoral-level board certified behavior analyst whose research focuses on behavioral assessment and intervention strategies for individuals with autism and other developmental disabilities. He is currently an associate editor for the *Journal of Applied Behavior Analysis (JABA)* and has served on the editorial boards of *Behavior Analysis in Practice*.

Claudia List Hilton   is an occupational therapist, has served on the occupational therapy faculties at Washington University and Saint Louis University in St. Louis, Missouri, and has completed a postdoctoral fellowship in the Department of Psychiatry at Washington University School of Medicine. Her research has focused on relationships between ethnicity, sensory responsiveness, and social and motor impairment. She currently serves on the occupational therapy and psychiatry faculties at Washington University School of Medicine in St. Louis, Missouri.

Steve Holburn   is head of the Intervention Research Laboratory at the New York State Institute for Basic Research in Developmental Disabilities, a board certified behavior analyst and a behavioral consultant at AHRC, New York City. He has worked in the field of developmental services for over 30 years and has authored books, chapters, and articles in a variety of areas, including person-centered planning, quality of life, health promotion, assistive technology, self-injurious behavior, and parents with intellectual disabilities.

Julie K. Irwin   is a graduate student in the Clinical Neuropsychology Program at the University of Victoria. She is interested in intelligence and in the development of executive functions, attention, language, and memory and the impact of aerobic exercise on cognitive, social, psychological, and behavioral outcomes in typically and atypically developing children.

Aaron A. Jones   received his master's degree in behavior analysis from the University of North Texas in 2007. He has worked as a behavior analyst for 10 years serving various populations, including individuals with developmental disabilities and child victims of abuse and neglect. He is an active member of the Association for Behavior Analysis International. He specializes in teaching behavior analysis and is also involved in efforts to increase employment opportunities for behavior analysts in the United Kingdom and Europe.

Kimberly A. Kerns   is an associate professor in the Psychology Department, Clinical Neuropsychology Program, at the University of Victoria. Her research interests are in developmental and pediatric clinical neuropsychology, the development of aspects of cognitive processing including attention, executive functions, and memory, in both typically and atypically developing children including children with prenatal alcohol exposure, attention deficit hyperactivity disorder, autism, and acquired brain injury. Primary clinical interests include the pediatric cognitive rehabilitation and remediation and social and emotional functioning of families and children with atypical development.

Alison M. Kozlowski received her Bachelor of Arts degree in psychology from Boston University. She was then employed at the May Institute, Randolph, Massachusetts, as the head teacher of a classroom for children with autism spectrum disorders. She subsequently enrolled in Louisiana State University's Clinical Psychology Doctoral Program. Her current clinical and research interests are the assessment and treatment of individuals with autism spectrum and other developmental disabilities, with a particular emphasis on challenging behaviors and communication training.

Giulio E. Lancioni is professor in the Department of Psychology at the University of Bari, Italy. His research interests include the development and evaluation of assistive technologies, social skills training, and strategies for examining and teaching choice and preference with individuals with severe/profound and multiple disabilities.

Debomoy K. Lahiri is professor of neurobiology, psychiatry and molecular genetics at Indiana University School of Medicine, Indianapolis. He has published over 225 papers on molecular genetics, neurobiology, and Alzheimer's disease and is the editor-in-chief of *Current Alzheimer Research*. He recently has authored *Protective Strategies for Neurodegenerative Diseases* published by the New York Academy of Sciences.

Geraldine Leader is lecturer in psychology at the National University of Ireland, Galway, where she directs the M.Sc. in applied behavior analysis and launched the structured Ph.D. in applied behavior analysis in 2008. Geraldine was the founding chair of the Division of Behaviour Analysis in the Psychological Society of Ireland and a member of the International Association for Behavior Analysis (ABA) and the European Association of Behaviour Analysis (EABA). Her research interests lie in the field of applied behavior analysis with a special interest in autism.

Luc Lecavalier is associate professor of psychology and psychiatry at the Ohio State University. He is a clinical psychologist and directs an outpatient treatment unit for children with developmental disabilities and behavior problems at the Nisonger Center. His research interests include diagnosis and measurement and behavior/psychiatric problems. In 2008, he was recipient of the Early Career Awards given by the American Association on Intellectual and Developmental Disabilities and Division 33 of the American Psychological Association. He currently serves on the editorial board of the *Journal of Autism and Developmental Disorders*.

Sophie E. Lind is lecturer in psychology at Durham University, United Kingdom, and holds a 3-year grant from the Economic and Social Research Council to explore episodic memory, episodic future thinking, imagination, and spatial navigation in autism. Prior to this, she was a member of the Autism Research Group at City University London, where she completed her Ph.D. and her subsequent Autism Speaks (USA)-funded postdoctoral fellowship. Her research focuses on a range of cognitive abilities in autism including memory, theory of mind, self-awareness, temporal cognition, and language.

Jennifer MacSween is a graduate student in the Clinical Neuropsychology Program at the University of Victoria. Her research interests are in the development of executive functions, attention, and memory and how cognitive functions might be improved in children with autism, fetal alcohol syndrome disorder, epilepsy, and attention hyperactivity disorder. Jennifer has worked with Dr. Kerns and the Department of Computer Science at University of Victoria designing new computerized training tasks that improve working memory and attentional abilities.

Lisa Madden is currently completing her Ph.D. in school/applied child psychology at McGill University, where her research focuses on parenting stress and behavioral difficulties. She has worked in the field of autism for over 10 years in both clinical and research capacities.

Sara Mahan is currently pursuing her doctoral degree in clinical psychology at Louisiana State University. Her research focuses on symptom presentation, assessment, psychotropic medication use, and intervention in autism spectrum disorder across the life span. Her clinical experience focuses on the assessment and intervention of those with intellectual disability and/or autism spectrum disorders. She has experience working with people who live at home with family, community homes, and developmental centers.

Garry L. Martin is a distinguished professor emeritus in psychology at the University of Manitoba, Canada. He has co-authored 8 books and over 150 scientific papers on autism, developmental disabilities, and sport psychology. His co-authored book on behavior modification is used as a primary text in many universities in 14 countries and has been translated into Spanish, Italian, Portuguese, Chinese, and Korean. He has received numerous honors and awards including induction into the Royal Society of Canada and the 2010 Award from the Canadian Psychological Association for Distinguished Contributions to Education and Training in Psychology.

Harald Martinsen is licensed as psychologist and professor at the Institute of Special Needs Education, University of Oslo, Norway. He has published approximately 250 scientific and professional books, articles, and papers on disabilities, in particular autism. He was head of the Autism Program (1993–1997) and the Autism Network (1998–2006), established to enhance professional competence and improve the development and provision of services in Norway.

Johnny L. Matson has spent his career as a researcher and is academically involved in the training of doctoral-level clinical psychologists specializing in developmental disabilities. He is the major professor of 48 Ph.D.s, many of whom have served as professors in major universities. He is the founding editor and editor-in-chief of *Research in Autism Spectrum Disorders* and *Research in Developmental Disabilities*. He has authored over 600 publications, including 34 books and 16 tests. He previously served on the psychology and psychiatric faculties at the University of Pittsburg. For the last 23 years he has been a professor at Louisiana State University. He is currently a professor and distinguished research master and director of clinical training in the Department of Psychology at Louisiana State University.

Jane McCarthy is consultant psychiatrist for the Mental Health in Learning Disability Service, South London, and Maudsley National Health Service Foundation Trust, Guy's Hospital, London, and lead for Research and Development, Estia Centre, Health Service and Population Research Department, Institute of Psychiatry. Her main areas of research are the mental health needs of people with intellectual disability including those with autism spectrum conditions. She is secretary to European Association for Mental Health in Intellectual Disability and co-editor of *Advances in Mental Health and Intellectual Disabilities Journal*.

Sarah Mohiuddin is an instructor in the Department of Psychiatry, University of Michigan, Ann Arbor, and director of Consultation-Liaison Psychiatry at the University of Michigan Medical Center, Ann Arbor.

Lauren Moskowitz is a doctoral candidate in clinical psychology at Stony Brook University (SBU). She studied under the late Dr. Edward (Ted) Carr and is currently a clinician and supervisor at Stoney Brook University's Psychological Center and Anxiety Clinic. She served as an adjunct lecturer at Hunter College.

Nathalie Nader-Grosbois is professor in the Catholic University of Louvain, Belgium. She focuses her studies on dysfunction in cognitive, communicative, emotional development in children and adolescents with intellectual disability, autism, or behavior disorders in the areas of self-regulation, self-concept, the Theory of Mind, socio-emotional competences, and resilience in these people. Her work focuses on the links between research and intervention. She is the author of 5 books, 30 chapters in joint publication, and about 40 manuscripts in peer-reviewed journals.

Nozomi Naoi is a postdoctoral fellow of Okanoya Emotional Information Project, Exploratory Research for Advanced Technology Japan Agency of Science and Technology at Kyoto University, Japan. She received her Ph.D. from Keio University, Tokyo, in 2009. Her research interests include the effect of behavioral intervention on brain plasticity in children with autism spectrum disorders, the development of behavioral intervention strategies targeting pre-verbal social skills, such as joint attention and imitation, and also finding early indicators of autism spectrum disorders.

Megan Norris is a postdoctoral fellow at the University of Rochester Medical Center, USA. She earned her doctorate degree from the Intellectual and Developmental Disabilities Psychology Program at Ohio State University. She has conducted research on psychopathology in children and adolescents with intellectual disability, the structure of autism spectrum disorder symptoms, assessment of dual diagnosis, and instrument development and refinement.

Kyle Pushkarenko is an instructor in the Department of Kinesiology at Medicine Hat College, Alberta, Canada. He has extensive experience working as a physical educator, classroom teacher, behavior therapist, educator, caseworker and recreation therapist working with children with autism spectrum and other developmental disorders. Kyle is also a volleyball coach at the varsity level and last season received recognition as coach of the year in the Alberta Colleges Athletic Conference.

Dennis H. Reid is director of the Carolina Behavior Analysis and Support Center in Morganton, North Carolina, USA. He has over 35 years experience as a supervisor, consultant, and clinician working with individuals who have autism and other developmental disabilities and their support staff. He is a fellow of the Association for Behavior Analysis International and 2006 recipient of the American Association on Intellectual and Developmental Disabilities Research Award. Dr. Reid is also the senior author of the AAIDD *Supervisor Training Curriculum: Evidence-Based Ways to Promote Work Quality and Enjoyment Among Support Staff.*

Greg Reid is professor in the Department of Kinesiology and Physical Education, McGill University. He has been involved with adapted physical activity for over 30 years and has supervised numerous graduate students whose research has been related to motor development and teaching strategies for individuals with autism and developmental disorders. He is the former editor of *Adapted Physical Activity Quarterly* and past-president of the International Federation of Adapted Physical Activity. He is an international fellow of the American Academy of Kinesiology and Physical Education and fellow of the North American Society of Health, Physical Education, Recreation, Sport, and Dance.

Joel E. Ringdahl is assistant professor in the Department of Pediatrics' Division of Psychology at the University of Iowa's Carver College of Medicine. His clinical work and research focuses on the behavior analytic approach to the assessment and treatment of severe behavior disorders exhibited by children and adults with developmental disabilities.

Laura Schreibman is a distinguished professor of psychology at the University of California, San Diego, and directs the University of California, San Diego, Autism Intervention Research Program, a Federally funded research program focusing on the experimental analysis and treatment of autism. Her research interests include naturalistic behavioral interventions, such as pivotal response training, development of individualized treatment protocols, translation of empirically based treatments into community settings, generalization of behavior change, and parent training. She is co-investigator on the University of California, San Diego, Autism Center of Excellence and a grant from the U.S. Department of Education. She is the author of 3 books, including *The Science and Fiction of Autism* (2005) published by Harvard University Press, and over 140 research articles and book chapters.

Laura J. Seiverling recently completed her doctorate of philosophy in learning processes and behavior analysis at the Graduate Center, City University of New York. Her doctoral dissertation involved training parents to conduct a procedure to decrease food selectivity in children with autism spectrum disorders. Currently, she is a postdoctoral fellow at the Westchester Institute for Human Development in Westchester, New York.

Tyra P. Sellers is a board certified behavior analyst with a master's degree in special education from San Francisco State University and a law degree from the University of San Francisco. She has 19 years experience working with individuals with disabilities in a variety of settings. She is currently pursuing her Ph.D. in special education/disabilities disciplines with an emphasis in applied behavior analysis at Utah State University.

Stacy Shumway is a postdoctoral research fellow at the National Institutes of Health. She is a speech-language pathologist by training and has several years experience working with young children with autism spectrum disorders. Her research interests include improving early identification and intervention for children with communication delays, particularly children with autism.

Judy Singh is a research scientist at ONE Research Institute in Midlothian, Virginia, USA. Her current interests are in program evaluation, personal narratives, and the use of mindfulness in daily life.

Nirbhay N. Singh is a senior scientist at ONE Research Institute in Midlothian, Virginia, USA. His current interests are in developing and evaluating mindfulness-based service delivery systems.

Marlena N. Smith is a research and development assistant at the Center for Autism and Related Disorders. Her current research interests include early detection, assessment, and behavioral interventions for autism spectrum disorders.

Anne V. Snow is a postdoctoral associate at the Yale Child Study Center. She earned her doctoral degree from a joint program in clinical psychology and intellectual and developmental disabilities at Ohio State University. Her research interests include early identification of the signs of autism spectrum disorders, the development of more refined screening measures, and understanding the trajectory of ASD symptoms throughout early development. Her clinical work focuses on diagnostic assessments of young children with ASDs.

Deborah K. Sokol is associate professor of neurology at Indiana University School of Medicine, Indianapolis, USA. She has published over 50 articles within the fields of pediatric neuropsychology and pediatric neurology.

Kerri L. Staples is an assistant professor in the Faculty of Kinesiology and Health Studies at the University of Regina, Saskatchewan, Canada. She has over 12 years of experience providing individualized instruction to children in a variety of adapted physical education and inclusive programs. Her research focuses on how children with autism spectrum disorders learn, plan, and perform fundamental movement skills, the acquisition of movement skills, and promotion of successful experiences in the physical activity domain for children of all ability levels.

Peter Sturmey is professor of psychology at Queens College and The Graduate Center, City University of New York, and a member of the Learning Processes and Behavior Analysis and Neuropsychology doctoral programs at City University of New York. He has published over 150 articles and 15 books on developmental disabilities. His current research focuses on applied behavior analysis and staff and parent training.

Jonathan Tarbox is the director of research and development at the Center for Autism and Related Disorders. He currently serves on the board of editors for the *Journal of Applied Behavior Analysis*, *The Analysis of Verbal Behavior*, and *Behavior Analysis in Practice* and is the president of the Nevada Association for Behavior Analysis. His primary research interests include verbal behavior, rule-governed behavior, private events, and recovery from autism.

Kendra Thomson has co-authored a number of scientific papers on discrete trials teaching with children with autism, preference assessment research, and sport psychology. She has also given 11 presentations at international psychology conferences and held a fellowship from the Social Sciences and Humanities Research Council of Canada during her Ph.D. program.

Audrey Thurm is a licensed child clinical psychologist and a staff scientist in the Pediatrics and Developmental Neuroscience Branch, part of the Intramural Research Program of the National Institute of Mental Health. She specializes in assessment of autism spectrum disorders and other neurodevelopmental disorders. Her research interests include longitudinal studies of the early diagnosis of autism and specific subtypes and onset patterns of autism. Dr. Thurm has served as an investigator on research projects focusing on clinical investigations and novel treatments for autism.

Elias Tsakanikos is lecturer and course director for the M.Sc. mental health in learning disabilities at Kings' College London. His background is in individual differences and neuropsychology and his current research activities on co-morbid psychopathology and care pathways in adults with autism fall within the Estia Centre and the Department of Forensic and Neurodevelopmental Science, Institute of Psychiatry, King's College London.

Jenny E. Tuzikow is senior behavior analyst in the Applied Behavior Analysis Laboratory at the New York State Institute for Basic Research in Developmental Disabilities and a licensed psychologist, school psychologist, and board certified behavior analyst. She has provided assessment and treatment to individuals with developmental disabilities in outpatient, inpatient, and educational settings for 10 years and has presented internationally on the assessment and treatment of problem behaviors displayed by individuals with autism.

Lisa Underwood is a health service researcher from the United Kingdom with a background in psychology. Having previously worked at the Royal College of Psychiatrists and the Institute of Education, she is now based at the Estia Centre, Institute of Psychiatry, King's College London, United Kingdom, specializing in research on the mental health of people with intellectual and developmental disabilities. Her research interests include mental health and service use of adults with autism and intellectual disability.

Kerri Walters is a Ph.D. candidate in psychology at the University of Manitoba, Canada. She has co-authored a number of scientific papers in the area of developmental disabilities, including generalization programming, preference assessment research, and the assessment of basic learning abilities. She has also given 24 presentations at international and local psychology conferences and held a fellowship from the Social Sciences and Humanities Research Council of Canada during her Ph.D. program.

John Ward-Horner is a doctoral candidate in the Learning Processes and Behavior Analysis psychology subprogram at Queens College and The Graduate Center of the City University of New York. His research interests include training parents and employees to teach individuals with developmental disabilities and conducting component analyses of behavioral treatment packages.

David M. Williams is lecturer in psychology at Durham University, United Kingdom. In 2008, he gained his Ph.D. from the Institute of Psychiatry in London, before completing postdoctoral fellowships at the Institute of Child Health, London, and City University London, United Kingdom. He has published work on self-awareness, theory of mind, inner speech use, and language impairment in autism spectrum disorder and was awarded the 2010 Young

Investigator (Behavioral–clinical) Award by the International Society for Autism Research. He is currently researching prospective memory in autism spectrum disorder, as part of a grant awarded by the Economic and Social Research Council, UK.

Keith E. Williams is an associate professor of pediatrics at the Penn State College of Medicine and director of the Feeding Program at the Penn State Hershey Medical Center. He is a licensed psychologist and a board certified behavior analyst and has published over 30 articles on childhood feeding problems and pediatric nutrition.

Alan S.W. Winton is a senior lecturer in the Department of Psychology at Massey University in Palmerston North, New Zealand. His current research interests are in mindfulness procedures and their application for service delivery.

Julie A. Worley is a doctoral student in clinical psychology at Louisiana State University. She has conducted research on children and adults diagnosed with intellectual and other developmental disabilities, including challenging behaviors, symptoms of co-morbid psychopathology, medical problems, such as seizure disorders and extrapyramidal side effects resulting from psychotropic medication use.

J. Helen Yoo is a board certified behavior analyst and a research scientist at the New York State Institute for Basic Research, where she serves as the head of the Applied Behavior Analysis Laboratory. She received her Ph.D. in developmental and child psychology from the University of Kansas. Her research interests include behavioral assessment and intervention of challenging behaviors in individuals with autism and developmental disabilities and drug–behavior interaction in the treatment of challenging behaviors.

C.T. Yu is professor of psychology at the University of Manitoba, Canada, and director of the St. Amant Research Centre. He has co-authored numerous scientific papers on autism and intellectual disabilities. He received the Outstanding Achievement Award from the University of Manitoba for exceptional contributions to research in 2008 and the Outstanding Mentorship Award from the Association for Behavior Analysis International in 2009.

About the Editors

Johnny L. Matson has spent his career as a researcher and is academically involved in the training of doctoral-level clinical psychologists specializing in developmental disabilities. He is the major professor of 48 Ph.D.s, many of whom have served as professors in major universities. He is the founding editor and editor-in-chief of *Research in Autism Spectrum Disorders* and *Research in Developmental Disabilities.* He has authored over 600 publications, including 34 books and 16 tests. He previously served on the psychology and psychiatric faculties at the University of Pittsburg. For the last 23 years he has been a professor at Louisiana State University. He is currently a professor and distinguished research master and director of clinical training in the Department of Psychology at Louisiana State University.

Peter Sturmey is professor of psychology at Queens College and The Graduate Center, City University of New York, and a member of the Learning Processes and Behavior Analysis and Neuropsychology doctoral programs at City University of New York. He has published over 150 articles and 15 books on developmental disabilities. His current research focuses on applied behavior analysis and staff and parent training.

History and Evolution of the Autism Spectrum Disorders

Julie K. Irwin, Jennifer MacSween, and Kimberly A. Kerns

Autistic spectrum disorders (ASDs) are characterized by impaired social interactions and communication, as well as restricted and repetitive behaviors and interests. Impairment in each of these dimensions can vary in severity, and symptomatologies among individuals with ASDs are often quite diverse. Over the past 20 years, there has been a marked increase in the diagnosis of individuals with ASDs. In 1966, Lotter undertook the first epidemiological study of autism, estimating the prevalence of autism disorder to be 4.5/10,000. Two decades later, the estimate rose to 10.1/10,000 (Bryson, Clark, & Smith, 1988). Currently, the community prevalence of ASDs is estimated to be *at least* 36.4/10,000 (Fombonne, 2005b), with some estimates as high as 67/10,000 (Bertrand et al., 2001). It has been suggested that this increase in the number of cases of ASDs is due, at least in part, to more inclusionary definitions of disorders within the autism spectrum (Fombonne, 2005a). While more in-depth discussion of this increase in ASD prevalence can be found in Chapter 3 of this volume, there is at least some suggestion that changes in prevalence may be due to changes in, and broadening of, the diagnostic conceptualization of ASD. Indeed over the 60 years that autism has been recognized, there have been many changes in our understanding of this disorder. The historical changes in the conception of autism and other pervasive developmental disorders are outlined below.

In 1943, Dr Leo Kanner, an Austrian child psychiatrist at John Hopkins University, published the paper "Autistic Disturbances of Affective Contact," where he described the behavior of 11 children. Observing one of the children, Kanner remarked "He does not observe the fact that anyone comes or goes, and never seems glad to see father or mother or any playmate… he seems almost to draw into his shell and live within himself" (1943, p. 218). Prior to Kanner's

case studies, children with similar behaviors were likely seen as being either mentally retarded or insane. Indeed, since Kanner (1943) first published case studies of these children whom he labeled "autistic," there have been several re-interpretations of historical accounts of "odd," emotionally disturbed, or mentally retarded children, who may, in fact, have been autistic. For example, Uta Frith (1989) has suggested that Victor, the "wild boy of Aveyron," showed signs of autism, including abnormal nonverbal expression and impaired attachment to his caregivers (based on the writings of Bonnaterre, 1800). Similarly, it may be that the children Henry Maudsley (1867) labeled as having "instinctive insanity" had autism. However, it was not until Kanner that an attempt to classify autistic children was made, with explicit criteria with which to identify them.

Kanner's detailed description of the 11 children in his landmark paper asserted that these children had a condition that differed "markedly and uniquely from anything reported so far" (p. 217). He borrowed the term "autism" from Bleuler (1911), a Swiss psychiatrist, who also coined the word "schizophrenia." From the Greek *autos* (self) and *ismos* (a suffix of state or action), "autistic" was used to describe the autocentric thinking and apparent withdrawal from the social world by children with schizophrenia. It was also a defining trait of the children Kanner studied and gradually the adjective, "autistic," led to the noun, "autism."

Kanner (1943) postulated that the fundamental disorder in children with autism was an "inability to relate themselves in the ordinary way to people and situations from the beginning of life" (p. 242). They were characterized by the following: (i) an "autistic aloneness"; (ii) a failure to use language to effectively communicate (e.g. mutism, echolalia, and overly literal language); (iii) repetitive, constricted activity and an "anxiously obsessive desire for the maintenance of sameness" (p. 245); and (iv) "good cognitive potential" shown in "excellent rote memory" (p. 243) and on performance tests. Indeed many of these distinctive and unusual behaviors described by Kanner remain cardinal to our definition and understanding of the disorder.

K.A. Kerns (✉)
Department of Psychology, University of Victoria, Victoria, BC, Canada V8W3P5
e-mail: kkerns@uvic.ca

J.L. Matson, P. Sturmey (eds.), *International Handbook of Autism and Pervasive Developmental Disorders*, Autism and Child Psychopathology Series, DOI 10.1007/978-1-4419-8065-6_1, © Springer Science+Business Media, LLC 2011

After publishing this first account, Kanner continued to work with autistic children, observing up to 120 further cases at Johns Hopkins Hospital. In 1956, he and Leon Eisenberg co-authored a paper revising what had come to be called early infantile autism. The authors proposed that the two defining features of autism were "extreme self-isolation" and an "obsessive insistence on sameness," believing autism could be reliably identified by these two characteristics alone. The non-communicative use of language, or its delay or failure to develop in autistic children, was seen as a direct result of a lack of relatedness with other people. As such, language impairment was originally seen as neither a core characteristic nor a reliable indicator of autism. Michael Rutter (1978) would later argue that language and prelanguage impairments are essential deficits of autism, asserting that this should be included as a diagnostic criterion along with the impairments in social relationships and insistence on sameness suggested by Eisenberg and Kanner.

In his earlier paper, Kanner (1943) also noted that the parents of the children he studied were highly intelligent, cold, and tended to be uninterested in people. However, since autistic aloneness was present from early infancy, he concluded that children with autism were born with no innate ability to form emotional connections with people. Later, Kanner (1949) assumed a much greater role of what was to be called the non-emotional "refrigerator mother" in the withdrawal of autistic children, a notion that fit well within the psychoanalytic zeitgeist current at the time. Indeed, while Kanner and Eisenberg (1956) acknowledged that outright rejection, neglect, or abuse of autistic children by their parents was rare, they viewed children with autism as experiencing "emotional refrigeration" by cold, unaffectionate, and mechanical parents and wrote that they could not dismiss the home environment as playing a role in the "genesis" of the disorder. However, since both still believed autism to be present from birth or very near to it, they also recognized that emotionally distant parenting alone was not sufficient to produce the disorder. Instead, they suggested that autism was the result of biological, psychological, and social factors (1956). Nonetheless, in an interview, Kanner (as cited in Thomas, 1960) still suggested that "refrigerator mothers" were a factor in the etiology of autism and proclaimed that parents of children with autism were so cold that they "just happen[ed] to defrost long enough to produce a child." Ironically, Kanner (1941) had earlier written a book called "In Defense of Mothers," subtitled, "How to Bring Up Children in Spite of the More Zealous Psychologists."

It was, however, Bettelheim's work that served to widely disseminate the "refrigerator mother" theory of the etiology of autism in the medical field, and even popularized it in the public sphere. Bettelheim, an Austrian-born American child psychologist, was the most well-known proponent of the view that autism was due to unemotional or unavailable mothers. Bettelheim's "Feral Children and Autistic Children" (1959) outlines the cases of Kamala and Amala, the "wolf girls" of Midnapore, India. The girls, aged eight and one and a half years old when found, were thought to have been raised by a she-wolf, demonstrating many "wolf-like behaviors." As has been done retrospectively with other feral children, Bettelheim speculated that these girls had actually been severely autistic. He argued that all parents of autistic children viewed these children as "unacceptable" and "wished to be rid of them." He reasoned that the girls had probably been emotionally, if not physically, abandoned. Bettelheim believed that being in the company of a wolf had little to do with Kamala and Amala's "animal" behavior and outlined cases of autistic children whose behavior paralleled that of these feral children in the absence of physical abandonment. Bettelheim asserted that both types of children displayed the same behaviors because they had both been subjected to extreme emotional isolation in combination with experiences interpreted as threatening to the self, stating "feral children seem to be produced not when wolves behave like mothers but when mothers behave like non-humans" (1959, p. 467).

Bettelheim's own life experiences deeply influenced his theories about autism. He had been detained in Nazi concentration camps, afterward writing about the loss of humanity he had witnessed in response to extreme situations (1943). In *The Empty Fortress: Infantile Autism and the Birth of the Self* (1967), Bettelheim likened the plight of autistic children to that of prisoners in German concentration camps. Autism, he contended, was a state of mind developed in reaction to "extreme situations," created by maternal rejection and hostility. Such situations left children feeling hopeless, anxious, apathetic, and increasingly unable to communicate with the outside world. In response, they withdrew from reality into themselves.

A serious challenge to this psychoanalytic view of autism, as purported by Bettelheim, came with Rimland's book, *Infantile Autism: The Syndrome and Its Implications for a Neural Theory of Behavior* (1964). The parent of an autistic son himself, Rimland argued convincingly that there was no evidence to support a psychogenic theory of autism. Instead, he believed there was a neurological basis for the disorder. In contrast to the unsubstantiated psychoanalytic theories, Rimland's arguments were based on empirical research and strongly influenced the field of autism research.

In Kanner's original description of autistic children (1943), he differentiated autism from schizophrenia, especially since some children with autism had been previously diagnosed with the latter disorder. He recognized that children with schizophrenia experienced some normal development before their behavior changed. Importantly, they withdrew from *previously existing* social relationships, while autistic children, he thought, failed from birth to ever form these social relationships. He viewed children with schizophrenia as trying to solve their problems by withdrawing from a world with which they had been engaged. Conversely, children with autism would cautiously begin to engage *more* with that world as they grew older.

Early researchers such as Bender (1947) and Kanner (1949; influenced by Despert) argued that autism was likely an early form of adult schizophrenia and some used "childhood schizophrenia" instead of "early infantile autism" to reflect the belief that these children were displaying the earliest expression of the adult disorder. Indeed, Creak (1961) described the results of a "working party" whose aims were to "discuss the present confused terminology and perhaps reach some clearer definition" (p. 501) for the number of children presenting with symptomatology variously classified as "autistic," "schizophrenic," and "atypical." Due to these overlapping descriptions, variations of the terms "autism," "childhood psychosis," and "schizophrenia" were used interchangeably by many clinicians and researchers at the time. Given the initial use of "autistic" as a descriptor of social withdrawal in individuals with schizophrenia, it is perhaps unsurprising that autism and schizophrenia remained linked in the literature until the 1970s. Indeed, Creak (1961) described nine criteria for "schizophrenic syndrome in childhood," which was the working party's agreed upon term for labeling "childhood psychosis," and represented his belief that these disorders were a childhood form of the later adult disorder. Interestingly, there is a high degree of overlap in these nine criteria and current diagnostic criteria for autistic disorder.

Kolvin and colleagues (Kolvin, 1971; Kolvin, Ounsted, Humphrey, & McNay, 1971) provided clear evidence that age of onset could be used to distinguish between autism and childhood schizophrenia. To reinforce this point, Rutter (1972) used the term *schizophrenic psychosis in childhood* to denote the child-onset type of schizophrenia as it is known today. He contrasted this with early infantile autism with an onset prior to age 3. Rutter (1968) also argued that autism could, in fact, be differentiated from schizophrenia, citing a number of factors such as the higher male-to-female incidence, the absence of delusions or hallucinations, and the overall stable course of autism in comparison to schizophrenia.

During the 1970s, those who researched autism's etiology focused increasingly on biological factors, including genetic ones. Examinations of gross chromosomal abnormalities (Böök, Nichtern, & Gruenberg, 1963), twin concordance rates (Rutter, 1967), and family studies (Lowe, 1966) were conducted during the 1960s. These failed to uncover a clear genetic basis of autism, though Folstein and Rutter (1977), in a study of 21 twins with autism, suggested that the inheritance of a cognitive abnormality, with or without perinatal brain damage, may lead to autism. This was

arguably the strongest evidence at the time of a genetic basis for the disorder, though Spence (1976) had already concluded that inheritance of autism was likely to be polygenic or multifactorial, and thus would be difficult to ascertain.

As evidence for biological explanations of autism mounted, psychogenic theories of the disorder lost credibility. Many alternative mechanisms and causes of autistic features were also proposed including, but not limited to, seizures (Schain & Yannet, 1960; Rutter & Lockyer, 1967), congenital defects of the reticular formation leading to hyperoxia (Rimland, 1964), very early developmental insults in utero (Walker, 1977), prenatal and perinatal complications (Lobascher, Kingerlee, & Gubbay, 1970; Taft & Goldfarb, 1964), and organic brain abnormality (Rutter, 1967). Most researchers agreed that they were searching for multiple and interacting causal factors of the disorder (Rutter, 1968), consistent with current biopsychosocial theories for the majority of mental disorders.

While Kanner is credited with first documenting children with autistic features, around the same time that he published his first account of autistic children, a German psychiatrist, Asperger, published a paper describing children he had been observing with similar characteristics (1944). Coincidentally, Asperger also used the label "autistic" for these children, calling their disorder "autistic psychopathy." The use of "psychopathy" was meant in the sense of an abnormality of personality. In choosing Bleuler's term "autism," Asperger, like Kanner, drew parallels between the behavior of the children he observed and that of adult patients with schizophrenia. Again he noted that those with schizophrenia and those with autistic psychopathy shared common features; they had all shut off relations between the self and the outside world to some degree. However, he did not think children with autistic psychopathy were psychotic or showed the "disintegration of personality" apparent in schizophrenia; their symptoms had not developed but had been present from birth (Asperger, 1944, as translated by Frith, 1991).

In addition to this broad characterization, Asperger (1944) described the children not only as (1) poor in social and emotional relationships and (2) showing a narrow, limited, and intense focus on special interests but also as (3) often extraordinary in some cognitive domain (e.g. mathematics); (4) having no obvious delay in language acquisition; (5) sometimes possessing excellent linguistic skills but with some abnormalities of speech and nonverbal communication; and (6) clumsy and uncoordinated (as noted in Frith, 1991). Asperger noticed that parents of many of the children he observed had similar personality characteristics and so thought it likely the traits were constitutional.

Asperger's work, originally published in German, did not come to be widely recognized in English-speaking countries until the 1980s; nearly four decades after Kanner first published, Asperger's original paper was translated into English by Frith (1991). Wing (1981), however, wrote about his work earlier than this, though she chose the more neutral term "Asperger's syndrome" (AS) as "psychopathy" was popularly associated with sociopathy. After presenting a summary of Asperger's original findings, Wing noted certain additional features she had observed in children with AS, namely that young infants with the disorder tended not to enjoy human interaction and made fewer social overtures (babbling, smiling, showing, and engaging in joint attention). These infants also showed a lack of imaginative pretend play; if it was present, it tended to be limited and repetitive.

From Wing's observations of these children, she disagreed with Asperger on two major points. First, Asperger (1944) thought that speech consistently developed before walking in his sample and wrote that many of the children he observed were very strong linguistically. In contrast, Wing (1981) found inconsistencies in whether these milestones were met on time. Upon careful analysis of the speech of children with AS, she found several peculiarities within the content, such as the inappropriate use of words, which often appeared to have been copied verbatim from a source. Second, though Asperger contended that many of those with AS were of high intelligence, he did not test this formally. Wing reasoned it was probable that the appearance of high intelligence was based mostly on excellent rote memory with little comprehension underlying this "knowledge" and noted that those with Asperger's syndrome showed a marked lack of common sense. Wing (1981) concluded by suggesting that those with AS could be identified by the presence of autistic features in combination with grammatical speech and less impaired social functioning.

In 1979, Wing and Gould published their findings from a large epidemiological study of children with any known impairments living in an area outside London, UK. They identified children under age 15 who had any features which were frequently associated with autism. Analysis from this study suggested a "triad of impairments" with deficits in social communication, verbal and nonverbal communication, and imagination (a lack of symbolic play) often found together. These impairments tended to be combined with narrow and repetitive routines and/or interests. In clustering children together by symptoms and the degree to which they displayed them, Wing and Gould (1979) suggested that these sub-groups did not represent distinct categories of disorder but rather a "continuum" of similar symptoms varying in severity. This, along with Wing's (1981) paper describing "Asperger's syndrome," was the first formal suggestion that autism was not a discrete, categorical disorder but represented a continuum of impairments and competencies. A review of the literature revealed that the first published mention of the "autism spectrum disorders" (ASDs) followed shortly (Tsai, Stewart, & August, 1981). Thereafter, the concept of an autistic spectrum took on vigor in the scientific

literature. Rutter (2005) notes that even in the 1960s, clinicians were aware of "children who showed disorders that were closely comparable to autism but did not quite meet the prevailing diagnostic criteria" (p. 4). Indeed, he contends that the broadening of the diagnostic concept of autism was brought about by four different causes: (1) epidemiological evidence has highlighted that there is a high frequency of autistic-like problems in children with severe or profound intellectual disability and that intellectual disability does not preclude autism; (2) there is a sizeable proportion of children with autism who were shown to have a diagnosable somatic disease or disorder that previously would have excluded the diagnosis of autism; (3) twin and family studies showing the high frequency of autistic-like features in relatives of individuals with autism leading to a "broader phenotype" of autism; and (4) the recognition of features of Asperger syndrome.

While Kanner's original description of autism was made in 1943, autism was not listed as a disorder in the first Diagnostic and Statistical Manual of Mental Disorders (DSM-I) published in 1952 (American Psychological Association). Children with autistic symptoms instead would have been diagnosed as exhibiting "schizophrenic reaction, childhood type," reflecting the mentality and belief that behaviors of children with autism were most similar to, and were likely an early manifestation of, adult schizophrenia. By the release of the DSM-II in 1968, despite Rimland's work, the increasing understanding of the biological nature of the disorder, and evidence suggesting children with autism had a "distinct" disorder, they were still diagnosed as "schizophrenic, childhood type." Features of the disorder were listed as "autistic, atypical, and withdrawn behavior," "general unevenness, gross immaturity, and inadequacy in development," and "failure to develop identity separate from the mother's" (APA, 1968). The latter criterion may be a reflection of psychodynamic theories at the time, wherein mental disorders were seen as caused by broad underlying conflicts or maladaptive reactions to life problems.

It was not until 1980, in the DSM-III (American Psychiatric Institute), that "infantile autism" was listed as a separate diagnostic category. The publishing of the DSM-III marked a radical reorganization of psychiatry and mental illness, with the role of diagnosis changing from marginal to being the basis of the specialty (Mayes & Horowitz, 2005). The DSM-III, which heralded the "medicalization" of mental illness, also introduced a system of five axes or dimensions for assessing all aspects of an individual's mental and emotional health. Autism was originally coded on Axis II, which included disorders of development and personality disorders. Infantile autism was listed as one of two "pervasive developmental disorders" (PDDs). Coined for use in the DSM-III, the term PDD was chosen for two main reasons. First, it was meant to subsume both autism and a number of conditions that shared some features with it. Second, it was meant to convey the broad extent (i.e. pervasiveness) of impairment across different domains in the disorders it encompassed (Volkmar & Cohen, 1991). One fundamental new aspect in the DSM-III was its use of categorical, symptom-based diagnosis to define mental illnesses. The criteria for a diagnosis of infantile autism included the following: (a) an onset before 30 months of age; (b) pervasive lack of responsiveness to other people; (c) gross deficits in language development; (d) if speech is present, peculiar speech patterns such as immediate and delayed echolalia, metaphorical language, and pronominal reversal; (e) bizarre responses to various aspects of the environment (e.g. resistance to change, peculiar interest in, or attachments to, animate or inanimate objects); and (f) absence of delusions, hallucinations, loosening of associations, and incoherence as in schizophrenia. The other diagnosis in the PDD category was pervasive developmental disorder – not otherwise specified (PDD-NOS) whose diagnostic criteria included the following: (a) gross and sustained impairment in social relationships; (b) three features from a list including excessive anxiety, constricted or inappropriate affect, resistance to change, oddities of motor movement, abnormalities of speech, hypo- or hypersensitivities, or self-mutilation; and (c) an onset of the full syndrome after 30 months of age and before 12 years of age with the absence of delusions, hallucinations, incoherence, or marked loosening of associations.

A major revision of the DSM was published in 1988 (DSM-III-R) wherein autistic disorder (299.00) was listed as the primary diagnosis still within the category of pervasive developmental disorders on Axis II. Diagnostic criteria were greatly expanded such that individuals had to exhibit at least two specific behaviors (listed within the criteria) from each of three broad categories: (a) qualitative impairments in reciprocal social interaction; (b) qualitative impairments in verbal and nonverbal communication and in imaginative activity; (c) markedly restricted repertoire of activities and interests, and an onset during infancy or early childhood. The second diagnosis within the category remained "pervasive developmental disorder – not otherwise specified" (PDD-NOS; 299.80), which included children with qualitative impairments in reciprocal social interactions and verbal and nonverbal communication skills but who did not meet the full criteria for autistic disorder.

The introduction of the DSM-IV in 1994, our current diagnostic criteria, represented another major shift in the conceptualization of the diagnosis of autism. First, autistic disorder was re-classified onto Axis I, as a clinical disorder, with Axis II diagnoses limited to coding intellectual disabilities (recognizing the independent nature of autism and intellectual capacity) and personality disorders. Second, PDD was reconceptualized as including a greater number of disorders, now frequently referred to as autistic spectrum disorders (ASDs) in the literature, which are defined as disorders primarily impacting social interaction. Interestingly, while commonly used, the term ASD does not actually appear in any version of the DSM (which instead uses the PDD designation) but is nonetheless widely used in the scientific literature, and even in clinical settings. Indeed, the social deficits in ASD are now viewed as forming a continuum from severe to relatively mild and are not necessarily correlated with the individual's language skills or intellectual capacity (Constantino, Przybeck, & Friesen, 2000; Posserud, Lundervold, & Gillberg, 2006). The category of PDD expanded to include autistic disorder, Asperger's disorder, Rett's disorder, childhood disintegrative disorder, and pervasive developmental disorder – not otherwise specified. While this grouping includes several disorders with many similar characteristics, it does not include all disorders which lead to a pervasive, lifelong developmental disorder (e.g. disorders such as fragile X and Landau–Kleffner syndromes were not included despite their impact on social interaction). Likewise, some have argued that Rett's disorder and childhood disintegrative disorder, while sharing some features with autistic disorders, are likely "separate" disorders and are perhaps best conceptualized of as including "autistic-like features" (Ozonoff, Goodlin-Jones, & Solomon, 2007; Rutter, 2005).

Rett's syndrome (RS) was first described in 1966 by Andreas Rett, a pediatrician working in Vienna. He wrote, in German, about the cases of 31 girls who had showed a regressive decline in mental ability early in life. In addition to mental retardation, they all showed behavioral abnormalities, stereotypic hand wringing, and also evidenced hand and gait apraxia. Rett also used the term "autism" as a descriptor of the disorder (Rett, 1966, as described by Hagberg, 1993). It was almost two decades later, when a publication of the disorder was made in English (Hagberg, Aicardi, Dias, & Ramos, 1983), that the disorder became a focus of study with the first set of diagnostic criteria for Rett's syndrome established in 1984 (Hagberg, Goutières, Hanefeld, Rett, & Wilson, 1985). The infant with RS characteristically develops typically for the first 5 months of life, followed by a noted deceleration in head growth between 6 months and 4 years of age, and a regression of already developed skills, including use of hands, motor coordination and gait, as well as communication skills. Mutations in the *MECP2* gene have been identified as a cause of RS (Amir et al., 1999) and are detected in most individuals with RS (Percy, 2008), though importantly these mutations do not appear to play a role in autism (Beyer et al., 2002). Indeed, some researchers have noted qualitative differences in the social behavior of individuals with RS and those with autism (Dahlgren Sandberg, Ehlers, Hagberg, & Gillberg, 2000; Olsson & Rett, 1987). Others have even argued that criteria for autistic disorder are frequently not met in those with RS and that it should be seen as a possible "co-morbid" diagnosis for some individuals

(Wulffaert, VanBerckelaer-Onnes, & Scholte, 2009) as, given current DSM-IV (TR) criteria (APA, 2000), individuals with RS cannot be separately diagnosed with autistic disorder.

Childhood disintegrative disorder (CDD), otherwise known as Heller syndrome or disintegrative psychosis, was first described by Heller in 1908. Heller described six cases of children who, after a normal developmental period of 3–4 years, showed a severe developmental regression. He proposed the term *dementia infantilis* for the condition. Diagnostic guidelines were subsequently set (Heller, 1930, as described by Volkmar, 1992) and included the following: (1) age of onset between 3 and 4 years; (2) loss or impairment of speech at onset with progressive intellectual and behavioral deterioration; (3) affective symptoms (fear, overactivity) and possible hallucinations; and (4) an absence of obvious markers of neurologic dysfunction (e.g. facial abnormalities). In comparison to autism, the most typical onset for CDD is between 2 and 4 years of age and is characterized by a substantial period of normal development followed by a profound developmental regression. Children affected by CDD can lose all of their language, toileting abilities, self-care skills, and interest in their environment, at which point the behaviors seen in affected children mimic those seen in autistic disorder. CDD does differ from autism in the pattern of onset, course, and aspects of outcome. In fact, estimates based on four surveys of individual ASD found fewer than 2 children per 100,000 could be classified as having CDD (Frombonne, 2002). Additional studies comparing children with autism and CDD have found that children with CDD have a significantly higher rate of epilepsy (Hendry, 2000; Kurita, Osada, & Miyake, 2004; Mouridsen, Rich, & Isager, 1998), and in one study, children with AD had significantly more even levels of intellectual functioning, and a tendency for less abnormality in auditory responsiveness than did children with CDD (Kurita et al., 2004). As noted by Rutter (2005), it remains unknown whether CDD "constitutes an unusual variant of autism or is something quite different" (p. 5).

Since Kanner's original characterization of autism, a fairly broad range of disorders with social interaction impairment at their core have been seen as being part of a broader phenotype, now labeled "autistic spectrum disorders." More recently, advances in genetic analysis, neuroimaging, and more refined descriptions of neurobehavioral symptomatology have allowed a better characterization of disorders such as Rett's disorder and CDD which, while sharing features of autism, certainly appear to have a very different etiology and course. While this may arguably preclude them from categorization as being autistic spectrum disorders, there is also a question of the utility and validity of identifying "separate disorders" in children who often present with such significant overlaps in behavioral symptomatology.

Indeed, during a discussion of the inclusion of Asperger's syndrome as a diagnosis, Schopler (1985) stated that AS was actually a "higher level" (i.e. higher functioning) autism. Wing (1981) originally agreed with this and formally suggested that either "AS or high-functioning autism" be placed at the mild end of the autistic spectrum (1991). Stemming from considerable overlap between Asperger's syndrome and autism, controversy still exists regarding whether AS is a distinct diagnostic category or whether it is indistinguishable from high-functioning autism (HFA). Furthermore, if they are meaningfully "separate" disorders, there still remains a question of the utility of treating them as such. Modern diagnostic systems have been categorical, though recently there has been a shift toward a dimensional classification system, given the significant occurrence of both co-morbid mental disorders and the overlap of symptomatology across diagnostic categories. It is argued that a dimensional approach is more suited to capture the entire range of severity and symptomatology of a disorder and to allow for greater flexibility in diagnosis (Kraemer, Noda, & O'Hara, 2004; MacCallum, Zhang, Preacher, & Rucker, 2002).

According to DSM-IV (TR) criteria (APA, 2000), a primary feature that distinguishes autism from AS is a language delay. Thus, a child is given a diagnosis of autism only if typical language milestones are not met, such as the use of single words by age 2 and meaningful phrases by age 3. However, research has shown that in some cases, children who have received diagnoses of autism demonstrate symptoms that are more consistent with AS, with the sole exception of the language criterion (Prior et al., 1998). Also, not all individuals with diagnoses of HFA demonstrate a severe language delay (Miller & Ozonoff, 2000). Furthermore, when children with autism or AS are grouped according to early language history, no other significant differences exist between the groups (Manjiviona & Prior, 1999). An additional study found that language ability measured in 6–8-year olds accounted for greater variability in later adaptive behavior and autism severity than the presence of an early language delay (Bennett et al., 2008). Overall, this research suggests that the presence of a language delay may not truly differentiate between HFA and AS and calls into question the diagnostic utility of differentiating AS as a separate disorder rather than as a variable expression of the symptomatology of autism. Indeed, questions about the importance and utility of the early language deficits were noted early on by Kanner and colleagues.

Contrary to these findings, other researchers have found support for the notion that groups of children with HFA and AS are indeed distinguishable on the basis of their early language developmental histories. In one study, a group of children with HFA displayed more severe behavioral symptoms in general and within the language domain had longer delays in language development, more impaired conversation abilities, and a higher use of stereotyped, repetitive, or idiosyncratic language (Ozonoff, South, & Miller, 2000). Similarly, another study demonstrated that children with HFA had more severe impairments in early developmental communication skills, reciprocal social interaction, and a greater degree of stereotyped behavior than did children with AS (Gilchrist et al., 2001). A noted difficulty in making conclusions from these types of studies is that the groups are often compared on the same variables that were originally used to differentiate the groups, creating a confounding tautology. Given that disturbed language development is a cardinal diagnostic feature of HFA in comparison to AS, post hoc group comparisons on the basis of specific language features would be anticipated to differ between the groups (diagnostic reliability) and thus offer no independent evidence of differentiation of the disorders. Given this, it is indeed interesting that in the Gilchrist et al.'s study (2001) comparison of the children with AS and HFA in adolescence found that, at this age, the communication differences between the groups no longer existed. Similarly, Howlin (2003) compared adults with HFA to those with AS and found no differences on ratings of social outcome or measures of language comprehension and expression. Thus, although there may be some support for distinguishing between HFA and AS on the basis of developmental language delay, this language differentiation may not be valid over time since there is a lack of association between a delayed onset of language and later language outcomes.

Less confounded have been studies which have attempted to differentiate children with HFA from those with AS in terms of other cognitive skills, social abilities, and specific behaviors. For example, Ehlers and colleagues (1997), looking at broader patterns of cognitive abilities, found that school-age children with HFA generally had poor verbal ability and strong perceptual ability, while the reverse pattern was true for school-age children diagnosed with AS. Szatmari, Archer, Fisman, Streiner, and Wilson (1995) compared abilities in a group of high-functioning children with PDD differentiated into HFA or AS categories (based on the Autism Diagnostic Interview conducted as a part of the study). Those identified as having autism (HFA) exhibited more social impairment than did children identified as having AS and although there were no differences on individual verbal and nonverbal communication items, the total communication score was significantly lower for the children with HFA. Additionally, while the groups were similar in the types of restrictive behaviors exhibited, the children with HFA also engaged in repetitive behaviors at a higher frequency and intensity than did those with AS. Likewise, Klin and colleagues (1995) compared individuals (age range extending from childhood through young adulthood) diagnosed by the investigators as having either HFA or AS (based

on ICD-10 criteria; all participants had an IQ over 70 for inclusion) on a range of neuropsychological measures. They found that individuals with AS in general had stronger verbal than performance ability scores (on measures of IQ), while individuals with HFA showed no consistent pattern of differences between verbal and performance abilities. In addition, individuals with AS scored higher on individual measures of auditory perception, verbal memory, articulation, vocabulary, and verbal output, while those with HFA scored higher on measures of fine and gross motor skills, visual–motor integration, visual–spatial perception, visual memory, and nonverbal concept formation. It is important to note, however, that part of the diagnostic criteria for AS included delayed motor milestones and presence of motor "clumsiness." Overall, while in general this study provides support for differentiation between AS and HFA in terms of a differential pattern of abilities, the authors do note that "this is a more complex issue, however, given that these two conditions could still share the same etiology or other pathogenetic processes while having phenotypic difference solely accounted for by neuropsychological differences" (p. 1138), much as the diversity seen in neuropsychological abilities between those with low- and high-functioning autism.

While there are a number of studies providing support either for or against the establishment of HFA and AS as distinct disorders, currently, there appears to be insufficient evidence to establish the validity of the distinction. As noted by Lord (in Wallis, 2009), "Nobody has been able to show consistent differences between what clinicians diagnose as Asperger's syndrome and what they diagnose as mild autistic disorder." Therefore, it is possible that in the upcoming revision of the DSM, AS may not be seen as a different disorder but as a milder variant of ASD (Wallis, 2009). The question of the validity of HFA and AS as separate disorders is of considerable importance to many, from insurance companies, service providers, and school districts to individuals whose "personal identities" are tied to their diagnostic categorization.

There is ample speculation that the upcoming DSM-V will embrace an alternative dimensional approach rather than its traditional classification method. Utilizing a dimensional approach for the diagnosis of autistic spectrum disorders would place low-functioning individuals at one end (identified by issues such as lower IQ, more frequent and severe symptoms, and less adaptive functioning) and high-functioning individuals at the opposite end of the spectrum (with higher IQ, fewer and milder symptoms, and overall, less disability). This conceptualization would be consistent with evidence that low-functioning individuals have more frequent and more extreme behavioral symptoms than do high-functioning individuals (Freeman et al., 1981). Szatmari (2000) has noted three potential issues that would arise with the use of a dimensional diagnostic system.

First, there are currently no accepted definitions for high- or low-functioning individuals; cutoffs need to be developed to determine the point at which an individual is considered high or low functioning. Second, research has not yet established the reliability and validity of this approach over time, as it is unknown whether development alters the placement of an individual on the spectrum. Third, this approach assumes that individuals comprising this scale will differ along one underlying dimension, specifically, symptom severity. However, nonverbal individuals cannot demonstrate symptoms such as echolalia and impaired conversation, and thus would be scored as exhibiting fewer symptoms (despite significantly more "language impairment"). This inverse relationship between number of symptoms and symptom severity may indicate the need for a scale that has multiple dimensions. According to Szatmari (2000), one dimension should indicate symptom severity, while a separate dimension reflects the individual's level of functioning. Overall, a number of systems which currently operate on the basis of a categorical approach to diagnosis would need to be changed in the event of a dimensional approach to diagnosis. Clearly, such a paradigm shift in conceptualizing diagnosis will have a major impact on existing systems, diagnostic and support services, and individuals affected by ASDs.

Given the extensive, negative impact of ASD on normal development, functional adaptation, social interaction, and ability to benefit from educational services, the development of interventions for individuals impacted by ASD has been pursued with intensity. While a thorough review of intervention approaches is beyond the scope of this chapter, there are several past treatments which are important to the history of autism. Over the past several decades, many different treatments have been proposed as bringing about significant improvements for individuals with autism. While many intervention approaches have been developed and marketed, most lack empirical support through the use of controlled studies of any kind, and for those that have undergone appropriate research, unfortunately, the results are frequently far from positive.

Early intervention approaches for autism derived from the previously discussed notion that autism was caused by a natural reaction to emotional isolation (Bettelheim, 1967; Eisenberg & Kanner, 1956). Thus, initial psychoanalytic approaches worked on "curing" autism. Bettelheim thought that "trying to rehabilitate autistic children while they continue to live at home, or by treating mother and child simultaneously, is a questionable procedure" (1967, p. 407) and advocated "parentectomy" which involved removing the autistic child from the home with the goal of teaching the autistic child that relationships could result in love and acceptance. Of course, given the misguided understanding of the "cause" of autism, these approaches at intervention had little success in the treatment of autism; the disorder was assumed to be "immutable" (Eisenberg & Kanner, 1956).

As autism began to be increasingly recognized as a "behavioral" disorder and as the zeitgeist of mental health treatment focused more on behavioral issues than on psychogenic underpinnings, behavioral interventions became more frequent in the treatment of individuals with ASD. Commonly cited as the first study to apply behavioral theory to autistic children, Ferster and DeMyer's (1961) seminal research demonstrated that reinforcements such as candy and toys increased the frequency that children with autism would press a key. This study was one of the first to demonstrate that, like adults with schizophrenia, the behavior of the autistic child could be brought under control via rewards and that autistic children were capable of being influenced by external environmental events.

This empirical evidence fuelled the development of many behavioral interventions, including widespread use of applied behavior analysis (ABA), which involves identifying target behaviors to increase or decrease in frequency, while simultaneously evaluating the resulting behavioral changes over time. In 1964, Wolf, Risley, and Mees used ABA to extend Ferster and DeMyer's (1961) findings to behaviors of more practical importance. An operant conditioning procedure was employed with the goal of decreasing temper tantrum behavior; negative reinforcement involved isolating the child each time a temper tantrum occurred. Over a period of 6 months, the frequency of tantrums was significantly reduced, with the gains still present an additional 6 months after intervention. To increase the robustness of therapeutic gains, the intervention was delivered in natural settings, such as the child's home and school (Nordquist & Wahler, 1973). Also, parents and teachers were successfully trained in behavior modification therapy (Koegel, Glahn, & Nieminen, 1978; Koegel, Russo, & Rincover, 1977). Overall, there is strong support for the use of behavioral therapy with autistic individuals, including reduced problem behaviors (Lovaas, 1987; Lovaas, Koegel, Simmons, & Long, 1973), IQ gains and reductions in symptom severity (Sheinkopf & Siegel, 1998), and improved language and adaptive behavior (Eikeseth, Smith, Jahr, & Eldevik, 2002).

One specific intervention grounded in behavioral theory is that of discrete trial teaching (DTT), a method that follows a prescribed order of events to teach a child a new skill. DTT involves presenting a stimulus, which is followed by a consequence dependent on whether the child's response to the stimulus is correct, incorrect, or no response was made. Smith's (2001) review concluded that DTT is an effective method for teaching new behaviors. However, limitations include a failure for new behaviors to generalize in the absence of cues and the time-intensive nature of the program required for DTT to be effective (Lovaas, 1987).

Historically noteworthy has been the very early, intensive behavioral interventions of Lovaas and his colleagues (Lovaas, 1993, 1996). Original research reported that this intervention approach resulted in major changes in children with an ASD diagnosis. Indeed claims were made that approximately 40% of the children who had received the early intensive behavioral intervention were "indistinguishable" from normally developing peers of the same age, promoting ideas of a cure. As well, there were reported significant increases in cognitive ability following intervention on the order of one to two standard deviations. These gains were claimed to be long-lasting as long as children were treated prior to age 5 (Lovaas, 1993). However, these claims have been disputed and criticized due to research and statistical issues which could have impacted the results (Magiati & Howlin, 2001). Furthermore, re-analysis of Lovaas' data suggests that claims of children attaining normal functioning were not substantiated, and while participants did make gains, none truly "recovered" from their autism (Shea, 2004).

Pivotal response training (PRT), originally the "natural language teaching paradigm," attempts to improve language skills in autistic children by motivating and naturally reinforcing skills in pivotal behaviors such as joint attention, self-monitoring, and self-initiation (Koegel, O'Dell, & Koegel, 1987). Positive results have been demonstrated for social communication (Pierce & Schreibman, 1995) and general social behavior (Koegel & Frea, 1993; Pierce & Schreibman, 1997). The PRT method has also been adapted to target symbolic play. Researchers indicated benefits in level and complexity of symbolic play, as well as improved interaction skills (Stahmer, 1995). Thus, there is some limited support for the use of PRT in treating autism. The Treatment and Education of Autistic and Related Communication Handicapped Children (TEACCH) focuses on structured teaching to enhance the learning of children with autism (Schopler & Reichler, 1971). The treatment targets social, communication, and motor skills. Behavioral and cognitive strategies are used to establish appropriate routines in the home in a manner such that the routines can be easily generalized across settings, including the school environment (Schopler, 1994). One of the few studies examining the TEACCH program showed significantly higher gains after 4 months of intervention on cognitive and developmental measures (Ozonoff & Cathcart, 1998). However, substantial methodological concerns compromised the validity of the conclusions (Gresham, Beebe-Frankenberger, & MacMillan, 1999).

The use of medication for children with autism is controversial and has been the topic of much debate, primarily due to limited empirical support but long-standing historical use. Antipsychotics have a long history of use to manage behavioral problems. Conventional antipsychotics can be differentiated from the newer, atypical antipsychotics on the basis of lessened or eliminated side effects (Barnard, Yong, Pearson, Geddes, & O'Brien, 2002). Such medication has been reported to reduce aggressive behavior (Horrigan & Barnhill, 1997), as well as increase adaptive behavior in children with autism (Williams et al., 2006). However, in a comprehensive review, Barnard et al. (2002) concluded that evidence supporting the viability of antipsychotics for autism treatment remains scarce and inadequate. Selective serotonin re-uptake inhibitors (SSRIs) are frequently used to treat anxiety, aggression, depression, and obsessive–compulsive symptoms in children with autism. Studies have demonstrated improvements in irritability, lethargy, stereotyped behavior, and inappropriate speech (Fatemi, Realmuto, Khan, & Thuras, 1998) as well as reductions in repetitive behaviors (Hollander et al., 2005). Another study concluded, based on measures of intellectual achievement, that the majority of children had excellent or good response (69%) after 36–76 months of SSRI treatment (DeLong, Ritch, & Burch, 2002). A summary review on the treatment of children with autism using SSRIs concluded that these drugs demonstrate some success in treating severity of autistic symptoms but that currently, research evidence is inadequate to make definitive conclusions about their efficacy (West, Brunssen, & Waldrop, 2009). Stimulants target issues of hyperactivity, impulsiveness, and inattention. Interestingly, certain stimulants have more robust effects depending on whether the individual is high or low functioning (Tsai, 2000). Studies have demonstrated positive results of stimulant use, including decreased ratings of hyperactivity, stereotypies, and inappropriate speech, with few side effects, indicating the potential for stimulants as a suitable treatment option (Handen, Johnson, & Lubetsky, 2000; Quintana et al., 1995).

Secretin, a gastrointestinal peptide hormone, is purported to treat autism by remedying gastrointestinal difficulties, which in turn reduces the prevalence of problematic behaviors (Kern, Miller, Evans, & Trivedi, 2002). In the late 1990s, media coverage promoting secretin as a cure for autism created substantial hype among parents of autistic children who hoped to attain secretin. The craze went so far as to cause secretin to become part of the black market in the United States of America (Volkmar, Lord, Bailey, Schultz, & Klin, 2004). However, many studies have failed to find any treatment benefits of secretin (Chez et al., 2000; Dunn-Geier et al., 2000; Handen & Hofkosh, 2005). One further study found that over the course of secretin treatment, the frequency of maladaptive behaviors actually increased (Carey et al., 2002). Thus, there is little clinical evidence to support the efficacy of secretin as a treatment for autism.

Due to the lack of treatment options that have been shown efficacious in all children, a number of alternative interventions have been developed and often heavily marketed for the treatment of children with autism. The amount of empirical support varies for each of the following therapies, and while some children with autism have reportedly benefited greatly, the great majority of children have not. Multivitamin therapy, originally introduced as orthomolecular psychiatric therapy in 1968 (Pauling), is based on the theory that the best treatment for mental illness is to provide the brain with the optimal molecular concentrations of nutrients. There were a few early studies published supporting the use of multivitamins in the reduction of autistic behavior and symptoms, particularly the use of vitamin B and magnesium (Lelord et al., 1981; Rimland, Callaway, & Dreyfus, 1978). While a research review concluded that vitamin B6 and magnesium therapy might be beneficial when used in combination with other interventions, more research is required (Pfeiffer, Norton, Nelson, & Shott, 1995). The gluten- and casein-free diet was developed, in part, from animal experiments that linked high levels of opiates to behavioral problems, supposedly similar to those exhibited by autistic children (Panksepp, 1979). Excessive opioid activity is thought to be linked to an over-abundance of opioid peptides from gluten and casein. Some have suggested that abnormal opioid activity leads not only to behavioral problems (Reichelt, Knivsberg, Lind, & Nødland, 1991) but also to deficits in brain maturation, attention, learning, and social communication (Knivsberg, Reichelt, Nødland, & Høien, 1995), characteristic of autism. In fact, abnormally high levels of these peptides have been found in the urine and cerebrospinal fluid of individuals with autism (Israngkun, Newman, Patel, DuRuibe, & Abou-Issa, 1986; Reichelt, Knivsberg, Lind, & Nødland, 1991). Thus, it was hypothesized that a diet free from casein and gluten would decrease opioid activity and improve symptoms of autism. Several studies reported positive results for autistic children after being placed on the restricted diet, including developmental gains, and parent- and teacher-reported behavioral improvements, and gains in social communication and interaction (Knivsberg, Reichelt, Høien, & Nødland, 2002; Whiteley, Rodgers, Savery, & Shattock, 1999). However, Elder and colleagues (2006), in one of the only studies to employ a double-blind manipulation, found no significant differences in autism severity between an experimental gluten- and casein-free diet group and a regular diet group (although notably, parents continued to report improvements).

Auditory integration therapy (AIT) targets auditory processing abnormalities and sensitivities to sound by having the child listen to music at modified frequencies. Rimland and Edelson (1995) reported gains in adaptive behavior, though there was no change in decreasing overall sound sensitivity. Dawson and Watling (2000) reviewed five studies of auditory integration and concluded that there is no support for the effectiveness of AIT in treating autism. The "Son-Rise Program" (Kaufman, 1994) was created by parents who claim to have cured their autistic child. The premise of this

intervention is that no expectation or judgment is placed on the child; rather, the child is given unconditional acceptance and approval. In one of the few studies to examine the efficacy of the program, parental report measures indicated more drawbacks than benefits, primarily due to the time-intensive nature of the program and the resulting negative effects this had on the rest of the family (Williams & Wishart, 2003). Finally, researchers concluded that, although the program has received support from case studies and testimonials, the effectiveness of the program has not yet been formally evaluated (Heflin & Simpson, 1998).

Finally, there are a few treatments still available which have no empirical support. There have been concerns that autism is the result of mercury poisoning, hypothesized to occur through administration of childhood vaccines which contain mercury as a preservative in the form of thiomersal (Bernard, Enayati, Redwood, Roger, & Binstock, 2001). Chelation, an invasive, chemical detoxification treatment that removes heavy metals, including mercury, from the body, has been touted as a treatment. Chelation therapy has not been shown to demonstrate any cognitive or behavioral benefits to individuals with autism (Dietrich et al., 2004; Rimland, 2000). Facilitated communication (FC) purportedly permits individuals with limited language abilities to communicate by having a facilitator physically support the arm or hand to enable pointing or typing. By providing physical support, researchers have found that the child is able to construct sentences by pointing at or typing words (Biklen & Schubert, 1991). However, multiple studies have failed to find any support for facilitated communication (Montee, Milterberger, & Wittrock, 1995; Regal, Rooney, & Wandas, 1994). In fact, one study demonstrated that autistic individuals typed the correct answer only if the facilitator knew the answer, indicating facilitators were responsible for the communication (Eberlin, McConnachie, Ibel, & Volpe, 1993). Currently, there is not enough support for the use of FC in autism.

In summary, the interventions presented above are not cures. Rather, for those interventions which are effective, they are merely methods that alleviate, to varying degrees, some of the deficits demonstrated by a child with autism. Some of the presented intervention strategies have weak theoretical or empirical foundations, others have not been thoroughly evaluated, while others clearly lack efficacy. As these therapies are often applied to young and vulnerable individuals, it is important that future therapies be thoroughly and empirically validated.

Autism has been re-defined many times since Kanner's (1943) original publication. It has subsequently been recognized, not as a uniform, categorical disorder but as a pervasive disability with characteristically heterogeneous manifestations. Although the latter idea has been epitomized by the concept of an autism spectrum, controversy remains as to what should be included on this continuum of autism.

Furthermore, despite several revisions of diagnostic criteria for autism and other pervasive developmental disorders, their validity and utility are yet to be satisfactorily established. This issue is not a trivial one; resource allocation, research, and clinical decisions rest on having the ability to accurately diagnose and treat individuals with any of the autism spectrum disorders. Furthermore, in order to assess potential new interventions for the ASDs, researchers must be able to clearly delineate clinical groups for whom a treatment is intended. As noted earlier in this chapter, such empirical validation of treatments is a necessity in the face of commercialization and media involvement which often accompany proposed treatments for these disorders that affect so many. Finally, with the apparent rise in the prevalence of ASDs, it has become even more important for those who work with individuals with ASDs to understand the history of these disorders. Having knowledge of how ASDs have come to be defined will be necessary to appreciate the changes in how we view these disorders that are certain to come.

References

American Psychiatric Association (1968). Committee on nomenclature and statistics. In *Diagnostic and statistical manual of mental disorders* (2nd ed.). Washington, DC: American Psychiatric Press.

American Psychiatric Association (1980). *Diagnostic and statistical manual of psychiatric disorders* (3rd ed.). Washington, DC: American Psychiatric Press.

American Psychiatric Association (2000). *Diagnostic and statistical manual of mental disorders* (4th ed., TR). Washington, DC: American Psychiatric Association.

Amir, R. E., Van den Veyver, I. B., Wan, M., Tran, C. Q., Francke, U., & Zoghbi, H. Y. (1999). Rett syndrome is caused by mutations in X-linked *MECP2*, encoding methyl-CpG-binding protein 2. *Nature Genetics, 23*, 185–188.

Asperger, H. (1944). Die autistichen psychopathen im kindersalter. *Archive fur psychiatrie und Nervenkrankheiten, 117*, 76–136.

Barnard, L., Yong, A. H., Pearson, J., Geddes, J., & O'Brien, G. (2002). A systematic review of the use of atypical antipsychotics in autism. *Journal of Psychopharmacology, 16*, 93–101.

Bender, L. (1947). Childhood schizophrenia, clinical study of one hundred schizophrenic children. *American Journal of Orthopsychiatry, 17*, 40–56.

Bennett, T., Szatmari, P., Bryson, S., Volden, J., Zwaigenbaum, L., Vaccarella, L., et al. (2008). Differentiating autism and Asperger syndrome on the basis of language delay or impairment. *Journal of Autism and Developmental Disorders, 38*, 616–625.

Bernard, S., Enayati, A., Redwood, L., Roger, H., & Binstock, T. (2001). Autism: A novel form of mercury poisoning. *Medical Hypotheses, 68*, 462–471.

Bertrand, J., Mars, A., Boyle, C., Bove, F., Yeargin-Allsopp, M., & Decoufle, P. (2001). Prevalence of autism in a United States population: The brick township, New Jersey, investigation. *Pediatrics, 108*, 1155–1161.

Bettelheim, B. (1943). Individual and mass behavior in extreme situations. *The Journal of Abnormal and Social Psychology, 38*, 417–452.

Bettelheim, B. (1959). Feral children and autistic children. *The American Journal of Sociology, 64*, 455–467.

Bettelheim, B. (1967). *The empty fortress: Infantile autism and the birth of the self*. London: Collier-Macmillan.

Beyer, K. S., Blasi, F., Bacchelli, E., Klauck, S. M., Maestrini, E., & Poustka, A. (2002). Mutation analysis of the coding sequence of the *MECP2* gene in infantile autism. *Human Genetics, 111*, 305–309.

Biklen, D., & Schubert, A. (1991). New words: The communication of students with autism. *Remedial and Special Education, 12*, 46–57.

Bleuler, E. (1911). Dementia praecox oder gruppe der schizophrenien. In G. Aschaffenburg (Ed.), *Handbuch der Psychiatrie. Spezieller Teil. 4. Abteilung. 1. Hälfte*. Leipzig und Wien: Franz Deuticke.

Bonnaterre, P. J. (1800). *Notice Historique sur le sauvage de l'Aveyron*. Paris: Pancoucke.

Böök, J. A., Nichtern, S., & Gruenberg, E. (1963). Cytogenetical investigation in childhood schizophrenia. *Acta Psychiatrica Scandinavica, 39*, 309–323.

Bryson, S. E., Clark, B. S., & Smith, I. M. (1988). First report of a Canadian epidemiological study of autistic syndromes. *Journal of Child Psychology and Psychiatry, 4*, 433–445.

Carey, T., Ratliff-Schaub, K., Funk, J., Weinle, C., Myers, M., & Jenks, J. (2002). Double-blind placebo-controlled trial of secretin: Effects on aberrant behavior in children with autism. *Journal of Autism and Developmental Disorders, 32*, 161–167.

Chez, M. G., Buchanan, C. P., Bagan, B. T., Hammer, M. S., McCarthy, K. S., Ovrutskaya, I., et al. (2000). Secretin and autism: A two-part clinical investigation. *Journal of Autism and Developmental Disorders, 30*, 87–94.

Constantino, J. N., Przybeck., T., & Friesen., D. (2000). Reciprocal social behavior in children with and without pervasive developmental disorders. *Journal of Developmental Behavior Pediatrics, 21*, 2–11.

Creak, M. (1961). Schizophrenia syndrome in childhood: Progress report of a working party. *Cerebral Palsy Bulletin, 3*, 501–504.

Dahlgren Sandberg, A., Ehlers, S., Hagberg, B., & Gillberg, C. (2000). The Rett Syndrome complex: Communicative functions in relation to developmental level and autistic features. *Autism, 4*, 249–267.

Dawson, G., & Watling, R. (2000). Interventions to facilitate auditory, visual, and motor integration in autism: A review of the evidence. *Journal of Autism and Developmental Disorders, 30*, 415–421.

DeLong, G. R., Ritch, C. R., & Burch, S. (2002). Fluoxetine response in children with autistic spectrum disorders: Correlation with familial major affective disorder and intellectual achievement. *Developmental Medicine and Child Neurology, 44*, 652–659.

Dietrich, K. N., Ware, J. H., Salganik, M., Radcliffe, J., Rogan, W. J., Rhoads, G. G., et al. (2004). Effect of chelation therapy on the neuropsychological and behavioral development of lead-exposed children after school entry. *Pediatrics, 114*, 19–26.

Dunn-Geier, J., Ho, H. H., Auersperg, E., Doyle, D., Eaves, L., Matsubu, C., et al. (2000). Effect of secretin on children with autism: A randomized controlled trial. *Developmental Medicine and Child Neurology, 42*, 796–802.

Eberlin, M., McConnachie, G., Ibel, S., & Volpe, L. (1993). Facilitated communication: A failure to replicate the phenomenon. *Journal of Autism and Developmental Disorders, 23*, 507–530.

Ehlers, S., Nyden, A., Gillberg, C., Sandberg, A. D., Dahlgren, S. -O., Hjelmquist, E., et al. (1997). Asperger syndrome, autism and attention disorders: A comparative study of the cognitive profiles of 120 children. *Journal of Child Psychology and Psychiatry, 38*, 207–217.

Eikeseth, S., Smith, T., Jahr, E., & Eldevik, S. (2002). A 1-year comparison controlled study. *Behavior Modification, 26*, 49–68.

Eisenberg, L., & Kanner, L. (1956). Early infantile autism, 1943–1955. *American Journal of Orthopsychiatry, 35*, 221–234.

Elder, J. H., Shankar, M., Shuster, J., Theriaque, D., Burns, S., & Sherrill, L. (2006). The gluten free, casein-free diet in autism: Results of a preliminary double blind clinical trial. *Journal of Autism and Developmental Disorders, 36*, 413–420.

Fatemi, S. H., Realmuto, G. M., Khan, L., & Thuras, P. (1998). Fluoxetine in treatment of adolescent patients with autism: A longitudinal open trial. *Journal of Autism and Developmental Disorders, 28*, 303–307.

Ferster, C. B., & DeMyer, M. K. (1961). The development of performances in autistic children in an automatically controlled environment. *Psychiatry, 13*, 312–345.

Folstein, S., & Rutter, M. (1977). Infantile autism: A genetic study of 21 twin pairs. *Journal of Child Psychology and Psychiatry, 18*(4), 297–321.

Fombonne, E. (2005a). Epidemiology of autistic disorder and other pervasive developmental disorders. *Journal of Clinical Psychiatry, 66*(suppl. 10), 3–8.

Fombonne, E. (2005b). Epidemiological studies of pervasive developmental disorders. In F. R. Volkmar, R. Paul, A. Klin, & D. Cohen (Eds.), *Handbook of autism and pervasive developmental disorders* (pp. 42–69). Hoboken, NJ: Wiley.

Freeman, B. J., Ritvo, E. R., Schroth, P. C., Tonick, I., Gutherie, D., & Wake, L. (1981). Behavioral characteristics of high- and low-autistic children. *American Journal of Psychiatry, 138*, 25–29.

Frith, U. (1989). *Autism: Explaining the enigma.* Oxford: Blackwell.

Frith, U. (1991). *Autism and Asperger syndrome.* Cambridge: Cambridge University Press.

Frombonne, E. (2002). Prevalence of childhood disintegrative disorder. *Autism, 6*, 149–157.

Gilchrist, A., Green, J., Cox, A., Burton, D., Rutter, M., & Le Couteur, A. (2001). Development and current functioning in adolescents with Asperger syndrome: A comparative study. *Journal of Child Psychology and Psychiatry, 42*, 227–240.

Gresham, F. M., Beebe-Frankenberger, M. E., & MacMillan, D. L. (1999). A selective review of treatments for children with autism: Description and methodological considerations. *School Psychology Review, 28*, 559–575.

Hagberg, B. (1993). Introduction. In B. Hagberg, M. Anvret, & J. Wahlström (Eds.), *Rett syndrome: Clinical & biological aspects* (pp. 1–3). London: Mac Keith Press.

Hagberg, B., Aicardi, J., Dias, K., & Ramos, O. (1983). A progressive syndrome of autism, dementia, ataxia, and loss of purposeful hand use in girls: Rett's syndrome: Report of 35 cases. *Annals of Neurology, 14*, 471–479.

Hagberg, B., Goutières, F., Hanefeld, F., Rett, A., & Wilson, J. (1985). Rett syndrome: Criteria for inclusion and exclusion. *Brain and Development, 7*, 372–373.

Handen, B. L., & Hofkosh, D. (2005). Secretin in children with autistic disorder: A double-blind, placebo-controlled trial. *Journal of Developmental and Physical Disabilities, 17*, 95–106.

Handen, B. L., Johnson, C. R., & Lubetsky, M. (2000). Efficacy of methylphenidate among children with autism and symptoms of attention-deficit hyperactivity disorder. *Journal of Autism and Developmental Disorders, 30*, 245–255.

Heflin, L. J., & Simpson, R. L. (1998). Interventions for children and youth with autism: Prudent choices in a world of exaggerated claims and empty promises. Part 1: Intervention and treatment option review. *Focus on Autism and Other Developmental Disabilities, 13*, 194–211.

Heller, T. (1908). Dementia infantilis. *Zeitschrift fur die Erforschung und Behandlung des Jugenlichen Schuachsinns, 3*, 141–165.

Heller, T. (1930). Uber dementia infantilis. *Zeitschrift fur Schwachsinns, 2*, 17–28.

Hendry, C. N. (2000). Childhood disintegrative disorder: Should it be considered a distinct diagnosis? *Clinical Psychology Review, 20*, 77–90.

Hollander, E., Phillips, A., Chaplin, W., Zagursky, K., Novotny, S., Wasserman, S., et al. (2005). A placebo-controlled crossover trial of liquid fluoxetine on repetitive behaviors in childhood and adolescent autism. *Neuropsychopharmacology, 30*, 582–589.

Horrigan, J. P., & Barnhill, L. J. (1997). Risperidone and explosive aggressive autism. *Journal of Autism and Developmental Disorders, 27*, 313–323.

Howlin, P. (2003). Outcome in high-functioning adults with autism with and without early language delays: Implications for the differentiation between autism and Asperger syndrome. *Journal of Autism and Developmental Disorders, 33*, 3–13.

Israngkun, P. P., Newman, H. A., Patel, S. T., DuRuibe, V. A., & Abou-Issa, H. (1986). Potential biochemical markers for infantile autism. *Neurochemical Pathology, 5*, 51–70.

Kanner, L. (1941). *In defense of mothers: How to bring up children in spite of the more zealous psychologists.* Springfield, IL: Charles C. Thomas.

Kanner, L. (1943). Autistic disturbances of affective contact. *Nervous Child, 2*, 217–250.

Kanner, L. (1949). Problems of nosology and psychodynamics in early infantile autism. *American Journal of Orthopsychiatry, 19*, 416–426.

Kanner, L., & Eisenberg, L. (1956). Early infantile autism, 1943–1955. *American Journal of Orthopsychiatry, 26*, 55–65.

Kaufman, B. (1994). *Son-Rose: The miracle continues.* Tiburon, CA: H.J. Kramer, Inc.

Kern, J. K., Miller, V. S., Evans, P. A., & Trivedi, M. H. (2002). Efficacy of porcine secretin in children with autism and pervasive developmental disorder. *Journal of Autism and Developmental Disorders, 32*, 153–160.

Klin, A., Volkmar, F. R., Sparrow, S. S., Cicchetti, D. V., & Rourke, B. P. (1995). Validity and neuropsychological characterization of Asperger syndrome: Convergence with nonverbal learning disabilities syndrome. *Journal of Child Psychology and Psychiatry, 36*, 1127–1140.

Knivsberg, A., Reichelt, K., Høien, T., & Nødland, M. (2002). A randomized, controlled study of dietary intervention in autistic syndromes. *Nutritional Neuroscience, 5*, 251–260.

Knivsberg, A., Reichelt, K. L., Nødland, M., & Høien, T. (1995). Autistic syndromes and diet: A follow-up study. *Scandinavian Journal of Educational Research, 39*, 222–236.

Koegel, R. L., & Frea, W. D. (1993). Treatment of social behavior in autism through the modification of pivotal social skills. *Journal of Applied Behavior Analysis, 26*, 369–377.

Koegel, R. L., Glahn, T. J., & Nieminen, G. S. (1978). Generalization of parent-training results. *Journal of Applied Behavior Analysis, 11*, 95–109.

Koegel, R. L., O'Dell, M. C., & Koegel, L. K. (1987). A natural language teaching paradigm for nonverbal autistic children. *Journal of Autism and Developmental Disorders, 17*, 187–200.

Koegel, R. L., Russo, D. C., & Rincover, A. (1977). Assessing and training teachers in the generalized use of behavior modification with autistic children. *Journal of Applied Behavior Analysis, 10*, 197–205.

Kolvin, I. (1971). Studies in the childhood psychoses: I. Diagnostic criteria and classification. *British Journal of Psychiatry, 118*, 381–384.

Kolvin, I., Ounsted, C., Humphrey, M., & McNay, A. (1971). Studies in the childhood psychoses: II. The phenomenology of childhood psychoses. *British Journal of Psychiatry, 118*, 385–395.

Kraemer, H. C., Noda, A., & O'Hara, R. (2004). Categorical versus dimensional approaches to diagnosis: Methodological challenges. *Journal of Psychiatric Research, 38*, 17–25.

Kurita, H., Osada, H., & Miyake, H. (2004). External validity of childhood disintegrative disorder in comparison with autistic disorder. *Journal of Autism and Developmental Disorders, 34*, 355–362.

Lelord, G., Muh, J. P., Barthelemy, C., Martineau, J., Garreau, B., & Callaway, E. (1981). Effects of pyridoxine and magnesium on autistic symptoms – Initial observations. *Journal of Autism and Developmental Disorders, 11*, 219–230.

Lobascher, M. E., Kingerlee, P. E., & Gubbay, S. S. (1970). Childhood autism: An investigation of aetiological factors in twenty-five cases. *British Journal of Psychiatry, 117*, 525–529.

Lotter, V. (1966). Epidemiology of autistic conditions in young children: I. Prevalence. *Social Psychiatry, 1*, 124–137.

Lovaas, O. I. (1987). Behavioral treatment and normal educational and intellectual functioning in young autistic children. *Journal of Consulting and Clinical Psychology, 55*, 3–9.

Lovaas, O. I. (1993). The development of a treatment – research project for developmentally disabled and autistic children. *Journal of Applied Behavioral Analysis, 26*, 617–630.

Lovaas, O. I. (1996). The UCLA young autism model of service delivery. In C. Maurice (Ed.), *Behavioral intervention for young children with autism* (pp. 241–250). Austin: Pro-Ed.

Lovaas, O. I., Koegel, R., Simmons, J. Q., & Long, J. S. (1973). Some generalization and follow-up measures on autistic children in behavior therapy. *Journal of Applied Behavior Analysis, 6*, 131–165.

Lowe, L. H. (1966). Families of children with early childhood schizophrenia. *Archives of General Psychiatry, 14*, 26–30.

MacCallum, R. C., Zhang, S., Preacher, K. J., & Rucker, D. D. (2002). On the practice of dichotomization of quantitative variables. *Psychological Methods, 7*, 19–40.

Magiati, I., & Howlin, P. (2001). Monitoring the progress of preschool children with autism enrolled in early intervention programmes: Problems in cognitive assessment. *Autism, 5*, 399–406.

Manjiviona, J., & Prior, M. (1999). Neuropsychological profiles of children with Asperger syndrome and autism. *Autism, 3*, 327–356.

Maudsley, H. (1867). Insanity of early life. In H. Maudsley (Ed.), *The physiology and pathology of the mind* (pp. 259–386). New York: Appleton.

Mayes, R., & Horowitz, A. V. (2005). DSM-III and the revolution in the classification of mental illness. *Journal of the History of the Behavioral Sciences, 41*, 249–267.

Miller, J. N., & Ozonoff, S. (2000). The external validity of Asperger disorder: Lack of evidence from the domain of neuropsychology. *Journal of Abnormal Psychology, 2*, 227–238.

Montee, B. B., Milterberger, R. G., & Wittrock, D. (1995). An experimental analysis of facilitated communication. *Journal of Applied Behavior Analysis, 28*, 189–200.

Mouridsen, S. E., Rich, B., & Isager, T. (1998). Validity of childhood disintegrative psychosis. General findings of a long-term follow-up study. *The British Journal of Psychiatry, 172*, 263–267.

Nordquist, V. M., & Wahler, R. G. (1973). Naturalistic treatment of an autistic child. *Journal of Applied Behavior Analysis, 6*, 79–87.

Olsson, B., & Rett, A. (1987). Autism and Rett syndrome: Behavioural investigations and differential diagnosis. *Developmental Medicine and Child Neurology, 29*, 429–441.

Ozonoff, S., & Cathcart, K. (1998). Effectiveness of a home program intervention for young children with autism. *Journal of Autism and Developmental Disorders, 28*, 25–32.

Ozonoff, S., Goodlin-Jones, B. L., & Solomon, M. (2007). Autism spectrum disorder. In E. J. Mash & R. A. Barkley (Eds.), *Assessment of childhood disorder* (4th ed., pp. 478–508). New York: Guilford Press.

Ozonoff, S., South, M., & Miller, J. N. (2000). DSM-IV-defined Asperger syndrome: Cognitive, behavioral and early history differentiation from high-functioning autism. *Autism, 4*, 29–46.

Panksepp, J. A. (1979). A neurochemical theory of autism. *Trends Neuroscience, 2*, 174–177.

Pauling, L. (1968). Orthomolecular psychiatry. *Science, 160*, 265–271.

Percy, A. K. (2008). Rett Syndrome: Recent research progress. *Journal of Child Neurology, 23*, 543–549.

Pfeiffer, S. I., Norton, J., Nelson, L., & Shott, S. (1995). Efficacy of vitamin B6 and magnesium in the treatment of autism: A methodology review and summary of outcomes. *Journal of Autism and Developmental Disorders, 25*, 481–493.

Pierce, K., & Schreibman, L. (1995). Increasing complex social behaviors in children with autism: Effects of peer-implemented pivotal response training. *Journal of Applied Behavior Analysis, 28*, 285–295.

Pierce, K., & Schreibman, L. (1997). Multiple peer use of pivotal response training to increase social behaviors of classmates with autism: Results from trained and untrained peers. *Journal of Applied Behavior Analysis, 30*, 157–160.

Posserud, M. B., Lundervold, A. J., & Gillberg, C. (2006). Autistic features in a total population of 7–9-year-old children assessed by the ASSQ (Autism Spectrum Screening Questionnaire). *Journal of Child Psychology & Psychiatry, 47*, 167–175.

Prior, M., Eisenmajer, R., Leekam, S., Wing, L., Gould, J., Ong, B., et al. (1998). Are there subgroups within the autistic spectrum? A cluster analysis of a group of children with autistic spectrum disorders. *Journal of Child Psychology and Psychiatry, 39*, 893–902.

Quintana, H., Birmaher, B., Stedge, D., Lennon, S., Freed, J., Bridge, J., et al. (1995). Use of methylphenidate in the treatment of children with autistic disorder. *Journal of autism and developmental disorders, 25*, 283–294.

Regal, R. A., Rooney, J. R., & Wandas, T. (1994). Facilitated communication: An experimental evaluation. *Journal of autism and developmental disorders, 24*, 345–355.

Reichelt, K. L., Knivsberg, A., Lind, G., & Nødland, M. (1991). Probable etiology and possible treatment of childhood autism. *Brain Dysfunction, 4*, 308–319.

Rett, A. (1966). Ueber ein eigenartiges hirnatrophisches syndrom bei hyperammoniamie im kindesalter. *Wiener Medizinische Wochenschrift, 116*, 723–738.

Rimland, B. (1964). *Infantile autism*. London: Methuen.

Rimland, B. (2000). "Garbage science" Brick walls, crossword puzzles, and mercury. *Autism Research Review International, 14*, 3.

Rimland, B., Callaway, E., & Dreyfus, P. (1978). The effect of high doses of vitamin B6 on autistic children: A double-blind crossover study. *American Journal of Psychiatry, 135*, 472–475.

Rimland, B., & Edelson, S. M. (1995). Brief report: A pilot study of auditory integration training in autism. *Journal of Autism and Developmental Disorders, 25*, 61–70.

Rutter, M. (1967). Psychotic disorders in early childhood. In A. J. Coppen & A. Walk (Eds.), *Recent developments in Schizophrenia: A symposium* (pp. 133–158). London: R.M.P.A.

Rutter, M. (1968). Concepts of autism: A review of research. *Journal of Child Psychology and Psychiatry, 9*, 1–25.

Rutter, M. (1972). Childhood schizophrenia reconsidered. *Journal of Autism and Childhood Schizophrenia, 2*, 315–337.

Rutter, M. (1978). Diagnosis and definition. In M. Rutter & E. Schopler (Eds.), *Autism: A reappraisal of concepts and treatment* (pp. 1–25). New York: Plenum Press.

Rutter, M. (2005). Incidence of autism spectrum disorders: Changes over time and their meaning. *Acta Pediatrica, 94*, 2–15.

Rutter, M., & Lockyer, L. A. (1967). A five to fifteen year follow-up study of infantile psychosis. I. Description of the sample. *British Journal of Psychiatry, 113*, 1169–1182.

Schain, R. J., & Yannet, H. (1960). Infantile autism: An analysis of fifty cases and a consideration of certain neurophysiologic concepts. *Journal of Pediatrics, 57*, 560–567.

Schopler, E. (1985). Convergence of learning disability, higher-level autism, and Asperger's syndrome. *Journal of Autism and Developmental Disorders, 15*, 359–360.

Schopler, E. (1994). Behavioral priorities for autism and related developmental disorders. In E. Schopler & G. B. Mesibov (Eds.), *Behavioral issues in autism* (pp. 55–80). New York: Plenum Press.

Schopler, E., & Reichler, R. J. (1971). Parents as cotherapists in the treatment of psychotic children. *Journal of Autism and Childhood Schizophrenia, 1*, 87–102.

Shea, V. (2004). A perspective on the research literature related to early intensive behavioural intervention (Lovaas) for young children with autism. *Autism, 8*, 349–367.

Sheinkopf, S. J., & Siegel, B. (1998). Home-based behavioral treatment of young children with autism. *Journal of Autism and Developmental Disorders, 28*, 15–23.

Smith, T. (2001). Discrete trial training in the treatment of autism. *Focus on Autism and Other Developmental Disabilities, 16*, 86–92.

Spence, M. A. (1976). Genetic studies. In E. Ritvo (Ed.), *Autism: Diagnosis, current research and management* (pp. 169–174). New York: Halstead/Wiley.

Stahmer, A. C. (1995). Teaching symbolic play skills to children with autism using pivotal response training. *Journal of Autism and Childhood Schizophrenia, 25*, 123–141.

Szatmari, P. (2000). The classification of autism, Asperger's syndrome, and pervasive developmental disorder. *Canadian Journal of Psychiatry, 45*, 731–738.

Szatmari, P., Archer, L., Fisman, S., Streiner, D. L., & Wilson, F. (1995). Asperger's syndrome and autism: Differences in behavior, cognition, and adaptive functioning. *Journal of the American Academy of Child and Adolescent Psychiatry, 34*, 1662–1671.

Taft, L. T., & Goldfarb, W. (1964). Prenatal and perinatal factors in childhood schizophrenia. *Developmental Medicine & Child Neurology, 6*, 32–43.

Thomas, C. C. (1960, July 25). Medicine: The child is father. *Time, 111*, 167.

Tsai, L. (2000). Children with autism spectrum disorder: Medicine today and in the new millennium. *Focus on Autism and Other Developmental Disabilities, 15*, 138–145.

Tsai, L., Stewart, M. A., & August, G. (1981). Implication of sex differences in the familial transmission of infantile autism. *Journal of Autism and Developmental Disorders, 11*, 165–173.

Volkmar, F. (1992). Childhood disintegrative disorder: Issues for the DSM-IV. *Journal of Autism and Developmental Disorders, 22*, 625–645.

Volkmar, F. R., & Cohen, D. J. (1991). Debate and argument: The utility of the term pervasive developmental disorder. *Journal of Child Psychology and Psychiatry, 32*, 1171–1172.

Volkmar, F. R., Lord, C., Bailey, A., Schultz, R. T., & Klin, A. (2004). Autism and pervasive developmental disorders. *Journal of Child Psychology and Psychiatry, 45*, 135–170.

Walker, H. A. (1977). Incidence of minor physical anomaly in autism. *Journal of Autism and Childhood Schizophrenia, 7*, 165–176.

Wallis, C. (2009, November 2). A powerful identity, a vanishing diagnosis. *The Wall Street Journal*, pp. D1.

West, L., Brunssen, S. H., & Waldrop, L. (2009). Review of the evidence for treatment of children with autism with selective serotonin reuptake inhibitors. *Journal for Specialists in Pediatric Nursing, 14*, 183–191.

Whiteley, P., Rodgers, J., Savery, D., & Shattock, P. (1999). A gluten-free diet as an intervention for autism and associated spectrum disorders: Preliminary findings. *Autism, 3*, 45–65.

Williams, S. K., Scahill, L., Vitiello, B., Aman, M. G., Arnold, E., McDougle, J., et al. (2006). Risperidone and adaptive behavior in children with autism. *Journal of the American Academy of Child Adolescent and Psychiatry, 45*, 431–439.

Williams, K. R., & Wishart, J. G. (2003). The son-rise program intervention for autism: An investigation into family experiences. *Journal of Intellectual Disability Research, 47*, 291–299.

Wing, L. (1981). Asperger's syndrome: A clinical account. *Psychological Bulletin, 11*, 115–129.

Wing, L. (1991). The relationship between Asperger's syndrome and Kanner's autism. In U. Frith (Ed.), *Autism and Asperger syndrome* (pp. 93–121). Cambridge: Cambridge University Press.

Wing, L., & Gould, J. (1979). Severe impairments of social interaction and associated abnormalities in children: Epidemiology and classification. *Journal of Autism and Developmental Disorders, 9*(1), 11–29.

Wolf, M. M., Risley, T., & Mees, H. (1964). Application of operant conditioning procedures to the behavior problems of an autistic child. *Behavior Research and Therapy, 1*, 305–312.

Wulffaert, J., VanBerckelaer-Onnes, A. I., & Scholte, E. M. (2009). Autistic disorder symptoms in Rett syndrome. *Autism, 13*, 567–581.

Diagnostic Systems

Christopher L. Gillberg

Diagnosis and epidemiology are core topics in psychiatry and developmental medicine. There can be no clinical medical work without diagnosis. There can be no medical epidemiological study of psychiatric disorder without a consideration of diagnostic boundaries.

While both clinical medical diagnostic practice and medical epidemiology have separate roots, purposes, and methods, a number of points of contact can be identified. Modern approaches to medical/psychiatric diagnostic description have made possible the design of potent tools for epidemiological surveys, and results from such surveys are contributing to the refinement of diagnostic profiles. The current international psychiatric and developmental diagnostic systems, including multiaxial formulations, not only of illness but also of the bigger picture of the patient's clinical condition, offer challenging opportunities for interaction and progress.

Diagnostic systems in psychiatric medicine are overarching models of symptoms, problems, functional restrictions, impairments, traits, signs, and biological test markers that constitute a particular disease, disorder, or group of disorders. Among these are factor analytic models, signal detection models, continuous distribution models with statistically pre-determined cutoff arbiters, artificial network models, and clinically based models such as the *International Classification of Diseases and Disorders* [*ICD*; World Health Organization (WHO), 1993] and, for psychiatric disorders, the *Diagnostic and Statistical Manual of Mental Disorders* [*DSM*; American Psychiatric Association (APA), 1980, 1987, 1994, 2000, 2010]. A distinction is made in this chapter between such modeling issues and specific tests and procedures used to make a particular diagnosis such as autism. The latter topic will be covered in other chapters.

C.L. Gillberg (✉)
Gillberg Neuropsychiatry Centre, Gothenburg University, Gothenburg, Sweden
e-mail: christopher.gillberg@pediat.gu.se

Factor Analytic and Latent Class Models

Several different types of factor analytic models have been applied to the field of child and adolescent psychiatric diagnosis. There are various ways in which factor analysis can be carried out, including exploratory and confirmatory techniques, and also a related but not identical procedure, referred to as principal component analysis. Factor analytic models can be conceptualized as subclasses of latent variable models, which also include latent trait, latent profile, and latent class analyses (used separately or in combination with the so-called Rasch model).

Perhaps the most illustrative example of how factor analysis has been applied in clinical child and adolescent psychiatric/developmental diagnosis comes from the much researched – and used – material developed by Thomas Achenbach (originally with colleague Edelbrock), often referred to as the "child behavior checklist" (CBCL) or the Achenbach System of Empirically Based Assessment (ASEBA; Achenbach et al., 2008).

The CBCL/1.5-5 and the CBCL/6-18 include 99 and 118 problem items, respectively, that can be scored by parents of children aged 1–18 years. The items refer to problem behaviors and emotions often encountered in children. A total problem score (comprising an internalizing and an externalizing score) is computed by adding scores for individual items. Subscores for aggressive behavior; anxious/depressed; attention problems; rule-breaking behavior; social problems; somatic complaints; thought problems; and withdrawn/depressed can also be calculated. The six DSM-oriented scales are affective problems; anxiety problems; somatic problems; attention deficit/hyperactivity problems; oppositional defiant problems; and conduct problems. The preschool 99-item version for 1.5–5-year olds also has a DSM-oriented scale for autism/"pervasive developmental disorder." In addition to the CBCL for parent rating, there is a related Teacher Report Form (TRF) and a Youth Self-Report (YSR) for 11–18-year olds.

Each item on the CBCL is given the same weight in the scoring system. The various subscales have been developed on the basis of factor and principal component analytic studies, and the DSM-oriented scales have been developed on the basis of a combination of statistical and clinical studies. One of the problems with the factor analytic approach relates to the fact that many of the individual items are completely unrelated and clearly do not have the same clinical weight. In fact, it can be argued that the individual items represent 118 different problems and that the subscales, to a considerable extent, represent artificial statistically derived constructs that do not necessarily correspond to recognizable clinical entities (in spite of having been assigned names that would suggest a clear correlation between the research and the clinical concept). This problem is not unique to the development of the CBCL (and related material) but applies equally to a number of other much used scales, including the Strengths and Difficulties Questionnaire (SDQ; Goodman, 1999) and the Autism Spectrum Screening Questionnaire (ASSQ; Ehlers & Gillberg, 1993).

A good example of how factor analytic models can be used to increase precision and understanding of a heterogeneous clinical psychiatric concept such as obsessive–compulsive disorder is given in a paper by Mataix-Cols and co-workers (Mataix-Cols, Rosario-Campos, & Leckman, 2005).

Signal Detection Models and Receiver Operating Characteristic (ROC)

Many diagnostic systems are used to distinguish between two classes of events, essentially "signals" and "noise," or "diagnosis" and "no diagnosis." For such systems, analysis in terms of the "relative (or receiver) operating characteristic" (ROC) of signal detection theory provides a fairly precise and valid measure of diagnostic accuracy. It is uninfluenced by decision biases and prior probabilities, and it puts the performances of diverse systems on a common, easily interpreted scale.

The ROC model applied to a diagnostic screening instrument with a wide range of possible scores (such as the CBCL, the SDQ or the ASSQ) is best presented in a graph detailing the true-positive rate (TPR = sensitivity) on the y-axis and the false-positive rate (FPR = 1 minus specificity) on the x-axis. The best trade-off for diagnostic purposes is usually seen at the point where the TPR is the highest and the FPR the lowest, i.e., at the inflection point on the curve. The value of TPR times FPR at this point represents the area under the curve (AUC). When the AUC approaches 1.0, the diagnostic precision of the screening instrument is excellent, but when it approaches 0.5, the precision is extremely poor. The use of the AUC concept as a measure in the evaluation

of new diagnostic screening tools has become something of a "gold standard" in recent years. It is important to understand that the inflection point of the ROC curve might not always be the preferred cutoff point for "diagnosis" according to a particular scale in all instances. Depending on the purpose of a study or on clinical praxis, having an extremely low FPR (i.e., minimizing the risk for overdiagnosis) might be of utmost importance, whereas in other instances, high TPR might be regarded essential (i.e., minimizing the risk for underdiagnosis).

Continuous Distribution Models

Most diagnostic systems, explicitly or implicitly, are, to some extent, based on notions of "normality" and "abnormality." Many human traits, functions, or markers of functional systems can be construed as existing on a normal distribution scale which will be relatively smooth when the range of possible scores is large. "Abnormality" is often defined as a specified distance from the mean or the median score of such a scale (for example (plus) minus two standard deviations from the mean or under or over the 2nd/98th percentile). A disease or a pathological state can then, for instance, be construed as existing when the value of a marker for a biological function is below a specified level (such as in pathological shortness or "dwarfism"), or above a set limit (such as in hyperthyroidism).

Much can be said for diagnosing a number of psychiatric disorders along continuous distribution curves. ADHD and ASD are but two examples of "disorders" that can, in many instances, be seen as extremes of "conditions" that exist along a normally/continuously distributed spectrum (Posserud, Lundervold, & Gillberg, 2006). However, problems arise when it comes to specificity and determining exactly which specific trait should be considered the key marker function for the disorder. For instance, in ADHD, it is still not possible to determine whether attention, activity, or impulsivity aspects/functions should be considered core features of the "disorder." Similarly, in ASD, it is not possible to assess the core quality of repetitive behaviors or, for that matter, perceptual functions, when it comes to delineating the "syndrome" of ASD. In the latter case – to "fully cover" the clinical spectrum of the "autistic state" in a given individual – it might be necessary to provide centile values for three or more continuous distribution curves, e.g., empathy, central coherence, and rigidity–flexibility, and this would entail a great deal of conceptual and practical problems in clinical practice.

There are other problems with the continuous distribution model. First, it is as difficult to reasonably determine cutoff for abnormality under this model as it is in the general medical model of categorical disorders. Second, there are quite a number of instances, for instance, in autism, when the model is totally inappropriate. It would not be correct or logical to categorize a case of autism caused by herpes encephalitis as being on a distribution curve shading into "normality." Third, and not least, there is a need for quick and dirty labels such as autism and ADHD, much like there is a need for terms like "fever" and "pneumonia" (imprecise and even more vague terms than those used in neuropsychiatry). One of the most important features of a diagnostic label is its "door-opening" quality; by having a label you will have easy access to knowledge. Having been given a percentage on a normal distribution curve, or worse, multiple different percentages on different curves, will possibly be closer to "the truth" but will often lead to more confusion than clarity. Having said this, the continuous distribution model has much to offer in second-level diagnostics: once a diagnosis of, for instance, autism has been made, providing information about the individual's level of functioning on a number of continuous distribution curves might actually help create a much more detailed (and holistic) view of that person's functioning.

The ICD

The evolution of diagnostic criteria is not simply a theoretical exercise but reflects empirically or historically based assumptions about the nature of the underlying pathology and the relationships between different disorders. Furthermore, these criteria determine which subjects are included in research and in clinical trials so that they shape the further development of psychiatric classification systems.

The ICD-10 was endorsed in 1990 and came into use in WHO member states in 1994. The ICD classification system has its origin in the 1850s. The first edition was adopted by the International Statistical Institute in 1893 ("List of Causes of Death"). The WHO took over the responsibility for the ICD at its creation in 1948. In 1967 the World Health Assembly adopted the WHO Nomenclature Regulations that stipulate the use of ICD in its most current revision for mortality and morbidity statistics by all member states.

The ICD is the international standard diagnostic classification for epidemiological, health management purposes, and in clinical practice. These include the analysis of the general health of population groups and the monitoring of prevalence of disorders and other health problems.

The ICD-10 has a section for psychiatric disorder (including for autism or "pervasive developmental disorders") that is similar but not identical to that of the DSM-IV which was published at about the same time as the ICD-10. Attempts were made during the development of the psychiatric section of the ICD-10 and the DSM-IV to streamline the two manuals. This was partly successful, but there are still considerable differences across the text, criteria and algorithms for diagnosing particular disorders, and some disorders appear in only one of the manuals.

Given that the DSM, compared to the ICD, has a much longer history when it comes to developing and analyzing operationalized criteria for psychiatric disorder, there will be a more detailed focus on the DSM-IV than on the ICD-10 in the present chapter. Much of what will be said about the DSM-IV (and the development of the DSM-V) applies in principle to the ICD-10 (and the development of the ICD-11, which is scheduled for publication in late 2013).

The DSM, Its History and Development with a Particular Focus on Autism

The Diagnostic and Statistical Manual of Mental Disorders is published by the American Psychiatric Association and provides diagnostic criteria for psychiatric disorders. It is used across the world, by clinicians, researchers, psychiatric drug regulation agencies, health insurance companies, pharmaceutical companies, and policy makers.

The *DSM-V* is currently under development and expected to be published in the spring of 2013. The *DSM-IV* – and the *DSM-IV Text Revision* (with virtually identical diagnostic operationalized criteria) – will then have been in use in clinical and research practice for almost two decades, which is considerably longer than the two 7-year periods of the forerunners *DSM-III* and *DSM-III-R*.

The DSM system is probably the most widely used diagnostic system for psychiatric and developmental disorders in the Western world. This has meant relative stability in the way psychiatric disorders have been conceptualized over several decades. However, as more and more research has documented the dimensional nature of so many of the core psychiatric disorders (including autism), the rigid structure and the algorithmic nature of the DSM have come under increasing criticism. The inclusion of dimensional elements in the psychiatric diagnostic systems has been advocated for many years. However it has been resisted due to concerns about clinical utility. Recent suggestions have been for a combination of categorical and dimensional data in future diagnostic classification systems.

The History of the DSM

In 1949, the WHO published the sixth revision of the ICD, which included a section on mental disorders for the first time. The *DSM-I* was published in 1952. Although the publisher of the *DSM-I*, the APA, was closely involved in the next significant revision of the mental disorder section of the ICD (version 8 in 1968), it also decided to go ahead with a revision of the DSM. The *DSM-II* was also published in 1968, was 134 pages long, and listed 182 disorders. Both the *DSM-I* and the *DSM-II* reflected the predominant psychodynamic psychiatry, although they also included biological perspectives and concepts from Kraepelin's system of classification. Symptoms were not operationalized in detail for specific disorders. Many were seen as reflections of broad underlying conflicts or maladaptive reactions to life problems, rooted in a distinction between "neurosis" and "psychosis." Sociological and biological knowledge was also incorporated in a model that did not emphasize a clear boundary between normality and abnormality.

In 1974, the decision to create a new revision of the DSM was taken, and Robert Spitzer was selected as chairman of the task force. The initial impetus was to make the DSM nomenclature consistent with that of the ICD. The revision took on a wider mandate under the influence and control of Spitzer. One goal was to improve the uniformity and validity of psychiatric diagnosis. There was also a need to standardize diagnostic practices after research had shown that psychiatric diagnoses differed markedly across Europe and the USA. The establishment of the DSM criteria was also an attempt to facilitate the pharmaceutical regulatory process.

The criteria adopted for many of the mental disorders were taken from the Research Diagnostic Criteria (RDC) and the Feighner Criteria, which had recently been developed by a group of research-orientated psychiatrists based primarily at Washington University in St. Louis and at the New York State Psychiatric Institute. Other criteria, and potential new categories of disorder, were established by consensus during meetings of the committee, as chaired by Spitzer. A key aim was to base categorization on descriptive language rather than assumptions of etiology. The psychodynamic and physiologic views were largely abandoned. A new "multiaxial" system attempted to yield a "bigger picture," more consistent with clinical reality than the "box-approach only" which would be the result of using the "superficial" operationalized diagnosis without further qualification.

The first draft of the *DSM-III* was prepared in 1975. Field trials sponsored by the US National Institute of Mental Health (NIMH) were conducted between 1977 and 1979 to test the reliability of the new diagnoses. When published in 1980, the *DSM-III* was almost 500 pages long and listed 265 diagnostic categories. It rapidly came into widespread international use by multiple stakeholders and has been termed a revolution or transformation in psychiatry.

In 1987 the *DSM-III-R* was published as a revision of *DSM-III*, under the direction of Spitzer. Categories were renamed, reorganized, and significant changes in criteria were made. Six categories were deleted, while others were added. The *DSM-III-R* contained 292 diagnoses and was 70 pages longer than the *DSM-III*.

In 1994, the *DSM-IV* was published, listing almost 300 disorders in just under 900 pages. The task force was chaired by Allen Frances. A steering committee was introduced, including a small number of psychologists. The steering committee created 13 work groups of 5–16 members. Each work group had approximately 20 advisers. The work groups conducted a three-step process. First, each group conducted literature reviews of their diagnoses. Then they requested data from researchers, conducting analyses to determine which criteria required change, with instructions to be conservative. Finally, they conducted field trials relating diagnoses to clinical practice. A change from previous versions was the inclusion of a clinical significance criterion to about half of the categories.

A "text revision" of the *DSM-IV*, known as the *DSM-IV-TR*, was published in 2000. The diagnostic categories and the vast majority of the specific criteria for diagnosis were unchanged. The text sections giving extra information on each diagnosis were updated, as were some of the diagnostic codes in order to maintain consistency with the ICD.

The *DSM-V*, under the chairmanship of David Kupfer, is currently expected to be published in 2013, months before the envisaged publication of the ICD-11 (Kupfer D and Sartorius N, Personal communication about DSM-V and ICD-11). Several of the personality disorder categories will be gone and a few new categories of psychiatric disorder will be included. It is expected that autism will be one category (not referred to as pervasive developmental disorder) and that subgrouping will be done on the basis of a number of "non-autism" demographics such as level of IQ, language competence, and severity.

The Categorical Nature of the DSM System

The categories in DSM are prototypes, and a patient with a close approximation to the prototype is said to have that disorder. Each category of disorder has a numeric code taken from the ICD coding system, used for administrative purposes (including insurance). One problem with this approach to diagnosis is that it does not properly deal with all those instances when a patient is severely impaired but does not meet *all* the criteria for a given discrete disorder. Everyday in clinical practice (and in research), this is illustrated by diagnosis in the field of autism and related disorders. Many Western societies now have legislation specifically for autism. This means that having a "correct" diagnosis (i.e., one that fits with federal legislation) is extremely important. In needy clinical patients and in research prevalence studies, the categorical nature of the DSM system can be the arbiter between help and no help in terms of service provision, and between case and non-case in epidemiological studies.

Why Do We Need a Cross-cultural Diagnostic Manual – Such as the DSM – for Autism and Related Disorders?

Clinical work – not least assessment, diagnosis, and clinical research – with children and adolescents suffering from mental health problems or psychiatric disorder is challenging and complex. Medical doctors must take into account children's vulnerabilities and respect their rights, regardless of legal barriers or developmental limitations.

Despite the fact that during the last 65 years a number of diagnostic systems and clinical models of autism have been proposed, defining this psychiatric/developmental disorder in a manner acceptable in both clinical and research settings remains one of the most difficult tasks in psychiatry and developmental medicine. While the description of symptoms and signs of autism has remained largely unchanged over the years, the way in which authors have articulated the multiple manifestations of autism has differed over time. Progress has been made in recent years, and this has brought about a convergence on a shared definition of autism, including methods of assessment that are acceptable to workers from clinical and research centers across the world. Structured interviews (e.g., the DISCO-11, the ADI-R, and the ASDI) and observation schedules (including the ADOS-G) have brought organizational focus to the traditional psychiatric interview and developmental assessment. Such methods have provided a stricter format and directions to the interviewer, which, in turn, have enabled systematic assessment of *all* the criteria necessary for a diagnosis according to the given diagnostic (e.g., DSM) system. Having a consensually shared set of diagnostic criteria as well as structured assessment devices has helped ensure a more common unit of analysis in clinical practice and research across the globe. Though most workers would consider the operationalization of diagnostic criteria as an advance in psychiatry and developmental medicine, there remain concerns about the impact that the quest for increased diagnostic reliability might have on validity. Given that the ultimate goal of any diagnostic system is to provide insights into the causes and treatment of a disorder, examining various alternative diagnostic constructs and their validity is still an important area of autism research.

Comorbidity and the DSM System

The term "comorbidity" was introduced in medicine by Feinstein (1970) to denote those cases in which a "distinct additional clinical entity" occurred during the clinical course of a patient having an index disease. This term has recently become very fashionable in psychiatry and developmental medicine to indicate not only those cases in which a patient receives both a psychiatric and a general medical diagnosis

(e.g., autism and tuberous sclerosis) but also those cases in which a patient receives two or more psychiatric diagnoses (e.g., autism and Tourette syndrome). This co-occurrence of two or more psychiatric diagnoses ("psychiatric comorbidity") has been reported to be very frequent. For instance, in a general population study, 85% of young children with ADHD had at least one additional DSM diagnosis leading to impairment (Kadesjo & Gillberg, 2001). In the case of severe autism, I would be surprised to find one single case in which there was no other mental or physical disorder. If a diagnosis of autistic disorder is made, you would have to be on the lookout for mental retardation/learning disability, epilepsy, a medical disorder such as tuberous sclerosis or 22q11deletion syndrome, a neuropsychiatric disorder such as Tourette syndrome or ADHD, a mood disorder, an anxiety disorder, an eating disorder, a sleep disorder, or a specific developmental disorder such as developmental coordination disorder.

This use of the term "comorbidity" to indicate the co-occurrence of two or more psychiatric diagnoses appears to be logically incorrect because in most cases it is unclear whether the concomitant diagnoses actually reflect the presence of distinct clinical entities or refer to multiple manifestations of a single clinical entity. Because "the use of imprecise language may lead to correspondingly imprecise thinking" (Lilienfeld, Waldman, & Israel, 1994), this usage of the term "comorbidity" should probably best be avoided.

Nevertheless, the co-occurrence of multiple psychiatric diagnoses is now much more frequent than just 10 years ago. This is to some extent due to the use of standardized diagnostic interviews, which help to identify several clinical aspects that in the past remained unnoticed after the principal diagnosis had been made. Fragmenting a complex clinical condition into several pieces may prevent a holistic approach to the individual.

An obvious determinant of the emergence of the phenomenon of "psychiatric comorbidity" (see below) has been the proliferation of diagnostic categories in recent classifications. If demarcations are made where they do not "really" exist, the probability that several diagnoses have to be made in an individual case will obviously increase.

A coveted tradition in psychiatry and developmental medicine has been to establish a hierarchy of diagnostic categories so that, for example, if autism were present, the possibly concomitant anxiety, depression, or ADHD would not be diagnosed because they would be regarded as part of the clinical picture of autism.

Because we now use operationalized diagnostic criteria, diagnoses such as autistic disorder are regarded as more reliable than traditional clinical diagnoses. The old clinical descriptions provided a gestalt of each diagnostic entity. Different emphasis was put on the various clinical aspects, whereas current operational definitions usually give equal weight to a variety of clinical manifestations, *counting* symptoms rather than *weighing* them. Traditional clinical assessment demanded arbiter differential diagnosis, whereas current operational definitions encourage multiple diagnoses, possibly in part because they are less able to convey the "essence" of each diagnostic entity.

The frequent co-occurrence of the mental disorders included in current diagnostic systems has been taken as evidence against the idea that these disorders represent discrete disease entities (Cloninger, 2002). The point has been made that psychopathology is usually complex and variable and that what is currently conceptualized as the co-occurrence of multiple disorders could be better reformulated as the complexity of many psychiatric conditions (with increasing complexity being a predictor of greater severity, disability, and service utilization). Even Kraepelin in one of his later works dismissed the model of discrete disease entities even for dementia praecox and manic–depressive disorder (Kraepelin, 1920).

However, an alternative possibility is that psychopathology does consist of discrete entities but that these entities are not well delineated by current diagnostic categories. If this is the case, then current clinical research on "psychiatric comorbidity" may be helpful in the search for "true" disease entities, contributing in the long term to a rearrangement of present classifications.

There is, of course, a third possibility, viz. that the nature of psychopathology is intrinsically heterogeneous, consisting partly of disease entities and categorical disorders, and partly of maladaptive response patterns or of exaggeration of traits that are more or less normally distributed in the general population.

The DSM as Used in Clinical Practice and Research

The DSM is much the most widely distributed diagnostic manual in psychiatry, both in research and clinical practice. In clinical work, it is used to determine and help doctors communicate a patient's diagnosis after an evaluation.

The DSM is primarily concerned with the symptoms and behavioral manifestation of mental disorders. With the exception of a small number of disorders (including "reactive attachment disorder"), it does not generally attempt to analyze or explain the conditions included in the manual.

The DSM-IV organizes each psychiatric diagnosis into five levels (axes) relating to different aspects of disorder or disability:

* *Axis I*: Clinical disorders, including major mental disorders, and learning disorders (very often the only axis that is thoroughly checked in clinical work and research). Axis I disorders include autistic disorder, Asperger's disorder, ADHD, oppositional defiant disorder, depression, anxiety disorders, Tourette's disorder, selective mutism bipolar disorder, phobias, schizophrenia, anorexia nervosa, and a whole host of other named disorders.
* *Axis II*: "Underlying" personality disorders and mental retardation ("learning disability" in European parlance).
* *Axis III*: Acute medical conditions and physical disorders, including brain injury syndromes, cerebral palsy, epilepsy, and other medical/physical disorders which may aggravate existing diseases or present symptoms similar to Axis I or Axis II disorders.
* *Axis IV*: psychosocial and environmental factors contributing to the Axis I disorder.
* *Axis V*: Global Assessment of Functioning (GAF) or Children's Global Assessment Scale (CGAS) for children and teenagers under the age of 18 years.

Appropriate use of the DSM diagnostic criteria requires extensive clinical training, and its contents cannot be applied in a cookbook fashion. There is a clear risk that patients and non-medical professionals may use the DSM in a checklist fashion and make "diagnosis" according to the number of checked symptoms. It needs to be stressed that the DSM is a manual for medical psychiatric diagnosis. In practice this should be taken to mean that the diagnostic criteria can be used only for making a definitive clinical diagnosis by highly skilled professionals (medical doctors with specialist training in psychiatry and for some disorders, including autism, ADHD and DCD, those with training in neurology and developmental medicine).

In clinical research, the manual is often used by other highly skilled professionals, including psychologists and speech language therapists with specialist training. However, research diagnoses should not uncritically be equated with clinical diagnoses, and if a psychiatrist or other specifically trained medical doctor has not been involved in the diagnostic process, the "DSM diagnosis" (which, in such cases, is not a DSM diagnosis in the intended sense of the word) should not be considered a psychiatric or a medical diagnosis.

The *DSM-V* published proposed diagnostic criteria in 2010. There was opportunity for specialists and the general public to react to these, and criteria were revised in the process. Once this was accomplished, the criteria were then tested in field trials. The results of these trials are not at hand at the publication of this volume. The process of work groups proposing criteria and the research community and general public reacting before final revision and field trials has been adhered to in the development of the DSM over the past 30 years. Even though this is in no way a guarantee that the criteria, once published, are "right," it is possibly the best that can be achieved at a time when there is still no litmus test for psychiatric disorder. In the future, when genetics and proteomics and neuropsychology and personal account will have helped define psychiatric disorder in a more rational fashion, this DSM approach to diagnosis will possibly be looked upon as undistinguished.

It has been argued that the DSM (and the ICD) is a system of classification that makes unjustified categorical distinctions between disorders, and between normal and abnormal. Although the *DSM-V* may move away from this categorical approach in some limited areas, some argue that a fully dimensional spectrum or complaint-oriented approach would better reflect the evidence (Krueger, Watson, & Barlow, 2005). Also, the level of impairment is sometimes not correlated with symptom counts and can stem from a variety of individual and psychosocial factors, increasing risk of producing "false-positive" cases. Nevertheless, it is very difficult to envisage an overall change, leading to fully dimensional diagnostics in psychiatry, given that it would not only be very difficult in practice but also entail a break with the tradition of categorical medical diagnosis that has a history of thousands of years.

Both the DSM and the ICD have been criticized as having a US slant. However, in the case of autism (and the more common symptom cluster referred to as ADHD), studies in many different countries and cross-cultural comparison across the US and Europe have shown that the phenotype of both autism and ADHD looks the same and has the same comorbidity and effects regardless of the cultural context in which it is studied.

Autism in the DSM-IV and the DSM-V

The *DSM-IV* comprised five different autism spectrum disorder categories: autistic disorder, Asperger's disorder, childhood disintegrative disorder (CDD), pervasive developmental disorder, not otherwise specified (PDD-NOS), and Rett syndrome. Rett syndrome was felt by most authorities to be misplaced from the start and it is now not even specifically mentioned in the *DSM-V*. The *DSM-V* contains only one autism category, incorporating autistic disorder, Asperger's disorder, CDD, and PDD-NOS into one common coded condition, referred to as "ASD" (see Box 2.1).

Box 2.1 Proposed DSM-V Criteria for Autism

Must meet criteria 1, 2, and 3:
1. Clinically significant, persistent deficits in social communication and interactions, as manifested by *all* of the following:
   a. Marked deficits in nonverbal and verbal communication used for social interaction;
   b. Lack of social reciprocity;
   c. Failure to develop and maintain peer relationships appropriate to developmental level.

2. Restricted, repetitive patterns of behavior, interests, and activities, as manifested by at least *two* of the following:
   a. Stereotyped motor or verbal behaviors, or unusual sensory behaviors;
   b. Excessive adherence to routines and ritualized patterns of behavior;
   c. Restricted, fixated interests.
3. Symptoms must be present in early childhood (but may not become fully manifest until social demands exceed limited capacities).

The change reflects increasing awareness that much of the *DSM-IV* subgrouping of autism was based on attitudes and personal stance rather than empirical evidence. For instance, most systematic studies have not found support for a clear distinction between autistic disorder and Asperger's disorder. It is also unclear to what extent CDD should be seen as different from autistic disorder with regression and whether or not "mild" or highly atypical cases of PDD-NOS are really related to autistic disorder at all.

Table 2.1 compares the *DSM-IV* and *DSM-V* criteria for autistic disorder/ASD. There are only six symptoms in the *DSM-V* as compared with twelve in the *DSM-IV*. There are only two subgroups of symptoms rather than three. The change to just half the number of symptoms superficially gives the impression of a major reconceptualization of the whole category. However, on closer inspection, what has been achieved is a pruning of four symptoms (that were felt by many to be vague and relatively unimportant or to be hallmarks of other conditions, such as severe learning disability or severe expressive language disorder) and a collapsing of four of the remaining eight into two. Also, the social and

Table 2.1 Comparison of DSM-IV and proposed DSM-V criteria for autism

DSM-IV criterion	Corresponding criterion in DSM-V
1a	1a
1b	1c
1c	–
1d	1b
2a	–
2b	1a
2c	2a
2d	–
3a	2c
3b	2b
3c	2a
3d	–

communication categories have been collapsed into one. This mirrors the now generally accepted notion that at the root of both the social and communication problems in autism is a shared deficit in intuitive understanding of the meaning of reciprocity. Finally, the three specific social–communication symptoms in the *DSM-V* must all be met for a diagnosis to be considered (compared to only two out of four in the *DSM-IV*), and there must be at least five of the six total number of symptoms met (compared to "only" six of the twelve autistic disorder criteria in the *DSM-IV*). Interestingly, there is also again referral to the unusual sensory behaviors that are almost universally encountered in autism but that were not specifically mentioned under the *DSM-IV*. The age criterion has been changed from delay or abnormal functioning being evident before age 3 years (*DSM-IV*) to symptoms having been present from early childhood (*DSM-V*).

Taken together, it would seem that the *DSM-V* might actually restrict somewhat the number of cases of autistic disorder meeting full criteria for autism spectrum disorder compared to the *DSM-IV*. Also, many of the cases meeting Asperger's disorder symptom criteria (only three symptoms in total needed in the *DSM-IV*) and PDD-NOS "criteria" (that are really extremely vague) would probably fall short of diagnostic status under the *DSM-V*. The Gillberg's Asperger syndrome category would, on the other hand, at least at a glance, usually meet criteria for ASD under the *DSM-V*. However, all of this is, of course, pure speculation at the present time. Changing the diagnostic criteria, as will happen with the introduction of the *DSM-V* (ICD-11), will definitely lead to changes in numbers of cases diagnosed. This, in the case of autism, will, almost certainly, lead to claims of "autism epidemics" or "autism disappearing?" in the headlines of many major newspapers from about 2015 onwards. This is the extent of what can be reasonably predicted as a result of the introduction of the new diagnostic manuals.

References

Achenbach, T. M., Becker, A., Dopfner, M., Heiervang, E., Roessner, V., Steinhausen, H. C., et al. (2008). Multicultural assessment of child and adolescent psychopathology with ASEBA and SDQ instruments: Research findings, applications, and future directions. *Journal of Child Psychology and Psychiatry, 49*, 251–275.

American Psychiatric Association (1980). *The diagnostic and statistical manual of mental disorders* (3rd ed.). Washington: Author.
American Psychiatric Association (1987). *The diagnostic and statistical manual of mental disorders* (Rev. 3rd ed.). Washington: Author.
American Psychiatric Association (1994). *The diagnostic and statistical manual of mental disorders* (4th ed.). Washington: Author.
American Psychiatric Association (2000). *The diagnostic and statistical manual of mental disorders* (Text Rev. 4th ed.). Washington: Author.
American Psychiatric Association (2010). dsm5.org
Cloninger, C. R. (2002). The discovery of susceptibility genes for mental disorders. *Proceedings of the National Academy of Sciences of the United States of America, 99*(21), 13365–13367.
Ehlers, S., & Gillberg, C. (1993). The epidemiology of Asperger syndrome. A total population study. *Journal of Child and Psychology and Psychiatry, 34*(8), 1327–1350.
Feinstein, A. R. (1970). The pre-therapeutic classification of co-morbidity in chronic disease. *Journal of Chronic Diseases, 23*(7), 455–468.
Goodman, R. (1999). The extended version of the strengths and difficulties questionnaire as a guide to child psychiatric caseness and consequent burden. *Journal of Child and Psychology and Psychiatry, 40*, 791–799.
Kadesjo, B., & Gillberg, C. (2001). The comorbidity of ADHD in the general population of Swedish school-age children. *Journal of Child and Psychology and Psychiatry, 42*, 487–492.
Kraepelin, E. (1920). Die Erscheinungsformen des Irreseins. *Zeitschrift für die gesamte Neurologie und Psychiatrie, 62*, 1–29.
Krueger, R. F., Watson, D., & Barlow, D. H. (2005). Introduction to the special section: Toward a dimensionally based taxonomy of psychopathology. *Journal of Abnormal Psychology, 114*(4), 491–493.
Lilienfeld, S. O., Waldman, I. D., & Israel, A. C. (1994). A critical examination of the use of the term and concept of comorbidity in psychopathology research. *The Clinical Psychologist: Science Practice, 1*, 71–83.
Mataix-Cols, D., Rosario-Campos, M. C., & Leckman, J. F. (2005). A multidimensional model of obsessive–compulsive disorder. *The American Journal of Psychiatry, 162*, 228–238.
Posserud, M. B., Lundervold, A. J., & Gillberg, C. (2006). Autistic features in a total population of 7–9-year-old children assessed by the ASSQ (Autism Spectrum Screening Questionnaire). *Journal of Child and Psychology and Psychiatry, 47*, 167–175.
World Health Organisation. (1993). *International classification of diseases and disorders* (10th ed.). Geneva: Author.

Colin Andrew Campbell, Sahar Davarya, Mayada Elsabbagh,
Lisa Madden, and Eric Fombonne

Determining the prevalence of autism spectrum disorders (ASDs) and monitoring it over time is important to ensure the training of ASD diagnosticians, to improve access to necessary interventions, and to understand causal mechanisms of ASDs. However, since an ASD is a behaviorally defined disorder, determining its prevalence is more difficult than for a disorder where clear biological markers exist. The symptoms of ASD vary in severity and may present differently in children with a mixture of cognitive abilities (King & Bearman, 2009). Furthermore, how the data are gathered, analyzed, and interpreted impacts the conclusions made regarding the prevalence of ASD (Fombonne, Quirke, & Hagen, 2011). As a result, there is controversy surrounding the prevalence of ASD, in particular, whether the recent rise in reports of the disorder are due to a true increase in incidence or whether there are other confounding factors that could be impacting the reports.

This chapter reports on an up-to-date review of the prevalence of ASDs and discusses the limitations and difficulties in interpreting the reports. Note ASDs and pervasive developmental disorders (PDDs) are used interchangeably in various articles, but are very similar in meaning. For this chapter, we will use ASD as the term of choice.

Prevalence Estimations

In order to estimate the current prevalence of ASDs, the studies selected for this review were based on prior reviews (Fombonne, 2003, 2005; Fombonne et al., 2011; Williams, Brayne, & Higgins, 2006). Studies not published in the English language or studies that utilized only questionnaire-based surveys to define caseness (e.g., Ghanizadeh, 2008)

were excluded since the validity of the diagnosis is uncertain in the questionnaire-based studies (for more information on the selection criteria, see Fombonne et al., 2011).

In total, 61 studies published between 1966 and 2010 were selected, with over half ($N = 36$) published in the last decade. The size of the population surveyed varied greatly (range: 826–4.95 million, median: 44,900). The studies were conducted in 18 different countries. Twenty-six percent of the studies were from the UK and 21% were from the USA. Of the 61 studies selected (see Table 3.1), 48 studies reported the prevalence on autistic disorder, 13 studies on Asperger syndrome (AS), 12 studies on childhood disintegrative disorder (CDD), and 27 studies provided information on the prevalence of all ASDs combined. The best current prevalence estimate of each of these disorders and the samples used to derive these rates are described below.

Autistic Disorder

The best current prevalence estimate of autistic disorder is 22/10,000 (interquartile range: 13–30/10,000; Table 3.2), which equates to 1 in 455 individuals (Fombonne et al., 2011). This rate was established based on 21 of the 48 studies because the prevalence rates of all 48 studies on autism were negatively correlated with sample size (Spearman's r: –0.71; $p < 0.001$) and positively correlated with year of publication (Spearman's r: 0.69; $p < 0.001$). Therefore, only studies published after 1999 with an adequate sample size were included. The 21 studies all used the modern diagnostic criteria for determining caseness (i.e., DSM-IV or ICD-10). The size of the population surveyed in each study varied from 8,896 to 4.95 million. The age ranged from 3 to 15, with a median age of 8.5 years. The male/female ratio averaged 5:1.

E. Fombonne (✉)
Department of Psychiatry, Montreal Children's Hospital, Montreal, QC, Canada H3Z 1P2
e-mail: eric.fombonne@mcgill.ca

J.L. Matson, P. Sturmey (eds.), *International Handbook of Autism and Pervasive Developmental Disorders*,
Autism and Child Psychopathology Series, DOI 10.1007/978-1-4419-8065-6_3, © Springer Science+Business Media, LLC 2011

Table 3.1 Prevalence surveys of ASD, autism, AS, and CDD

	Authors	Country	Size of target population	Age	Diagnostic criteria	Autism prevalence rate/10,000 (95% CI)	AS prevalence rate/10,000 (95% CI)	ASD prevalence rate/10,000 (95% CI)	CDD prevalence rate/10,000 (95% CI)
1	Lotter (1966)	UK	78,000	8–10	Kanner	4.1 (2.7–5.5)			
2	Brask (1972)	Denmark	46,500	2–14	Kanner	4.3 (2.4–6.2)			
3	Treffert (1970)	USA	899,750	3–12	Kanner	0.7 (0.6–0.9)			
4	Wing et al. (1976)	UK	25,000	5–14	Kanner (24 items)	4.8 (2.1–7.5)			
5	Hoshino et al. (1982)	Japan	609,848	0–18	Kanner	2.33 (1.9–2.7)			
6	Bohman et al. (1983)	Sweden	69,000	0–20	Rutter criteria	5.6 (3.9–7.4)			
7	McCarthy et al. (1984)	Ireland	65,000	8–10	Kanner	4.3 (2.7–5.9)			
8	Steinhausen et al. (1986)	Germany	279,616	0–14	Rutter	1.9 (1.4–2.4)			
9	Burd et al. (1987)	USA	180,986	2–18	DSM-III	3.26 (2.4–4.1)			0.11 (0.01–0.34)
10	Matsuishi et al. (1987)	Japan	32,834	4–12	DSM-III	15.5 (11.3–19.8)			
11	Tanoue et al. (1988)	Japan	95,394	7	DSM-III	13.8 (11.5–16.2)			
12	Bryson et al. (1988)	Canada	20,800	6–14	DSM-III-R	10.1 (5.8–14.4)			
13	Sugiyama and Abe (1989)	Japan	12,263	3	DSM-III	13.0 (6.7–19.4)			
14	Cialdella and Mamelle (1989)	France	135,180	3–9	DSM-III-like	4.5 (3.4–5.6)			
15	Ritvo et al. (1989)	USA	769,620	3–27	DSM-III	2.47 (2.1–2.8)			
16	Gillberg et al. (1991)	Sweden	78,106	4–13	DSM-III-R	9.5 (7.3–11.6)			
17	Fombonne and du Mazaubrun (1992)	France	274,816	9 & 13	Clinical ICD-10-like	4.9 (4.1–5.7)			
18	Wignyosumarto et al. (1992)	Indonesia	5,120	4–7	CARS	11.7 (2.3–21.1)			
19	Honda et al. (1996)	Japan	8,537	5	ICD-10	21.08 (11.4–30.8)			
20	Fombonne et al. (1997)	France	325,347	8–16	Clinical ICD-10-like	5.35 (4.6–6.1)			
21	Webb et al. (1997)	UK	73,301	3–15	DSM-III-R	7.2 (5.3–9.3)			
22	Arvidsson et al. (1997)	Sweden	1,941	3–6	ICD-10	46.4 (16.1–76.6)			
23	Sponheim and Skjeldal (1998)	Norway	65,688	3–14	ICD-10	5.2 (3.4–6.9)	0.3		0.15 (0.00–0.85)
24	Taylor et al. (1999)	UK	≈490,000	0–16	ICD-10	8.7 (7.9–9.5)	1.4		
25	Kadesjö et al. (1999)	Sweden	826	6.7–7.7	DSM-III-R/ICD-10 Gillberg's criteria (Asperger syndrome)	72.6 (14.7–130.6)	48.4		
26	Baird et al. (2000)	UK	16,235	7	ICD-10	30.8 (22.9–40.6)	3.1	57.9 (46.8–70.9)	
27	Powell et al. (2000)	UK	25,377	1–4.11	Clinical/ICD-10/ DSM-IV/DSM-III-R	7.8 (5.8–10.5)			
28	Kielinen et al. (2000)	Finland	27,572	5–7	DSM-IV	20.7 (15.3–26.0)			

Table 3.1 (continued)

	Authors	Country	Size of target population	Age	Diagnostic criteria	Autism prevalence rate/10,000 (95% CI)	AS prevalence rate/10,000 (95% CI)	ASD prevalence rate/10,000 (95% CI)	CDD prevalence rate/10,000 (95% CI)
29	Bertrand et al. (2001)	USA	8,896	3–10	DSM-IV	40.5 (28.0–56.0)		67.4 (51.5–86.7)[a]	
30	Fombonne et al. (2001)	UK	10,438	5–15	DSM-IV/ICD-10	26.1 (16.2–36.0)			
31	Magnússon and Saemundsen (2001)	Iceland	43,153	5–14	Mostly ICD-10	13.2 (9.8–16.6)			0.23 (0.03–0.84)
32	Chakrabarti and Fombonne (2001)	UK	15,500	2.5–6.5	ICD-10/DSM-IV	16.8 (10.3–23.2)	8.4	61.9 (50.2–75.6)	0.65 (0.02–3.59)
33	Davidovitch et al. (2001)	Israel	26,160	7–11	DSM-III-R/DSM-IV	10 (6.6–14.4)			
34	Croen et al. (2002)	USA	4,950,333	5–12	CDER "full syndrome"	11 (10.7–11.3)			
35	Madsen et al. (2002)	Denmark	63,859	8	ICD-10	7.2 (5.0–10.0)		30.0 (–)	
36	Scott et al. (2002)	UK	33,598	5–11	ICD-10			58.3[a] (50–67)[a]	
37	Gurney et al. (2003)	USA	–	8–10	–			52.0[b] 66 (–)	
38	Yeargin-Allsopp et al. (2003)	USA	289,456	3–10	DSM-IV			34.0 (32–36)	
39	Icasiano et al. (2004)	Australia	≈ 54,000	2–17	DSM-IV			39.2 (–)	
40	Tebruegge et al. (2004)	UK	2,536	8–9	ICD-10	23.7 (9.6–49.1)		82.8 (51.3–126.3)	
41	Chakrabarti and Fombonne (2005)	UK	10,903	4–7	ICD-10/DSM-IV	22.0 (14.4–32.2)	11.0	58.7 (45.2–74.9)	0.92 (0.00–5.86)
42	Barbaresi et al. (2005)	Minnesota, USA	37,726	0–21	DSM-IV	29.7 (24.0–36.0)			
43	Honda et al. (2005)[c]	Japan	32,791	5	ICD-10	37.5 (31.0–45.0)			
44	Fombonne et al. (2006)	Canada	27,749	5–17	DSM-IV	21.6 (16.5–27.8)	10.1	64.9 (55.8–75.0)	0.36 (0.00–2.00)
45	Gillberg et al. (2006)	Sweden	102,485	7–12	Gillberg's criteria	20.5		53.3	0.02
46	Baird et al. (2006)	UK	56,946	9–10	ICD-10	38.9 (29.9–47.8)		116.1 (90.4–141.8)	
47	Harrison et al. (2006)	UK	134,661	0–15	ICD-10, DSM-IV			44.2[d] (39.5–48.9)	
48	CDC (2007a)	USA	187,761	8	DSM-IV-TR			67 (–)	
49	CDC (2007b)	USA	407,578	8	DSM-IV-TR			66 (63–68)	
50	Ellefsen et al. (2007)	Denmark	7,689	8–17	ICD-10, DSM-IV, Gillberg's criteria for AS	16 (7.0–25.0)	26.0	53.3 (36.0–70.0)	0 (–)
51	Oliveira et al. (2007)	Portugal	67,795	6–9	DSM-IV	16.7 (14.0–20.0)			
52	Latif and Williams (2007)	UK	39,220	0–17	ICD-10, DSM-IV, Kanner's and Gillberg's criteria	12.7 (9.0–17.0)	35.4	61.2 (54–69)[a]	
53	Kawamura et al. (2008)	Japan	12,589	5–8	DSM-IV			181.1 (158.5–205.9)[a]	0 (–)
54	Nicholas et al. (2008)	USA	47,726	8	DSM-IV-TR			62 (56–70)	

Table 3.1 (continued)

	Authors	Country	Size of target population	Age	Diagnostic criteria	Autism prevalence rate/10,000 (95% CI)	AS prevalence rate/10,000 (95% CI)	ASD prevalence rate/10,000 (95% CI)	CDD prevalence rate/10,000 (95% CI)
55	Williams et al. (2008)	UK	14,062	11	ICD-10	21.6 (13.9–29.3)	16.6	61.9 (48.8–74.9)	0 (–)
56	Wong & Hui (2008)	China	4,247,206	0–14	DSM-IV			16.1 (1986–2005), 30.0 (2005)	
57	Baron-Cohen et al. (2009)	UK	8,824	5–9	ICD-10			94[e] (75–116)	
58	Kogan et al. (2007)	USA	77,911	3–17	–			110 (94–128)	
59	Van Balkom et al. (2009)	Netherlands	13,109	0–13	DSM-IV	19.1 (12.3–28.1)	1.5	52.6 (41.0–66.6)	0
60	CDC (2009)	USA	307,790	8	DSM-IV			89.6 (86–93)	
61	Lazoff et al. (2010)	Canada	23,635	5–17	DSM-IV	25.4 (19.0–31.8)	11.8	79.1 (67.8–90.4)	0.42 (0.00–2.40)

[a]Calculated by the author.

[b]These are the highest prevalences reported in this study of time trends. The prevalence in 10-year-olds is for the 1991 birth cohort, and that for 8-year-olds for the 1993 birth cohort. Both prevalences were calculated in the 2001–2002 school year.

[c]This figure was calculated by the author and refers to prevalence data (not cumulative incidence) presented in the chapter.

[d]Estimated using a capture–recapture analysis, the number of cases used to calculate prevalence was estimated to be 596.

[e]Rate based on Special Education Needs register. A figure of 99/10,000 is provided from a parental and diagnostic survey. Other estimates in this study vary from 47 to 165/10,000 deriving from various assumptions made by the authors.

Table 3.2 Best current estimates of ASDs

ASD subtype	Mean rate/10,000	Number of studies used in analysis	Range of rates	Gender ratio (male:female)
Autism	21.6	21	7.2–40.5	5:1
AS[a]	10.5	13	0.3–48.4	
CDD	0.2	12	0.0–0.9	9:1
ASD	69.2	27	30.0–181.1	5.5:1

[a]No gender ratio for Asperger's is reported in the meta-analysis.

Asperger Syndrome and Childhood Disintegrative Disorder

The prevalence of ASDs other than autistic disorder such as Asperger syndrome (AS) and childhood disintegrative disorder (CDD) has been less thoroughly examined. Therefore, caution must be taken in interpreting these prevalence reports because of the rarity of the disorders and the heterogeneity of data. For example, AS was not recognized as a separate diagnostic category until the early 1990s. Currently, there is disagreement on whether AS should be considered a separate category from high-functioning autism. As a result, there are few studies that report the prevalence of AS as distinct from autistic disorder.

The best current prevalence estimate of AS is 11/10,000 (interquartile range: 2–28/10,000), or 1 in 909 individuals (Fombonne et al., 2011). This estimate (see Table 3.2) is based on 13 studies published since 1998, and the variability of this estimate is evidenced by the 160-fold variation in the prevalence rates (range: 0.3–48.4/10,000). The number of children with AS was consistently lower than that with autistic disorder in all but one study (i.e., Latif & Williams, 2007). With regard to the Latif and Williams (2007) study, it is questionable whether high-functioning autism was included in the reported prevalence of AS (Fombonne et al., 2011), possibly contributing to the high rate in AS prevalence. The size of the population ranged from 826 to 490,000, with a mean of 60,385. The median age was 8 years.

The prevalence of CDD is much lower than that of autistic disorder and of AS, with the best current estimate as 0.2 per 10,000 (interquartile range: 0.0–0.4/10,000; see Table 3.2), or 1 in 50,000 individuals (Fombonne et al., 2011). This rate is based on 12 studies. There was not much variability in the number of cases, and the total number of cases was sparse due to the rarity of the disorder. Four of the 12 studies reported no cases, and none of the studies reported more than 2 cases. In total, there were 11 identified cases out of a surveyed population of 560,000 children. The prevalence estimate ranged from 0 to 0.92/10,000. The male/female ratio was 9:1.

Combined ASDs

The best current estimate of the prevalence of all ASDs combined, which includes autistic disorder, AS, PDD-NOS, and CDD is 70/10,000 (interquartile range: 53–80/10,000) (Fombonne et al., 2011) or 1 in 143 individuals. All 27 studies were published after 1999 in 8 different countries. The mean sample size was 243,156 (range: 2,536–4,247,206) and the median age was 8.0 years (range: 5.0–12.5). The mean male/female ratio was 5.5:1 and ranged from 2.7:1 to 15.7:1.

Conclusion

Based on current best estimates of the prevalence of ASD, rates derived from studies written in English and published in the last decade show that the current prevalence of autistic disorder is approximately 22/10,000, while the prevalence rate for all ASDs is approximately 70/10,000. Rates of AS and CDD have been more difficult to calculate because of the rarity of the disorder, especially CDD, or the lack of clear differentiation of the clinical phenotype within the spectrum of ASDs, especially for AS. For each specific ASD, males outnumbered females. Considering the current rates of all ASDs, the following sections of this chapter outline controversy surrounding them and trends that show an increase in ASDs over the past 5 decades.

Is There an Autism Epidemic?

The recent Centre for Disease Control and Prevention (CDC) reports indicate a clear rise in prevalence of ASDs in recent years. News reports and parents groups have called this an "Autism Epidemic," with the recent CDC estimates suggesting that 1 in 110 children 8 years of age have an ASD (CDC, 2009). To verify this report, we used the autistic disorder prevalence data to graph a scatterplot of autism prevalence by year of publication (see Fig. 3.1). There is a curvilinear increase in these data, and when testing different plots, the square root of the prevalence best fits the data by year of publication (Fig. 3.2). Based on these data alone, there is clear support for the claim for a rise in prevalence reported for autistic disorder over time. This leads to the next questions:

1. Can one imply a rise in the incidence of ASDs from these data?
2. Is this a true increase in prevalence or are there other potential confounding factors that have impacted the data such that, when accounted for in the statistics, they take away this linear curve and level the ASD prevalence over time?

The next sections will attempt to evaluate these questions.

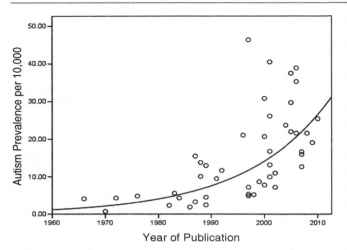

Fig. 3.1 Studies showing the prevalence of autism by year, 1966–2010

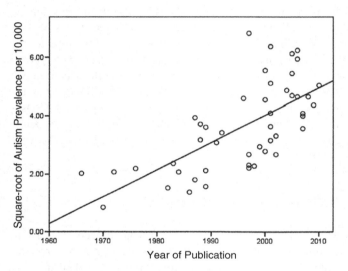

Fig. 3.2 Square root of studies showing the prevalence of autism by year, 1966–2010

Prevalence vs. Incidence

Distinguishing *prevalence* from *incidence* is important in understanding the methodologies used to collect data and making conclusions based on the statistical analyses of the studies presented. Prevalence is the proportion of individuals in a population who suffer from a defined disorder at any point in time, while incidence is the number of new cases occurring in a population over a period of time. Incidence does not include individuals with ongoing treatment of the condition, only the new cases occurring during a certain time period. Prevalence is useful for estimating needs and planning services. Causal research can only be investigated through incidence rates. An increase in incidence does not necessarily mean an increase in prevalence and vice versa

because prevalence is the cumulative sum of past and current incidence in that time period.

In the case of the ASD prevalence reports, one cannot imply incidence from prevalence data because they require different methodologies and analysis. Also, there are various problems with interpreting and comparing prevalence data that include different definitions, different methodologies, different sources, and different time periods. Awareness of autism, advocacy groups, and changes in policy may also impact prevalence data, since as more people learn and seek help for autism, prevalence data will report a higher number of cases with ASD over time.

Controversies Surrounding Interpreting Prevalence

Case Definition

Studies reporting the prevalence of ASDs have been carried out in numerous countries and during various time periods. Differences in the way these studies defined ASD, called *case definition,* and identified their cases, called *case identification,* make it difficult to compare between studies and report on the changes in prevalence over time. Variation exists in the ways that studies have defined ASDs. Some of the earliest studies were conducted in the 1960s and 1970s, using Leo Kanner's (1943) definition for the diagnosis of autism. He is typically credited with the first thoroughly written account of autism, called "early infantile autism" (Kanner, 1943), which focused on the severely impaired. The diagnostic criteria for autism emerged with the ICD-9 (World Health Organization [WHO], 1977), followed by the DSM-III (American Psychiatric Association [APA], 1980), the DSM-III-R (APA, 1987), and more recently the ICD-10 (WHO, 1992), DSM-IV (APA, 1994), and DSM-IV-TR (APA, 2000). In the more recent diagnostic criteria, autism has expanded into a broader class of ASDs. Unlike before, autism occurring without co-morbid mental retardation and separate diagnostic categories for Asperger disorder (AS) and pervasive developmental disorder not otherwise specified (PDD-NOS) are also recognized. If historical trends are any indication, the ASD criteria will likely continue to expand and modify (Fombonne et al., 2011). For example, individuals who exhibit specific traits of a broader autism phenotype but fail to meet current criteria for a specific diagnosis of an ASD may be included in a category such as "broader autism phenotype" in future editions of the DSM or ICD.

The evolution of the case definition of autism into a spectrum disorder has created a challenge in examining prevalence rates between studies, especially over time (Fombonne, 2003). In the 1960s and 1970s, surveys only dealt with the narrow definition of autism disorder using Kanner's (1943) descriptions. Thus, the closest estimate of ASD prevalence available in the late 1970s was 20 per 10,000 in a survey from the UK that was limited to severely impaired children (Wing & Gould, 1979). Clearly, this estimate is far lower than the rates reported today, indicating an increase. Thus, the change in definition should be accounted for in analysis of time trends.

Diagnostic Substitution and Accretion

The modifications in the diagnostic criteria of autism to a spectrum disorder may be impacting more recent prevalence reports because it is possible that some of the cases currently with an ASD diagnosis may not have received a diagnosis previously using older diagnostic criteria. More specifically, *diagnostic substitution,* when a case receives one diagnosis at one point and then later receives a different diagnosis, may be playing a role (Shattuck, 2006). For example, some cases may have received a diagnosis of mental retardation when they were younger, and then later received an ASD diagnosis because of the change in diagnostic criteria. It is also possible that some cases diagnosed with one disorder earlier in time may later acquire a co-morbid diagnosis that includes ASD, called *diagnostic accretion.* For example, other cases may have received a diagnosis of mental retardation when they were younger, and then later received a co-morbid diagnosis including autism.

Prevalence of time trends may be confounded when studies do not control for diagnostic substitution and accretion in their analysis. Using the California DDS Client Development and Evaluation Report data, King and Bearman (2009) reported that the chance of a patient acquiring a diagnosis of autism was elevated during periods for which the practices for diagnosing autism changed. More specifically, they reported that 26.4% of the increase in autism caseload was associated with diagnostic change in individuals previously diagnosed with mental retardation. Likewise, Shattuck (2006) reported that a relatively high proportion of children previously diagnosed as having mental retardation were later identified as having a PDD diagnosis based on an analysis of Department of Education data in 50 US states. He demonstrated that the growing prevalence of ASD was directly associated with decreasing prevalence of the diagnosis of learning disability and mental retardation within states. One study in the UK reported that 34.2% of adults initially diagnosed with a developmental language disorder as a child would have met diagnostic criteria for an ASD, confirmed by both the ADI-R and ADOS-G (Bishop, Whitehouse, Watt, & Line, 2008). These reports suggest that diagnostic substitution and accretion may have impacted widely used data to report prevalence, and care must be taken in interpretation of prevalence.

Variability in Case Ascertainment Methods

The studies that report on prevalence use a variety of methods, and each of these methods have their own limitations in reporting prevalence. Also, the unique design features between studies could also be impacting the prevalence variations, making it particularly difficult to compare published prevalence rates over time. Following is a discussion of the various case ascertainment methods.

Pre-existing databases. Some studies use pre-existing databases, such as service provider databases (Croen, Grether, Hoogstrate, & Selvin, 2002), special educational databases (Fombonne, Zakarian, Bennett, Meng, & McLean-Heywood, 2006; Gurney et al., 2003; Lazoff, Zhong, Piperni, & Fombonne, 2010), or national registers (Madsen et al., 2002), to identify cases. Utilizing these databases to report prevalence excludes individuals who have the disorder but are not in contact with the agency maintaining the database. This results in an underestimation of the true prevalence. In addition, many of these pre-existing databases are not set up specifically for epidemiological studies, so the reliability and rigor in systematically ascertaining cases may not have been followed in the same regard.

With the pre-existing databases, confounding variables must be taken into account in time trend analysis. Other factors such as heightened public awareness, decreasing age at diagnosis, and changes in diagnostic concepts and practices may also play a role in the increasing numbers in these pre-existing databases (Fombonne, 2009). For example, upward trends reported using the California Developmental Database Services (CDDS 1999; CDDS, 2003) database may suggest that those children identified were only a subset of the population prevalence pool and that the increasing numbers actually reflect an increasing proportion of children receiving services. Unfortunately, the CDDS data have been misused and result in imperfect statistics. For more information, see Fombonne et al. (2011).

Multi-stage screening surveys. Another method used for case ascertainment includes a multi-stage approach, which involves a screening stage followed by a more in-depth stage. The goal of the screening stage is to identify an exhaustive list of cases possibly affected with an ASD, leaving the comprehensive diagnostic assessment to the next stage. The number of data sources, the type of screening scale used, and the response rate influence the number of cases selected in the first stage, which then impacts the number of cases in the second stage. Studies utilizing the multi-stage approach have varied in these details within their methodology. For example, studies have varied in how they screened cases, from sending letters to using reliable screening scales requesting school and health professionals or other data sources to identify possible cases of ASDs.

The cases identified as positive screens in the first stage go through the second stage to finalize their case status.

Methodological variability may also occur at this stage. The source of information used to determine cases usually involves a combination of data from different informants (e.g., medical records, other health professionals) and data sources. When subjects are directly examined, the assessments are conducted using various diagnostic instruments, ranging from a typical unstructured examination by a clinical expert (but without demonstrated psychometric properties) to the use of a battery of standardized measures by trained research staff such as the Autism Diagnostic Interview (LeCouteur et al., 1989) and/or the Autism Diagnostic Observational Schedule (Lord et al., 2000).

Not all studies, such as the large-scale studies conducted by the Center for Disease Control (CDC; 2007a, 2007b, 2009) or in national registers (Madsen et al., 2002), include a direct assessment of the person with autism. Direct assessment of all subjects can be costly and require manpower, which is very difficult for large-scale studies. However, investigators in the CDC studies could generally confirm the accuracy of their final cases by conducting a more complete diagnostic work-up on a randomly selected subsample (Fombonne et al., 2011). There is still question regarding the reliability of gathering cases across sites. For example, one would expect comparable prevalence rates for studies conducted during the same year and using similar methods of case ascertainment. But, for example, in the recent CDC reports (CDC, 2007b) there was huge variation of rate by state. One plausible explanation is that some states have more services and awareness toward ASD, creating higher rates of prevalence for those states. Fombonne et al. (2011) also found that up to a third of prevalence cases may be missed by an ascertainment source, evidenced by Harrison and colleagues (2006), leading toward an underestimation in prevalence and an increase in rate over the years especially as services increase.

The Public Health Response, Public Awareness, and Policy Changes

Tracking the prevalence has become a national priority in a few countries where such estimates are used in service planning and development. In the USA, research funding for autism, as well as the number of autism research grants, has increased steadily over the past decade (Singh, Illes, Lazzeroni, & Hallmayer, 2009). Recently, CDC estimates suggested that 1 in 110 children 8 years of age has an ASD (CDC, 2009), which is a huge rise compared to previous studies conducted in the 1980s and early 1990s. While these findings have often been described as an autism "epidemic," there is no doubt that increase in public awareness, access to services, and improved identification of autism in primary health care has contributed toward the increase in prevalence and may also account for regional variation within the USA.

Changes in funding policies and government regulations could also have an impact on prevalence estimates. For example, the US federal Individual with Disabilities Educational Act (IDEA), formerly known as the Education of All Handicapped Children Act and designed to protect the rights of students with disabilities, only included ASDs as of 1990 (Silverstein, 2005). Gurney et al. (2003) found that the inclusion of ASDs in IDEA may be influencing some of the upward trends reported in the prevalence data. Croen et al. (2002) and Shattuck (2006) supported these findings in their respective analyses of the California Department of Developmental Services data and of the US Department of Education data. Such changes in policy may also have an impact through diagnostic substitution. For example, with the introduction of publicly funded programs such as the Early Intervention and special education programs, it is possible that some children with developmental delay, mental retardation, and learning disabilities may have been initially classified as having an ASD to facilitate receipt of needed services (Shattuck, 2006).

Reports of the increasing prevalence of ASDs in the research literature as well as by the media have helped to raise awareness in the general population, and especially among parents of affected children. Parent groups have been discussing the rising rates of ASDs all over the USA and Canada, as well as many other nations. Government officials are taking notice of the public response. April 2, 2008, was the first international World Autism Awareness Day, as designated by the United Nations National Assembly. In New York, senators have recently called for a council to discuss specific issues surrounding autism in response to this report. In Canada, federal legislation has been proposed that would ensure that behavioral treatments for autism are covered under each province's respective healthcare plans. Often, the raising prevalence of ASDs is cited by legislators and politicians as part of the reason for moving forward with plans such as the ones listed.

Conclusion

As shown in this review, current estimates for the prevalence of autistic disorder is 1 in 455 individuals (Fombonne et al., 2011), and the prevalence of all ASDs combined is approximately 1 in 143 individuals. Additionally, comparisons of prevalence studies by year indicate a distinct trend of increasing rates of prevalence. However, whether this increase is the sign of a true ASD epidemic or not is subject to debate. Many factors, such as changes in the diagnostic criteria for ASD included in the DSM and ICD over time, diagnostic substitution and accretion, and the variability in case ascertainment across studies, can explain at least some of the reasons for increasing prevalence rates of ASD. Despite alternate explanations for the increasing prevalence of autism, the public has taken hold of this information. Parents and autism interest groups have used the autism epidemic to improve the plight of individuals with ASD, which has led to the discussion of autism by governmental bodies, which regardless of the nature of the increase of ASD has been beneficial to those affected by it. In conclusion, it appears as though increasing rates of ASD can be explained by factors associated with the collection of data, and not necessarily by an actual increase in incidence although the latter possibility remains to be further investigated.

References

American Psychiatric Association. (1980). *Diagnostic and statistical manual of mental disorders* (3rd ed.). Washington, DC: Author.

American Psychiatric Association. (1987). *Diagnostic and statistical manual of mental disorders* (3rd ed., revised). Washington, DC: Author.

American Psychiatric Association. (1994). *Diagnostic and statistical manual of mental disorders* (4th ed.). Washington, DC: Author.

American Psychiatric Association. (2000). *Diagnostic and statistical manual of mental disorders* (4th ed., TR). Washington, DC: Author.

Arvidsson, T., Danielsson, B., Forsberg, P., Gillberg, C., Johansson, M., & Kjellgren, G. (1997). Autism in 3–6 year-old in a suburb of Goteborg, Sweden. *Autism, 2*, 163–173.

Baird, G., Charman, T., Baron-Cohen, S., Cox, A., Swettenham, J., Wheelwright, S., et al. (2000). A screening instrument for autism at 18 months of age: A 6 year follow-up study. *Journal of the American Academy of Child and Adolescent Psychiatry, 39*, 694–702.

Baird, G., Simonoff, E., Pickles, A., Chandler, S., Loucas, T., Meldrum, D., et al. (2006). Prevalence of disorders of the autism spectrum in a population cohort of children in South Thames: The special needs and autism project (SNAP). *Lancet, 368*, 210–215.

Barbaresi, W. J., Katusic, S. K., Colligan, R. C., Weaver, A. L., & Jacobsen, S. J. (2005). The incidence of autism in Olmsted County, Minnesota, 1976–1997: Results from a population-based study. *Archives of Pediatric Adolescent Medicine, 159*, 37–44.

Baron-Cohen, S., Scott, F. J., Allison, C., Williams, J., Bolton, P., Matthews, F. E., & Brayne, C. (2009). Autism Spectrum Prevalence: A school-based U.K. population study. *British Journal of Psychiatry, 194*, 500–509.

Bertrand, J., Mars, A., Boyle, C., Bove, F., Yeargin-Allsopp, M., & Decoufle, P. (2001). Prevalence of autism in a United States population: The Brick Township, New Jersey, investigation. *Pediatrics, 108*, 1155–1161.

Bishop, D. V., Whitehouse, A. J., Watt, H. J., & Line, E. A. (2008). Autism and diagnostic substitution: Evidence from a study of adults with a history of developmental language disorder. *Developmental Medicine & Child Neurology, 50*(5), 341–345.

Bohman, M., Bohman, I., Bjorck, P., & Sjoholm, E. (1983). Childhood psychosis in a northern Swedish county: Some preliminary findings from an epidemiological survey. In M. Schmidt, & H. Remschmidt (Eds.), *Epidemiological approaches in child psychiatry* (pp. 164–173). Stuttgart: Georg Thieme Verlag.

Brask, B. (1972). *A prevalence investigation of childhood psychoses.* Paper presented at the Nordic symposium on the care of psychotic children, Oslo.

Bryson, S. E., Clark, B. S., & Smith, I. M. (1988). First report of a Canadian epidemiological study of autistic syndromes. *Journal of Child Psychology & Psychiatry & Allied Disciplines, 29*, 433–445.

Burd, L., Fisher, W., & Kerbeshan, J. (1987). A prevalance study of pervasive developmental disorders in North Dakota. *Journal of the American Academy of Child and Adolescent Psychiatry, 26*, 700–703.

California Department of Developmental Services. (1999). *Changes in the population of persons with autism and pervasive developmental disorders in California's developmental services system: 1987 through 1998.* Report to the Legislature, March 1, 1999, p. 19.

California Department of Developmental Services. (2003, April). Autism spectrum disorders: Changes in the California caseload – an update 1999 through 2002. http://www.dds.ca.gov/Autism/pdf/AutismReport2003.pdf

Center for Disease Control. (2007a). Prevalence of autism spectrum disorders–autism and developmental disabilities monitoring network, six sites, United States, 2000. *Morbidity and Mortality Weekly Report Surveillance Summaries, 56*(1), 1–11.

Center for Disease Control. (2007b). Prevalence of autism spectrum disorders–autism and developmental disabilities monitoring network, 14 sites, United States, 2002. *Morbidity and Mortality Weekly Report Surveillance Summaries, 56*(1), 12–28.

Center for Disease Control. (2009). Prevalence of autism spectrum disorders– autism and developmental disabilities monitoring network, United States, 2006. *Morbidity and Mortality Weekly Report Surveillance Summary, 58*, 1–14.

Chakrabarti, S., & Fombonne, E. (2001). Pervasive developmental disorders in preschool children. *Journal of the American Medical Association, 285*, 3093–3099.

Chakrabarti, S., & Fombonne, E. (2005). Pervasive developmental disorders in preschool children: Confirmation of high prevalence. *American Journal of Psychiatry, 162*, 1133–1141.

Cialdella, P., & Mamelle, N. (1989). An epidemiological study of infantile autism in a French department (Rhone): A research note. *Journal of Child Psychology & Psychiatry & Allied Disciplines, 30*, 165–175.

Croen, L. A., Grether, J. K., Hoogstrate, J., & Selvin, S. (2002). The changing prevalence of autism in California. *Journal of Autism and Developmental Disorders, 32*, 207–215.

Davidovitch, M., Holtzman, G., & Tirosh, E. (2001). Autism in the Haifa area – an epidemiological perspective. *Israeli Medical Association Journal, 3*, 188–189.

Ellefsen, A., Kampmann, H., Billstedt, E., Gillberg, I. C., & Gillberg, C. (2007). Autism in the Faroe islands: An epidemiological study. *Journal of Autism and Developmental Disorders, 37*, 437–444.

Fombonne, E. (2003). The prevalence of autism. *Journal of the American Medical Association, 289*(1), 1–3.

Fombonne, E. (2005). Epidemiology of autistic disorder and other pervasive developmental disorders. *Journal of Clinical Psychiatry, 66*(Suppl 10), 3–8.

Fombonne, E. (2009). Commentary: On King and Bearman. *International Journal of Epidemiology, 38*(5), 1241–1242.

Fombonne, E., & du Mazaubrun, C. (1992). Prevalence of infantile autism in four French regions. *Social Psychiatry & Psychiatric Epidemiology, 27*, 203–210.

Fombonne, E., du Mazaubrun, C., Cans, C., & Grandjean, H. (1997). Autism and associated medical disorders in a French epidemiological survey. *Journal of the American Academy of Child & Adolescent Psychiatry, 36*, 1561–1569.

Fombonne, E., Simmons, H., Ford, T., Meltzer, H., & Goodman, R. (2001). Prevalence of pervasive developmental disorders in the British nationwide survey of child mental health. *Journal of the American Academy of Child & Adolescent Psychiatry, 40*, 820–827.

Fombonne, E., Quirke, S., & Hagen, A. (2011). Epidemiology of pervasive developmental disorders. In D. G. Amaral, G. Dawson, & D. H. Geschwind (Eds.), *Autism spectrum disorders.* Oxford University Press.

Fombonne, E., Zakarian, R., Bennett, A., Meng, L., & McLean-Heywood, D. (2006). Pervasive developmental disorders in Montreal, Quebec, Canada: Prevalence and links with immunizations. *Pediatrics, 118*(1), 139–150.

Ghanizadeh, A. (2008). A preliminary study on screening prevalence of pervasive developmental disorder in school children in Iran. *Journal of Autism and Developmental Disorders, 38*(4), 759–763.

Gillberg, C., Cederlund, M., Lamberg, K., & Zeijlon, L. (2006). Brief report: "The autism epidemic". The registered prevalence of autism in a Swedish urban area. *Journal of Autism and Developmental Disorders, 36*, 429–435.

Gillberg, C., Steffenburg, S., & Schaumann, H. (1991). Is autism more common now than ten years ago? *British Journal of Psychiatry, 158*, 403–409.

Gurney, J. G., Fritz, M. S., Ness, K. K., Sievers, P., Newschaffer, C. J., & Shapiro, E. G. (2003). Analysis of prevalence trends of autism spectrum disorder in Minnesota.[comment]. *Archives of Pediatrics & Adolescent Medicine, 157*(7), 622–627.

Harrison, M. J., O'Hare, A. E., Campbell, H., Adamson, A., & McNeillage, J. (2006). Prevalence of autistic spectrum disorders in Lothian, Scotland: An estimate using the "capture-recapture" technique. *Archives of Disease in Childhood, 91*(1), 16–19.

Honda, H., Shimizu, Y., Misumi, K., Niimi, M., & Ohashi, Y. (1996). Cumulative incidence and prevalence of childhood autism in children in Japan. *British Journal of Psychiatry, 169*, 228–235.

Honda, H., Shimizu, Y., & Rutter, M. (2005). No effect of MMR withdrawal on the incidence of autism: A total population study. *Journal of Child Psychology & Psychiatry, 46*, 572–579.

Hoshino, Y., Kumashiro, H., Yashima, Y., Tachibana, R., & Watanabe, M. (1982). The epidemiological study of autism in Fukushima-Ken. *Folia Psychiatrica et Neurologica Japonica, 36*, 115–124.

Icasiano, F., Hewson, P., Machet, P., Cooper, C., & Marshall, A. (2004). Childhood autism spectrum disorder in the Barwon region: A community based study. *Journal of Paediatric Child Health, 40*, 696–701.

Kadesjö, B., Gillberg, C., & Hagberg, B. (1999). Brief report: Autism and Asperger syndrome in seven-year-old children: A total population study. *Journal of Autism and Developmental Disorders, 29*, 327–331.

Kanner, L. (1943). Autistic disturbances of affective contact. *Nervous Child, 2*, 217–250.

Kawamura, Y., Takahashi, O., & Ishii, T. (2008). Reevaluating the incidence of pervasive developmental disorders: Impact of elevated rates of detection through implementation of an integrated system of screening in Toyota, Japan. *Psychiatry and Clinical Neuroscience, 62*, 152–159.

Kielinen, M., Linna, S.-L., & Moilanen, I. (2000). Autism in northern Finland. *European Child and Adolescent Psychiatry, 9*, 162–167.

King, M., & Bearman, P. (2009). Diagnostic change and the increase in prevalence of autism. *International Journal of Epidemiology, 38*(5), 1224–1234.

Kogan, M. D., Blumberg, S. J., Schieve, L. A., Boyle, C. A., Perrin, J. M., Ghandour, R. M., et al. (2007). Prevalence of parent-reported diagnosis of autism spectrum disorder among children in the US. *Pediatrics, 124*, 1395–1403.

Latif, A. H. A., & Williams, W. R. (2007). Diagnostic trends in autism spectrum disorders in the South Wales valleys. *Autism, 11*, 479–487.

Lazoff, T., Zhong, L. H., Piperni, T., & Fombonne, E. (2010). Prevalence of pervasive developmental disorders among children at the English Montreal School Board. *Canadian Journal of Psychiatry, 55*(11), 715–720.

LeCouteur, A., Rutter, M., Lord, C., Rios, P., Robertson, S., Holdgrafer, M., et al. (1989). Autism diagnostic interview: A standardized investigator-based instrument. *Journal of Autism and Developmental Disorders, 19*, 363–387.

Lord, C., Risi, S., Lambrecht, L., Cook, E. H., Leventhal, B. L., DiLavore, P. C., et al. (2000). The autism diagnostic observation schedule-generic: A standard measure of social and communication deficits associated with the spectrum of autism. *Journal of Autism and Developmental Disorders, 30*, 205–223.

Lotter, V. (1966). Epidemiology of autistic conditions in young children: I. Prevalence. *Social Psychiatry, 1*, 124–137.

Madsen, K. M., Hviid, A., Vestergaard, M., Schendel, D., Wohlfahrt, J., Thorsen, P., et al. (2002). A population-based study of measles, mumps, and rubella vaccination and autism. *New England Journal of Medicine, 347*(19), 1477–1482.

Magnússon, P., & Saemundsen, E. (2001). Prevalence of autism in Iceland. *Journal of Autism and Developmental Disorders, 31*, 153–163.

Matsuishi, T., Shiotsuki, M., Yoshimura, K., Shoji, H., Imuta, F., & Yamashita, F. (1987). High prevalence of infantile autism in Kurume city, Japan. *Journal of Child Neurology, 2*, 268–271.

McCarthy, P., Fitzgerald, M., & Smith, M. (1984). Prevalence of childhood autism in Ireland. *Irish Medical Journal, 77*, 129–130.

Nicholas, J. S., Charles, J. M., Carpenter, L. A., King, L. B., Jenner, W., & Spratt, E. G. (2008). Prevalence and characteristics of children with autism-spectrum disorders. *Annals of Epidemiology, 18*, 130–136.

Oliveira, G., Ataide, A., Marques, C., Miguel, T. S., Coutinho, A. M., Mota-Vieira, L., et al. (2007). Epidemiology of autism spectrum disorder in Portugal: Prevalence, clinical characterization, and medical conditions. *Developmental Medicine and Child Neurology, 49*, 726–733.

Powell, J., Edwards, A., Edwards, M., Pandit, B., Sungum-Paliwal, S., & Whitehouse, W. (2000). Changes in the incidence of childhood autism and other autistic spectrum disorders in preschool children from two areas of the West Midlands, UK. *Developmental Medicine and Child Neurology, 42*, 624–628.

Ritvo, E., Freeman, B., Pingree, C., Mason-Brothers, A., Jorde, L., Jenson, W., et al. (1989). The UCLA-University of Utah epidemiologic survey of autism: Prevalence. *American Journal of Psychiatry, 146*, 194–199.

Scott, F. J., Baron-Cohen, S., Bolton, P., & Brayne, C. (2002). Brief report: Prevalence of autism spectrum conditions in children aged 5–11 years in Cambridgeshire, UK. *Autism, 6*, 231–237.

Shattuck, P. T. (2006). The contribution of diagnostic substitution to the growing administrative prevalence of autism in US special education. *Pediatrics, 117*(4), 1028–1037.

Silverstein, R. (2005). *A user's guide to the 2004 IDEA reauthorization* (P.L. 108-446 and the conference report). Washington, DC: Consortium for Citizens with Disabilities.

Singh, J., Illes, J., Lazzeroni, L., & Hallmayer, J. (2009). Trends in US autism research funding. *Journal of Autism and Developmental Disorders, 39*, 788–795.

Sponheim, E., & Skjeldal, O. (1998). Autism and related disorders: Epidemiological findings in a Norwegian study using ICD-10 diagnostic criteria. *Journal of Autism and Developmental Disorders, 28*, 217–227.

Steinhausen, H.-C., Gobel, D., Breinlinger, M., & Wohlloben, B. (1986). A community survey of infantile autism. *Journal of the American Academy of Child Psychiatry, 25*, 186–189.

Sugiyama, T., & Abe, T. (1989). The prevalence of autism in Nagoya, Japan: A total population study. *Journal of Autism and Developmental Disorders, 19*, 87–96.

Tanoue, Y., Oda, S., Asano, F., & Kawashima, K. (1988). Epidemiology of infantile autism in southern Ibaraki, Japan: Differences in prevalence in birth cohorts. *Journal of Autism and Developmental Disorders, 18*, 155–166.

Taylor, B., Miller, E., Farrington, C., Petropoulos, M.-C., Favot-Mayaud, I., Li, J., et al. (1999). Autism and measles, mumps, and rubella vaccine: No epidemiological evidence for a causal association. *The Lancet, 353*, 2026–2029.

Tebruegge, M., Nandini, V., & Ritchie, J. (2004). Does routine child health surveillance contribute to the early detection of children with pervasive developmental disorders? An epidemiological study in Kent, UK. *BMC Pediatrics, 4*, 4.

Treffert, D. A. (1970). Epidemiology of infantile autism. *Archives of General Psychiatry, 22*, 431–438.

Van Balkom, I. D. C., Bresnahan, M., Vogtlander, M. F., van Hoeken, D., Minderaa, R. B., Susser, E., et al. (2009). Prevalence of treated autism spectrum disorders in Aruba. *Journal of Neurodevelopmental Disorders, 1*, 197–204.

Webb, E., Lobo, S., Hervas, A., Scourfield, J., & Fraser, W. (1997). The changing prevalence of autistic disorder in a Welsh health district. *Developmental Medicine and Child Neurology, 39*, 150–152.

Williams, J. G., Brayne, C. E., & Higgins, J. P. (2006). Systematic review of prevalence studies of autism spectrum disorders. *Archives of Disease in Childhood, 91*, 8–15.

Williams, E., Thomas, K., Sidebotham, H., & Emond, A. (2008). Prevalence and characteristics of autistic spectrum disorders in the ALSPAC cohort. *Developmental Medicine and Child Neurology, 50*, 672–677.

Wignyosumarto, S., Mukhlas, M., & Shirataki, S. (1992). Epidemiological and clinical study of autistic children in Yogyakarta, Indonesia. *Kobe Journal of Medical Sciences, 38*, 1–19.

Wing, L., & Gould, J. (1979). Severe impairments of social interactions and associated abnormalities in children: Epidemiology and classification. *Journal of Autism and Developmental Disorders, 9*, 11–29.

Wing, L., Yeates, S., Brierly, L., & Gould, J. (1976). The prevalence of early childhood autism: Comparison of administrative and epidemiological studies. *Psychological Medicine, 6*, 89–100.

Wong, V. C., & Hui, S. L. (2008). Epidemiological study of autism spectrum disorder in China. *Journal of Child Neurology, 23*, 67–72.

World Health Organization. (1977). *Manual of the international statistical classification of diseases, injuries, and causes of death* (Vol. 1). Geneva: World Health Organization.

World Health Organization. (1992). *The ICD-10 classification of mental and behavioural disorders: Clinical descriptions and diagnostic guidelines.* Geneva: World Health Organization.

Yeargin-Allsopp, M., Rice, C., Karapurkar, T., Doernberg, N., Boyle, C., & Murphy, C. (2003). Prevalence of autism in a US metropolitan area. *Journal of the American Medical Association, 289*, 49–55.

Autism Spectrum Disorders and Intellectual Disability

4

Luc Lecavalier, Anne V. Snow, and Megan Norris

Introduction

There is a significant overlap between autism spectrum disorders (ASDs) and intellectual disability (ID). In this chapter, we review this co-occurring relationship. We choose to tackle this task by examining issues related to definition and classification, biological underpinnings, and epidemiology. We then discuss the impact of level of functioning on the presentation of ASDs and their associated features as well as the similarities and differences between the two disabilities in terms of psychopathology and adaptive behavior. This chapter is not meant to be a comprehensive review of the literature. Rather, it is meant to provide a summary of relevant and contemporary studies on these selected themes.

Definition and Classification

The term "autism spectrum disorders" (ASDs) is used by researchers and clinicians to describe a group of neurodevelopmental disorders characterized by qualitative impairments in social-communicative behaviors and repetitive and restrictive behaviors and interests. In the latest edition of the *Diagnostic and Statistical Manual of Mental Disorders* (DSM-IV-TR; APA, 2000), ASDs belong to the pervasive developmental disorder (PDD) category and are found on Axis I. The term PDD has recently fallen out of favor; ASD is more recognizable to parents and perhaps more accurate in that impairments are not always pervasive.

ASDs are used to describe three diagnostic groups, namely autistic disorder, Asperger's disorder, and pervasive developmental disorder not otherwise specified (PDDNOS). Current conceptualizations view ASDs as distributed along a continuum, with autistic disorder representing the most severe form at one end of the spectrum, and PDDNOS representing milder variants at the other. The communality across subtypes is the qualitative impairment in social interactions. At the time of this writing, there are indications that the next edition of the DSM will move toward subsuming all three subtypes under one category called "autism spectrum disorders." Level of intellectual functioning will most likely be used as a clinical specifier and/or associated feature to further describe individuals, which is quite germane to this chapter.

ASDs present quite heterogeneously from a clinical standpoint. There is tremendous variability in terms of intellectual and language abilities. In addition, symptoms change with development and level of functioning. Diagnostic disagreements and related philosophical issues tend to be the most pronounced at the extremes of the life span and cognitive spectrum. Behaviors that are very common among preschoolers and/or those with severe cognitive delays may not be as common in older, higher functioning people with ASDs. Although major diagnostic systems attempt to allow for these variations, they have no systematic way of doing so. This extreme heterogeneity leads to important challenges for diagnosis and classification, for epidemiology, and in terms of unraveling the pathogenesis of the disorders.

In contrast to ASDs which are defined by deviances from the norm, ID is a particular state of functioning characterized by concurrent deficits (usually defined as two standard deviations below the population average) in intellectual and adaptive functioning. ID is found on Axis II in the DSM. Qualitative deviances from normative behavior and delays in functioning can (and do) co-occur, but should not be misconstrued to be synonyms. Levels of intellectual and adaptive functioning are measured with standardized instruments, and objective (but arbitrary) cutoffs are used to establish delays. This is not the case when evaluating the core behavioral features of ASDs. Diagnoses are based implicitly on normative behavior, but quantitatively based cutoffs are not used. In other words, deviances from normative social behavior are not defined statistically. Despite this important difference,

L. Lecavalier (✉)
Ohio State University, Columbus, OH 43210, USA
e-mail: luc.lecavalier@osumc.edu

J.L. Matson, P. Sturmey (eds.), *International Handbook of Autism and Pervasive Developmental Disorders*, Autism and Child Psychopathology Series, DOI 10.1007/978-1-4419-8065-6_4, © Springer Science+Business Media, LLC 2011

there is significant overlap between the two developmental disabilities.

At the heart of it all, both ASDs and ID are defined by problems in social competence. Social competence is a subjective judgment about how effectively an individual performs social tasks. This global appraisal of social functioning is based on a collection of discrete behaviors. It is a multidimensional construct that includes socially oriented adaptive skills (e.g., expressing self, interacting with others, playing and leisure skills) and peer relationship variables such as popularity and friendship. We contrast social competence with social skills which are specific measurable interpersonal behaviors (e.g., establishing eye contact, smiling, turn taking). None of these specific behaviors are necessary for a diagnosis of ASD or ID, but they permeate most aspects of functioning and determine a range of adaptive outcomes. Indeed, ASDs can be viewed primarily as disorders of social relatedness (Klin, Jones, Schultz, & Volkmar, 2003) and the construct of social competence has been central to the definition and classification of ID for decades (Lecavalier & Butter, 2010).

Biological Underpinnings of ASD

Both ASDs and ID are defined behaviorally and have an onset in the period of development. They share common descriptive elements and characteristics and are associated with a myriad of poorly understood environmental and biological factors. They have many different etiologies and are seen as the final pathway of different pathological processes (e.g., Abrahams & Geschwind, 2008; Levis, Mandell, & Schultz, 2009; Matson & Shoemaker, 2009; Skuse, 2007).

Tremendous progress has been made in the biological understanding of ASDs. This is quite remarkable, given that as recently as a few decades ago there was a virtual absence of any biological understanding of ASDs. We now know that defined mutations, genetic syndromes, and de novo copy number variations (CNVs) account for about 10–20% of ASD cases (Abrahams & Geschwind, 2008). Almost all of the CNVs are deletions, with many fragments containing several genes. CNVs seem to be strongly associated with ID and dysmorphology.

None of these known biologic causes account for more than a small percentage of ASD cases (Levis et al., 2009). This is quite reminiscent of ID for which there is no single major genetic cause, but rather many relatively rare mutations. In other words, none of the genetic causes are specific to the disorder. Rather, they are specific to a range of phenotypes, including ID. The most common causes include fragile X syndrome (about 3%), tuberous sclerosis (about 2%), and various cytogenetic abnormal findings such as

maternal duplication of 15q1-q13 (roughly 2%) and deletions and duplications of 16p11 (about 1%).

Even in the last 10 years, there have been radical changes in our understanding of the genetics of ASDs. Previously, the field was guided almost exclusively by the common disorder–common gene model, proposing that many genes frequently identified in the general population each confers small-to-moderate effects on the phenotype. Only a few common variants have been identified as possible candidate genes in linkage studies and many of these have not been verified in subsequent independent replication studies, pointing to the difficulty of finding common causes in such a heterogeneous disorder. The failure of linkage studies to reveal consistent signals is probably related in part to the reliance on categorical diagnoses for the selection of participants. After all, why would our genes follow DSM nosology?

A better understanding of the relationship between ASDs and ID has implications for studying the causes of ASDs. The great deal of overlap between the two disorders suggests possible genetic similarities. Indeed, genetic disorders that are characterized in part by ID have also been demonstrated to occur at higher rates in individuals with ASDs as compared to the general population (e.g., Bailey et al., 1993; Smalley, 1998). A significant overlap between ASDs and ID would argue for a search of genes influencing both traits, whereas a limited association would argue for separate genetic influences on specific traits. A recent study speaks to this association. Hoekstra, Happé, Baron-Cohen, and Ronald (2009) reported on the association between autistic traits and ID in a population-based sample of 11,652 children aged between 7 and 9 years. Only modest correlations were found between IQ and autistic traits (correlations varying between –0.01 and –0.40). The association was driven by communication problems characteristic of autism and suggested that autistic traits are substantially genetically independent of ID.

Some have proposed that the genetic risks for autism and ID may be distinctly different, and it is the combination of these conditions that leads to a recognizable ASD (Skuse, 2007). According to this view, individuals who are genetically susceptible to ASDs who also have adequate cognitive skills can compensate for the social–cognitive deficits that are associated with the genetic vulnerability toward autism. Individuals with the same genetic risk for ASD who function at a lower level are more likely to develop an ASD due to the absence of protective cognitive skills and the increased likelihood of clinical identification.

Although there has been remarkable progress in the understanding of the biological and genetic underpinnings of ASDs, much work remains to be done. One thing is clear: the genetic basis of ASDs is complex, with multiple genes contributing to ASD susceptibility.

Epidemiology of ASDs and ID

The overlap between ASDs and ID is quite apparent when one considers epidemiological data. The epidemiology of disorders could be approached in two ways: by examining rates of ASDs in people with ID or by looking at rates of ID in people with ASDs. No matter how the topic is approached, rates vary significantly based on a number of methodological factors, including the design of the studies, the definitions of ASDs and ID, and the ascertainment methods used.

Because the criteria used to assess ID are objective, one might suspect that rates would be straightforward to establish. This has not been the case, with rates varying significantly across studies from 0.5 to 3% (Roeleveld, Zielhuis, & Gabreels, 1997). The IQ cutoff used to define ID illustrates well the impact definitions have on prevalence rates. Based on normal distributions, the following rates are obtained with different cutoffs: IQ ≤ 75, 5.48%; IQ < 75, 4.75%, IQ ≤ 70, 2.68%, and IQ < 70, 2.28%.

In their review of studies published between 1981 and 1995 that examined prevalence data of ID in young people, Roeleveld et al. (1997) concluded that rates were about 0.4% for individuals with IQs < 50 and about 0.5% for individuals with IQs between 50 and 70. Rates were much more variable for individuals functioning in the mild range of ID. More recent North American and European surveys converge with these estimates and support the general conclusion that combined rates for all levels of ID fall just below 1% (Bryson, Bradley, Thompson, & Wainwright, 2008; Lee et al., 2001; Westerinen, Kaski, Virta, Almqvist, & Livanainen, 2007). The situation is more complex when it comes to identifying individuals with mild ID. Adaptive skills are more variable for this subgroup and many individuals are less likely to be captured in surveys due to successful integration policies. In addition, individuals with mild ID are less likely to be identified in the school system unless presenting with behavioral problems, which biases ascertainment rates.

Turning to the rates of ASDs in ID populations, the literature contains a wide range of estimates, with most varying from 5% to more than 50% (see Bryson et al., 2008; De Bildt, Sytema, Kraijer, & Monderra, 2005). The varying rates are explained partly by the different populations sampled and the different assessment methods used. In one of the earlier influential reports, Wing and Gould (1979) reported that 40% of their sample showed the "triad of autistic impairments" (social reciprocity, communication, and imagination and behavioral flexibility). The sample was composed largely of individuals with severe ID and it is unclear how the triad of autistic impairments would map on the current DSM, although presumably a large proportion of the identified cases would meet current criteria for autistic disorder. Nordon and Gillberg (1996) reported a

rate of 19.8% for all ASDs and 8.9% for autistic disorder in a population-based study of Swedish preschoolers and school-age children with ID. ASD criteria were based on the DSM-III-R and the *Childhood Autism Rating Scale*. In their study of Dutch children and adolescents with ID, De Bildt et al. (2005) reported a rate of 16.7% for all ASDs. Rates varied from 7.8 to 19.8%, depending on the instrument and definition of ASDs used. The rate of 16.7% was considered the best estimate as it was based on multiple informants and time points. It could be broken down further into 8.8% for autistic disorder and 7.9% for PDDNOS. Rates were lower for youngsters with mild ID (9.3%) compared to those with moderate to profound ID (26.1%). Finally, in their epidemiological study of 14- to 20-year-old Canadians with ID, Bryson et al. (2008) reported a rate of 28% for autistic disorder. The *Autism Diagnostic Interview-Revised* (ADI-R; Lord, Rutter, & LeCouteur, 1994) was used in this study to confirm the presence of autism. Unlike other studies, the authors reported that autism was more equally distributed among those with mild ID (24%) or severe ID (32%).

The broadened conceptualization of ASDs in more recent studies can certainly help to explain some of the discrepancy in prevalence rates across studies. Many earlier studies only included autistic disorder and did not include PDDNOS in their conceptualization of ASDs. The higher rates in the more recent studies may also note a greater willingness to note comorbidity, a notion that has taken on greater importance (Matson & Nebel-Schwalm, 2007; Matson & Shoemaker, 2009; Rutter, 2009).

Epidemiological rates of ASDs have been the object of heated controversy in recent years. Studies vary significantly in terms of sample characteristics, conceptualization of ASDs, and ascertainment methods (Fombonne, 2005a). While most studies have a screening and direct assessment phase, some have ascertained cases based on existing medical or education records (e.g., Yeargin-Allsopp et al., 2003) and others have done so based on parent report. In one recent study (Kogan et al., 2009), a child was considered to have an ASD if a parent/guardian reported that a healthcare provider had ever said that the child had an ASD and if the child currently had the condition. The weighted ASD point-prevalence for this study was 110 per 10,000.

Taken as a whole, recent surveys have suggested rates of about 60/10,000 for all ASDs combined (Fombonne, 2003). The reported proportion of children with ASDs who also have ID varies widely, ranging between 26 and 68% of cases (Fombonne, 2005b). How ASDs and ID are defined in these studies is critical in interpreting results. In one epidemiological study, Chakrabarti and Fombonne (2001) reported that 26% of preschool-aged children with any ASD met criteria for ID as defined by IQ < 70. However, when data were examined by ASD subtype, 69% of those who met strict criteria for autistic disorder also met criteria for ID. In another study with similar methods, the same authors confirmed their previous findings (Chakrabarti & Fombonne, 2005). They reported that 30% of preschoolers with any ASD met criteria for ID. Again, rates of ID differed significantly among ASD subtypes, with 67% of the autistic disorder group meeting criteria for ID. While it is believed that most children on the autism spectrum do not function in the range of ID, it is estimated that autistic disorder is associated with ID in about 70% of the cases (Bryson & Smith, 1998; Fombonne, 2003). These rates vary according to the level of intellectual impairments, with approximately 30% having mild to moderate impairments and 40% having severe to profound impairments.

The more recent rates represent noticeable increase from earlier reports. Indeed, studies published after 2000 have generally yielded significantly higher rates (Fombonne, 2005c). According to the Center for Disease Control's Autism and Developmental Disabilities Monitoring Network (2009), rates have increased 57% between 2002 and 2006 with some parts of the USA seeing much higher rates than others (CDC, 2009). For example, the rate of 8 year olds diagnosed with an ASD is almost three times higher in Arizona than in Florida.

Although there is little doubt that the prevalence of ASDs has increased over the past 30 years, the reasons for such increases remain uncertain. Changes in our conceptualizations of ASDs to include children from all levels of functioning and those with other neuropsychiatric and medical disorders have contributed to this increase. In addition, a number of legislation and social/educational policy changes have contributed to increased referral rates. The introduction of the 1990 Individual Disabilities Educational Act (IDEA) in the USA was followed by diagnostic practice changes, whereby children previously diagnosed with ID were now diagnosed with ASDs, either with (accretion) or without (substitution) a co-occurring diagnosis of ID. Several authors have reported evidence of simultaneous decreases in the population prevalence of ID along with increases in ASDs (Croen, Grether, Hoogstrate, & Selvin, 2002; Shattuck, 2006). Recently, King and Bearman (2009) analyzed data from the California Department of Developmental Services (DDS) database. They found that children previously classified with "mental retardation" account for one-quarter of the measured increase in autism prevalence in the DDS between 1992 and 2005. Of course, this leaves 75% of the increase due to other factors. It is certainly possible that children who in the past would have received a diagnosis of ID would receive an ASD diagnosis in more recent times when presenting with the same behaviors. Relying on existing data sets for estimates of prevalence leads to a host of interpretation difficulties (e.g., see Charman et al., 2009). Although informative, administrative data sets do not allow us to conclude on whether or not there has been a rise in the incidence of ASDs.

Several studies have pointed to other social influences involved in the epidemiology of ASDs (e.g., Palmer, Blanchard, Jean, & Mandell, 2005; Van Meter et al., 2010). For instance, Palmer et al. (2005) examined data on the number of children identified with ASDs in the Texas Education Agency database and found that the proportion of economically disadvantaged children per district was inversely associated with the proportion of autism cases. The prevalence estimates for the top decile of revenue (21 children per 10,000) were six times higher than for the bottom decile (3.5 children per 10,000). The ability to navigate convoluted bureaucracies to be deemed eligible for services can impact identification rates and advantage families of higher socioeconomic status. The interesting parallel here is the well-known fact that the prevalence of mild ID is higher in families of lower socioeconomic status (e.g., Leonard et al., 2005).

Despite the varying estimates and heated controversies, the overlap between ASDs and ID is clear based on epidemiological surveys. Only large-scale prospective epidemiological/longitudinal studies with consistent definitions and robust assessment procedures will lead to satisfying answers on the true epidemiology of ASDs and ID.

Impact of IQ on the Presentation of ASD and Associated Features

The complex relationship between ASDs and ID obscures the distinction between them and our understanding of pathogenesis. The literature shows that the clinical presentation of individuals with ASDs varies with respect to level of functioning. IQ has been shown to moderate the presentation of core ASD symptoms as well as associated features such as sex differences, comorbid psychiatric and behavior problems, and medical conditions. In addition, IQ is an important variable in understanding the course of ASD and response to treatment. Furthermore, IQ has been the most consistently reported indicator of differences between ASD subtypes. In the following sections, we describe the impact of IQ on the presentation of ASDs.

IQ and Core ASD Symptoms

Several emerging lines of evidence point to a relationship between level of functioning and the severity of ASD symptomatology. First, correlational and cross-sectional analyses of IQ and ASD symptoms consistently demonstrate a significant association between these two variables. Studies have found evidence for negative correlations between level of functioning and a number of symptoms in all three of the ASD core symptom domains. IQ has also been shown to be associated with measures of the broad autism phenotype. Dawson et al. (2007) reported that IQ was significantly negatively correlated with social and communication scores on the *Broader Phenotype Autism Symptoms Scale* (BPASS). Another measure of the broad autism phenotype, the *Social Responsiveness Scale* (SRS; Constantino, 2002), was reported to have insignificant correlations with IQ (Constantino et al., 2003). However, the SRS has been shown to be negatively correlated with the *Vineland Adaptive Behavior Scales* (VABS) composite score (Pine, Luby, Abbacchi, & Constantino, 2006).

Within the domains of social and communication impairment, lower verbal IQ (VIQ) and nonverbal IQ (NVIQ) have been associated with higher levels of ASD symptoms (DiLavore, Lord, & Rutter, 1995; Spiker, Lotspeich, Dimiceli, Myers, & Risch, 2002). In a study that aimed to delineate the behavioral phenotype of sibling pairs with autism, Spiker et al. (2002) found that ASD symptoms and NVIQ represented parallel dimensions of severity. Children with lower NVIQs also tended to have the most severe ASD symptoms, particularly in the social-communication domains. Evidence of the relationship between verbal skills and social-communication symptoms of ASDs also comes from the initial reliability and validity studies of the *Pre-Linguistic Autism Diagnostic Observation Schedule* (PL-ADOS; DiLavore et al., 1995). The initial validity study of the PL-ADOS indicated that the optimal scoring algorithm correctly classified 89% (16/18) of the nonverbal children with autism, but misclassified all three of the verbal children with autism. Verbal status in this study was defined as the child using short phrases as well as single-word utterances. It appears that even elementary verbal skills can influence the symptom expression of ASDs.

We now turn to the relationship between IQ and restrictive repetitive behaviors and interests (RRBIs). Recent empirical studies have proposed two main groups of RRBIs (Cuccaro et al., 2003; Szatmari et al., 2006). On the one hand, there are "lower order" sensory motor behaviors such as hand/finger mannerisms, unusual sensory interests, repetitive use of objects/parts of objects, and rocking. On the other hand, there are "higher order" behaviors related to rigidity or resistance to change which include difficulties with changes in routine, resistance to trivial changes in environment, and compulsions/rituals. The two broad groups of RRBIs seem to have different relationships with level of functioning. Both Cuccaro et al. (2003) and Szatmari et al. (2006) reported that composite adaptive behavior scores were negatively correlated with repetitive sensory and motor behaviors. In contrast, scores on items measuring rigidity or resistance to change were not significantly related to overall functioning.

In one of the largest studies of this type, Bishop, Richler, and Lord (2006) examined the relationship between RRBIs, age, and NVIQ in children with ASDs ($n = 830$) who ranged in age from 15 months to 11 years and 11 months. There was a significant interaction between NVIQ and chronological age, such that NVIQ was more strongly related to the prevalence of several RRBIs in older children. The prevalence of a number of repetitive behaviors (e.g., repetitive use of objects, hand and finger mannerisms) was negatively associated with IQ. However, the prevalence of certain behaviors (e.g., circumscribed interests) was positively associated with NVIQ, which provides additional support for the idea of different classes of RRBIs.

The role of IQ in moderating ASD symptoms has also been examined by comparing individuals who have been grouped into high- and low-IQ groups (Ben Itzchak, Lahat, Burgin, & Zachor, 2008; Matson, Dempsey, LoVullo, & Wilkins, 2008). Ben Itzchak et al. (2008) grouped 44 preschoolers with autism by cognitive level into normal (IQ > 90), borderline (70 < IQ < 89), and impaired (50 < IQ < 69) groups and compared *Autism Diagnostic Observation Schedule* (ADOS; Lord et al., 2000) scores. Compared to the two other groups, the impaired group had significantly higher scores in the reciprocal social interaction domain. The impaired group also had higher scores than the borderline group in the stereotyped behavior domain. Differences were not found between the borderline and the normal groups.

There is some evidence suggesting that the effect of IQ on ASD symptoms may be specific to diagnostic groups. Matson, Dempsey, et al. (2008) compared adults with ID, autism, or PDDNOS on the *Autism Spectrum Disorders-Diagnosis for Intellectually Disabled Adults* (ASD-DA; Matson, Wilkins, & Gonzalez, 2007). The three diagnostic groups were further separated into high- and low-IQ groups, based on scores from two adaptive behavior instruments. ASD symptoms were compared between diagnostic groups and within groups, based on IQ classification. In the ID and PDDNOS groups, those in the low-IQ group had more severe social and communication impairments and higher rates of repetitive and restricted behaviors than their counterparts in the high-IQ groups. Individuals diagnosed with autism did not show differences in any of the three symptom domains as a function of IQ. These results indicated that for adults with ID, IQ appears to have a significant effect on the presence of ASD symptoms. This effect was also present to a moderate degree in individuals with PDDNOS, but it was not evident in individuals with autism. The authors concluded that IQ might be useful in the differential diagnosis between ASDs and ID.

Other attempts to elucidate the association between IQ and ASD symptom presentation have focused on the impact of uneven intellectual abilities on core symptoms (Black, Wallace, Sokoloff, & Kenworthy, 2009; Joseph, Tager-Flusberg, & Lord, 2002). Joseph et al. (2002) found that for preschool and school-age children with autism, discrepantly high nonverbal skills were associated with greater deficits in social skills. As the NVIQ > VIQ discrepancy increased, so did the degree of social impairment. Black et al. (2009) examined this trend in a sample of 78 high-functioning (NVIQ > 70) children with ASDs. ASD symptoms were measured using a composite of ADI-R and ADOS scores. In contrast to the results of Joseph et al. (2002), this group found that a discrepancy in IQ in either direction (NVIQ < VIQ or VIQ > NVIQ) was associated with greater social impairment.

Examining classification systems and diagnostic instruments is another way to shed some light on the relationship between IQ and core ASD features. IQ has also been shown to modulate the sensitivity of DSM-IV criteria for autistic disorder (Buitelaar, Van der Gaag, Klin, & Volkmar, 1999). Using the DSM-IV field trial data, Buitelaar et al. (1999) reported that 8 of the 12 symptom criteria were associated with higher sensitivity for individuals with more severe degrees of ID. In other words, two-thirds of the diagnostic criteria for autism showed higher frequencies in individuals with lower IQs. It has been noted elsewhere that the current DSM diagnostic criteria, as well as the most frequently used diagnostic and screening instruments for ASDs, are most effective when applied to individuals who also have moderate ID (Lord & Corsello, 2005).

The range of intellectual and language skills found in people with ASDs is one of the major challenges in developing sound diagnostic instruments. Despite this challenge, two of the most widely used and rigorously studied instruments, the ADI-R and ADOS, have demonstrated very good diagnostic validity (e.g., de Bildt et al., 2004). While the ADOS addresses different levels of functioning through the use of different modules (with module 1 being appropriate for young children or individuals with limited-to-no speech), the ADI-R is designed for individuals with a mental age of 2 years or older. There is some evidence that both instruments perform well in lower functioning individuals (de Bildt et al., 2004).

Norris and Lecavalier (2010) recently reviewed the diagnostic validity of five Level 2 ASD caregiver-completed rating scales. Of these, only the *Gilliam Autism Rating Scale* (Gilliam, 2006) was developed for all levels of functioning, and it demonstrated lackluster accuracy. The *Social Communication Questionnaire* (SCQ; Berument, Rutter, Lord, Pickles, & Bailey, 1999) is the most widely studied ASD screening instrument and seems to perform best in those above the age of 7 years (Norris & Lecavalier, 2010). By comparison, the *Autism Spectrum Disorders-Diagnosis for Intellectually Disabled Adults* (ASD-DA; Matson et al., 2007), a 31-item rating scale designed to assist with the differential diagnosis of ASDs, is one of the few instruments that has been studied largely among very low functioning adults (Matson, Boisjoli, Gonzalez, Smith, & Wilkins, 2007; Matson, Wilkins, Boisjoli, & Smith, 2008).

IQ and Sex Differences

Level of functioning has also been shown to impact sex differences in ASDs. The characteristic male-to-female ratio in ASDs is 4:1 (Fombonne, 2003). However, it has long been reported that this ratio varies as a function of IQ (Lord, Schopler, & Revicki, 1982). Early reports suggested that at the lower IQ range (IQ < 35), the proportion of females with autism increased. More recent epidemiological studies have replicated and extended these findings (Bryson et al., 2008; Scott, Baron-Cohen, Bolton, & Brayne, 2002; Sponheim & Skjeldal, 1998). These studies have shown that the sex ratio approaches equality at the level of moderate to severe ID. For example, Sponheim and Skjedal (1998) found a sex ratio of 1:1 in individuals with ASDs who had moderate to severe intellectual deficits. In the higher functioning groups, the sex ratio was 9:0 for individuals with autism and 5:2 for those with PDDNOS or Asperger's disorder. It appears that the well-documented sex differences characteristic of ASDs are not evident in lower functioning individuals, where the sex ratio approaches equality.

A possible explanation for the interaction between gender, IQ, and risk for ASDs is that males and females have different thresholds for the genetic liability to autism (Skuse, 2006). While males and females are at equal genetic risk for autism, females may have genetic or hormonal protective factors that enable them to compensate for such risk. As such, females are more resistant to the genetic determinants of autism and need a higher genetic load to overcome the protective effect and become affected. This might imply that autism in females is associated with more severe genetic abnormalities, which would presumably result in more severe cognitive impairments.

IQ and Psychopathology

It has been well documented that individuals with ASDs present with high rates of behavior problems (e.g., Brereton, Tonge, & Einfeld, 2006; Lecavalier, 2006) as well as psychiatric disorders (Gadow, DeVincent, Pomeroy, & Azizian, 2005; Lecavalier, Gadow, DeVincent, & Edwards, 2009; Matson & Nebel-Schwalm, 2007; Simonof et al., 2008). Commonly reported behavior problems include self-injurious behaviors, tantrums, aggression, and property destruction (Lecavalier, 2006). Commonly reported psychiatric symptoms include those of attention deficit hyperactivity disorder (ADHD) (Gadow et al., 2005; Gillberg & Billstedt, 2000), obsessive-compulsive disorder (McDougle et al., 1995), mood disorder (Lainhart & Folstein, 1994), and anxiety and fears (Sukhodolsky et al., 2008; Weisbrot, Gadow, DeVincent, & Pomeroy, 2005).

Level of functioning has been shown to moderate levels of behavior problems in children with ASDs. Lecavalier (2006) examined the association between adaptive behavior scores and behavior problems in children with ASDs. In this study, children with more impaired adaptive skills had significantly more problems on most of the prosocial and problem behavior subscales of the *Nisonger Child Behavior Rating Form* (Aman, Tassé, Rojahn, & Hammer, 1996).

The trend of greater behavior problems in lower functioning individuals is also true for adolescents and adults with ASDs. In their longitudinal study of behavior problems in individuals with ASDs ($n = 241$), Shattuck and colleagues (2007) found that individuals with comorbid ID had more behavior problems than those without ID. Furthermore, the rates of behavior problems in individuals with comorbid ID improved less over a period of 4.5 years as compared to those without ID.

Several studies have examined the effect of level of functioning on psychiatric problems in individuals with ASDs. In one such study, Kim, Szatmari, Bryson, Streiner, and Wilson (2000) examined differences in anxiety and mood symptoms between children with Asperger's disorder and autistic disorder. The authors did not find evidence that NVIQ or VIQ alone predicted anxiety symptoms. However, they did find that a higher VIQ–NVIQ split accounted for a portion of the variance in anxiety and mood symptoms. Sukhodolsky et al. (2008) also found that higher levels of anxiety were associated with higher IQs in their sample of children with ASDs. Similar results were also reported in a study using the *Developmental Behavior Checklist* (DBC) to examine psychiatric symptoms in children and adolescents with ASDs (Brereton et al., 2006). Individuals with an IQ in the average range scored higher on the DBC depression subscale than those with intellectual deficits.

Similar results were reported in a study examining how IQ could predict psychiatric symptoms in a sample of school-age children with ASDs (Estes, Dawson, Sterling, & Munson, 2007). In this study, children classified as higher functioning (based on IQ and adaptive behavior scores) at the age of 6 years demonstrated increased internalizing symptoms at age 9. Those classified as low functioning displayed higher rates of hyperactivity, attention problems, and irritability at age 9.

Witwer and Lecavalier (2010) used the Parent version of the *Children's Interview for Psychiatric Symptoms* (P-ChIPS), a structured interview based on the DSM, to compare psychiatric symptom endorsement rates of children with ASDs. They found that children with an IQ < 70 had fewer reported symptoms than those with an IQ ≥ 70. Individuals with IQ < 70 were more likely to be subsyndromal for generalized anxiety disorder and nonverbal individuals were more likely to be subsyndromal for oppositional defiant disorder. Symptom endorsement also varied based on language levels.

Contrasting results to the previous studies were found in one study examining risk factors for psychiatric disorders in a sample of 112 children with ASD who were aged 10–14 years (Simonoff et al., 2008). Neither IQ nor adaptive behavior scores were associated with increased rates of psychiatric disorders. Simonoff et al. explained the lack of association between IQ and psychiatric disorders as possibly indicating that ASDs "trump" other risk factors, whereby the influence of IQ is diminished in this population due to the more potent risk factor of ASD itself.

IQ and Epilepsy

In addition to behavior and psychiatric problems, ASDs are associated with several medical conditions. One of the more commonly reported co-occurring medical problems is epilepsy (Caniato, 2007; Tuchman & Rapin, 2002). Whereas the prevalence of epilepsy in the general population is 0.5–1%, the prevalence in ASDs ranges from 5 to 40% (Caniato, 2007; Hauser, Annegers, & Kurland, 1991). ID has been identified as one factor that may account for this variability in prevalence. The literature examining the relationship between epilepsy and intellectual functioning in individuals with ASD was synthesized in a meta-analysis by Amiet and colleagues (2008). The authors concluded that the prevalence of epilepsy was higher in individuals with ASDs and ID as compared to those without ID. Pooled prevalence rates indicated a rate of 21.4% for individuals with autism and ID vs 8% in individuals with autism without ID. Additionally, it was reported that within the sample of individuals with comorbid ID, the prevalence of epilepsy increases with the severity of ID.

IQ and Outcome/Response to Treatment

The long-term course of ASDs is generally understood to involve lifelong impairments with a modest trend toward improvement (Seltzer, Shattuck, Abbeduto, & Greenberg, 2004). However, individual characteristics such as severity of cognitive deficits influence the trajectory of the disorder and its eventual outcome. The most frequently cited characteristics that influence the course of ASDs are comorbid ID and overall language ability (Szatmari, Bryson, Boyle, Streiner, & Duku, 2003; Tager-Flusberg & Joseph, 2003; Volkmar, 2002). The absence of ID and the presence of better language skills have been consistently associated with greater likelihood of improvement over time.

Szatmari et al. (2003) examined the role of ID and language ability in determining outcome in young children with high-functioning autism or Asperger's disorder. Results indicated that nonverbal cognitive skills as well as early language skills predicted better outcome in adaptive behavior and ASD symptoms at a 2- to 6-year follow-up. Along the same lines, in another study, language abilities from the age of 3 years were shown to predict NVIQ, VIQ, expressive and receptive language outcomes, as well as composite scores on the ADI-R and ADOS at age 9 (Luyster, Qiu, Lopez, & Lord, 2007). This study also indicated that the use of nonverbal communication skills, such as symbolic and communicative gestures, predicted VIQ, expressive language, and adaptive skills at age 9.

Studies examining the course of ASDs into adulthood have supported the role of cognitive and language ability in predicting improvement over time (Howlin, Goode, Hutton, & Rutter, 2004; McGovern & Sigman, 2005; Seltzer et al., 2004; Shattuck et al., 2007). For example, Shattuck et al. (2007) examined change in autism symptoms over a 4.5-year period in adolescents and adults with ASDs. Although the majority of the sample showed improvement, those individuals with comorbid ID improved less over time. In fact, the absence of ID was the most robust predictor of change in symptoms. Similarly, in a follow-up study of adults who met criteria for ASDs as children, Howlin et al. (2004) found that individuals with a childhood NVIQ of 70 or higher had a significantly better outcome in adulthood.

In terms of response to treatment, several studies have indicated that IQ is a strong predictor of response to early behavioral interventions (see Helt et al., 2008). For instance, Sallows and Graupner (2005) examined the predictors of best response to a 4-year applied behavioral analysis-based treatment for children with ASDs. Results indicated significantly higher pre-treatment NVIQs in children who attained optimal outcomes at the end of treatment. Similarly, a study of preschool children who received an early intensive behavioral intervention indicated that the best outcomes were achieved by those who had higher IQs and adaptive skills at baseline (Remington et al., 2007). Finally, Ben Itzchak and Zachor (2007) examined predictors of outcome of early behavioral intervention in preschool children with autism. Children with ID demonstrated slower acquisition of receptive and expressive language skills, play skills, and nonverbal communication skills after 1 year of treatment. In this study, the progress in receptive language domain was highly related to pre-treatment cognitive and social abilities. Children with higher pre-treatment cognitive levels or with better social reciprocal abilities made more gains in their receptive language compared to children with lower pre-treatment cognitive and social abilities.

IQ as a Basis for Subtyping ASDs

Taken together, the above evidence suggests that IQ plays a strong role in the clinical presentation of ASDs. It has been

argued that because IQ can account for a substantial amount of the heterogeneity in autism, it could be used to distinguish ASD subgroups. One recent study has examined the possibility that ASDs can be subtyped based on IQ. Munson et al. (2008) used latent class analysis and taxometric methods to classify 456 children with ASDs based on Mullen scores. The data suggested four groups that were characterized by overall level of functioning and the magnitude of discrepancy between verbal and nonverbal scores. The greatest impairments in adaptive functioning as well as autistic symptomology were in the group with the lowest overall level of cognitive functioning. Among the other three groups, severity of symptoms decreased as overall cognitive skills improved.

Further evidence for the role of IQ in distinguishing subtypes was provided in a review of the literature on the validity of the distinction between autism, PDDNOS, and Asperger's disorder (Witwer & Lecavalier, 2008a). The report contained a review of 22 studies published between 1994 and 2006 that compared subtypes on clinical and demographic characteristics, neuropsychological profiles, comorbidity, and prognosis. Results indicated few consistent differences across subtypes in terms of the variables reviewed. In fact, the most consistently reported indicator of differences between groups was IQ. Based on this review, it could be argued that IQ is a more valid indicator of subtype distinction as compared to current diagnostic groupings. It seems as though the next edition of the DSM is heading in this direction.

Taken as a whole, the literature suggests that the clinical presentation of individuals with ASDs varies significantly with respect to level of functioning. Using cognitive functioning in the classification of ASDs appears to be a worthwhile pursuit, as differences in intellectual ability help to explain some of the vast heterogeneity associated with ASDs. Steps that move the field closer to identifying meaningful subgroups of individuals with ASDs will contribute to the unraveling of the pathogenesis of this group of disorders.

Similarities and Differences Between ASDs and ID

The significant behavioral overlap between ASD and ID has long been known. In fact, in people with the most severe intellectual deficits, it can be quite challenging to make the determination as to whether or not the absence of social and communication skills and the presence of repetitive behaviors are attributable to gross cognitive impairment or an additional ASD (Bradley, Summers, Wood, & Bryson, 2004). Many would argue that the distinction is academic in that the overriding factor determining outcome and care will be the severity of cognitive delays.

In addition to the clinical heterogeneity associated with ASDs and their overlap with ID, the relationship with other neuropsychiatric conditions remains unclear. Social skills and social competence problems not only are related to ASDs and ID, but have also been associated with other mental health problems such as substance abuse, conduct problems, schizophrenia, ADHD, anxiety, and sexual disorders (Bellack & Hersen, 1998). Likewise, repetitive behaviors are not unique to ASDs and ID. They are also characteristic of other psychiatric disorders (e.g., schizophrenia, obsessive-compulsive disorder) and other neurological conditions (e.g., Tourette's syndrome, Parkinson's disease).

This section addresses similarities and differences between ID and ASDs in terms of psychopathology and adaptive behavior. One way to approach this topic is with the framework proposed by Robins and Guze (1970). According to this perspective, the validation of diagnostic groups is a process involving many steps. The first step consists of describing the clinical and associated features of disorders. Then, comparisons between clinical groups are made on external variables (e.g., psychological measures) and in terms of follow-up and family studies. Differences between clinical groups on these comparisons not only support their validity, but can provide valuable information in understanding their pathogenesis. The following sections present some studies that have adopted this framework by comparing individuals with ID, ASDs, or both in terms of psychopathology and adaptive behavior.

Psychopathology

We use the term psychopathology to encompass two related but distinct clinical phenomenon: psychiatric disorders such as those found in the DSM or ICD and behavior problems such as tantrums and aggression. We realize the distinction is not always clear-cut in that some instruments measure both behavior problems and psychiatric symptoms. We also realize that the conceptual distinction between psychopathology and ASDs can be quite muddy. Simply put, it remains unclear if some of the behavior and emotional problems experienced by so many are part of the ASD diathesis or separate clinical entities.

Witwer and Lecavalier (2008b) reviewed the child ID literature for risk markers and correlates of psychopathology and found three studies which compared children and adolescents with ID and autism to those with ID only (Eisenhower, Baker, & Blancher, 2005; Hastings, Daley, Burns, & Beck, 2006; Tonge & Einfeld, 2003). Overall, these studies indicated that children with ID and autism exhibited higher rates of psychopathology than those with ID only. One discrepant finding from the Eisenhower et al. (2005) study was that differences on *Child Behavior Checklist* scores between the

autism ($n = 14$) and non-differentiated ID group ($n = 43$) disappeared after controlling for maternal level of education. It is possible that the small sample could account for this outcome. Witwer and Lecavalier concluded that autism/ASD was a risk marker for psychopathology. McClintock, Hall, and Oliver (2003) conducted a similar review, examining risk markers for challenging behaviors within the ID literature. This review differed from Witwer and Lecavalier (2008b) in that it included all ages, focused on problem behaviors only (excluding psychiatric disorders), and included studies only if sufficient information was presented for the calculation of odds ratios. After examining 22 eligible studies, the authors concluded that autism was a risk factor for self-injurious behavior, aggression toward others, and property destruction. Lower cognitive functioning was a risk marker for self-injury and stereotypy, and communication deficits were a risk marker for self-injury. Findings from both reviews should be interpreted with caution given the relatively small number of studies with individuals with ASDs.

Psychiatric Symptoms

A number of studies examining differences between people with ASDs and ID have focused on psychiatric problems. Bradley et al. (2004) compared twelve 14- to 20-year-olds with ASDs and ID to 12 individuals with ID but no ASD. All participants had IQs below 40 and diagnoses were confirmed with the ADI-R. Both groups were matched in terms of age, gender, and NVIQ. Results indicated that participants with ASDs obtained higher scores on the *Diagnostic Assessment for the Severely Handicapped, Second Edition* (DASH-II). This was the case for the total score and for 7 out of 13 DASH-II subscales, including anxiety, PDD/autism, mania, depression, stereotypies/tics, sleep disorders, and organic syndromes. Also telling was the proportion of individuals with ASDs and ID who scored at or above clinical cut-offs on specific subscales compared to those with ID only. At least 50% of the ASD/ID group had clinically elevated scores for seven disorders (PDD/autism, mania, depression, stereotypies/tics, self-injury, eating disorders, sleep disorders), whereas the ID group reached this 50% criterion in only one area (self-injury).

Likewise, Hill and Furniss (2006) compared 8- to 29-year-olds with severe ID and ASDs ($n = 69$) to those with severe ID and no ASD ($n = 13$). Group membership was based on the PDD/autism subscale of the DASH-II. The ASD group was further separated into moderately autistic ($n = 34$) or severely autistic ($n = 35$) based on DASH-II PDD/autism subscale scores. *Aberrant Behavior Checklist* scores indicated that groups were comparable in terms of behavior problems. Overall, the severely autistic group scored the highest on the DASH-II subscales, followed by the moderately autistic group, with the ID only group scoring lowest. Significant differences were found on the anxiety, mood, mania, PDD/autism, stereotypies, and schizophrenia subscales, with both ASD groups scoring higher than the ID only group.

Bradley and Bolton (2006) focused on episodic psychiatric disorders in an epidemiological sample of individuals aged 14–20 years. Thirty-six individuals with ID (IQ < 75) and autism (as per ADI-R classification) were matched on age, gender, and NVIQ to 36 individuals with ID only. The *Schedule for the Assessment of Psychiatric Problems Associated with Autism* (SAPPA) was administered to informants. Results indicated that individuals with autism had more episodic disorders than their counterparts with ID only (47% of the ASD/ID group compared to 17% of the ID group). The most commonly endorsed category was mood disorders. This is one of the few studies to include the full range of ID (though the distribution of participants across levels is unclear), and interestingly, the disorders did not appear to be related to level of functioning.

Although in current versions of the DSM and ICD, ASDs are an exclusionary criteria for ADHD or hyperkinetic syndrome (HKS), many individuals on the autism spectrum present with symptoms of inattention, hyperactivity, and impulsivity (e.g., Gadow, DeVincent, Pomeroy, & Azizian, 2004; Gadow et al., 2005; Lecavalier, 2006). Bradley and Isaacs (2006) compared these symptoms in 31 pairs of teenagers, one set having autism and ID and the other having ID only. The ADI-R was used to establish presence/absence of autism and groups were matched on age, gender, and NVIQ. Based on clinician assessment of ADHD/HKS symptoms, logistic regressions indicated that participants with autism were more likely to present with hyperactivity and impulsivity (but not inattention) than those with ID only.

In contrast, Tsakanikos and colleagues (2006) challenged the conclusion that individuals with autism have higher rates of psychopathology. In this study, individuals aged 16–84 years with ID and autism (*n* = 147) or with ID only (*n* = 605) underwent a clinical assessment and ICD-10 diagnoses were assigned by clinicians. A subsample (55 with an ASD and ID and 172 with ID only) was also assessed with the *Psychopathology Assessment Schedule for Adults with Developmental Disabilities* (PAS-ADD) checklist. After controlling for the effects of age, gender, level of ID, and medication use, multivariate analyses did not indicate any significant differences between groups on the three PAS-ADD checklist subscales (affective/neurotic, possible organic, and psychotic disorders). The only difference found with respect to clinician-derived psychiatric diagnoses was that people with ASDs were less likely to be diagnosed with personality disorders. It is possible that the PAS-ADD checklist was not sensitive enough to detect differences between groups, as it is relatively short (29 items) and lumps several disorders on the same subscale. Additionally, more people in the autism group were taking psychotropic medicines (70 vs 57% in the ID group), which could suggest that psychopathology was well controlled in this group.

Behavior Problems

As mentioned previously, the distinction between certain behavior problems and core features of ASDs, particularly repetitive and stereotyped behaviors, can be blurred. Nonetheless, several studies have compared behavior problems in people with ASDs and ID. In a study of institutionalized adults with autism and ID matched on IQ to a sample of adults with ID only, Bodfish, Symons, Parker, and Lewis (2000) reported that while the occurrence of specific repetitive behaviors was high in both groups, nearly all of the behaviors examined occurred at a higher rate in individuals with autism. Carcani-Rathwell, Hasketh-Rabe, and Santosh (2006) performed a retrospective chart review to examine repetitive behaviors in individuals aged 1–18 years. Scores from the ADI-R, ADOS, and various IQ tests were used to classify individuals into three groups: those with ASDs and average intelligence (*n* = 319), those with ASD and ID (*n* = 183), and those with ID only (*n* = 119). Consistent with Bodfish and colleagues, individuals diagnosed with an ASD (with or without ID) had higher rates of repetitive and stereotyped behavior than those without ASDs.

Matson, Wilkins, and Ancona (2008) found that adults with severe to profound ID and ASDs had more impairment in social interaction and restricted and/or repetitive behaviors and interests than adults with ID only. Fifty-seven individuals in each group were matched on age, IQ, gender, and verbal skills. Logistic regressions indicated that several items from different scales accurately predicted group membership. Many of these items appeared to measure DSM autism symptoms (e.g., items related to avoidance of interaction with others, stereotypies, and a restricted range of interests). Interestingly, while items on three scales (the *Autism Spectrum Disorders-Diagnosis for Intellectually Disabled Adults* or ASD-DA, *Autism Spectrum Disorders-Problem Behaviors for Adults with Intellectual Disabilities* or ASD-PBA, and *Matson Evaluation of Social Skills for Individuals with Severe Retardation* or MESSIER) showed differences between groups, there were no significant differences between groups on adaptive behaviors as measured by the VABS communication, daily living skills, or socialization domains. One possible explanation is that all participants were very low functioning, which truncated scores. Differences between groups on adaptive behavior are further discussed below.

Brereton et al. (2006) used the DBC to compare behavior problems in children with ID and those with ASDs. Participants were 381 young people with autism (75% of whom had IQs below 70) and an epidemiological sample of 550 Australian young people with borderline IQ or ID aged 4–18 years (some of whom also had autism).

Results indicated that the youngsters in the autism group had significantly higher levels of psychopathology than those in the ID group (total DBC score of 61 vs 43). In fact, 73.5% of children and adolescents with autism had a total DBC score above the recommended clinical cutoff score.

Together these studies support the idea that while people with both ID and ASDs experience the full range of psychopathology, those with ASDs experience more of these problems than their counterparts with ID only. Specifically, individuals with ASDs have been found to experience more psychiatric symptoms, including those related to mood and anxiety disorders, schizophrenia, ADHD, and sleep disorders (Bradley & Bolton, 2006; Bradley & Isaacs, 2006; Bradley et al., 2004; Hill & Furniss, 2006). They are also more at risk for a variety of challenging behaviors like self-injurious behaviors, aggression, property destruction, and repetitive and stereotypical behaviors (Carcani-Rathwell et al., 2006; Matson, Dempsey et al., 2008; McClintock et al., 2003; Witwer & Lecavalier, 2008b). The higher prevalence of psychopathology in people with ASDs seems to hold true whether or not comorbid ID is also present and when level of functioning is accounted for in the research design or analyses.

Adaptive Behavior

As outlined above, impairments in adaptive behavior are required for a diagnosis of ID. Of interest is whether or not individuals with ASDs and ID have different adaptive behavior profiles. When validating the VABS-II (Sparrow, Cicchetti, & Balla, 2005), different clinical groups (aged 6 years and above) were compared, including a group of individuals with mild ID ($n = 79$), moderate ID ($n = 64$), and severe/profound ID ($n = 56$). In general, profiles for these ID groups were flat (i.e., domain scores were all depressed and had little scatter). There was also a trend for older subgroups (age 19 years and up) to score lower within groups compared to younger subgroups (aged 6–18 years). Two autism groups were also examined, a nonverbal group ($n = 31$) aged 2–10 years and a verbal group ($n = 46$) aged 3–19 years. Unlike the fairly flat profiles observed in individuals with ID, the two autism groups had more scatter across domains. Within the verbal group, socialization was the lowest domain score and motor skill was a relative strength. Within the nonverbal group, communication was the lowest domain score, followed by socialization and daily living skills, while motor skills again was a relative strength. Validation of the VABS-II notwithstanding, few studies have focused on differences between children with ID and ASD on adaptive behavior measures.

Matson, Rivet, Fodstad, Dempsey, and Boisjoli (2009) compared four groups of adults on the socialization, communication, and daily living skills domains of the VABS-II: ID and ASDs ($n = 60$); ID, ASDs, and Axis I disorders ($n = 30$); ID and Axis I disorders ($n = 37$); and those with ID only ($n = 250$). All but four participants were functioning in the severe ($n = 40$) or profound ($n = 312$) range of ID and groups were matched on gender and level of functioning. Axis I disorders included bipolar disorder, mood disorder not otherwise specified, depression, and stereotypic movement disorder. Results indicated that those with ID generally had more skills across domains than those with ID and ASDs. Individuals with ID, ASD, and Axis I disorders or with ID and Axis I disorders were similar to each other and demonstrated fewer skills than the other two groups, highlighting the additional impairment associated with Axis I disorders.

Matson, Dempsey, and Fodstad (2009) also examined adaptive behavior in 234 adults with ID (level unspecified) using the *Adaptive Behavior Task Analysis Checklist* (ABTAC). Participants were divided into three groups: autism ($n = 65$), PDDNOS ($n = 104$), and ID only ($n = 65$). Analyses revealed no differences between groups on the subscales of bathing, housekeeping, and meal preparation. On the dressing and hygiene domains, the autism and PDDNOS groups were more impaired than the ID group but did not differ from each other. On the grooming domain, the autism group was the most impaired, followed by the PDDNOS group, while the ID group was the least impaired.

Using the MESSIER and VABS socialization domain, Wilkins and Matson (2009) examined social skills profiles of 16- to 81-year-olds with autism and ID, PDDNOS and ID, and ID only. Seventy-two adults were in each group; authors matched individuals as closely as possible on age, gender, and verbal ability (i.e., verbal or nonverbal). The majority of the sample functioned within the profound range of ID and was nonverbal. While groups differed significantly on MESSIER subscales (generally less positive and more problem behaviors for ASD groups), no differences were observed on the VABS. It is possible that the VABS was not sensitive enough to detect differences with such impaired groups (Sparrow et al., 2005). Interestingly, no significant differences were found between the autism and PDDNOS groups on the measures.

In summary, while few studies have examined differences and similarities between ASDs and ID in terms of adaptive behavior, the studies available indicate that those with both ASDs and ID have significantly more deficits in adaptive behaviors compared to those with ID only. There is also evidence that comorbid psychiatric disorders negatively impact adaptive behavior in those with ID, regardless of the presence of an ASD. Unfortunately, too few studies have been performed to comment extensively on whether differences in adaptive behavior patterns exist and how they relate to treatment outcomes. In addition, studies have almost exclusively focused on adults.

Although the above-mentioned studies represent progress in better understanding the relationship between ID and

ASDs, important methodological points need to be kept in mind when interpreting findings. Several studies contained small samples, which reduces power of analyses and generalization of findings. This is understandable given the relatively low incidence of ID and ASDs in the population. Recruiting large samples can be time consuming and expensive, particularly if one desires homogeneous groups in terms of IQ and age. Conversely, when large samples are used, it is often at the expense of homogeneity which can make data more difficult to interpret. It is interesting to note that several studies have focused on adults with severe/profound ID. This may be due to the greater stability of ASD diagnoses post-childhood, but it remains to be seen if similar results would be found in younger individuals. Even though generalization of findings may be limited, targeting such a homogeneous subgroup has its advantages. Differential diagnosis is the most complex among the most severely impaired and such studies provide valuable insight in this difficult-to-diagnose subgroup. Finally, one needs to be cognizant about how clinical groups are defined; there is great variability in the instruments and procedures used across studies. In the absence of an "absolute" gold standard such as a biological marker to define groups, investigators need to accept the limitations of less-than-perfect diagnoses derived with current instruments and procedures.

Conclusion

There are vast literatures on ID and ASDs. The topics covered in this chapter highlight the significant overlap between disorders. They both are defined behaviorally and share common clinical features. They also share common genetic and neurodevelopmental pathways, although evidence also suggests independent genetic contributions. IQ is among the most robust predictors of the presentation, associated features, and outcome of ASDs. In addition, support exists for the use of IQ in the classification of ASDs. A better understanding of the relationship between ASD features, IQ, and age will facilitate the development of more accurate screening and diagnostic measures for use with special subgroups such as very young children or individuals with severe ID. The question of how these variables relate is also relevant to understanding the pathogenesis and course of the disorders. Much of the progress in the ASD field in the last 15 years has been made with people who function above the range of ID. However, ID might well be the most common co-occurring disorder with ASDs and a strong predictor of poor prognosis. There is a need for even greater efforts at understanding the relationship between the two disabilities.

References

Abrahams, B. S., & Geschwind, D. H. (2008). Advances in autism genetics: On the threshold of a new neurobiology. *Nature Reviews, Genetics, 9*, 341–355.

Aman, M. G., Tassé, M. J., Rojahn, J., & Hammer, D. (1996). The Nisonger CBRF: A child behavior rating form for children with developmental disabilities. *Research in Developmental Disabilities, 17*, 41–57.

American Psychiatric Association. (2000). *Diagnostic and statistical manual of mental disorders* (4th ed., Text Revisions). Washington, DC: Author.

Amiet, C., Gourfinkel-An, I., Bouzamondo, A., Tordjman, S., Baulac, M., Lechat, P., et al. (2008). Epilepsy in autism is associated with intellectual disability and gender: Evidence from a meta-analysis. *Biological Psychiatry, 64*, 577–582.

Bailey, A., Bolton, P., Butler, L., Le Couteur, A., Murphy, M., Scott, S., et al. (1993). Prevalence of the Fragile X anomaly amongst autistic twins and singletons. *Journal of Child Psychology and Psychiatry, 34*, 673–688.

Bellack, A. S., & Hersen, M. (1998). *Behavioral assessment: A practical handbook* (4th ed.). Needham Heights, MA: Allyn & Bacon.

Ben Itzchak, E., Lahat, E., Burgin, R., & Zachor, A. D. (2008). Cognitive, behavior, and intervention outcome in young children with autism. *Research in Developmental Disabilities, 29*, 447–458.

Ben Itzchak, E., & Zachor, A. D. (2007). The effects of intellectual functioning and autism severity on outcome of early behavioral intervention for children with autism. *Research in Developmental Disabilities, 28*, 287–303.

Berument, S. L., Rutter, M., Lord, C., Pickles, A., & Bailey, A. (1999). Autism screening questionnaire: Diagnostic validity. *British Journal of Psychiatry, 175*, 444–451.

Bishop, S. L., Richler, J., & Lord, C. (2006). Association between restricted and repetitive behaviors and nonverbal IQ in children with autism spectrum disorders. *Clinical Neuropsychology, 12*, 247–267.

Black, D. O., Wallace, G. L., Sokoloff, J. L., & Kenworthy, L. (2009). Brief report: IQ split predicts social symptoms and communication abilities in high-functioning children with autism spectrum disorders. *Journal of Autism and Developmental Disabilities, 39*, 1613–1619.

Bodfish, J. W., Symons, F. J., Parker, D. E., & Lewis, M. H. (2000). Varieties of repetitive behaviors in autism: Comparisons to mental retardation. *Journal of Autism and Developmental Disorders, 30*, 237–243.

Bradley, E. A., & Bolton, P. (2006). Episodic psychiatric disorders in teenagers with learning disabilities with and without autism. *British Journal of Psychiatry, 189*, 361–366.

Bradley, E. A., & Isaacs, B. J. (2006). Inattention, hyperactivity, and impulsivity in teenagers with intellectual disabilities, with and without autism. *Canadian Journal of Psychiatry, 51*, 598–606.

Bradley, E. A., Summers, J. A., Wood, H. L., & Bryson, S. E. (2004). Comparing rates of psychiatric and behavior disorders in adolescents and young adults with severe intellectual disability with and without autism. *Journal of Autism and Developmental Disorders, 34*, 151–161.

Brereton, A. V., Tonge, B. J., & Einfeld, S. L. (2006). Psychopathology in children and adolescents with autism compared to young people with intellectual disability. *Journal of Autism and Developmental Disorders, 36*, 863–870.

Bryson, S. E., Bradley, E. A., Thompson, A., & Wainwright, A. (2008). Prevalence of autism among adolescents with intellectual disabilities. *The Canadian Journal of Psychiatry, 53*, 449–459.

Bryson, S. E., & Smith, I. M. (1998). Epidemiology of autism: Prevalence, associated characteristics, and implications for research and service delivery. *Mental Retardation and Developmental Disabilities Research Reviews, 4,* 97–103.

Buitelaar, J. K., Van der Gaag, R., Klin, A., & Volkmar, F. R. (1999). Exploring the boundaries of pervasive developmental disorder not otherwise specified: Analyses of data from the DSM-IV autistic disorder field trial. *Journal of Autism and Developmental Disorders, 29,* 33–43.

Caniato, R. (2007). Epilepsy in autism spectrum disorders. *European Child and Adolescent Psychiatry, 16,* 61–66.

Carcani-Rathwell, I., Hasketh-Rabe, S., & Santosh, P. J. (2006). Repetitive and stereotyped behaviors in pervasive developmental disorders. *Journal of Child Psychology and Psychiatry, 47,* 573–581.

Center for Disease Control and Prevention. (2009). *Autism and developmental disorders monitoring network.* Retrieved March 18, 2010, from http://www.cdc.gov/ncbddd/autism/addm.html

Chakrabarti, S., & Fombonne, E. (2001). Pervasive developmental disorders in preschool children. *Journal of the American Medical Association, 285,* 3093–3099.

Chakrabarti, S., & Fombonne, E. (2005). Pervasive developmental disorders in preschool children: Confirmation of high prevalence. *American Journal of Psychiatry, 162,* 1133–1141.

Charman, T., Pickles, A., Chandler, S., Wing, L., Bryson, S., Simonoff, E., et al. (2009). Commentary: Effects of diagnostic thresholds and research vs service and administrative diagnosis on autism prevalence. *International Journal of Epidemiology, 38,* 1234–1238.

Constantino, J. (2002). *The social responsiveness scale.* Los Angeles: Western Psychological Services.

Constantino, J. N., Davis, S. A., Todd, R. D., Schindler, M. K., Gross, M. M., Brophy, S. L., et al. (2003). Validation of a brief quantitative measure of autistic traits: Comparison of the social responsiveness scale with the Autism Diagnostic Interview-Revised. *Journal of Autism and Developmental Disorders, 33,* 427–433.

Croen, L. A., Grether, J. K., Hoogstrate, J., & Selvin, S. (2002). The changing prevalence of autism in California. *Journal of Autism and Developmental Disorders, 32,* 207–215.

Cuccaro, M. L., Shao, Y., Grubber, J., Slifer, M., Wolpert, C. M., Donnelly, S. L., et al. (2003). Factor analysis of restricted and repetitive behaviors in autism using the Autism Diagnostic Interview – R. *Child Psychiatry and Human Development, 34,* 3–17.

Dawson, G., Estes, A., Munson, J., Schellenberg, G., Bernier, R., & Abbott, R. (2007). Quantitative assessment of autism symptom-related traits in probands and parents: Broader phenotype autism assessment scale. *Journal of Autism and Developmental Disorders, 37,* 523–536.

de Bildt, A., Sytema, S., Ketelaars, C., Kraijer, D., Mulder, E., Volkmar, F., et al. (2004). Interrelationship between the Autism Diagnostic Observation Schedule-Generic (ADOS-G), Autism Diagnostic Interview-Revised (ADI-R), and the Diagnostic and Statistical Manual of Mental Disorders (DSM-IV-TR) classification in children and adolescents with mental retardation. *Journal of Autism and Developmental Disorders, 34,* 129–137.

De Bildt, A., Sytema, S., Kraijer, D., & Monderra, R. (2005). Prevalence of pervasive developmental disorders in children and adolescents with mental retardation. *Journal of Child Psychology and Psychiatry, 46,* 275–286.

DiLavore, P. C., Lord, C., & Rutter, M. (1995). The prelinguistic autism diagnostic observation schedule. *Journal of Autism and Developmental Disorders, 25,* 355–379.

Eisenhower, A. S., Baker, B. L., & Blancher, J. (2005). Preschool children with intellectual disability: Syndrome specificity, behavior problems, and maternal well-being. *Journal of Intellectual Disability Research, 49,* 657–671.

Estes, A. M., Dawson, G., Sterling, L., & Munson, J. (2007). Level of intellectual functioning predicts patterns of associated symptoms in school-age children with autism spectrum disorder. *American Journal on Mental Retardation, 112,* 439–449.

Fombonne, E. (2003). Epidemiological surveys of autism and other pervasive developmental disorders: An update. *Journal of Autism and Developmental Disorders, 33,* 365–382.

Fombonne, E. (2005a). Epidemiological studies of pervasive developmental disorders. In F. R. Volkmar, R. Paul, A. Klin, & D. Cohen (Eds.), *Handbook of autism and pervasive developmental disorders* (pp. 42–69). Hoboken, NJ: Wiley.

Fombonne, E. (2005b). Epidemiology of Autistic Disorder and other pervasive Developmental Disorders. *Journal of Clinical Psychiatry, 66*(Supplement 10), 3–8.

Fombonne, E. (2005c). The changing epidemiology of autism. *Journal of Applied Research in Intellectual Disabilities, 18,* 281–294.

Gadow, K. D., DeVincent, C. J., Pomeroy, J., & Azizian, A. (2004). Psychiatric symptoms in preschool children with PDD and clinic and comparison samples. *Journal of Autism and Developmental Disorders, 34,* 379–393.

Gadow, K. D., DeVincent, C. J., Pomeroy, J., & Azizian, A. (2005). Comparison of DSM-IV symptoms in elementary school-age children with PDD versus clinic and community. *Autism, 9,* 392–415.

Gillberg, C., & Billstedt, E. (2000). Autism and Asperger's syndrome: Coexistence with other clinical disorders. *Acta Psychiatrica Scandanavia, 102,* 321–330.

Gilliam, J. E. (2006). *Gilliam autism rating scale* (2nd ed.). Austin: ProEd.

Hastings, R. P., Daley, D., Burns, C., & Beck, A. (2006). Maternal distress and expressed emotion: Cross-sectional and longitudinal relationships with behavior problems of children with intellectual disabilities. *American Journal on Mental Retardation, 111,* 48–61.

Hauser, W. A., Annegers, J. F., & Kurland, L. T. (1991). Prevalence of epilepsy in Rochester, Minnesota: 1940–1980. *Epilepsia, 32,* 429–445.

Helt, M., Kelley, E., Kinsbourne, M., Pandey, J., Boorstein, H., Herbert, M., et al. (2008). Can children with autism recover? If so, how? *Neuropsychology Review, 18,* 339–366.

Hill, J., & Furniss, F. (2006). Patterns of emotional and behavioral disturbance associated with autistic traits in young people with severe intellectual disabilities and challenging behaviors. *Research in Developmental Disabilities, 27,* 517–528.

Hoekstra, R. A., Happé, F., Baron-Cohen, S., & Ronald, A. (2009). Association between extreme sutistic traits and intellectual disability. *British Journal of Psychiatry, 195,* 531–536.

Howlin, P., Goode, S., Hutton, J., & Rutter, M. (2004). Adult outcome for children with autism. *Journal of Child Psychology and Psychiatry, 45,* 212–229.

Joseph, R. M., Tager-Flusberg, H., & Lord, C. (2002). Cognitive profiles and social-communication functioning in children with autism spectrum disorder. *Journal of Child Psychology and Psychiatry, 43,* 807–821.

Kim, J. A., Szatmari, P., Bryson, S. E., Streiner, D. L., & Wilson, F. J. (2000). The prevalence of anxiety and mood problems among children with autism and Asperger syndrome. *Autism, 4,* 117–132.

King, M., & Bearman, P. (2009). Diagnostic change and the increased prevalence of autism. *International Journal of Epidemiology, 38,* 1224–1234.

Klin, A., Jones, W., Schultz, R., & Volkmar, F. R. (2003). The enactive mind, or from actions to cognition: Lessons from autism. *Philosophical Transactions of the Royal Society of London – Series B: Biological Sciences, 358,* 345–360.

Kogan, M. D., Blumberg, S. J., Schieve, L. A., Boyle, C. A., Perrin, J. M., Ghandour, R. M., et al. (2009). Prevalence of parent-reported diagnosis of autism spectrum disorder among children in the US, 2007. *Pediatrics.* doi:10.1542/peds.2009-1522.

Lainhart, J. E., & Folstein, S. E. (1994). Affective disorders in people with autism: A review of published cases. *Journal of Autism and Developmental Disorders, 24*, 587–601.

Lecavalier, L. (2006). Behavioral and emotional problems in young people with pervasive developmental disorders: Relative prevalence, effects of subject characteristics, and empirical classification. *Journal of Autism and Developmental Disorders, 36*, 1101–1114.

Lecavalier, L., & Butter, E. M. (2010). Assessment of social skills and intellectual disability. In D. Nangle, D. Hansen, C. Erdley, & P. J. Norton (Eds.), *Practitioner's guide to empirically-based measures of social skills* (pp. 179–192). New York: Association for the Advancement of Behavior Therapy and Springer.

Lecavalier, L., Gadow, K., DeVincent, C. J., & Edwards, M. C. (2009). Validation of DSM-IV model of psychiatric syndromes in children with autism spectrum disorders. *Journal of Autism and Developmental Disorders, 39*, 278–289.

Lee, J. H., Larson, S. A., Lakin, C., Anderson, L., Nohoon, K. L., & Anderson, D. (2001). Prevalence of mental retardation and developmental disabilities: Estimates from the 1994/1995 national health interview survey disability supplements. *American Journal on Mental Retardation, 106*, 231–252.

Leonard, H., Petterson, B., De Clerk, N., Zubrick, S. R., Glasson, E., Sanders, R., et al. (2005). Association of sociodemographic characteristics of children with intellectual disability in Western Australia. *Social Science & Medicine, 60*, 1499–1513.

Levis, S. E., Mandell, D. S., & Schultz, R. T. (2009). Autism. *Lancet, 374*, 1627–1638.

Lord, C., & Corsello, C. (2005). Diagnostic instruments in autistic spectrum disorders. In F. R. Volkmar, R. Paul, A. Klin, & D. Cohen (Eds.), *Handbook of autism and pervasive developmental disorders* (pp. 730–771). Hoboken, NJ: Wiley.

Lord, C., Risi, S., Lambrecht, L., Cook, E. H., Leventhal, B. L., DiLavore, P. C., et al. (2000). The Autism Diagnostic Observation Schedule-Generic: A standard measure of social and communication deficits associated with the spectrum of autism. *Journal of Autism and Developmental Disorders, 30*, 205–223.

Lord, C., Rutter, M., & LeCouteur, A. (1994). *The Autism Diagnostic Interview-Revised*: A revised version of a diagnostic interview for caregivers of individuals with possible pervasive developmental disorders. *Journal of Autism and Developmental Disorders, 24*, 659–685.

Lord, C., Schopler, E., & Revicki, D. (1982). Sex differences in autism. *Journal of Autism and Developmental Disorders, 12*, 317–330.

Luyster, R., Qiu, S., Lopez, K., & Lord, C. (2007). Predicting outcomes of children referred for autism using the MacArthur-Bates communication inventory. *Journal of Speech, Language, and Hearing Research, 50*, 667–681.

Matson, J. L., Boisjoli, J. A., Gonzalez, M. L., Smith, K. R., & Wilkins, J. (2007). Norms and cut off scores for the autism spectrum disorders diagnosis for adults (ASD-DA) with intellectual disability. *Research in Autism Spectrum Disorders, 1*, 330–338.

Matson, J. L., Dempsey, T., & Fodstad, J. C. (2009). The effect of autism spectrum disorders on adaptive independent living skills in adults with severe intellectual disability. *Research in Developmental Disabilities, 30*, 1203–1211.

Matson, J. L., Dempsey, T., LoVullo, S. V., & Wilkins, J. (2008). The effects of intellectual functioning on the range of core symptoms in autism spectrum disorders. *Research in Developmental Disabilities, 29*, 341–350.

Matson, J. L., & Nebel-Schwalm, M. S. (2007). Comorbid psychopathology with autism spectrum disorder in children: An overview. *Research in Developmental Disabilities, 28*, 341–352.

Matson, J. L., Rivet, T. T., Fodstad, J. C., Dempsey, T., & Boisjoli, J. A. (2009). Examination of adaptive behavior differences in adults with autism spectrum disorders and intellectual disability. *Research in Developmental Disabilities, 30*, 1317–1325.

Matson, J. L., & Shoemaker, M. (2009). Intellectual disability and its relationship to autism spectrum disorders. *Research in Developmental Disabilities, 30*, 1107–1114.

Matson, J. L., Wilkins, J., & Ancona, M. (2008). Autism in adults with severe intellectual disability: An empirical study of symptom presentation. *Journal of Intellectual and Developmental Disability, 33*, 36–42.

Matson, J. L., Wilkins, J., Boisjoli, J. A., & Smith, K. R. (2008). The validity of the autism spectrum disorders-diagnosis for intellectually disabled adults (ASD-DA). *Research in Developmental Disabilities, 29*, 537–546.

Matson, J. L., Wilkins, J., & Gonzalez, M. L. (2007). Reliability and factor structure of the Autism Spectrum Disorders–Diagnosis for Intellectually Disabled Adults (ASD-DA). *Journal of Developmental and Physical Disabilities, 1*, 565–577.

McClintock, K., Hall, S., & Oliver, C. (2003). Risk markers associated with challenging behaviors in people with intellectual disabilities: A meta-analytic study. *Journal of Intellectual Disability Research, 47*, 405–416.

McDougle, C. J., Kresch, L. E., Goodman, W. K., Naylor, S. T., Volkmar, F. R., Cohen, D. J., et al. (1995). A case-controlled study of repetitive thoughts and behavior in adults with autistic disorder and obsessive-compulsive disorder. *American Journal of Psychiatry, 152*, 772–777.

McGovern, C. W., & Sigman, M. (2005). Continuity and change from early childhood to adolescence in autism. *Journal of Child Psychology and Psychiatry, 46*, 401–408.

Munson, J., Dawson, G., Sterling, L., Beauchaine, T., Zhou, A., Koehler, E., et al. (2008). Evidence for latent classes of IQ in young children with autism spectrum disorder. *American Journal on Mental Retardation, 113*, 439–452.

Nordin, V., & Gillberg, C. (1996). Autism spectrum disorders in children with physical or mental disability or both. I: Clinical and epidemiological aspects. *Developmental Medicine and Child Neurology, 38*, 297–313.

Norris, M., & Lecavalier, L. (2010). Screening accuracy of level 2 Autism Spectrum Disorder rating scales: A review of selected instruments. *Autism, 14*, 263–284.

Palmer, R. F., Blanchard, S., Jean, C. R., & Mandell, D. S. (2005). School district resources and identification of children with autistic disorder. *American Journal of Public Health, 95*, 125–130.

Pine, E., Luby, J., Abbacchi, A., & Constantino, J. N. (2006). Quantitative assessment of autistic symptomatology in preschoolers. *Autism, 10*, 344–352.

Remington, B., Hastings, R. P., Kovshoff, H., degli Espinosa, F., Jahr, E., Brown, T., et al. (2007). Early intensive behavioral intervention: Outcomes for children with autism and their parents after two years. *American Journal on Mental Retardation, 112*, 418–438.

Robins, E., & Guze, S. B. (1970). Establishment of diagnostic validity in psychiatric illness: Its application to schizophrenia. *American Journal of Psychiatry, 126*, 983–987.

Roeleveld, N., Zielhuis, G. A., & Gabreels, F. (1997). The prevalence of mental retardation: A critical review of recent literature. *Developmental Medicine and Child Neurology, 39*, 125–132.

Rutter, M. (2009). Commentary: Fact and artifact in the secular increase in the rate of autism. *International Journal of Epidemiology, 38*, 1238–1239.

Sallows, G. O., & Graupner, T. D. (2005). Intensive behavioral treatment for children with autism: Four-year outcome and predictors. *American Journal on Mental Retardation, 110*, 417–438.

Scott, F. J., Baron-Cohen, S., Bolton, P., & Brayne, C. (2002). Brief report: Prevalence of autism spectrum conditions in children aged 5–11 years in Cambridgeshire, UK. *Autism, 6*, 231–237.

Seltzer, M. M., Shattuck, P., Abbeduto, L., & Greenberg, J. S. (2004). Trajectory of development in adolescents and adults with autism. *Mental Retardation and Developmental Disabilities Research Reviews, 10,* 234–247.

Shattuck, P. T. (2006). The contribution of diagnostic substitution to the growing administrative prevalence of autism in US special education. *Pediatrics, 117,* 1028–1037.

Shattuck, P. T., Seltzer, M. M., Greenberg, J. S., Orsmond, G. I., Bolt, D., Kring, S., et al. (2007). Change in autism symptoms and maladaptive behaviors in adolescents and adults with an autism spectrum disorder. *Journal of Autism and Developmental Disorders, 37,* 1735–1747.

Simonoff, E., Pickles, A., Charman, T., Chandler, S., Loucas, T., & Baird, G. (2008). Psychiatric disorders in children with autism spectrum disorders: Prevalence, comorbidity, and associated factors in a population-derived sample. *Journal of the American Academy of Child and Adoelscent Psychiatry, 47,* 921–929.

Skuse, D. H. (2006). Genetic influences on the neural basis of social cognition. *Philosophical Transactions of the Royal Society of London Biological Sciences, 361,* 2129–2141.

Skuse, D. H. (2007). Rethinking the nature of genetic vulnerability to autistic spectrum disorders. *Trends in Genetics, 8,* 387–395.

Smalley, S. L. (1998). Autism and tuberous sclerosis. *Journal of Autism and Developmental Disorders, 28,* 407–414.

Sparrow, S. S., Cicchetti, D. V., & Balla, D. A. (2005). *Vineland adaptive behavior scales – Second edition: Survey forms manual.* Circle Pines, MN: AGS Publishing.

Spiker, D., Lotspeich, L. J., Dimiceli, S., Myers, R. M., & Risch, N. (2002). Behavioral phenotypic variation in autism multiplex families: Evidence for a continuous severity gradient. *American Journal of Medical Genetics (Neuropsychiatric Genetics), 114,* 129–136.

Sponheim, E., & Skjeldal, O. (1998). Autism and related disorders: Epidemiological findings in a Norwegian study using ICD-10 diagnostic criteria. *Journal of Autism and Developmental Disorders, 28,* 217–227.

Sukhodolsky, D. G., Scahill, L., Gadow, K. G., Arnold, L. E., Aman, M. G., McDougle, C. J., et al. (2008). Parent-rated anxiety symptoms in children with pervasive developmental disorders: Frequency and association with core autism symptoms and cognitive functioning. *Journal of Abnormal Child Psychology, 36,* 117–128.

Szatmari, P., Bryson, S. E., Boyle, M. H., Streiner, D. L., & Duku, E. (2003). Predictors of outcome among high functioning children with autism and Asperger syndrome. *Journal of Child Psychology and Psychiatry, 44,* 520–528.

Szatmari, P., Georgiades, S., Bryson, S., Zwaigenbaum, L., Roberts, W., Mahoney, W., et al. (2006). Investigating the structure of the restricted, repetitive behaviors and interests domain of autism. *Journal of Child Psychology and Pscyiatry, 47,* 582–590.

Tager-Flusberg, H., & Joseph, R. M. (2003). Identifying neurocognitive phenotypes in autism. *Philosophical Transactions of the Royal Society of London, Biological Science, 358,* 303–314.

Tonge, B. J., & Einfeld, S. L. (2003). Psychopathology and intellectual disability: The Australian child to adult longitudinal study. *International Review of Research in Mental Retardation, 26,* 61–91.

Tsakanikos, E., Costello, H., Holt, G., Bouras, N., Sturmey, P., & Newton, T. (2006). Psychopathology in adults with autism and intellectual disability. *Journal of Autism and Developmental Disorders, 36,* 1123–1129.

Tuchman, R., & Rapin, I. (2002). Epilepsy in autism. *Lancet Neurology, 1,* 352–358.

Van Meter, K. C., Christiansen, L. E., Delwiche, L. D., Azari, R., Carpenter, T. E., & Hertz-Picciotto, I. (2010). Geographic distribution of autism in California: A retrospective birth cohort analysis. *Autism Research.* doi:10.1002/aur.110.

Volkmar, F. R. (2002). Predicting outcome in autism. *Journal of Autism and Developmental Disorders, 32,* 63–64.

Wesibrot, D. M., Gadow, K. D., DeVincent, C. J., & Pomeroy, J. (2005). The presentation of anxiety in children with pervasive developmental disorders. *Journal of Child and Adolescent Psychopharmacology, 15,* 477–496.

Westerinen, H., Kaski, M., Virta, L., Almqvist, F., & Livanainen, M. (2007). Prevalence of intellectual disability: A comprehensive study based on national registers. *Journal of Intellectual Disability Research, 51,* 715–725.

Wilkins, J., & Matson, J. L. (2009). A comparison of social skills profiles in intellectually disabled adults with and without ASD. *Behavior Modification, 33,* 143–155.

Wing, L., & Gould, J. (1979). Severe impairments of social interaction and associated abnormalities in children: Epidemiology and classification. *Journal of Autism and Developmental Disorders, 9,* 11–29.

Witwer, A. N., & Lecavalier, L. (2008a). Validity of autism spectrum disorder subtypes. *Journal of Autism and Developmental Disorders, 38,* 1611–1624.

Witwer, A. N., & Lecavalier, L. (2008b). Psychopathology in children with intellectual disability: Risk markers and correlates. *Journal of Mental Health Research and Intellectual Disabilities, 1,* 75–96.

Witwer, A. N., & Lecavalier, L. (2010). Validity of comorbid psychiatric disorders in children with autism spectrum disorders. *Journal of Developmental and Physical Disabilities, 22,* 367–380.

Yeargin-Allsopp, M., Rice, C., Karapurkar, T., Doernberg, N., Boyle, C., & Murphy, C. (2003). Prevalence of autism in a US metropolitan area. *Journal of the American Medical Association, 289,* 49–55.

Psychiatric Disorders in People with Autism Spectrum Disorders: Phenomenology and Recognition

5

Sissel Berge Helverschou, Trine Lise Bakken, and Harald Martinsen

The prevalence and incidence rates of psychiatric disorders are higher in people with autism spectrum disorders (ASD) than in the general population (Bradley, Summers, Hayley, & Bryson, 2004; Brereton, Tonge, & Einfeld, 2006; Clarke, Baxter, Perry, & Prasher, 1999; Ghaziuddin & Greden, 1998; Ghaziuddin, 2005; Ghaziuddin, Alessi, & Greden, 1995; Ghaziuddin, Tsai, & Ghaziuddin, 1992; Glenn, Bihm, & Lammers, 2003; Howlin, 1997, 2000; Howlin, Goode, Hutton, & Rutter, 2004; Lainhart, 1999; Leyfer et al., 2006; Matson & Nebel-Schwalm, 2007; Morgan, Roy, & Chance, 2003; Simonoff et al., 2008; Tsakanikos et al., 2006). Individuals with ASD are believed to be especially vulnerable to psychiatric problems; however, psychiatric disorders are frequently overlooked in this group and psychiatric symptoms are attributed to the disability itself (Borthwick-Duffy, 1994; Ghaziuddin, 2005; Glenn et al., 2003; Howlin, 2002; Jacobsen, 1999; Jopp & Keys, 2001; Lainhart, 1999; Mason & Scior, 2004; Matson & Boisjoli, 2008; Wing, 1996). This chapter describes the manifestation of four major psychiatric disorders in ASD – anxiety disorders, psychoses, depression, and obsessive-compulsive disorder (OCD) – and discusses how these disorders may be recognized and defined in this population.

Identification of Psychiatric Disorders in People with Autism Spectrum Disorders

It has proved difficult to identify psychiatric disorders in people with ASD. This is reflected in the varying prevalence estimates reported, which range from 9 to 89% (Howlin, 2002). This wide variation indicates that psychiatric disorders are both under- and over-diagnosed in people with ASD.

In general, it is difficult to distinguish between the symptoms of a psychiatric disorder and autistic behavior (Clarke et al., 1999; Clarke, Littlejohns, Corbett, & Joseph, 1989; Ghaziuddin et al., 1995, 1992; Kobayashi & Murata, 1998; Lainhart, 1999; Long, Wood, & Holmes, 2000; McDougle, Kresch, & Posey, 2000; Reaven & Hepburn, 2003; Volkmar & Cohen, 1991). Four main problems make this task difficult. First, the criteria for the level of the patient's adjustment problems and discomfort may be set too low, in order to diagnose a psychiatric disorder. Second, the characteristics of people with ASD make it difficult to employ the diagnostic criteria for psychiatric disorders and ordinary diagnostic procedures. Third, autistic traits and symptoms of psychiatric disorders co-occur. Finally, different types of psychiatric disorders also co-occur.

Individuals with a psychiatric disorder may have severe difficulties in coping with the challenges of daily life. Core symptoms of the disorder interfere with everyday functioning and general adjustment problems develop, such as psychosomatic disturbances, sleeping and eating problems, passivity, restlessness, irritability, aggression, social withdrawal, and self-injurious behavior. Prominent general adjustment problems have been shown to be present in the mental illness of both people with average IQ (Gelder, Lopez-Ibor, & Andreasen, 2003) and people with intellectual disability (ID; Gustafsson & Sonnander, 2004, 2005). Adjustment problems are correlated with symptom scores for psychosis, anxiety, depression, and OCD in individuals with ASD and ID (Helverschou, Bakken, & Martinsen, 2009) and adjustment problems can be used as a suitable indicator when screening for possible psychiatric disorders in people with ASD (Bakken et al., 2010). Because of their co-occurrence with symptoms of psychiatric disorders, the presence of severe adjustment problems is widely used as a criterion of mental illness in addition to high "symptom burden," the extent of negative impact, created by the core symptoms (American Psychiatric Association [APA], 2000; Sadock, 2005; World Health Organization [WHO], 2001). If the criteria for degree of symptom burden and co-occurring adjustment problems

S.B. Helverschou (✉)
The National Autism Unit, Rikshospitalet, Oslo University Hospital, 0027 Oslo, Norway
e-mail: s.b.helverschou@rikshospitalet.no

J.L. Matson, P. Sturmey (eds.), *International Handbook of Autism and Pervasive Developmental Disorders*, Autism and Child Psychopathology Series, DOI 10.1007/978-1-4419-8065-6_5, © Springer Science+Business Media, LLC 2011

are set too low, it may be difficult to identify psychiatric disorders. This is a particular problem with OCD and anxiety disorders (Eknes, 2008). For example, there is a diagnostic prerequisite that obsessions and compulsions should be experienced as problematic in order to be diagnosed as OCD. In clinical work, emphasis is usually given to the intention behind the behavior, which may result in diagnosing OCD in people who do not experience obsession or compulsions.

Individuals with ASD and most individuals with ID have severe language and communication problems, which make it difficult or impossible for some people with ASD and ID to report their feelings and experiences. This constitutes a major problem for the identification of psychiatric disorders, especially in people with ASD and ID, since the diagnostic criteria for psychiatric disorders are largely based on self-report (Sadock, 2005). The problem is exacerbated in people with ASD, since even those with the best communication and language skills have difficulty in self-reporting and making themselves understood by others. Individuals with ASD often do not understand social contexts, intentions, their own and other people's feelings, ambiguous or vague concepts, and social relations. In addition, their idiosyncratic language may cause other people to misunderstand what they say. Thus, communication with people with ASD concerning their emotional lives is challenging.

It may also be difficult to distinguish between the symptoms of ASD and a psychiatric disorder (Clarke et al., 1989, 1999; Ghaziuddin et al., 1995, 1992; Kobayashi & Murata, 1998; Lainhart, 1999; Long et al., 2000; McDougle et al., 2000; Reaven & Hepburn, 2003; Volkmar & Cohen, 1991) because of overlap between ASD criteria and criteria for other disorders; thus, other disorders may be overlooked or wrongly attributed to ASD. Symptom overlap between autism and psychiatric disorders is considerable (Clarke et al., 1989, 1999; Ghaziuddin et al., 1995, 1992; Kobayashi & Murata, 1998; Lainhart, 1999; Long et al., 2000; McDougle et al., 2000; Reaven & Hepburn, 2003; Volkmar & Cohen, 1991; Wing, 1996) and most clearly found for ASD and schizophrenia and ASD and OCD. The ritualistic and repetitive behaviors that are one of the core characteristics of ASD may also be symptoms of OCD. Lack of social interaction is both a feature of ASD and a symptom of schizophrenia. In addition, signs of anxiety are characteristic of ASD (Lainhart, 1999; MacNeil, Lopes, & Minnes, 2009; Tsai, 2006), indeed, co-occurrence between anxiety and ASD is so high that Kanner (1943, 1944) emphasized anxiety reactions in his first description of children with autism. The diagnostic criteria for depression do not overlap with the characteristics of ASD, but symptoms of depression may be overlooked in individuals with ASD (Gillberg & Billstedt, 2000). Mood changes, which are among the main symptoms of depression, may be especially difficult

to observe (Perry, Marston, Hinder, Munden, & Roy, 2001). Symptoms of depression may also be overshadowed by and wrongly attributed to ASD, since social withdrawal, limited facial expression, and flattered affect may be indicators of both disorders (Skokauskas & Gallagher, 2010). Similarly, sleeping and eating problems may be interpreted as related to ASD or as symptoms of depression (Perry et al., 2001).

Individuals with ASD who develop an additional psychiatric disorder seem to show more autistic behavior than they did previously, which makes it likely that the psychiatric symptoms will be attributed to the autistic condition (Lainhart, 1999). For example, idiosyncratic speech described in psychotic patients increases, and repetitive and ritualistic behavior becomes more frequent in individuals with an anxiety disorder. Both characteristics of ASD (Lainhart, 1999; Stavrakiki, 1999; Tantam, 2000) and autistic traits (Tantam, 2000; Wing, 1996) appear to increase in frequency. Autistic traits include ritual arrangement of objects, moving furniture and other objects back to where they were placed earlier, rituals connected with eating and going to bed (Kanner, 1943, 1944; Prior & Macmillan, 1973; Rumsey, Rapoport, & Sceery, 1985), as well as rocking back and forth, waving of arms or hands, eye-ball pressing, head banging, and posturing.

The main reason that different psychiatric disorders are confounded is that reactions shown by individuals with a disorder, which are similar across different psychiatric disorders, are used as diagnostic criteria of *specific* disorders. For example, the negative symptoms of schizophrenia overlap with the defining criteria of depression, and withdrawal is both a defining criterion of social phobia and a typical behavioral feature of psychotic individuals. Similarly, many diagnostic instruments use the presence of typical adjustment problems as symptoms of the disorder in question. An example is the use of low activity level, apathy, and lack of initiative as depressive symptoms. Psychosomatic reactions are an important source of confounding, since they may be caused by stress, which is linked with all types of psychiatric disorders. In addition, psychiatric disorders are associated with different medical conditions that may themselves cause stress in patients.

Comorbidity of Psychiatric Disorders in ASD

Studies of clinical samples, mainly children and intellectually higher functioning individuals, suggest that between 50 and 70% of individuals with ASD have additional psychiatric disorders (Ghaziuddin & Zafar, 2008). Depression is the most frequent disorder, often combined with anxiety disorders (Ghaziuddin & Greden, 1998; Ghaziuddin et al., 1992,

1995; Howlin, 1997, 2000; Howlin et al., 2004; Lainhart, 1999; Schopler & Mesibov, 1994; Tantam, 2000). Although the reported prevalence rates are lower in recent studies of community samples, they point to depression and anxiety disorders being the most frequent comorbid psychiatric disorder in people with ASD (Hutton, Goode, Murphy, Couteur, & Rutter, 2008; Melville et al., 2008; Morgan et al., 2003). Anxiety disorders are not addressed in all studies, but are the most common disorder identified in the studies that include anxiety disorders and phobias (Bradley et al., 2004; Leyfer et al., 2006).

Despite the large variation and somewhat inconsistent findings regarding the prevalence rates of psychiatric disorders in individuals with ASD in general, lower prevalence rates are found for OCD and psychosis (Howlin et al., 2004; Lainhart, 1999). In people with ASD, the reported OCD rates vary between 0 and 37% (Leyfer et al., 2006; Melville et al., 2008), and in some studies OCD has been reported as being the second most common disorder (Hutton et al., 2008; Leyfer et al., 2006). The probability of developing schizophrenia seems to be similar to the risk in the general population (Cederlund, Hagberg, Billstedt, Gillberg, & Gillberg, 2008; Ghaziuddin et al., 1992, 1995; Howlin, 1997, 2000; Howlin et al., 2004; Lainhart, 1999; Schopler & Mesibov, 1994; Tantam, 2000); however, higher prevalence rates of psychotic disorders have been reported in recently published studies (Bradley et al., 2004; Morgan et al., 2003; Mouridsen, Rich, Isager, & Nedergaard, 2008; Tsakanikos et al., 2006), and psychotic depression was the most common psychiatric diagnosis reported in a review of case studies (Howlin, 2002). This may indicate that the majority of individuals with autism who become psychotic develop an affective type of psychosis.

Individuals with psychiatric disorders often display symptoms of more than one disorder, and co-occurrence of disorders has been found in ASD populations (Ghaziuddin, 2005; Howlin, 2002; Lainhart, 1999). For example, in two studies conducted in community-based samples, Leyfer and colleagues (2006) reported a median number of three psychiatric diagnoses per child, and Simonoff and colleagues (2008) identified two or more disorders in 41% of those who were identified as having a psychiatric disorder. The co-occurrence of more than one psychiatric disorder seems to be high among individuals with both ASD and ID. In a screening study, a representative sample of individuals with ASD and ID was compared with a representative sample of persons with ID only (Bakken et al., 2010). Fifty-five percent of the ASD group and 70% of the ID-only group obtained scores indicating more than one psychiatric disorder in those who screened positive for a psychiatric disorder. In both groups, a mean number of 2.1 disorders was found.

The degree of overlap seems to vary according to the psychiatric disorder. Anxiety and depression, which are the most prevalent disorders, often co-occur (Howlin, 2000) and these disorders most often overlap with other disorders as well (Bakken et al., 2010); however, the likelihood of overlap seems higher for OCD and psychosis. This is illustrated by the Bakken et al.'s (2010) finding that individuals identified as having OCD had an average of 2.1 other comorbid disorders, and those with psychosis an average of 1.9 other comorbid disorders whereas individuals identified as having anxiety and depression had 1.5 and 1.3 other comorbid disorders, respectively. In general, there is a positive association between comorbidity and the severity of the psychopathological condition (Clarke et al., 1999). Accordingly, individuals with psychosis, which is traditionally regarded as the most severe of these four disorders, and individuals with OCD, which is especially related to autism (Scahill et al., 2006; Tantam, 2000), had severe adjustment problems and higher degrees of overlap than individuals with depression and anxiety (Bakken et al., 2010).

There is reason to assume that there are some similarities or standard trajectories in the development of comorbid psychiatric disorders. For example, it has been argued that depression is often followed by OCD, but OCD very seldom precedes depression (Eknes, 2008) and 40–50% of persons with social phobia later develop depression (Alden & Crozier, 2001). In people with Asperger syndrome, long-standing anxiety may lead to depression (Tantam, 2000). This suggests that anxiety may have a central role in the development of psychiatric disorders in people with ASD and is in line with our clinical experience from adolescents and young adults with Asperger syndrome; after several years with anxiety problems, they eventually develop depression in 20–30% of the cases. In a relatively few cases, psychosis follows thereafter. In general, anxiety symptoms are likely to co-occur with severe mental illness (Alden & Crozier, 2001; Coplan, Pine, Papp, & Gorman, 1997; Davidson, 2002; Gelder et al., 2003; Heim & Nemeroff, 1999; Lindenmayer et al., 2004; Regier, Rae, Narrow, Kaelber, & Schatzberg, 1998; Schneier, Johnson, Hornig, Liebowitz, & Weissman, 1992; Schneier, Martin, Liebowitz, Gorman, & Fyer, 1989), and there is a close association between anxiety and other psychiatric disorders in individuals with ASD with or without ID (Dekker & Kooth, 2003; Ghaziuddin, 2005; Helverschou et al., 2009; Kim, Szatmari, Bryson, Streiner, & Wilson, 2000; Lainhart, 1999; Matson et al., 2000; Matson, Gardner, Coe, & Sovner, 1991; Moss et al., 2000; Rutter, Tizard, Yule, Graham, & Whitmore, 1976). Furthermore, anxiety is strongly associated with depression and OCD in both Asperger syndrome and other clinical groups (Glenn et al., 2003).

Adjustment Problems and Psychiatric Disorders in ASD

ASD as a Developmental Risk Factor

A disability is defined as having problems in coping with the challenges of everyday life (WHO, 2001, 2007). A disability that is present from birth or the early months of life will most likely influence the formative development of a child, create adjustment challenges, and may, in addition to the direct effects of the disability, be regarded as a *developmental* risk (Martinsen & Tellevik, 2001). The magnitude of the risk varies for the different disabilities. Being born blind or losing one's sight in the first few months of life is an example of a very severe developmental risk, since more than 40% of these people have been reported as having severe developmental problems, most of them satisfying the criteria of ASD (Brandsborg, 1993). ASD is a *pervasive* developmental disorder, which means that it persistently affects central functions such as the ability to communicate and understand social interaction, and must be recognized as a more severe developmental risk than most other disabilities (Martinsen & Tellevik, 2001; Wing & Gould, 1979).

Adjustment Problems in ASD

The symptoms that characterize individuals with ASD are associated with a number of problems and considered general risk factors when they occur in the general population. Thus, the characteristics of ASD seem to imply a significant vulnerability for developing adjustment problems (Clarke et al., 1999; Lainhart, 1999). Most individuals with ASD have difficulties in social interaction and in understanding social rules and conventions, many have unusual interests, and, due to their communication and interpretation difficulties, many become confused about what is going to happen during the day. They often find the environment unpredictable and confusing, and the struggle of understanding other people's expectations frequently leads to cognitive overload. Negative reactions to novelty exacerbate the stress of everyday life. Each day they may be confronted with challenges they find difficult to cope with, and consequently, they may experience dramatic reactions to these challenges.

Many of the large number of problems linked with ASD may be regarded as stressors. The magnitude of stress problems was demonstrated in a study of children, adolescents, and adults with ASD ($N = 226$), mainly recruited from schools for pupils with ASD, where both biological and situational stressors were assessed (Martinsen & Hildebrand, in preparation). A factor analysis of biological stressors yielded a two-factor solution: named somatic stressors and sensitivity. The somatic stressors included digestive problems, fluctuations in regulation of biological functions, eating problems, sleeping problems, and frequent expressions of pain. The sensitivity factor included sensitivity to sensory stimulation and sensitivity to pain. Most of the persons with ASD showed problems with more than one of the variants of the two factors. About 80% had severe problems connected with at least one of the somatic stressors (factor I) and 74% with at least one of the variants of sensitivity (factor II). Overall, 82.9% had severe problems related to at least one of the biological stressors.

A factor analysis of situational stressors was also performed. Three factors were found and named "sameness," "social pressure," and "personal contact." Sameness, which included structure-dependent and negative reactions to novelty, was a serious problem for about 9%, and social pressure, which included being in the focus of other persons, pressure, nagging, and demands, was a serious problem for about 14%. The third factor, personal contact included negative reactions to adults and negative reactions to children and was a serious problem for about 18% of the participants. In all, one or more of the situational stressors was a serious problem for 31% of the group. The overlap between the stressors was very high: Approximately 83% had problems with at least one of the biological or situational stressors. Since the sample studied was not a representative sample, the percentages are not estimates of the prevalence of stressors; nevertheless, the findings demonstrate that there are high frequencies of biological and situational stressors in some groups of people with ASD that may create adjustment problems.

Adjustment problems were also assessed in a screening study in two representative samples of adolescents and adults with ASD and ID and with ID only (Bakken et al., 2010; Martinsen, Bakken, Helverschou, & von Tetzchner, 2008). Raters collected data on these problems using a four-point rating scale in which the four points were labeled no problem (1); minor problem (2); moderate problem (3); and severe problem (4). Table 5.1 displays the adjustment problems assessed in the ASD and ID group and ID-only group. In the two right-hand columns the percentage of participants with a severe adjustment, defined as an average score of 2.0 or greater, in the total samples is displayed for each problem. At the bottom of these two columns the total percentage of individuals in both groups identified as having severe adjustment problems is displayed.

The frequency of severe adjustment problems was higher for all problems in the ASD group than in the ID-only group. The average adjustment problems score was also higher in the ASD and ID group ($M = 2.1$), than in the ID-only group ($M = 1.7$) (t [192] $= 5.3$, $p < 0.0005$). This replicates other studies that have also shown higher rates of adjustment problems among individuals with ASD. The problems in question appear to be *general* adjustment problems as demonstrated in

Table 5.1 Adjustment problems in the ASD plus ID groups and in the ID-only group. Analysis based on data from Bakken et al. (2010)

Type of problem	Severe problems (%)[a]			
	Total samples		Individuals with severe adjustment problems[b]	
	ASD + ID (N = 62)	ID only (N = 132)	ASD + ID (N = 35)	ID only (N = 30)
Violent behavior	11.1	3.0	19	17
Breaking items	6.3	3.7	11	22
Self-injurious behavior	9.5	3.0	17	17
Passivity	12.7	9.0	19	22
Lack of initiative	31.7	16.4	39	48
Restlessness	15.9	6.0	28	35
Irritability**	30.2	6.7	50	26
Withdrawal (avoiding social settings)	15.9	6.7	28	26
Obsessed with confirmation	41.3	17.9	58	44
Rituals and compulsive behavior**	11.1	1.5	19	0
Sleep problems	9.5	5.2	14	13
Complaints about pain**	6.3	6.0	3	22
Total with severe adjustment problems	57.1	17.2	–	–

** = $p < 0.05$, t-test, two-tailed.
[a]Severe problems = percentage of participants with scores of 2.0 or greater.
[b]Participants with scores above the defined pathological cutoff = average score of 2.0 or greater on all problems, named severe adjustment problems.

the two columns to the left in Table 5.1. This table displays the percentage of each problem among the participants who were identified as having severe adjustment problems.

The table illustrates that problems were not consistently higher in the ASD and ID than in the ID-only group. The group showing the highest frequency varied with the problem in question. There were only three significant group differences: The ASD and ID group was more irritable and showed more rituals and compulsive behavior than the ID-only group, while the ID-only group complained more about pain; however, these differences may reflect ASD

characteristics. Rituals and compulsive behavior are a defining criterion of ASD, and irritability may reflect anxiousness, which has been regarded as an ASD characteristic since the earliest descriptions of autism (Kanner, 1943, 1944). The relative lack of complaints about pain might reflect a low expression of pain among individuals with ASD and difficulties other people have in reading cues about pain in people with ASD.

Adjustment Problems and Psychiatric Disorders

It is well established that the presence of adjustment problems is linked to having a psychiatric disorder. According to the World Health Organization (2001) and the American Psychiatric Association (2000), a psychological or behavioral condition or disorder is only a psychiatric disorder when it causes a significant degree of distress and impairment of the person's performance of everyday activities or suffering or significant loss of freedom. Thus, in clinical practice, the diagnosis of a psychiatric order is contingent on a person having distress, impairment or suffering, etc. Individuals who master their everyday challenges do not meet the criteria for a psychiatric disorder, even if they show some psychiatric symptoms and appear uncomfortable. Adjustment problems are found in people of average intelligence with a psychiatric disorder (Gelder et al., 2003) and in people with an ID who become mentally ill (Gustafsson & Sonnander, 2004, 2005). Adjustment problems are typically associated with most psychiatric disorders in individuals with ID (Reiss, 1988), and indicators of general adjustment problems may be necessary to identify anxiety and other psychiatric problems in individuals with ASD (Ghaziuddin, 2005; Lainhart, 1999; Stavrakiki, 1999).

In the pilot study and the first validation of the psychopathology in autism checklist (Helverschou et al., 2009), psychiatric disorders and adjustment problems were related. The scores of adults with ASD and ID previously identified as having co-occurring psychosis, depression, anxiety, or OCD were compared with the scores of adults with ASD and ID without psychiatric diagnoses. The adults with ASD and co-occurring psychiatric disorders have significantly higher average scores than the autism-only group on general adjustment problems (robust rank-order test, one-tailed probabilities: psychosis $\alpha = 81$, $p < 0.01$; depression $\alpha = 45$, $p < 0.01$; anxiety disorder $\alpha = 3.00$, $p < 0.025$; OCD $\alpha = 3$, $p < 0.025$). The scores of the psychiatric subgroups were approximately twice as high as the adults with ASD without an additional psychiatric diagnosis. All adults in the autism-only group obtained a score of less than the subsequently defined pathological cutoff value. Thus, a high prevalence of severe adjustment problems was found in the group with co-occurring psychiatric disorders, while no severe adjustment problems were found in the autism-only group. These findings were replicated in a screening study of the whole population of adolescents and adults with autism and ID in Norway's Nordland County (Bakken et al., 2010) and only approximately 3% were identified as having severe adjustment problems without concurrent psychiatric problems. Furthermore, adjustment problems were highly correlated with psychosis, depression, anxiety, and OCD disorder scores.

Anxiety and Autism Spectrum Disorders

Anxiousness is a continuum from calm, to insecurity, via anxiousness and restlessness, to anxiety and panic. Anxiousness is characterized by weaker reactions than anxiety; includes shyness, embarrassment, and inhibition; and is a reaction most people experience (Crozier & Alden, 2001). The prevalence of social anxiousness is between 50 and 60%. Surveys suggest an increase in the incidence (Crozier & Alden, 2001). Anxiety disorders are among the most common psychiatric disorders, with lifetime incidence estimates in the USA of approximately 30% among women and approximately 20% among men (Kessler et al., 1994). Because of the differences in severity and frequency, it is important to distinguish anxiousness from anxiety disorders.

Both fear and anxiety are characterized by bodily preparedness and physiological arousal. What differentiates between the conditions is whether the reactions are linked to a known object or not. When people experience fear, they know what they are afraid of whereas anxiety is characterized by an arousal the individual is unable to explain (Martinsen, Laneskog, & Duckert, 1979).

The symptoms of anxiety fall into two main categories: cognitive and somatic (Doctor, Kahn, & Adamec, 2008; ICD-10; DSM-IV). Somatic symptoms are signs of physiological arousal, and subjective and emotional feelings of uneasiness and discomfort are the cognitive aspect of anxiety (Norwegian Board of Health Supervision, 2000). Somatic symptoms, such as hyperventilation, sweating, and shivering, are relatively easy to recognize by an observer (Doctor et al., 2008); however, the only true measure of cognitive anxiety, such as personal distress and worry, is the person's own report of feelings of uneasiness and discomfort.

In typically developing children there seems to be an interaction between biologically rooted early temperament and their interaction with their social environment, which presages later anxiousness and anxiety problems (Alden, 2001). Some children seem to have an inborn vulnerability for developing anxiousness and anxiety (Kagan & Snidman, 2004; Kagan, 1994). According to Kagan (1998), fearfulness and shyness are included in the broader temperament category of behavioral inhibition, and an inhibited temperament is vulnerability for developing anxiety problems. Inhibited children tend to develop social anxiety and other anxiety disorders later in life more often than other children (Hirschfeldt et al., 1992; Kagan & Snidman, 2004; Kagan, 1998; Turner, Beidel, & Wolff, 1996).

Anxiety in Children and Adults with Autism Spectrum Disorder

Anxiety disorders in people with ASD may be unrecognized or mislabeled (Lainhart, 1999; MacNeil et al., 2009; Tsai, 2006). For example, distress and panic attacks are sometimes interpreted as behavioral problems and/or as related to autism (Tsai, 2006). On the other hand, common ASD behavior such as verbal rituals, abnormal communication, or frequent and repetitive questioning may be interpreted as signs of anxiety (Ghaziuddin et al., 1995). Helverschou, Bakken and Martinsen (2008) illustrated the difficulty of differentiating between symptoms of autism and of anxiety. They used a panel of clinicians to investigate which symptoms clinicians use to discriminate between autism and four major psychiatric disorders – psychosis, depression, anxiety disorder, and OCD. The result was a set of symptoms rated as specific to a psychiatric disorder and not characteristic of autism. Of the four disorders examined, anxiety disorder obtained the lowest scores and the lowest degree of agreement among the raters. Thus, even experienced clinicians seem uncertain of whether symptoms are characteristics of anxiety or of ASD, illustrating the difficulty of differentiating between the two disorders (Lainhart, 1999; MacNeil et al., 2009; Tsai, 2006). Nevertheless, these results demonstrated the possibility of differentiating between the symptoms of the two disorders and to identify indicators of anxiety and other psychiatric disorders that do not overlap with autism. The results support an interpretation of anxiety as a separate disorder from autism (Bellini, 2006; Ghaziuddin, 2005; Gillott & Stranden, 2007; Goldstein et al., 1994; Lainhart, 1999; Morgan, 2006; Steingard, Zimnitzky, DeMaso, Bauman, & Bucci, 1997).

Nervousness and anxiety symptoms were included in the earliest descriptions of autism. Kanner (1943/1968) described how anxiety related to changes in routines or furniture arrangements was "an anxiously obsessive desire for the maintenance of sameness" (p. 130) and that panic attacks could be the consequences of such changes. Anxiety and ASD seem to be intertwined to such a degree that it has been suggested that anxiety is an integral component of autism (Weisbrot, Gadow, DeVincent, & Pomeroy, 2005). Some have argued that generalized anxiety is so common in individuals with ASD that it should not be diagnosed as a separate disorder (Bellini, 2006; Ghaziuddin, 2005; Gillott & Stranden, 2007; Goldstein et al., 1994; Lainhart, 1999; Morgan, 2006; Steingard et al., 1997), despite the fact that anxiety symptoms are not included in the symptoms that define autism.

The high prevalence of anxiety symptoms and disorders reported in the last decade may have contributed to a growing awareness of the presence of anxiety in individuals with ASD (Green, Gilchrist, Burton, & Cox, 2000; Lainhart, 1999; Luscre & Center, 1996; Matson & Nebel-Schwalm, 2007; Schopler & Mesibov, 1994; Tantam, 2000). A review of 13 studies on anxiety in ASD conducted between 1995 and 2008 (MacNeil et al., 2009) suggested that children and adolescents with ASD show higher levels of anxiety than typical community samples. Comparisons with clinically anxious groups have demonstrated similar levels of anxiety, while higher levels have been demonstrated in people with ASD than in people with conduct or language disorders, and different patterns of anxiety have been demonstrated in samples with Down syndrome and people with ID without ASD (Evans, Canavera, Kleinpeter, Maccubbin, & Taga, 2005; Gillott, Furniss, & Walter, 2001; Green et al., 2000). Reports of such high prevalence emphasize the importance for the conceptualization and treatment of these individuals of identifying anxiety problems in addition to the diagnosis of ASD (Gillott et al., 2001; Green et al., 2000; Kim et al., 2000; Luscre & Center, 1996; MacNeil et al., 2009; Matson & Nebel-Schwalm, 2007; White, Oswald, Ollendick, & Schahill, 2009).

Comparisons across ASD subtypes have yielded conflicting results. Most studies suggest that cognitively more able children and adolescents with Asperger syndrome and pervasive developmental disorder not otherwise specified (PDD-NOS) may experience more anxiety symptoms than individuals with autistic disorder and ID (Gillott et al., 2001; Kim et al., 2000; MacNeil et al., 2009; Sukhodolsky et al., 2008). These findings may indicate that anxiety problems are related to cognitive ability and ASD subgroup (White et al., 2009); however, the special difficulties encountered when identifying anxiety in individuals with ASD and ID (Green et al., 2000; Lainhart, 1999; Luscre & Center, 1996; Matson & Nebel-Schwalm, 2007; Schopler & Mesibov, 1994; Tantam, 2000) may have resulted in failure to recognize anxiety and under-reporting in individuals with more severe cognitive impairments. In particular, it is difficult to recognize the cognitive aspect of anxiety in individuals who are not able to report on their feelings of uneasiness, worry, and discomfort. In individuals with ASD and ID, physiological arousal may not be as readily observable as previously assumed (Helverschou & Martinsen, 2011) and there is a lack of methods for assessing anxiety in people with ASD (MacNeil et al., 2009). Thus, these two factors may explain why fears, phobias, and anxiety among people with ASD have been ignored in the literature (Green et al., 2000; Lainhart, 1999; Luscre & Center, 1996; Matson & Nebel-Schwalm, 2007; Schopler & Mesibov, 1994; Tantam, 2000).

Common Characteristics of Anxiety and Autism Spectrum Disorders

Diagnostic overshadowing refers to the tendency to attribute psychiatric symptoms, such as anxiety, to ASD rather than the psychiatric disorder (Lainhart, 1999; MacNeil et al., 2009; Tsai, 2006). As Table 5.2 demonstrates, this may be a common problem with people with ASD. Table 5.2 includes problems frequently reported in anxious children (Evans, 2001) with our clinical experience of typical reactions in individuals with ASD and with typical reactions in individuals with ASD who additionally have a psychiatric disorder. The resemblance between problems reported in anxious, typically developing children and individuals with ASD is striking, showing that similar problems occur in both groups. This resemblance to anxious children may indicate sub-clinical anxiety problems leveling people with ASD, and perhaps reflects their special vulnerability to anxiety problems (Gillott & Stranden, 2007). In contrast, individuals with ASD and co-occurring psychiatric disorders have similar but more frequent problems, which may reflect the fact that anxiety is a problem in their everyday life. This is consistent with the moderate levels of anxiety demonstrated in many individuals with ASD, ID, and co-occurring psychosis, depression, or OCD (Helverschou et al., 2009). Thus, anxiety does not seem to be an intrinsic feature of autism (Bellini, 2006; Helverschou et al., 2008; Lainhart, 1999), but is more likely to be a problem for those individuals with combined ASD and mental health problems (Bakken et al., 2010; Ghaziuddin, 2005; Gillott & Stranden, 2007; Goldstein et al., 1994; Steingard et al., 1997).

Anxiety as a Reaction to Everyday Challenges in ASD Individuals

Individuals with ASD seem especially vulnerable to developing anxiety, which may be related to life problems associated with ASD (Gillott & Stranden, 2007). The cognitive comprehension difficulties that characterize individuals with ASD may lead to confusion and coping difficulties: Their negative reactions to environmental change often result in bodily preparedness and distress, and difficulties in arousal regulation may lead to a reduced capacity for coping with stress (Bellini, 2006; Goldstein et al., 1994; Steingard et al., 1997). Thus, most of the problems that characterize autism, such as difficulties in communication, comprehension, and social interaction, are biologically rooted and influence their interplay with the environment and represent vulnerability factors. In addition, poor social skills, misunderstandings, confusion, and insecurity concerning their own achievements may make children with ASD more vulnerable to anxiousness and anxiety (Bellini, 2006; Bruch, 2001;

Table 5.2 Problems in anxious non-ASD children, typical reactions in children and adults with ASD, and typical reactions in ASD individuals with psychiatric comorbidity

Problems/symptoms	Anxious typical children*	Children and adults with ASD**	Children and adults with ASD + psych. comorbidity**
Sleeping problems	++	+	++
Problems with separation	++	+	++
Insecurity	+	+	++
Anxiousness with strangers	+	+	++
Shyness in interplay with peers	+	+	++
Mainly alone in activities	+	+	++
Answers questions "don't know"	+	+	++
Observers to others	+	+	++
Do not ask for help, not even when in pain	+	+	++
Do not interrupt others	+	+	++
Dislike being in focus	+	+	++
Negative reactions to novelty	+	+	++
Temper tantrums when change in routines	+	++	++
Resistance to new activities or clothes	+	++	++
Dressing in fixed order	+	++	++
Dislike of loud noises	+	++	++
Complains about noisy peers	+	+	++
Sensitive about food	+	+	++
Prefers order and rules	+	++	++
Strong sense of morals	+	++	++
Negative reactions to events experienced as positive by others	+	+	++

Rating scale: + occurs, ++ occurs in at least 50% of the individuals.
*Ratings based on interviews with parents about their everyday experiences with their anxious children (Warnke & Evans, as cited in Evans, 2001).
**Ratings based on the authors' broad clinical experience.

Gillott & Stranden, 2007; Goldstein et al., 1994; Steingard et al., 1997). It is likely that children with ASD, who have an inhibited temperament, as well as those who react strongly to novelty and have particular difficulty with arousal regulation, are especially at risk of developing anxiety problems.

Some of the features that characterize ASD, such as rituals and repetitive behavior, have also been regarded as related to anxiety or as strategies for coping with anxiety, since such behaviors may function to reduce anxiety or regulate arousal (Ghaziuddin et al., 1995; Howlin, 1997). Thus, anxiety in individuals with ASD has been interpreted as an effect of having ASD as well as causing some of the characteristics of autism (Ghaziuddin et al., 1995; Gillott et al., 2001; Howlin, 1997). Moreover, treatment procedures typically recommended for individuals with ASD, such as the creation of structure and predictability, include strategies similar to those recommended for preventing and reducing anxiety (Helverschou, 2006).

Obsessions and Compulsions in People with Autism Spectrum Disorders

In the general population, there seems to be a continuous distribution of obsessiveness, with no obvious break between a normal and a pathological condition. Between 80 and 99% of people sometimes experience unwanted thoughts (Niehous & Stein, 1997) and about 15% have periods of obsessive thoughts and compulsive behavior resembling OCD, but not in a very troublesome way. The prevalence of OCD is approximately 1.6% with a lifetime incidence of approximately 2.5% (Karno, Goldin, Sorenson, & Burnam, 1988; Osborn, 1998; Rasmussen & Eisen, 1998), but estimates differ depending on the diagnostic criteria used (Stein, 2002). A distinguishing feature of OCD is to experience distress and discomfort while having obsessive thoughts or compulsive behavior as those thoughts or compulsions are egodystonic. It is also a diagnostic requirement that the individuals themselves have recognized that the obsessions or compulsions cause distress; however, young children are exempt from this requirement, and McDougle et al. (2000) argue that this criterion should also be waived for individuals with ID. Rapoport, Swedo, and Leonard's (1992) study of children with OCD found that compulsions were more frequent than obsessions, and that *pure* obsessives were much less frequent than *pure* compulsives, whereas compulsions are readily observable behavior, obsessions imply an awareness of and ability to describe intrusive thoughts and ideas.

Repetitive Thoughts and Behavior in Autism Spectrum Disorders

When Kanner (1943, 1944) used "obsessive insistence of sameness" as a cardinal symptom of autism he listed uncommon interests, negative reactions to novelty, such as changes in daily routines and in the physical environment and repetition of words, sentences. and questions. Notably, he also listed lack of flexibility in the performance of activities and with respect to what is right and wrong. Since then, obsessiveness and inflexibility have colored the view of ASD and have been included in the diagnostic criteria (APA, 1994, 2000; WHO, 1992, 1993). Repetitive behavior, which is common in people with ASD, includes ritualistic movements, performing activities in a similar, fixed way, arranging objects in patterns, moving furniture and objects back to where they were before being moved by others, and eating and going to bed rituals. Stereotyped movements such as bizarre posturing, weaving, grimacing, head banging, waving of fingers and hands, flicking the fingers before the eyes, touching or stroking parts of the body, body-rocking, twirling, eye-poking, and self-injurious behavior (SIB) are also often included in descriptions of repetitive behavior among persons with ASD (Hoder & Cohen, 1983; Rumsey et al., 1985).

It is usually important to individuals with ASD that the environment is arranged in a particular way. Some people with ASD arrange toys and other objects in patterns and sort them according to attributes such as size and color instead of using them as others do. For some, this is linked with very strong affect, and they may become disturbed and agitated if, for example, a window hasp is not closed in the correct way. Most people with ASD are also strongly interested in what is going to happen in the course of the day and in the near future and may repeatedly ask about what they are about to do. For some people with ASD it may be very important that familiar activities occur in a fixed order, in a similar way, and that they are performed at the same place as they usually are. Some people with ASD are also very concerned with who their companions will be, what they and each of their companions will do together; some children with ASD want to do specific things with one particular companion and other things with others. Various terms have been used to describe these phenomena (McDougle et al., 2000). This is sometimes referred to as "maintenance of sameness" and "resistance to change" (McDougle, 1998; McDougle, Kresch, Goodman, & Naylor, 1995).

There are two main problems with using repetitive thought and behavior as part of the definition of ASD. First, it is necessary to infer the presence of obsessions from how persons with ASD act and communicate. Second, repetitive behavior is frequently also shown by typical infants (Thelen, 1979), by many people with ID without ASD (Baumeister & Forehand, 1972) and by people with visual impairments (Martinsen, 1977) and thus may not necessarily indicate the presence of obsessions.

Comparison of ASD and OCD

ASD and OCD overlap since ritualistic and repetitive behaviors are core symptoms of both ASD and defining criteria of OCD (Ghaziuddin, 2005; Scahill et al., 2006); thus, it is difficult to diagnose OCD in individuals with ASD using unmodified ICD (WHO, 1993) or DSM criteria (APA, 1994, 2000). Some individuals with ASD will be incorrectly diagnosed with OCD whereas in other cases a diagnosis of OCD will be missed if the clinician strictly applies the criterion of the individual having insight into his/her obsessive thoughts or compulsive behavior.

Nevertheless, the compulsion-driven quality that characterizes OCD goes beyond the core features of autism (Ghaziuddin, 2005; Lainhart, 1999; Scahill et al., 2006). In general, the experiences of the individual make it possible to differentiate between compulsive behavior in OCD and ritualistic behavior in ASD. Typical ritualistic behavior among individuals with, for example, Asperger syndrome is not unwanted and linked with distress, and in most cases is coherently argued for by the person (Ghaziuddin, 2005; Szatmari, 1991). Thus, the compulsions associated with ASD do not seem to occur against the person's will, in contrast to uncontrollable and unpleasant compulsions associated with OCD (Scahill et al., 2006). In our experience, individuals with Asperger syndrome and OCD are greatly discomforted by their obsessions and compulsions, and they typically want to hide their symptoms and seek help to get rid of them. It is the use of the criterion of being "compelled" to perform compulsive acts, and "to do things against their own will" that distinguishes individuals who additionally have OCD from the majority of individuals with ASD (Ghaziuddin, 2005; Lainhart, 1999; Scahill et al., 2006).

Thus, despite the difficulties in diagnosing OCD in people with ASD, specialists in the field of autism should be able to recognize individuals who differ from most people with ASD by being significantly more obsessive and compulsive and who seem to perform the compulsions against their own will. One example is a young man with autism and ID who was so obsessed with naked female shoulders that once he was unable to stop looking at the shoulder of a woman sitting next to him, although he urgently needed to urinate. When the young man cried in pain, and a bystander covered the shoulder with a handkerchief, he ran sobbing to the toilet. Repetitive routines and rituals are frequent in ASD (Kobayashi & Murata, 1998), and often identical to those seen in OCD (Bejerot, 2007), but the behavior pattern seems to differ in some respects. In ASD, some types of behavior seem to occur more often and others more seldom. A study by McDougle and colleagues (1995) investigated repetitive thoughts and behavior in adults with ASD compared with adults with OCD. Fifty patients between the ages of 18 and 53 with a diagnosis of ASD and 50 patients with OCD, who were matched on age and sex, were compared. In the ASD group, 35 had ID and 15 of them did not speak. A somewhat altered version of the Yale-Brown Compulsive Scale Symptom Checklist (Y-BOCS SCL) (Goodman, Price, Rasmussen, Mazure, Fleichman, et al., 1989; Goodman, Price, Rasmussen, Mazure, Delgado, et al., 1989) was used. The diagnostic criterion of insight for OCD was disregarded. The McDougle group concluded that the findings indicated that adults with ASD and OCD might be distinguished from those with OCD only based on their types of repetitive thoughts and behavior. Compared with the OCD group, the patients with ASD were significantly less likely to have aggressive, contamination, sexual, religious, symmetry, and somatic thoughts. Repetitive ordering, hoarding, touching, tapping, or rubbing, and self-damaging or self-mutilating behaviors were reported significantly more often in the patients with ASD, whereas cleaning, checking, and counting behaviors were less frequent in the group with ASD compared with the patients with OCD.

Bejerot, Nylander and Lindstrøm (2001) described autistic traits among 64 patients with OCD and identified three of them as having Asperger syndrome. In a later paper, Bejerot (2007) suggested that OCD is related to ASD and summarized her postulated differences between "pure OCD" and "OCD with autistic traits." Table 5.3 builds on the findings of the McDougle group (1995) and the proposals of Bejerot (2007) and illustrates the differences in symptomatology between individuals with OCD and ASD.

The McDougle group's data illustrate that "touching" and "ordering," and to a lesser degree, "repeating," "need to know," and "self-damaging" are more frequent in individuals with ASD, while "aggressive," "contamination," "sexual," "cleaning," "checking," and "need to tell or ask" are the most prevalent in OCD. The group differences in "contamination," "touching," and "self-damaging" are confirmed by Bejerot's proposals. In contrast to McDougle and colleagues, however, Bejerot proposed that "hoarding" is most often found among persons with OCD, while "symmetry" and "counting" characterize persons who have autistic traits. Thus, the characteristics that distinguish ASD from OCD in Table 5.3 also seem to be in line with clinical knowledge about typical autistic behavior.

Dimensions of Obsessive and Compulsive Behavior in ASD

In a study of a large group of children, adolescents, and adults with ASD, mainly recruited from schools for pupils with

Table 5.3 Repetitive thoughts and behavior in ASD and OCD

	After McDougle et al. (1995)		After Bejerot (2007)	
	ASD	OCD	OCD + autistic traits	OCD
Repetitive thoughts				
Aggressive	+	+++		
Contamination	++	+++	+	++
Sexual	–	+	–	–
Religious	–	+		
Symmetry	–	++	+++	+
Somatic	–	+		
Need to know	++	+		
Repetitive behavior				
Cleaning	++	+++		
Checking	+	++		
Repeating	+++	++		
Counting	–	+	+++	+
Hoarding	++	++	+	++
Ordering	+++	+		
Need to tell or ask	+	++		
Touching	+++	–	+++	++
Self-damaging	+	–	++	–

In Bejerot: – rarely present, + present to a limited extent, ++ often present, +++ very often present.
In McDougle et al.: – present in <10%, + present in 11–30%, ++ present in 31–50, +++ present in >50.

ASD (Martinsen et al., in preparation), 20 items assessing obsessive and compulsive behavior were included in a factor analysis. The analysis gave a five-factor solution. The factors and measures with high factor loads on the five-factor measures are shown in Table 5.4.

The first three factors are behavior that usually occurs in individuals with ASD and related to "obsessive insistence on sameness." The most interesting point is that they are divided into three different factors. The fourth factor is related to the first three, but reflects more obsessiveness. The importance of performing activities correctly may be recognized in clinical descriptions of Asperger syndrome, related to "doing right," with a focus on justice and fairness by the most literal individuals, but is not usually emphasized as different from the first three factors. Only the fifth factor resembles OCD.

Depression in People with Autism Spectrum Disorder

Persons with ASD are prone to depressive episodes, especially after puberty. Clinic-based studies suggest that depression is the most common psychiatric disorder in persons with ASD during their life span. A recent study gave a lifetime rate

Table 5.4 Dimensions of obsessive and compulsive behavior

Factor	Measure	LOADS
I. Importance of familiar situational structure	Important that activities have fixed locations	0.806
	Dependent on environment being arranged in a particular way to perform an activity	0.682
	Important that objects have fixed locations	0.649
	Negative reactions to change of routines	0.646
	Negative reactions to unstructured situations	0.625
	Negative reactions when the order of daily activities is changed	0.520
II. Concern about the structure of daily activities	Concerned about what is going to happen during the day	0.901
	Concerned about what he himself is going to do during the day	0.884
	Concerned about who he is going to be together with during the day	0.866
III. Negative reactions to newness	Negative reactions to new places	0.768
	Negative reactions to unknown individuals	0.756
	Negative reactions to new objects	0.631
	Negative reactions to new activities	0.622
IV. Importance of correct performance of activities	Dependent on starting an activity in the same way every time it is performed	0.719
	Negative reactions when the activities in a particular situation are changed	0.660
	Dependent on former activity being correctly ended in order to perform a new activity	0.634
	Difficulty in starting an activity before the surroundings are "correctly" arranged	0.573
V. Self-disruption	Disrupts himself to perform an act or movement which is not a part of the activity	0.838
	Disrupts himself to repeat parts of the activity several times	0.763
	Disrupts himself before finishing some activity which he is motivated to perform	0.711

of 53% for mood disorders in consecutively recruited adults with ASD (Hofvander et al., 2009). Compared to community matched children, high-functioning children with autism or Asperger's syndrome (AS) (IQ > 70) may have higher rates of anxiety and mood conditions, which often occur together (Kim et al., 2000). Previous estimates of comorbid depression in ASD ranged from 4 to 38% (Lainhart, 1999). When DSM-IV criteria for major depressive disorder were utilized, Leyfer and colleagues found a rate of 10% in children with autism using a modified Kiddie Schedule for Affective Disorders and Schizophrenia (Leyfer et al., 2006); the rate was 20% in a cross-sectional study of adolescents and young adults with Asperger's syndrome (Shtayermman, 2007); however, most reports are derived from small, clinical samples that are often seen in tertiary care centers. Large-scale epidemiologic studies have not been done.

Core Symptoms

In contrast to transient states of depressed mood, depression is a distinct medical condition characterized by a combination of psychological and physical symptoms. These consist of persistently depressed mood, loss of interest in pleasurable activities, a tendency to focus on negative aspects of life, excessive preoccupation with sad themes, and recurrent thoughts of self-harm and death. Other features include problems with attention and concentration, distractibility, impairment of short-term memory, and self-blame and ruminations of guilt. From a social point of view, depressed patients tend to isolate themselves, often do not interact with others, and have difficulties with relationships and employment. Severe cases may lead to suicidal attempts.

Table 5.5 Symptoms of depression in ASD

	Number of cases
Core symptoms of depression	
Depressed mood	13
Diminished interest or pleasure in almost all activities	7
Significant weight loss or gain, or change in appetite	9
Insomnia/hypersomnia	11
Psychomotor agitation/retardation	2
Fatigue or loss of energy	1
Feelings of worthlessness, or excessive or inappropriate guilt	1
Diminished ability to think/concentrate or indecisiveness	2
Recurrent thoughts of death, suicidal ideation, suicidal attempt, or plan	2
Symptoms associated with depression	
Decrease in self-care	4
Decrease/regression in speech	2
New onset/exacerbation of maladaptive behavior like self-injury or aggression	8
Increase in stereotypes	1

Based on a review of 15 case studies by Stewart et al. (2006).
Number of cases = number of cases where this symptom was described in the published study.

In persons with ASD the presentation of depression depends mainly on the level of cognitive functioning. In those individuals who are lower functioning, the main features consist of a change in behavior, such as regression of skills, weight loss, and mutism. In those who are higher functioning, that is, individuals who have relatively good language, the clinical features are the same as those in depressed persons in the general population. Anhedonia is often present. Stewart and colleagues (2006) reviewed the presentation of depression in 15 case studies in ASD. The results are presented in Table 5.5. They found that depressed mood was reported by subject report or observation in 13 of 15 cases and that loss of interest was mentioned as a prominent feature in 7 of the 15 reports. In addition, in persons with ASD certain special features are associated with depression. These often consist of an increase in or new onset of maladaptive behavior like self-injury or aggression, in 8 of the 15 case reports, decrease in self-care or speech, or a change in the tone and flavor of autistic preoccupations, such as the patient previously obsessed with meterology who lost interest when he became depressed (Gillberg, 1985).

Identification of Depression in ASD

There are no universally recognized scales to assess for depression in this population (Stewart et al., 2006). Communication difficulties in many individuals with ASD limit the ability to ascertain an internal mood state by self-report (Skokauskas & Gallagher, 2010). While verbally intact patients may be reliably diagnosed with a comorbid mood condition, clinicians may be reluctant to diagnose mood disorders in individuals with greater communication impairment. Due to the inherent challenges in diagnosing comorbid affective conditions, treatment may be delayed for years despite frequent medical evaluations and visits. Depression can impair family activities and relationships (Kim et al., 2000). The development of catatonia, a potentially life-threatening condition, may be attributable to life events or depression (Wing, 2000). As such, a high index of suspicion for depression is advised and, if found, can have considerable prognostic implication.

To sum up, depression frequently occurs in ASD. Several factors may contribute to the occurrence of depression in ASD. Excessive negative life events may precede depression similar to that seen in the general population (Ghaziuddin et al., 1995). In general, two types of stressors seem to contribute to the emergence of depressive symptoms: exposure to general life events (that is, events that are common to all and that are known to be associated with depression, such as bereavement and parental divorce, and exposure to specific life events, that is, life events that are unique to people with ASD, such as change of schools, problems with dating, and socializing). Associated medical conditions, such as seizure disorder, increase the risk of all forms of psychopathology in persons with ASD, including depression. Genetic factors may also account for the occurrence of depression in persons with ASD. For example, depressed children with ASD are more likely to have parents with depression (Lainhart, 1999; Mazefsky, Folstein, & Lainhart, 2008).

Schizophrenia and ASD

Psychotic patients live in a splintered and chaotic world. They may be disorganized and socially withdrawn. Having audible thoughts, hearing voices commenting on or discussing them, thought withdrawal, delusions about their thoughts being broadcast, experiences of their body being influenced by external forces, and delusional perception have traditionally been regarded as first-rank symptoms of schizophrenia (Schneider, 1950). These, together with additional negative symptoms, constitute the criteria for schizophrenia. The course of the illness is characterized by remissions and relapses, and schizophrenia usually has a more chronic course than other psychotic disorders (Gelder,

Harrison, & Cowen, 2006). Like other people, individuals with ASD may become psychotic.

The characteristics of schizophrenia and ASD resemble each other. *No close friends or confidants, odd, eccentric, or curious behavior or speech, inappropriate or constricted affect* are among features that have been used to screen for schizophrenia among adolescents (Diforio, Walker, & Kestler, 2000). These are criteria that also may fit well with a diagnosis of PDD-NOS or even Asperger syndrome, in children and adults alike (Nylander, Lugnegård, & Hallerback, 2008). Generally, the characteristics of their language and communication make it difficult to employ the usual criteria for assessing a schizophrenic disorder in individuals with ASD, even in those with an IQ within the average range.

The age of onset and developmental course differ between schizophrenia and ASD. ASD is present from birth in most cases, and it was made clear early on, that autism present from birth did not later develop into psychosis (Eisenberg & Kanner, 1956; Eisenberg, 1956; Kanner, Rodriguez, & Ashenden, 1972; Lotter, 1974); however, a distinction was made between autism with onset in the first 2 years of life and so-called childhood psychosis, with an onset after 30 months of life. Later it was argued that the two categories did not differ clearly in appearance or prognosis (DeMyer et al., 1973; Rutter, 1970), and childhood psychosis was incorporated into childhood autism. In DSM-III (APA, 1980), infantile autism was defined as a pervasive developmental disorder with an early onset and an absence of hallucinations, delusions, and incoherence.

Psychosis with clearly recognizable primary symptoms of schizophrenia is typically shown from adolescence, but also occurs, though infrequently, in childhood. Very early onset schizophrenia (VEOS) is defined as having an onset before the age of 11. Thus, a gradual unfolding of deterioration, beginning in infancy, is reported (Watkins, Asarnow, & Tanguay, 1988). Immature language development makes it difficult or impossible to diagnose positive symptoms of schizophrenia in young children less than 5 years of age or in adults with severe ID (Werry, 1992).

There are several reasons that schizophrenia may be both under- and over-diagnosed in people with ASD: Schizophrenia may not be recognized because the symptoms are interpreted as autistic characteristics. The person may lack language skills. Pre-morbid signs of VEOS or schizophrenia may not recognized. Symptoms are wrongly perceived as age-typical understanding and use of language in young children; symptoms of schizophrenia are wrongly attributed to signs of another psychiatric disorder. An incorrect diagnosis of schizophrenia is made because autistic characteristics are wrongly perceived to be schizophrenia symptoms, because pre-morbid signs of schizophrenia are wrongly believed to be present or because VEOS is wrongly diagnosed. Finally, an incorrect diagnosis of schizophrenia is

made because age-typical understanding and use of language in young children are interpreted as symptoms of schizophrenia. Thus, there are many reasons why schizophrenia may be misdiagnosed in people with ASD.

Core Symptoms

Schizophrenia is currently referred to as a multi-dimensional disorder that includes at least three symptom dimensions: positive, negative, and disorganization (Breier & Berg, 1999; Lenzenweger & Dworkin, 1996). This is the most common and accepted view in the field, but there are still discussions about the definitions of the diagnosis of schizophrenia (Deutsch & Davis, 1983; van Os & Kaour, 2009). Although patients with schizophrenia share some common core features, a central point to the discussion is that they are extremely different from each other with respect to the type and intensity of symptoms, duration of episodes, and number of relapses (Bentall, 2003). The three dimensions of schizophrenia include the core symptoms of delusions, hallucinations, disorganized speech (formal thought disorder), disorganized behavior, and negative symptoms. Besides core symptoms, a decline in global functioning, including self-care, task solving, and maintenance of relationships, is also used as a criterion when diagnosing schizophrenia (APA, 1994).

Positive schizophrenia symptoms, delusions and hallucinations, will for the most part not be reported from individuals with ASD who also have significantly below average intelligence. More cognitively able individuals with Asperger syndrome or PDD-NOS are able to report such experiences, but their idiosyncratic language, ideas, and behavior may regularly be misinterpreted as delusions. In people with ASD who also have significantly below average intellectually lower functioning, one may expect some sort of altered behavior indicating auditory hallucinations (Bakken, Friis, Lovoll, Smeby, & Martinsen, 2007; Hurley, 1996). In patients with ASD and moderate, severe, or profound ID, psychotic hallucinatory or delusional symptoms will usually remain undetected, even if the patients display hallucinatory behavior like staring at fixed points and covering their ears while screaming (Bakken et al., 2007).

Whether disorganization is really a manifestation of thought disorder or whether disorganized speech can be regarded as a speech disorder has been discussed; however, patients with disordered speech also show distorted responses to reality testing, strange non-verbal behavior, and distorted thinking (Harrow et al., 2003). Such results are consistent with earlier assumptions of disordered speech as a manifestation of thought disorder. Since Kraeplin and Bleuler, strange behavior and bizarre motor activity has been associated with schizophrenia (Bentall, 2003). The strange and altered behavior displayed by persons with schizophrenia has not been examined to the same degree as their speech (Breier & Berg, 1999; Flaum & Schultz, 1996).

Disorganization, in both speech and behavior, may be identified in individuals with ASD and ID; however, disorganized speech will be observable only in patients with a minimal amount of verbal skills. Because disorganized behavior is observable and can therefore be used when diagnosing possible psychosis in individuals who talk only to a limited amount, it is important to demonstrate its link to thought disorder, which is considered a core symptom of schizophrenia (Andreasen, 1979; Flaum & Schultz, 1996; Kerns & Berenbaum, 2002). Both people with ASD and people with schizophrenia will show features of thought disorder, but adults with schizophrenia will tend to show more incoherent speech, pressure of speech, and derailment, whereas adults with ASD will exhibit more impoverished speech, deviant responses, and inappropriate thinking (Konstantareas & Hewitt, 2001; O'Dwyer, 2000; Rumsey, Andreasen, & Rapoport, 1986).

Negative symptoms like fatigue, lack of motivation, and social withdrawal may for the most part be regarded as behaviorally equivalent at all levels of ID additional to ASD; however, negative symptoms in patients with a severe level of ID have not been studied thoroughly to date (O'Dwyer, 2000). In a study with a sample of convenience, eight subjects with ASD and schizophrenia who were investigated all showed considerable aggravated social withdrawal (Bakken et al., 2007).

People with ASD and people with schizophrenia both struggle to maintain social relationships. In people with schizophrenia, social withdrawnness typically increases slightly with increasing symptoms, while social skills in ASD are more stable or may even increase with training. The social withdrawnness and social passivity shown by individuals with schizophrenia do not include the idiosyncratic social behavior that might be seen in those with ASD, for example, greeting rituals including pirouettes, touching, and smelling other people.

Identification of Schizophrenia in ASD

The features that distinguish ASD from schizophrenia or related disorders have been discussed in follow-up studies of children with ASD (Clarke et al., 1989; DeMyer et al., 1973; Eisenberg & Kanner, 1956; Eisenberg, 1956; Kanner et al., 1972; Lotter, 1974; Petty, Ornitz, Michelman, & Zimmerman, 1984; Rumsey et al., 1985; Rutter, 1970), comparisons of individuals with ASD and schizophrenia (Bakken et al., 2007; Konstantareas & Hewitt, 2001; Nylander et al., 2008; Werry, 1992), comparative studies of children with early and late onset (Howells & Guirguis, 1984; Kolvin,

Ounsted, Humphrey, & McNay, 1971), descriptions of ASD (Caplan & Tanguay, 2002; Dykens, Volkmar, & Glick, 1991; Kanner, 1943), follow-up and retrospective studies of individuals with schizophrenia (Jones, Rodgers, Murray, & Marmot, 1994; Malmberg, Lewis, David, & Allenbeck, 1998), and studies describing or comparing the characteristics of schizophrenia with early and late onset (Done, Crow, Johnstone, & Sacket, 1994; Garralda, 1984). Although some contradictions are found, a consistent picture emerges. In Table 5.6 the most important features distinguishing between ASD and schizophrenia are evaluated and listed.

The problem that many individuals with both ASD and ID face, who lack language skills and are unable to talk about their experiences and discomfort, was addressed in a series of studies investigating the possibility of using disorganized behavior as an indicator of schizophrenia in these individuals (Bakken, Eilertsen, Smeby, & Martinsen, 2008a; Bakken, Eilertsen, Smeby, & Martinsen, 2009; Bakken et al., 2007). First, behavioral disorganization occurred significantly more often in patients with schizophrenia than among individuals with plain ASD and patients with non-psychotic psychiatric disorders additional to ASD (Bakken et al., 2007). Second, behavioral disorganization could be reliably assessed by systematic observation of daily activity and social interaction in individuals with schizophrenia, ASD, and ID (Bakken, Eilertsen, Smeby, & Martinsen, 2008b; Bakken et al., 2008a). Finally, behavioral disorganization for the most part occurred concurrently with disorganized speech in one adult woman with autism, schizophrenia, and ID (Bakken et al., 2009). The findings suggest disorganized behavior as an equivalent and alternative measure to disorganized speech, which is commonly regarded as a sign of thought disorder. Thus, it seems that observation of behavior and social interaction may be used to assess schizophrenia in individuals with ASD and ID.

Confounding of schizophrenia symptoms and age-typical understanding and use of language in young children can be avoided only if detailed knowledge of child development is available in the diagnostic process. The diagnosis of psychotic phenomena is not possible without considering the developmental limitations, and that identification of schizophrenia symptoms loses reliability in a chronological age of less than 7 years (Volkmar & Tsatsanis, 2002). Accordingly, alternative developmentally normal mental phenomena may often explain a suspected psychotic disorder in children under the age of 10 years (Dossetor, 2007). Concrete thinking in younger children is so common that the initial use of abstract words after 6–7 years of age has traditionally been called the *concrete abstract shift* in child development (Barenboim, 1981; Erwin, 1993). Preschool children attribute feelings to wants or intentions, for example, believing that one is made happy when something turns out in a wanted or intended way and sad if something else happens (Gnepp, Klayman, & Trabasso, 1982; Harris &

Table 5.6 Distinguishing features of ASD and schizophrenia

Characteristics	ASD	Schizophrenia
Onset before 30 months of age	+++[*]	0
Deterioration in 24–36 months of age[a]	+++	+
Low intellectual functioning	+++	+
Late or deviant early cognitive development	+++	+
Ability to articulate own problems and distress	0	+++
Positive schizophrenia symptoms in adolescence or adulthood	+	+++[*]
Hallucinations	+	+++[*]
Delusions	+	+++[*]
Thought disorder	+	+++[*]
Disorganized/incoherent speech	+	+++[*]
Disorganized behavior	+	+++[*]
Derailment	+	+++[*]
Cognitive slippage	+	+++[*]
Perceptual distortion	+	+++[*]
Illogicality	+	+++[*]
Concrete thinking	+++	+++
Seemingly delusional thought related to the context	+++	+
Immature beliefs and naivety	+++	+
Obliviousness	+++	+++
Withdrawal	++	+++
Negative symptoms of schizophrenia	+++	+++[*]
Low energy level	++	+++[*]
Apathy	+	++[*]
Affective flattening	++	+++
Language problems	+++[*]	++
Late acquisition of speech	+++	+
Echolalia	+++	+
Idiosyncratic speech	+++	++
Neologisms	+++	+++
Poor communication	+++	++
Non-verbal communication difficulties	+++	+++
Social problems	+++	+++
Unusual preoccupations or interests	+++[*]	+
Lack of ability to relate normally to other people	+++[*]	+
Lack of interest in social interaction with other people	++[b,c]	+++
Diminished social skills	+++[*]	+++

Table 5.6 (continued)

Characteristics	ASD	Schizophrenia
Problems with social interaction	+++	+++
Self-isolating behavior	++[c]	++
Solitary play	+++	++
Withdrawal from initially present relationship	+	+++
Gaze avoidance	++	++
Inappropriate behavior	+++	+++
Resistance to change/negative reactions to novelty	++[c]	+
Sensory preoccupation	+++	+
Oversensitivity to sensory stimulation	+++	++
Anxiousness in social situations	+++	++
Anxiety disorder	++	+
Depressive disorder	+	+
Hostility	+	++
Motor problems	++	+
Hyperactivity	++	+
Problems with activity control	++	+

[a]Previously called childhood psychosis, now incorporated in autism.
[b]Earlier defining criteria (Kanner, 1943), not pathognomic to ASD.
[c]After infancy and the toddler age.
[*] Defining criteria; 0 not present; + present, but seldom, <20%; ++ prominent, estimated, prevalence/incidence >20%; +++ very prominent, estimated prevalence/incidence >50%.

Saarni, 1989). The problem of differentiating between normal language and schizophrenia is increased by the fact that there is a high prevalence of language problems in the very early onset of schizophrenia.

Hallucinations are hardly ever reported in children under the age of 8 (Caplan, 1994). Hallucinations and delusions have to be distinguished from pretend/imaginary friends, relationships with a transitional object, such as treating a toy as if it were a real friend, stereotypic preoccupations, concrete externalizations of thoughts or consciousness, and pseudo-hallucinations. Pretend friends are common in childhood, reported by 25–65% of children (Taylor, Carlson, Bayto, Geron, & Charley, 2004) and may persist in primary school and adolescence. In many cases, the presence of pretend friends in children with ASD, which are pseudo-hallucinations, may be wrongly perceived as a sign of psychosis. Nevertheless, the ability to discriminate between what is fantasy and what is real is typically present from age 3 (Wellman & Estes, 1986); it is most evident from how children talk about things and events (Schatz, Wellman, & Silber, 1983).

Communication impairment in ASD may include echolalia, repetition of words or phrases, detailed explanatory language, idiosyncratic use of words or expressions and literal interpretation (Howlin, 2002). As showed in Table 5.6, these features may be shared with features of schizophrenia. Even when the form of speech is less grossly distorted, there are disturbances in conceptualization and the logic of thought and association, which renders it more or less incomprehensible to others. Words may be used idiosyncratically or condensed and distorted to create neologisms in both individuals with ASD and schizophrenia. Problems arise when one relies on neologisms or thought disorder as characteristic features of schizophrenia (Caplan & Tanguay, 2002). In a study of 11 individuals with ASD, without a control but with a reference group, more poverty of speech for ASD and also lower illogicality were found (Dykens et al., 1991). High-functioning adults with ASD and patients with schizophrenia both had similar problems with cognitive slippage, perceptual distortion, and reality testing. Rumsey and colleagues (1985) found affect flattening and concrete thinking, regarded as negative schizophrenia symptoms, in men previously diagnosed with ASD. Some parents reported immature beliefs and naivety such as beliefs in fictional characters like Santa Claus until late adolescence.

In a comparative study of males with ASD and with schizophrenia, some of the most visible symptoms of ASD were also those that best differentiate the two groups, such as stereotypical and inappropriate behavior, resistance to change, sensory preoccupations, and difficulty with non-verbal communication (Konstantareas & Hewitt, 2001).

To sum up, schizophrenia occurs in persons with ASD, with or without additional ID. Aetiology has not been investigated and is probably exceptionally complex. ASD and schizophrenia have a number of overlapping symptoms. Delusions and hallucinations may be confused with autistic characteristics such as idiosyncratic language, bizarre behavior, and uncommon interests. Likewise, concrete thinking, lack of communication skills, and literalness may be misinterpreted as signs of schizophrenia. Negative schizophrenia symptoms such as low social activity, little use of speech, lack of motivation, and limited expressions of feelings and affect, including a low degree of facial mimicry, may be confused with characteristics of ASD.

Recognition of Psychiatric Disorders in People with Autism Spectrum Disorders

People with ASD may develop psychiatric disorders in the same way as other people. It is reasonable to suppose that they may experience the same psychiatric disorders as the general population and that the disorders have the same core characteristics (Clarke et al., 1999; Kobayashi & Murata, 1998; Lainhart, 1999; Moss, 1999; Volkmar & Cohen, 1991). There is no reason to believe that ASD is a protective factor against developing psychiatric illness, as

evidenced by several studies describing psychiatric symptoms in individuals with ASD not related to autism (Bradley et al., 2004; Clarke et al., 1999; Ghaziuddin, 2005; Howlin, 2000; Lainhart, 1999; Leyfer et al., 2006; Matson & Nebel-Schwalm, 2007; Reaven & Hepburn, 2003; Tantam, 2000; Wing, 1996). On the contrary, ASD seems to represent an increased vulnerability for mental health disorders (Clarke et al., 1999; Ghaziuddin, 2005; Lainhart, 1999).

The manifestations of psychiatric disorders in individuals with ASD, however, may be different from individuals without ASD. Psychiatric symptoms may appear in atypical or idiosyncratic ways in this group, for example, in the form of self-injury, irritability, aggression, bizarre movements, and strange behavior (Ghaziuddin, 2005; Hutton et al., 2008). In case studies of individuals with ASD, idiosyncratic and atypical psychiatric symptoms have frequently been reported (Lainhart, 1999; Myers & Winters, 2002; Stavrakiki, 1999; Tantam, 2000). For example, challenging behavior like self-injury and aggressive behavior has been reported as a sign of depression (Myers & Winters, 2002; Stewart et al., 2006), and more intense rumination and an increase in typical autism symptoms like repetitive and ritualistic behavior have been described when individuals with ASD develop psychiatric disorders (Tantam, 2000; Wing, 1996). The challenges of recognition are also increased by the fact that people with ASD seem to show more symptoms and more severe symptoms of ASD when they develop a psychiatric disorder. Nevertheless, by using indicators of psychiatric disorders that do not overlap with the core characteristics of ASD, it is possible to differentiate between individuals with ASD and ID who have a psychiatric disorder and those who do not (Helverschou et al., 2009). Furthermore, in a study on the manifestation of anxiety in individuals with ASD and ID, an examination was made of the sort of anxiety symptoms most frequently reported in clinical anxiety assessment, i.e., typical anxiety symptoms or more unusual expressions (Helverschou & Martinsen, 2011). The proportion of such symptoms was lower than expected, and most anxiety symptoms reported were typical of those found in individuals with anxiety disorders without ASD. The higher rates of idiosyncratic and atypical symptoms reported in other studies may be due to such symptoms being more easily recognized than typical anxiety symptoms because they are more usual and therefore more visible.

As previously stated, the occurrence of anxiety and depression in people with ASD seems to be especially high. The close association between anxiety and depression, the special relationship between anxiety and autism, and the potential central role of anxiety in the development of psychiatric disorders among individuals with ASD highlight the importance of recognizing anxiety in this population. Anxiety may be recognized by symptoms similar to those in individuals without ASD (Helverschou et al., 2008,

2009); however, it may be difficult to recognize specific signs of arousal, which is called for in a diagnosis of anxiety (Helverschou & Martinsen, 2011). An educational perspective seems indicated in order to teach care staff and professionals to be more aware of anxiety symptoms in this population.

The resemblance of the diagnostic criteria and patients' symptoms seems to make it exceptionally difficult to recognize schizophrenia among individuals with ASD. When a psychotic condition is suspected in individuals with ASD, it is essential to investigate the following: the degree of decline in global functioning, the level of additional adjustment problems, the presence of psychotic disorganized speech or disorganized behavior, and aggravated social withdrawal and apathy. Hallucinatory behavior and delusions must be considered in the light of the person's developmental history from childhood with regard to idiosyncrasies.

There seems to be general agreement that accurate diagnostic assessment of psychiatric disorders in people with ASD depends on distinguishing between symptoms that represent the autistic condition and symptoms that represent other psychiatric conditions (Ghaziuddin, 2005; Lainhart, 1999; Tsai, 1996). Thus, the diagnostics should be based on identifying qualitative changes in long-standing symptomatology in the individual's pre-morbid features of autism, conventional diagnostic criteria related to specific disorders, and the interpretation of idiosyncratic or atypical symptoms (Ghaziuddin, 2005; Lainhart, 1999).

It is very important to co-operate with the family and others who know the person well in order to obtain information on well-being or uneasiness, changes in relation to pre-morbid or typical patterns of behavior and mood, to provide information on idiosyncratic or atypical symptoms, and to consider the information according to diagnostic criteria (Bradley et al., 2004; Howlin, 1997; Lainhart, 1999; Matson & Boisjoli, 2008). For example, the probability of false positives increases if anxiety is identified by observation alone (Matson, Smiroldo, Hamilton, & Baglio, 1997) and that information from caregivers was needed to ensure that the participants' statements were not rated as delusions or hallucinations (Konstantareas & Hewitt, 2001).

It is also important that those responsible for the diagnostic process know both individuals with ASD and individuals with psychiatric disorders well; however, this might be difficult, since those who are specialized in schizophrenia and other psychiatric illnesses are with few exceptions specialists in adult psychiatry with psychopathology as their main interest, while those who are specialized in ASD are child experts, often with an interest in cognition (Nylander et al., 2008).

The course of the illness may provide essential information about the correct diagnosis. For example, it is possible to distinguish very early onset schizophrenia from ASD only by making a careful developmental history of the details of onset and pattern of autistic impairment in communication, social reciprocity, and interests/behavior (Hollis, 2002). Changes in behavior and severe adjustment problems may reflect a psychiatric disorder. Probably both changes in adjustment problems and disorder-specific signs should be focused on. For example, a high presence of compulsive behavior in individuals with ASD does not necessarily lead to an inordinately high occurrence of OCD.

There are conflicting findings as to whether individuals with ASD and ID are more prone to develop psychiatric disorders than those with ID alone (Bradley et al., 2004; Melville et al., 2008; Morgan et al., 2003; Mouridsen et al., 2008; Tsakanikos et al., 2006). In a screening study, a comparison was made of two representative samples of adolescents and adults with ASD and ID and with ID only (Bakken et al., 2010). In this study, ASD had a marked effect on the prevalence of psychiatric disorders. The occurrence of a psychiatric disorder was approximately 2.5 times higher in the ASD and ID group than in the ID-only group, and the diagnosis–psychiatric disorder interaction was highly significant. A relatively high prevalence of anxiety disorder was especially linked to ASD. If individuals with ASD and ID are more prone to psychiatric disorders than individuals with only ID, a need for greater attention to the recognition of psychiatric disorders in this population is indicated.

References

Alden, L. E. (2001). Interpersonal perspectives on social phobia. In W. R. Crozier & L. E. Alden (Eds.), *International handbook of social anxiety. Concepts, research and interventions relating to the self and shyness* (pp. 381–404). London: Wiley.

Alden, L. E., & Crozier, W. R. (2001). Social anxiety as a clinical condition. In W. R. Crozier & L. E. Alden (Eds.), *International handbook of social anxiety: Concepts, research and interventions relating to the self and shyness* (pp. 327–334). London: Wiley.

American Psychiatric Association. (1980). *Diagnostic and statistical manual of mental disorders* (3rd ed., DSM-III). Washington, DC: Author.

American Psychiatric Association. (1994). *Diagnostic and statistical manual of mental disorders* (4th ed., DSM-IV). Washington, DC: Author.

American Psychiatric Association. (2000). *Diagnostic and statistical manual of mental disorders* (4th ed., text revision, DSM-IV-TR). Washington, DC: Author.

Andreasen, N. C. (1979). Thought, language, and communication disorders. *Archives of General Psychiatry, 36*, 1315–1321.

Bakken, T. L., Eilertsen, D. E., Smeby, N. A., & Martinsen, H. (2008a). Effective communication related to psychotic disorganized behavior in adults with intellectual disability and autism. *Nordic Journal of Nursing Research and Clinical Studies, 28*, 9–13.

Bakken, T. L., Eilertsen, D. E., Smeby, N. A., & Martinsen, H. (2008b). Observing communication skills in staffs interacting with adults suffering from intellectual disability, autism and schizophrenia. *Nordic Journal of Nursing Research and Clinical Studies, 28*, 30–35.

Bakken, T. L., Eilertsen, D. E., Smeby, N. A., & Martinsen, H. (2009). The validity of disorganized behavior as an indicator of psychosis in adults with autism and intellectual disability: A single case study. *Mental Health Aspects of Developmental Disabilities, 12*, 17–22.

Bakken, T. L., Friis, S., Lovoll, S., Smeby, N. A., & Martinsen, H. (2007). Behavioral disorganization as an indicator of psychosis in adults with intellectual disability and autism. *Mental Health Aspects of Developmental Disabilities, 10*, 37–46.

Bakken, T. L., Helverschou, S. B., Eilertsen, D. E., Hegglund, T., Myrbakk, E., & Martinsen, H. (2010). Psychiatric disorders in adolescents and adults with autism and intellectual disability: A representative study in one county in Norway. *Research in Developmental Disabilities, 31*, 1669–1677.

Barenboim, C. (1981). The development of person perception in childhood and adolescence: From behavioral comparisons to psychological constructs to psychological comparisons. *Child Development, 52*, 129–144.

Baumeister, A. A., & Forehand, R. (1972). Effects of contingent shock and verbal command on stereotyped body rocking of retardates. *Journal of Clinical Psychology, 28*, 586–590.

Bejerot, S. (2007). An autistic dimension. A proposed subtype of obsessive-compulsive disorder. *Autism, 11*, 101–110.

Bejerot, S., Nylander, L., & Lindström, E. (2001). Autistic traits in obsessive-compulsive disorder. *Nordic Journal of Psychiatry, 55*, 169–176.

Bellini, S. (2006). The development of social anxiety in adolescents with autism spectrum disorders. *Focus on Autism and Other Developmental Disabilities, 21*, 138–145.

Bentall, R. (2003). *Madness explained: Psychosis and human nature.* London: The Penguin Press.

Borthwick-Duffy, S. A. (1994). Epidemiology and prevalence of psychopathology in people with mental retardation. *Journal of Consulting and Clinical Psychology, 62*, 17–27.

Bradley, E. A., Summers, J. A., Hayley, L., & Bryson, S. E. (2004). Comparing rates of psychiatric and behavior disorders in adolescents and young adults with severe intellectual disability with and without autism. *Journal of Autism and Developmental Disorders, 34*, 151–161.

Brandsborg, K. (1993). *Blindfødte barns psykososiale utvikling. En undersøkelse av utbredelse av avvikende utvikling og en diskusjon av synstap som utviklingsrisiko* [The psychosocial development of children born blind. An exploration of the extent of deviant development and discussion of loss of vision as a developmental risk]. Prosjektrapport i *Synspunkt* [Project report] nr. 1, 3–23. Melhus, Norway: Tambartun kompetansesenter.

Breier, A., & Berg, P. H. (1999). The psychosis of schizophrenia: Prevalence, response to atypical antipsychotics, and prediction of outcome. *Biological Psychiatry, 46*, 361–364.

Brereton, A. V., Tonge, B. J., & Einfeld, S. L. (2006). Psychopathology in children and adolescents with autism compared to young people with intellectual disability. *Journal of Autism and Developmental Disability, 36*, 863–870.

Bruch, M. A. (2001). Shyness and social interaction. In W. R. Crozier & L. E. Alden (Eds.), *International handbook of social anxiety. Concepts, research and interventions relating to the self and shyness* (pp. 195–215). London: Wiley.

Caplan, R. (1994). Thought disorder in middle childhood. *Journal of American Academy of Child and Adolescent Psychiatry, 33*, 605–615.

Caplan, R., & Tanguay, P. (2002). Development of psychotic thinking. In M. Lewis (Ed.), *Child and adolescent psychiatry* (pp. 359–365). Philadelphia, PA: Lippincott Williams & Wilkins.

Cederlund, M., Hagberg, B., Billstedt, E., Gillberg, I. C., & Gillberg, C. (2008). Asperger syndrome and autism: A comparative longitudinal follow-up study more than 5 years after original diagnosis. *Journal of Autism and Developmental Disorders, 38*, 72–85.

Clarke, D., Baxter, M., Perry, D., & Prasher, V. (1999). The diagnosis of effective and psychotic disorders in adults with autism: Seven case reports. *Autism, 3*, 149–164.

Clarke, D. J., Littlejohns, C. S., Corbett, J. A., & Joseph, S. (1989). Pervasive developmental disorders and psychoses in adult life. *British Journal of Psychiatry, 155*, 692–699.

Coplan, J. D., Pine, D. S., Papp, L. A., & Gorman, J. M. (1997). A view on noradrenergic, hypothalamic-pituitary-adrenal axis and extra hypothalamic corticotrophin-releasing factor function in anxiety and affective disorders: The reduced growth hormone response to clonidine. *Psychopharmacology Bulletin, 33*, 193–204.

Crozier, W. R., & Alden, E. A. (2001). The social nature of social anxiety. In W. R. Crozier & L. E. Alden (Eds.), *International handbook of social anxiety. Concepts, research and interventions relating to the self and shyness* (pp. 1–20). London: Wiley.

Davidson, R. J. (2002). Anxiety and affective style: Role of prefrontal cortex and amygdala. *Biological Psychiatry, 51*, 68–80.

Dekker, M., & Kooth, H. M. (2003). DSM-IV Disorders in children with borderline to moderate intellectual disability. I: Prevalence and impact. *Journal of the American Academy of Child and Adolescent Psychiatry, 42*, 915–922.

DeMyer, M. K., Barton, S., DeMyer, W. E., Norton, J. A., Allen, J., & Steel, R. (1973). Prognosis in autism: A follow-up study. *Journal of Autism and Childhood Schizophrenia, 3*, 199–246.

Deutsch, S., & Davis, K. L. (1983). Schizophrenia: A review of diagnostic and biological issues I. Diagnosis and prognosis. *Hospital and Community Psychiatry, 34*, 313–322.

Diforio, D., Walker, E. F., & Kestler, L. P. (2000). Executive functions in adolescents with schizotypal personality disorder. *Schizophrenia Research, 42*, 125–134.

Doctor, R. M., Kahn, A. P., & Adamec, C. (2008). *The encyclopaedia of phobias, fears, and anxieties* (3rd ed.). New York: Fact on File.

Done, J. D., Crow, T. J., Johnstone, E., & Sacket, A. (1994). Childhood antecedents of schizophrenia and affective illness: Social adjustment at ages 7 and 11. *British Medical Journal, 309*, 699–703.

Dossetor, D. R. (2007). 'All that glitters is not gold': Misdiagnosis of psychosis in pervasive developmental disorders – A case series. *Clinical Child Psychology and Psychiatry, 12*, 537–548.

Dykens, E., Volkmar, F., & Glick, M. (1991). Thought disorder in high functioning autistic adults. *Journal of Autism and Developmental Disorders, 23*, 291–301.

Eisenberg, L. (1956). The autistic child in adolescence. *American Journal of Psychiatry, 112*, 607–612.

Eisenberg, L., & Kanner, L. (1956). Early infantile autism: 1943–55. *American Journal of Orthopsychiatry, 26*, 556–566 (Reprinted from *Psychopathology: A source book,* pp. 3–14, by C. F. Reed, I. E. Alexander, & S. S. Tomkins, Eds., Cambridge, MA: Harvard University Press).

Eknes, J. (2008). Diagnostisering av tvangslidelse hos personer med utviklingshemning (Diagnosing OCD in individuals with ID). In J. Eknes, T. L. Bakken, J. A. Løkke, & I. Mæhle (Eds.), *Utredning og diagnostisering. Utviklingshemning, psykiske lidelser og atferdsvansker* [Assessment and diagnostics. ID, Psychiatric disorders and behavior problems] (pp. 182–196). Oslo, Norway: Universitetsforlaget.

Erwin, P. (1993). *Friendship and peer relations in children.* Chichester: Wiley.

Evans, M. A. (2001). Shyness in the classroom and home. In W. R. Crozier & L. E. Alden (Eds.), *International handbook of social anxiety. Concepts, research and interventions relating to the self and shyness* (pp. 159–183). London: Wiley.

Evans, D. W., Canavera, K., Kleinpeter, F. L., Maccubbin, E., & Taga, K. (2005). The fears, phobias and anxieties of children with autism spectrum disorders and down syndrome: Comparisons with developmentally and chronologically age matched children. *Child Psychiatry and Human Development, 36*, 3–26.

Flaum, M., & Schultz, S. K. (1996). The core symptoms of schizophrenia. *Annual Medicine, 28*, 525–531.

Garralda, M. E. (1984). Hallucinations in children with conduct and emotional disorders. I. The clinical phenomena. *Psychological medicine, 14*, 589–596.

Gelder, M., Harrison, P., & Cowen, P. (2006). *Shorter Oxford textbook of psychiatry* (5th ed.). Oxford: Oxford University Press.

Gelder, M., Lopez-Ibor, J., & Andreasen, N. (2003). *New Oxford textbook of psychiatry*. Oxford: Oxford University Press.

Ghaziuddin, M. (2005). *Mental health aspects of autism and Asperger syndrome*. London: Jessica Kingsley.

Ghaziuddin, M., Alessi, N., & Greden, J. F. (1995). Life events and depression in children with pervasive developmental disorders. *Journal of Autism and Developmental Disorders, 25*, 495–502.

Ghaziuddin, M., & Greden, J. F. (1998). Depression in children with autism/pervasive developmental disorders: A case-control family history study. *Journal of Autism and Developmental Disorders, 28*, 111–115.

Ghaziuddin, M., Tsai, L., & Ghaziuddin, N. (1992). Comorbidity of autistic disorder in children and adolescents. *European Child and Adolescent Psychiatry, 1*, 209–213.

Ghaziuddin, M., & Zafar, S. (2008). Psychiatric comorbidity of adults with autism spectrum disorders. *Clinical Neuropsychiatry, 5*, 9–12.

Gillberg, C. (1985). Asperger syndrome and recurrent psychosis: A case study. *Journal of Autism and Developmental Disorders, 15*, 389–397.

Gillberg, C., & Billstedt, E. (2000). Autism and Asperger syndrome: Coexistence with other clinical disorders. *Acta Psychiatrica Scandinavia, 102*, 321–330.

Gillott, A., Furniss, F., & Walter, A. (2001). Anxiety in high-functioning children with autism. *Autism, 5*, 277–286.

Gillott, A., & Stranden, P. J. (2007). Levels of anxiety and sources of stress in adults with autism. *Journal of Intellectual Disabilities, 11*, 359–370.

Glenn, E., Bihm, E. M., & Lammers, W. (2003). Depression, anxiety, and relevant cognitions in persons with mental retardation. *Journal of Autism and Developmental Disorders, 33*, 69–76.

Gnepp, J., Klayman, J., & Trabasso, T. (1982). A hierarchy of information sources for inferring emotional reactions. *Journal of Experimental Child Psychology, 33*, 111–123.

Goldstein, R. B., Weissman, M. M., Adams, P. B., Horwath, E., Lish., J. D., Charney, D., et al. (1994). Psychiatric disorders in relatives of probands with panic disorder and/or major depression. *Archives of General Psychiatry, 51*, 383–394.

Goodman, W. K., Price, L. H., Rasmussen, S. A., Mazure, C., Delgado, P., Heninger, G. R., et al. (1989). The Yale-Brown Compulsive Scale (Y-BOCS): Part II: Validity. *Archives of General Psychiatry, 46*, 1012–1016.

Goodman, W. K., Price, L. H., Rasmussen, S. A., Mazure, C., Fleischmann, R. L., Hill, C. L., et al. (1989). The Yale-Brown Compulsive Scale (Y-BOCS): Part I: Development, use, and reliability. *Archives of General Psychiatry, 46*, 1006–1011.

Green, J., Gilchrist, A., Burton, D., & Cox, A. (2000). Social and psychiatric functioning in adolescents with Asperger syndrome compared with conduct disorder. *Journal of Autism and Developmental Disorders, 30*, 279–293.

Gustafsson, C., & Sonnander, K. A. (2004). Occurrence of mental health problems in Swedish samples of adults with intellectual disabilities. *Social Psychiatry and Psychiatric Epidemiology, 39*, 448–456.

Gustafsson, C., & Sonnander, K. A. (2005). A psychometric evaluation of a Swedish version of the psychopathology inventory for mentally retarded adults (PIMRA). *Research in Developmental Disabilities, 26*, 183–201.

Harris, P. L., & Saarni, C. (1989). Children's understanding of emotion: An introduction. In C. Saarni & P. L. Harris (Eds.), *Children's understanding of emotion*. New York: Cambridge University Press.

Harrow, M., O'Connel, E., Herbener, E. S., Altman, A. M., Kaplan, K. J., & Jobe, T. H. (2003). Disordres verbalization in Schizophrenia: A speech disturbance or thought disorder? *Comprehensive Psychiatry, 44*, 353–359.

Heim, C., & Nemeroff, C. B. (1999). The impact of early aversive experiences on brain systems involved in the pathophysiology of anxiety and affective disorders. *Biological Psychiatry, 46*, 1509–1522.

Helverschou, S. B. (2006). Struktur, forutsigbarhet og tegnopplæring som emosjonsregulerende og angstregulerende strategier [Structure, predictability and manual sign teaching as strategies in regulation of emotions and anxiety]. In S. von Tetzchner, E. Grindheim, J. Johannessen, D. Smørvik, & V. Yttterland (Eds.), *Biologiske forutsetninger for kulturalisering* [Biological presuppositions to culturalization]. Oslo, Norway: Autismeforeningen og Universitetet i Oslo [The autism society and University of Oslo].

Helverschou, S. B., Bakken, T. L., & Martinsen, H. (2008). Identifying symptoms of psychiatric disorders in people with autism and intellectual disability: An empirical conceptual analysis. *Mental Health Aspects of Developmental Disabilities, 11*, 105–115.

Helverschou, S. B., Bakken, T. L., & Martinsen, H. (2009). The Psychopathology in Autism Checklist (PAC): A pilot study. *Research in Autism Spectrum Disorders, 3*, 179–195.

Helverschou, S. B., & Martinsen, H. (2011). Anxiety in people diagnosed with autism and intellectual disability: Recognition and phenomenology. *Research in Autism Spectrum Disorders, 5*, 377–387.

Hirschfeld, D. R., Rosenbaum, J. F., Biederman, J., Bolduc, E. A., Faraone, S. V., Snidman, N., et al. (1992). Stable behavioral inhibition and its association with anxiety disorder. *Journal of American Academy and Child and Adolescent Psychiatry, 31*, 103–111.

Hoder, E. L., & Cohen, D. J. (1983). Repetitive behavior patterns in childhood. In M. Levine & W. Carey (Eds.)., *Developmental-behavioral pediatrics* (pp. 607–622). Philadelphia, PA: Saunders.

Hofvander, B., Delorme, R., Chaste, P., Nyden, A., Wentz, E., Stahlberg, O., et al. (2009). Psychiatric and psychosocial problems in adults with normal-intelligence autism spectrum disorders. *BMC Psychiatry, 9*, 35.

Hollis, C. (2002). Schizophrenia and allied disorders. In M. Rutter & E. Taylor (Eds.), *Child and adolescent psychiatry* (pp. 612–635). Oxford: Blackwell.

Howells, J. G., & Guirguis, W. R. (1984). Childhood schizophrenia 20 years later. *Archives of General Psychiatry, 41*, 123–128.

Howlin, P. (1997). *Autism: Preparing for adulthood*. London: Routledge.

Howlin, P. (2000). Outcome in adult life for more able individuals with autism or Asperger syndrome. *Autism, 4*, 63–83.

Howlin, P. (2002). Autistic disorders. In P. Howlin & O. Udwin (Eds.), *Outcomes in neurodevelopmental and genetic disorders*. Cambridge: Cambridge University Press.

Howlin, P., Goode, S., Hutton, J., & Rutter, M. (2004). Adult outcome for children with autism. *Journal of Child Psychology and Psychiatry, 45*, 212–229.

Hurley, A. D. (1996). The misdiagnosis of hallucinations and delusions in persons with mental retardation: A neurodevelopmental perspective. *Seminars in Clinical Neuropsychiatry, 1*, 122–133.

Hutton, J., Goode, S., Murphy, M., Couteur, A. L., & Rutter, M. (2008). New-onset psychiatric disorders in individuals with autism. *Autism, 12*, 373–390.

Jacobsen, J. (1999). Dual diagnosis services: History, progress and perspectives. In N. Bouras (Ed.), *Psychiatric and behavioral disorders in developmental disabilities and mental retardation*. Cambridge: Cambridge University Press.

Jones, P., Rodgers, B., Murray, R., & Marmot, M. (1994). Child development risk factors for adult schizophrenia in the British 1946 cohort. *Lancet, 344*, 1398–1402.

Jopp, A. D., & Keys, C. B. (2001). Diagnostic overshadowing reviewed and reconsidered. *American Journal on Mental Retardation, 106*, 416–433.

Kagan, J. (1994). *Galen's prophecy*. New York: Basic Books.

Kagan, J. (1998). The biology of the child. In N. Eisenberg (Ed.), *Handbook of child psychology: Vol. 3. Social, emotional and personality development* (pp. 177–235). New York: Wiley.

Kagan, J., & Snidman, N. (2004). *The long shadow of temperament*. Cambridge: Harvard University press.

Kanner, L. (1943). Autistic disturbances of affective contact. *Nervous Child, 2*, 217–250 (Reprinted from *Acta Paedopsychiatrica*, 1968, *35*, 100–136).

Kanner, L. (1944). Early infantile autism. *The Journal of Pediatrics, 25*, 211–217.

Kanner, L., Rodriguez, A., & Ashenden, B. (1972). How far can autistic children go in matters of social adaptation? *Journal of Autism and Childhood Schizophrenia (Now titled: Journal of Autism and Developmental Disorders), 2*, 9–33.

Karno, M., Goldin, J. M., Sorenson, S. B., & Burnam, M. A. (1988). The epidemiology of obsessive-compulsive disorders in five US communities. *Archives of General Psychiatry, 45*, 1094–1099.

Kerns, J. G., & Berenbaum, H. (2002). Cognitive impairments associated with formal thought disorder in people with schizophrenia. *Journal of Abnormal Psychology, 111*, 211–224.

Kessler, R. C., McGonagle, K. A., Zhao, S., Nelson, C. B., Hughes, M., Eshleman, S., et al. (1994). Lifetime and 12-month prevalence of DSM-III-R psychiatric disorders in the United States: Results from the national comorbidity survey. *Archives of General Psychiatry, 51*, 8–19.

Kim, J. A., Szatmari, P., Bryson, S. E., Streiner, D. L., & Wilson, F. J. (2000). The prevalence of anxiety and mood problems among children with autism and Asperger syndrome. *Autism, 4*, 117–132.

Kobayashi, R., & Murata, T. (1998). Behavioral characteristics of 187 young adults with autism. *Psychiatry and Clinical Neuroscience, 52*, 383–390.

Kolvin, I., Ounsted, C., Humphrey, M., & McNay, A. (1971). Studies in the childhood psychoses: II. The phenomenology of childhood psychoses. *British Journal of Psychiatry, 118*, 385–395.

Konstantareas, M. M., & Hewitt, T. (2001). Autistic disorder and schizophrenia: Diagnostic overlaps. *Journal of Autism and Developmental Disorders, 31*, 19–28.

Lainhart, J. E. (1999). Psychiatric problems in individuals with autism, their parents and siblings. *International Review of Psychiatry, 11*, 278–298.

Lenzenweger, M. F., & Dworkin, R. H. (1996). The dimensions of schizophrenia phenomenology: Not one or two, at least three perhaps four. *British Journal of Psychiatry, 168*, 432–440.

Leyfer, O. T., Folstein, S. E., Bacalman, S., Davis, N. O., Dinh, E., Morgan, J., et al. (2006). Comorbid psychiatric disorders in children with autism: Interview development and rates of disorders. *Journal of Autism and Developmental Disorders, 36*, 849–861.

Lindenmayer, J. P., Brown, E., Baker, R. W., Schuh, L. M., Shao, L., Tohen, M., et al. (2004). An excitement subscale of the positive and negative syndrome scale. *Schizophrenia Research, 68*, 331–337.

Long, K., Wood, H., & Holmes, N. (2000). Presentation, assessment and treatment of depression in a young woman with learning disability and autism. *British Journal of Learning Disabilities, 28*, 102–108.

Lotter, V. (1974). Factors related to outcome in autistic children. *Journal of Autism and Childhood Schizophrenia, 4*, 263–277.

Luscre, D., & Center, D. B. (1996). Procedures for reducing dental fear in children with autism. *Journal of Autism and Developmental Disorders, 26*, 547–556.

MacNeil, B. M., Lopes, V. A., & Minnes, P. M. (2009). Anxiety in children and adolescents with autism spectrum disorders. *Research in Autism Spectrum Disorders, 3*, 1–21.

Malmberg, A., Lewis, G., David, A., & Allenbeck, P. (1998). Premorbid adjustment and personality in people with schizophrenia. *British Journal of Psychiatry, 172*, 308–315.

Martinsen, H. (1977). *Development of passivity and occurrence of stereotyped activities in congenitally blind children. Presentation of a model* [Monograph]. Institute of Psychology, University of Oslo, Norway.

Martinsen, H., Bakken, T. L., Helverschou, S. B., & von Tetzchner, S. (2008). Tilspasningsproblemer hos mennesker med ASD. (Adjustment problems in people with ASD). In H. Martinsen & S. O. Vea (Eds.), *Spesialisert men nært. Autismeteamet i Nordland* [Specialized but close. The Autism Team in Nordland] (pp. 167–186). Bodø, Norway: Nordlandssykehuset.

Martinsen, H., Eknes, J., Bakken, T. L., Helverschou, S. B., Hildebrand, K., & Nærland, T. (in preparation). Obsessive and compulsive behavior among persons with autism.

Martinsen, H., & Hildebrand, K. (in preparation). Stress in autism.

Martinsen, H., Laneskog, J., & Duckert, M. (1979). Angst: Emosjonelle reaksjoner hos folk som er fysiologisk aroused, men ikke i stand til å forklare hvorfor [Anxiety: Emotional reactions in persons who are psychologically aroused, but not able to explain why]. *Impuls, 33*, 6–21.

Martinsen, H., & Tellevik, J. M. (2001). Autisme – en spesialpedagogisk utfordring [Autism – A challenge to special needs education]. In E. Befring & R. Tangen (Eds.), *Spesialpedagogikk* [Special needs education] (pp. 337–355). Oslo, Norway: Cappelen Akademisk.

Mason, J., & Scior, K. (2004). Diagnostic overshadowing amongst clinicians working with people with intellectual disability in the UK. *Journal of Applied Research in Intellectual Disabilities, 17*, 85–90.

Matson, L., Bamburg, J. W., Mayville, E. A., Pinkston, J., Bielecki, J., Kuhn, D., et al. (2000). Psychopharmacology and mental retardation: A 10-year review (1990–1999). *Research in Developmental Disabilities, 21*, 263–296.

Matson, J. L., & Boisjoli, J. A. (2008). Autism spectrum disorders in adults with intellectual disability and comorbid psychopathology: Scale development and reliability of the ASD-CA. *Research in Autism Spectrum disorders, 2*, 276–287.

Matson, J. L., Gardner, W. I., Coe, D. A., & Sovner, R. (1991). A scale for evaluating emotional disorders in severely and profoundly mentally retarded persons. Development of the diagnostic assessment for the severely handicapped (DASH) scale. *British Journal of Psychiatry, 159*, 404–409.

Matson, J. L., & Nebel-Schwalm, M. S. (2007). Comorbid psychopathology with autism spectrum disorder children: An overview. *Research in Developmental Disabilities, 28*, 341–352.

Matson, J. L., Smiroldo, B. B., Hamilton, M., & Baglio, C. S. (1997). Do anxiety disorders exist in persons with severe and profound mental retardation? *Research in Developmental Disabilities, 18*, 39–44.

Mazefsky, C. A., Folstein, S. E., & Lainhart, J. E. (2008). Overrepresentation of mood and anxiety disorders in adults with autism and their first-degree relatives: What does it mean? *Autism Research, 1*, 193–197.

McDougle, C. J. (1998). Repetitive thought and behavior in pervasive developmental disorders. Phenomenology and pharmacology. In E. Schopler, G. Mesibov, & L. Kunce (Eds.), *Asperger syndrome or high-functioning autism?* (pp. 293–316). New York: Plenum Press.

McDougle, C. J., Kresch, L. E., Goodman, W. K., & Naylor, S. T. (1995). A case-controlled study of repetitive thoughts and behavior in adults with autistic disorder and obsessive-compulsive disorder. *American Journal of Psychiatry, 152*, 772–777.

McDougle, C. J., Kresch, L. E., & Posey, D. J. (2000). Repetitive thoughts and behavior in pervasive developmental disorders: Treatment with serotonin reuptake inhibitors. *Journal of Autism and Developmental Disorders, 30*, 427–435.

Melville, C. A., Cooper, S. A., Morrison, J., Smiley, J., Allan, L., Jackson, A., et al. (2008). The prevalence and incidence of mental ill-health in adults with autism and intellectual disability. *Journal of Autism and Developmental Disorders, 38*, 1676–1688.

Morgan, K. (2006). Is autism a stress disorder? What studies of nonautistic populations can tell us. In M. G. Baron, J. Groden, G. Groden, & L. P. Lipsitt (Eds.), *Stress and coping in autism* (pp. 129–182). Oxford: Oxford University Press.

Morgan, C. N., Roy, M., & Chance, P. (2003). Psychiatric comorbidity and medication use in autism: A community survey. *Psychiatric Bulletin, 27*, 378–381.

Moss, S. (1999). Assessment: Conceptual issues. In N. Bouras (Ed.), *Psychiatric disorders in developmental disabilities and mental retardation*. Cambridge: Cambridge University Press.

Moss, S., Emerson, E., Kiernan, C., Turner, S., Hatton, C., & Alborz, A. (2000). Psychiatric symptoms in adults with learning disability and challenging behavior. *British Journal of Psychiatry, 177*, 452–456.

Mouridsen, S. E., Rich, B., Isager, T., & Nedergaard, N. J. (2008). Psychiatric disorders in individuals diagnosed with infantile autism as children: A case study. *Journal of Psychiatric Practice, 14*, 5–12.

Myers, K., & Winters, N. C. (2002). Ten-year review of rating scales, II: Scales for internalizing disorders. *Journal of the American Academy of Child and Adolescent Psychiatry, 41*, 634–659.

Niehous, D. J. H., & Stein, D. J. (1997). Obsessive-compulsive disorder: Diagnosis and assessment. In I. E. Hollander & D. J. Stein (Eds.), *Obsessive-compulsive disorders: Diagnosis, etiology, treatment*. New York: Marchel Dekker.

Norwegian Board of Health Supervision. (2000). *Anxiety disorders – Clinical guidelines for assessment and treatment*. (Statens helsetilsyn: *Angstlidelser – kliniske retningslinjer for utredning og behandling*). Report 4:99. Oslo, Norway.

Nylander, L., Lugnegård, T., & Hallerback, M. U. (2008). Autism spectrum disorders and schizophrenia spectrum disorders in adults – Is there a connection? A literature review and some suggestions for future clinical research. *Clinical Neuropsychiatry, 5*, 43–54.

Osborn, I. (1998). *Tormenting thoughts and secret rituals*. New York: Dell.

O'Dwyer, J. M. (2000). Autistic disorder and schizophrenia: Similarities and differences and their co-existence in two cases. *Mental Health Aspects of Developmental Disabilities, 3*, 121–131.

Perry, D. W., Marston, G. M., Hinder, S. A. J., Munden, A. C., & Roy, A. (2001). The phenomenology of depressive illness in people with a learning disability and autism. *Autism, 5*, 265–275.

Petty, L. K., Ornitz, E. M., Michelman, J. D., & Zimmerman, E. G. (1984). Autistic children who become schizophrenic. *Archives of General Psychiatry, 41*, 129–135.

Prior, M., & MacMillan, M. (1973). Maintenance of sameness in children with Kanner's syndrome. *Journal of Autism and Childhood Schizophrenia, 3*, 154–167.

Rapoport, J. L., Swedo, S. E., & Leonard, H. L. (1992). Childhood obsessive-compulsive disorder. *Journal of Clinical Psychiatry, 56*, 11–16.

Rasmussen, S. A., & Eisen, J. L. (1998). The epidemiology and clinical features of obsessive-compulsive disorders. In M. A. Jenike & W. E. Minichello (Eds.), *Obsessive-compulsive disorders: Practical management*. St. Louis, MO: Mosby.

Reaven, J., & Hepburn, S. (2003). Cognitive-behavioral treatment of obsessive-compulsive disorder in a child with Asperger syndrome. *Autism, 7*, 145–164.

Regier, D. A., Rae, D. S., Narrow, W. E., Kaelber, C. T., & Schatzberg, A. F. (1998). Prevalence of anxiety disorders and their comorbidity with mood and addictive disorders. *British Journal of Psychiatry, 173*, 24–28.

Reiss, S. (1988). Dual diagnosis in the United States, Australia and New Zealand. *Journal of Developmental Disabilities, 14*, 43–48.

Rumsey, J. M., Andreasen, N. C., & Rapoport, J. L. (1986). Thought, language, communication and affective flattening in autistic adults. *Archives of General Psychiatry, 43*, 771–777.

Rumsey, J. M., Rapoport, J. L., & Sceery, W. R. (1985). Autistic children as adults: Psychiatric, social, and behavioral outcomes. *Journal of the American Academy of Child and Adolescent Psychiatry, 24*, 465–473.

Rutter, M. (1970). Autistic children: Infancy to adulthood. *Seminar in Psychiatry, 2*, 435–450.

Rutter, M., Tizard, J., Yule, W., Graham, P., & Whitmore, K. (1976). Isle of wight studies, 1964–1974. *Psychological Medicine, 6*, 313–332.

Sadock, B. J. (2005). Signs and symptoms of psychiatry. In B. J. Kaplan & V. A. Sadock (Eds.), *Comprehensive textbook of psychiatry* (8th ed., pp. 847–860). Philadelphia, PA: Lippincott, Williams & Wilkins.

Scahill, L., McDougle, C. J., Williams, S. K., Dimitropoulos, A., Aman, M. G., McCracken, J. T., et al. (2006). Children's yale-brown obsessive compulsive scale modified for pervasive developmental disorders. *Journal of American Academy of Child and Adolescent Psychiatry, 45*, 1114–1123.

Schatz, M., Wellman, H. M., & Silber, S. (1983). The acquisition of mental verbs: A systematic investigation of the first reference to mental state. *Cognition, 14*, 301–321.

Schneider, K. (1950). *Klinische Psychopathologie* (8th ed.). Stuttgart, Germany: Thieme.

Schneier, F. R., Johnson, J., Hornig, C. D., Liebowitz, M. R., & Weissman, M. M. (1992). Social phobia: Comorbidity and morbidity in an epidemiological sample. *Archives of General Psychiatry, 49*, 282–288.

Schneier, F. R., Martin, L. Y., Liebowitz, M. R., Gorman, J. M., & Fyer, A. J. (1989). Alcohol abuse in social phobia. *Journal of Anxiety Disorders, 3*, 15–23.

Schopler, E., & Mesibov, G. B. (Eds.). (1994). *Behavioral issues in autism*. New York: Plenum Press.

Shtayermman, O. (2007). Peer victimization in adolescents and young adults diagnosed with Asperger's syndrome: A link to depressive symptomatology, anxiety symptomatology and suicidal ideation. *Issues in Comprehensive Pediatric Nursing, 30*, 87–107.

Simonoff, E., Pickles, A., Charman, T., Chandler, S., Loucas, T., & Baird, G. (2008). Psychiatric disorders in children with autism spectrum disorders: Prevalence, comorbidity, and associated factors in a population-derived sample. *Journal of American Academy of Child and Adolescent Psychiatry, 47*, 921–929.

Skokauskas, N., & Gallagher, L. (2010). Psychosis, affective disorders and anxiety in autistic spectrum disorder: Prevalence and nosological considerations. *Psychopathology, 43*, 8–16.

Stavrakiki, C. (1999). Depression, anxiety and adjustment disorders in people with developmental disabilities. In N. Bouras (Ed.), *Psychiatric disorders in developmental disabilities and mental retardation* (pp. 175–187). Cambridge: Cambridge University Press.

Stein, D. J. (2002). Obsessive-compulsive disorder. *The Lancet, 360*, 397–405.

Steingard, R. J., Zimnitzky, B., DeMaso, D. R., Bauman, M. L., & Bucci, J. P. (1997). Sertraline treatment of transition-associated anxiety and agitation on children with autistic disorder. *Journal of Child and Adolescent Psychopharmacology, 7*, 9–15.

Stewart, M. E., Barnard, L., Pearson, J., Hasan, R., & O'Brien, G. (2006). Presentation of depression in autism and Asperger syndrome: A review. *Autism, 10*, 103–116.

Sukhodolsky, D. G., Schahill, L., Gadow, K. D., Arnold, L. E., Aman, M. G., McDougle, C. J., et al. (2008). Parent-rated anxiety symptoms in children with pervasive developmental disorders: Frequency and association with core autism symptoms and cognitive functioning. *Journal of Abnormal Child Psychology, 36*, 117–128.

Szatmari, P. (1991). Asperger's syndrome: Diagnosis, treatment, and outcome. *Psychiatric Clinics of North America, 14*, 81–93.

Tantam, D. (2000). Psychological disorder in adolescents and adults with Asperger syndrome. *Autism, 4*, 47–62.

Taylor, M., Carlson, M., Bayto, M., Geron, L., & Charley, C. (2004). The characteristics and correlates of fantasy in school-age children: Imaginary companions, impersonation and social understanding. *Developmental Psychology, 40*, 1173–1187.

Thelen, E. (1979). Rhythmical stereotypies in normal human infants. *Animal Behavior, 27*, 699–715.

Tsai, L. Y. (1996). Brief report: Comorbid psychiatric disorders of autistic disorder. *Journal of Autism and Developmental Disorders, 26*, 159–163.

Tsai, L. (2006). Diagnosis and treatment of anxiety disorders in individuals with autism spectrum disorders. In M. G. Baron, J. Groden, G. Groden, & L. P. Lipsitt (Eds.), *Stress and coping in autism* (pp. 388–440). Oxford: Oxford University Press.

Tsakanikos, E., Costello, H., Holt, G., Bouras, N., Sturmey, P., & Newton, T. (2006). Psychopathology in adults with autism and intellectual disability. *Journal of Autism and Developmental Disorders, 36*, 1123–1129.

Turner, S. M., Beidel, D. C., & Wolff, P. L. (1996). Is behavioral inhibition related to the anxiety disorders? *Clinical Psychology Review, 16*, 157–172.

Van Os, J., & Kaour, S. (2009). Schizophrenia. *Lancet, 374*, 635–645.

Volkmar, F. R., & Cohen, D. J. (1991). Comorbid association of autism and schizophrenia. *American Journal of Psychiatry, 148*, 1705–1707.

Volkmar, F., & Tsatsanis, K. (2002). Childhood schizophrenia. In M. Lewis (Ed.)., *Child and adolescent psychiatry* (pp. 745–754). Philadelphia, PA: Lippincott Williams & Wilkins.

Watkins, J. M., Asarnow, R. F., & Tanguay, P. E. (1988). Symptom development in childhood onset schizophrenia. *Journal of Child Psychology and Psychiatry, 29*, 865–878.

Weisbrot, D. M., Gadow, K. D., DeVincent, C. J., & Pomeroy, J. (2005). The presentation of anxiety in children with pervasive developmental disorders. *Journal of Child and Adolescent Psychopharmacology, 15*, 477–496.

Wellman, H. M., & Estes, D. (1986). Early understanding of mental entitles: A re-examination of childhood realism. *Child Development, 57*, 910–923.

Werry, J. S. (1992). Child and adolescent (early onset) schizophrenia: A review in light of DSM-III-R. *Journal of Autism and Developmental Research, 22*, 601–624.

White, S. W., Oswald, D., Ollendick, T., & Schahill, L. (2009). Anxiety in children and adolescents with autism spectrum disorders. *Clinical Psychology Review, 29*, 216–229.

Wing, L. (1996). *The autistic spectrum: A guide for parents and professionals.* London: Constable.

Wing, L. (2000). Past and future of research on Asperger syndrome. In A. Klin, F. Volkmar, & S. Sparrow (Eds.), *Asperger syndrome* (pp. 418–432). New York: Guildford Press.

Wing, L., & Gould, J. (1979). Severe impairment of social interaction and associated abnormalities in children: Epidemiology and classification. *Journal of Autism and Developmental Disorders, 9*, 11–29.

World Health Organization. (1992). *The ICD-10 classification of mental and behavioral disorders. Clinical descriptions and diagnostic guidelines.* Geneva: Author.

World Health Organization. (1993). *The ICD-10 classification of mental and behavior disorders. Diagnostic criteria for research.* Geneva: Author.

World Health Organization. (2001). *International classification of functioning. Introduction.* Geneva: Author.

World Health Organization. (2007). *International classification of functioning. Disability and health.* Geneva: Author.

The Genetics of Autism

6

Deborah K. Sokol and Debomoy K. Lahiri

This chapter is written to make the fast-paced, expanding field of the genetics of autism accessible to those practitioners who help children with autism. New genetic knowledge and technology have quickly developed over the past 30 years, particularly within the past decade, and have made many optimistic about our ability to explain autism. Among these advances include the sequencing of the human genome (Lander et al., 2001) and the identification of common genetic variants via the HapMap project (International HapMap Consortium, 2005), and the development of cost-efficient genotyping and analysis technologies (Losh, Sullivan, Trembath, & Piven, 2008). Improvement in technology has led to improved visualization of chromosomal abnormality down to the molecular level. The four most common syndromes associated with autism include fragile X syndrome, tuberous sclerosis, 15q duplications, and untreated phenylketonuria (PKU; Costa e Silva, 2008). FXS and 15q duplications are discussed within the context of cytogenetics. TSC is illustrated within the description of linkage analysis.

As recently reviewed (Li & Andersson, 2009), the first inkling of chromosomal anomaly causing clinical pathology occurred in 1959 when an extra copy of chromosome 21 was associated with the Down syndrome phenotype. Shortly thereafter, chromosomal abnormality was recognized for Patau's syndrome (trisomy 13) and Edward's syndrome (trisomy 18). The chromosomal banding technique developed in 1970 led to the identification of many structural chromosomal abnormalities associated with clinical conditions. The discovery that genes located close to each other on a chromosome are often inherited together led to linkage analysis in the 1970s and 1980s. Linkage techniques related chromosomal abnormalities with known genetic anomalies using an affected sibling–pair design in multiplex (having more than one affected member) families. This led to the identification of chromosomal abnormalities in such conditions as neurofibromatosis, tuberous sclerosis, and dyslexia (Smith, 2007). Improving technology in the 1990s enabled the detection of small genomic alterations of 50–100 kb and the direct visualization of these alterations in uncultured cells via fluorescent in situ hybridization (FISH). This technique ushered in the field of molecular genetics (Li & Andersson, 2009) and allowed the identification of chromosomal microdeletions and duplications in areas of the chromosome where there is already high suspicion that abnormality would exist. FISH enables prenatal and cancer genetics screening and has led to the identification of genetic aberrations associated with Angelman's and Prader Willi syndromes.

In the past decade, microarray cytogenetics has permitted the study of the entire genome on a single chip with resolution as fine as a few hundred base pairs (Li & Andersson, 2009). Such microarray technology represents a union between molecular genetics and classical cytogenetics. Two types of microarray technology are used clinically: comparative genomic hybridization (CGH) and single-nucleotide polymorphism (SNP) analysis. CGH directly measures copy number differences between a patient's DNA and a normal reference DNA spanning known genes, chromosomal regions, or across the entire genome. SNP analysis, on the other hand, provides identification of a single point mutation via sequencing the gene in areas of suspected abnormality, previously identified via CGH or FISH. Another offshoot of microarray technology is submicroscopic chromosome copy number variation (CNV) analysis, in which deletions or duplications involving > 1-kb DNA have been detected in patients with mental retardation, autism, and multiple congenital anomalies.

There are several recent, detailed reviews of the genetics of autism (Abrahams & Geschwind, 2008; Li & Andersson, 2009; Losh et al., 2008; O'Roak & State, 2008) and this chapter summarizes those reviews. The reader is encouraged to first review the overview of gene expression (Box 6.1) and

D.K. Sokol (✉)
Department of Neurology, Riley Hospital for Children, Indiana University School of Medicine, Indianapolis, IN 46202, USA
e-mail: dksokol@iupui.edu

J.L. Matson, P. Sturmey (eds.), *International Handbook of Autism and Pervasive Developmental Disorders*,
Autism and Child Psychopathology Series, DOI 10.1007/978-1-4419-8065-6_6, © Springer Science+Business Media, LLC 2011

essential nomenclature used in genetics (Box 6.2). In addition, one must understand basic concepts pertinent to brain development (Box 6.3) and to the neurobiology of autism (Box 6.4) in order to understand its genetics. For example, there is a compelling rationale that genetically directed mechanisms that regulate the assembly of the brain during embryogenesis, when gone awry, may cause autism (Costa e Silva, 2008).

Box 6.1 Overview of DNA Replication and Gene Expression*

Genes. A gene is a unit of hereditary material located in a specific place (locus) on a chromosome. Most genes carry the instructions for producing a specific protein. A protein-coding human gene will have a coding sequence, which contains the information for protein production. The coding sequence may be broken up into several sub-sequences, or exons, which are separated by noncoding DNA sequences, or introns. The coding sequence is flanked by a promoter and (usually) a 5′-untranslated region (5′-UTR) that occur immediately before the coding sequence and by a 3′-UTR and a terminator that occur immediately after the coding sequence. Promoters, terminators, UTRs, and introns can regulate the activity of a given gene. At a molecular level, chromosomes are composed of long chains of deoxyribonucleic acid (DNA) upon which genes are linearly arranged. The DNA exists in a double helix and the helical strands are usually wrapped around histone proteins. In addition to DNA and histones, chromosomes contain scaffolding proteins that provide structural support and may also participate in gene regulation. DNA is a molecule composed of a chain of four different types of nucleotides. It is the sequence of these nucleotides that is the genetic information that organisms inherit. DNA is double stranded with nucleotides on each strand complementary to each other. Each strand acts as a template for creating a new partner strand. This is the physical method for making copies of genes that are inherited. Both individual DNA nucleotides and DNA-associated proteins can be chemically modified to produce epigenetic variation that may be in response to environmental conditions and might or might not be inherited in any individual case. Epigenetic variation can significantly alter the expression level of a gene without changing its basic genetic code.

DNA replication. During DNA replication, a DNA strand is produced from component nucleotides using its partner strand as a template. This is done by DNA polymerases that "proofread" to ensure accuracy and repair when necessary. Despite these safeguards, errors called mutations can occur during the polymerization of this second strand. A mutation is any nucleotide sequence in a DNA molecule that does not match its original DNA molecule from which it is copied. Radiation, such as ultraviolet rays and X-rays, viruses, and errors that occur during meiosis or during DNA replication can cause errors in DNA molecules. These mutations can have an impact on the phenotype of an organism, especially when they occur within the protein-coding sequence of the gene. Kinds of mutations include the following:

Frameshift Mutation: One or more bases are inserted or deleted. This can alter the entire amino acid sequence of a protein or introduce aberrant RNA splicing.

Deletion. Missing DNA sequences can range from a single base pair to longer deletions involving many genes in the chromosome.

Insertion. Additional nucleotides are inserted in the DNA sequence and can result in a nonfunctional protein.

Duplication (or gene amplification). Multiple copies of a complete gene or genes, increasing the dosage of genes located within chromosomes.

Inversion. DNA sequence of nucleotides is reversed, either among a few bases within one gene or among longer DNA sequences containing several genes.

Point mutations. Known as substitutions, this is a replacement of a single base nucleotide with another nucleotide.

Missense mutations. A point mutation where a single nucleotide is changed to cause substitution of a different amino acid.

Nonsense mutation. A point mutation that results in a premature stop codon in the transcribed mRNA and possibly a nonfunctional protein product.

RNA splicing mutation. A point mutation that inserts or deletes an intron/exon border necessary for splicing of heterogeneous nuclear RNA to mRNA.

Silent mutation. A point mutation that does not alter the amino acid coding for that codon.

Gene expression is the process in which genes express their functional effect through the production of proteins which are responsible for most functions of the cell. The DNA sequence of a gene is used to produce a specific protein through a ribose nucleic acid (RNA) intermediate. Gene DNA is the map which directs the production of the protein, normally following a one-way pathway:

	$\rightarrow$		$\rightarrow$		$\rightarrow$	
DNA		hnRNA		mRNA		Protein
	Transcription		Splicing		Translation	

Gene regulation gives the cell control over structure and function and is the basis for cellular differentiation and adaptability of any organism. Gene regulation is controlled by noncoding DNA sequences, such as the promoter, terminator, or introns, and by epigenetic variation, such as differences in DNA methylation and histone acetylation. This entire process takes place within the cell in the vicinity of the nucleus, where DNA is housed and hnRNA is spliced, and in the cytoplasm, where ribosomes are located along the rough endoplasmic reticulum. Some proteins are further processed in the Golgi apparatus if they are to be exported from the cell. The correspondence between nucleotide and amino acid sequence is known as the genetic code.

RNA transcription. In transcription, DNA is used as a blueprint for the production of RNA. Transcription is performed by RNA polymerase which adds one ribonucleotide to a growing RNA strand, complimentary to the DNA nucleotide being transcribed. This product is heterologous nuclear RNA (hnRNA).

RNA splicing. In splicing, hnRNA is processed within the nucleus to remove introns which may function to partially regulate transcription and join exons, which code for the actual protein product. The product of slicing is mRNA.

Translation. Translation is the production of proteins by decoding the mRNA that was produced by transcription and splicing. The mRNA sequence is the template that guides the production of a chain of amino acids that form a protein.

*Pack (2002)

Box 6.2 Genetic Terms**

Allele. This is an alternate DNA sequence at the same physical gene locus which may represent different phenotypes. For example, for ABO blood type, there are three alleles, I^0, I^A, and I^B. Any individual has one of six genotypes (AA, AO, BB, BO, AB, and OO) that produce four phenotypes: "A" (produced by AA homozygous and AO heterozygous genotypes), "B" (produced by BB homozygous and BO heterozygous genotypes), "AB" heterozygotes, and "O" homozygotes.

Association Study. A test to determine whether a particular variant (allele) of a marker or a gene occurs more frequently in those with the disorder than in those without the disorder. It detects effects in much smaller regions of the genome than linkage.

Comparative genomic hybridization (CGH). A microarray technique that directly measures copy number differences between a patient's DNA and a normal reference DNA spanning known genes, chromosomal regions, or across the entire genome.

Copy number variation (CNV) analysis. This technique is an offshoot of microarray technology in which 0, 1, or 3 copies, defined as deletions or duplications involving >1 kb DNA, are detected in patients with mental retardation, autism, and multiple congenital anomalies.

Cytogenetics. Study of the structure and function of a cell as it relates to the chromosomes

Fluorescent in situ hybridization (FISH). This is a molecular genetic technique which allows direct visualization of microdeletions and duplications of 50–100 kb of a specific chromosome region in uncultured cells. FISH has enabled prenatal screens for chromosomal abnormality and developmental conditions such as Angelman's and Prader Willi syndromes and postnatal screening for cancer. FISH can only probe specific sequences that are known and suspected to be associated with known syndromes.

Genome. The full set of hereditary material in an organism – usually the combined DNA sequences of all chromosomes. Genome-wide association studies (GWAS) compare genetic risk factors in the form of specific genetic markers in cases and controls. These markers are distributed across the entire genome rather than limited to specific gene regions such as in the sib–pair method.

Genotype: A pair of two alleles which can be the same (homozygous) or different (heterozygous). Genotype interactions between the two alleles at a locus can be dominant (where the heterozygote is indistinguishable from one of the homozygotes), recessive (the allele which is under expressed if mixed with a dominant allele), semi-dominant (where the heterozygote resembles the homozygote dominant more than it does the homozygote recessive but does not have the full homozygote dominant trait), or co-dominant (when both alleles contribute equally to a phenotype that is distinct from either homozygote). In the case of human blood types, for example, I^A and I^B are each dominant over I^0, while I^A and I^B have co-dominance with each other.

Linkage Study. A test to determine where genetic markers are inherited along with a given disorder. When genes are located together on a chromosome, they are often inherited together. Finding a marker linked to a disorder gives the approximate location of a risk gene for that disorder. In the sib–pair linkage study method, siblings with autism are evaluated to determine whether they share any region of the genome more frequently than would be expected by chance.

Mendelian locus. A single gene variant sufficient to completely explain a phenotypic trait, such as a disorder. Examples of pathogenic variations or mutations of single genes include PKU, sickle cell, and Angelman's syndrome.

Mendelian transmission. A condition that is inherited via autosomal dominant, recessive, or sex-linked transmission.

Microarray technology. Developed within the last decade, this technique enables examination of the whole human genome on a single chip with a resolution as high as a few hundred base pairs. This resolution is at least 10-fold greater than the best prometaphase chromosomal analysis and therefore, it is the most sensitive for whole genome screen for deletions and duplications.

Penetrance. The proportion of individuals carrying a particular variation of a gene that also expresses an associated trait. For example, if a mutation has 95% penetrance, then 95% of those with the mutation will develop the syndrome, while 5% will not.

Quantitative trait locus (QTL). A gene variant that is expressed along a continuous phenotype, whose extreme end may produce the disorder such as hypertension, reading disability, or attention-deficit disorder with hyperactivity (ADHD).

Recessive genetic disorders. A number of genetic disorders are caused when an individual inherits two recessive alleles for a single gene trait, such as with cystic fibrosis, PKU, or albinism. Recessive alleles can be located on the X chromosome so that males are more affected than females (hemizygous), such as in fragile X.

Single-nucleotide polymorphism (SNP) analysis. A microarray technique that identifies a single point mutation via sequencing the gene in areas of suspected abnormality as identified via CGH or FISH. This looks at a smaller region with greater detail than does CGH.
**Solomon, Berg, and Martin (2008)

Box 6.3 Normal Brain Development

During embryologic development, the brain emerges from the neural tube, an early embryonic structure. The anterior neural tube expands rapidly due to cell proliferation and eventually gives rise to the brain. Cells stop dividing and differentiate into neurons and glial cells, the main cellular components of the brain. The neurons must migrate to different parts of the developing brain to self-organize into different brain structures. The neurons grow connections (axons and dendrites) which often must span long distances to reach their target cells. Growth cones are the highly motile filamentous connections that eventually form more stable synapses between neurons. Neurons communicate with other neurons via these synapses. This communication leads to the establishment of functional neural circuits that mediate sensory–motor processing and behavior.

Associated with this period of synaptogenesis is a brief period of "programmed" cell death, a pruning process in which cells succumb during natural development (Mattson & Furukawa, 1998). Migration of cells from the ventricular zone lining the central canal of the neural tube to the developing cortex next takes place followed by a more protracted period of pruning (Volpe, 2001). One mechanism that allows cells to detach and migrate away from each other appears to be regulated by a "molecular switch" regulated by catenin adhesion proteins (DiCicco-Bloom, 2006). Neuroligin, recently described in autism research, is a cell adhesion molecule found in the postsynaptic membrane. Also, brain-derived neurotrophic factor (BDNF) is produced by the brain and regulates several functions within the developing synapse, including enhancement of neurotransmitter release.

Activity at the CNS synapses occurs over the life span and is thought to underlie learning and memory. The excitatory neurotransmitter glutamate and its receptors, particularly the N-methyl-D-aspartate (NMDA) receptor, initiate synaptogenesis through activation of downstream products. At the CNS synapse, a nerve terminal is separated from the post-synaptic membrane by a cleft containing specialized extracellular material. Localized vesicles are at the active sites and clustered receptors are at the postsynaptic membrane with glial cells that encapsulate the entire synaptic cleft. There is differentiation of the pre- and postsynaptic membrane following initial contact between two cells. This includes the clustering of receptors, localized upregulation of protein synthesis at the active sites, and continued neuronal pruning through synapse elimination. Neurons within the CNS receive multiple inputs that must be processed and integrated for successful transfer of information. The multiple inputs physically represent the plasticity of the brain.

Box 6.4 Neurobiology of Autism

Macrocephaly has been one of the "most widely replicated biological findings in autism" (McCaffery & Deutsch, 2005), affecting up to 20% of all children with autism. Several reports have shown increased brain volume (macroencephaly/megalencephaly) in both white and grey matter with results varying as a function of age. MRI volumetric studies have showed increased brain volume in younger (total ages 2–21) subjects compared to older (total ages 5–21) subjects (Courchesne, Carper, & Akshoomoff, 2003; Sokol & Edwards-Brown, 2004; Sparks et al., 2002). To explain the relevance of brain volume enlargement in autism, it has been proposed that brain "growth without guidance" occurs in young autistic children (Courchesne et al., 2001) with premature expansion and overgrowth of neural elements and dendritic connections. Indeed, brain enlargement appears to develop postnatally, arising before or during the early recognition of autistic behaviors – between 18 months and 3 years (Courchesne et al., 2003).

Proposed mechanisms underlying brain enlargement include overproduction of synapses, failure of synaptic pruning, excessive neurogenesis, gliogenesis, or reduction in cell death (McCaffery & Deutsch, 2005). The mechanisms underlying the tremendous growth of the typically developing embryonic brain, compared to the relatively more limited postnatal and adult brain growth, have been implicated in the brain enlargement seen in autism. This leads to the proposal that overstimulation of nuclear receptor-mediated gene transcription may increase neural progenitor cells that generate marked increases in cortical surface area

(McCaffery & Deutsch, 2005). Therefore, the number of neurons in the young cortex is a function of the number of proliferative cells present at the onset of neurogenesis. Tumor suppressor genes which control brain growth and migration, when defective, could contribute to macrocephaly of failure in synaptic pruning. This explains the great interest in tumor suppressor genes such as *PTEN* as candidate genes for autism.

Recently, neuronal cell adhesion has been proposed as another mechanism involved in brain overgrowth in autism. Cell adhesion suppresses brain growth, while abnormalities in adhesion promote growth or contribute to aberrant growth. It is believed that heterogeneous causes of autism may be associated with alterations in adhesion molecules of the synapse or cytoplasmic molecules associated with synaptic receptors. Indeed, recent genetic evidence has found associations between autism susceptibility and other neuronal cell adhesion molecules, such as NLGN1 and ASTN2 and specific cadherins.

There is an emerging theory, as recently reviewed in Geschwind (2009), that short-range brain connections may be overgrown and longer range brain connections between different brain lobules are reduced in autism. In autism, there has been a noted reduction in the size of the corpus callosum which connects the two cerebral hemispheres and reduced connectivity between the frontal and temporal lobes of the brain, locations responsible for language and social judgment. The preservation of normal short-range connections could explain some of the preserved processing functions such as visual perception or attention to detail experienced by many with autism (Geschwind, 2009).

Indirect Evidence of Heritability

Three lines of research indirectly attest to the heritability of autism: twin studies, family studies, and the fact that autism affects more boys than girls. In general, hereditability appears to be greater when a broader definition of autism (including individuals with cognitive deficits and/or social impairment) instead of the specific DSM-IV criteria for autism is used.

Twin Studies

In the first twin study of autism (Folstein & Rutter, 1977), the concordance rate in monozygotic (MZ) pairs (36%) was significantly greater than that found in dizygotic (DZ) pairs (0%). If the phenotype was expanded to include a cognitive or a language disorder, the concordance rates were 82 and 10%, respectively. Two subsequent studies found an MZ/DZ concordance rate of 91–0% (Steffenburg et al., 1989) or 60–5% utilizing the specific phenotype, and 90% vs. 10% using the broader phenotype which included social or cognitive deficits (Bailey et al., 1995). Across twin studies of autism, the difference between MZ and DZ concordance rates is sizable, averaging roughly 10:1 (Pennington, 2009). This rate is greater than that for other psychiatric disorders such as depression, bipolar disorder, and schizophrenia (between 2:1 and 4:1), indicating a high heritability for autism (Pennington, 2009). On the other hand, there was great variability in IQ and clinical behaviors in the 16 MZ pairs concordant for autism in the (Bailey et al., 1995) study. In other words, there was no more similarity for these traits within MZ pairs than that between individuals picked at random from different MZ pairs who also had autism. As interpreted by Pennington (2009), this finding suggests that although autism is heritable, the genes may not dictate the exact phenotype. Nonadditive interaction among genes (epistasis) and nonshared environmental influences likely contribute to these differences in phenotypes. Further, the large disparity between the MZ and the DZ concordance rates has been attributed to epistasis (Pennington, 2009). Alternatively, rare gene variants causing a common disorder (autism), as described below, could contribute to this large MZ/DZ discordance.

Familiarity

Individuals with autism rarely marry and have children so that vertical transmission of the diagnosis from parent to child is rarely observed (Pennington, 2009). However, genetic transmission is still possible as parents can transmit genetic risk factors without having the diagnosis themselves. Family studies (cited in Geschwind & Konopka, 2009; Pennington, 2009) suggest that the risk of autism is 20–60% higher in siblings compared to the incidence of autism in the general population, and to that of other psychiatric disorders. Several studies have shown that a broad autism phenotype is transmitted in families of individuals with autism (Piven, 1999; Rutter, 2000). For example, first-degree relatives of individuals with autism were shown to be shy, aloof, and have problematic pragmatic language (Rutter, 2000). This pattern is consistent with the segregation of sub-threshold traits within these families (Abrahams & Geschwind, 2008).

Gender Differences

Finally, autism affects more boys than girls (4:1), a finding which has remained constant since Kanner's first description of autism in 1945, and despite the increasing incidence of this diagnosis. The predominantly male ratio has been attributed to an abnormality on the X chromosome (discussed below), or to sex linkage or genomic imprinting (Lintas & Persico, 2009; Marco & Skuse, 2006). Sex linkage involves a gene on the X chromosome transmitted from the mother to the son. As the son has only one X chromosome, this gene would be expressed. Since the mother's daughter has two copies of the X chromosome – one from her father and one from her mother – the daughter likely would not express the abnormal phenotype. The most well-known example of a sex-linked disorder is hemophilia, which is on the X chromosome. Genomic imprinting, on the other hand, is an epigenetic phenomenon wherein chemical modification of DNA that does not alter the basic DNA sequence or modification of the DNA-associated histone proteins determines whether the maternal or the paternal copy of a specific gene is expressed. Genomic imprinting has been determined for Prader Willi and Angelman's syndrome.

Finally, increased risk for autism has been identified in the offspring of older fathers (Reichenberg et al., 2006). Therefore, the gender and age of the parent may confer risk for offspring with autism.

Genetic Models of Autism

The conclusion drawn from indirect evidence is that autism is the most heritable and familial neurodevelopmental disorder (Pennington, 2009). With rare exceptions, however, autism does not appear to be the action of a single gene inherited in a strictly Mendelian pattern (autosomal dominant, recessive, or X-linked; Gupta & State, 2007; O'Roak & State, 2008). Rather, there are reports of multiple, distinctly rare changes in the genetic code in small subsets of individuals that cause or contribute to autism. There may be multiple gene variants – "a conspiracy of multiple genes" (Gupta & State, 2007) – that converge leading to a given phenotype.

Despite the indirect evidence for heritability and recent genetic technological advances, a genetic cause can be attributed to only 10–20% of all cases (reviewed in Abrahams & Geschwind, 2008), with a recent report suggesting a genetic cause can be uncovered in up to 40% of cases (Schaefer & Lutz, 2006). Further, Abraham and Geschwind (2008) state that no single genetic cause accounts for more than 1–2% of cases – similar to what is seen in mental retardation, another condition without a single genetic cause. While numerous studies identifying candidate genes or makers have been reported, very few studies have been replicated (Losh et al., 2008). Reasons to explain why candidates have not been agreed upon include the initial lack of uniform diagnostic criteria (strict vs. broad definition), limited power, varying methodology (Losh et al., 2008), and neglect of epigenetic factors modeling the disorder (Lahiri, Maloney, & Zawia, 2009). Further, as with other conditions with a strong heritable component, it appears that different genes may contribute to distinct components of the condition which gives rise to the full disorder through concerted actions (Losh et al., 2008; Pickles et al., 1995). Consequently, it has been said that linkage technology has not "found the autism gene," but rather it demonstrated that more powerful technology is necessary to explain the multiple genes associated with autism (Abrahams & Geschwind, 2008). No one knows just how heterogeneous the syndrome is likely to be, that is,

how many genes or regions of DNA (loci) may contribute either within a single individual or among the entire group of affected individuals. Some of the chromosomal regions and genes that have been associated with autism are summarized in Table 6.1 and will be addressed herein.

In addition, it is important to distinguish between locus heterogeneity, which refers to a variation at many different genes or loci resulting in a similar phenotype, and allelic heterogeneity, which refers to different variations or mutations at the same locus leading to an identical or overlapping clinical picture. Accumulating evidence suggest that both play a role in autism (O'Roak & State, 2008).

Recently, a rare-variant common disease model has been introduced (O'Roak & State, 2008). In this model, rare genes explain the common disease of autism. This makes sense in the Darwinian tradition that a deleterious change

Table 6.1 The polygenetics of autism, selected chromosomal regions, and genes

Chromosome and location[a]	Specific gene (if applicable)	Gene name (if applicable)	Normal protein function (if applicable)	Autism-associated endophenotypes (if applicable)	References
2p16.3	NRXN1	Neurexin 1	Cell adhesion, receptor, nervous system		Lintas and Persico (2009), Etherton et al. (2009); Szatmari et al. (2007)
2q					IMGSAC (1998), (2001b)
2q37					Costa de Silva (2008); Schaefer and Mendelsohn (2008)
5p15					Weiss et al., 2009
5p15.2	SEMA5A	Sema domain, seven thrombospondin repeats (type 1 and type 1-like), transmembrane domain (TM), and short cytoplasmic domain (semaphorin) 5A	Involved in axonal guidance during neural development		Weiss et al. (2009)
6q27					Weiss et al. (2009)
7q				Specific language impairment	Losh et al. (2008)
7q21-22					IMGSAC (1998), (2001a)
7q22	RELN	Reelin	Controls cell–cell interactions critical for cell positioning and neuronal migration during brain development		Ashley et al. (2007); Persico et al. (2002); Zhang et al. (2002)
7q31	FOXP2	Forkhead box P2	Development of speech and language regions of the brain during embryogenesis	Specific language impairment	Konopka et al. (2009); Lai et al. (2001); O'Brien et al. (2003)
7q31					Vincent et al. (2002)

Table 6.1 (continued)

Chromosome and location[a]	Specific gene (if applicable)	Gene name (if applicable)	Normal protein function (if applicable)	Autism-associated endophenotypes (if applicable)	References
7q31.1-31.3	ST7	Suppression of tumorigenicity 7	Function not determined		Vincent et al., 2002
7q31.2	WNT2	Wingless-type MMTV integration site family member 2	Implicated in oncogenesis and in several developmental processes		Wassink et al. (2004) Lai et al. (2001)
7q32-36					IMGSAC (1998); CLSA (1999)
7q35-36	CNTNAP2	Contactin-associated protein-like 2	Cell adhesion, local axonal differentiation	Autism language phenotype	Strauss et al. (2006), Jackman et al. (2009), Alarcon et al. (2008)
9q34	TSC1	Tuberous sclerosis 1	Growth inhibitory protein		Au et al. (2004); Fryer et al. (1987)
10q23.3	PTEN	Phosphatase and tensin homolog	Tumor suppressor, negatively regulates AKT/PKB signaling	Macrocephaly	Kwon et al. (2006); Butler et al. (2005), Herman et al. (2007a)
11q12-p13					Szatmari et al. (2007)
11q13	NRXN2	Neurexin 2	Cell adhesion, receptor, nervous system		Lintas and Persico (2009)
13q21				Specific language impairment	Bartlett et al. (2002), (2004)
14q31	NRXN3	Neurexin 3	Cell adhesion, receptor, nervous system		Feng et al. (2006)
15q11-13				Mental retardation, motor impairment, seizure, impairment in communication, restrictive and repetitive behavior	Cook et al. (1997); Schroer et al. (1998); Shao et al. (2003)
16p13.3	TSC2	Tuberous sclerosis 2	Tumor suppressor, stimulates specific GTPases		Au et al. (2004)
16q24				Specific language impairment	SLI Consortium (2002), (2004)
17p11					Costa e Silva (2008); Schaefer and Mendelsohn (2008)
17q11-17					Cantor et al. (2005)
17q11.1-q12	SLC6A4	Solute carrier family 6 (neurotransmitter transporter, serotonin), member 4	Transports serotonin into presynaptic neurons		Losh et al. (2008)
18q21.2-22.3					Mahr et al. (1996)
19q13				Specific language impairment	SLI Consortium (2002), (2004)
20p13					Weiss et al. (2009)
21q21.2-21.3	APP	Amyloid beta (A4) precursor protein	Neurite outgrowth, cell adhesion	Self-injurious and aggressive behavior	Bailey et al. (2008); Sokol et al. (2006)

Table 6.1 (continued)

Chromosome and location[a]	Specific gene (if applicable)	Gene name (if applicable)	Normal protein function (if applicable)	Autism-associated endophenotypes (if applicable)	References
22q11					Costa e Silva (2008); Schaefer and Mendelsohn (2008); Sykes and Lamb (2007)
22q13					Costa e Silva (2008); Schaefer and Mendelsohn (2008); Sykes and Lamb (2007)
22q13.3	SHANK3	SH3 and multiple ankyrin repeat domains 3	Connects neurotransmitter receptors, ion channels, and other membrane proteins to the actin cytoskeleton and G protein-coupled signaling pathways, and plays a role in synapse formation and dendritic spine maturation		Durand et al. (2007); Moessner et al. (2007)
Xp					Schaefer and Mendelsohn (2008)
Xq13.1	NLGN3	Neuroligin 3	Formation and remodeling of central nervous system synapses		Jamain et al. (2003)
Xq22.31-32	NLGN4X	Neuroligin 4, X-linked	Formation and remodeling of central nervous system synapses		Jamain et al. (2003), Laumonnier et al. (2004); Lawson-Yuen et al. (2008)
Xq27.3	FMR1	Fragile X mental retardation 1	mRNA translation regulation	Gaze avoidance, stereotypic movements, echolalia, ritualistic behaviors	Einfeld et al. (1989); Maes et al. (1993)
Xq28	MECP2	Methyl-CpG-binding protein 2	Binds to methyl-CpG in methylation regulation of gene expression	Mental retardation, female only	Lintas and Persico (2009)
XY mosaicism					Costa e Silva (2008); Sykes and Lamb (2007); Schafer and Mendelsohn (2008)
XYY					Costa e Silva (2008); Schaefer and Mendelsohn (2008)

[a]Chromosome location, gene symbol, gene name, and protein function are from the NCBI Entrez gene database (http://www.ncbi.nlm.nih.gov/gene/), accessed 1 January 2010.

in the human genome leads to reduced fitness and that this would not be likely to propagate within a population. Autism fits the rare gene-common disease model as it begins early in life, impairs social interactions, and is associated with mental retardation which impacts reproductive fitness (O'Roak & State, 2008). The large difference seen between monozygotic and dizygotic concordance rates is consistent with de novo (rare gene) mutation. It appears that simplex families demonstrate de novo mutations more frequently – with one family member with autism (Sebat et al., 2007) – whereas multiplex families demonstrate transmitted variants (Bakkaloglu et al., 2008). The search for rare variants has led to the study of families that are genetically isolated, with shared ancestry and prone to consanguinity (Morrow et al., 2008; Strauss et al., 2006) to locate recessive alleles. Finally, rare sequence variations have been detected, thanks to improved technology such as CNV analysis. Indeed within the last 5–10 years, 20 bona fide risk genes have been identified due to the improved technology developed after the linkage method (Abrahams & Geschwind, 2008). Several of these risk genes will be discussed in the following sections.

Genetic Research

Abrahams and Geschwind (2008) write that two views underlie genetic autism research. The first is that rare variants involve an abnormality in a single molecule causing the clinical pathology in autism. Mendelian inheritance (autosomal dominant vs. recessive) takes this form. Technology compatible with this approach includes cytogenetics (including karyotyping and FISH), gene association studies (analysis of genes and protein system from less complex genetic syndromes similar to autism such as Rett and fragile X syndromes), linkage studies (including genome screens in affected sibling pairs), microarray technology, and CNV analysis. The second view involves the study of independent hereditary endophenotypes representing the core features of autism. An endophenotype is an operationally defined behavioral feature such as age of first spoken word. Although there is a general consensus regarding endophenotypes commonly seen in autism, the behaviors may not be specific to autism, as delay in language acquisition accompanies many developmental disorders. Ideally, endophenotypes represent discreet behaviors which do not overlap with other behaviors from the autism core domains (i.e., language, socialization, and rigid behavior). For example, poor eye contact, representing a deficit with socialization, is construed as being independent of repetitive behaviors, thought to represent the rigid behavior domain. Genetic study of these discreet endophenotypes, largely undertaken via linkage studies, narrows the scope of analysis (Losh et al., 2008; O'Roak & State, 2008).

Cytogenetics: Rare Mutations

Reports of chromosomal abnormalities detected by karyotyping first demonstrated that rare variants may contribute to autism (Vorstman et al., 2006). Estimates of chromosomal abnormalities in autism range from 6 to 40% (Abrahams & Geschwind, 2008; Marshall et al., 2008; Pennington, 2009; Schaefer & Lutz, 2006) so that genetic workup is now being recommended for all children diagnosed with autism (Pennington, 2009; Schaefer & Mendelsohn, 2008).

Chromosome 15q11-13

Chromosomal studies have produced a great interest in chromosome 15q11-13, the site of the most frequent chromosomal anomaly seen in autism (reviewed in Veenstra-VanderWeele & Cook, 2004). The maternally derived duplication of this region involves an imprinting mechanism. Maternal interstitial duplication or supernumerary inverted duplication of 15q11-13 is seen in 1–3% of patients (Cook et al., 1990; Schroer et al., 1998). Clinical features of chromosomal derangement in this region include mental retardation, motor impairment, seizure disorder, and impairment in communication, in some but not all with autism or attention-deficit hyperactivity disorder (ADHD; Cook et al., 1997; Schroer et al., 1998).

The duplication of 15q11-13 seen in some cases of autism is the opposite of deletions from the same region seen in Angelman's syndrome (if inherited from the mother) or Prader Willi syndrome (if inherited from the father). Angelman's syndrome, known as the "happy puppet" phenotype, involves mental retardation, epilepsy, ataxia, lack of speech, predominant laughing and smiling, and a high rate of autism. Prader Willi syndrome associated with mental retardation and hyperphagia is only occasionally associated with autism. Presently, there is ongoing research regarding how duplications and deletions in this gene region lead to an increased risk of autism (Veenstra-VanderWeele & Cook, 2004). This region, however, has not been identified as one of interest in whole genome searches, perhaps due to its rarity (Pennington, 2009). Still, FISH analysis of chromosome 15q11-13 is often performed in evaluation of children with autism. Recently, FISH is being replaced by CGH due to improved detection of abnormality within the 15q11-13 region.

Fragile X Syndrome

Cytogenetic approaches provided the first evidence for an autism gene 40 years ago when Lubs (1969) identified an abnormal or "fragile" site on the long arm of chromosome X in four males with mental retardation, leading to the recognition of fragile X syndrome (FXS). This syndrome, associated with mental retardation and autistic features, is more severely expressed in males. FXS is caused by a deficiency of the fragile X mental retardation protein (FMRP), resulting from little or none of the disease gene fragile X mental retardation 1 (*FMR1*) mRNA. The *FMR1* gene mutation consisting of expanded CGG repeats of > 200 at chromosome site Xq27.3 is considered the origin of FXS. Autism, using the broad definition, has been reported in up to 30% of males with FXS, and FXS can be found in as many as 7–8% of individuals with autism (Muhle, Trentacoste, & Rapin, 2004).

Later studies, using DNA measures of the fragile X mutation rather than cytogenetics and strict autism criteria, have found a smaller association between FXS and autism (Pennington, 2009). Two investigations, however, which studied carefully controlled groups of FXS-negative and FXS-positive males matched on intelligence, found higher rates of the following autistic symptoms in FXS males: gaze avoidance and hand flapping (Einfeld, Molony, & Hall, 1989) and stereotypic movements (including hand flapping, rocking, and hitting, scratching, or rubbing their own bodies), echolalia, gaze avoidance, and ritualistic behaviors (Maes, Fryns, Van Walleghem, & Van den Berghe, 1993). Studies of endophenotype behaviors rather than the strict autism criteria are more likely to uncover robust similarities between FXS and autism.

Exploring similarities between rare sub-groups of patients with a known disorder and those with a more common disorder (autism) provides a window into the shared biology between the disorders. FMRP has been shown to interact with multiple transcripts in repressing metabotropic glutamate receptor-5 (mGluR$_5$) signaling activity which regulates long-term depression (LTD) associated with synaptic elimination. Without FMRP acting as a "brake," mGluR–LTD is enhanced (Bear, Huber, & Warren, 2004). This favors an anabolic state which could contribute to the key features of FXS such as epilepsy, cognitive impairment, loss of motor coordination, and increased density of thin, long, dendritic spines in neurons (Bear, 2005). These observations have invited drug trials of glutamate receptor antagonists to reduce the expression of mGluR$_5$ (Dolen et al., 2007) in individuals with FXS and in individuals with autism.

Investigation of Candidate Genes Contributing to Biochemical Pathways

Other genes contributing to medical conditions such as Alzheimer's disease are under investigation to determine if they, too, share biology with autism and FXS. The discovery of fragile X ataxia syndrome (FXTAS) provides a precedent to study the relationship of developmental conditions across the life span within and between families. FXTAS is an adult-onset ataxia/dementia syndrome found in older family members of individuals with FXS (Hagerman, 2002; Hagerman et al., 2001). In contrast to what is found in FXS, FXTAS occurs with a rise in *FMR1* mRNA level (Hagerman, 2006), fewer than 200 repeats (Basehore & Friez, 2009), and hypomethylation (Berry-Kravis, Potanas, Weinberg, Zhou, & Goetz, 2005) in the FMR1 CGG section on the X chromosome. This association of two clinically divergent disorders, regulated by the same gene produced in different doses, sets the stage for the investigation of the shared biology between autism, FXS, and other genes related to Alzheimer's disease such as amyloid precursor protein (APP).

Amyloid Precursor Protein

APP, which is encoded by a gene on chromosome 21, is a large (695–770 amino acid) glycoprotein produced in several central nervous system (CNS) cell types including microglia, astrocytes, oligodendrocytes, and neurons. After protein processing, mature APP is axonally transported and can be released from axon terminals in response to electrical activity. APP is believed to play an important role in neuronal maturation and in synaptogenesis as reviewed by Lahiri, Farlow, Greig, Giacobini, and Schneider (2003). APP is of great interest because processing products of APP can include the insoluble 40–42-amino acid amyloid β-peptide (Aβ-40 and Aβ-42, respectively), the principal component of the cerebral plaques associated with memory and cognitive decline in Alzheimer's disease (Alley et al., 2010). Recent research linking APP to autism illustrates how association studies enable the generation of new hypotheses about the biology of autism and ultimately advance our understanding of this disorder. Recently, we found evidence to support an association between autism and one of the APP pathways established for Alzheimer's disease. In contrast to the upregulation of the amyloidogenic pathway as seen in Alzheimer's disease, we found evidence that there may be an upregulation of the nonamyloidogenic (α-secretase amyloid precursor protein, sAPPα) pathway in a small sample of children with severe autism associated with self-injurious and aggressive behavior. That is, children with severe autism expressed total sAPP (representing the combined amyloidogenic and nonamyloidogenic pathways) at two or more times the levels of children without autism and up to four times the levels of children with mild autism (Sokol et al., 2006). Overall, there was a trend toward higher sAPPα within the children with autism. One of the severely autistic children in this study had FXS. High levels of sAPPα have also been found in a sample of children with autism from an independent laboratory (Bailey et al., 2008). High levels of sAPPα imply an increased α-secretase pathway in autism (anabolic), opposite to what is seen in Alzheimer's disease. This would be consistent with the brain overgrowth hypothesis attributed to autism, in contrast to the brain atrophy seen with the deposition of amyloid plaque in Alzheimer's disease. Coincidentally, via animal studies, Westmark and Malter (2007) concluded that FMRP binds to and regulates translation of APP mRNA through mGLuR$_5$, providing a potential link between neuronal proteins associated with AD and FXS. By way of mGluR$_5$, FMRP provides the "brake," which if unchecked in conditions such as FXS would favor high levels of APP. Further, high levels of APP have been found in another study of FMR1 knockout mice (D'Agata et al., 2002). These findings have led to enticing speculation that the APP gene may influence several neurodevelopmental disorders across the life span.

Chromosome 7q

Both chromosomal inversions and translocations have been reported near 7q31 in boys with autism. One of these translocation breakpoints identified the deranged gene as RAY1/ST7 (FAM4A1), a putative tumor suppressor gene (Vincent et al., 2002), and work in this region is ongoing. Mutations leading to amino acid changes have been found on the *WNT2* gene on 7q31 in two families with autism, and one affected parent transmitting the mutation to two affected children (Li et al., 2004; Wassink, Brzustowicz, Bartlett, & Szatmari, 2004). The *FOXP2* gene on 7q31 was found to be disrupted in one family with an autosomal dominant form of specific language impairment (SLI) (Lai, Fisher, Hurst, Vargha-Khadem, & Monaco, 2001), and this was replicated in a larger study of SLI (O'Brien, Zhang, Nishimura, Tomblin, & Murray, 2003), although initial studies failed to associate this with autism (Newbury et al., 2002; Wassink et al., 2001). Recently, FOXP2 differences in gene expression were found between chimp and human cell cultures (Konopka et al., 2009). Compared to chimps, in human culture, the *FOXP2* gene affected transcription upregulation in 61 genes and downregulation in 55 genes. Further, the *FOXP2* gene was shown to regulate downstream effects involving cerebellar motor function, craniofacial formation, and cartilage and connective tissue formation required for expressive language. As discussed in section "Endophenotype," there is a suspected association between the chromosome 7q region and speech abnormality seen in autism.

The *RELN* gene maps to chromosome 7q22. This gene encodes a protein that controls intercellular interactions involved in neuronal migration and positioning in brain development. A large polymorphic trinucleotide repeat in the 5′-YTR of the *RELN* gene has been implicated in autism in several studies (Ashley-Koch et al., 2007; Persico et al., 2002; Zhang et al., 2002). Further support for this candidate gene comes from the RELN mouse model which carries a large deletion in RELN and shows atypical cortical organization similar to cytoarchitectural pathological anomalies reported in the brains of individuals with autism (Bailey et al., 2008).

Phosphatase and Tensin Homolog Gene (PTEN)

PTEN is a tumor suppressor gene located on chromosome 10q23. This gene influences the cell–cell arrest cycle and apoptosis or programmed cell death (Lintas & Persico, 2009). PTEN inactivation causes excessive growth of dendrites and axons, with an increased number of synapses (Kwon et al., 2006). Mutations in PTEN cause Cowden's syndrome (macrocephaly, hamartomas, and autism). This gene has been of interest to autism researchers as macrocephaly has been considered to be one of the "most widely replicated biological findings in autism" affecting up to 20% of all children with the condition (McCaffery & Deutsch, 2005). Butler et al. (2005) examined the *PTEN* gene in 18 individuals with autism and macrocephaly. They discovered three with *PTEN* missense mutations. Others have found PTEN mutations in macrocephalic patients with autism (Herman et al., 2007a, 2007b).

Other Cytogenetic Regions

Cytogenic abnormalities have included deletions and duplications involving 2q37, 22 q13, 22q11, 17p11, 16p11.2,18q, Xp, and sex chromosome aneuploidies (47, XYY and 45, X/46, and XY mosaicism) (Costa e Silva, 2008; Mendelsohn & Schaefer, 2008; Schaefer & Mendelsohn, 2008; Sykes & Lamb, 2007). These genetic findings have generated interest in testing the association of a number of candidate genes in these regions via linkage and animal studies.

Autism and Synapse Formation (Synaptogenesis) Overview

Accumulating evidence points to the involvement of three genes (neuroligin, SHANK3, and neurexin) in the synapse formation of glutamate neurons. Glutamate is an excitatory neurotransmitter and aberrant glutamate function has long been suspected to contribute to autism. Neuroligins induce presynaptic differentiation in glutamate axons. SHANK3 encodes for a postsynaptic scaffolding protein which regulates the structural organization of dendritic spines in neurons. Consequently, SHANK3 is a binding partner of neuroligins. Neurexin induces glutamate postsynaptic differentiation in contacting dendrites. Altogether, these genes appear to contribute to glutamatergic synapse formation.

Neuroligin Genes (NLGN3 and NLGN4)

Neuronal cell adhesion is important in the development of the nervous system, contributing to axonal guidance, synaptic formation and plasticity, and neuronal–glial interactions (Glessner et al., 2009; Lien, Klezovitch, & Vasioukhin, 2006). Derangement in cell adhesion could contribute to migrational abnormalities including brain overgrowth. Neuroligins are cell-adhesion molecules localized postsynaptically at both glutamatergic (NLGN1, NLGN3, NLGN4, NLGN4Y) and γ-aminobutyric acidergic (NLGN2) synapses (Lintas & Persico, 2009). Neuroligins trigger the formation of functional presynaptic structures in contacting axons. As mentioned above, they interact with postsynaptic scaffolding proteins such as SHANK3 (see below). The *NLGN3* and *NLGN4* genes are located at chromosomes Xq13 and Xq22, 33, respectively, and mutations here have been associated with autism Jamain et al. (2003). Extensive genetic screens conducted by several research groups have confirmed the low frequency of neuroligin mutations among individuals with autism (Lintas & Persico, 2009). For example, Jamain et al. (2003) found a frameshift mutation in NLGN4 and a missense mutation in NLGN3 in two unrelated Swedish families, inherited from unaffected mothers. Laumonnier et al. (2004) reported a frameshift mutation in NLGN4 in 13 affected male members of a single pedigree. Lawson-Yuen, Saldivar, Sommer, and Picker (2008) found a deletion of exons 4–6 of NLGN4 in a boy with autism and in his brother with Tourette syndrome whose mother showed psychiatric problems and also carried the mutation. Neuroligin mutation carriers, however, display a variety of syndromes, such as X-linked mental retardation without autism (Laumonnier et al., 2004), Asperger's syndrome, autistic disorder of variable severity, and PDD-NOS (Yan et al., 2005). The symptoms may be slow, or abrupt and associated with regression. Despite intensive investigation, the low frequency of neuroligin mutations and the lack of similar phenotypes have led to the recommendation that neuroligins should not be included in widespread screens for individuals with nonsyndromic autism (Lintas & Persico, 2009).

SH3 Multiple Ankyrin Repeat Domains 3 Gene (SHANK3)

The *SHANK3* gene is located on chromosome 22q13.3 which encodes for a scaffolding protein found in the postsynaptic density complex of excitatory synapses binding to neuroligins. Recently, two studies have reported a correlation between mutations affecting SHANK3 and an autism phenotype characterized by severe verbal and social deficits (Durand et al., 2007; Moessner et al., 2007). Of the seven patients reported with the *SHANK3* gene mutations, five were deletions, one was a missense, and another a frameshift mutation. In addition, rare SHANK3 variations were present in the autism group, but not in the control group. These variations were inherited from healthy parents and they were present in unaffected siblings, perhaps demonstrating incomplete penetrance. Another interesting observation is that in both studies (Durand et al., 2007; Moessner et al., 2007), the SHANK3 deletion was

inherited via a paternal balanced translocation. Further, in both studies, siblings of the probands with SHANK3 abnormalities had partial 22q13 trisomy that resulted in attention-deficit hyperactivity disorder (Moessner et al., 2007) and Asperger's syndrome with early language development (Durand et al., 2007). Like neuroligins, SHANK3 mutations are very rare. However, because of the robust genotype–phenotype correlation reported in two studies (Durand et al., 2007; Moessner et al., 2007), it has been recommended that children with severe language and social impairment obtain SHANK3 mutation screening (Lintas & Persico, 2009).

Neurexin Genes

Presynaptic neurexins influence postsynaptic differentiation in contacting dendrites by interactions with postsynaptic neuroligins. Three neurexin genes (*NRXN1*, *NRXN2*, and *NRXN3*) are located on chromosome loci 2q32, 11q13, and 14q24.3-q31.1, respectively. Again, neurexin mutations are very rare. For example, two missense mutations were present in 4 of 264 (1.5%) individuals with autism compared to none in 729 controls (Feng et al., 2006). However, in this study, missense mutations also occurred in first-degree relatives who displayed heterogeneous phenotypes such as hyperactivity, depression, and learning problems. Incomplete penetrance may explain these findings, or autism may be caused by neurexin acting synergistically with other susceptibility genes. Neurexin-1α is being intensely studied in mice as deletion in this molecule resulted in increased repetitive behavior, whereas social behavior was relatively intact (Etherton, Blaiss, Powell, & Sudhof, 2009). This implies an animal model for a discreet feature of autistic behavior (endotype), as discussed below.

Contactin-associated protein-like 2 (CNTNAP2) is a member of the neurexin superfamily which involves a recessive frameshift mutation on chromosome 7q35. It is one of the largest genes of the human genome and encodes CASPR2, a transmembrane scaffolding protein. CNTNAP2 has been associated with cortical dysplasia–focal epilepsy in an Old Order Amish community (Strauss et al., 2006). Autism was present in up to 67% of these individuals. We recently reported CNTNAP2 in an Amish girl with epilepsy and autism who also showed hepatosplenomegaly (Jackman, Horn, Molleston, & Sokol, 2009). CNTNAP2 has been associated with an autism language phenotype in large studies of non-Amish individuals (Alarcon et al., 2008). Further, stage two of this investigation showed that CNTNAP2 was expressed in the language centers (frontal and anterior temporal lobes) of fetal brain (Alarcon et al., 2008). It has been recommended that Amish children presenting with autism should be tested for *CNTNAP2* gene mutation (Strauss, personal communication). This work again supports a language function associated with chromosome 7.

The Methyl-CpG-Binding Protein 2 Gene

Methyl-CpG-binding protein 2 (MeCP2) works as a transcriptional repressor within gene-promoting regions involved in chromatin repression. This gene is located on chromosome Xq28 and shows mutation in 80% of females with Rett syndrome (pervasive developmental disorder, acquired microcephaly, epilepsy, and loss of hand function). This gene has been studied in children with autism, and MeCP2 mutations are considered to be rare (0.8–1.3%) in females with autism. Interestingly, autism and Rett syndrome share some similarities at the phenotypic and pathogenic levels, and both disorders were proposed to result from disruption of postnatal or experience-dependent synaptic plasticity (Zoghbi, 2003). Among the Rett mutations reported are a frameshift mutation, a nonsense mutation, and additional introns (Lintas & Persico, 2009). Schaefer and Mendelsohn (2008) observe that MeCP2 has not been associated with idiopathic autism in males so that this gene test is recommended only for females with autism.

Linkage Studies

Linkage studies involve determining whether the transmission of a chromosomal segment from one generation to another coincides with the presence of the phenotype of interest (Gupta & State, 2007). Linkage can be utilized in Mendelian inherited conditions and can also be used to study complex conditions such as in autism when Mendelian inheritance is unlikely, and there is no hypotheses regarding the specific nature of transmission.

Linkage studies can be grouped into two types – the conventional study of a chromosomal region of interest in affected sibling–pairs from multiplex families and the more recent genome-wide linkage analysis in which every chromosome is evaluated simultaneously. In the sib–pair study method, siblings with autism are evaluated to determine whether they share any regions of the genome more frequently than would be expected by chance.

Genomic wide association studies compare genetic risk factors in the form of specific genetic markers in cases and controls. These markers are distributed within the entire genome rather than limited to specific gene regions such as in the sib–pair method. This enables a more unbiased ascertainment of regions of interest (Losh et al., 2008). Several genome-wide scans of individuals with autism have been reported and evidence in favor of linkage has been determined for the majority of chromosomes (Gupta & State,

2007). The trouble with these studies is that the evidence has not reached statistical significance and there is lack of replication for many of these findings. Statistical significance is calculated by a logarithm of the odds (LOD) score. This score represents the logarithm of the likelihood ratio of observing the data under a model of linkage to observing the data under a model of free recombination (no linkage). An LOD score of 3.5 in a sib–pair analysis is considered to be a significant linkage (Lander & Kruglyak, 1995). Suggestive linkage is an LOD score of 2.2, and a highly significant LOD score is 5.4. For replication studies, the replication threshold is considered to be 1.4 (Lander & Kruglyak, 1995). By chance, one would expect to see a suggestive linkage peak once every genome scan or a significant peak once every 20 scans (Gupta & State, 2007).

Most linkage studies have identified linkage regions reaching the level of suggestive linkage at best (Freitag, 2007). Despite large increases in the size of patient cohorts, linkage signals have not increased significantly with sample size (Abrahams & Geschwind, 2008). Only three loci (2q, 7q, and 17q11-17) have been replicated for nonsyndromic autism and are considered to have genome-wide significance. Genomic-wide screens have engendered great interest in chromosome 7q with distinctive peaks involving two distinct regions: 7q21-22 and 7q32-36 (International Molecular Genetic Study of Autism Consortium-IMGSAC, 1998; Collaborative Linkage Study of Autism, 2001). As chromosome 7q has been discussed in section "Cytogenetics: Rare Mutations," chromosome 2 and then 17q11 will follow the description of how linkage studies led to the discovery of the gene loci for a syndromic form of autism: tuberous sclerosis complex (TSC). The sibling–pair from multiplex family design has been used to study autism within many genetic loci, including those involved in TSC; the genome-wide linkage analysis has detected linkage on chromosomes 7q, 2q, 17q11, and novel loci.

Tuberous Sclerosis Complex

Tuberous sclerosis complex (TSC) is a neurodevelopmental disorder characterized by cognitive delay, epilepsy, and neurocutaneous growths including hamartomas (i.e., tubers) within the central nervous system and other organs. Up to 60% of individuals with TSC have autism. The first suspicion of a chromosomal abnormality associated with TSC originated from a linkage study of 26 protein markers within 19 multigenerational families affected with TSC (Fryer et al., 1987). In eight of the families, ABO blood group gene mapped to chromosome 9q34.3. Many groups corroborated these results using larger numbers of families (Au, Williams, Gambello, & Northrup, 2004). These linkage studies established the *TSC1* gene, later discovered to encode hamartin, a growth suppressor protein.

Another TSC gene site was discovered via linkage studies on chromosome 16p13.3, known as TSC2. This gene produces the tumor suppressor protein tuberin. Further evidence showed that hamartin works together with tuberin in several cell-signaling pathways including a growth and translation regulatory pathway (P13K/PKB), a cell adhesion/migration/protein transportation pathway [glycogen synthase kinase 3 (GSK3)/β-catenin/focal adhesion kinase/Ras-related homolog (Rho) pathway], and a cell growth and proliferation pathway [mitogen-activated protein kinase (MAPK)]. The tuberin–hamartin complex affects mTOR kinase activity (Au et al., 2004), promoting tumor growth. This discovery has led to the study of rapamycin, a drug used in organ transplant and cancer treatment, as a therapy for suppressing growth of tumors in TSC (Kenerson, Aicher, True, & Yeung, 2002).

Other growth-promoting genes such as *PTEN* have been linked to the tuberin–hamartin gene complex as contributors to the general overgrowth in TSC. As previously discussed, *PTEN* is a gene of interest in autism.

Chromosome 2q

Buxbaum et al. (2007), together with the Seaver Autism Research Center (SARS), reported a two-point dominant LOD score of 2.25 on chromosome 2q in 35 affected sibling pairs. In a second-stage screening which employed 60 families with autism probands, the strongest linkage was at this same location. The IMGSAC study showed a strong linkage to 7q as described above, but also found linkage to 2q (IMGSAC, 1998), with a more recent study also providing evidence for linkage to 2q (IMGSAC, 2001b).

Chromosome 17q

Early recognition of the need for large patient cohorts and substantial genetic heterogeneity led to the establishment of the autism genetic resource exchange (AGRE) composed of over 500 families. AGRE is a publically available resource of phenotypic data and biomaterials. Genomic scan linkage analysis was performed on 109 autistic sibling pairs from 91 AGRE families together with analysis of those pairs from an independent sample of 345 families from the same AGRE cohort (Cantor et al., 2005). When families with autism were stratified into only those with affected males, there was significant linkage at 17q11-21 in both samples. The LOD score for this replicated work was at genome-wide level of significance (LOD score > 1.4). One positional candidate gene close to this region is the serotonin transporter gene

(*SLC6A4*) which codes for a protein controlling the reuptake of serotonin in the synapse. This was exciting as elevated levels of serotonin have been determined in 25–30% of cases of autism (Cook et al., 1990). Indeed, relationship between the SLC6A4 site and a repeat polymorphic region in its promoter region (5HTTLPR) recently has been independently investigated (Losh et al., 2008). The chromosome 17q locus, however, has not been uniformly observed in subsequent, large-scale studies (Schellenberg et al., 2006) which may be due to phenotypic heterogeneity.

Novel Loci for Autism

A very recent genome-wide linkage mapping study in a sample of 1,031 multiplex autism families (Weiss, Arking, Daly, & Chakravarti, 2009) identified significant linkage on chromosome 20p13 and suggestive linkage on chromosome 6q27. In this study, no associations meeting criteria for genome-wide significance were found, suggesting there are not many common loci of moderate to large effect size. However, replication data revealed a novel SNP locus on chromosome 5p15. This region was adjacent to SEMA5A, a member of the semaphoring axonal guidance protein family which has been shown to be downregulated in transformed B lymphocytes from autism samples (Weiss et al., 2009). The authors further demonstrated lower *SEMA5A* gene expression in autism brain tissue. This finding is in keeping with the suspected derangement in the migration of cortical neurons during embryogenesis in autism.

Microarray Technology

Microarray technology is transforming the identification of chromosome duplications and deletions (Gupta & State, 2007). This new technology, known as high-density, oligonucleotide-based array comparative genomic hybridization (aCGH), is now available for widespread use. This technique uses patient DNA and control DNA, each labeled with a fluorescent tag (red or green). Equal amounts of DNA from patient and control are hybridized to known regions of the human genome pre-arrayed on a slide. If patient and control have equal copy numbers at a given locus, the color turns yellow, representing an equal measure of DNA. If the patient has lost (deleted) a locus, only the control color is visualized. If the patient has an extra copy at a locus (duplication), the patient color predominates. The aCGH probe may be enriched for known genes or specific chromosomal regions for known syndromes, or distributed evenly across the whole genome. This new technique is now available at all major medical centers and through Signature Genomic Laboratories (www.signaturegenomics.com).

Single-nucleotide polymorphism (SNP) analysis probes thousands of SNPs and provides data about copy number and genotype (Li & Andersson, 2009). The genotype can be used to study uniparental disomy (UPI) seen in imprinting disorders and consanguinity. This technique is better at focused study of specific gene regions instead of the whole genome. Additionally, SNP analysis uses pre-established laboratory standards rather than intraexperimental controls. Both SNP analysis and aCGH map produce copy number variation, and it is common for labs to first perform aCGH and follow up with SNP in specific regions of interest.

Today, CNV from several thousand nucleotides can be identified, greatly improving upon the sensitivity of conventional cytogenetics. Sebat et al. (2007) showed that CNVs were present in 10% of affected individuals from single-incidence autism families (i.e., sporadic cases), contrasting with substantially lower rates observed in controls (1%) and autism cases from multiplex families (3%). This has led to the general expectation that de novo CNVs are more likely to be found in sporadic (and as it turns out, dysmorphic) cases. Jacquemont et al., 2006 reported CNV rearrangements in 8 (27.5%) of 29 patients with syndromic autism (including facial dysmorphism, limb or visceral malformations, and growth abnormalities). There were no reoccurrence or overlap in these variants for the eight children. Chromosome 11q12-p13 and neurexins were implicated in a linkage study using SNP–CNV in 1,181 families with at least two affected individuals through the Autism Genome Project (Szatmari et al., 2007).

Microarray technology, however, comes with the realization that typically developing individuals have more structural variants than previously imagined (Sebat et al., 2007). There is growing concern that CNV irregularities may not be pathological and therefore not be a cause of autism (Tabor & Cho, 2007). These authors note that using diagnostic tools prematurely in a clinical context may be "unethical, either because of over-treatment, under-treatment, unwarranted labeling and stigmatization, or a false sense of security." Certainly, further studies on large cohorts of children with the same deletion/duplication are necessary to enable clinical application of this technology.

Endophenotypes

Due to the phenotypic heterogeneity of autism and the lack of finding a specific gene, researchers have narrowed the scope of analysis to more pure, operationally defined behaviors/traits. Endophenotypes are behavioral, physiological, and/or neuropsychological markers that are present in both affected and unaffected individuals. Rather than searching for "autism genes," endophenotype investigations search for smaller grouping of genes that contribute to discreet

phenotypes (Losh et al., 2008). This approach allows for measurement of "dosage" of a trait and can be applied to affected as well as unaffected individuals.

Specific Language Impairment

Specific language impairment (SLI) is defined as the failure of normal development of language without hearing loss, mental retardation, or oral motor, neurological, or psychiatric impairment. This affects approximately 7% of children entering school (Tomblin et al., 1997). Individuals with SLI perform poorly on phonologically based tasks and many go on to develop dyslexia (Stothard, Snowling, Bishop, Chipchase, & Kaplan, 1998). There appears to be neurostructural association between SLI and autism (Herbert et al., 2002; 2004), and there is an associated finding of language delay in relatives of probands with autism (Wassink et al., 2004). Several investigations have found strong linkage of SLI to chromosome 13q21 (Bartlett et al., 2002; 2004) and to chromosomes 16q and 19q (SLI Consortium, 2002, 2004). This finding is noteworthy as it directly overlies the 16q locus linked to autism (Wassink et al., 2004). A specific language marker, age of first word, has shown significant linkage to chromosome 7 observed by five separate investigators (Losh et al., 2008). The 7q region has been the subject of intense investigation, as described above, and may be the loci associated with autism language.

Restrictive and Repetitive Behavior

The restricted and repetitive behavior (RRB) endophenotype in children with autism is receiving attention (Morgan, Wetherby, & Barber, 2008). RRB comprises one prong of the autism clinical triad (language deficit, social deficit, and RRB). Cuccaro et al. (2003) identified two factors underlying RRB as measured by the Autism Diagnostic Interview-Revised (ADI-R): repetitive sensory motor actions and resistance to change. This is of interest as a genetic linkage signal has been reported for resistance to change on chromosome 15 (Shao et al., 2003). It appears that the analysis of phenotypic homogeneous subtypes may be a powerful tool for mapping of candidate genes in complex traits such as autism.

Clinical Genetics Evaluation

The recent marked increase in the incidence and awareness of autism has resulted in an increase in the number of children sent for diagnostic evaluation. The general consensus within the literature is that genetic consultation should be conducted on all persons with the confirmed diagnosis of autism. While referral for genetic consult is often preferred, often the primary practitioner, pediatrician, and/or pediatric neurologist are in a position to conduct the initial evaluation. Further, clinical geneticists may not be available, particularly in underserved areas of the country, or a timely genetic evaluation may not be possible due to lengthy waiting lists. Therefore, the clinician taking care of a child with autism may wish to initiate the genetic evaluation.

Recently, sequential guidelines for clinical genetics evaluation in autism have been published by Schaefer, Mendelsohn, and the Professional Practice and Guidelines Committee (2008) (see Box 6.5). These evidence-based guidelines have evolved from an original retrospective study of patients referred for clinical genetics evaluation between the years 2002 and 2004 at the University of Nebraska Medical Center (Schaefer & Lutz, 2006). The guidelines are dynamic rather than static and have been updated, for example, as aCGH has become more available. The stepwise approach was designed to balance cost with the expected yield of the tests. Further, there is a pyramidal effect so that "earlier tiers have a greater expected diagnostic yield, lower invasiveness of testing, better potential of intervention, and easier overall practicality" (Schaefer & Mendelsohn, 2008). Summarizing the diagnostic yields expected for the following investigations (high-resolution chromosome studies, 5%; aCGH – beyond that detected by chromosome analysis – 10%; fragile X, 5%; MECP2, 5% women only; PTEN, 3% if head circumference >2.5 SD; other, 10%), it was predicted that utilization of these guidelines would lead to diagnosis in 40% of cases (Schaefer, Mendelsohn, and the Professional Practice and Guidelines Committee (2008). Finally, this stepwise approach has met the approval of third-party payers and families (Schaefer & Lutz, 2006).

Box 6.5 Template for the Clinical Genetic Diagnostic Evaluation of Autism Spectrum Disorders
Pre-evaluation
   Confirmation of diagnosis of autism by trained professional using objective criteria and tools
   Sensory screening (complete audiogram)
   Electroencephalogram – if clinical suspicion of seizures
   Cognitive testing
Verify results of newborn screening
   (High-resolution chromosomal analysis and fragile X studies may be performed before referral)
First tier
   Initial evaluation to identify known syndromes or associated conditions

   Examination with special attention to dysmorphic features
      Should include Wood's lamp evaluation
   If specific diagnosis is suspected, proceed with targeted testing
      Rubella titers – if clinical indicators present
      "Standard" metabolic screening – if clinical indicators present and if suspected condition was not assessed by newborn screening
   Urine mucopolysaccharides and organic acids
   Serum lactate, amino acids, ammonia, and acylcarnitine profile
   High-resolution chromosomal analysis – if not already performed.
Second tier
   Fibroblast karyotype if leukocyte karyotype is normal and clonal pigmentary abnormalities are noted
   Comparative genomic hybridization (chromosomal microarray)
   MECP2 gene testing (females only)
   PTEN gene testing (if head circumference is 2.5 SD greater than the mean)
Third tier
   Brain magnetic resonance imaging
   Serum and urine uric acid
   If elevated, hypoxanthine–guanine phosphoribosyltransferase (HgPRT) and
   Phosphoribosylpyrophosphate (PRPP) synthetase superactivity testing
   If low, purine/pyrimidine panel (uracil excretion, xanthine, and hypoxanthine)
   If severe language deficit, check for *Shank3* mutation*
Extracted from Shaefer, GB, Mendelsohn, NJ & the Professional Practice and Guidelines Committee (2008). Clinical genetics evaluation in identifying the etiology of autism spectrum disorders. *Genetics in Medicine, 10*, 301–305 and used with the authors' permission.
*Recommended by Sokol and Lahiri

Pre-evaluation

This initial step includes confirming the diagnosis of autism using objective (DSM-IV) criteria and/or standardized objective measures such as those discussed in Chapter 15. An audiogram is obtained to rule out hearing loss and an electroencephalogram (EEG) is obtained if there is a clinical suspicion of seizures. Cognitive testing, when appropriate, can determine mental retardation. Finally, verifying the results of the newborn screen can help rule out rubella and PKU.

Tier 1

Initial assessment involves a standard clinical genetic history and physical exam to identify known syndromes or associated conditions. Included would be a Wood's lamp examination of the skin to help rule out neurocutaneous conditions such as TSC. Also, for suspected diagnoses, standard metabolic screening is performed to check for urine mucopolysaccharides and organic acids as well as serum lactate, amino acid, ammonia, and acylcarnitine profile. If not already performed, high-resolution chromosomal analysis and DNA for fragile X is sent.

Tier 2

If the studies in the first tier are unrevealing, the second tier checks for aCGH duplications and deletions. For patients with pigmentary abnormalities on exam but with a normal leukocyte karyotype, skin biopsy can be obtained to obtain a fibroblast karyotype. For females, MECP2 gene testing is obtained; for children with head circumference greater than 2.5 SD from the mean, PTEN gene testing is recommended.

Tier 3

Lower yield tests have been reserved for this level: brain magnetic resonance imaging and serum and urine uric acid. Further tests are outlined depending on the results (high or low) of the uric acid tests. We would add here that if a child has significant language impairment, a Shank3 mutation should be ruled out.

Finally, new susceptibility loci that can contribute to the autism phenotype are continually identified and catalogued in the Online Mendelian Inheritance in Man (OMIM) database (http//www.ncbi.nlm.nih.gov/sites/entrez). Using this search engine, a patient's phenotype including dysmorphic features can be entered into the program to generate a list of possible genetic diagnoses.

Counseling

Most clinical geneticists work with genetic counselors who interpret the findings into recurrent risks for full siblings. The tiered clinical genetics evaluation should identify two groups of individuals: those with and those without an identifiable etiology for autism. For those without an identifiable etiology, counseling should be provided according to multifactorial inheritance (Schaefer & Mendelsohn, 2008). That is, 4% recurrence rate if the proband is a girl and 7% if the proband is a boy. If a second child has autism, a reasonable recurrence rate, based upon published reports, is 30%.

Acknowledgment Thanks to Bryan Maloney, M.S. for his help in editing this manuscript.

References

Abrahams, B. S., & Geschwind, D. H. (2008). Advances in autism genetics: On the threshold of a new neurobiology. *Nature Reviews Genetics, 9*(5), 341–355.

Alarcon, M., Abrahams, B. S., Stone, J. L., Duvall, J. A., Perederiy, J. V., Bomar, J. M., et al. (2008). Linkage, association, and gene-expression analyses identify CNTNAP2 as an autism-susceptibility gene. *American Journal of Human Genetics, 82*(1), 150–159.

Alley, G. M., Bailey, J. A., Chen, D. -M., Ray, B., Puli, L. K., Tanila, H., et al. (2010). Memantine lowers amyloid-beta peptide levels in neuronal cultures and in APP/PS1 transgenic mice. *Journal of Neuroscience Research, 88*, 143–154.

Ashley-Koch, A. E., Jaworski, J., Ma de, Q., Mei, H., Ritchie, M. D., Skaar, D. A., et al. (2007). Investigation of potential gene–gene interactions between APOE and RELN contributing to autism risk. *Psychiatric Genetics, 17*, 221–226.

Au, K. S., Williams, A. T., Gambello, M. J., & Northrup, H. (2004). Molecular genetic basis of tuberous sclerosis complex: From bench to bedside. *Journal of Child Neurology, 19*, 699–709.

Bailey, A. R., Giunta, B. N., Obregon, D., Nikolic, W. V., Tian, J., Sanberg, C. D., et al. (2008). Peripheral biomarkers in autism: Secreted amyloid precursor protein-alpha as a probable key player in early diagnosis. *International Journal of Clinical Experimental Medicine, 1*, 338–344.

Bailey, A., Le Couteur, A., Gottesman, I., Bolton, P., Simonoff, E., Yuzda, E., et al. (1995). Autism as a strongly genetic disorder: Evidence from a British twin study. *Psychological Medicine, 25*, 63–77.

Bakkaloglu, B., O'Roak, B. J., Louvi, A., Gupta, A. R., Abelson, J. F., Morgan, T. M., et al. (2008). Molecular cytogenetic analysis and resequencing of contactin associated protein-like 2 in autism spectrum disorders. *American Journal of Human Genetics, 82*, 165–173.

Bartlett, C. W., Flax, J. F., Logue, M. W., Smith, B. J., Vieland, V. J., Tallal, P., et al. (2004). Examination of potential overlap in autism and language loci on chromosomes 2, 7, and 13 in two independent samples ascertained for specific language impairment. *Human Hereditary, 57*, 10–20.

Bartlett, C. W., Flax, J. F., Logue, M. W., Vieland, V. J., Bassett, A. S., Tallal, P., et al. (2002). A major susceptibility locus for specific language impairment is located on 13q21. *American Journal of Human Genetics, 71*, 45–55.

Basehore, M. J., & Friez, M. J. (2009). Molecular Analysis of Fragile X Syndrome. *Current Protocols in Human Genetics, 63* (Chapter 9, Unit 9).

Bear, M. F. (2005). Therapeutic implications of the mGluR theory of fragile X mental retardation. *Genes Brain & Behavior, 4*, 393–398.

Bear, M. F., Huber, K. M., & Warren, S. T. (2004). The mGluR theory of fragile X mental retardation. *Trends in Neuroscience, 27*, 370–377.

Berry-Kravis, E., Potanas, K., Weinberg, D., Zhou, L., & Goetz, C. G. (2005). Fragile X-associated tremor/ataxia syndrome in sisters related to X-inactivation. *Annals of Neurology, 57,* 144–147.

Butler, M. G., Dasouki, M. J., Zhou, X. P., Talebizadeh, Z., Brown, M., Takahashi, T. N., et al. (2005). Subset of individuals with autism spectrum disorders and extreme macrocephaly associated with germline PTEN tumour suppressor gene mutations. *Journal of Medical Genetics, 42,* 318–321.

Buxbaum, J. D., Cai, G., Chaste, P., Nygren, G., Goldsmith, J., Reichert, J., et al. (2007). Mutation screening of the PTEN gene in patients with autism spectrum disorders and macrocephaly. *American Journal of Medical Genetics, 144B,* 484–491.

Cantor, R. M., Kono, N., Duvall, J. A., Alvarez-Retuerto, A., Stone, J. L., Alarcon, M., et al. (2005). Replication of autism linkage: Fine-mapping peak at 17q21. *American Journal of Human Genetics, 76,* 1050–1056.

Collaborative Linkage Study of Autism (CLSA). (1999). An autosomal genomic screen for autism. *American Journal of Medical Genetics, 88,* 609–615.

Collaborative Linkage Study of Autism. (2001). An autosomal genomic screen for autism. *American Journal of Medical Genetics, 105,* 609–615.

Cook, E. H., Jr., Leventhal, B. L., Heller, W., Metz, J., Wainwright, M., & Freedman, D. X. (1990). Autistic children and their first degree relatives: Relationships between serotonin and norepinephrine levels and intelligence. *The Journal of Neuropsychiatry and Clinical Neurosciences, 2,* 268–274.

Cook, E. H., Jr., Lindgren, V., Leventhal, B. L., Courchesne, R., Lincoln, A., Shulman, C., et al. (1997). Autism or atypical autism in maternally but not paternally derived proximal 15q duplication. *American Journal of Human Genetics, 60,* 928–934.

Costa e Silva, J. A. (2008). Autism, a brain developmental disorder: Some new pathophysiologic and genetics findings. *Metabolism, 57*(Suppl 2), S40–S43.

Courchesne, E., Carper, R., & Akshoomoff, N. (2003). Evidence of brain overgrowth in the first year of life in autism. *Journal of the American Medical Association, 290,* 337–344.

Courchesne, E., Karns, C. M., Davis, H. R., Ziccardi, R., Carper, R. A., Tigue, Z. D., et al. (2001). Unusual brain growth patterns in early life in patients with autistic disorder: An MRI study. *Neurology, 57,* 245–254.

Cuccaro, M. L., Shao, Y., Grubber, J., Slifer, M., Wolpert, C. M., Donnelly, S. L., et al. (2003). Factor analysis of restricted and repetitive behaviors in autism using the autism diagnostic interview-R. *Child Psychiatry and Human Development, 34,* 3–17.

DiCicco-Bloom, E. (2006). Neuron, know thy neighbor. *Science, 311,* 1560–1562.

Dolen, G., Osterweil, E., Rao, B. S., Smith, G. B., Auerbach, B. D., Chattarji, S., et al. (2007). Correction of fragile X syndrome in mice. *Neuron, 59,* 955–962.

Durand, C. M., Betancur, C., Boeckers, T. M., Bockmann, J., Chaste, P., Fauchereau, F., et al. (2007). Mutations in the gene encoding the synaptic scaffolding protein SHANK3 are associated with autism spectrum disorders. *Nature Genetics, 39,* 25–27.

D'Agata, V., Warren, S. T., Zhao, W., Torre, E. R., Alkon, D. L., & Cavallaro, S. (2002). Gene expression profiles in a transgenic animal model of fragile X syndrome. *Neurobiology of Disease, 10,* 211–218.

Einfeld, S., Molony, H., & Hall, W. (1989). Autism is not associated with the fragile X syndrome. *American Journal of Medical Genetics, 34,* 187–193.

Etherton, M. R., Blaiss, C. A., Powell, C. M., & Sudhof, T. C. (2009). Mouse neurexin-1alpha deletion causes correlated electrophysiological and behavioral changes consistent with cognitive impairments. *Proceedings of the National Academy of Sciences, 106,* 17998–18003.

Feng, J., Schroer, R., Yan, J., Song, W., Yang, C., Bockholt, A., et al. (2006). High frequency of neurexin 1beta signal peptide structural variants in patients with autism. *Neuroscience Letters, 409,* 10–13.

Folstein, S., & Rutter, M. (1977). Infantile autism: A genetic study of 21 twin pairs. *Journal of Child Psychology and Psychiatry, 18,* 297–321.

Freitag, C. M. (2007). The genetics of autistic disorders and its clinical relevance: A review of the literature. *Molecular Psychiatry, 12,* 2–22.

Fryer, A. E., Chalmers, A., Connor, J. M., Fraser, I., Povey, S., Yates, A. D., et al. (1987). Evidence that the gene for tuberous sclerosis is on chromosome 9. *Lancet, 1,* 659–661.

Geschwind, D. H. (2009). Advances in autism. *Annual Review of Medicine, 60,* 367–380.

Geschwind, D. H., & Konopka, G. (2009). Neuroscience in the era of functional genomics and systems biology. *Nature, 461,* 908–915.

Glessner, J. T., Wang, K., Cai, G., Korvatska, O., Kim, C. E., Wood, S., et al. (2009). Autism genome-wide copy number variation reveals ubiquitin and neuronal genes. *Nature, 459,* 569–573.

Gupta, A. R., & State, M. W. (2007). Recent advances in the genetics of autism. *Biological Psychiatry, 61,* 429–437.

Hagerman, R. J. (2002). The physical and behavioral phenotype. In R. J. Hagerman & P. J. Hagerman (Eds.), *Fragile X syndrome: Diagnosis, treatment, and research* (3rd ed., pp. 3–109). Baltimore: Johns Hopkins University Press.

Hagerman, R. J. (2006). Lessons from fragile X regarding neurobiology, autism, and neurodegeneration. *Journal of Developmental Behavioral Pediatrics, 27,* 63–74.

Hagerman, R. J., Leehey, M., Heinrichs, W., Tassone, F., Wilson, R., Hills, J., et al. (2001). Intention tremor, parkinsonism, and generalized brain atrophy in male carriers of fragile X. *Neurology, 57,* 127–130.

Herbert, M. R., Harris, G. J., Adrien, K. T., Ziegler, D. A., Makris, N., Kennedy, D. N., et al. (2002). Abnormal asymmetry in language association cortex in autism. *Annals of Neurology, 52,* 588–596.

Herbert, M. R., Ziegler, D. A., Makris, N., Filipek, P. A., Kemper, T. L., Normandin, J. J., et al. (2004). Localization of white matter volume increase in autism and developmental language disorder. *Annals of Neurology, 55,* 530–540.

Herman, G. E., Butter, E., Enrile, B., Partore, M., Prior, T. W., & Sommer, A. (2007b). Increasing knowledge of PTEN germline mutations: Two additional patients with autism and macrocephaly. *American Journal of Medical Genetics, 143,* 589–593.

Herman, G. E., Henninger, N., Ratliff-Schaub, K., Pastore, M., Fitzgerald, S., & MCBride, K. L. (2007a). Genetic testing in autism: How much is enough? *Genetics in Medicine, 9,* 268–273.

International HapMap Consortium. (2005). A haplotype map of the human genome. *Nature, 437,* 1299–1320.

International Molecular Genetic Study of Autism Consortium (IMGSAC). (1998). A full genome screen for autism with evidence for linkage to a region on chromosome 7q. International molecular genetic study of autism consortium. *Human Molecular Genetics, 7,* 571–578.

International Molecular Genetic Study of Autism Consortium (IMGSAC). (2001a). Further characterization of the autism susceptibility locus AUTS1 on chromosome 7q. *Human Molecular Genetics, 10,* 973–982.

International Molecular Genetic Study of Autism Consortium (IMGSAC). (2001b). A genomewide screen for autism: Strong evidence for linkage to chromosomes 2q, 7q, and 16p. *American Journal of Human Genetics, 69,* 570–581.

Jackman, C., Horn, N. D., Molleston, J. P., & Sokol, D. K. (2009). Gene associated with seizures, autism, and hepatomegaly in an Amish girl. *Pediatric Neurology, 40,* 310–313.

Jacquemont, M. L., Sanlaville, D., Redon, R., Raoul, O., Cormier-Daire, V., Lyonnet, S., et al. (2006). Array-based comparative genomic hybridisation identifies high frequency of cryptic chromosomal rearrangements in patients with syndromic autism spectrum disorders. *Journal of Medical Genetics, 43*, 843–849.

Jamain, S., Quach, H., Betancur, C., Rastam, M., Colineaux, C., Gillberg, I. C., et al. (2003). Mutations of the X-linked genes encoding neuroligins NLGN3 and NLGN4 are associated with autism. *Nature Genetics, 34*, 27–29.

Kenerson, H. L., Aicher, L. D., True, L. D., & Yeung, R. S. (2002). Activated mammalian target of rapamycin pathway in the pathogenesis of tuberous sclerosis complex renal tumors. *Cancer Research, 62*, 5645–5650.

Konopka, G., Bomar, J. M., Winden, K., Coppola, G., Jonsson, Z. O., Gao, F., et al. (2009). Human-specific transcriptional regulation of CNS development genes by FOXP2. *Nature, 462*, 213–217.

Kwon, C. H., Luikart, B. W., Powell, C. M., Zhou, J., Matheny, S. A., Zhang, W., et al. (2006). Pten regulates neuronal arborization and social interaction in mice. *Neuron, 50*, 377–388.

Lahiri, D. K., Farlow, M. R., Greig, N. H., Giacobini, E., & Schneider, L. S. (2003). A critical analysis of new molecular targets and strategies for drug developments in Alzheimer's disease. *Current Drug Targets, 4*, 97–112.

Lahiri, D. K., Maloney, B., & Zawia, N. H. (2009). The LEARn model: An epigenetic explanation for idiopathic neurobiological diseases. *Molecular Psychiatry, 14*, 992–1003.

Lai, C. S., Fisher, S. E., Hurst, J. A., Vargha-Khadem, F., & Monaco, A. P. (2001). A forkhead-domain gene is mutated in a severe speech and language disorder. *Nature, 413*, 519–523.

Lander, E., & Kruglyak, L. (1995). Genetic dissection of complex traits: Guidelines for interpreting and reporting linkage results. *Nature Genetics, 11*, 241–247.

Lander, E. S., Linton, L. M., Birren, B., Nusbaum, C., Zody, M. C., Baldwin, J., et al. (2001). Initial sequencing and analysis of the human genome. *Nature, 409*, 860–921.

Laumonnier, F., Bonnet-Brilhault, F., Gomot, M., Blanc, R., David, A., Moizard, M. P., et al. (2004). X-linked mental retardation and autism are associated with a mutation in the NLGN4 gene, a member of the neuroligin family. *American Journal of Human Genetics, 74*, 552–557.

Lawson-Yuen, A., Saldivar, J. S., Sommer, S., & Picker, J. (2008). Familial deletion within NLGN4 associated with autism and Tourette syndrome. *European Journal of Human Genetics, 16*, 614–618.

Li, M. M., & Andersson, H. C. (2009). Clinical application of microarray-based molecular cytogenetics: An emerging new era of genomic medicine. *Journal of Pediatrics, 155*, 311–317.

Li, J., Nguyen, L., Gleason, C., Lotspeich, L., Spiker, D., Risch, N., et al. (2004). Lack of evidence for an association between WNT2 and RELN polymorphisms and autism. *American Journal of Medical Genetics, 126B*, 51–57.

Lien, W. H., Klezovitch, O., & Vasioukhin, V. (2006). Cadherin–catenin proteins in vertebrate development. *Current Opinion Cell Biology, 18*, 499–506.

Lintas, C., & Persico, A. M. (2009). Autistic phenotypes and genetic testing: State-of-the-art for the clinical geneticist. *Journal of Medical Genetics, 46*, 1–8.

Losh, M., Sullivan, P. F., Trembath, D., & Piven, J. (2008). Current developments in the genetics of autism: From phenome to genome. *Journal of Neuropathological Exp Neurology, 67*, 829–837.

Lubs, H. A. (1969). A marker X chromosome. *Am J Hum Genet, 21*(3), 231–244.

Maes, B., Fryns, J. P., Van Walleghem, M., & Van den Berghe, H. (1993). Fragile-X syndrome and autism: A prevalent association or a misinterpreted connection? *Genetic Counseling, 4*, 245–263.

Mahr, R. N., Moberg, P. J., Overhauser, J., Strathdee, G., Kamhoampbell, J., Loevner, L. A. et al. (1996). Neuropsychiatry of 18q-. *American Journal of Medical Genetics, 67*, 172C–178C.

Marco, E. J., & Skuse, D. H. (2006). Autism-lessons from the X chromosome. *Social Cognitive and Affective Neuroscience, 1*, 183–193.

Marshall, C. R., Noor, A., Vincent, J. B., Lionel, A. C., Feuk, L., Skaug, J., et al. (2008). Structural variation of chromosomes in autism spectrum disorder. *American Journal of Human Genetics, 82*, 477–488.

Mattson, M. P., & Furukawa, K. (1998). Signaling events regulating the neurodevelopmental triad. Glutamate and secreted forms of beta-amyloid precursor protein as examples. *Perspectives on Developmental Neurobiology, 5*, 337–352.

McCaffery, P., & Deutsch, C. K. (2005). Macrocephaly and the control of brain growth in autistic disorders. *Progress in Neurobiology, 77*, 38–56.

Mendelsohn, N. J., & Schaefer, G. B. (2008). Genetic evaluation of autism. *Seminars in Pediatric Neurology, 15*, 27–31.

Moessner, R., Marshall, C. R., Sutcliffe, J. S., Skaug, J., Pinto, D., Vincent, J., et al. (2007). Contribution of SHANK3 mutations to autism spectrum disorder. *American Journal of Medical Genetics, 81*, 1289–1297.

Morgan, L., Wetherby, A. M., & Barber, A. (2008). Repetitive and stereotyped movements in children with autism spectrum disorders late in the second year of life. *Journal of Child Psychology & Psychiatry, 49*, 826–837.

Morrow, E. M., Yoo, S. Y., Flavell, S. W., Kim, T. K., Lin, Y., Hill, R. S., et al. (2008). Identifying autism loci and genes by tracing recent shared ancestry. *Science, 321*, 218–223.

Muhle, R., Trentacoste, S. V., & Rapin, I. (2004). The genetics of autism. *Pediatrics, 113*, 472–486.

Newbury, D. F., Bonora, E., Lamb, J. A., Fisher, S. E., Lai, C. S., Baird, G., et al. (2002). FOXP2 is not a major susceptibility gene for autism or specific language impairment. *American Journal of Human Genetics, 70*, 1318–1327.

O'Brien, E. K., Zhang, X., Nishimura, C., Tomblin, J. B., & Murray, J. C. (2003). Association of specific language impairment (SLI) to the region of 7q31. *American Journal of Human Genetics, 72*, 1536–1543.

O'Roak, B. J., & State, M. W. (2008). Autism genetics: Strategies, challenges, and opportunities. *Autism Research, 1*, 4–17.

Pack, P. (2002). *Biology (Cliffs AP)* (2nd ed.). Hoboken, NJ: Wiley.

Pennington, B. F. (2009). *Diagnosing learning disorders: A neuropsychological framework*. New York: Guilford Press.

Persico, A. M., Pascucci, T., Puglisi-Allegra, S., Militerni, R., Bravaccio, C., Schneider, C., et al. (2002). Serotonin transporter gene promoter variants do not explain the hyperserotonemia in autistic children. *Molecular Psychiatry, 7*, 795–800.

Pickles, A., Bolton, P., Macdonald, H., Bailey, A., Le Couteur, A., Sim, C. H., et al. (1995). Latent-class analysis of recurrence risks for complex phenotypes with selection and measurement error: A twin and family history study of autism. *American Journal of Human Genetics, 57*, 717–726.

Piven, J. (1999). Genetic liability for autism: The behavioral expression in relatives. *International Review of Psychiatry, 11*, 299–308.

Reichenberg, A., Gross, R., Weiser, M., Bresnahan, M., Silverman, J., Harlap, S., et al. (2006). Advancing paternal age and autism. *Archives of General Psychiatry, 63*, 1026–1032.

Rutter, M. (2000). Genetic studies of autism: From the 1970s into the millennium. *Journal of Abnormal Child Psychiatry, 28*, 3–14.

Schaefer, G. B., & Lutz, R. E. (2006). Diagnostic yield in the clinical genetics evaluation of autism spectrum disorders. *Genetics in Medicine, 8*, 549–556.

Schaefer, G. B., & Mendelsohn, N. J. (2008). Genetics evaluation for the etiologic diagnosis of autism spectrum disorders. *Genetics in Medicine, 10*, 4–12.

Schaefer, G. B., & Mendelsohn, N. J., Professional Practice and Guidelines Committee. (2008). Clinical genetics evaluation in identifying the etiology of autism spectrum disorders. *Genetics in Medicine, 10*, 301–305.

Schellenberg, G. D., Dawson, G., Sung, Y. J., Estes, A., Munson, J., Rosenthal, E., et al. (2006). Evidence for multiple loci from a genome scan of autism kindreds. *Molecular Psychiatry, 11*, 1049–1060.

Schroer, R. J., Phelan, M. C., Michaelis, R. C., Crawford, E. C., Skinner, S. A., Cuccaro, M., et al. (1998). Autism and maternally derived aberrations of chromosome 15q. *American Journal of Medical Genetics, 76*, 327–336.

Sebat, J., Lakshmi, B., Malhotra, D., Troge, J., Lese-Martin, C., Walsh, T., et al. (2007). Strong association of de novo copy number mutations with autism. *Science, 316*, 445–449.

Shao, Y., Cuccaro, M. L., Hauser, E. R., Raiford, K. L., Menold, M. M., Wolpert, C. M., et al. (2003). Fine mapping of autistic disorder to chromosome 15q11-q13 by use of phenotypic subtypes. *American Journal of Medical Genetics, 72*, 539–548.

SLI Consortium. (2002). A genomewide scan identifies two novel loci involved in specific language impairment. *American Journal of Human Genetics, 70*, 384–398.

SLI Consortium. (2004). Highly significant linkage to the SLI1 locus in an expanded sample of individuals affected by specific language impairment. *American Journal of Human Genetics, 74*, 1225–1238.

Smith, S. D. (2007). Genes, language development, and language disorders. *Mental Retardation and Developmental Disabilities Research Reviews, 13*, 96–105.

Sokol, D. K., Chen, D., Farlow, M. R., Dunn, D. W., Maloney, B., Zimmer, J. A., et al. (2006). High levels of Alzheimer beta-amyloid precursor protein (APP) in children with severely autistic behavior and aggression. *Journal of Child Neurology, 21*, 444–449.

Sokol, D. K., & Edwards-Brown, M. (2004). Neuroimaging in autistic spectrum disorder (ASD). *Journal of Neuroimaging, 14*, 8–15.

Solomon, E., Berg, L., & Martin, D. W. (2008). *Biology* (8th ed.). San Francisco: BrooksCole.

Sparks, B. F., Friedman, S. D., Shaw, D. W., Aylward, E. H., Echelard, D., Artru, A. A., et al. (2002). Brain structural abnormalities in young children with autism spectrum disorder. *Neurology, 59*, 184–192.

Steffenburg, S., Gillberg, C., Hellgren, L., Andersson, L., Gillberg, I. C., Jakobsson, G., et al. (1989). A twin study of autism in Denmark, Finland, Iceland, Norway and Sweden. *Journal Child Psychology &Psychiatry, 30*, 405–416.

Stothard, S. E., Snowling, M. J., Bishop, D. V., Chipchase, B. B., & Kaplan, C. A. (1998). Language-impaired preschoolers: A follow-up into adolescence. *Journal of Speech, Language, and Hearing Research, 41*, 407–418.

Strauss, K. A., Puffenberger, E. G., Huentelman, M. J., Gottlieb, S., Dobrin, S. E., Parod, J. M., et al. (2006). Recessive symptomatic focal epilepsy and mutant contactin-associated protein-like 2. *New England Journal of Medicine, 354*, 1370–1377.

Sykes, N. H., & Lamb, J. A. (2007). Autism: The quest for the genes. *Expert Reviews in Molecular Medicine, 9*, 1–15.

Szatmari, P., Paterson, A. D., Zwaigenbaum, L., Roberts, W., Brian, J., Liu, X. Q., et al. (2007). Mapping autism risk loci using genetic linkage and chromosomal rearrangements. *Nature Genetics, 39*, 319–328.

Tabor, H. K., & Cho, M. K. (2007). Ethical implications of array comparative genomic hybridization in complex phenotypes: Points to consider in research. *Genetics in Medicine, 9*, 626–631.

Tomblin, J. B., Records, N. L., Buckwalter, P., Zhang, X., Smith, E., & O'Brien, M. (1997). Prevalence of specific language impairment in kindergarten children. *Journal of Speech, Language and Hearing Research, 40*, 1245–1260.

Veenstra-VanderWeele, J., & Cook, E. H., Jr. (2004). Molecular genetics of autism spectrum disorder. *Molecular Psychiatry, 9*, 819–832.

Vincent, J. B., Petek, E., Thevarkunnel, S., Kolozsvari, D., Cheung, J., Patel, M., et al. (2002). The RAY1/ST7 tumor-suppressor locus on chromosome 7q31 represents a complex multi-transcript system. *Genomics, 80*, 283–294.

Volpe, J. J. (2001). *Neurology of the newborn* (4th ed.). Philadelphia: WB Saunders.

Vorstman, J. A., Staal, W. G., van Daalen, E., van Engeland, H., Hochstenbach, P. F., & Franke, L. (2006). Identification of novel autism candidate regions through analysis of reported cytogenetic abnormalities associated with autism. *Molecular Psychiatry, 11*(1), 18–28.

Wassink, T. H., Brzustowicz, L. M., Bartlett, C. W., & Szatmari, P. (2004). The search for autism disease genes. *Mental Retardation Developmental Disabilities Research Review, 10*, 272–283.

Wassink, T. H., Piven, J., Vieland, V. J., Huang, J., Swiderski, R. E., Pietila, J., et al. (2001). Evidence supporting WNT2 as an autism susceptibility gene. *American Journal of Medical Genetics, 105*, 406–413.

Weiss, L. A., Arking, D. E., Daly, M. J., & Chakravarti, A. (2009). A genome-wide linkage and association scan reveals novel loci for autism. *Nature, 461*, 802–808.

Westmark, C. J., & Malter, J. S. (2007). FMRP mediates mGluR5-dependent translation of amyloid precursor protein. *Public Library of Science Biology, 5*, e52.

Yan, D., Oliveira, G., Coutinho, A., Yang, C., Feng, J., Katz, C., et al. (2005). Analysis of the neuroligin 3 and 4 genes in autism and other neuropsychiatric patients. *Molecular Psychiatry, 10*, 329–332.

Zhang, H., Liu, X., Zhang, C., Mundo, E., Macciardi, F., Grayson, D. R., et al. (2002). Reelin gene alleles and susceptibility to autism spectrum disorders. *Molecular Psychiatry, 7*, 1012–1017.

Zoghbi, H. Y. (2003). Postnatal neurodevelopmental disorders: Meeting at the synapse? *Science, 302*, 826–830.

Behavioural, Biopsychosocial, and Cognitive Models of Autism Spectrum Disorders

Sophie E. Lind and David M. Williams

Introduction

Autism spectrum disorder (ASD) comprises a range of developmental disorders including autistic disorder, Asperger's disorder, and pervasive developmental disorder not otherwise specified/atypical autism, each of which is characterized by a triad of impairments in social interaction, communication, and restricted, repetitive behaviours and interests (RRBIs) (American Psychiatric Association, 2000; World Health Organization, 1993). ASD was originally identified and described in 1943 by Kanner, who believed the disorder to be biologically based. However, in the following decades, psychosocial explanations for ASD began to gain influence. Most notably, Bettelheim (1967) attributed the development of ASD as a response to emotionally "cold" parenting. Although this theory was influential for a significant period of time, it has not received empirical support, and it is now widely agreed that ASD is a biologically based disorder. Twin studies have consistently indicated that ASD is a highly heritable disorder (e.g. Bailey et al., 1995; Folstein & Rutter, 1977; Steffenburg, Hellgren, Gillberg, Jakobsen, & Bohman, 1989). Furthermore, although molecular genetic studies have not yet established a set of necessary and sufficient genes that cause the disorder, they have begun to identify a set of genes that are reliably associated with ASD (International Molecular Genetic Study of Autism Consortium, 1998, 2001, 2005).

Thus, ASD is a behaviourally defined disorder with a biological basis. The behavioural definition and the (presumably forthcoming) identification of a set of genetic or neurobiological markers for ASD represent *descriptive* models of the disorder. Morton and Frith (1995) have argued that in order to develop a *causal* model of ASD, a third level of

explanation – the cognitive or psychological level – is necessary to bridge the gap between the biological and behavioural levels. In other words, in order to understand the mechanisms by which genes and neurobiology influence behaviour, it is necessary to understand the cognitive processes that mediate that behaviour – there is arguably no direct link between biology and behaviour in ASD. For this reason, cognitive accounts are essential to our understanding of the disorder.

This chapter reviews three of the most influential accounts (as well as some of their variants/alternatives) and their respective relationships to brain function and behaviour, in the spirit of the causal modelling approach. We will begin by describing the theory of mind hypothesis of ASD – a domain-specific, "social" account – and go on to discuss the executive dysfunction and weak central coherence hypotheses – domain-general, broadly "non-social" accounts. Evidence for and against each of the theories will be considered, as well as issues of universality, specificity, and relationships to ASD diagnostic features. The chapter concludes with a section considering future directions for cognitive explanations of ASD.

The Theory of Mind Hypothesis

According to the original definition, a "theory of mind" (ToM) should be credited to any individual who attributes mental states (such as beliefs, desires, and intentions) to self and others in order to explain and predict behaviour (Premack & Woodruff, 1978). In everyday life, attributing mental states to people is a swift, frequently non-conscious activity. For this reason the term "mentalizing", which places less emphasis on the conscious, deliberate acquisition of any *theory* about the mind, is preferred to the term ToM by some researchers (e.g. Frith, 2003). From a cognitive science perspective, the computational underpinnings of ToM/mentalizing are complex. According to Leslie (1987), in the first year and a half of life, typically developing infants possess only primary representations of the

S.E. Lind (✉)
Department of Psychology, Durham University, Science Site, South Road, Durham, DH1 3LE, UK
e-mail: sophie.lind@durham.ac.uk

world. During these early months, reality (objects, people, events, etc.) is represented purely veridically. At approximately 18 months of age, however, infants develop the capacity to form second-order representations that are "decoupled" from reality. According to Leslie, these representations are no longer of/about the world (as primary representations are), but of/about one's (primary) representation of the world – they are representations *of* representations, or "M-representations" (Leslie & Roth, 1993). Because the infant can now represent representations (rather than just reality), they can begin to think about other people's (mental) representations and manipulate their own representations, as reflected in the act of pretence, which typically emerges at around 18 months of age. According to Leslie, M-representations are innately specified by a "theory of mind mechanism", which is damaged in ASD. With a diminished ability to form M-representations, children with ASD are limited largely to representing their own and others' behaviour, but not the mental states that underlie behaviour.

Intuitively, the ToM theory makes sense of the specific profile of everyday behaviour characteristically diminished amongst people with ASD, who rarely tell jokes, understand or use sarcasm, tell lies or deceive others, or communicate important information to other people. In one way or another, each of these behaviours appear to require the recognition that it is possible to hold a mental perspective on reality, which is separate from reality itself. Likewise, two cardinal features of ASD are potentially explained in the same way; a limited propensity to initiate, or respond to, joint attention can be explained by a failure to recognize that other people hold a mental perspective that is different from one's own (Leslie & Happé, 1989). Also, the fact that children with ASD tend not to understand pretend play in others, or engage in pretend play themselves, can be explained by a limited ability to form M-representations. For example, to understand that a banana can be used as a telephone (or anything else) during pretend play arguably requires the ability to recognize the distinction between reality (that the banana is a banana) and one's own and others' pretend representations of reality (Leslie, 1987). From a clinical perspective, then, the ToM theory of ASD parsimoniously explains many of the social and communicative difficulties that are core features of ASD.

Evidence for the ToM Hypothesis

This version of the ToM hypothesis of ASD has the advantage of being very well specified and providing clear, testable predictions as to the kinds of activity and understanding individuals with ASD should show limitations in. Specific empirical evidence for the hypothesis came from a series of landmark studies, beginning in the mid-1980s, which found

that children with ASD had significant difficulties with recognizing that other people can hold false beliefs about the world. For example, Baron-Cohen, Leslie, and Frith (1985) gave children with and without ASD a "location change" false belief task (Wimmer & Perner, 1983) in which a scenario is presented where one character, Sally, places her marble in a basket, and then leaves the vicinity. While Sally is out of sight, another character, "naughty Anne", removes the marble from the basket and places it in a nearby box. Participants were then asked a ToM test question regarding which location Sally will look for her marble when she returns to collect it. A correct answer requires the participant to recognize that Sally will act on the basis of her belief (that the marble is in the basket), rather than reality (that the marble is in the box). Strikingly, Baron-Cohen et al. found that 80% of the children with ASD failed this question, despite the fact that, on average, they had a mental age of 5.5 years, which is 1.5 years higher than the age at which typically developing children reliably pass false belief tasks (Wellman, Cross, & Watson, 2001). The fact that participants with ASD succeeded on a number of carefully designed control tasks ensured that failure on the ToM test question was not merely the result of difficulties with memory or general logical reasoning. Children with ASD seemed to have a specific problem with recognizing mental states, as the ToM theory predicted would be the case.

Baron-Cohen et al.'s (1985) study formed the cornerstone for a further two decades of research into ToM in ASD, which has consistently revealed deficits in the ability of affected individuals to explicitly understand a variety of mental states, including beliefs (Happé, 1995), intentions (Williams & Happé, 2010), knowledge and ignorance (Lind & Bowler, 2010), and deception (Sodian & Frith, 1992) in others or in self (see Williams, Lind, & Happé, 2009). For example, in one experiment, Sodian and Frith asked children to keep a piece of candy safe by placing it in an opaque box. The children were then introduced to two puppets – a "nasty thieving wolf" and a "nice friendly seal". The participants' task was to prevent the wolf from getting the candy, since he would steal it. Instead, the children had to ensure that the seal found the candy so that they received a reward of two pieces of candy. In one condition, participants could achieve these goals by lying to the wolf and telling him that the box did not contain candy, but telling the seal the truth about the contents of the box. In this "deception" condition, for the children to achieve their goals they needed to *induce a false belief* in the wolf, which clearly requires a ToM. In another condition, participants could achieve their goals by physically locking the box whenever the wolf appeared, but simply leaving the box unlocked whenever the seal appeared. In this "sabotage" condition, participants only needed to understand a chain of physical causation; locking the box prevented a puppet from getting the candy, whereas leaving the box unlocked allowed the puppet to obtain the contents. Sodian and Frith found that whereas all participants, including those with ASD, performed very well in the sabotage condition, children with ASD were unique in performing poorly in the deception condition, highlighting the specificity of the mentalizing deficits in ASD.

The ToM theory has also received support from neurobiological studies, which have identified a "core ToM network" of brain regions amongst typically developing children. Areas of the brain reliably recruited specifically for the purpose of solving ToM tasks include the medial prefrontal cortex and orbitofrontal region, anterior- and paracingulate cortices, superior temporal sulcus, and temporoparietal junction (e.g. Gallagher et al., 2000). Indeed, in a recent meta-analysis focusing on neurobiological studies of ToM in typical development, the medial prefrontal cortex was associated with ToM task performance in 37/40 studies (Carrington & Bailey, 2009). Supporting the ToM theory of ASD, several studies have now shown that this core ToM network – particularly the medial prefrontal cortex – is under-activated amongst individuals with ASD during ToM tasks (e.g. Castelli, Frith, Happé, & Frith, 2002; Kana, Keller, Cherkassky, Minshew, & Just, 2009; see also Zilbovicius, Meresse, Chabane, Brunelle, & Samson, 2006). At a minimum, these studies confirm that ToM difficulties in ASD are *associated* consistently with specific neurobiological abnormalities. However, it is important to note that these findings do not necessarily indicate that the neural *basis* of ToM impairments in ASD has been uncovered. The brain regions that comprise the core ToM network have a protracted development amongst typically developing individuals, not reaching full maturity until late adolescence or early adulthood (see Dumontheil, Burgess, & Blakemore, 2008). As such, it may be that these regions *become* specialized for mentalizing, rather than being "pre-wired" for such a function as Leslie's 1987 theory might predict.

Challenges to the ToM Hypothesis

Despite the fact that the ToM theory of ASD has intuitive appeal and is supported by a significant body of empirical evidence from both cognitive and neurobiological studies, it has been challenged in several ways in recent years. The first challenge to the theory concerns the *universality* of the ToM impairment in ASD. Even from the earliest cognitive studies of ToM, it was clear that not all children with ASD failed traditional ToM tasks. In a meta-analysis of 13 studies of false belief understanding in ASD, Happé (1995) found participant success rates ranged from 16.6 to 60%. Across studies, 17 out of 70 (20%) children with ASD passed all false belief test questions. This compared with 20 out of 34 (58.8%) participants with moderate learning disability (MLD), who did not have ASD. Clearly, on a strong version of the ToM

hypothesis, if an impairment in ToM is the underlying cognitive cause of the social–communicative features of ASD, then impairments on false belief tasks should be universal in ASD, assuming these tasks are valid measures of ToM.

Additionally, some have claimed that a further problem for the ToM hypothesis concerns the *diagnostic specificity* of the ToM impairment in ASD. Several studies have now shown that a proportion of children with other disorders manifest difficulties on traditional measures of ToM. Hence, children with congenital deafness who are born to hearing parents show diminished performance on false belief tasks (e.g. Peterson & Seigal, 1995), as do children with congenital blindness (e.g. Peterson, Peterson, & Webb, 2000), or generalized intellectual disability (Yirmiya, Erel, Shaked, & Solomonica-Levi, 1998). The fact that children with developmental disorders other than ASD show impaired ToM task performance, but generally not the social–communicative difficulties associated with ASD, presents an additional challenge to the ToM account of ASD.

Although the issues of universality and diagnostic specificity are apparent challenges to the ToM account of ASD, we are not inclined to view them as particularly persuasive ones. In our view, as highlighted above, it is essential to distinguish surface-level behaviour (in this case, task performance) from the cognitive underpinnings of behaviour. The same behaviour may have different underlying cognitive causes in different disorders (Morton & Frith, 1995). In particular, several researchers have argued that, whereas children with ASD fail traditional false belief tasks because they have diminished ToM competence as a result of a faulty underlying cognitive mechanism, children without ASD fail such tasks because of extraneous (performance) factors. In other words, children without ASD possess the basic underlying cognitive mechanism responsible for ToM, but fail to utilize this mechanism appropriately during ToM tasks. One way to test whether poor task performance has the same underlying cognitive cause across disorders is to manipulate the task of interest in systematic ways and investigate whether the manipulations affect performance in a comparable way in each disorder. If the underlying causes of ToM task success and failure are different amongst individuals with ASD than amongst children without ASD, then the issues of universality and diagnostic specificity do not provide strong challenges to the ToM account of ASD.

Adopting this approach, several studies have indicated that, in fact, different manipulations to false belief tasks affect the performance of children with different disorders in different ways. For example, Surian and Leslie (1999) found that asking children with ASD where Sally would look for her marble *first* (as opposed to merely asking where she would look) on a location change false belief task made no difference to their task performance. By contrast, this manipulation significantly increased the performance of typically developing 3-year-olds, as it also did in a study by Siegal and Beattie (1991). Conversely, Williams and Happé (2009a) found that if children with ASD were not allowed to verbalize their own false belief in an "unexpected contents" false belief task (Hogrefe, Wimmer, & Perner, 1986), then their performance on the subsequent "self test question" (which assessed awareness of own false beliefs) was significantly poorer than their performance on the "other-person test question", which assesses awareness of another person's false belief. In contrast, parallel performance across the self and other-person test questions was observed amongst both children with intellectual disability and young typically developing children, regardless of whether or not they verbalized their own false belief. Furthermore, Peterson, Wellman, and Lui (2005) found that children with ASD were unique in finding false belief tasks significantly more difficult than a task requiring the identification of a hidden emotion (e.g. in an individual who pretends not to be embarrassed, when they really are). Both typically developing and congenitally deaf children showed the opposite pattern of performance, finding it more difficult to identify a hidden emotion than a false belief.

These studies suggest that the underlying cognitive causes of false belief task *failure* amongst children with ASD are somewhat different to the causes underlying task failure amongst children without ASD. As such, the issue of diagnostic specificity of diminished ToM task performance is not such a challenge to the ToM account of ASD. Conversely, other studies suggest that *success* on traditional ToM tasks also has different causes in children with and without ASD. Several studies have observed a close connection between verbal ability and success on traditional false belief tasks. In particular, grammatical knowledge appears strongly tied to successful performance amongst children with ASD, but significantly less so (Fisher, Happé, & Dunn, 2005), or not at all (Lind & Bowler, 2009) amongst children with intellectual disability. This has led to the claim that children with ASD employ compensatory strategies to "hack out" solutions to ToM tasks in the absence of true ToM competence (Bowler, 1992; Happé, 1995). Supporting this possibility, Senju, Southgate, White, and Frith (2009) found that adults with ASD who pass traditional, *explicit* false belief tasks nonetheless perform atypically on a measure of *implicit* ToM that requires attention to be spontaneously deployed on the basis of another person's mental state. This suggests that explicit knowledge of mental states amongst verbally able individuals with ASD has been acquired in an atypical fashion and *not* primarily via the ToM mechanism. As such, the finding that some individuals with ASD perform well on traditional ToM tasks does not necessarily challenge the ToM account.

A third challenge to the ToM account concerns the fact that evidence for a direct link between ToM task performance

and severity of clinical features in ASD is somewhat mixed. In two studies of general adaptive behaviour amongst individuals with ASD, significant differences in specific aspects of social behaviour were observed between those individuals who passed ToM tasks and those who did not (see Fombonne, Siddons, Achard, Frith, & Happé, 1994; Frith, Happé, & Siddons, 1994). Frith et al. interviewed parents about their children with ASD using, amongst other measures, an "Active and Interactive Sociability Scale". The Active Sociability subscale consisted of questions concerning social skills that were *not* thought to rely on mentalizing (e.g. saying "please" when requesting something; playing board games). The Interactive Sociability subscale consisted of questions concerning social skills that *were* thought to rely on mentalizing (e.g. keeping secrets; apologizing for hurting another's feelings). In addition, the children with ASD, themselves, were given two standard false belief tasks. Frith et al. found that while there were no differences on the Active Sociability subscale between ToM passers and ToM failers, differences were observed on the Interactive Sociability subscale. Hence, on average, children who passed the false belief tasks were rated as showing superior interactive social skills than children who failed the false belief tasks. This supports the ToM account. However, Frith et al. also found that the real-life social skills of a significant proportion of children in the study could not be distinguished by false belief task performance. Hence, a number of children who passed the false belief tasks nonetheless displayed diminished interactive social skills, suggesting that ToM is not closely related to severity of clinical features.

The results of Frith et al. (1994) were replicated and extended by Fombonne et al. (1994), providing only partial support for the ToM account. However, caution needs to be taken when drawing absolute conclusions from these studies. As highlighted above, some individuals with ASD may well hack out solutions to traditional ToM tasks, using intellectual strategies. Therefore, performance on false belief tasks may not relate to severity of social–communication deficits amongst individuals with ASD because performance on the false belief tasks may not always tap true ToM competence. It is essential that future studies of the relation between ToM and feature severity in ASD employ implicit measures of mentalizing ability, the solutions to which are not easily hacked out by explicit problem-solving strategies (e.g. Senju et al., 2009). For the ToM account of ASD to be plausible, a relation must be observed between implicit awareness of mental states on these tasks and severity of social–communication impairments in ASD.

Even if the ToM account can ultimately explain the social–communication deficits in ASD, it is less likely to explain adequately the repetitive and stereotyped behaviours and interests that characterize the disorder. Although repetitive behaviours and interests could be considered a reaction to anxiety and confusion caused by social incomprehension (caused ultimately by a ToM deficit; see Happé, Ronald, & Plomin, 2006). Turner (1999) has argued that this is unlikely to be the case. As she points out, repetitive behaviours have both an *arousing* and a calming function amongst many individuals with ASD. Thus, they are unlikely to be merely a coping strategy employed to deal with social–communication problems. As such, it seems that the ToM account may not be able to explain fully the whole range of clinical features in ASD.

Alternatives to the ToM Hypothesis

Arguably, one of the most significant challenges to the ToM account of ASD is to explain those core social features of ASD that do not obviously require the high-level representation of mental states. Manifestations of primary inter-subjectivity, such as social smiling, social orienting, and the maintenance of eye contact – all of which are diminished in ASD – do not seem to require high-level mentalizing. Rather, one might intuitively suppose that difficulties with spontaneous orienting to and establishing coordination with others are related to, or perhaps even underpin, difficulties with representing mental states in people. Indeed, Hobson (1989, 1993, 2002) has argued persuasively that difficulties with establishing and maintaining affective engagement with others *lead to*, rather than *result from*, a diminished ToM (related, but subtly different, accounts are provided by Loveland, 1991; Klin, Jones, Schultz, & Volkmar, 2003). Hobson suggests that in typical development, young infants have a biologically based predisposition to "identify" with the bodily expressed stances and attitudes of others. For example, even from the earliest weeks of life, infants have been shown to coordinate their own feelings closely with those of others (Haviland & Lelwica, 1987). According to Hobson, it is through this (preconceptual, initially non-representational) process of being continually moved between different perspectives throughout early development that leads typically developing children to eventually *recognize* the distinction between perspective and reality (i.e. develop a ToM). According to Hobson, the diagnostic deficits in social–communication in ASD, as well as the characteristic deficits in ToM, are a consequence of an innately reduced propensity to identify with others.

Hobson's (1989, 1993, 2002) theory shares characteristics with the ToM account of ASD. It is "domain-specific", in that it places social deficits at the core of the disorder, and it emphasizes children's difficulty with representing mental states as a cause of the characteristic features of the disorder (e.g. deficits in pretend play). Arguably, however, it has the advantage of being able to account, in principle, for difficulties with primary inter-subjectivity, as well as with ToM,

amongst people with ASD. Hobson's theory has not gone unchallenged by ToM theorists, however, who have argued that his theory fails to account for exactly how concepts of mind emerge from the pre-conceptual process of identification (see Hobson, 2002; Leslie & Frith, 1990, pp. 255–260). Also, like the ToM account, Hobson's theory has difficulty explaining the apparently "non-social" repetitive behaviours and interests that characterize ASD. To explain these deficits, alternative cognitive accounts may be necessary.

The Executive Dysfunction Hypothesis

Although the definition of executive function is hotly debated (Jurado & Rosselli, 2007), the term is commonly used to refer to a broad range of high-level cognitive functions, primarily underpinned by the frontal lobes (Stuss et al., 2002), such as planning, cognitive flexibility/set-shifting, inhibitory control, working memory, and generativity (Hill, 2004). Neuropsychological patients with specific damage to the frontal lobes show inflexibility of cognition and behaviour that is reminiscent of that observed amongst individuals with ASD. This led to an early hypothesis that executive functions would be impaired in ASD and that this impairment could underpin the behavioural features of the disorder (e.g. Hughes, Russell, & Robbins, 1994; Pennington & Ozonoff, 1996).

The executive dysfunction hypothesis makes intuitive sense of the restricted, repetitive, and stereotyped patterns of behaviour in ASD. A difficulty in generating, planning, and controlling behaviour would likely result in a tendency to engage in only a limited number of activities that would be repeated over and over again, with limited imagination or variation (e.g. Turner, 1999). The theory also has the potential to explain deficits in joint attention associated with ASD. Joint attention requires the disengagement of attention from one's current focus and a shifting of attention to the object or event in the world that is the focus of another person's attention. As such, joint attention deficits in ASD might result from executive difficulties with set-shifting/cognitive flexibility (e.g. McEvoy, Rogers, & Pennington, 1993), rather than a failure to recognize mental states in others (e.g. Leslie & Happé, 1989). In a similar vein, some researchers have argued that deficits in pretend play are most parsimoniously explained by a limited ability to *generate* pretend scenarios (Jarrold, 2003), rather than an inability to *form* M-representations, as the ToM hypothesis suggests (Leslie, 1987). Some theorists have gone further than this, however, and suggested that executive dysfunction could have cascading effects that result in the full range of social–communication deficits, as well as repetitive behaviours, in ASD.

Arguably the most theoretically developed executive dysfunction account of ASD was provided by Russell (e.g. 1996). According to Russell, the most basic executive function is the ability to monitor one's actions. Russell and Hill (2001, p. 317) define action monitoring as "the mechanisms that ensure that agents know, without self-observation, (a) for which changes in perceptual input they are responsible and (b) what they are currently engaged in doing". Therefore, effective action monitoring allows an individual to distinguish between "self-caused" and "world-caused" changes in experience and hence, in Russell's (1996) theory, gives rise to an experience of *agency*. This "sub-personal", nonconscious process, which is a pre-requisite for all other (higher) components of executive functioning (e.g. planning), is thought to involve generating a visual ("efference") copy of a motor intention for action and then monitoring this copy in relation to the sensory consequences of one's action (e.g. Wolpert, Ghahramani, & Jordan, 1995). According to Russell, a primary deficit in action monitoring results in a failure to develop higher forms of executive functioning, which contributes to repetitive behaviours and interests in ASD. More importantly, in Russell's theory a deficit in action monitoring leads to a failure amongst individuals with ASD to experience their agency. As a developmental consequence, infants with ASD fail to recognize *others* as agents (with mental states), which directly causes their diagnostic social–communication impairments.

Evidence for the Executive Dysfunction Hypothesis

Consistent with the executive dysfunction theory, several higher components of executive functioning have been shown to be diminished in ASD. For instance, planning ability is assessed most frequently using the Tower of London task (Shallice, 1982). This task involves moving beads across pegs from an initial starting position to match a particular specified end-state in as few moves as possible. Several studies have shown that individuals with ASD perform less well than matched comparison participants on this task, requiring a greater number of moves to complete the puzzle (e.g. Bennetto, Pennington, & Rogers, 1996; Ozonoff, Pennington, & Rogers, 1991; Pellicano, 2007).

Another component of executive functioning that appears reliably impaired amongst individuals with ASD is cognitive flexibility, which is traditionally assessed using the Wisconsin Card Sorting Test (WCST) (Heaton, 1981). In this test, participants are presented with four *stimulus* picture cards depicting (a) one red triangle, (b) two green stars, (c) three yellow crosses, and (4) four blue circles, respectively, as well as a deck of *response* picture cards that vary on the dimensions of number, colour, and shape. The participant is

required to match the response cards to one of the stimulus cards according to one dimension specified by a particular unspoken rule (e.g. match according to colour). Although the experimenter does not explicitly state the sorting rule, he/she provides corrective feedback for each of the participant's card placements. On the basis of this feedback, the participant must deduce the nature of the rule. Once the participant has provided 10 consecutive correct responses, unbeknownst to him/her, the experimenter changes the unspoken rule. Thus, in order to continue providing correct responses he/she must flexibly shift to the new rule (e.g. sort according to number). Individuals with ASD typically show significantly more perseverative errors on the WCST (e.g. Ambery, Russell, Perry, Morris, & Murphy, 2006; Dichter & Belger, 2007; Ozonoff et al., 1991; Rumsey, 1985). Such findings are generally taken as evidence for impaired set-shifting/cognitive flexibility in ASD. However, it is also possible that difficulties with other components of executive functioning, such as working memory and/or inhibition, contribute to such perseveration.

Inhibitory control refers to "the ability to suppress the activation, processing, or expression of information that would otherwise interfere with the efficient attainment of a cognitive or behavioral goal" (Christ, Holt, White, & Green, 2007, p. 1156). In ASD, it has been most commonly assessed using Stroop (Stroop, 1935) and go/no-go (Drewe, 1975) tasks. Standard Stroop tasks require participants to identify the colour of the ink in which stimulus words are presented. In the key inhibitory control condition, the stimulus words are colour names printed in incongruent ink colours (e.g. "red" displayed in green font). In order to successfully name the colour of the ink, the participant must inhibit the automatic behaviour of simply reading the word. Studies have overwhelmingly shown intact Stroop performance in ASD (e.g. Ambery et al., 2006), notably, even when participants with ASD have significantly lower IQs than typical comparison participants (e.g. Christ et al., 2007; Ozonoff & Jensen, 1999).

In go/no-go tasks, participants are repeatedly presented with two different stimuli (e.g. a square and a circle), one at a time, in a random order, and asked to respond to only one of them (e.g. by pressing the spacebar). Hence, they might be asked to press the spacebar when they see a square (go trials) but not when they see a circle (no-go trials). Hence, on the no-go trials they must inhibit their motor response. Thus, the key variable of interest is the commission error rate on no-go trials. The majority of studies employing well-matched groups suggest unimpaired performance amongst individuals with ASD (e.g. Geurts, Begeer, & Stockmann, 2009; Happé, Booth, Charlton, & Hughes, 2006; Schmitz et al., 2006). Despite the fact that individuals with ASD have few difficulties on classic test of inhibition such as the Stroop and go/no-go tasks, they show impairments on tasks which require the inhibition of *prepotent responses* (Hill, 2004). For example, Hughes and Russell (1993) assessed this type of inhibition using a "detour reaching task", which involved retrieving a marble from a platform inside a box. Reaching directly for the marble caused an infrared light beam to be broken resulting in the marble dropping through a trapdoor, rendering it inaccessible. Therefore, to perform successfully on the task, the participant had to inhibit this prepotent response. Instead, they needed to either flick a switch on the side of box in order to turn off the beam of light and then directly pick up the marble, or turn a knob that caused the marble to descend down a chute from which they could safely retrieve it. It was found that participants with ASD were significantly impaired on this task, finding it difficult to inhibit the impulse to reach directly for the marble.

Working memory is another executive function that has been the focus of many studies of ASD. Working memory is a term used to refer to "a limited capacity system allowing the temporary storage and manipulation of information" (Baddeley, 2000, p. 418). Working memory can be measured using "*n*-back" tasks, which involve both the short-term storage *and* manipulation of information. Here, participants are asked to monitor a continuous sequence of stimuli (e.g. letters) and respond when the presented stimulus matches one presented *n* trials previously, where *n* is typically pre-specified as 1, 2, or 3 (Owen, McMillan, & Laird, 2005). Studies involving zero-back (where the target is the first item in the stimulus sequence), one-back, and two-back conditions have shown that individuals with ASD are unimpaired (Koshino et al., 2005; Ozonoff & Strayer, 2001; Williams, Goldstein, Carpenter, & Minshew, 2005). However, ceiling effects may have obscured possible group differences in these studies – the error rate was very low in each case. Indeed, it should be noted that the zero-, one-, and two-back conditions used in each of these experiments may have lacked the sensitivity needed to detect possible group differences in working memory – in other words the tasks were not taxing enough to reveal group differences if present. Indeed, Hockey and Geffen (2004) have argued that *n*-back tasks only involve a significant working memory load when *n* equals three or more.

Computerized box search tasks, such as the spatial working memory task from the Cambridge Neuropsychological Test Automated Battery (Cambridge Cognition, 1996), have also been used to assess working memory in ASD. In this type of task, participants must search through an array of boxes in order to retrieve hidden tokens. Importantly, they are asked to avoid opening boxes that they have already searched – tokens never appear in the same box more than once. The key dependent measure in such tasks is the number of search errors in which participants re-search an already searched box for a particular target token. The majority of studies indicate that individuals with ASD show significantly more search errors than age- and IQ-matched comparison individuals (Landa & Goldberg, 2005; Sinzig, Morsche, Bruning, Schmidt, & Lehmkuhl, 2008; Steele, Minshew, Luna, & Sweeney, 2007; but see Edgin & Pennington, 2005; Happé et al., 2006). Consistent with the suggestion made above, in relation to methodological weaknesses in *n*-back studies, Steele et al. (2007) found that ASD-specific working memory impairments were load-dependent, such that difficulties only began to emerge in high-load conditions. Thus, the evidence regarding working memory in ASD is equivocal – some studies find impairments, others do not. Further research using more demanding tasks will be required to resolve the debate.

It should be clear from this brief review of the literature that ASD does not involve blanket executive function deficits – some aspects appear to be impaired while others appear to be intact, and results are variable across studies. But what is the neural basis of those deficits that are present? Since the late 1970s, it has been hypothesized that specific abnormalities within the frontal lobes have a causal role in ASD (Damasio & Maurer, 1978) and such hypothesized abnormalities could potentially account for executive dysfunction. Indeed, a number of functional neuroimaging studies have indicated functional abnormalities within the frontal lobes of individuals with ASD during executive tasks (Di Martino et al., 2009). Unfortunately, many of these studies are not able to directly address the question of whether frontal lobe dysfunction underlies executive dysfunction in ASD. A number of investigations have demonstrated different levels and patterns of neural activity during executive task performance amongst individuals with ASD but this is alongside *intact* behavioural performance on those executive tasks (e.g. Gilbert, Bird, Brindleya, Frith, & Burgess, 2008; Kana, Keller, Minshew, & Just, 2007; Koshino et al., 2005; Schmitz et al., 2006). While such findings are interesting in their own right, they tell us little about the neural basis of executive function *impairments*. However, at least two functional imagining studies have established functional abnormalities in the presence of behavioural impairments. For example, Luna et al. (2002) found that individuals with ASD showed reduced levels of activation within the dorsolateral prefrontal cortex and posterior cingulate cortex during a spatial working memory task. Furthermore, Just, Cherkassky, Keller, Kana, and Minshew (2007) observed similar levels of activation between participants with and without ASD but reduced functional connectivity between frontal and parietal areas during the Tower of London planning task. Findings such as these provide a plausible explanation for why some individuals with ASD experience executive dysfunction. However, in order to further clarify these issues, it will be important for imaging researchers to carefully select behavioural paradigms that are robustly found to be problematic for individuals with ASD.

One significant strength of the executive dysfunction hypothesis is that it potentially explains the RRBIs that characterize ASD. Although there have been some negative or mixed findings (e.g. Dichter et al., 2009; South, Ozonoff, & McMahon, 2007), a number of studies have reported significant correlations between executive dysfunction and level of RRBIs. For example, Lopez, Lincoln, Ozonoff, and Lai (2005) found that cognitive flexibility, working memory, and inhibition (but not planning or fluency) were significantly related to RRBIs. In another study, Boyd, McBee, Holtzclaw, Baranek, and Bodfish (2009) assessed the relationship between executive dysfunction and repetitive behaviours using the Behavior Rating Inventory of Executive Function (BRIEF) (Gioia, Isquith, Guy, & Kenworthy, 2000) and the Repetitive Behavior Scale-Revised (RBS-R) (Bodfish, Symons, & Lewis, 1999; Lam & Aman, 2007). The BRIEF is a questionnaire that yields both a composite score and two separate indices: behavioural regulation (subscales: inhibition, shifting attention, and emotional control) and metacognition (subscales: initiating, working memory, planning/organizing, organization of materials, and monitoring). The RBS-R is a questionnaire that assesses various repetitive behaviours across six subscales (stereotypy, self-injurious behaviour, compulsions, rituals, sameness, and restricted interests). Boyd et al. found that RBS-R total score was significantly correlated with the BRIEF behavioural regulation score but not BRIEF metacognition or composite scores. These findings suggest that the executive dysfunction theory offers a credible explanation for at least some of the clinical features of ASD.

Challenges to the Executive Dysfunction Hypothesis

Despite the evidence discussed in support of the executive dysfunction account, several challenges have been made to the account in recent years. First, although some higher-order components of executive functioning are impaired in ASD, basic action monitoring skills appear to be preserved, contrary to Russell's (1996) central claim. Williams and Happé (2009b) explored action monitoring amongst children with autism, using a task adapted from Russell and Hill (2001). In this task, participants needed to judge which one of several coloured squares on a computer screen was under their intentional control (through movements of the mouse) and which "distractor" squares were under the control of the computer. So, although all of the squares on the screen were activated when the mouse was moved, only one of the squares behaved directly in accordance with the participant's movements. The movements of the other squares were randomly generated by the computer. Ensuring that participants could not solve the task by visually comparing the movements of

their hand with the movements of the squares on the screen (i.e. through self-observation), their hand was located inside a box while they moved the mouse. Therefore, to recognize the square that they were controlling, participants needed to monitor accurately an efference copy of their motor command and compare this to the visual input from the computer screen (i.e. to detect their own agency). Williams and Happé found that adolescents with ASD performed well on this task and not significantly differently from closely matched comparison participants. Moreover, Williams (2010) confirmed that participants with ASD in Williams and Happé's study showed significantly diminished ToM. Therefore, there was no evidence either that action monitoring was impaired in ASD, or that awareness of one's own agency resulting from action monitoring is sufficient to recognize others as agents with mental states (see also David et al., 2008; Frith & Hermelin, 1969).

Although these findings provide strong evidence against Russell's (1996) version of the executive dysfunction account of ASD, they do not necessarily show that impairments in other components of executive functioning are not a primary cognitive deficit in ASD. This latter suggestion is challenged by other findings, however. First, although diminished cognitive flexibility/set-shifting, inhibition of a prepotent response, and working memory (see above) have been observed in children with ASD from around 5.5 years of age (e.g. Dawson, Meltzoff, Osterling, & Rinaldi, 1998; McEvoy et al., 1993), studies of younger children with ASD have failed to find evidence of deficits in any of these areas. In studies by Dawson et al. (2002) and Griffith, Pennington, Wehner, and Rogers (1999), children with ASD between the ages of 3 and 5 years were tested on a variety of executive functioning tasks that are suitable for young children and on which impairments are seen in monkeys with lesions in the prefrontal cortex (e.g. Diamond & Goldman-Rakic, 1989). In particular, in contrast to studies involving older children with ASD, no differences were seen between children with and without ASD on a spatial reversal task (assessing cognitive flexibility and inhibition of a prepotent response), the A not B task (assessing working memory and inhibition of a prepotent response), or boxes tasks (assessing working memory).

These findings amongst young, preschool children with ASD cast doubt on the hypothesis that impairments in (at least these components of) executive functioning represent a primary cognitive deficit in ASD. Arguably, a parsimonious interpretation is that executive dysfunction *emerges* with age in ASD and is a secondary consequence of other deficits in this disorder. Establishing this possibility will, ultimately, require longitudinal studies of executive functioning in ASD, using a variety of measures that are sensitive to executive dysfunction.

Consideration of universality and specificity is also pertinent when evaluating the executive dysfunction hypothesis. With regard to universality, it is clear that results are mixed, with many studies obtaining null results. Even within those studies that have found executive difficulties on the group level, there is still considerable variability *within* the groups. For example, Pellicano, Maybery, Durkin, and Maley (2006) found that only 48% of children with ASD fell at least one standard deviation below the mean of the comparison group on the Tower of London planning task, and only 55% on a set-shifting task similar to the WCST. It should also be noted that executive dysfunction is certainly not specific to ASD – it is common in other disorders such as attention deficit hyperactivity disorder (ADHD) and Tourette syndrome, which involve a very different set of behavioural impairments to those seen in ASD. However, what may prove to be specific to ASD is the executive dysfunction *profile* that characterizes the disorder (Happé et al., 2006; Ozonoff & Jensen, 1999).

The Weak Central Coherence Hypothesis

The weak central coherence hypothesis of autism was originally proposed by Frith (1989, 2003). The hypothesis draws on ideas from gestalt psychology and assumes that while typically developing individuals have "a built-in propensity to form coherence over as wide a range of stimuli as possible, and to generalize over as wide a range of contexts as possible" (Frith, 2003, pp. 159–160), individuals with ASD have a diminution in this propensity. Metaphorically, according to Frith's original weak central coherence account, children with ASD are unable to "see the wood for the trees". Weak central coherence was originally conceptualized as a core *deficit* in extracting meaning and processing wholes. However, more recent versions of the theory have adopted the idea that weak central coherence is a "cognitive style" rather than a cognitive deficit (Happé, 1999). According to this view, individuals can fall anywhere on the continuum of central coherence, ranging from preferential processing of parts – local bias – to preferential processing of wholes – global bias. Thus, individuals with ASD tend to show a cognitive style that falls towards the "local" end of the continuum.

Weak central coherence was originally thought to contribute to the social features of ASD and Frith (1989) hypothesized that weak central coherence may underlie ToM impairments in the disorder. However, more recent versions of the theory have retracted from this argument, instead focusing on the theory's potential to account for non-social features and perceptual anomalies (Happé & Frith, 2006). For example, the hypothesis is consistent with Kanner's (1943) early observation that individuals with autism show an "inability to experience wholes without full attention to the constituent parts" (p. 246) and clinical observations that children with autism tend to be pre-occupied with parts of objects (e.g. spinning the wheels on toy cars) and show increased sensitivity to minute changes in the environment.

Evidence for the Weak Central Coherence Hypothesis

Although there are a number of contradictory findings, several sources of evidence suggest that individuals with ASD show *superior* performance when tasks depend on processing of local features but *inferior* performance when tasks depend on processing of global features, providing support for the weak central coherence hypothesis (see Happé & Frith, 2006, for a review). Studies of block design represent one particularly compelling source of evidence for the hypothesis. The block design test is a subtest from the Wechsler Intelligence Scales (e.g. Wechsler Intelligence Scale for Children, Wechsler, 2004) and requires participants to reproduce two-dimensional, red and white, geometric patterns using a set of three-dimensional cubes, which have two red, two white, and two diagonally oriented half-red and half-white sides. Although there are a handful of contrary findings (e.g. Bölte, Holtman, Poustka, Scheurich, & Schmidt, 2007), it is generally accepted that individuals with ASD show superior performance on the block design test (e.g. Caron, Mottron, Berthiaume, & Dawson, 2006). According to the weak central coherence hypothesis, this performance peak is attributable to the fact that individuals with ASD process the two-dimensional patterns in a piecemeal fashion, automatically focusing on the constituent parts of the design.

Support for this interpretation was provided in a landmark study by Shah and Frith (1993). Both low- and high-functioning adolescents/young adults with autism were asked to complete two different versions of the block design task: the standard "un-segmented" version and a "pre-segmented" version in which the constituent blocks were shown spaced apart in the two-dimensional design to be copied. It was found that participants with autism showed significantly superior performance (i.e. construction times were significantly faster) only in the un-segmented version of the task. The authors argued that the pre-segmented version effectively eliminated the advantage that individuals with ASD had over typical individuals in the un-segmented version by removing the global image and highlighting the constituent parts (already apparent to participants with ASD) to the non-autistic participants. These findings have recently been replicated by Caron et al. (2006) in a sample of high-functioning adults with autism. However, Kaland, Mortensen, and Smith (2007) reported no significant group differences in either segmented or un-segmented block design between high-functioning adolescents with autism/Asperger's syndrome and typical adolescents (matched on chronological age, VIQ, PIQ, and FSIQ). In fact, the ASD group was a little slower than the comparison group in each case.

Research using the embedded figures test (Witkin, Oltman, Raskin, & Karp, 1971) has also been cited in support of the weak central coherence hypothesis. Here, the task is to search for and identify a simple hidden target shape within a more complex picture (e.g. a triangle within a picture of a pram). Shah and Frith (1983) found that low-functioning children with ASD achieved significantly higher accuracy on this task than age- and non-verbal mental age-matched comparison children with intellectual disability (55%) and non-verbal mental age-matched typically developing children. In a later study of high-functioning adults with autism or Asperger's syndrome, Jolliffe and Baron-Cohen (1997) found that although all groups showed a similar level of *accuracy*, while typical participants took an average of 53 s to locate the hidden figures, participants with autism or Asperger's syndrome (matched for age, VIQ, PIQ and FSIQ) took only 29 and 32 s, respectively.

Shah and Frith argued that individuals with ASD experience less "capture by meaning". In other words, individuals with ASD are faster or more accurate on the task because they are unhindered by the overall global meaning of the picture (e.g. the fact that it is a picture of a *pram*). Although a number of studies have replicated the finding that individuals with ASD outperform matched comparison individuals on the embedded figures test (Edgin & Pennington, 2005; Jarrold, Gilchrist, & Bender, 2005; Pellicano et al., 2006), there have also been a number of contrary findings (Bölte et al., 2007; Kaland et al., 2007; Morgan, Maybery, & Durkin, 2003; Schlooz et al., 2006).

Susceptibility to visual illusions is also thought to be mediated by central coherence. Happé (1996) found that low-functioning children with autism were less likely to succumb to visual illusions such as the Müller-Lyer figures and Kanizsa triangle than comparison children (matched for age and verbal IQ). Confirming this finding, a recent study by Bölte et al. (2007) revealed that high-functioning adults with autism were less susceptible to visual illusions than typical comparison adults (matched on verbal IQ, performance IQ, and age). Other studies have failed to find evidence for decreased susceptibility to visual illusions in ASD (Hoy, Hatton, & Hare, 2004; Ropar & Mitchell, 1999; Ropar & Mitchell, 2001). However, each of the studies that obtained null results failed to include comparison groups that were closely matched on age and intellectual ability. For example, in the Hoy et al. study, the autism group was younger and less verbally able than the comparison group. Indeed, the effect sizes for the differences between the autism and comparison groups on age (Cohen's $d = 1.05$) and verbal mental age (Cohen's $d = 0.54$) were large and moderate, respectively,

indicating that the groups were not closely matched. The validity of these findings is therefore questionable.

Studies of homograph reading are another key source of evidence that is consistent with the weak central coherence hypothesis. Homographs are words with one spelling but multiple pronunciations and meanings (e.g. "She had a pink *bow*" versus "She made a deep *bow*"). In homograph reading tasks, participants are required to read aloud sentences that include homographs (e.g. "It was *lead* in the box that made it so heavy"). In such tasks, the correct pronunciation for the homograph can only be ascertained through considering the overall context of the sentence. It has been consistently found that children (Frith & Snowling, 1983, Experiment 5), adolescents (Happé, 1997; López & Leekam, 2003), and adults (Jolliffe & Baron-Cohen, 1999, Experiment 1) with ASD are significantly more likely to mispronounce homographs, tending to adopt the most common pronunciation without taking into account the sentence context. Frith and Snowling suggest that the tendency to mispronounce homographs in context arises from using a word-by-word reading strategy – evidence for weak central coherence.

By and large evidence from block design, embedded figures, visual illusions, and homograph reading is consistent with the idea that weak central coherence can result in either inferior or superior performance, depending upon the particular task demands. Superior block design/embedded figures test performance and decreased susceptibility to visual illusions, alongside inferior homograph reading, suggest that weak central coherence operates at both the perceptual and the conceptual levels.

Challenges to the Weak Central Coherence Account of ASD

As is the case for impaired ToM and executive dysfunction, weak central coherence does not appear to be universal in ASD. Teunisse, Cools, van Spaendonck, Aerts, and Berger (2001), for example, found that although weak central coherence was more common in ASD, it was not universally found – only 57% (20/35) of young adults with ASD showed this cognitive style. On the other hand, Pellicano et al. (2006) found that 92% of children with ASD were more than one standard deviation quicker than the mean of the matched comparison children on the embedded figures test. There are also questions over the diagnostic specificity of weak central coherence to ASD. For example, in their study of visual illusions, Bölte et al. (2007) found that adults with depression or schizophrenia were less susceptible to visual illusions than typical adults and did not significantly differ from participants with ASD in terms of level of susceptibility.

Perhaps more importantly, the explanatory power of the weak central coherence hypothesis is rather limited. At best, it is likely to explain only limited aspects of the behavioural phenotype. Although few studies have empirically assessed the relationship between weak central coherence and the clinical features of ASD, these have generally failed to find significant relationships with either social impairments (Teunisse et al., 2001) or RRBIs (South et al., 2007). This would seem to suggest that weak central coherence should be viewed as largely an explanation of non-triad features of ASD, which affect some individuals but not others. Intriguingly, however, research employing a *non*-clinical sample indicates a positive relationship between weak central coherence and levels of autistic-like traits (Stewart, Watson, Allcock, & Yaqoob, 2009).

Alternative Explanations for Weak Central Coherence "Effects"

One of the main limitations of the weak central coherence account is that it remains largely descriptive – no specific cognitive or neural mechanisms for local bias are posited. Alternative accounts for weak central coherence "effects" have gone some way towards specifying the underlying mechanisms responsible.

The enhanced perceptual functioning theory (Mottron & Burack, 2001; Mottron, Dawson, Soulieres, Hubert, & Burack, 2006) is probably the most influential alternative explanation for weak central coherence "effects". According to this theory, individuals with ASD do not show deficits in global processing or a bias towards local processing (as suggested by the weak central coherence account) but, rather, show *enhanced* perceptual processing, which results in a local bias. Here, perception is broadly defined and is said to range from "feature detection up to and including pattern recognition" (Mottron et al., 2006, p. 28).

In terms of their neurobiological basis, Brock, Brown, Boucher, and Rippon (2002) have hypothesized that weak central coherence effects in ASD are underpinned by a deficit in temporal binding. Thus, the brain activity of individuals with ASD is characterized by diminished temporal synchronization of neuronal activity between functionally specialized local neural networks. Brock et al. argue that individuals with ASD therefore show diminished performance on experimental tasks that require the integration of information from different functionally specialized local networks but undiminished performance on tasks that depend only upon isolated local networks. In a similar vein, Just, Cherkassky, Keller, and Minshew (2004) propose that underconnectivity – diminished coordination and communication – between brain regions underlies weak central coherence effects. Like the temporal binding hypothesis, the underconnectivity hypothesis also predicts that individuals with ASD should

perform well when tasks do not require coordination of disparate cortical regions but poorly when tasks depend upon the multiple cortical regions. Data from a number of fMRI studies do seem to suggest reduced functional connectivity in ASD (Castelli et al., 2002; Just et al., 2004).

The Future of Psychological Theories of ASD: Multiple or Single Deficit Accounts and the Possible Fractionation of the Triad

Cognitive theories of ASD have generally attempted (with varying degrees of success) to identify a *single* primary cognitive deficit as the causal factor underlying the complete triad of behavioural impairments that characterize ASD. However, it is becoming clear that, standing alone, none of the existing cognitive theories (the most influential of which have been described above) provide a satisfactory explanation for the full range of behavioural deficits seen in ASD. For this reason, the trend towards *multiple* deficit accounts is now gaining momentum (Bishop, 1989; Boucher, 2006; Goodman, 1989; Happé, Ronald, & Plomin, 2006). Researchers have also begun to question whether the domains of the triad of impairments are separable. If they are separable, then arguably we already have adequate theoretical explanations for the individual triad domains. For example, Happé and Ronald (2008) suggest that while ToM impairments may account for social and communication impairments, executive dysfunction may account for RRBIs. On the other hand, if the triad of impairments is not fractionable, it is clear that we have a lot of theory building left to do. Thus, the future of psychological models of ASD will critically depend on the outcome of research investigating the relations amongst the triad of impairments.

The earliest study to address this question was conducted by Wing and Gould (1979). They selected a sample of 132 children from a "psychiatric and mental retardation register", who had severe intellectual disability (mental retardation) or one or more of the following clinical features: (a) impairment of social interaction; (b) impairment of verbal and non-verbal communication; (c) repetitive, stereotyped activities. On the basis of clinical assessments, Wing and Gould established that impairments in each domain tended to cluster together within individuals. For example, of the 74 children with social impairment, 55% had no speech, and 72% showed RRBIs. However, we can only draw limited conclusions from these findings, given that definitions and criteria for ASD have changed so significantly since 1979 (Happé & Ronald, 2008). Another notable disadvantage of this study is that the sample was drawn from a register of psychiatric patients – a population that is likely to show higher rates of co-morbidity (e.g. between each domain of the triad) than community samples. This sampling method may therefore artificially elevate the number of individuals in the sample who have impairments across multiple domains (Caron & Rutter, 1991).

More recent research has overcome this limitation by employing population-based community samples and "bottom-up" factor analytic techniques. This type of research takes a dimensional rather than categorical approach to the ASD triad and assumes that autistic-like traits within each of the triad domains vary continuously in the general population (Baron-Cohen, Wheelwright, Skinner, Martin, & Clubley, 2001; Constantino & Todd, 2003). Here, sub-clinical levels of autistic-like traits are referred to as the "broader autism phenotype". Using this type of approach, Constantino, Przybeck, Freisen, and Todd (2000) assessed 287 school-aged typically developing children and 158 child psychiatric patients using the Social Reciprocity Scale (SRS) (now referred to as the "Social *Responsiveness* Scale"; Constantino, 2002) – a 65-item, parent/teacher-rated quantitative scale, measuring autistic-like traits. A factor analysis revealed that a single factor (rather than three factors as would be expected if the triad is fractionable) explained 70% of the variance in SRS scores.

However, studies using other measures of autistic-like traits have generally found multiple factor solutions, ranging from 2 to 8 factors (Auyeung, Baron-Cohen, Wheelwright, & Allison, 2005; see Happé & Ronald, 2008, for a review; Hoekstra, Bartels, Cath, & Boomsma, 2008). For example, Austin (2005) assessed 201 undergraduate students using the autism-spectrum quotient (AQ) (Baron-Cohen et al., 2001) – a 50-item self-report questionnaire – and found that a three-factor model explained 28% of the variance in scores. These findings were closely replicated in a recent study of 1,005 psychology undergraduate students (Hurst, Mitchell, Kimbrel, Kwapil, & Nelson-Gray, 2007). However, it should be noted that each of these studies used an oblique rotation method, which allows factors to be correlated. Neither study reported the inter-factor correlations, making it difficult to judge the degree of independence amongst the factors. A recent study by Stewart and Austin (2009), employing a sample of 536 university students, reported a four-factor solution, accounting for 29% of the variance in AQ scores. These factors were labelled as follows: (1) socialness, (2) patterns, (3) understanding others/communication, and (4) imagination. The correlations between each pair of factors ranged from 0.00 to 0.22, with the highest correlation being between socialness and understanding others/communication.

Clearly, there is a great deal of variation in results both within and between the different types of measure of autistic traits. Overall, these findings call into question the notion of a *triad* of domains of autistic-like impairments in the general population, with the majority of studies suggesting either fewer or a greater number of domains. What is also unclear is the degree to which these domains are correlated with one another. Studies of clinical populations provide equally variable results, with some studies suggesting a single factor (e.g. Constantino et al., 2004; Szatmari et al., 2002) and others suggesting multiple factors (e.g. Dworzynski, Happé, Bolton, & Ronald, 2009; Mandy & Skuse, 2008). One point to bear in mind when considering the results of these studies is that factor structure may be an artefact of the particular *measure* used rather than a reflection of any objectively independent causal factors.

The question of whether or not ASD involves a triad of independent impairments is yet to be definitively answered. Undoubtedly, there will be an intensive research effort to this end in the coming years. This research will have clear implications for psychological accounts of ASD, which will need to be refined according to the outcome of this research effort. Equally, a better understanding of the cognitive basis/bases of ASD could help to shape our understanding of the aetiology of the disorder. For example, Bishop (e.g. 2006) has argued that one way for genetic studies to circumvent the difficulties associated with defining the behavioural phenotype is to "cut loose from conventional clinical criteria for diagnosing disorders and to focus instead on measures of underlying cognitive mechanisms. Psychology can inform genetics by clarifying what the key dimensions are for heritable phenotypes" (p. 1153). By developing a finer-grained understanding of cognition in ASD, it might be possible to focus on a set of genes that are reliably associated with a specific cognitive endophenotype in ASD (as has been done in other disorders; e.g. SLI Consortium, 2004). Vice versa, such genetic studies may also clarify the nature of cognition in developmental disorders like ASD (e.g. Bishop et al., 1999). Either way, we believe that a complete account of ASD will require an understanding of the cognitive underpinnings of the disorder.

References

Ambery, F. Z., Russell, A. J., Perry, K., Morris, R., & Murphy, D. G. (2006). Neuropsychological functioning in adults with Asperger syndrome. *Autism, 10*, 551–564.

American Psychiatric Association. (2000). *Diagnostic and statistical manual of mental disorders* (4th ed., text revision). New York: American Psychiatric Association.

Austin, E. J. (2005). Personality correlates of the broader autism phenotype as assessed by the Autism Spectrum Quotient (AQ). *Personality and Individual Differences, 38*, 451–460.

Auyeung, B., Baron-Cohen, S., Wheelwright, S., & Allison, C. (2005). The Autism Spectrum Quotient: Children's version (AQ-Child). *Journal of Autism and Developmental Disorders, 38*, 1230–1240.

Baddeley, A. (2000). The episodic buffer: A new component of working memory? *Trends in Cognitive Sciences, 4*, 417–423.

Bailey, A., LeCouteur, A., Gottesman, I., Bolton, P., Simonoff, E., Yuzda, E., et al. (1995). Autism as a strongly genetic disorder: Evidence from a British twin study. *Psychological Medicine, 25*, 63–77.

Baron-Cohen, S., Leslie, A. M., & Frith, U. (1985). Does the autistic child have a theory of mind? *Cognition, 21*, 37–46.

Baron-Cohen, S., Wheelwright, S. J., Skinner, R., Martin, J., & Clubley, E. (2001). The autism-spectrum quotient (AQ): Evidence from Asperger syndrome/high-functioning autism, males and females, scientists and mathematicians. *Journal of Autism and Developmental Disorders, 31*, 5–17.

Bennetto, L., Pennington, B. F., & Rogers, S. J. (1996). Intact and impaired memory functions in autism. *Child Development, 67*, 1816–1835.

Bettelheim, B. (1967). *The empty fortress: Infantile autism and the birth of self*. New York: The Free Press.

Bishop, D. V. M. (1989). Autism, Asperger's syndrome and semantic-pragmatic disorder: Where are the boundaries? *International Journal of Language and Communication Disorders, 24*, 107–121.

Bishop, D. V. M. (2006). Developmental cognitive genetics: How psychology can inform genetics and vice versa. *Quarterly Journal of Experimental Psychology, 59*, 1153–1168.

Bishop, D. V. M., Bishop, S. J., Bright, P., James, C.,Delaney, T., & Tallal, P. (1999). Different origin of auditory and phonological processing problems in children with language impairment: Evidence from a twin study. *Journal of Speech, Language and Hearing Research, 42*, 155–168.

Bodfish, J. W., Symons, C. S., & Lewis, M. H. (1999). *The Repetitive Behavior Scales (RBS)*. Western Carolina Center Research Reports.

Bölte, S., Holtman, M., Poustka, F., Scheurich, A., & Schmidt, L. (2007). Gestalt perception and local-global processing in high-functioning autism. *Journal of Autism and Developmental Disorders, 37*, 1493–1507.

Boucher, J. (2006). Is the search for a unitary explanation of autistic spectrum disorders justified? *Journal of Autism and Developmental Disorders, 36*, 289.

Bowler, D. M. (1992). 'Theory of mind' in Asperger's syndrome. *Journal of Child Psychology and Psychiatry, 33*, 877–893.

Boyd, B. A., McBee, M., Holtzclaw, T., Baranek, G. T., & Bodfish, J. W. (2009). Relationships among repetitive behaviors, sensory features, and executive functions in high functioning autism. *Research in Autism Spectrum Disorders, 3*, 959–966.

Brock, J., Brown, C. C., Boucher, J., & Rippon, G. (2002). The temporal binding deficit hypothesis of autism. *Development and Psychopathology, 14*, 209–224.

Cambridge Cognition. (1996). *CANTAB®*. Cambridge: Cambridge Cognition Limited.

Caron, M. J., Mottron, L., Berthiaume, C., & Dawson, M. (2006). Cognitive mechanisms, specificity and neural underpinnings of visuospatial peaks in autism. *Brain, 129*, 1789–1802.

Caron, C., & Rutter, M. (1991). Comorbidity in child psychopathology: Concepts, issues and research strategies. *Journal of Child Psychology and Psychiatry, 32*, 1063–1080.

Carrington, S. J., & Bailey, A. J. (2009). Are there theory of mind regions in the brain? A review of the neuroimaging literature. *Human Brain Mapping, 30*, 2313–2335.

Castelli, F., Frith, C., Happe, F., & Frith, U. (2002). Autism, Asperger syndrome and brain mechanisms for the attribution of mental states to animated shapes. *Brain, 125*, 1839–1849.

Christ, S. E., Holt, D. D., White, D. A., & Green, L. (2007). Inhibitory control in children with autism spectrum disorder. *Journal of Autism and Developmental Disorders, 37*, 1155–1165.

Constantino, J. N. (2002). *The social responsiveness scale*. Los Angeles: Western Psychological Services.

Constantino, J. N., Gruber, C. P., Davis, S., Hayes, S., Passanante, N., & Przybeck, T. (2004). The factor structure of autistic traits. *Journal of Child Psychology and Psychiatry, 45*, 719–726.

Constantino, J., Przybeck, J., Freisen, D., & Todd, R. D. (2000). Reciprocal social behavior in children with and without pervasive developmental disorders. *Journal of Developmental & Behavioral Pediatrics, 21*, 2–11.

Constantino, J. N., & Todd, R. D. (2003). Autistic traits in the general population: A twin study. *Archives of General Psychiatry, 60*, 524–530.

Damasio, A. R., & Maurer, R. G. (1978). Neurological model for childhood autism. *Archives of Neurology, 35*, 777–786.

David, N., Gawronski, A., Santos, N. S., Huff, W., Lehnardt, F., Newen, A., & Vogeley, K. (2008). Dissociation between key processes of social cognition in autism: Impaired mentalizing but intact sense of agency. *Journal of Autism and Developmental Disorders, 38*, 593–605.

Dawson, G., Meltzoff, A. N., Osterling, J., & Rinaldi, J. (1998). Neuropsychological correlates of early symptoms of autism. *Child Development, 69*, 1276–1285.

Dawson, G., Munson, J., Estes, A., Osterling, J., McPartland, J., Toth, K., Carver, L., & Abbott, R. (2002). Neurocognitive function and joint attention ability in young children with autism spectrum disorder versus developmental delay. *Child Development, 73*, 345–358.

Di Martino, A., Ross, K., Uddin, L. Q., Sklar, A. B., Castellanos, F. X., & Milham, P. (2009). Functional brain correlates of social and nonsocial processes in autism spectrum disorders: An activation likelihood estimation meta-analysis. *Biological Psychiatry, 65*, 63–74.

Diamond, A., & Goldman-Rakic, P. (1989). Comparison of human infants and rhesus monkeys on Piaget's A not B task: Evidence for dependence on dorsolateral prefrontal cortex. *Experimental Brain Research, 74*, 24–40.

Dichter, G. S., & Belger, A. (2007). Social stimuli interfere with cognitive control in autism. *Neuroimage, 35*, 1219–1230.

Dichter, G. S., Radonovich, K. J., Turner-Brown, L. M., Lam, K. S. L., Holtzclaw, Y. N., & Bodfish. J. W. (2009). Performance of children with autism spectrum disorders on the dimension-change card sort task. *Journal of Autism and Developmental Disorders*. Advance online publication. doi: 10.1007/s10803-009-0886-1.

Drewe, E. (1975). Go-no go learning after frontal lobe lesions in humans. *Cortex, 11*, 8–16.

Dumontheil, I., Burgess, P. W., & Blakemore, S. J. (2008). Development of rostral prefrontal cortex and cognitive and behavioural disorders. *Developmental Medicine and Child Neurology, 50*, 168–181.

Dworzynski, K., Happé, F., Bolton, P., & Ronald, A. (2009). Relationship between symptom domains in autism spectrum disorders: A population based twin study. *Journal of Autism and Developmental Disorders, 39*, 1197–1210.

Edgin, J., & Pennington, B. (2005). Spatial cognition in autism spectrum disorders: Superior, impaired, or just intact? *Journal of Autism and Developmental Disorders, 35*, 729–745.

Fisher, N., Happé, F., & Dunn, J. (2005). The relationship between vocabulary, grammar, and false belief task performance in children with autistic spectrum disorders and children with moderate learning difficulties. *Journal of Child Psychology and Psychiatry, 46*, 409–419.

Folstein, S., & Rutter, M. (1977). Infantile autism: A genetic study of 21 twin pairs. *Journal of Child Psychology and Psychiatry, 18*, 297–321.

Fombonne, E., Siddons, F., Achard, S., Frith, U., & Happé, F. (1994). Adaptive behaviour and theory of mind in autism. *European Child and Adolescent Psychiatry, 3*, 176–186.

Frith, U. (1989). *Autism: Explaining the enigma*. Oxford: Blackwell.

Frith, U. (2003). *Autism: Explaining the enigma* (2nd ed.). Oxford: Blackwell.

Frith, U., Happé, F., & Siddons, F. (1994). Autism and theory of mind in everyday life. *Social Development, 2*, 108–124.

Frith, U., & Hermelin, B. (1969). The role of visual and motor cues for normal, subnormal and autistic children. *Journal of Child Psychology and Psychiatry, 10*, 153–163.

Frith, U., & Snowling, M. (1983). Reading for meaning and reading for sound in autistic and dyslexic children. *British Journal of Developmental Psychology, 1*, 329–342.

Gallagher, H. L., Happé, F., Brunswick, N., Fletcher, P. C., Frith, U., & Frith, C. D. (2000). Reading the mind in cartoons and stories: An fMRI study of 'theory of mind' in verbal and nonverbal tasks. *Neuropsychologia, 38*, 11–21.

Geurts, H., Begeer, S., & Stockmann, L. (2009). Brief report: Inhibitory control of socially relevant stimuli in children with high functioning autism. *Journal of Autism and Developmental Disorders, 39*, 1603–1607.

Gilbert, S. J., Bird, G., Brindleya, R., Frith, C., & Burgess, P. W. (2008). Atypical recruitment of medial prefrontal cortex in autism spectrum disorders: An fMRI study of two executive function tasks. *Neuropsychologia, 46*, 2281–2291.

Gioia, G. A., Isquith, P. K., Guy, S., & Kenworthy, L. (2000). *BRIEF: The behavior rating inventory of executive function*. Odessa, FL: Psychological Assessment Resources.

Goodman, R. (1989). Infantile autism: A syndrome of multiple primary deficits? *Journal of Autism and Developmental Disorders, 19*, 409–424.

Griffith, E. M., Pennington, B. F., Wehner, E. A., & Rogers, S. J. (1999). Executive functions in young children with autism. *Child Development, 70*, 817–832.

Happé, F. G. E. (1995). The role of age and verbal ability in the theory of mind task performance of subjects with autism. *Child Development, 66*, 843–855.

Happé, F. G. E. (1996). Studying weak central coherence at low levels: Children with autism do not succumb to visual illusions. A research note. *Journal of Child Psychology and Psychiatry, 37*, 873–877.

Happé, F. G. E. (1997). Central coherence and theory of mind in autism: Reading homographs in context. *British Journal of Developmental Psychology, 15*, 1–12.

Happé, F. (1999). Autism: Cognitive deficit of cognitive style. *Trends in Cognitive Sciences, 3*, 216–222.

Happé, F. G. E., Booth, R., Charlton, R., & Hughes, C. (2006). Executive function deficits in autism spectrum disorders and attention-deficit/hyperactivity disorder: Examining profiles across domains and ages. *Brain and Cognition, 61*, 25–39.

Happé, F. G. E., & Frith, U. (2006). The weak coherence account: Detail-focused cognitive style in autism spectrum disorders. *Journal of Autism and Developmental Disorders, 36*, 5–25.

Happé, F., & Ronald, A. (2008). The 'fractionable autism triad': A review of evidence from behavioural, genetic, cognitive and neural research. *Neuropsychological Review, 18*, 287–304.

Happé, F., Ronald, A., & Plomin, R. (2006). Time to give up on a single explanation for autism. *Nature Neuroscience, 9*, 1218–1220.

Haviland, J. M., & Lelwica, M. L. (1987). The induced affect response: 10 week-old infants' responses to three emotional expressions. *Developmental Psychology, 23*, 97–104.

Heaton, R. K. (1981). *Wisconsin card sorting test manual*. Odessa, FL: Psychological Assessment Resources.

Hill, E. L. (2004). Evaluating the theory of executive dysfunction in autism. *Developmental Review, 24*, 189–233.

Hobson, R. P. (1989). Beyond cognition: A theory of autism. In G. Dawson (Ed.), *Autism: Nature, diagnosis and treatment* (pp. 22–48). New York: Guildford.

Hobson, R. P. (1993). *Autism and the development of mind*. Oxford University Press: Oxford.

Hobson, R. P. (2002). *The cradle of thought: Exploring the origins of thinking*. London: Macmillan.

Hockey, A., & Geffen, G. (2004). The concurrent validity and test-retest reliability of a visuospatial working memory task. *Intelligence, 32*, 591–605.

Hoekstra, R. A., Bartels, M., Cath, D. C., & Boomsma, D. I. (2008). Factor structure, reliability and criterion validity of the autism spectrum quotient (AQ): A study in Dutch population and patient groups. *Journal of Autism and Developmental Disorders, 38*, 1555–1566.

Hogrefe, G. -J., Wimmer, H., & Perner, J. (1986). Ignorance versus false belief: A developmental lag in attribution of epistemic states. *Child Development, 57*, 567–582.

Hoy, J. A., Hatton, C., & Hare, D. (2004). Weak central coherence: A cross-domain phenomenon specific to autism? *Autism, 8*, 267–281.

Hughes, C. H., & Russell, J. (1993). Autistic children's difficulties with mental disengagement from an object: Its implications for theories of Autism. *Developmental Psychology, 29*, 498–510.

Hughes, C., Russell, J., & Robbins, T. W. (1994). Evidence for executive dysfunction in autism. *Neuropsychologia, 32*, 477–492.

Hurst, R. M., Mitchell, J. T., Kimbrel, N. A., Kwapil, T. K., & Nelson-Gray, R. O. (2007). Examination of the reliability and factor structure of the Autism Spectrum Quotient (AQ) in a non-clinical sample. *Personality and Individual Differences, 43*, 1938–1949.

International Molecular Genetic Study of Autism Consortium. (1998). A full genome screen for autism with evidence for linkage to a region on chromosome 7q. *Human Molecular Genetics, 7*, 571–578.

International Molecular Genetic Study of Autism Consortium. (2001). Further characterization of the autism susceptibility locus AUTS1 on chromosome 7q. *Human Molecular Genetics, 10*, 973–982.

International Molecular Genetic Study of Autism Consortium. (2005). Analysis of IMGSAC autism susceptibility loci: Evidence for sex limited and parent origin specific effects. *Journal of Medical Genetics, 42*, 132–137.

Jarrold, C. (2003). A review of research into pretend play in autism. *Autism, 7*, 379–390.

Jarrold, C., Gilchrist, I. D., & Bender, A. (2005). Embedded figures detection in autism and typical development: Preliminary evidence of a double dissociation in relationships with visual search. *Developmental Science, 8*, 344–351.

Jolliffe, T., & Baron-Cohen, S. (1997). Are people with autism and Asperger syndrome faster than normal on the embedded figures test. *Journal of Child Psychology and Psychiatry, 38*, 527–534.

Jolliffe, T., & Baron-Cohen, S. (1999). A test of central coherence theory: Linguistic processing in high-functioning adults with autism or Asperger syndrome: Is local coherence impaired? *Cognition, 71*, 149–185.

Jurado, M., & Rosselli, M. (2007). The elusive nature of executive functions: A review of our current understanding. *Neuropsychology Review, 17*, 213–233.

Just, M. A., Cherkassky, V. L., Keller, T. A., Kana, R. K., & Minshew, N. J. (2007). Functional and anatomical cortical underconnectivity in autism: Evidence from an fMRI study of an executive function task and corpus callosum morphometry. *Cerebral Cortex, 17*, 951–961.

Just, M. A., Cherkassky, V. L., Keller, T. A., & Minshew, N. J. (2004). Cortical activation and synchronization during sentence comprehension in high-functioning autism: Evidence of underconnectivity. *Brain, 127*, 1811–1821.

Kaland, N., Mortensen, E. L., & Smith, L. (2007). Disembedding performance in children and adolescents with Asperger syndrome or high-functioning autism. *Autism, 11*, 81–92.

Kana, R. K., Keller, T. A., Cherkassky, V. L., Minshew, N. J., & Just, M. A. (2009). Atypical frontal-posterior synchronization of theory of mind regions in autism during mental state attribution. *Social Neuroscience, 4*, 135–152.

Kana, R. K., Keller, T. A., Minshew, N. J., & Just, M. A. (2007). Inhibitory control in high-functioning autism: Decreased activation and underconnectivity in inhibition networks. *Biological Psychiatry, 62*, 198–206.

Kanner, L. (1943). Autistic disturbances of affective contact. *Nervous Child, 2*, 217–250.

Klin, A., Jones, W., Schultz, R., & Volkmar, F. (2003). The enactive mind, or from actions to cognition: Lessons from autism. *Philosophical Transactions of the Royal Society B-Biological Sciences, 358,* 345–360.

Koshino, H., Carpenter, P. A., Minshew, N. J., Cherkassky, V. L., Keller, T. A., & Just, M. A. (2005). Functional connectivity in an fMRI working memory task in high-functioning autism. *Neuroimage, 24,* 810–821.

Lam, K. S. L., & Aman, M. G. (2007). The repetitive behavior scale-revised: Independent validation in individuals with autism spectrum disorders. *Journal of Autism and Developmental Disorders, 37,* 855–866.

Landa, R. J., & Goldberg, M. C. (2005). Language, social, and executive functions in high functioning autism: A continuum of performance. *Journal of Autism and Developmental Disorders, 35,* 557–573.

Leslie, A. M. (1987). Pretense and representation: The origins of theory of mind. *Psychological Review, 94,* 412–426.

Leslie, A. M., & Frith, U. (1990). Prospects for a cognitive neuropsychology of autism: Hobson's choice. *Psychological Review, 97,* 122–131.

Leslie, A. M., & Happé, F. (1989). Autism and ostensive communication: The relevance of metarepresentation. *Development and Psychopathology, 1,* 205–212.

Leslie, A. M., & Roth, D. (1993). What autism teaches us about metarepresentation. In S. Baron-Cohen, H. Tager-Flusberg, & D. Cohen (Eds.), *Understanding other minds: Perspectives from autism* (pp. 83–111). Oxford: Oxford University Press.

Lind, S. E., & Bowler, D. M. (2009). Language and theory of mind in autism spectrum disorder: The relationship between complement syntax and false belief task performance. *Journal of Autism and Developmental Disorders, 39,* 929–937.

Lind, S. E., & Bowler, D. M. (2010). Impaired performance on see-know tasks amongst children with autism: Evidence of specific difficulties with theory of mind or domain general task factors? *Journal of Autism and Developmental Disorders, 40,* 479–484.

López, B., & Leekam, S. R. (2003). Do children with autism fail to process information in context? *Journal of Child Psychology and Psychiatry, 44,* 285–300.

Lopez, B. R., Lincoln, A. J., Ozonoff, S., & Lai, Z. (2005). Examining the relationship between executive functions and restricted, repetitive symptoms of autistic disorder. *Journal of Autism and Developmental Disorders, 35,* 445–460.

Loveland, K. A. (1991). Social affordances and interaction II: Autism and the affordances of the human environment. *Ecological Psychology, 3,* 99–119.

Luna, B., Minshew, N. J., Garver, K. E., Lazar, N. A., Thulborn, K. R., Eddy, W. F., et al. (2002). Neocortical system abnormalities in autism: An fMRI study of spatial working memory. *Neurology, 59,* 834–840.

Mandy, W. P. L., & Skuse, D. H. (2008). What is the association between the social-communication element of autism and repetitive interests, behaviours and activities? *Journal of Child Psychology and Psychiatry, 49,* 795–808.

McEvoy, R., Rogers, S. J., & Pennington, B. F. (1993). Executive function and social communication deficits in your autistic children. *Journal of Child Psychology and Psychiatry, 34,* 563–578.

Morgan, B., Maybery, M., & Durkin, K. (2003). Weak central coherence, poor joint attention, and low verbal ability: Independent deficits in early autism. *Developmental Psychology, 39,* 646–656.

Morton, J., & Frith, U. (1995). Causal modeling: A structural approach to developmental psychopathology. In D. Cicchetti & D. J. Cohen (Eds.), *Developmental psychopathology, volume 1, theory and methods* (pp. 357–390). New York: Wiley.

Mottron, L., & Burack, J. A. (2001). Enhanced perceptual functioning in the development of autism. In J. A. Burack, T. Charman, N. Yirmiya, & P. R. Zelazo (Eds.), *The development of autism: Perspectives from theory and research* (pp. 131–148). Mahwah, NJ: Erlbaum.

Mottron, L., Dawson, M., Soulieres, I., Hubert, B., & Burack, J. A. (2006). Enhanced perceptual functioning in autism: An update, and eight principles of autistic perception. *Journal of Autism and Developmental Disorders, 36,* 27–43.

Owen, A. M., McMillan, K. M., & Laird, A. R. (2005). N-back working memory paradigm: A meta-analysis of normative functional neuroimaging studies. *Human Brain Mapping, 25,* 46–59.

Ozonoff, S., & Jensen, J. (1999). Brief report: Specific executive function profiles in three neurodevelopmental disorders. *Journal of Autism and Developmental Disorders, 29,* 171–177.

Ozonoff, S., Pennington, B. F., & Rogers, S. J. (1991). Executive functioning deficits in high-functioning autistic individuals: Relationship to theory of mind. *Journal of Child Psychology and Psychiatry, 32,* 1081–1105.

Ozonoff, S., & Strayer, D. L. (2001). Further evidence of intact working memory in autism. *Journal of Autism and Developmental Disorders, 31,* 257–263.

Pellicano, E. (2007). Links between theory of mind and executive function in young children with autism: Clues to developmental primacy. *Developmental Psychology, 43,* 974–990.

Pellicano, E., Maybery, M., Durkin, K., & Maley, A. (2006). Multiple cognitive capabilities/deficits in children with an autism spectrum disorder: "Weak" central coherence and its relationship to theory of mind and executive control. *Development and Psychopathology, 18,* 77–98.

Pennington, B. F., & Ozonoff, S. (1996). Executive functions and developmental psychopathology. *Journal of Child Psychology and Psychiatry, 37,* 51–87.

Peterson, C. C., Peterson, J. L., & Webb, J. (2000). Factors influencing the development of a theory of mind in blind children. *British Journal of Developmental Psychology, 18,* 431–447.

Peterson, C. C., & Seigal, M. (1995). Deafness, conversation and theory of mind. *Journal of Child Psychology and Psychiatry, 36,* 459–474.

Peterson, C. C., Wellman, H. M., & Lui, D. (2005). Steps in theory-of-mind development for children with deafness or autism. *Child Development, 76,* 502–517.

Premack, D., & Woodruff, G. (1978). Does the chimpanzee have a theory of mind? *Behavioral and Brain Sciences, 1,* 515–526.

Ropar, D., & Mitchell, P. (1999). Are individuals with autism and Asperger's syndrome susceptible to visual illusions? *Journal of Child Psychology and Psychiatry, 40,* 1283–1293.

Ropar, D., & Mitchell, P. (2001). Susceptibility to illusions and performance on visuospatial tasks in individuals with autism. *Journal of Child Psychology and Psychiatry, 42,* 539–549.

Rumsey, J. M. (1985). Conceptual problem-solving in highly verbal, nonretarded autistic men. *Journal of Autism and Developmental Disorders, 15,* 23–36.

Russell, J. (1996). *Agency: Its role in mental development.* Hove: Lawrence Erlbaum Associates/Taylor and Francis.

Russell, J., & Hill, E. L. (2001). Action monitoring and intention reporting in children with autism. *Journal of Child Psychology and Psychiatry, 42,* 317–328.

Schlooz, W. A. J. M., Hulstijn, W., van den Broek, P. J. A., van der Pijll, A. C. A. M., Gabreëls, F., van der Gaag, R. J., et al. (2006). Fragmented visuospatial processing in children with pervasive developmental disorder. *Journal of Autism and Developmental Disorders, 36,* 1025–1037.

Schmitz, N., Rubia, K., Daly, E., Smith, A., Williams, S., & Murphy, D. G. M. (2006). Neural correlates of executive function in autistic spectrum disorders. *Biological Psychiatry, 59,* 7–16.

Senju, A., Southgate, V., White, S., & Frith, U. (2009). Mindblind eyes: An absence of spontaneous theory of mind in Asperger syndrome. *Science, 325,* 883–885.

Shah, A., & Frith, U. (1983). An islet of ability in autism: A research note. *Journal of Child Psychology and Psychiatry, 24*, 613–620.

Shah, A., & Frith, U. (1993). Why do autistic individuals show superior performance on the block design task? *Journal of Child Psychology and Psychiatry, 34*, 1351–1364.

Shallice, T. (1982). Specific impairments in planning. *Philosophical Transactions of the Royal Society of London, Series B, 298*, 199–209.

Siegal, M., & Beattie, K. (1991). Where to look first for children's knowledge of false beliefs. *Cognition, 38*, 1–12.

Sinzig, J., Morsche, P. A., Bruning, N., Schmidt, M. H., & Lehmkuhl, G. (2008). Inhibition, flexibility, working memory and planning in autism spectrum disorders with and without comorbid ADHD-symptoms. *Child and Adolescent Psychiatry and Mental Health, 2*, 4.

SLI Consortium. (2004). Highly significant linkage to the *SLI1* locus in an expanded sample of individuals affected by specific language impairment. *American Journal of Human Genetics, 74*, 1225–1238.

Sodian, B., & Frith, U. (1992). Deception and sabotage in autistic, retarded and normal children. *Journal of Child Psychology and Psychiatry, 33*, 591–605.

South, M., Ozonoff, S., & McMahon, W. M. (2007). The relationship between executive functioning, central coherence, and repetitive behaviors in the high-functioning autism spectrum. *Autism, 11*, 437–451.

Steele, S. D., Minshew, N. J., Luna, B., & Sweeney, J. A. (2007). Spatial working memory deficits in autism. *Journal of Autism and Developmental Disorders, 37*, 605–612.

Steffenburg, S., Hellgren, L. A. L., Gillberg, I. C., Jakobsen, G., & Bohman, M. (1989). A twin study of autism in Denmark, Finland, Iceland, Norway and Sweden. *Journal of Child Psychology and Psychiatry, 30*, 405–416.

Stewart, M. E., & Austin, E. J. (2009). The structure of the Autism-Spectrum Quotient (AQ): Evidence from a student sample in Scotland. *Personality and Individual Differences, 47*, 224–228.

Stewart, M. E., Watson, J., Allcock, A. –J., & Yaqoob, T. (2009). Autistic traits predict performance on the block design. *Autism, 13*, 133–142.

Stroop, J. R. (1935). Studies of interference in serial verbal reactions. *Journal of Experimental Psychology, 18*, 613–662.

Stuss, D. T., Alexander, M. P., Floden, D., Binns, M. A., Levine, B., McIntosh, A. R., et al. (2002). Fractionation and localization of distinct frontal lobe processes: Evidence from focal lesions in humans. In D. T. Stuss & R. T. Knight (Eds.), *Principles of frontal lobe function* (pp. 392–407). New York: Oxford University Press.

Surian, L., & Leslie, A. M. (1999). Competence and performance in false belief understanding: A comparison of autistic and normal 3-year-old children. *British Journal of Developmental Psychology, 17*, 141–155.

Szatmari, P., Merrette, C., Bryson, S. E., Thivierge, J., Roy, M. A., Cayer, M., et al. (2002). Quantifying dimensions in autism: A factor-analytic study. *Journal of the American Academy of Child & Adolescent Psychiatry, 41*, 467–474.

Teunisse, J. -P., Cools, A. R., van Spaendonck, K. P. M., Aerts, F. H., & Berger, H. J. (2001). Cognitive styles in high-functioning adolescents with autistic disorder. *Journal of Autism and Developmental Disorders, 31*, 55–66.

Turner, M. (1999). Repetitive behaviour in autism: A review of psychological research. *Journal of Child Psychology and Psychiatry, 40*, 839–849.

Wechsler, D. (2004). *Wechsler intelligence scale for children* (4th UK ed.). London: Harcourt Assessment.

Wellman, H., Cross, D., & Watson, J. (2001). Meta-analysis of theory of mind development: The truth about false belief. *Child Development, 72*, 655–684.

Williams, D. L., Goldstein, G., Carpenter, P. A., & Minshew, N. J. (2005). Verbal and spatial working memory in autism. *Journal of Autism and Developmental Disorders, 35*, 747–756.

Williams, D. M., & Happé, F. (2009a). What did I say? versus What did I think?: Attributing false beliefs to self amongst children with and without autism. *Journal of Autism and Developmental Disorders, 39*, 865–873.

Williams, D., & Happé, F. (2009b). Pre-conceptual aspects of self-awareness in autism spectrum disorder: The case of action monitoring. *Journal of Autism and Developmental Disorders, 39*, 251–259.

Williams, D. M., & Happé, F. (2010). Representing intentions in self and others: Studies of autism and typical development. *Developmental Science, 13*, 307–319.

Williams, D. M. (2010). Theory of own mind in autism: Evidence of a specific deficit in self-awareness? *Autism, 14*, 474–494.

Williams, D. M., Lind, S. E., & Happé, F. G. E. (2009). Metacognition may be more impaired than mindreading in autism. *Behavioral and Brain Sciences, 32*, 162–163.

Wimmer, H., & Perner, J. (1983). Beliefs about beliefs: Representation and constraining function of wrong beliefs in young children's understanding of deception. *Cognition, 13*, 103–128.

Wing, L., & Gould, J. (1979). Severe impairments of social interaction and associated abnormalities in children: Epidemiology and classification. *Journal of Autism and Childhood Schizophrenia, 9*, 11–29.

Witkin, H. A., Oltman, P. K., Raskin, E., & Karp, S. (1971). *A manual for the embedded figures test*. Palo Alto, CA: Consulting Psychologists Press.

Wolpert, D. M., Ghahramani, Z., & Jordan, M. I. (1995). An internal model for sensorimotor integration. *Science, 269*, 1880–1882.

World Health Organization. (1993). *International classification of diseases* (10th ed.). Geneva: World Health Organization.

Yirmiya, N., Erel, O., Shaked, M., & Solomonica-Levi, D. (1998). Meta-analyses comparing theory of mind abilities of individuals with autism, individuals with mental retardation, and normally developing individuals. *Psychological Bulletin, 124*, 283–307.

Zilbovicius, M., Meresse, I., Chabane, N., Brunelle, F., Samson, Y., et al. (2006). Autism, the superior temporal sulcus and social perception. *Trends in Neuroscience, 29*, 359–366.

Nosology and Theories of Repetitive and Restricted Behaviours and Interests

Eynat Gal

Introduction

Repetitive and restrictive behaviours and interests (RRBI) are defining core features of autism spectrum disorders (ASD), described in Kanner's original paper (1943). They are also one of three behavioural domains – the other being deficits in social interaction and deficits in communication required for the current diagnosis of autism (ICD-10, World Health Organization, 1990; DSM-IV, American Psychiatric Association, 1994). These behaviours often look bizarre, grotesque and inappropriate to others and interfere with everyday functions. Accordingly they are of specific concern for parents and clinicians who live and work with people with ASD.

This chapter describes the various rituals, special interests and other repetitive behaviours and movements and reviews their incidence and prevalence across the various ASD. In addition it surveys the effects of intellectual disability, obsessive compulsive behaviours and other comorbid disorders on the rate and type of rituals and repetitive behaviours.

Repetitive Behaviours – What Are They?

'Repetitive and restrictive behaviours and interests' (RRBI) is an umbrella term for the broad class of behaviours linked by repetition, rigidity, invariance and inappropriateness to the place and context (Turner, 1997). In autism they include rituals and routines, narrow and circumscribed interests, repetitive use of language, stereotyped motor movements, repetitive manipulation of objects and repetitive self-injurious behaviour (Lewis & Boucher, 1988; Schopler, 1995; Turner, 1999).

E. Gal (✉)
Department of Occupational Therapy, University of Haifa,
Haifa 31905, Israel
e-mail: egal@univ.haifa.ac.il

Rituals and Routines

Many people with ASD appear to adhere inflexibly to routines, will not tolerate changes in routine and suffer from subsequent anxiety when novel events unexpectedly occur. Changes in the routine, such as in the route to work, in the usual furniture arrangement or in school activities, may cause extreme distress. Insistence on inflexible routines may reflect the need present in many people with ASD for predictability and structure.

Along with the adherence to routines, many people with ASD perform ritualistic behaviours which are often compulsive in nature such as demanding consistency in their environment or an apparent compulsion always to act in exactly the same way at a specific time (Schopler, 1995). This may be irrelevant and inappropriate to the environment's needs and demands. For example, a child with ASD may feel compelled to close the door behind him and turn off the lights every time he leaves a room even if other people are still using it. Another may have a strong need to put things away even when they are still needed. Many insist on eating the same foods, at the same time, and sitting in precisely the same place at the table every day. A minor change in their physical environment or their routine such as a tilted picture on the wall or a change of school's schedule may be extremely upsetting.

These behaviours may create great difficulties for the people around such a person, may prevent him from being involved in more appropriate play/work activities, and may negatively affect his ability to participate in extended family events and cultural and community life.

Narrow and Circumscribed Interests

The development of unusual, narrow and circumscribed interests or an obsession or fascination with a particular topic is a hallmark symptom of people on the autism spectrum. Individuals with ASD, both children and adults, often develop intense interest in restricted subjects and can talk, often for hours, about their interest. For children, one way that these interests are shown is attachment to a specific object. Unlike typical young children who often form attachments to soft and cuddly transitional objects, attachments to objects in young children with ASD are almost always 'different'. The attachment may be to hard objects (e.g. metal cars) or to a class of objects rather than a specific object (e.g. a magazine of a certain type but not a specific magazine) (Volkmar, 2005). Some children will carry these objects around and refuse to part with them. Others may show an extreme reaction that looks bizarre whenever they come into contact with a particular object. Later in life children with ASD may develop specific interests or a peculiar fascination with subjects rather than objects. Typical examples are phone numbers, the many varieties of electric fans (or anything else), birth dates, weather reports and commercials. Such interests might be more complex, such as diagrams, maps or stories by a specific writer (Schopler, 1995).

The narrow and circumscribed interests may present both a challenge and an advantage for the person with ASD: for children with autism, obsessive interests become all-consuming and they may talk about little else. The narrow interests, often pursued to the exclusion of other more appropriate behaviours, can substantially interfere with social functioning and academic success. Coupled with impairments in social development, which is a clear mark of the disorder, the narrow interests will create further 'weirdness' as someone on the autism spectrum will have difficulties judging when a listener is not interested in the endless wealth of information about a specific topic of interest. It also may affect participation as a child may sit and think about her topic of interest when she is expected to be engaged in other activities, such as playing on the playground or doing homework.

But among the positive possibilities is the development in some children on the Autism spectrum of lifelong interests, which if directed, guided and expanded could evolve into a career. For example, a child who obsesses on weather patterns may mature into a meteorologist as an adult; one interested in books or fascinated by dates and other numbers may find future career working in a library.

Repetitive Use of Language

Repetitive use of language, such as the repetition of favourite sounds, words, sentences or songs, or asking the same question over and over again, is also a common form of ritualized behaviour.

Repetitive verbalization can have a non-communicative purpose, where a response is not expected. Alternatively, perseverative speech may be communicative in nature, representing the child's processing difficulties and/or his emotional state; often it relates to his anxiety due to routine and change of routine issues, for example, a child may say repeatedly 'go to gym' when a gym class has been cancelled. Clearly, repetitive verbalization can interfere with social interaction, and it is often exasperating to other people.

Stereotyped Motor Movements

Stereotyped movements (SMs) or stereotypies have been described as patterned movements which are highly consistent, invariant and repetitious, excessive in rate, frequency and/or amplitude and are inappropriate, odd and lack an obvious goal (Dantzer, 1986; Turner, 1999). Typical examples of these movements are rhythmic body rocking in a sitting or standing position, head bobbing, various arm and hand movements such as arm waving and hand flapping, eye rolling, finger wiggling, finger waving (in front or at the sides of the face), repetitive pacing and jumping and hair twirling (Schopler, 1995). Movements last from seconds to minutes and may appear multiple times a day. Each child has his/her own repertoire, which can evolve with time. Nevertheless, several primary movements, such as bilateral flapping or rotating the hands, fluttering fingers in front of the face, flapping/waving arm movements and head nodding, tend to predominate (Singer, 2009). Stereotyped movements vary in many ways. They differ in the body parts that are involved, and the same person may show more than one stereotyped movement, involving a few different body parts (Mason & Turner, 1993), and they differ in how often they are repeated. Bouts of SM may be long or short, with few or many repetitions (Turner, 1999), and the bouts themselves vary in how often they recur. Some stereotyped movements may be repeated many times a day, in a variety of different circumstances, while others are much more limited in the circumstances in which they are performed. They may differ in their degree of 'inappropriateness' or 'oddness'. For example, repetitive leg movement, with concentration, might look more 'appropriate' than flipping hands in front of the eyes or intensive rocking movements while standing and talking. This criterion, of course, is prone to subjective and cultural-oriented judgment.

The movements which are defined as stereotyped within disabled populations, according to the various above-mentioned criteria, are challenging for the person who performs them in the cognitive, social and functional aspects of his life. They differ significantly from aimed and planned movements shown along a lifespan in typically developed people. As such, they strongly influence the social life of the person who performs them. Stereotyped movements are problematic for the observer or the intervener, but they also constitute a significant barrier for the individual exhibiting them, the person struggling to live a life as productive and independent as possible. Stereotyped movements often engage the child's attention totally, so that he or she is unlikely to take notice of possible alternative pursuits. They are often highly reinforcing, and more attractive to the child than their alternatives (Wing, 1976), hence are often refractory to treatment (Bodfish et al., 1995). Accordingly, stereotyped movements are perceived as a major problem for parents, educators and clinicians who work with children with ASD. This is attested by the attention of both clinicians and literature to the attenuation of such movements.

Repetitive Manipulation of Objects

Repetitive manipulation of objects relates to the repetition of the same motor activity used to manipulate the physical environment. Typical repetitive manipulation of objects among individuals with ASD may include lining up objects, flicking light switches, or displaying repetitive manipulation of an object such as a string, rubber tubing, or a toy. A child may stack blocks over and over again without demonstrating pride in the accomplishment, dump toys or turn light switches on and off repeatedly. When repetitive manipulation of objects relates to toys, it is often called 'stereotypic/repetitive play'. Repetitive play often replaces imaginative play in a child with ASD. Most typically developing children at the age of 2 and up will use their imagination to pretend and create new uses for an object (e.g. will use stones as food for the doll). The child with ASD, however, rarely pretends. That child may be preoccupied with spinning the wheels on a toy car rather than playing a racing or driving game. Rather than rocking a doll she may simply hold it, smell it or spin it for hours. The repetitive play has been suggested as representing difficulty in forming a visual perception of an object and abstracting its potential uses (Ayres, 1979), lack of curiosity and incapability of a more advanced spontaneous symbolic play (Roeyers & Van Berckelaer-Onnes, 1994).

Repetitive Self-Injurious Behaviours (SIB)

According to an earlier definition, self-injury is any of a number of behaviours whereby the individual causes physical damage to his/her own body (Tate & Baroff, 1966). Apart from their capacity to cause harm, the self-injurious behaviours of people with developmental disorders, including autism (Baumeister & Forehand, 1973; Baumeister, 1978; Berkson, 1983; Tate & Baroff, 1966; Tröster, Brambring, & Beelmann, 1991; Turner, 1999), appear to have nothing in common with the self-harming behaviour of other clinical groups (Alderman, 1997; Baroff,

1974; Briere & Gil, 1998; Favazza, 1996; Schroeder, Schroeder, Smith, & Dalldorf, 1978). Rather, as Matson et al. (1997) noted, the self-injurious behaviour of people with developmental disorders is frequently rhythmic and repetitive: it closely resembles the repetitive and stereotyped movements that are a defining characteristic of autism.

Repetitive self-injurious behaviours in autism and other developmental disabilities can cause tissue damage (bruises, redness, open wounds) and often include head banging or hitting, hand-biting, compulsive scratching or rubbing, eye gouging, teeth grinding (bruxism), wound picking and breath holding (Alderman, 1997; Favazza, 1996).

Until recently, self-injurious and other stereotyped movements were included together in a class of RRBI, behaviours marked by repetition, rigidity, invariance and inappropriate continuation (Baumeister & Rolling, 1976; de Lissavoy, 1961; Turner, 1997; Wing, 1976), and classified as a 'substrate of stereotyped behaviours' (Gorman-Smith & Matson, 1985). More recently self-injurious behaviours, with aggressive/destructive behaviour and noncompliance, have been construed as distinct subcategories of 'problem' (Rojahn, Matson, Lott, Esbensen, & Smalls, 2001) or 'challenging' behaviour (Matson & Nebel-Schwalm, 2007), and self-injury is nowadays excluded from some definitions of RRBI (Leekam et al., 2007).

Self-injury in people with autism can become an intransigent and lifelong problem, as both epidemiological and intervention studies have demonstrated (Murphy, Hall, Oliver, & Kissi-Debra, 1999). It may cause differing degrees of harm to the person who performs it, from bruises due to slapping and calluses due to biting to open wounds and haematomas that may be life endangering (Carr, 1977).

In addition to the obvious physical distress and danger that these behaviours may cause to the individual, SIB has social psychological and educational implications, as peers, parents and staff members dealing with it are often reluctant to place demands on the child for fear of precipitating a SIB episode (Carr, 1977). Under such circumstances the child misses important opportunities for productive interaction with his/her social and physical environment (Schreibman, 1988). Due to the overwhelming and sometimes life-threatening nature of SIB and the barrier it poses to social and intellectual development, treatment efforts have been numerous over the years, but not always successful (Romanczyk, Ekdahl, & Lockshin, 1992).

Incidence and Prevalence of Repetitive Behaviours Across the Various ASD

Being defining core features of ASD, some repetitive behaviours and movements, rituals or special interests are prevalent across all people with ASD. Diagnostic criteria for autism require, however, only the presence of one behaviour out of any of the four repetitive-behaviour categories: (a) narrow, circumscribed patterns of interests that are intensely pursued; (b) preoccupation with parts of objects or non-functional objects; (c) stereotyped motor mannerisms; and (d) insistence on sameness. Obviously, while all of these involve repetitiveness and persistence, they are heterogeneous behaviours, which the literature tries to distinguish in various ways. First, it suggests that some of these behaviours are more prevalent than others. Second, there is the question of how stable the prevalence of these behaviours is across lifespan, and third, some studies have investigated whether these core features vary across the diverse disorders on the autism spectrum.

Studying the symptoms of ASD manifested by 405 individuals aged between 10 and 53 years, Seltzer et al. (2003) used the Autism Diagnostic Interview-Revised (ADI-R) to assess the patterns of various autism symptoms in adolescence and adulthood. They centred on seven items in the restricted, repetitive behaviours and interests domain: circumscribed interests, unusual preoccupations, compulsions, hand and finger mannerisms, other complex mannerisms and body movements, repetitive use of objects and unusual sensory interests.

These authors found that repetitive movements and mannerisms were more prevalent in people with ASD during their lifespan than rituals and compulsions: 46% of their sample showed repetitive use of objects, 23.8% demonstrated hand and finger mannerisms and 33% showed other complex mannerisms and body movements. However, only 13.9% showed verbal rituals and 9.8% compulsions; and 6% were reported ever showing circumscribed interests.

As for the consistency of specific repetitive-behaviour symptoms across one's lifespan, this, like the stability of ASD diagnosis, is a relatively unexplored area. However, some studies on this issue usually address its stability in early childhood or from adolescence to adulthood (Morgan, Wetherby, & Barber, 2008).

Studies using home videotapes as a primary data source have provided little or no indication that repetitive behaviour is an important discriminating variable in children younger than 2 years (Baranek, 1999; Osterling, Dawson, & Munson, 2002). However, a number of studies that utilized retrospective parent reports from the Autism Diagnostic Interview-Revised have indicated such discrimination (Richler, Bishop, Kleinke, & Lord, 2007; Watson et al., 2007; Werner, Dawson, Munson, & Osterling, 2005).

While repetitive symptoms have been identified as differentiating children with ASD from those with typical development and developmental disabilities as early as 6 months old, some studies suggest that these behaviours may not be fully developed until at least 3 years of age (Lord, 1995; Moore &

Goodson, 2003; Stone et al., 1999) and indicate that repetitive behaviours generally increase from age 2 to 4 (Cox et al., 1999; Moore & Goodson, 2003; Stone et al., 1999).

Studies seeking evidence of repetitive behaviours from early childhood to late adolescence suggest both continuity and change in the developmental trajectory of children with autism. Mesibov, Schopler, Schaffer and Michal (1989) and Eaves and Ho (1996) report stability of the diagnosis of autism from childhood to adolescence, but with a change in the intensity of symptoms and an amelioration of autistic symptoms prior to the age 10 years and then again after age 13. However, these are not specific to RRBI. In fact, comparing parents' reports of autistic symptom expression in their adolescent and young adult children with retrospective reports when their children were aged 5, Piven and colleagues reported a decrease of social and communicative symptoms, but not repetitive behaviours and stereotyped interest from childhood to adolescence (Piven, Harper, Palmer, & Arndt, 1996). In their aforementioned study, Seltzer et al. (2003) found that the adults were less symptomatic than the adolescents at both time points with respect to restricted, repetitive behaviours and interests. These researchers concluded that the adults were more likely to improve in the restricted, repetitive behaviours and interests' domain.

The third issue that relates to prevalence of repetitive behaviours in people with ASD is the difference in the nature of these behaviours across various disorders on the autism spectrum. Their broad range is often subdivided into two categories: lower-level and higher-level repetitive behaviours. The former are characterized by repetition of movement (stereotyped movements, repetitive manipulation of objects, dyskinesias, tics and repetitive forms of self-injurious behaviour). The more complex higher-level repetitive behaviours include object attachments, insistence on the maintenance of sameness, repetitive language and circumscribed interests (Bodfish, Symons, Parker, & Lewis, 2000). Factor analyses of items from the Autism Diagnostic Interview-Revised (ADI-R) have indeed yielded two factors: 'repetitive sensory motor behaviour' and 'resistance to change', findings which indeed support this categorization (Cuccaro et al., 2003).

Turner (1999) reviewed repetitive behaviours in autism and noted that motor behaviours – stereotyped movements in particular, the most widely studied form of repetitive behaviours in autism – are generally believed to index low cognitive ability. In contrast, higher-level repetitive behaviours, such as circumscribed interests, are more commonly observed in higher functioning individuals. Turner's review suggests that repetitive behaviours are not unidimensional and may serve as an index of ability or severity of autism.

The view that classification of repetitive phenomena into higher-order and lower-order categories, with the suggestion that these categories are differentially associated with IQ (lower-order behaviours are more typically associated with reduced IQ), was also supported by Schopler (1995), who related the various types of repetitive behaviours to the level of the person's developmental function. Specifically he suggested that at an early developmental level, stereotyped behaviours merely involve sensory peculiarities like excessive licking, smelling or making odd sounds and stereotyped movements such as hand flapping, finger twisting, twirling and spinning of objects. At a higher level of development, preoccupations may include repetitive manipulation of objects showing attachment to an object like a string, rubber tubing or a toy; obsessive interests may be more prevalent also.

Studies have aimed not only to differentiate between lower to higher functioning children with autism but also to assess differences between various disorders at the high end of the spectrum by means of repetitive behaviours. Specifically, various attempts have been made to differentiate Asperger syndrome from high-functioning autism (HFA). The results are mixed: Gilchrist et al. (2001), based on parents' report using the ADI-R, suggested that young children with HFA were more likely to demonstrate unusual attachments and sensory interests, compulsions and rituals, and body rocking than children with Asperger syndrome, but that by adolescence the groups differed only in a specific stereotyped movement, namely body rocking (Gilchrist et al., 2001). Similarly Starr, Szatmari, Bryson, and Zwaigenbaum (2003) applied the ADI and found that participants with HFA differed from participants with Asperger syndrome in that the latter made consistently lower mean scores on the ADI repetitive domain score.

Other studies suggest that no differences exist between these groups in repetitive behaviours (Cuccaro et al., 2007; Howlin, 2003), specifically in circumscribed interests (South, Ozonoff, & McMahon, 2005); they are similar in the presence of repetitive behaviours as well as in their intensity or severity. This finding reduces support for application of this symptom as a diagnostic marker for Asperger syndrome.

Studies with samples of individuals with ASD with IQ above 70 identified all forms of repetitive behaviours, including lower-order ones such as stereotyped movements and repetitive manipulation of objects (Cuccaro et al., 2007; Gal, 2006). This suggests that lower-order repetitive behaviours are not specific to low-functioning individuals with ASD.

The upshot of these studies is that grouping behaviours in such broad categories poses challenges for a categorical diagnostic approach. Consequently, the categorization of repetitive behaviours according to functional level must be used with caution. Additionally, the effects of intellectual disability, obsessive compulsive behaviours, and other comorbid disorders should be taken into account. Although repetitive behaviours are one of the defining characteristics of ASD, they are not exclusive to this population. Comorbidity, in relation to the assessment of ASD as a whole, and specifically to repetitive behaviours, is therefore a topic of importance.

In the context of discussions of ASD, comorbidity has most often been related to intellectual disability (ID), first because with the exception of Asperger syndrome these two conditions co-occur frequently: 75% of persons with autism show some level of ID (Croen, Grether, & Selvin, 2002), and second because symptoms of autism, particularly language delays, stereotyped movements and self-injury, increase as the severity of ID increases (Gal, Dyck, & Passmore, 2009; Matson & Nebel-Schwalm, 2007; Wing & Gould, 1979).

The terms 'repetitive behaviour' and 'repetitive movements' are also employed in respect of many other different populations. Repetitive behaviours, particularly repetitive movements, are seen in young children with typical development (Bodfish et al., 2000; Evans et al., 1997; Thelen, 1979) as well as in those with neuro-psychological sensory and developmental disorders (Baumeister & Forehand, 1973; Berkson, 1983; Freeman et al., 1981; Frith & Done, 1990; McKenna, Thornton, & Turner, 1998). Various studies have attempted to identify the nature of repetitive behaviours within and between populations. Certain classes of repetitive behaviours have been described as non-specific to autism, while others have been deemed particularly significant for the disorder.

Mostly, higher-level repetitive behaviours are considered particularly significant for ASD, often being described as autism specific; lower-level repetitive behaviours are often seen as not especially prevalent, severe or characteristic in autism. These include various classes of repetitive motor behaviour such as stereotyped movements, spontaneous dyskinesias, tics or repetitive self-injury (Turner, 1999).

Stereotyped Movements: Specificity to ASD?

The literature on stereotyped movements makes little or no distinction between such behaviours in autistic and non-autistic individuals and has tended to foster the assumption that low-level repetitive motor behaviour is non-specific to autism (Turner, 1999).

This notion is supported by the high prevalence of repetitive motor movements in normally developing infants and young children (Evans et al., 1997; Thelen, 1979) and in other developmental, sensory and psychiatric conditions such as Tourette's syndrome, fragile X syndrome, Rett syndrome, Parkinson's disease and schizophrenia (Freeman et al., 1981; Frith & Done, 1990; Gal et al., 2009; McKenna et al., 1998).

Repetitive Movements in Typical Populations

Movements labelled repetitive/stereotyped are variable and wide ranging in typical populations. In infants and young children they tend to be motor activities such as head nodding, arm flapping, finger wiggling and body rocking. They are taken to be a common feature in the normal development of infants (Piek, 1995; Thelen, 1979); earlier literature suggested that they marked transitions in motor growth (Lourie, 1949). Thelen further suggested that these movements follow a predictable course of development which mirrors the stages of neuromuscular maturation, and as such each has a characteristic age of onset. She later hypothesized that an infant's spontaneous movements form the neuromuscular bases on which higher skills such as sitting and walking are built, and that SMs appear in typically developing children when they are progressing through transitional stages in motor development (Thelen, 1996).

Typically, stereotyped motor movements begin during the first 3 years of life. In a group of normal children with motor stereotypies, about 80% began before age 24 months, 12% between 24 and 35 months and 8% at 36 months or older (Harris, Mahone, & Singer, 2008). In fact, 90% of the general population demonstrates body rocking as part of typical motor development (Berkson, Tupa, & Sherman, 2001).

However, repetitive movements do not characterize only typically developed babies and youngsters; interestingly, these movements which supposedly indicate a neurological maturation process often appear in typically developed and healthy adults as well (Werry, Carlielle, & Fitzpatrick, 1983). In college students they include nail biting, tapping the feet or a pencil, hair twirling and smoking (Harris et al., 2008). Other typical examples later in life are leg rocking or pacing back and forth in times of stress, boredom or discomfort. In some societies specific repetitive movements are a part of the culture or religious habits. This may be seen in some very repetitive African dances or in the typical upper-body rocking movements of praying in some communities.

Repetitive Movements in Populations with Disabilities

The persistence or recurrence of repetitive patterns of movements after childhood and into later life stages is most often associated, in addition to ASD, with various psychiatric, sensory and neurological disorders and developmental disabilities such as intellectual handicaps (Baumeister & Forehand, 1973; Berkson, 1983).

The literature suggests that intellectual level serves as a major contributor to repetitive movements. Various studies confirm a high presence of repetitive movements in children with intellectual handicaps (Bartak & Rutter, 1976;

Rojahn & Sisson, 1990), one-third to two-thirds of whom display them (Rojahn & Sisson, 1990). While this number can be explained in that one-third of children with an intellectual disability also have a pervasive developmental disorder (Kraijer, 1997), studies suggest that intellectual disability in itself also contributes to the prevalence and type of repetitive movement and manipulation of objects. Gal (2006), who assessed the profiles of repetitive movements of children with and without an intellectual handicap, identified various stereotyped movements which are displayed significantly more in children with low intellectual abilities than in those with high intellectual abilities with or without disabilities. Children with intellectual disabilities were significantly different in object manipulation; rhythmic rocking; repetitive operation of light switches, taps and toilet flushing; repetitive object mouthing; and pacing in a repetitive manner. The severity of repetitive movements was also attributed to the interaction between diagnosis and intellectual level, suggesting that intellectual disabilities interact with other problems to amplify stereotyped movements (Gal et al., 2009).

Indeed, various genetic syndromes often also associated with intellectual disabilities demonstrate an association with repetitive movements. These include Angelman, Cornelia de Lange, Cri-du-Chat, fragile X, Prader–Willi, Lowe and Smith-Magenis syndromes and Rett syndrome. A review of repetitive behaviours in these syndromes suggests extreme heterogeneity of repetitive behaviours across genetic syndromes, with clearly diverse syndrome-specific profiles differing in amount and type of repetitive movement. For example, fragile X syndrome showed a variety of repetitive movements, Angelman syndrome showed a significantly lower probability of most behaviours, and Prader–Willi, Cri-du-Chat and Smith-Magenis syndromes showed unique profiles of repetitive behaviour (Moss, Oliver, Arron, Burbidge, & Berg, 2009). Canitano and Vivanti (2007) pointed an association between ASD and tics. They assessed the overlap between tics and other to repetitive movements and behaviours in ASD and found that in individuals with ASD 22% presented tic disorders: 11% with Tourette's disorder (TD) and 11% with chronic motor tics. This suggests that the association between tics and ASD is more frequent than would be expected by chance.

Intellectual disability is not the only factor that contributes to the presence of repetitive movements. Other populations with disabilities demonstrate repetitive movements which differ in amount and type from those observed in a typical population. Sensory loss and severe sensory processing dysfunction have been identified as affecting the presence of stereotyped movements as well (Gabriels et al., 2008; Gal, Dyck, & Passmore, in press).

Stereotyped movements are a frequent phenomenon in children suffering from sensory loss such as blindness and visual impairment. Studies revealed that most blind children display at least one stereotyped movement, often more. Body rocking and eye poking were the most commonly displayed movements, while object manipulation, noise making, finger sucking and arm and hand flapping were also common (Tröster et al., 1991; Gal & Dyck, in press).

As stated, other repetitive motor behaviours such as spontaneous dyskinesias and self-injury are non-specific to ASD and were suggested to be similar in both topography and prevalence to those described for individuals with schizophrenia and learning disabilities (Freeman et al., 1981; McKenna et al., 1998).

To conclude, researchers suggests that low-level repetitive behaviours such as stereotyped movements, object manipulation, self-injury, tics and spontaneous dyskinesias are not restricted to the autism syndrome but are prevalent in varying degree and form in typical people (stereotyped movements) as well as those with various disabilities (all low-level repetitive behaviours). Various classes of repetitive motor behaviour may be related to factors such as intellectual level, sensory disabilities or the presence of specific organic pathology.

Higher-Level Repetitive Behaviour: Specificity to ASD

While lower-level repetitive behaviours are shown to be non-specific to ASD, there is some evidence that certain classes of higher-level behaviours are particularly characteristic of them. One of them, namely circumscribed interests, is reported to be prevalent in as many as 86–95% of children on the autism spectrum with normal intelligence and above (Kerbeshian, Burd, & Fisher, 1990; Szatmari, Bartolucci, & Bremner, 1989; Tantam, 1991). Insistence on various routines and rituals constitutes another class of repetitive behaviours, which although non-specific to ASD and also prevalent in individuals with learning difficulties (Lewis, Bodfish, Powell, & Golden, 1994) and Tourette's syndrome (Grad, Pelcovitz, Olson, Matthews, & Grad, 1987; Swedo, Rapoport, Leonard, Lenane, & Cheslow, 1989), proved more prevalent and marked in individuals with autism than in age- and ability-matched control subjects (Bartak & Rutter, 1976; Lord & Pickles, 1996). These differences were supported by Wing and Gould (1979), who reported elaborate routines in 94% of individuals in their sample who had ASD, in comparison with only 2% of those who did not.

Similarly, 'insistence on sameness' has been considered especially prevalent in ASD (Szatmari et al., 1989). However, like stereotyped movements, this behaviour was suggested also as characteristic of normally developing children aged between 2 and 4 years (e.g. insisting that foods must be placed in a certain arrangement on the plate). This

indicates that this behaviour serves as an adaptive function in typical development (Evans et al., 1997).

However, not all high-level repetitive behaviours are considered specific to or mainly prevalent in people with ASD. Perhaps more than any other disorder, concern about whether ASD can be separated from obsessive compulsive disorder (OCD) has been debated (Matson & Nebel-Schwalm, 2007). Zandt, Prior, and Kyrios (2007) compared children with ASD and children with OCD on a range of repetitive behaviours. Both groups were found to show more compulsions and obsessions than a typically developing comparison group, although types of compulsions and obsessions tended to be less sophisticated in children with ASD than in those with OCD.

To conclude, the literature suggests that like lower-level repetitive behaviours, higher-level ones are not specific to ASD. However, they characterize children with ASD much more than typically developed children or children with other disabilities.

What is unique to repetitive behaviours of people with ASD? Although RRBI, including repetitive movements, do not occur exclusively on the autism spectrum and are known to appear in various populations of people with disabilities, they seem to assume different forms and characteristics in each population and to have unique forms which distinguish those with ASD from those without them. Differences have been described in the topography of movements, number of behaviours and their rate, frequency and severity.

Bodfish et al. (2000) compared specific repetitive behaviours in adults with autism and mental retardation with a group of individuals diagnosed with mental retardation alone and matched for age, gender and IQ. The autism group exhibited a significantly higher number of stereotyped movements and compulsions, and more severe compulsions, than the mental retardation group. There was also a positive relationship between the number of stereotyped movements and compulsions and autism severity.

Higher rates and range of repetitive behaviour have been shown to distinguish individuals with ASD from individuals with a variety of other conditions (Bodfish et al., 2000; Lewis & Bodfish, 1998; Prior & Macmillan, 1973; Rojahn et al., 2001; Turner, 1997).

The topography of repetitive movements has been reported to vary across populations, although it does not clearly distinguish them. For example, eye poking is considered very specific to blind people (Fraiberg, 1977; Gal & Dyck, 2009; Tröster et al., 1991) and repetitive self-hugging may be unique to Smith-Magenis syndrome. People with this condition also compulsively lick their fingers (Smith, Dykens, & Greenberg, 1998).

No stereotyped movements are described as specific to ASD, but some are more prevalent in ASD than others, for example, rhythmic body rocking, arm or hand flapping and finger waving in front of the face (Schopler, 1995). While in typically developed children stereotyped movements might seem like typical, albeit exaggerated behaviour, usually directly associated with external stresses, the stereotyped movements associated with children with ASD often look bizarre and grotesque, differing significantly from normal 'play behaviour' associated with normal childhood (Schopler, 1995). Additionally, while in non-autistic individuals stereotyped movements are firmly associated with intellectual level (Smith & Van Houten, 1996), individuals with autism engage in more frequent, more severe and longer bouts of stereotyped movements than do age- and ability-matched controls (Freeman et al., 1981; Lord & Pickles, 1996; Lord, 1995); within children with ASD, even those with high intellectual level show stereotyped movements (Gal, 2006; Szatmari et al., 1989).

The evidence suggests that important differences in the display of some other forms of repetitive behaviours in autistic and non-autistic populations as well. For example, while people with ASD and with OCD display similarities in some behaviours, the latter tend to show mainly obsessions and compulsions. Also, they appear to have a bimodal pattern of onset, with the first peak occurring around puberty and the second in early adulthood (Zohar, 1999). In children with ASD a much wider range of repetitive behaviours has been described (Smith, Magyar, & Arnold-Saritepe, 2002), and the behaviours appear to change in presentation over time; younger children with autism (2–4 years) engaged in more low-level motor repetitive behaviours, while older children (7–11 years) engaged in more complex behaviours (Militerni, Bravaccio, Falco, Fico, & Palermo, 2002).

Children with ASD differ from others in their response to changes in their routines or to attempts to stop their repetitive behaviours: the extreme distress and catastrophic reaction shown by many autistic people in response to changes in routine is rarely described in non-autistic individuals (Turner, 1996).

Some of the differences possibly lie in the definition itself: the term repetitive behaviour refers to a wide range of behaviours that are performed often and in an invariant manner and that are inappropriate or odd (Turner, 1997).

The repetitive movements of those with ASD indeed differ from other disabilities in their range, frequency and consistency. But probably the most distinctive feature of repetitive behaviours of people with ASD as against typically developed people is their oddness and inappropriateness: the repetitive behaviours of those with ASD are ill adapted to social norms. While typical people may use more normative repetitive behaviours that are not perceived as aberrant, such as leg rocking, those with ASD may perform movements that more directly serve their current inner needs regardless of their unsuitability for social norms and specific situations. A first-hand account written by Luke Jackson, a 13-year-old

youth with Asperger syndrome, supports this view: 'People (with ASD) often flap their hands or do things that may seem weird to other people. These are all very satisfying and comforting things to do actually, but generally not accepted in our wonderful world... Personally it doesn't bother me who flaps and jumps. All this stuff is about "appearing normal" and really no one should ever have to do that...' (Jackson & Attwood, 2002, p. 24).

It should not be assumed that typical people and people with ASD differ in regard to repetitive movements only because of lack of adaptability. We should not assume that the 'need' to perform those movements is equal in all human beings, but rather some people are able to adapt them to social expectations and others cannot. The basic 'need' to perform repetitive movements may differ in different populations, in different individuals sharing the same diagnosis and in the same individual at different times or in different situations. While by definition, RRBI lack of an obvious goal, there is evidence that they do, in fact, have a function, as for the individual who performs them: RRBI and specifically stereotyped movements are often highly reinforcing and more attractive to the child with ASD than goal-oriented movements involved in play, learning and daily activities. They are difficult to abolish either by punishment or by various positive reinforcements (Bodfish et al., 1995; Wing, 1976). Additionally, people with ASD who engage in RRBI seem driven to carry them out in a specific way, and if interfered with, a range of problem behaviours may precipitate (Schopler & Mesibov, 1995). These may serve as evidences that these behaviours are, in fact, rewarding for people with ASD. Interestingly, as opposed to clinicians who often perceive RRBI as interfering with participation in daily activities, and therefore disruptive, individuals with autism describe them as their unique trait often being the key to bring discomfort and difficulties under control, and as a result free the autistic individual to gain pleasure and enjoyment from other experiences, such as social contact, allowing, in fact, better participation in everyday activities (Jones, Quigney, & Huws, 2003).

The mechanisms underlying repetitive behaviours are unclear, although the literature has sought to explain the existence of repetitive behaviour in autism, suggesting various explanations. It has been hypothesized that core neurocognitive deficits, such as weak central coherence, that is the ability to understand context, underlie the disorder (Frith, 2003), impaired neurobiological mechanisms (Markram, Rinaldi, & Markram, 2007; Maurer & Damasio, 1982) or impaired executive functioning (Turner, 1997). Other theories suggest that some repetitive movements serve as a general homeostatic mechanism or alternatively a specific coping mechanism directed to the regulation of one sensory modality (Gal, Dyck, & Passmore, 2002, 2009).

While it is not clear yet what these mechanisms exactly are, these theories may shed some light on behaviours that otherwise may be viewed just as 'aberrant' and 'inappropriate', and to explain, why, in fact, repetitive behaviours may be adaptive to the neurological system of those with ASD. It is of importance, therefore, to clinically address them in a sensitive and respectful way aimed at finding an optimal match between the needs of the person with ASD and those of the social environment.

References

Alderman, T. (1997). *The scarred soul: Understanding & ending self-inflicted violence*. Oakland, CA: New Harbinger.

American Psychiatric Association. (1994). *Diagnostic and statistical manual of mental disorders* (4th ed., DSM-IV). Washington, DC: Author.

Ayres, J. (1979). *Sensory integration and the child*. Los Angeles: Western Psychological Services.

Baranek, G. T. (1999). Autism during infancy: A retrospective video analysis of sensory-motor and social behaviours at 9–12 months of age. *Journal of Autism and Developmental Disorders, 29*, 213–224.

Baroff, G. S. (1974). *Mental retardation: Nature, cause, and management*. Washington, DC: Hemisphere.

Bartak, L., & Rutter, M. (1976). Differences between mentally retarded and normally intelligent autistic children. *Journal of Autism and Developmental Disorders, 6*, 109–120.

Baumeister, A. A. (1978). Origins and control of stereotyped movements. In C. E. Meyers (Ed.), *Quality of life in severely and profoundly mentally retarded people: Research foundations for improvement* (Monograph No.3). Washington, DC: American Association for Mental Deficiency.

Baumeister, A. A., & Forehand, R. (1973). Stereotyped acts. In N. R. Ellis (Ed.), *International review of research in mental retardation* (pp. 55–96). New York: Academic Press.

Baumeister, A. A., & Rolling, J. P. (1976). Self-injurious behaviour. In N. R. Ellis (Ed.), *International review of research in mental retardation*. New York: Academic Press.

Berkson, G. (1983). Repetitive stereotyped behaviours. *American Journal of Mental Deficiency, 88*, 239–246.

Berkson, G., Tupa, M., & Sherman, L. (2001). Early development of stereotyped and self-injurious behaviours: I. Incidence. *American Journal on Mental Retardation, 106*, 539–547.

Bodfish, J. W., Crawford, T. W., Powell, S. B., Parker, D. E., Golden, R. N., & Lewis, M. H. (1995). Compulsions in adults with mental retardation: Prevalence, phenomenology, and comorbidity with stereotypy and self-injury. *American Journal of Mental Retardation, 100*, 183–192.

Bodfish, J. W., Symons, F. J., Parker, D. E., & Lewis, M. H. (2000). Varieties of repetitive behaviour in autism: Comparisons to mental retardation. *Journal of Autism and Developmental Disorders, 30*, 237–243.

Briere, J., & Gil, E. (1998). Self-mutilation in clinical and general population samples: Prevalence, correlates, and functions. *American Journal of Orthopsychiatry, 68*, 609–620.

Canitano, R., & Vivanti, G. (2007). Tics and Tourette syndrome in autism spectrum disorders. *Autism, 11*, 19–28.

Carr, E. G. (1977). The motivation of self-injurious behaviour: A review of some hypotheses. *Psychological Bulletin, 84*, 800–816.

Cox, A., Klein, K., Charman, T., Baird, G., Baron-Cohen, S., Swettenham, J., et al. (1999). Autism spectrum disorders at 20 and 42 months of age: Stability of clinical and ADI-R diagnosis. *The Journal of Child Psychology and Psychiatry, 40*, 719–732.

Croen, L. A., Grether, J. K., & Selvin, S. (2002). Descriptive epidemiology of autism in a California population: Who is at risk? *Journal of Autism and Developmental Disorders, 32*, 217–224.

Cuccaro, M. L., Nations, L., Brinkley, J., Abramson, R. K., Wright, H. H., Hall, A., et al. (2007). A comparison of repetitive behaviours in Asperger's disorder and high functioning autism. *Child Psychiatry Human Development, 37*, 347–360.

Cuccaro, M. L., Shao, Y., Grubber, J., Slifer, M., Wolpert, C. M., Donnelly, S. L., et al. (2003). Factor analysis of restricted and repetitive behaviours in autism using the autism diagnostic interview-R. *Child Psychiatry and Human Development, 34*, 3–17.

Dantzer, R. (1986). Behavioural, physiological and functional aspects of stereotyped behaviour: A review and a re-interpretation. *Journal of Animal Science, 62*, 1776–1786.

de Lissavoy, V. (1961). Head banging in early childhood. *The Journal of Pediatrics, 58*, 803–805.

Eaves, L. C., & Ho, H. H. (1996). Brief report: Stability and change in cognitive and behavioural characteristics of autism through childhood. *Journal of Autism and Developmental Disorders, 26*, 557–569.

Evans, D. W., Leckman, J. F., Carter, A., Reznick, J. S., Henshaw, D., King, R. A., et al. (1997). Ritual, habit, and perfectionism: The prevalence and development of compulsive-like behaviour in normal young children. *Child Development, 68*, 58–68.

Favazza, A. R. (1996). *Bodies under siege: Self-mutilation and body modification in culture and psychiatry* (2nd ed.). Baltimore: Johns Hopkins University Press.

Fraiberg, S. (1977). *Insights from the blind: Comparative studies of blind and sighted infants*. New York: Basic Books.

Freeman, B. J., Ritvo, E. R., Schroth, P. C., Tonick, I., Guthrie, D., & Wake, L. (1981). Behavioural characteristics of high- and low-IQ autistic children. *American Journal of Psychiatry, 138*, 25–29.

Frith, U. (2003). *Autism: Explaining the enigma*. Malden: Blackwell.

Frith, C. D., & Done, D. J. (1990). Stereotyped behaviour in madness and in health. In S. J. Cooper & C. T. Dourish (Eds.), *Neurobiology of stereotyped behaviour* (pp. 232–259). Oxford: Clarendon Press.

Gabriels, R. L., Agnew, J. A., Miller, L. J., Gralla, J., Pan, Z., Goldson, E., et al. (2008). Is there a relationship between restricted, repetitive, stereotyped behaviours and interests and abnormal sensory response in children with autism spectrum disorders? *Research in Autism Spectrum Disorders, 2*, 660–670.

Gal, E. (2006). *An investigation of the relationship of sensory differences and intellectual level to stereotyped and self injurious movements in children*. Unpublished dissertation, Curtin University, Australia.

Gal, E., & Dyck, M. (2009). Stereotyped movements among children who are visually impaired or blind. *Journal of Visual Impairment and Blindness, 103*, 754–765.

Gal, E., Dyck, M., & Passmore, A. (2002). Sensory differences and stereotyped movements in children with autism. *Behaviour Change, 4*, 207–219.

Gal, E., Dyck, M. J., & Passmore, A. (2009). The relationship between stereotyped movements and self-injurious behaviour in children with developmental or sensory disabilities. *Research in Developmental Disabilities, 30*, 342–352.

Gilchrist, A., Green, J., Cox, A., Burton, D., Rutter, M., & Le Couteur, A. (2001). Development and current functioning in adolescents with Asperger syndrome: A comparative study. *The Journal of Child Psychology and Psychiatry, 42*, 227–240.

Gorman-Smith, D., & Matson, J. L. (1985). A review of treatment research for self-injurious and stereotyped responding. *Journal of Mental Deficiency Research, 29*, 295–308.

Grad, L. R., Pelcovitz, D., Olson, M., Matthews, M., & Grad, G. J. (1987). Obsessive-compulsive symptomatology in children with Tourette's syndrome. *Journal of American Academy of Child & Adolescent Psychiatry, 26*, 69–73.

Harris, K. M., Mahone, E. M., & Singer, H. S. (2008). Nonautistic motor stereotypies: Clinical features and longitudinal follow-up. *Pediatric Neurology, 38*, 267–272.

Howlin, P. (2003). Outcome in high-functioning adults with autism with and without early language delays: Implications for the differentiation between autism and Asperger syndrome. *Journal of Autism and Developmental Disorders, 33*, 3–13.

Jackson, L., & Attwood, T. (2002). *Freaks, geeks and Asperger syndrome: A user guide to adolescence.* London: Jessica Kingsley.

Jones, R. P., Quigney, C., & Huws, J. C. (2003). First-hand accounts of sensory perceptual experiences in autism: A qualitative analysis. *Journal of Intellectual and developmental Disability, 28*, 112–121.

Kanner, L. (1943). Autistic disturbances of affective contact. *Nervous Child, 2*, 217–250.

Kerbeshian, J., Burd, L., & Fisher, W. (1990). Asperger's syndrome: To be or not to be? *The British Journal of Psychiatry, 156*, 721.

Kraijer, D. (1997). *Autism and autistic-like conditions in mental retardation.* Lisse: Swets & Zeitlinger.

Leekam, S., Tandos, J., McConachie, H., Meins, E., Parkinson, K., Wright, C., et al. (2007). Repetitive behaviours in typically developing 2-year-olds. *Journal of Child Psychology & Psychiatry, 48*, 1131–1138.

Lewis, M. H., & Bodfish, J. W. (1998). Repetitive behaviour disorders in autism. *Mental Retardation and Developmental Disabilities Research Reviews, 4*, 80–89.

Lewis, M. H., Bodfish, J. W., Powell, S. B., & Golden, R. N. (1994). Compulsive and stereotyped behaviour disorders in mentally retarded patients. *Biological Psychiatry, 35*, 643–644.

Lewis, V., & Boucher, J. (1988). Spontaneous, instructed and elicited play in relatively able autistic children. *British Journal of Developmental Psychology, 6*, 325–339.

Lord, C. (1995). Follow-up of two-year-olds referred for possible autism. *Journal of Child Psychology and Psychiatry, 36*, 1365–1382.

Lord, C., & Pickles, A. (1996). Language level and nonverbal social-communicative behaviours in autistic and language-delayed children. *Journal of American Academy of Child & Adolescent Psychiatry, 35*, 1542–1550.

Lourie, R. S. (1949). The role of rhythmic patterns in childhood. *American Journal of Psychiatry, 105*, 653–660.

Markram, H., Rinaldi, T., & Markram, K. (2007). The intense world syndrome – an alternative hypothesis for autism. *Frontiers in Neuroscience, 1*, 77–96.

Mason, G. J., & Turner, M. A. (1993). Mechanisms involved in the development and control of stereotypies. In P. P. G. Bateson, P. H. Klopfer, & N. S. Thompson (Eds.), *Perspectives in ethology* (pp. 53–85). New York: Plenum.

Matson, J. L., Hamilton, M., Duncan, D., Bamburg, J., Smiroldo, B., Anderson, S., et al. (1997). Characteristics of stereotypic movement disorder and self-injurious behaviour assessed with the diagnostic assessment for the severely handicapped (DASH-II). *Research in Developmental Disabilities, 18*, 457–469.

Matson, J. L., & Nebel-Schwalm, M. (2007). Assessing challenging behaviours in children with autism spectrum disorders: A review. *Research in Developmental Disabilities, 28*, 567–579.

Maurer, R. G., & Damasio, A. R. (1982). Childhood autism from the point of view of behavioral neurology. *Journal of Autism and Developmental Disorders, 12*, 195–205.

McKenna, P. J., Thornton, A., & Turner, M. A. (1998). Catatonia in and outside schizophrenia. In C. Williams & A. Simms (Eds.), *Disorders of volition and action in psychiatry* (pp. 105–135). Leeds: University of Leeds Press.

Mesibov, G. B., Schopler, E., Schaffer, B., & Michal, N. (1989). Use of the childhood autism rating scale with autistic adolescents and adults. *Journal of American Academy of Child & Adolescent Psychiatry, 28*, 538–541.

Militerni, R., Bravaccio, C., Falco, C., Fico, C., & Palermo, M. T. (2002). Repetitive behaviours in autistic disorder. *European Child & Adolescent Psychiatry, 11*, 210–218.

Moore, V., & Goodson, S. (2003). How well does early diagnosis of autism stand the test of time? *Autism, 7*, 47–63.

Morgan, L., Wetherby, A. M., & Barber, A. (2008). Repetitive and stereotyped movements in children with autism spectrum disorders late in the second year of life. *Journal of Child Psychology and Psychiatry, 49*, 826–837.

Moss, J., Oliver, C., Arron, K., Burbidge, C., & Berg, K. (2009). The prevalence and phenomenology of repetitive behaviour in genetic syndromes. *Journal of Autism and Developmental Disorders, 39*, 572–588.

Murphy, G., Hall, S., Oliver, C., & Kissi-Debra, R. (1999). Identification of early self-injurious behaviour in young children with intellectual disability. *Journal of Intellectual Disability Research, 43*, 149–163.

Osterling, J. A., Dawson, G., & Munson, J. A. (2002). Early recognition of 1-year-old infants with autism spectrum disorder versus mental retardation. *Development and Psychopathology, 14*, 239–251.

Piek, J. P. (1995). The contribution of spontaneous movements in the acquisition of motor coordination in infants. In D. J. Glencross & J. P. Piek (Eds.), *Motor control and sensory integration* (pp. 199–230). Amsterdam: Elsevier.

Piven, J., Harper, J., Palmer, P., & Arndt, S. (1996). Course of behavioural change in autism: A retrospective study of high IQ adolescents and adults. *Journal of the American Academy of Child and Adolescent Psychiatry, 35*, 523–529.

Prior, M., & Macmillan, M. B. (1973). Maintenance of sameness in children with Kanner's syndrome. *Journal of Autism and Developmental Disorders, 3*, 154–167.

Richler, J., Bishop, S. L., Kleinke, J. R., & Lord, C. (2007). Restricted and repetitive behaviours in young children with autism spectrum disorders. *Journal of Autism and Developmental Disorders, 37*, 73–85.

Roeyers, H., & Van Berckelaer-Onnes, I. A. (1994). Play in autistic children. *Communication & Cognition, 27*, 349–359.

Rojahn, J., Matson, J. L., Lott, D., Esbensen, A. J., & Smalls, Y. (2001). The behaviour problems inventory: An instrument for the assessment of self-injury, stereotyped behaviour, and aggression/destruction in individuals with developmental disabilities. *Journal of Autism and Developmental Disorders, 31*, 577–588.

Rojahn, J., & Sisson, L. A. (1990). Stereotyped behaviour. In J. L. Matson (Ed.), *Handbook of behaviour modification with the mentally retarded* (2nd ed., pp. 181–217). New York: Plenum Press.

Romanczyk, R. G., Ekdahl, M., & Lockshin, S. B. (1992). Perspectives on research in autism: Current trends and future directions. In D. E. Berkell (Ed.), *Autism: Identification, education and treatment* (pp. 21–51). Hillsdale, NJ: Erlbaum.

Schopler, E. (1995). *Parent survival manual.* New York: Plenum.

Schopler, E., & Mesibov, G. B. (1995). *Learning and cognition in autism.* New York: Plenum Press.

Schreibman, L. (1988). *Autism.* Newbury Park, CA: Sage.

Schroeder, S. R., Schroeder, C. S., Smith, B., & Dalldorf, J. (1978). Prevalence of self-injurious behaviours in a large state facility for the retarded: A three-year follow-up study. *Journal of Autism and Developmental Disorders, 8*, 261–269.

Seltzer, M. M., Krauss, M. W., Shattuck, P. T., Orsmond, G., Swe, A., & Lord, C. (2003). The symptoms of autism spectrum disorders in adolescence and adulthood. *Journal of Autism and Developmental Disorders, 33*, 565–581.

Singer, H. S. (2009). Motor stereotypies. *Seminars in pediatric neurology*, *16*(2), 77–81.

Smith, A. C. M., Dykens, E., & Greenberg, F. (1998). Behavioural phenotype of Smith-Magenis syndrome (del 17p11.2). *American Journal of Medical Genetics*, *81*, 179–185.

Smith, T., Magyar, C., & Arnold-Saritepe, A. (2002). Autism spectrum disorder. In D. T. Marsh & M. A. Fristad (Eds.), *Handbook of serious emotional disturbance* (pp. 131–148). New York: Wiley.

Smith, E. A., & Van Houten, R. (1996). A comparison of the characteristics of self-stimulatory behaviours in "normal" children and children with developmental delays. *Research in Developmental Disabilities*, *17*, 253–268.

South, M., Ozonoff, S., & McMahon, W. M. (2005). Repetitive behaviour profiles in Asperger syndrome and high-functioning autism. *Journal of Autism and Developmental Disorders*, *35*, 145–158.

Starr, E., Szatmari, P., Bryson, S., & Zwaigenbaum, L. (2003). Stability and change among high-functioning children with pervasive developmental disorders: A 2-year outcome study. *Journal of Autism and Developmental Disorders*, *33*, 15–22.

Stone, W. L., Lee, E. B., Ashford, L., Brissie, J., Hepburn, S. L., Coonrod, E. E., et al. (1999). Can autism be diagnosed accurately in children under 3 years? *Journal of Child Psychology and Psychiatry*, *40*, 219–226.

Swedo, S. E., Rapoport, J. L., Leonard, H., Lenane, M., & Cheslow, D. (1989). Obsessive-compulsive disorder in children and adolescents: Clinical phenomenology of 70 consecutive cases. *Archives of General Psychiatry*, *46*, 335–341.

Szatmari, P., Bartolucci, G., & Bremner, R. (1989). Asperger's syndrome and autism: Comparison of early history and outcome. *Developmental Medicine and Child Neurology*, *31*, 709–720.

Tantam, D. (1991). Asperger syndrome in adulthood. In U. Frith (Ed.), *Autism and Asperger syndrome* (pp. 147–183). Cambridge: Cambridge University Press.

Tate, B. G., & Baroff, G. S. (1966). Aversive control of self-injurious behaviour in a psychotic boy. *Behaviour Research and Therapy*, *4*, 281–287.

Thelen, E. (1979). Rhythmical stereotypies in normal human infants. *Animal Behaviour*, *27*, 699–715.

Thelen, E. (1996). Motor development: A new synthesis. *American Psychologist*, *50*, 79–95.

Tröster, H., Brambring, M., & Beelmann, A. (1991). Prevalence and situational causes of stereotyped behaviours in blind infants and preschoolers. *Journal of Abnormal Child Psychology*, *19*, 569–590.

Turner, M. A. (1996). *Repetitive behaviour and cognitive functioning in autism*. Unpublished PhD thesis, University of Cambridge, Cambridge, UK.

Turner, M. A. (1997). Towards an executive dysfunction account of repetitive behaviour in autism. In J. Russell (Ed.), *Autism as an executive disorder* (pp. 57–100). Oxford: Oxford University Press.

Turner, M. A. (1999). Annotation: Repetitive behaviour in autism: A review of psychological research. *The Journal of Child Psychology and Psychiatry*, *40*, 839–849.

Volkmar, F. R. (2005). *Handbook of autism and pervasive developmental disorders: Assessment, interventions, and policy*. Hoboken, NJ: Wiley.

Watson, L. R., Baranek, G. T., Crais, E. R., Reznick, J. S., Dykstra, J., & Perryman, T. (2007). The first year inventory: Retrospective parent responses to a questionnaire designed to identify one-year-olds at risk for autism. *Journal of Autism and Developmental Disorders*, *37*, 49–61.

Werner, E., Dawson, G., Munson, J., & Osterling, J. (2005). Variation in early developmental course in autism and its relation with behavioural outcome at 3–4 years of age. *Journal of Autism and Developmental Disorders*, *35*, 337–350.

Werry, J. S., Carlielle, J., & Fitzpatrick, J. (1983). Rhythmic motor activities (stereotypies) in children under five: Etiology and prevalence. *Journal of the American Academy of Child Psychiatry*, *22*, 329–336.

Wing, L. (1976). Diagnosis, clinical description and prognosis. In L. Wing (Ed.), *Early childhood autism: Clinical, educational and social aspects* (2nd ed.). Oxford: Pergamon Press.

Wing, L., & Gould, J. (1979). Severe impairments of social interaction and associated abnormalities in children: Epidemiology and classification. *Journal of Autism and Developmental Disorders*, *9*, 11–29.

World Health Organization. (1990). *International classification of diseases and related health problems – Tenth revision (ICD-10)*. Geneva: World Health Organization.

Zandt, F., Prior, M., & Kyrios, M. (2007). Repetitive behaviour in children with high functioning autism and obsessive compulsive disorder. *Journal of Autism and Developmental Disorders*, *37*, 251–259.

Zohar, A. H. (1999). The epidemiology of obsessive-compulsive disorder in children and adolescents. *Child and Adolescent Psychiatric Clinics of North America*, *8*, 445–460.

Emotional Cognition: Theory of Mind and Face Recognition

Nathalie Nader-Grosbois and James M. Day

Introduction

In the relevant literature, several authors[1] have described a variety of skills that are necessary to develop emotional competence and emotional self-efficacy, even psychological well-being, in social situations. We summarize these skills as follows:

- To be aware of one's emotional states that may be experienced in multiple ways (notably body feelings) and that may induce contradictory or mixed emotions simultaneously;
- To have an awareness that the emotion may activate an action, a behaviour;
- To express one's own emotions and feelings;
- To process the perceptions of others' faces and orient one's attention toward them;
- To identify emotional expressions in others, to discern and to interpret others' emotions, using physical, vocal, facial, social cues and human movements;
- To recognize that inner emotions and outer behavioural expressions of emotions do not necessarily correspond, either in oneself or others;
- To empathize with others;
- To use vocabulary about emotions and emotional verbal expressions in conventional ways;
- To regulate one's own emotions or emotional expressions, according to the context;
- To cope with aversive or distressing emotions;
- To know that the nature of social relationships is characterized largely by the quality of emotional communication experienced together in social interactions.

These skills reflect all the complexity of emotional competence and the indispensable contribution of cognitive abilities or strategies that are potentially mobilized by typical people in social situations. From infancy onwards and throughout the lifespan, emotional experiences, dynamic emotional processes and responses are contextually embedded in social interactions; emotions become meaningful in the interactions with other people, they are useful in social exchanges (varying according to the type and the requirements of context), and they contribute to create social relationships with others and vice versa (Dunn, 2003; Ekman, 1992; Halberstadt, Denham, & Dunsmore, 2001; Saarni, 1999; Salovey, 2003).

In order to approach the literature on specificities in emotional competence and in emotional cognition in children and adolescents with autism spectrum disorders (ASD),[2] we will refer, in this chapter, to these distinct skills and their links. Several areas, such as developmental psychology, psychopathology of development and neuropsychology, are the main framework of theoretical conceptions and of studies we consulted about emotional competence and emotional cognition in people with ASD. More particularly, we focus on the contribution of theory of mind (ToM) and of some cognitive theoretical models in order to describe and explain both deficits and specificities in emotional cognition in children and adolescents with ASD.

The "Theory of Mind": Several Approaches of People with ASD

First, we will give some landmarks regarding the theory of mind-related research and the understanding of emotions by typically developing (TD) children.

---

[1] Begeer et al. (2008), Celani et al. (1999), Dunn (2003), Ekman (1992), Luminet (2002), Mikolajczak et al. (2009), Mottron (2004), Philippot (2007), Rimé (2007), Saarni (1999), Salovey (2003).

[2] We will use "HFASD" to designate high-functioning individuals with ASD and "IDASD" to indicate intellectually disabled individuals with ASD.

N. Nader-Grosbois (✉)
Faculty of Psychology, Catholic University of Louvain, 1348 Louvain-la-Neuve, Belgium
e-mail: nathalie.nader@uclouvain.be

J.L. Matson, P. Sturmey (eds.), *International Handbook of Autism and Pervasive Developmental Disorders,* Autism and Child Psychopathology Series, DOI 10.1007/978-1-4419-8065-6_9, © Springer Science+Business Media, LLC 2011

In the psychology of human development, the theory of mind (ToM) refers to one's abilities to understand nine mental states of others including perceptive states (visual perception and attention), volitional and motivational states (desire and intention), epistemic states (beliefs and false beliefs), pretence, thinking and emotions (Emery, 2005; Flavell, 1999; Wellman, 1990, 1991). The ToM constitutes a corpus of knowledge about human mind because it corresponds to the individual's abilities to infer or attribute these mental states in other people in various social situations, throughout behaviour, multimodal expressions (Abbeduto & Murphy, 2004; Wellman, 1990, 2000). Therefore, this understanding of others' mental states can contribute to individuals' social adjustment, even if this understanding is moderated by the developmental age (Deneault & Morin, 2007; Mitchell, 1996; Nader-Grosbois, 2011; Thirion-Marissiaux & Nader-Grosbois, 2008a, 2008b, 2008c). Such ToM abilities are sometimes considered as "perspective taking", or a component of "social cognition". In several conceptions and empirical studies on social competence in TD and atypical children, the ToM represents an important component because each particular behaviour which is likely to be socially adequate or successful often depends on the current mental state of the person with whom the individual is interacting. Detecting others' mental states or taking the others' perspective not only helps to develop empathy towards others but also increases the probability of harmonious and reciprocal social interactions, and communication between individuals.

More specifically about the ToM relative to "emotions", it is important to distinguish, in TD and atypical children, their abilities in the understanding of causes of emotions (or prediction of emotions depending on the situation) and of consequences of emotions (or prediction of adequate behaviour depending on the felt emotions), particularly concerning the four primary emotions (joy, sadness, anger and fear) (Thirion-Marissiaux & Nader-Grosbois, 2008a, Nader-Grosbois, 2011). An appropriate social adjustment could be appreciated through the way in which children respond to negative emotions displayed by peers (Denham, 1998). It is essentially during preschool age in TD children that the development of these ToM "emotion" abilities occurs.

However, in the first 2 years of typical development, some signs of understanding emotions are already observed. TD infants who are 9 months old relate other people's emotional expressions to other people's actions (Barna & Legerstee, 2005). Starting at around 18 months, TD young children become knowledgeable about the connection between emotions and desires (Lagattuta, 2005; Repacholi & Gopnik, 1997; Wellman, Phillips, & Rodriguez, 2000). Generally, they begin to comment on their own and others' emotions when they start talking (Wellman, Harris, Banerjee, & Sinclair, 1995) and when they can evoke emotions during

pretend play (in imaging others' emotions and attributing emotions to a doll) (Deneault & Morin, 2007; Gordon, 1992; Harris, 2000; Harris, Johnson, Hutton, Andrews, & Cooke, 1989, 1991; Leslie, 1987). From 3 years of age, children distinguish emotions, they progressively discover that it is possible to have two emotions simultaneously and they begin to connect emotions to external causes (Rieffe, Meerum Terwogt, & Cowan, 2005).[3] For example, they understand that receiving a present could make someone happy or the death of a pet could make someone sad. So the development of the understanding of emotions is also closely related to the development of theory of mind, and of pretend play. In their imaginative games of make-believe, children show their ability to comprehend that others have wishes, beliefs and feelings as much as they have themselves (Harris et al., 1989). Preschoolers develop the knowledge that emotions are connected to a person's representations of objective situations (Cutting & Dunn, 1999; Wellman et al., 2000) and they progressively understand the situational causes and consequences of emotions. TD children from 4 to 6 years of age discover that it is not only objective situations that could provoke emotions (for example, receiving a present causes happiness or falling over make crying) but also mental states such as beliefs or desires (feeling happy when a person has what she want) (Harris et al., 1989). The understanding of these representations of objective situations or the ability to attribute mental states such as emotions, intentions, desires and beliefs to oneself and others correspond to ToM (Baron-Cohen, Tager-Flusberg, & Cohen, 2000; Leslie, 1987). At 5 years of age, children acknowledge the link between beliefs and emotions (Rieffe et al., 2005).

More precisely, researchers have described two orders of theory of mind ability corresponding to distinct levels of acquisition assessed by tasks of different complexity (Baron-Cohen, 1995). The level of first-order ToM refers to inferring the thoughts of another person. This level is achieved at around the age of 4 years in TD children. For example, a child could know what his or her friend might be going through after encountering a critical situation, such as losing his or her favourite toy. The level of second-order ToM refers to reasoning, that is, what another person (than self) thinks about the thoughts in another person. For example, a third child is watching the first two children and is reasoning what the first child would be thinking about the second child.

In this sense, ToM knowledge is particularly linked to the understanding of complex emotions (such as surprise, embarrassment, shame, guilt and pride) that cannot be acquired before children are about 4 years old, when their knowledge of mental states develops. When they are about 10–12

---

[3] Negative experiences are "bad" according to 2-year-old children; preschoolers differentiate between being "sad" and "angry".

years old, TD children easily use and understand various social emotions (Draghi-Lorenz, Reddy, & Costall, 2001; Frith, 2003; Gilbert, 2004; Mills, 2005; Saarni, 1999; Tracy, Robins, & Lagattuta, 2005).

What About Children and Adolescents with ASD?

In individuals with ASD, since they may and often do not understand that other people think differently from themselves, they encounter problems to get in touch with and communicate with other people. In various situations, they may not be able to anticipate what others will feel, do or say and therefore they appear to be uncaring toward others and self-centred.

By contrast to cognitive general models (which will be presented in a following section), the "theory of mind hypothesis" posits a domain-specific deficit in people with ASD. The numerous empirical studies and the development of theoretical conceptualizations of theory of mind in individuals with ASD show the essential interest of the abilities that the ToM implies when researchers want to examine emotional and social competence in these people (Dixon, Tarbox, & Najdowski, 2009).

Before the development of ToM abilities, several precursors have been examined in TD and atypical infants and children; the focusing on these precursors has led to some hypotheses about perceptual, cognitive and information processing aspects operating in the acquisition of ToM. In addition, several approaches of ToM have been developed and could offer different ways to apprehend specificities in people with ASD. Studies of brain imaging and the peculiar association between specific deficits in children with ASD have encouraged researchers and have given them information useful to elaborate models to explain their deficits in ToM. Some models suggest a modular approach of the ToM, and others models suggest a non-modular approach, explaining the deficits in ToM by means of more general cognitive models (presented in a next section) or also by specificities in socio-emotional interactions in young children with ASD. Here we will outline hypotheses and results of empirical studies that are more focused on processes implicated in the understanding of the mental state of emotions.

Deficits in Specialized Processes and Precursors of a Theory of Mind in People with ASD

Several authors emphasize that in children with ASD, there is a structural impairment of specialized processing of mental human states, notably of precursors of ToM, like specific information processing of face, of facial emotional

expressions and of gaze direction, reactivity or emotional and motivational reciprocity, empathy, detection of intentional movements, imitation, coupling action–perception between self and others, etc. At this level of functioning, studies examined anomalies in these primary processes leading potentially to deficits in the understanding of mental states, in ToM.

Information processing of face and of facial emotional expressions. The first models of ASD were based on neuropsychological data supporting early brain specialization of information processing of human faces (de Schonen, Mathivet, & Deruelle, 1989; Haxby, Hoffman, & Gobbini, 2000). Since the 1980s, several studies examining children with ASD detected specific deficits in information processing of faces. For example, some studies (Hobson, 1989, 1991, 1993; Langdell, 1978) emphasized their inability to apprehend the expressive dynamic of a face and of other emotional indicators that could impede their understanding of several mental states. In comparison with TD participants, matching on their non-verbal mental age (MA), children with ASD present more difficulties in tasks implying the association of facial cues of emotions and others cues (vocal, gesture and postural) of the same emotions. The multimodal association of these distinct kinds of information may be more problematic than only the processing of emotional expression itself. We will specify this next.

Early imitation as precursor of ToM. Amongst primary precursors of ToM, perturbed in ASD, there is also an emphasis of deficits in motor resonance in some aspects of imitation in children with ASD (Dawson & Adams, 1984; Heimann, 1998; Meltzoff & Gopnik, 1993; Nadel, 1998a) and in their sensory motor representations of self and others (Rogers & Penington, 1991). In the last decade, these approaches benefit from a revival of interest because of evolution of knowledge in brain biology of specific processes that could be implicated in imitation and simulation. They are founded on a modelling of early typical development of babies born with abilities of coupling multimodal perceptions provided from one's own actions and observations of similar actions accomplished by others (Meltzoff, 1999). In other words, imitative skills in babies could be a base allowing them to be open to other's perspective at 18 months and to capture other's goals and intentions for acting (it refers to simulation approach of the development of theory of mind). Deficits in these elementary mechanisms in young infants with ASD should lead to important dysfunction in communicative exchanges and in representations of self and of others, notably in the orientation of attention towards the most pertinent cues amongst the multiple stimuli emitted by people and in the taking into account of reciprocal mental states (detection of intentionality and of emotions, for example). But according to Smith and Bryson (1994), in the domain of imitation, empirical studies report heterogeneous findings on imitative skills in children with ASD; moreover, most studies elicit imitation on request in ways not best adapted to inform us about elementary motor resonance. Only some clinical descriptions of imitation in social interactions or trials of positive reinforcement of imitation in children with ASD showed that they are able to improve their imitative abilities (facilitating the communication) if they benefit from well-adjusted scaffolding; thus, interpersonal motor resonance might not be globally deficient and could need sustained scaffolding in these children (Dawson & Galpert, 1990a; Field, Field, Sanders, & Nadel, 2001; Nadel & Pezé, 1993).

Regarding neuronal aspects, some researchers postulate that these early skills of coupling interpersonal perceptions and actions are based on a system of mirror neurons, in the pre-motor cortex, that are activated when a person makes an intentional action or observes the same action produced by another person or when a person evokes a mental simulation of the action (by extension of what occurs in the animal world) (Decety, 2002; Iacobani & Dapretto, 2006). This could be interpreted as an essential functional basis for imitation and detection of others' intentions, considered as precursors of ToM development by simulation processes (Gallese & Goldman, 1998). In people with ASD, some studies, using EEG or imaging techniques, emphasized the sub-activation of this system of mirror neurons in tasks of reproduction or of observation of emotional expressions and the weakness of activation correlated with the intensity of autistic disorders (Dapretto et al., 2006; Oberman et al., 2005).

In addition, beyond considering imitation as a precursor of ToM development, some studies reported particularly strong links between imitative abilities and ToM in children with ASD; their impairment in imitation and in ToM conjointly discriminates them in comparison with TD or ID children (notably, Perra et al., 2008).

Detection of biological movements, gaze direction, joint attention and social referencing as precursors of ToM. Other early elementary processes are explored as innate potential components contributing to the access of ToM development, such as detection of biological movements (opposed to mechanic movements of physical entities) that help the perception of intentionality and specifically the detection of gaze direction that is useful to establish joint attention in TD children (Deneault & Morin, 2007; Tourrette, 1999; Tourrette, Recordon, Barbe, & Soares-Boucaud, 2000).

Results concerning people with ASD are heterogeneous regarding their impaired or non-impaired functioning of these types of detection; they vary depending on the children's age (Blake, Turner, Smoski, Pozdol, & Stone, 2003; Parron et al., 2008; Webster & Potter, 2008). More specifically, Baron-Cohen (1991c) emphasized that attention towards others in infants who are 7–9 months old constitutes potentially a "critical precursor" to the ToM development.

He explains this as follows. Decoding another's gaze direction and their attention oriented to an object or an event contributes to understand that the object or the event is the other's focus of interest. The gestural pointing (or "proto-declarative pointing") induces a share of attention between two individuals or "joint attention" and implicates that they could take into account each other's mental state. Baron-Cohen (1995) conceptualized this ability as a "shared attention mechanism" (SAM). So, this ability of joint attention (considered as early social references) attests to the interest towards another person and the establishment of shared interests in both persons; they are essential components for ToM development.

Numerous studies proved that these early joint attention behaviours (initiation, response or maintain) are impaired in children with ASD (Bono, Daley, & Sigman, 2004; Loveland & Landry, 1986; Mundy & Crowson, 1997; Mundy & Gomes, 1998; Smith, Mirenda, & Zaidman-Zait, 2007; Toth, Munson, Meltzoff, & Dawson, 2006; Vaughan et al., 2003) and they are a target of training (Hwang & Hughes, 2000; Jones, 2009; Jones & Carr, 2004; Jones, Carr, & Feeley, 2006; Jones & Feeley, 2007; Kasari, Freeman, & Paparella, 2001b, 2006; Whalen & Schreibman, 2003; Whalen, Schreibman, & Ingersoll, 2006). Some studies pointed out that their joint attention ability skills are positively linked to or are predictive of their skills in ToM (Baron-Cohen, 1991c, 1995; Gattegno, Ionescu, Malvy, & Adrien, 1999; Phillips, Baron-Cohen, & Rutter, 1992; Robertson, Tanguay, L'Ecuyer, Sims, & Waltrip, 1999; Tourrette et al., 2000; Yirmiya, Pilowsky, Solomonica-Levi, & Shulman, 1999).

A larger competence than joint attention is also evoked as a precursor of ToM development (Deneault & Morin, 2007; Tourrette, 1999), namely social referencing.[4] This competence also seems impaired in children with ASD;

---

[4] Social references refers to "the use of one's perceptions of another's interpretations of a situation to form one' own understanding of that situation" (Feinman, 1982, p. 445). In an interactive episode, this ability allows to seek out and use information in the reactions of others to guide one's own responding in the contents of uncertainty or ambiguity. It includes three components: (a) the referent or the ambiguous object or event that evokes the solicitation of social information in the form of another's response to that object or event; (b) the referrer or the individual who solicits the social information and whose behaviour is influenced by the social discriminative stimuli provided by another, and (c) the referee or the individual who provides discriminative stimuli in the presence of the referent, which influence the referrer's behaviour (Feinman et al., 1992). According to these authors, the social referencing conditions vary with modalities of communication (single, e.g. facial expression; or multiple, e.g. facial, verbal and gestural cues) and also with regard to the affective content of the referencing message conveyed by the referee concerning the referent [positive messages (e.g. joy) or negative messages (e.g. fear and disgust)]. After the communicated message, the person may display behaviour of approach, contact or affective responding.

certain components of social referencing, or this skill in its entirety, are the objects of training (Brim, Buffington Townsend, DeQuinzio, & Poulson, 2009; Buffington, Krantz, McClannahan, & Poulson, 1998; Gena, Krantz, McClannahan, & Poulson, 1996; Gewirtz & Pelaez-Nogueres, 1992; Sigman, Arbelle, & Dissanayake, 1995).

The "Theory of Mind Hypothesis": "Mind Blindness", "Modular" Approach and Metacognitive Deficit in People with ASD

To characterize children with ASD, a triad of disorders are recognized as specific; they present social impairment, reduced communication and lack of imaginative play (Wing, 1986). Baron-Cohen, Leslie, and Frith (1985) suggested that this combination of deficits related to these three areas could be explained by a single cognitive deficit corresponding to an inability to cognitively represent mental states, called a theory of mind.

The "theory of mind hypothesis" postulates a fundamental deficit in children with ASD in the ability to ascribe mental states to others. In other words, as they lack a ToM, they have difficulties understanding another's perspective, in order to appreciate someone else's mental states to make sense of and predict their behaviour in referring to these mental states; this is called "mind blindness" (Baron-Cohen, 1989a, 1989b, 1991a, 1991b, 1995; Baron-Cohen et al., 1985, 1986; Leslie & Thaiss, 1992; Perner, Frith, Leslie, & Leekam, 1989). In this perspective, researchers suggest that children with ASD do not understand others' minds because they do not develop a sense that they have their own mental states or they cannot appreciate the contents of their own mind. In addition, severe deficits in ToM in people with ASD are linked to their social and communicative abnormalities (Baron-Cohen, 1988, 1991c; Eisenmajer & Prior, 1991; Frith, 2003) and may influence their behaviour in social interaction situations (Baron-Cohen et al., 2000).

Authors who are in line with a cognitive module underlying the ToM have pointed out that ToM abilities appear to be dissociable from the development of other cognitive abilities in other domains. Even if children with ASD may lack a ToM, they may display good cognitive abilities in other respects (Baron-Cohen et al., 2000). For example, children with William's syndrome can show intact ToM despite a delay in other cognitive domains (Karmiloff-Smith, Klima, Bellugi, Grant, & Baron-Cohen, 1995).

According to Leslie (1987, 1991, 2000; Leslie & Roth, 2000), individuals with ASD present an impairment in a basic cognitive mechanism, such as the ability to elaborate metarepresentation. This deficient metacognition leads to their difficulty in constructing mental representations of what is going on in others' mental states and also in developing their pretend play. Leslie (2000) postulates that there is a "ToM mechanism" functioning jointly with a more general cognitive mechanism called "the selection processor", which together are activated by the child in order to solve ToM tasks ("beliefs" tasks or other mental state tasks). The specific brain area that is selectively responsible for understanding and interpreting mental states in TD children is impaired in individuals with ASD (Leslie, 1991).

In order to conceptualize this ToM hypothesis, a modular approach was also conceived by Baron-Cohen and his colleagues, as an innate conception of the ToM acquisition. The child has, at one's disposal at birth, specialized modules of information processing and in the course of neurological maturation he or she becomes progressively capable of attaining a certain level of understanding of the human world (Baron-Cohen, 1991a, 1991b, 1991c, 1995; Baron-Cohen et al., 1985; Deneault & Morin, 2007; Leslie, 2000). Based on his background in evolutionary biology and in developmental psychology, Baron-Cohen (1995, 1999, 2000) led several studies of children with ASD in order to validate his modular model including four innate mechanisms or subsystems allowing "mind reading". These four mechanisms are the "intentionality detector" (ID), the "eye direction detector" (EDD), the "shared attention mechanism" (SAM) and the "theory of mind mechanism" (ToMM). In children with ASD, these mechanisms may be particularly damaged.

The "ID" sub-system corresponds to a perceptual innate mechanism that interprets "primitive volitional" basic mental states (such as goal and desire) required for making sense of movements of organisms in the environment. The "EDD" has three basic functions: the detection of the presence of eye-like stimuli; the evaluation of whether eyes are oriented to it or to another direction and the interpretation of person's gaze as "seeing" in inferring from the observation that the person's eyes are directed at something else that it actually sees something. This last function contributes to mind-reading process because it allows the infant to attribute a specific perceptual state to the person or an organism. These first two sub-systems allow the infant to interpret observed behaviour as some mental states and to interpret behaviour at a dyadic level (between agent–infant, between agent–object he sees). The third sub-system, the "SAM", corresponds to a more complex skill that allows the child to conceptualize "triadic representations", in establishing relations between an agent, the self, and an object or another agent. The child is able to perceive the perceptual state in another agent and to compute shared attention, by comparing another agent's perceptual state with the self's current perceptual state. The "ToMM" is conceived as a system for inferring all epistemic mental states (believing, feeling, knowing, deceiving, imagining, dreaming, etc., alone or combined) from the observation of human and animal behaviour. It helps the child to elaborate an understanding of how a person's mental states are linked with their actions and relate to each other.

According to Baron-Cohen (1989a), the neurodevelopmental disorder in children with ASD restricts the maturation of this specific module; this explains failures met by children with ASD in ToM tasks when they are older than 4 years (contrary to what is observed in TD children). Globally, their social information processing should not be affected but it should be less efficient when the adjustment towards other people needs to take into account potentially their different beliefs, intentions or thinking than ones own. In a similar way, he suggests that the skills to detect emotions are not impaired when the emotional state is in adequation with the context and the other person's behaviour (expressions of internal state). By contrast, children with ASD could have difficulties when emotions are not congruent with the apparent context or when complex emotions involve a representational interpretation (for example, the surprise; Baron-Cohen, Spitz, & Cross, 1993).

In reference to this modular perspective, some studies in neuropsychology examined specific links with the solving of ToM tasks (eliciting these cognitive modules) and specific brain activation in TD participants[5] and participants with ASD[6]: it appeared that there is a functional sub-activation of similar brain regions in people with ASD.

Even numerous studies in developmental psychopathology have been founded on this modular approach in order to explain deficits in certain domains of development; the main criticism addressed to this conception is, on the one hand, the absence of evidence of exclusive deficit in ToM mechanism/ToMM in people with ASD and, on the other hand, the deficit of other cognitive functions (such as executive functions and language) (Baron-Cohen, 1995). Moreover, the conception of this unitary and innate metacognitive competence was criticized by searchers in developmental psychology who emphasize the progression in the construction of a ToM viewed as a multi-construct that could benefit from environmental and social interactions. Even in current theories evolved into constructs that imply, still, a relatively modular approach, there is less apparent delineation of functions. However, a purely neurobiological explanation could not completely explain the deficits in ToM in individuals with ASD even if there are definite genetic and biochemical influences.

Socio-affective Bases of ToM Development in Children with ASD

In the perspective developed by Hobson (1986a, 1986b, 1993), concerning deficits in ToM acquisitions in children with ASD, it was postulated that they result from a primary innate inability to interact in emotional ways with other people. Their relative incapacity for inter-subjective contact and engagement in social interactions and encounters with other people, and their problem of emotional connection with others implicate consequences in cognitive, linguistic and social domains (Hobson, 1993, p. 3) and constrain the development of the sense of self, their symbolization and the sense of others' attitudes and feelings (Hobson, 1993, p. 5). In other words, in individuals with ASD, the lack of understanding of others' feelings infringes on their understanding of their own emotions and vice versa; by implication, they are likely to have difficulty empathizing with other people and responding adequately to emotions expressed by others (Hobson, 1993). This author considers that there is a specific developmental delay in each stage of development that alters notably their progression in their joint attention behaviours which could induce their failure to elaborate a ToM. Studies led by Hobson and his colleagues showed that children with ASD (compared with TD and ID children, matched on their MA) present a disharmonic pattern in their performances when confronted with emotional, versus non-emotional, tasks, sustaining the hypothesis of their specific deficit in emotional processing (notably identifying auditory and visual emotional stimuli, and designating emotions) (Hobson, 1986a, 1986b, 1993; Hobson, Ouston, & Lee, 1988, 1989).

Studies of Understanding Emotions, ToM "Emotions" in Children with ASD

Whereas their impairments in ToM development of other mental states are well described in the literature, by the description of their pervasive deficits in their understanding of desires, thoughts and beliefs (Baron-Cohen, 2000; Yirmiya, Erel, Shaked, & Solomonica-Levi, 1998), there are fewer studies of ToM "emotions", the understanding of emotions, of their causes and consequences, or of the link between imagination and emotional competence in children with ID or ASD.

Some authors report that when explicit questions about emotions are asked to children around 10 years of age with IDASD and children matched on their MA, participants show, in prototypical situations (like birthdays or hurting

---

[5] For example, activation of prefrontal median cortex, temporal–parietal junction, temporal poles, amygdala (Apperly, Samson, & Humphreys, 2005; Gallagher & Frith, 2003; Saxe, Carey, & Kanwisher, 2004; Siegal & Varley, 2002; Völlm et al., 2006).

[6] Frontal brain regions are specifically more active during ToM tasks than during control tasks, but there is relatively little agreement on the exact sub-regions involved (Baron-Cohen et al., 1994; Fletcher et al., 1995). Baron-Cohen et al. (1994) reported an increased activation in the right orbito-frontal regions. Fletcher et al. (1995) used stories requiring mental state attribution, a skill difficult for even high-functioning children with ASD and found through PET imaging that left medial frontal regions were significantly more active during the task. See also the synthesis by Frith (2001).

yourself, or getting what you want), a similar understanding of simple emotions (Baron-Cohen, 1991b; Baron-Cohen et al., 1993; Fein, Lucci, Braverman, & Waterhouse, 1992).

Deficits are reported in some studies of children with IDASD, notably in their abilities to associate drawings of facial expressions or of emotional gestures according to adequate contexts or facial expressions with vocal information, and in their understanding of particular internal causes of emotions (Baron-Cohen, 1991b; Celani, Battacchi, & Arcidiacono, 1999; Hadwin, Baron-Cohen, Howlin, & Hill, 1996; Hobson, 1986a, 1986b; Loveland et al., 1995; Southam-Gerow & Kendall, 2002). Sigman, Kasari, Kwon, and Yirmiya (1992) found that children with IDASD ignore or do not recognize that adults felt negative emotions from their expressions, whereas TD and ID children are more receptive to them and understand adults' emotions well.

As they present impairments in ToM "beliefs" and "desires", it is comprehensible that emotions caused by these mental states are poorly understood in school-aged children with IDASD (Baron-Cohen, 1991b; Serra, Loth, van Geert, Hurkens, & Minderaa, 2002). In the use of complex emotions by preschoolers with IDASD, they are poorly interested in others' mental states: even if they displayed pride in similar situations as TD children, notably when mastering a new skill, they pass over the social function of pride because they did not monitor the reaction from their audience (Kasari, Sigman, Baumgartner, & Stipek, 1993b).

By contrast to TD preschoolers, children with IDASD clearly differ from controls matched on their MA. They seem to have difficulty improving their understanding of emotions through experience, because they display very little progress during the preschool years. Beyond the simple acknowledgement of prototypical causes of emotions, they fail to show a good understanding of causes and consequences of emotions in various situations, and their impairments could be related to their poor imagination and ToM development (Begeer, Koot, Rieffe, Meerum Terwogt, & Stegge, 2008).

Concerning children with HFASD at school age, they understand simple emotions according to contexts and causes, and even they refer to complex emotions such as pride or embarrassment at equivalent rates as their TD peers (Capps, Sigman, & Yirmiya, 1995; Capps, Yirmiya, & Sigman, 1992; Downs & Smith, 2004; Peterson, Wellman, & Liu, 2005), and they acknowledge that emotional states in others influence their behaviour (Begeer, Meerum Terwogt, Rieffe, Stegge, & Koot, 2007). However, they have difficulty acknowledging mixed emotions, particularly negative emotions (such as anger and sadness) displayed simultaneously (Rieffe, Meerum Terwogt, & Kotronopoulou, 2007). In comparison with TD children of similar chronological age (CA), they lack spontaneity and their comments on emotions are uninformative or lacking in pragmatics (Hadwin, Baron-Cohen, Howlin, & Hill, 1997), depending

on explicit contextual information (Begeer et al., 2007), superficial or scripted (Adams, Green, Gilchrist, & Cox, 2002; Hale & Tager-Flusberg, 2005), idiosyncratic, materialistic, including fewer references to social causes (Baron-Cohen, 1991b; Dennis, Lockyer, & Lazenby, 2000; Jaedicke, Storoschuk, & Lord, 1994; Losh & Capps, 2006; Rieffe, Meerum Terwogt, & Stockmann, 2000, 2007).

When they reach preadolescence, these abilities in ToM "emotions" improve over time and they usually acknowledge others' mental states (Baron-Cohen, Jolliffe, Mortimore, & Robertson, 1997b; Bauminger & Kasari, 1999; Bowler, 1992; Dahlgren & Trillingsgaard, 1996; Happé, 1995; Steele, Joseph, & Tager-Flusberg, 2003), even though they continue to have poor understanding of complex emotions like shame, embarrassment or jealousy. Some authors explain this by the fact that children with HFASD generally fail to imagine, during play, the content of others' mental states on reality and consequently fail to explain how complex emotions arise from these mental states (Bauminger, 2004; Buitelaar & van der Wees, 1997; Buitelaar, van der Wees, Swaab-Barneveld, & van der Gaag, 1999a). Even if they can explain, after an explicit question, the impact of an audience's perspective on their own actions, they do not spontaneously mention such audience effects when explaining self-conscious emotions (Baron-Cohen et al., 1993; Bauminger, 2002; Heerey, Keltner, & Capps, 2003; Hillier & Allinson, 2002). Whereas children with HFASD are able to explain conceptually emotional display rules, they fail to apply this knowledge in their explanations of specific situations. The developmental sequence of display rules in these children suggests strong reliance on rote responses (Dennis et al., 2000; Peterson et al., 2005). So, individuals with HFASD give atypical or theoretical responses to emotions. It seems that they infer responses to emotions not from their own personal experience but rather from verbal and conceptual information (Capps et al., 1992; Frith, 2004; Kasari, Chamberlain, & Bauminger, 2001a; Lindner & Rosen, 2006).

In children with HFASD or with IDASD, their levels in understanding of emotions are linked with their IQ or their cognitive abilities (Happé, 1995; Kasari et al., 2001a; Yirmiya, Sigman, Kasari, & Mundy, 1992). Their success in emotional tasks or ToM "emotion" tasks is also variable according to verbal or non-verbal competence (Buitelaar, van der Wees, Swaab-Barneveld, & van der Gaag, 1999b; Happé, 1995).

Even in the light of the theory of mind hypothesis, and of studies of the understanding of emotions in people with ASD, according to Mottron (2004), deficits in ToM could not be the only explanation for their difficulties in socio-emotional areas, including ToM, because it implies so many other perceptual, executive and cognitive abilities in information processing. In order to infer what other people think or feel, one needs, for example, the perception of subtlety of face, voice and body movements, the processing of various sources of information simultaneously, the selection of the most important and pertinent information in context and the inhibition of an already given response in a similar situation in order to find another more appropriate one. In addition, ToM development may also have an impact on cognitive processes.[7]

In the following sections, we will show how cognitive models could provide some explanations for deficits in ToM or in emotional cognition in individuals with ASD and also what are the specificities of information processing, of face recognition, of integration of socio-emotional cues and other emotional abilities in them.

Other Cognitive Models of People with ASD

In the literature, some cognitive-dominant models are advanced of the underlying cognitive deficit in individuals with ASD that help approach differently their ToM development or their social cognition: the "weak central coherence theory"; the "executive control dysfunction" hypothesis; "cognitive complexity and control theory" and more recently, "enactive mind" conception is offered to approach their "embodied" social cognition.

"Weak Central Coherence Theory"

The "weak central coherence (WCC) theory" (Frith & Happé, 1994; Frith, 2003; Happé, 1999) is founded on the concept of "central coherence", defined as the ability to draw together several bits of information in an environment, in a task aimed at constructing a high level of meaning in context. In other words, the ability of central coherence involves the viewing of a task, of an environment as a whole, rather than only specific isolated aspects. In this theory, the hierarchization of information processing implies that global analysis of stimuli usually precedes local analysis; it is called "global precedence".

In the late 1980s, Uta Frith first advanced the weak central coherence theory in order to explain that children with ASD actually perceive details better than do TD people. So, in children with ASD, this central coherence ability is

deficient because they privilege local information processing and they have difficulty in shifting between local aspects and global approach. Thus, in this perspective, their cognitive deficit in information processing and their weakness in central coherence disrupt their problem solving, requiring the establishment of interrelationships between social cues (for example, different parts of face) and the apprehension of material having semantic meaning (Frith & Happé, 1994; Happé, 2000).

But this theory explains some specificities of perceptual–cognitive style (towards both non-social and social aspects) that limits the understanding of context in people with ASD, in comparison with TD people, more than it explains their overall difficulties, notably in emotional and social areas (Rajendran & Mitchell, 2007). Certain studies outlined partial support about inter- and intra-individual variability in weak central coherence within individuals with ASD from childhood to adult age (notably, Noens & van Berckelaer-Onnes, 2008; van Lang, Bouma, Sytema, Kraijer, & Minderaa, 2006). According to Noens & van Berckelaer-Onnes (2008), the debate on the locus of WCC effects has been obscured by two problems: the definition of local and global varies across studies and distinguishing between two levels of information processing is probably insufficient to characterize the exact locus of WCC effects. They suggest that the differentiation of four levels of sense making (sensation, presentation, representation and metarepresentation) might offer an interesting starting point and also the distinction of specific subgroups within ASD.

An alternative approach of WCC theory was offered by Mottron and his colleagues (Mottron & Burack, 2001; Mottron, Dawson, Soulieres, Hubert, & Burack, 2006). They agreed with the approach of hierarchization of information processing of global and local analysis of stimuli and they recognized it could contribute to understand that people with ASD present information processing focused on local details but suggested that there is a deficit in handling the relation between the global and the local levels of analyses. In other words, individuals with ASD are able to have a global and a local information processing but the first one does not precede the second one; there are problems in the hierarchical organisation of information processing. Other authors suggested that there is instead an interference from local to global in attention tasks in individuals with ASD (Plaisted, Swettenham, & Rees, 1999; Rinehart, Bradshaw, Moss, Brereton, & Tonge, 2000) that may be explained by deficit of inhibition process; or there is a slow spread of their visual attention that makes difficult the integration of local aspects in global form in these people (Mann & Walker, 2003). In the next section, we will explain some implications these characteristics of information processing could have for facial emotional recognition and for the integration of several emotional cues in individuals with ASD.

---

[7] Recently, Le Sourn-Bissaoui, Caillies, Gierski, and Motte (2009) examined in which measure ToM competence (notably false belief) could play a role in processing of causal, predictive and pragmatic inferences in 10 adolescents with Asperger syndrome and 10 controls matched for CA, sex and verbal IQ. The adolescents with Asperger syndrome had greater difficulty processing inferences (both semantic and pragmatic) than did the controls, and their ToM could subtend inference drawing.

The "Executive Control Dysfunction" Hypothesis

Executive function designates neuropsychological processes allowing physical, emotional and social self-control necessary to maintain goal-oriented actions; it includes inhibition of responses, working memory, cognitive flexibility, planning of actions and fluency (Corbett, Constantine, Hendren, Rocke, & Ozonoff, 2009; Mottron, 2004; Ozonoff, Pennington, & Rogers, 1991; Rajendran & Mitchell, 2007).

According to the "executive control dysfunction" hypothesis in people with ASD, it was hypothesized that the deficit in their executive control system generates a set of problems in these people, including their poor flexibility in behaviour, their disorders in inhibition in their behaviour and of immediate goals, their deficits in planning, in strategy selection, in shifting attention (Corbett et al., 2009; Mottron, 2004; Ozonoff et al., 1991; Russell, 1997; Turner, 1997), and could create obstacles in several areas of development, notably in the construction of social cognition. Russell (1997) suggests that the early dysfunction of action-monitoring system, the developmental features of executive functioning and memory problems have an impact on children with ASD for their self-awareness, on the development of knowledge regarding their own actions, on their regulation through inner speech, on the imitation of others' actions, as well as on their understanding of others' intentions and minds.

Even if this hypothesis of dysfunction in executive control may help to explain several features of cognitive strategies and behaviour in people with ASD, there is variability in their profiles of executive functions and certain executive problems are not only specific to them but also shared by people presenting other disorders (Rajendran & Mitchell, 2007). Some researchers argue that executive abilities may be linked with the ToM and on the contrary, other researchers suggest that executive abilities are needed for the ToM. So there is a debate as to whether ToM tasks can be reduced to executive processes (e.g. Pellicano, 2007; Russell & Hill, 2001; Russell, 1997; Russell, Hala, & Hill, 2003; Russell, Mauthner, Sharpe, & Tidswell, 1991) or whether a ToM is required for executive control (e.g. Perner, Lang, & Kloo, 2002).

Pellicano's study (2007) investigated the relationship between ToM and executive functions in 30 children with ASD (5.6 years old) and in 40 TD children, matched on their CA, in order to examine issues of developmental primacy. These children were assessed by means of a battery of tasks measuring ToM (first- and second-order false belief tasks) and components of executive functioning (planning, set shifting and inhibition). A significant correlation was obtained between ToM and executive function components in the ASD group, independent of age and ability, while ToM and higher order planning ability remained significantly linked in the TD group. Examination of the relational pattern of ToM executive functioning impairments in the ASD group showed dissociations in only one direction: impaired ToM with intact executive functioning. Even if these results support the view that executive functioning may be an important factor in the acquisition of ToM in children with ASD, it cannot explain alone their difficulties in ToM. In their studies, Pellicano and his colleagues (2007; Pellicano, Maybery, Durkin, & Maley, 2006) showed that as executive functions are composed of several processes (assessed by means of a set of tasks) inducing non-unitary cognitive style in children with ASD, there are specific links between their particular executive (dys)function and their particular (dis)abilities in ToM.

"Cognitive Complexity and Control Theory"

Some authors elaborated a hybrid alternative approach, called "cognitive complexity and control (CCC) theory" (Frye, Zelazo, & Palfai, 1995; Zelazo & Frye, 1997; Zelazo, Burack, Boseovski, Jacques, & Frye, 2001, 2002). In the CCC theory, the executive functioning is related to ToM in TD and atypical people because both ToM and measures of executive functions include higher order rule use (leading to a correct judgement in belief tasks, for example). So the advantage of this CCC theory is that it is not based on arguments of "either-or" about the links between these domains but is founded rather on interrelations between them: whether executive abilities are required to perform ToM tasks or inversely, ToM understanding also helps in the mobilization of executive functions. Three main arguments are advanced by Zelazo et al. (2001) in favour of the potential utility of the CCC approach in order to understand people with developmental disorders. First, they argue that each developmental disorder may induce an impact on the consciousness, the control of behaviour and the rule complexity and the researchers should not neglect that specifically in people with ASD, a large proportion are intellectually impaired; this intellectual deficit may interact with other inabilities to implicate various findings observed in studies of both their executive functioning and their ToM development. Second, they suggest that the CCC conception allows identifying, in people presenting distinct disorders (including ASD), what the specificities are in particular components of executive functions and in ToM. Third, the CCC approach allows observing participants' performance on various tasks from different domains to be equated and consequently appreciates the specificity in each developmental disorder. Some empirical studies support the CCC conception. In their study of children with IDASD and Down syndrome, Zelazo et al. (2002) reported that individual differences in ToM are correlated with individual differences in performances on two tests of rule use, except in children with IDASD who present a severe intellectual deficit (VIQ <40). A replication of this study was made by Colvert, Custance, and Swettenham (2002) with other samples, children with HFASD compared with two TD groups.

Future research should investigate, in a nuanced way, specificities in subgroups of children and adolescents with distinct disorders (including comparison between participants presenting genetic syndromes, intellectual disabilities,[8] distinct profiles of ASD, language impairments, behaviour disorders), by using assessment measures taking into account several components of cognitive, executive functions of ToM and of socio-emotional areas and involving ecologically valid tasks (as it is also partially suggested by some authors in order to take into account the heterogeneity in ASD and their multiple-deficit accounts; Baron-Cohen & Swettenham, 1997a; Bishop, 1993; Happé, Ronald, & Plomin, 2006; Joseph, Tager-Flusberg, & Lord, 2002; Rajendran & Mitchell, 2007). This could yield specific guidelines to improve the efficiency of intervention towards subgroups of people more or less impaired in one domain or another (Teunisse, Cools, van Spaendonck, Aerts, & Berger, 2001a).

"Enactive Mind" Conception

Klin, Jones, Schultz, and Volkmar (2003) reconceptualised the ToM through the interesting "enactive mind" (EM) explanation. This conception is inspired by the "embodied cognitive science" that considers cognition as bodily experiences accrued as resulting from adaptive actions based on salient stimuli in the environment. These authors postulate that this "embodied" social cognition is deviant in the development of children with ASD, from an early age, because of a deficit in salience towards social stimuli, present at the same time as non-social stimuli. This developmental hypothesis considers what researchers know about specificities in perception and could explain why some people with ASD presenting no cognitive deficits are able to solve explicit social cognitive problems (e.g. succeed in ToM tasks) at a better level than the level of ability they attain when they are confronted with naturalistic social situations in everyday life. Klin et al. (2003) suggest that from the outset, the mind of individuals with ASD is not attuned to the social world. Whereas TD individuals seem to be constantly ready to interpret social stimuli and social meaning (even from non-living objects), individuals with ASD show they are not. Their arguments are based on observations about their gaze following patterns that differ from those operated by neurotypical people.

From their observations of a group of adolescents and adults with HFASD, another group with ASD, both compared with neurotypicals, who were asked to describe a silent animation of geometric objects interacting with each other, after which the researchers analysed the narratives (Klin, 2000). The neurotypical control group tried to find social meaning in the animation but the two groups with ASD gave descriptions in mainly geometric terms reflecting relations involving physical properties. In other studies (Klin, Jones, Schultz, Volkmar, & Cohen, 2002a, 2002b) of eye tracking in normative IQ adolescents and adults with ASD, some specificities were obtained in comparison with TD people. In a first study, Klin et al. (2002a) reported that adolescents and adults with ASD displayed unusual reactions (like not following the pointing gesture of a character in the video sequence,[9] using essentially verbal cues, and neglecting gestures), leading to an inefficient pursuit of the referenced painting, by contrast to young TD children who were able to use non-verbal cues and pointed immediately, ending up deliberately on the correct painting. In a second study, Klin et al. (2002b) observed discrepancies in viewing patterns in adolescents and adults with ASD, compared with the control groups (matched on age, IQ and gender), when they viewed a video sequence[10]: while participants with ASD directed their gaze to the slightly open mouth of the man, providing few expression cues in order to understand what was happening in the scene, the TD participants responded easily to the surprised look expressed by the man's eyes in focusing their gaze on pertinent social cues. The combination of the technology of eye tracking and of video sequencing in an eliciting situation seems to be a highly appropriate methodological approach for exploring socio-cognitive strategies in individuals with ASD and TD individuals towards dynamic social situations (replicating more proximally, naturalistic social situations) by contrast to the use of static pictures illustrating social situations. This last support was used by van der Geest, Kemner, Verbaten, and van Engeland (2002), who did not find differences in visual fixation patterns between participants with and without ASD.

According to this enactive mind hypothesis, as in social situations in everyday life, many pertinent social cues occur rapidly and sometimes simultaneously; failing to identify and to interpret them by individuals with ASD may lead them not to succeed in the appreciation of meaning in situations and to

---

[8] ID is the abbreviation to designate intellectual disabilities or intellectually disabled.

[9] In the video sequence, a young man enquires about a painting hanging on a distant wall. First, he points to a specific painting (among several paintings) on the wall and second he asks, by a general question, the older man who did the painting. The pointing specified which painting is evoked by the young man.

[10] This video sequence illustrates behaviour and expressions displayed by two characters (a man and a woman) notably showing surprise and horror in their eye expression (particularly in the man).

display social maladjustment (Klin et al., 2003). Their selective attention is more oriented towards physical non-social stimuli from things in the environment than to social stimuli from people and their interactions; so they benefit from a specialization of things helping them to acquire concepts but they have poor tools in order to interpret and solve naturalistic social situations. Several studies on face processing may nuance these observations; they will be presented in a next section.

Specificities in Emotional Recognition in People with ASD

In TD children's development, emotional competence is potentially influenced by age, intellectual ability and also by situational context; this has been widely examined in longitudinal and cross-sectional studies. TD children's evolution is described concerning their emotional expression, recognition, regulation and understanding (which will be summarized in this section). But about children and adolescents with ASD, there are fewer longitudinal studies that allow deducting similar precisions about how their emotional abilities progress over time (their course or their differentiated trajectories of development) and how IQ influences their emotional development (Bieberich & Morgan, 2004; Dissanayake, Sigman, & Kasari, 1996; McGovern & Sigman, 2005; Seltzer et al., 2003). Most studies on children and adolescents with ASD conducted in cross-sectional design include comparison with participants without ID or distinct level of functioning (e.g. with HFASD), in varying the matching of compared groups (their CA, their MA, their verbal or non-verbal developmental age), and sometimes, confusion is induced by this lack of differentiation between individuals with ASD with and without ID.

In this section, we will summarize specificities in emotional recognition in children and adolescents with ASD; some of them could be better understood according to their specificities in cognitive processes, in their ToM development and precursors we presented before in previous sections of this chapter.

Face Recognition, Facial Emotion Recognition and Face Reading

When an individual wants to infer information about other people's emotional states, he or she will decrypt their faces, voices, postures or gestures and all cross-modal interactions between these forms of expression (Ekman & Friesen, 1975). However, facial expressions of emotions have been more frequently studied than other modes of expressions. In typical development, here is the progression.

The study led by Field & Walden (1982) shows that very young infants are able to detect the difference between two facial expressions. At around 7 months, the infant begins to recognize and categorize facial expressions amongst several examples, as different models or variable levels of intensity (Nelson, 1987; Saarni, Mumme, & Campos, 1998). At the end of the first year of life, children become able to give meanings to facial expression to which they are sensitive and they discriminate a variety of facial emotional expressions (Gosselin, 1995; Luminet & Lenoir, 2006; Nelson, 1987). Progressively, they begin to understand the message transmitted by a person's emotional expression (Repacholi, 1998). At this period, in new or ambiguous situations, young children actively search emotional information from their surroundings, in order to adjust themselves to context. According to Feinman, Roberts, Hsieh, Sawyer, and Swanson (1992), it is from social references (related to joint attention evoked as necessary precursors of the acquisition of ToM development) that the children perform the discrimination of emotional expressions in faces and display their adaptation depending on emotional cues. Around the second year of life, when the child is able to verbalize, he or she is able to more clearly identify emotional states (Luminet & Lenoir, 2006, p. 283). Most authors point out that positive emotions (such as joy) are recognized (around 3 years) before the negative emotions (such as anger, sadness and fear) (Brun, 2001a; Cole, 1986; Denham, 1998; Field & Walden, 1982; Denham & Couchoud, 1990; Denham, McKinley, Couchoud, Holt, 1990; Denham et al., 2001, 2003; Leppanen & Hietanen, 2001; Saarni, 1999; Saarni et al., 1998). Other emotions, such as surprise and disgust, are recognized later, at around 5–6 years of age (Gosselin, 2005; Leppanen & Hietanen, 2001; Luminet & Lenoir, 2006; Widen & Russel, 2002). The ability to infer an emotional state from a facial expression and the ability to associate it to an emotional term emerge from 3 years onwards (Gosselin, 1995, p. 108). This emotional verbalization coincides with the better differentiation between facial expressions of joy, sadness and anger, at around the age of 4–5 years. Designating the expressions of disgust and surprise appears at 6–8 years.

Even if deficits in the perception of emotions are not explicitly specified in the diagnostic criteria for ASD, they could partially explain their impaired emotional competence in the DSM-IV criteria.

Children with IDASD could not be considered as being "blind" to emotional expressions because results of empirical studies do not establish a consistent link between these facial emotional recognition and other emotional abilities.

According to some authors, at 3–4 years and also at school age, children with IDASD recognize emotions in faces, distinguish between different emotions and are interested in realistic, moving images of emotions (Balconi & Carrera,

2006; Castelli, 2005; Davies, Bishop, Manstead, & Tantam, 1994; Dawson et al., 2002; Ozonoff, Pennington, & Rogers, 1990; Prior, Dahlstrom, & Squires, 1990).

By contrast, other authors emphasized difficulties in the recognition of emotions expressed by others and in their interpretation (Baron-Cohen, 1991b; Brun & Nadel, 1998; Celani et al., 1999; Jemel, Mottron, & Dawson, 2006; Loveland et al., 1995; MacDonald et al., 1989; Rieffe et al., 2000). In their study, de Wit, Falck-Ytter, and von Hofsten (2008) found that although the 3- to 6-year-old children with ASD looked less at feature areas of the face (eyes, mouth, nose) than did the 5-year-old TD children, both groups of children displayed differential scanning patterns for faces displaying positive and negative emotions. They increased scanning of the eye region when looking at faces displaying negative emotions. This study shows that although young children with ASD exhibit abnormal face scanning patterns, they do exhibit differential viewing strategies while scanning positive and negative facial expressions. Recently, Peterson and Slaughter (2009) emphasized significant correlational and predictive links between abilities in eye reading and in false belief in 22 children[11] with IDASD aged 6–13 and in control groups. Several studies have shown abnormalities displayed by individuals with ASD[12] in their visual scanning of faces, measured notably by eye tracking, including their focused attention on mouth region rather than eye region (Dawson, Webb, Carver, Panagiotides, & McPartland, 2004; Joseph & Tanaka, 2003; Klin et al., 2002b; Klin & Jones, 2008). So it seems that patterns of face processing may have an impact on the understanding of others' emotions or beliefs.

In addition, when they are asked to match and categorize faces on the basis of expressions (Braverman, Fein, Lucci, & Waterhouse, 1989; Celani et al., 1999) or across different modes (gestured, vocal or facial) of expression (Hobson, 1986a, 1986b; Hobson et al., 1988), they are less efficient than controls. In tasks of facial expression processing (pick the one that does not fit, amongst a set of emotions, and designate emotions) or tasks implying the dynamic of expressions (movements of face), some deficits in emotional recognition persist (Gepner, de Schonen, & Buttin, 1994, 2004; Tantam, Monaghan, Nicholson, & Stirling, 1989; van

der Geest et al., 2002). But variability in this processing may be obtained depending on some methodological aspects.

Some authors (Celani et al., 1999) also specify that according to the duration of presentation of stimuli to the participant, significant differences are obtained or not between performances displayed by participants with ASD and control group. In a condition of brief presentation of stimuli, participants with ASD, even without ID, perform significantly at a lower level than the control group, whereas they easily recognize emotions when the presentation is longer. In this study, the difference concerns essentially the spread of facial expression processing that may be due to the difficulty to rapidly explore the face, particularly in very short duration of exposition of stimuli. Tardif, Lainé, Rodriguez, and Gepner (2007) also found that children with ASD are more able to match emotions during slow presentations of stimuli including facial movements and vocal sounds. In another example, Gepner et al. (2004) assessed the influence of motion on facial expression recognition in 13 children with ASD (mean age of 69.38 months), matched for developmental level with 13 TD children (mean age of 40.53 months). They compared the ability of both groups for matching videotaped "still", "dynamic" and "strobe" emotional and non-emotional facial expressions with photographs. They observed that children with ASD do not perform significantly worse than their controls in any experimental condition. Compared to previous studies showing lower performance in autistic than in control children when presented with static faces, these data suggest that slow dynamic presentations facilitate facial expression recognition by children with ASD. In addition, during tasks of implicit or explicit judgments of emotional expressions, Critchley et al. (2000) reported that participants with ASD without ID presented differences in brain activations.

More specifically, individuals with HFASD, compared to TD controls matched on their CA, various observations are reported.

Most studies did not find any deficits in the perception of simple emotions by children with HFASD (Adolphs, Sears, & Piven, 2001; Capps et al., 1992; Gross, 2004; Grossman, Klin, Carter, & Volkmar, 2000; Ozonoff et al., 1990; Prior et al., 1990; Robel et al., 2004; Travis & Sigman, 1998), compared to TD children matched on their CA. On the contrary, some studies reported deviations in the perception of simple emotional expressions such as anger, happiness, sadness and fear in children with HFASD (Bolte & Poustka, 2003; Bormannkischkel, Vilsmeier, & Baude, 1995; Davies et al., 1994; Piggot et al., 2004). For example, in their study, Downs and Smith (2004) compared the identification of emotions in 10 children with HFASD who had average IQ to that in 16 children with attention deficit/hyperactivity disorder and oppositional defiant disorder and 10 TD children. They reported that whereas the children with HFASD present advanced ToM abilities, they continue to show deficits in

---

[11] Compared with 65 typical developers in three control groups (11 AC-matched primary schoolers; 37 ToM-matched preschoolers and 17 adults).

[12] Recent observations also found evidence for these effects in younger children; less scanning of the eyes was found in the case of a 15-month-old infant with ASD (Klin & Jones, 2008). Klin et al. (2002b) showed that adolescents with ASD scanned dynamic social scenes in a deviant way. Compared to controls, the group with ASD showed heightened scanning of the mouth, bodies and objects, at the expense of scanning of the eyes.

identifying emotions and displaying socially appropriate behaviour. Moreover, more difficulties were reported in the recognition of facial expressions when they are presented by means of photographs but not by means of drawings of faces, in comparison with 5–9-year-old TD children. Some studies indicated that children and adolescents with HFASD show a deficit in labelling, categorizing, matching or identifying static facial emotions (Gross, 2004; Tantam et al., 1989), dynamic expressions (Lindner & Rosen, 2006) for categorical perception of emotional expressions (Teunisse & de Gelder, 2001b).

Concerning young adolescents with HFASD, it is also reported that they have difficulty perceiving subliminally presented facial emotional expressions, (Kamio, Wolf, & Fein, 2006) and that they need more time to respond to facial expressions (Piggot et al., 2004), particularly when it could provoke anxiety in them (Ashwin, Wheelwright, & Baron-Cohen, 2006). The difficulty in identifying emotions, on the basis of eye cues, is also observed in individuals with HFASD (children, adolescents or adults), notably because they privilege focusing their attention on mouth region and develop a relative lipreading expertise (Bar-Haim, Shulman, Lamy, & Reuveni, 2006; Baron-Cohen & Hammer, 1997c; Baron-Cohen, Wheelwright, Hill, Raste, & Plumb, 2001; Grossman & Tager-Flusberg, 2008[13]; Klin et al., 2002b; Lahaie et al., 2006).

Some authors explain that even if HFASD children are sensitive to social or emotional facial cues, they sometimes misinterpret their meaning (Adolphs et al., 2001; Dawson, Webb, & McPartland, 2005; van der Geest et al., 2002; Yirmiya et al., 1992). Others explanations are based on the fact that there is a problem in HFASD children in their automatic sensitivity to facial expressions or in their intrinsic motivation to perceive emotions (Begeer, Rieffe, Meerum Terwogt, & Stockmann, 2006; Behrmann, Thomas, & Humphreys, 2006; Wang, Dapretto, Hariri, Sigman, & Bookheimer, 2004). In addition, their tendency to rely on specific features of a face, rather than globally processing facial information, could implicate weak emotion recognition (Gross, 2005). Deviations in the processing of emotional cues from faces may be consequences

from general perceptual problems towards face in people with ASD (Pelphrey et al., 2002; Sasson, 2006) or towards situational contexts.

Recently, Da Fonseca et al. (2009) examined in 19 children and adolescents with HFASD (compared to 19 TD controls matched on CA and gender) whether they were able to recognize facial expressions of emotion and objects missing on the basis of contextual cues. Participants with HFASD were able to use contextual cues to recognize objects but not emotions because they have difficulty extracting emotional information.

It seems that there is no unequivocal impairment in emotion perception in individuals with ASD (with or without ID). Results in these studies do not give a clear justification of certain differences: is it a difference linked to domain-specific processing of the human face or of facial expressions? Or, is it a difference relative to a more general problem in the nature of implicated perceptive processes? Is it a deficit in holistic or analytic processing? Indeed, some specificities in facial emotion recognition in people with ASD (with or without ID) may depend on their perceptive style, the types of processing (global versus local) of stimuli, the integration of the two processing or of cross-modal information (facial and vocal), particularities in their processing of social versus nonsocial stimuli (as it was evoked before in previous section of this chapter) and also motivational and contextual aspects. Moreover, the lack of convergence in results obtained in these studies could also be attributed to the unclear consensus about elementary perception of simple and complex emotions, the different methods used for their assessment (Hobson, 1991) and the different criteria for matching the comparison groups (CA or MA) (Nadel, 1998b).

Recognition of Vocal Emotional Intonation and Integration of Different Emotional Cues

Difficulties in emotional recognition are not limited in children and adolescents with ASD to facial expression processing because they appear in other contexts and towards other kinds of stimuli. Notably, they display difficulty in recognition of vocal intonations or deficient production, on request, of vocal emotional intonations in everyday life (Bacon, Fein, Morris, Waterhouse, & Allen, 1998). Even if children with ASD are sensitive to vocal cues, they present difficulty in interpreting them correctly (Boucher, Lewis, & Collis, 2000). According to Celani et al. (1999), the difficulty in the interpretation of facial expressions and in the integration of various cues (vocal, facial, bodily, situational cues) by children with ASD imply that they develop misunderstanding of the meaning of emotional expressions according to the contexts. By contrast, in 4-year-old children with ASD, Kahana-Kalman and Goldman (2008) do not observe a general inability to detect intermodal correspondences between

---

[13] Grossman & Tager-Flusberg (2008) explored the processing of pseudo-dynamic facial emotions and visual speech in 25 adolescents with ASD, compared with 25 typical adolescents, and examined their ability to recreate the sequences of four dynamic emotional facial expressions (happy, sad, disgust and fear) as well as four spoken words (with, bath, thumb and watch) using six still images taken from a video sequence. Typical adolescents performed significantly better at recreating the dynamic properties of emotional expressions than did those of facial speech, while the ASD group showed the reverse accuracy pattern. When the eye region was obscured, no significant difference appeared between the 22 adolescents with ASD and 22 typical controls. Specifically, fearful faces achieved the highest accuracy results among the emotions in both groups.

visual and vocal events (by using matching paradigm), but they explain that their ability to detect affective correspondences between facial and vocal expressions of emotions may be limited to familiar displays. Indeed, these children performed well in the detection of affective correspondences towards their mothers' portray, but not towards a stranger, and they showed a preference for sound-matched.

Specifically in individuals with HFASD, some deficits are observed when they must identify, on the basis of voice cues, complex emotions, such as pride or jealousy; this impairment is potentially generated by their poor understanding of subjective states (Alcantara, Weisblatt, Moore, & Bolton, 2004; Gervais et al., 2004; Golan, Baron-Cohen, & Hill, 2006a; Rutherford, Baron-Cohen, & Wheelwright, 2002). In children with HFASD, difficulties are also observed in the integration of information when vocal, facial, bodily and situational cues are presented simultaneously (Koning & Magill-Evans, 2001). This limited ability to integrate information has also been found when school-aged children with HFASD process information on single faces. When vocal cues or eye regions are presented, or when emotional expressions are shown in combination with contrasting emotion words, their difficulties are especially evident (Grossman et al., 2000).

Feeling and Expression of Emotions

Feeling and Expression of Emotions, and Links Between Emotion Recognition in Others and Emotion Expression, or Responding in Typical Children

In typical development, the expression of emotions and feelings appeared in early social interactions, through various cues that could induce reactions from the social environment, more particularly the caregivers. Just after birth, the TD baby expresses a cry, and during intervening months, he or she produces more discrete and differentiated expressions of emotions, such as interest, disgust, joy, sadness, anger and fear, that may be easily recognizable from the surrounding (Harris et al., 1989; Haynie & Lamb, 1995; Izard & Malatesta, 1987; Izard, Huebner, Risser, McGuinnes, & Dougherty, 1980; Lewis & Sullivan, 1996; Oster, 2003). From early infancy, TD children automatically respond to emotions and use these responses in their interactions with others. At the beginning of the second year of life, the child becomes able to express "social emotions" such as empathy (Lewis, Sullivan, Stanger, & Weiss, 1989). Progressively, during the first 3 years of life, infants increase their expressiveness of emotions and feelings and they begin to verbally express their emotional states (Harris et al., 1989; Malatesta-Magai, Leak, Tesman, & Shepard, 1994). At preschool

age, children express their positive emotions in a social context (Snow, Hertzig, & Shapiro, 1987). In the socialization process of emotional expressions, preschoolers express increasingly their own emotions in conformity with social rules (Saarni, 1999) and at 6 years of age, they are able to explain those behaviour (Kieras, Tobin, Graziano, & Rothbart, 2005). The expression of more complex emotions (e.g. shame, embarrassment and pride) starts during toddler hood (Saarni, 1999). In the next section, we will specify how emotion regulation develops.

Emotional Expression and Emotional Responding in Children with ASD

Because of late reliable diagnoses of ASD, studies on toddlers are relatively rare; it is usually at school age, around 6–12 years, that children with ASD are studied (Dumont-Mathieu & Fein, 2005). However, in order to study the expressive behaviour of young "autistic" infants, it is possible to use delayed diagnoses.

One-year-old children, later diagnosed with IDASD, show similar expressions of emotions to TD or ID children (Baranek, 1999; Palomo, Belinchon, & Ozonoff, 2006). During the first year of life, infants (later diagnosed as ASD and presenting various IQs) showed that they are less attentive to faces and their affective behaviour are less oriented to others, than control infants, in structured observations of their behaviour recorded in video (Baranek, 1999; Maestro et al., 2002, 2005; Osterling, Dawson, & Munson, 2002; Palomo et al., 2006; Werner, Dawson, Osterling, & Dinno, 2000). But it was observed that toddlers with ASD were sensitive to eye movement (Chawarska, Klin, & Volkmar, 2003). Saarni (1999) explained that children with ASD, because of their cognitive specificities or deficits in the way they interpret their own emotional experiences and those felt by others, are unlikely to convey their emotions conventionally. Even if children with ASD are sensible to emotional cues emitted by others, such as the distress (Nadel et al., 2000; Sigman et al., 1992), they have difficulties to product in an adequate way their emotional expressions (Brun, Nadel, & Mattlinger, 1998; Loveland et al., 1994; Snow et al., 1987; Yirmiya et al., 1992).

Preschoolers with IDASD, compared with children matching on their MA, display similar emotional expressiveness during social interactions, or when they were watching video sequences illustrating emotional expressions in others (Capps, Kasari, Yirmiya, & Sigman, 1993). By using "the Maximally Discriminative Facial Movement Coding System" (MAX) in order to code the units of facial expression movements, Yirmiya, Kasari, Sigman, & Mundy, 1989 observed that children with ASD show similar quantities of positive and negative emotions to TD children; however, their facial movements express more than one emotion, and they display more combinations of incongruous facial movements (for example, joy and sadness). By contrast, Snow et al. (1987) reported that young children with ASD display fewer expressions of positive emotions than do TD and ID children. Poor emotional expressiveness in children with ASD was emphasized, in comparison with TD and Down syndrome children (Kasari & Sigman, 1996; Loveland et al., 1994).

At around 2–5 years of age, children with ASD barely initiate shared attention with others and language (Mundy, Sigman, & Kasari, 1990; Travis, Sigman, & Ruskin, 2001; Warreyn, Roeyers, & De Groote, 2005). At preschool age, children with IDASD show poorer emotional coordination and timing of affect during social exchanges, in comparison with children matched on their MA and their CA (Scambler, Hepburn, Rutherford, Wehner, & Rogers, 2007). At school age, they respond, with less concern and comforting behaviour or empathic behaviour, to others' emotional expressions; they do not easily share their affects or their emotional states with a partner (Bacon et al., 1998; Corona, Dissanayake, Arbelle, Wellington, & Sigman, 1998; Dawson et al., 2004; Kasari, Sigman, Mundy, & Yirmiya, 1990; Sigman et al., 1992). This weak responsiveness to others' emotions remains stable over a 5-year period (Dissanayake et al., 1996). This lack of empathy in children and adolescents with ASD has been widely reported and sometimes empathic responses in social scenarios are specifically trained (Argott, Buffington Townsend, Sturmey, & Poulson, 2008; Charman et al., 1997, 1998; Dyck, Ferguson, & Shochet, 2001; Gena et al., 1996; Hudry & Slaughter, 2009; Sigman et al., 1992; Travis et al., 2001; Yirmiya et al., 1992). However, empathy behaviour may vary according to specific emotional context, as it was reported by parents (in their response to "Day-to-Day Child Empathy Questionnaire", DCEQ) who indicate that their children with ASD are more likely to display empathy towards familiar agent (Hudry & Slaughter, 2009), and inter-individual variability has also been shown (McGovern & Sigman, 2005).

At school age, by contrast to TD or ID children who spontaneously display their positive emotions in social interactions, children with IDASD share their emotional expressions with others in a less spontaneous way (Attwood, Frith, & Hermelin, 1988; Bieberich & Morgan, 2004; Snow et al., 1987), notably in unstructured situations, in the case where the caregiver does not initiate the interaction (Kasari, Sigman, & Yirmiya, 1993a). The combination between their emotional expression and eye contact and the reciprocal expressiveness face to their caregiver's expressions are also less displayed by them, in comparison with control groups (Dawson, Hill, Spencer, Galpert, & Watson, 1990b). So, they appear less expressive because they more often show neutral, flat or idiosyncratic expressions, in comparison with MA controls, and this continues later in their lives (Czapinski &

Bryson, 2003; Hobson & Lee, 1998; Kasari et al., 1990; Loveland et al., 1994; Yirmiya et al., 1989). For example, these children displayed less attention and less smiles when other children are laughing in play situations, than did children with Down syndrome (Reddy, Williams, & Vaughan, 2002). Sometimes, children with ASD more often display happy expressions in solitary or unpleasant situations than in social situations (Whitman, 2004).

As for feeling of complex emotions, it was reported that individuals with ASD do not experience certain complex emotions, such as embarrassment, pride and guilt, or do not experience, in the same way as TD people, these emotions (Grandin, 1995).

In addition, when individuals with ASD describe their own emotions, they seem to give scripted, less personally relevant and tangential responses (Kasari et al., 2001a); in adults with ASD, the lesser differentiation between felt emotions and their difficulty to describe them are also observed (Hill, Berthoz, & Frith, 2004).

In short, some differences in expression emotions seem to be observed in older children, adolescents and adults with IDASD than in youngest, when they are compared with participants matched on their MA.

More specifically concerning children, preadolescents and adolescents with HFASD, some studies observed that they have a relatively adequate expressiveness that does not differ clearly from MA-matched controls; notably, there are able to verbally express emotions (Jaedicke et al., 1994), and sometimes they may express more positive emotions (Capps et al., 1993). Another recent study emphasized that children with HFASD, who are 10 years old, are less aware of their own emotions, evoke to a lower degree, emotionally charged situations from their own social experience and more often explain they do not feel an emotion (Rieffe et al., 2007). These last authors observed notably that these children claimed not to feel anger in the condition in which anger is presented alone. Rieffe et al. (2007) suggest that the self-awareness of emotional states should be distinguished from the expressiveness of emotions, because a child may learn to recognize their emotions when parents designate them but that he or she should establish links between a physiologic state and an emotional situation. Concerning people with HFASD, research should continue to investigate similarities versus dissimilarities in emotional expressiveness (Begeer et al., 2008).

By contrast to children with IDASD, school-aged children with HFASD show that they are able to name others' emotions, can respond appropriately to emotional displays and take others' perspective (Capps et al., 1992; Peterson et al., 2005). Even if they are less spontaneously empathic or pro-social in their non-verbal and verbal behaviour towards a partner in distress, in comparison with TD children matched on their CA and MA, they can improve these reactions when they are prompted by another person (Bacon et al., 1998; Capps et al., 1993; Doussard-Roosevelt, Joe, Bazhenova, & Porges, 2003; Loveland & Tunali, 1991; Yirmiya et al., 1992). In the study led by Hilton, Graver, and LaVesser (2007), large number of significant correlations were obtained between the sensory profile (SP, Dunn, 1999)[14] and the social responsiveness scores (SRS, Constantino & Gruber, 2005) in children with HFASD between the ages of 6 and 10 years. These authors emphasized that the majority of these children were found to have some sensory processing difficulties, but this is often overlooked in examination of children with ASD. They consider that it is important to examine sensory processing in these children with HFASD, in link with their social responsiveness, and to take into account these processes in diagnostic procedure.

According to Begeer et al. (2008), in comparison with TD children, children with ASD should present similar elementary emotional expressiveness and experiences, but they should differ in the inter- and intra-personal integration of their emotions. These authors also specified that "empirical evidence found for the influence of age, intelligence and context factors on the level of emotional expressiveness in children and adolescents with ASD refines the marked impairments of emotional expressive behaviour that are suggested in the diagnostic manuals" (Begeer et al., 2008, p. 346).

Sensitivity and Physiological Responses Towards Others' Emotions in Children with ASD

Some studies found evidence for an impaired physiological basis to respond to emotions in individuals with ASD (with or without ID) but it is not generalized.

At school age, the arousal in children with IDASD, in response to pictures of distress in others, measured with heart rate or skin conductance responses, is similar to control children matched on their CA and MA (Blair, 1999). But preadolescents with IDASD show less arousal in response to another persons' distress (Corona et al., 1998) or eye gaze (Kylliainen & Hietanen, 2006). Concerning school-aged children with HFASD, they show lower heart rates than do TD controls in response to others' emotions (Corona et al.,

1998). However, impaired emotional responsiveness is not confirmed in skin conductance (Ben Shalom et al., 2006) or eye-blink magnitude (Bernier, Dawson, Panagiotides, & Webb, 2005) measured in preadolescents with HFASD. Even if the method of measuring physiological responses allows examining automatic response to emotions, current results have not indicated, in a congruent way, clear impairments in ASD.

The results obtained in these types of studies in this section confirm the general impairments, considered in the diagnostic of ASD, concerning their emotional sharing and emotional reciprocity. However, their performances in these domains could vary depending on their age, their IQ, their motivation and the explicitness of task demands and the condition of observations (spontaneous behaviour in unstructured situations or behaviour following explicit requests in structured situations), according to Begeer et al. (2008).

Emotional Regulation

Emotional regulation corresponds to a set of processes by which an individual assesses, control and modify his spontaneous emotional responses in order to accomplish his goals or in order to express socially adequate emotional behaviour (Eisenberg, Fabes, Guthrie, & Reiser, 2000, 2006, 2007; Gross & Thompson, 2007; Luminet, 2002; Mikolajczak, Quoidbach, Kotsou, & Nélis, 2009; Nader-Grosbois, 2009, 2011; Thompson, 1994). According to these authors, by his/her manner to mentally conceive an emotional situation, a person may modify the type of emotional states and the duration of emotional responses or their intensity: the regulation may amplify or inhibit emotional responses, by using varied strategies.[15] Various levels of regulation come into the picture: emotions may act as regulators, or they may be regulated or it could be desirable to regulate emotions in social interactions (Philippot, 2007; Rimé, 2007). So emotional regulation is included in emotional intelligence[16] that itself participates in the construction of social intelligence (Salovey, Hsee, & Mayer, 1993). Emotional regulation presents a value of social communication, in which emotions have a function of organizing relationships of individuals

---

[14] The SP (most appropriate for ages 5–10) is a 125-item questionnaire that describes responses to sensory events in daily life and measures the degree to which children exhibit problems in sensory processing, modulation, behavioural and emotional responses, and responsiveness to sensory events. The caregiver reports how frequently the child uses that response to particular sensory events and they are classified in comparison to how a typically developing child responds to the same sensory input.

[15] In this instance, the person may select the situation (according to the probability of desirable or non-desirable emotions); modify the situation (according to emotional impact); focus her attention only on particular aspects of the situation; operate a cognitive change about the meaning of this situation in order to appreciate her abilities to affront to it; and finally, regulate her emotional, behavioural, verbal and physiological responses (Eisenberg et al., 2006; Gross, 1998; Luminet, 2002; Philippot, 2007).

[16] Emotional intelligence corresponds to abilities of control, of discrimination of our own emotions, those in others and of the utilisation of these indications in order to guide our actions and thoughts.

to their environment, and is the basis of socialisation, and also of social sharing (Eisenberg et al., 2000, 2006; Rimé, 2007; Thompson, 1994). Indeed, the regulation contributing to individuals' adjustment to the environment activates internal and external processes responsible for supervising, assessing and modifying emotional reactions in the course of realization of goals (Brun, 2001b; Brun & Mellier, 2004[17]; Thompson, 1994).

During the first years of life, emotional regulation develops progressively and induces significant effects on child's behaviour. From the age of 3 years, the child starts to modify the intensity of her or his emotional expression depending on the situation, in conformity with social rules (Cole, 1986; Joseph, 1994). From preschool age, children intentionally control their emotional expressions in order to induct a false belief in their partner (Perron & Gosselin, 2004) or in order to avoid hurting others' sensibility or their own vulnerability (Saarni, 1999). Indeed, even if children develop skills to express their emotions, the imperatives of social life imply that they learn to dissimulate, control their own emotional states and regulate their expressive behaviour in particular contexts; children begin to distinguish real and apparent emotions at 3–4 years of age, and progressively the dissimulation of emotions develops from 6 to 10 years of age (Banerjee, 1997; Ceschi & Scherer, 2001; Gosselin, 2005; Harris et al., 1989; Josephs, 1994; Malatesta & Haviland, 1982; Perron & Gosselin, 2004; Sissons Joshi & McLean, 1994; Zeman, Cassano, Perry-Parrish, & Stegall, 2006). The development of emotional regulation has a potential role in social interactions between TD preschoolers and in the evolution of their social competence (Cole, Martin, & Dennis, 2004; Dennis, 2006; Dennis & Kelemen, 2009, Dennis, Malone, Chen, 2009; Eisenberg et al., 1995, 1997a, 1997b, 2006; Eisenberg & Spinrad, 2004; Fabes et al., 1999; Rieder, Perrez, Reicherts, & Horn, 2007; Spinrad et al., 2006). In other words, the children's abilities to regulate and to control their emotional and behavioural responses could help them to have good interactions with peers and could contribute to social adjustment, including in school (Eisenberg et al., 1995, 1997a, 1997b; Fabes et al., 1999). Social interactions with peers not only develop their cognitive, social and communicative abilities but offer opportunities to exercise their emotional regulation; emotional and behavioural

responses from peers should provide them feedback on their own abilities (Bronson, 2000; Dunn, 1996; Hartup, 1983; Parker & Asher, 1987). Through behaviour of social referencing and socio-cognitive development, the child acquires an understanding of emotions (causes and consequences), ToM emotions, and also a knowledge of social rules that allows him or her to determinate which emotion is to express when, towards who and in which circumstance. Social abilities in children are linked with their skills to express, to recognize emotions and to understand others' emotions and intentions (Cassidy et al., 1998; Denham et al., 2003; Dodge, Pettit, McClaskey, & Brown, 1986; Fabes et al., 1999). In addition, depending on contexts or situations of interaction, emotional regulation in preschoolers could potentially vary in order to adequately adjust their emotions. For example, during cooperative play between peers, children display exchanges, are emotionally expressive and positive, or are particularly engaged towards their partner and express joy (Broadhead, 2001; Gottman, 1986; Herbé, Tremblay, & Mallet, 2007; Nader-Grosbois, 2009). Emotional regulation comprises intra-individual processes related to cognitive and control processes (Dumas & Lebeau, 1998; Garitte, 2003; Harris et al., 1989; Stein, Trabasso, & Liwag, 1993) and inter-individual social processes (Campos, Campos, & Barret, 1989; Eisenberg & Fabes, 1992; Eisenberg et al., 1997a, 1997b, 2000; Walden & Smith, 1997), both of which play a basic role in the development of social competence.

What About Emotional Regulation in Children with ASD?

Studies focused on emotional regulation in atypical children are rare. However, poor emotional regulation is a characteristic frequently associated with autistic profiles (Southam-Gerow & Kendall, 2002). Tardif et al. (2007) reported that studies on emotional expressivity have emphasized in ASD children a deficit in expression, in modulation and in internal and external regulation of emotions. They are described as easily stressed, anxious and fearful. They have difficulty in self-regulating their emotions when their feelings become excessive (Whitman, 2004). At preschool age, children with IDASD barely modify their emotional reactions in response to others during social exchanges (Konstantareas & Stewart, 2006). Several authors postulate that there is an important impairment of emotional regulation, or more globally of self-regulation, that could explain a set of inabilities in children with ASD in their social interactions (Adrien, 1996; Konstantareas & Stewart, 2006; Trevarthen, 1989; Whitman, 2004).

Trevarthen (1989) suggests that autism is due to an early basic deficit in the production of emotions and of emotional regulation in reaction to environmental stimulations.

---

[17] Brun and Mellier (2004) conceived an evolution of three types of emotional regulation. First, the "intra-personal regulation" includes vigilance, regulation of stress and the application of emotional representations. Second, the "inter-individual regulation in imaginary situation" refers to the recognition of facial expressions, to evocation, to identification of mental states and to the understanding of emotional terms and it allows reflecting the child's level of emotional knowledge. Third, "the interpersonal regulation in interactive situation" concerns the emotional language, shared and joint attention, empathy and the searching of social reference on others' face.

He hypothesized a biological origin of this impairment: a dysfunction of central regulator systems. Children with ASD do not feel emotions related to exchanges initiated by others or to experiences they have towards objects. Moreover, poor or absent or paradoxically excessive emotion in children with ASD does not play its role of regulator, as search, product, maintain, inhibit and interrupt behaviours oriented to others or to objects (Tanguay, 1987).

In Adrien's perspective (1996), he proposes that this deficiency in emotionality in children with ASD appears more in situations requiring regulation: breaking off, maintaining, amplifying or reducing the emotional affects. They prefer to resist change and to conserve their initial state, notably in order to avoid different social situations which are sources of emotional amplifications or reductions, requiring regulation. This author designates all deficits in regulation processes in autism by the term of functional and developmental "dysregulation". Adrien's view (1996) is supported by results of some empirical studies and also by clinical observations, showing dysregulation in children with ASD not only in cognitive operations but also in socio-emotional problem solving or interactive situations (Huebner & Dunn, 2001; Nader-Grosbois, 2007a, 2007b; Paris, 2000; Seynhaeve & Nader-Grosbois, 2008a; Seynhaeve, Nader-Grosbois, & Dionne, 2008b).

In his model "the development of autism: a self-regulatory perspective", Whitman (2004) notably emphasized the essential role of self-regulation in several processes of development and of functioning in children with autism, including emotional and social areas. Whitman (2004, pp. 158–160) suggests that emotions and self-regulation must be considered in conjunction because they can be either risk or protective factors in social adjustment of children with or without ASD. He specified that children with ASD may be vulnerable to stress if their arousal and state regulation dysfunction, if their self-regulatory system is poorly developed and environmental stressors are too intense or prolonged. His theory also describes that the emotions in children with ASD indirectly influence the development of self-regulation through their impact on sensory, motor, social, cognitive and language or communicative processes. Not only these latter processes directly affect the development of self-regulatory behaviour (through the tools they provide for self-regulation) but also self-regulation provides individuals the capacity to control their emotions.

Future research should examine more specifically the links between emotional regulation, self-regulation in varied contexts and the understanding of emotions, the ToM development in children with ASD, in creating methodological design that should allow observing them in more "natural" contexts as possible.

Implications of ToM and Emotional Cognition Studies for Assessment and Intervention

In order to improve and integrate assessment and intervention towards individuals with ASD, we suggest several guidelines based on relevant literature cited in this chapter and structured in relationship to the components of three levels of social functioning included in the heuristic model of social competence developed by Yeates et al. (2007), in this case, social information processing, social interaction and social adjustment (Nader-Grosbois, 2011) (see Fig. 9.1). We propose to assess (by means of various methodologies: testing, relevant questionnaires completed by the surrounding, observations in naturalistic settings) and to train (see A in Fig. 9.1):

(a) their precursors of ToM and emotional cognition[18] from infancy and childhood: training for emotional recognition of diverse types of stimuli (facial, vocal, gestural, body movements) by using various supports (photographs,[19] videos, computer software[20]), of face processing, of early imitation, of joint attention[21] and social referencing[22];

(b) their socio-perceptive processing (towards social cues) and perceptive integration;

(c) their cognitive executive functions[23] and self-regulation strategies[24];

---

[18] Several tasks have been conceived in order to assess facial expression processing and face processing in people with developmental disorders in a battery of social and emotional cognition (Hippolyte, Barisnikov, Van der Linden, & Detraux, 2009).

[19] For training facial emotional recognition in children and adolescents with ASD (Swettenham, Baron-Cohen, Gomez, & Walsh, 1996).

[20] Several intervention programs towards people with ASD trained emotional recognition by using multimedia supports (Golan & Baron-Cohen, 2006b), for example "Gaining Face" (www.ccoder. com/GainingFace, Stone Mountain software), "Emotion Trainer" (Silver, 2000), "Mind Reading-Emotion Library" (Baron-Cohen, 2004), "VisTA" (Pollak & Sinha, 2002). Stewart and Singh (1995) trained facial emotional recognition in ID children by using the "Facial Action Coding System" (Ekman & Friesen, 1977, 1978).

[21] See Hwang & Hughes, 2000; Jones et al., 2006; Kasari et al., 2001b, 2006; Whalen & Schreibman, 2003; Whalen et al., 2006; Jones, 2009.

[22] See Brim et al., 2009.

[23] The combined training of executive function and ToM beliefs by using stories is efficient in TD preschoolers (Kloo & Perner, 2003) and children with ASD (Fisher & Happé, 2006).

[24] Cotugno (2009) assessed efficiency of a training of children's self-management abilities in solving conflicts between peers. See also Antonietti, Sempoi and Marchetti (2006); Nader-Grosbois (2007a, 2007b).

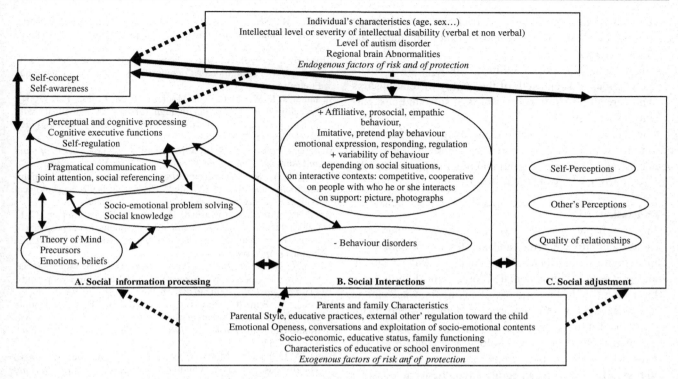

Fig. 9.1 Integrated model of socio-emotional cognition in ASD individuals (Nader-Grosbois & Day), inspired from model of social competences in children with brain disorder (Yeates et al., 2007)

(d) their development of social information processing and of social knowledge[25];

(e) their ToM abilities[26] (beliefs and emotions), notably their understanding of causes and of consequences of four basic emotions and of more complex emotions;

(f) their skills in socio-emotional problem solving or challenges and social scripts,[27] for the level of social interaction (see *B* in Fig. 9.1);

(g) their emotional expression, emotional regulation[28] and conventional responding towards others' emotions and

---

[25] Barisnikov, Hippolyte, Urben, and Pizzo (2009) developed a battery of social cognition assessment, adapted for individuals with ID, including several subtests.

[26] Multiple adaptations of classic ToM testing are elaborated in order to adjust them according to cultural environment and to functioning of atypical children or adolescents with developmental disorders (including ASD or ID; see Thirion-Marissiaux & Nader-Grosbois, 2008a, 2008b, 2008c). In addition, some instruments or standardized questionnaires used to evaluate child's social behaviours in daily life include items about ToM (for example, EASE; Hugues, Soares-Boucaud, Hochman, & Frith, 1997).

See Charlop-Christy and Daneshvar (2003); Feng, Lo, & Tsai, 2008; Gevers, Clifford, Mager, & Boer, 2006; Hadwin et al., 1996, 1997; LeBlanc et al., 2003; McGregor, Whiten, & Blackburn, 1998; Ozonoff & Miller, 1995; Parsons & Mitchell, 1999; Steerneman, Jackson, Pelzer, & Muris, 1996; Swettenham, 1996; Swettenham et al., 1996; Wellman, Hollander, & Schult, 1996, 2002 for efficient training of ToM abilities, with various tasks and supports. Howlin, Baron-Cohen and Hadwin (1999) developed the "Teaching Children with Autism to Mind-Read: A Practical Guide". Softwares are also used to train ToM emotions, notably "Emotion Trainer" (Silver & Oakes, 2001; Silver, 2000) and "Mind Reading: The Interactive Guide to Emotions – Learning Centre & Games Zone" (Baron-Cohen, 2004). During parent–child interactions, training conversations on mental states, beliefs and emotions (Cassidy et al., 1998; Dyer, Shatz, & Wellman, 2000; LaBounty, Wellman, & Olson, 2008; Nader-Grosbois, 2009, 2011; Ontai & Thompson, 2002; Peterson & Slaughter, 2003).

[27] "Social Responsiveness Scale" (SRS; Constantino & Gruber, 2005) includes items covering social cognition and social awareness in order to best discriminate social behaviours in ASD; a preschool version of SRS was conceived by Pine, Luby, Abbacchi, and Constantino (2006). Among the items of "Matson Evaluation of Social Skills with Youngsters" (MESSY; Matson, Rotatori, & Helsel, 1983) to read to the parents in an interview, it is also possible to emphasize some problematic behaviours in children with ASD related to emotional and social cognition, notably making eye contact, smiling at people they know, initiating social conversation and saying thank you. Barisnikov et al. (2009) elaborated subtests assessing knowledge of social rules and social problem solving in their battery. For training socio-emotional skills by scenarios, Gray (1994, 2004; Gray & Garand, 1993) elaborated "Comic Strip Conversations", "Social Stories"; McAfee (2001), "Navigating the Social World".

[28] Nader-Grosbois (2009) and her colleagues elaborated several instruments and designs to assess emotional regulation in children with and without developmental disorders and their parents' external regulation.

"The Incredible 5-point Scale: Assisting Students with Autism Spectrum Disorders" helps to understand social interactions and control their emotional responses (Buron & Curtis, 2004). Riggs, Greenberg, Kusche, and Pentz (2006) showed an improvement of self-control and a decreasing of behaviour disorders by applying the "Promoting Alternative Thinking Strategies" (PATHS, Kusché & Greenberg, 1994).

empathic behaviours[29] in various contexts and towards different persons, for the level of social adjustment (see *C* in Fig. 9.1);

(h) their social adaptive abilities, through their self-perceptions of social self, of the quality of relationships and perceptions from peers, adults of surroundings, parents or teachers.[30]

Considering both endogenous and exogenous factors as potential risk or protection factors in socio-emotional competence would seem to us essential in order to understand the variety of profiles in people with ASD.

Conclusion

In this chapter we have shown how the "theory of mind", cognitive models, and studies on emotions can meaningfully contribute to our understanding of autism and pervasive developmental disorders. In doing so, we have stressed the importance of taking into account in a complementary way research from models and methods rooted in developmental psychology, developmental psychopathology, neuropsychology and educational science. Moreover, we have emphasized how it is pertinent in research to conceive integrated hypotheses, to consider several levels of functioning in assessment and to interpret results of ASD people in the light of meaningful dynamic links between these levels. It would seem clear, on the basis of the research we have cited in this chapter and the perspective we have adopted in considering it, that such an approach could generate effective interventions contributing to the enhancement of human welfare.

References

Abbeduto, L., & Murphy, M. M. (2004). Language, social cognition, maladaptive behavior and communication in Down syndrome and Fragile X syndrome. In M. L. Rice & S. F. Warren (Eds.), *Developmental language disorders. From phenotypes to etiologies* (pp. 77–97). London: Lawrence Erlbaum Associates Publishers.

Adams, C., Green, J., Gilchrist, A., & Cox, A. (2002). Conversational behaviour of children with Asperger syndrome and conduct disorder. *Journal of Child Psychology and Psychiatry, 43*, 679–690.

---

[29] The "Social Skills Rating System" (SSRS; Gresham & Elliott, 1990) includes an area of ability of empathy. Parents may also complete the "Day-to-Day Child Empathy Questionnaire" (DCEQ, Hudry & Slaughter, 2009).

Valdivia-Salas, Luciano, Gutierrez-Martinez, and Visdomine (2009) provide a set of guidelines in order to sustain the development of empathy in a structured way, in referring to stages of empathy, on the basis of evoked experiences and events, and to facilitate the children's understanding of their own and others' emotions, and empathic behaviour.

[30] Gutstein (2000), in the "Solving the Relationship Puzzle", described method of scaffolding children with ASD in order to discover themselves in their daily life interactions and create significant relationships in which they may share their emotions with privileged people.

Adolphs, R., Sears, L., & Piven, J. (2001). Abnormal processing of social information from faces in autism. *Journal of Cognitive Neuroscience, 13*, 232–240.

Adrien, J. L. (1996). *Autisme du jeune enfant: Développement psychologique et régulation de l'activité*. Paris: Expansion Scientifique Française.

Alcantara, J. I., Weisblatt, E. J., Moore, B. C., & Bolton, P. F. (2004). Speech-in-noise perception in high functioning individuals with autism or Asperger's syndrome. *Journal of Child Psychology and Psychiatry, 45*, 1107–1114.

Antonietti, A., Sempoi, O. L., & Marchetti, A. (2006). *Theory of mind and language in developmental contexts*. New York: Springer.

Apperly, I. A., Samson, D., & Humphreys, G. W. (2005). Domain-specificity and theory of mind: Evaluating neuropsychological evidence. *Trends in Cognitive Sciences, 9*, 572–577.

Argott, P., Buffington Townsend, D., Sturmey, P., & Poulson, C. L. (2008). Increasing the use of empathic statements in the presence of a non-verbal affective stimulus in adolescents with autism. *Research in Autism Spectrum Disorders, 2*, 341–352.

Ashwin, C., Wheelwright, S., & Baron-Cohen, S. (2006). Attention bias to faces in Asperger syndrome: A pictorial emotion stroop study. *Psychological Medicine, 36*, 835–843.

Attwood, A., Frith, U., & Hermelin, B. (1988). The understanding and use of interpersonal gestures by autistic and Down's syndrome children. *Journal of Autism and Developmental Disorders, 18*, 241–257.

Bacon, A. L., Fein, D., Morris, R., Waterhouse, L., & Allen, D. (1998). The responses of autistic children to the distress of others. *Journal of Autism and Developmental Disorders, 28*, 129–142.

Balconi, M., & Carrera, A. (2006). Emotional representation in facial expression and script: A comparison between normal and autistic children. *Research in Developmental Disabilities, 28*, 409–422.

Banerjee, M. (1997). Hidden emotion: Preschoolers' knowledge of appearance-reality and emotion display rules. *Social Cognition, 15*, 107–132.

Bar-Haim, Y., Shulman, C., Lamy, D., & Reuveni, A. (2006). Attention to eyes and mouth in high-functioning children with autism. *Journal of Autism and Developmental Disorders, 36*, 2006.

Baranek, G. T. (1999). Autism during infancy: A retrospective video analysis of sensory-motor and social behaviours at 9–12 months of age. *Journal of Autism and Developmental Disorders, 29*, 213–224.

Barisnikov, K., Hippolyte, L., Urben, S., & Pizzo, R. (2009). *The knowledge of social rules: A developmental study*. Paper presented at the 11th Congress of the Swiss Psychological Society, August 19th–20th, University of Neuchâtel, Neuchâtel, Switzerland.

Barna, J., & Legerstee, M. (2005). Nine- and twelve-month-old infants relate emotions to people's actions. *Cognition & Emotion, 19*, 53–67.

Baron-Cohen, S. (1988). Social and pragmatic deficits in autism: Cognitive or affective? *Journal of Autism and Developmental Disorders, 18*, 379–402.

Baron-Cohen, S. (1989a). The autistic child's theory of mind: A case of specific developmental delay. *Journal of Child Psychology and Psychiatry, 30*, 285–298.

Baron-Cohen, S. (1989b). Are autistic children behaviourists? An examination of their mental–physical and appearance–reality distinctions. *Journal of Autism and Developmental Disorders, 19*, 579–600.

Baron-Cohen, S. (1991a). The development of a theory of mind in autism: Deviance and delay? *Psychiatric Clinics of North America, 14*, 33–51.

Baron-Cohen, S. (1991b). Do people with autism understand what causes emotion? *Child Development, 62*, 385–395.

Baron-Cohen, S. (1991c). Precursors to a theory of mind: Understanding attention in others. In A. Whiten (Ed.), *The emergence of mindreading: The evolution development, and simulation or second-order mental representation* (pp. 233–251). Oxford: Basil Blackwell.

Baron-Cohen, S. (1995). *Mindblindness: An essay on autism and theory of mind*. London: The MIT Press.

Baron-Cohen, S. (1999). La cécité mentale dans l'autisme. *Enfance, 3*, 285–293.

Baron-Cohen, S. (2000). From attention-goal psychology to belief-desire psychology: The development of a theory of mind and its dysfunction. In S. Baron-Cohen, H. Tager-Flusberg, & D. J. Cohen (Eds.), *Understanding other minds: Perspectives for autism* (pp. 59–82). Oxford: Oxford University Press.

Baron-Cohen, S. (2004). *Mind reading: The interactive guide to emotions. [computer software]*. London: Jessica Kingsley Publishers. http://www.jkp.com/mindreading

Baron-Cohen, S., & Hammer, J. (1997c). Parents of children with Asperger syndrome: What is the cognitive phenotype? *Journal of Cognitive Neuroscience, 9*, 548–554.

Baron-Cohen, S., Jolliffe, T., Mortimore, C., & Robertson, M. (1997b). Another advanced test of theory of mind: Evidence from very high functioning adults with autism or Asperger syndrome. *Journal of Child Psychology and Psychiatry, 38*, 813–822.

Baron-Cohen, S., Leslie, A. M., & Frith, U. (1985). Does the autistic child have a "theory of mind"? *Cognition, 21*, 37–46.

Baron-Cohen, S., Leslie, A. M., & Frith, U. (1986). Mechanical, behavioural and intentional understanding of picture stories in autistic children. *British Journal of Developmental Psychology, 4*, 113–125.

Baron-Cohen, S., Ring, H., Moriarty, J., Schmitz, B., Costa, D., & Ell, P. (1994). The brain basis of theory of mind: The role of the orbitofrontal region. *British Journal of Psychiatry, 165*, 640–649.

Baron-Cohen, S., Spitz, A., & Cross, P. (1993). Do children with autism recognize surprise? A research note. *Cognition and Emotion, 7*, 507–516.

Baron-Cohen, S., & Swettenham, J. (1997a). Theory of mind in autism: Its relationship to executive function and central coherence. In D. J. Cohen & F. R. Volkmar (Eds.), *Handbook for autism and pervasive developmental disorders* (pp. 880–893). New York: Wiley.

Baron-Cohen, S., Tager-Flusberg, H., & Cohen, D. J. (2000). *Understanding other minds: Perspectives from autism and developmental neuroscience* (2nd ed.). Oxford: Oxford University Press.

Baron-Cohen, S., Wheelwright, S., Hill, J., Raste, Y., & Plumb, I. (2001). The "Reading the Mind in the Eyes" Test revised version: A study with normal adults, and adults with Asperger syndrome or high-functioning autism. *Journal of Child Psychology and Psychiatry, 42*, 241–251.

Bauminger, N. (2002). The facilitation of social-emotional understanding and social interaction in high-functioning children with autism: Intervention outcomes. *Journal of Autism and Developmental Disorders, 32*, 283–298.

Bauminger, N. (2004). The expression and understanding of jealousy in children with autism. *Development and Psychopathology, 16*, 157–177.

Bauminger, N., & Kasari, C. (1999). Brief report: Theory of mind in high-functioning children with autism. *Journal of Autism and Developmental Disorders, 29*, 81–86.

Begeer, S., Koot, H. M., Rieffe, C., Meerum Terwogt, M., & Stegge, H. (2008). Emotional Competence in children with autism. Diagnostic criteria and empirical evidence. *Developmental Review, 28*, 342–369.

Begeer, S., Meerum Terwogt, M., Rieffe, C., Stegge, H., & Koot, J. M. (2007). Do children with autism acknowledge the influence of mood on behaviour? *Autism, 11*, 503–521.

Begeer, S., Rieffe, C., Meerum Terwogt, M., & Stockmann, L. (2006). Attention to facial emotion expressions in children with autism. *Autism, 10*, 37–51.

Behrmann, M., Thomas, C., & Humphreys, K. (2006). Seeing it differently: Visual processing in autism. *Trends in Cognitive Sciences, 10*, 258–264.

Ben Shalom, D., Mostofsky, S. H., Hazlett, R. L., Goldberg, M. C., Landa, R. J., Faran, Y., et al. (2006). Normal physiological emotions but differences in expression of conscious feelings in children with high-functioning autism. *Journal of Autism and Developmental Disorders, 36*, 395–400.

Bernier, R., Dawson, G., Panagiotides, H., & Webb, S. (2005). Individuals with autism spectrum disorder show normal responses to a fear potential startle paradigm. *Journal of Autism and Developmental Disorders, 35*, 575–583.

Bieberich, A. A., & Morgan, S. B. (2004). Self-regulation and affective expression during play in children with autism or Down syndrome: A short-term longitudinal study. *Journal of Autism and developmental Disorders, 34*(4), 439–448.

Bishop, D. V. M. (1993). Autism, executive functions and theory of mind – a neuropsychological perspective. *Journal of Child Psychology and Psychiatry and Allied Disciplines, 34*, 279–293.

Blair, R. J. R. (1999). Psychophysiological responsiveness to the distress of others in children with autism. *Personality and Individual Differences, 26*, 477–485.

Blake, R., Turner, L. M., Smoski, M. J., Pozdol, S. L., & Stone, W. L. (2003). Visual recognition of biological motion is impaired in children with autism. *Psychological Science, 14*, 151–157.

Bolte, S., & Poustka, F. (2003). The recognition of facial affect in autistic and schizophrenic subjects and their first-degree relatives. *Psychological Medicine, 33*, 907–915.

Bono, M. A., Daley, T., & Sigman, M. (2004). Relations among joint attention, amount of intervention, and language gain in autism. *Journal of Autism and Developmental Disabilities, 34*, 495–505.

Bormannkischkel, C., Vilsmeier, M., & Baude, B. (1995). The development of emotional concepts in autism. *Journal of Child Psychology and Psychiatry, 36*, 1243–1259.

Boucher, J., Lewis, V., & Collis, G. M. (2000). Voice processing abilities in children with autism, children with specific language impairments, and young typically developing children. *Journal of Child Psychology and Psychiatry, 41*, 847–857.

Bowler, D. M. (1992). "Theory of mind" in Asperger's syndrome. *Journal of Child Psychology and Psychiatry, 33*, 877–893.

Braverman, M., Fein, D., Lucci, D., & Waterhouse, L. (1989). Affect comprehension in children with pervasive developmental disorders. *Journal of Autism and Developmental Disorders, 19*, 301–316.

Brim, D., Buffington Townsend, D., DeQuinzio, J. A., & Poulson, C. L. (2009). Analysis of social referencing skills among children with autism. *Research in Autism Spectrum Disorders, 3*, 942–958.

Broadhead, P. (2001). Investigating sociability and cooperation in four and five years olds in reception class settings. *International Journal of Early Years Education, 9*, 23–35.

Bronson, M. B. (2000). *Self regulation in early childhood. Nature and nurture*. New York: Guildford Press.

Brun, P. (2001a). La vie émotionnelle de l'enfant: Nouvelles perspectives et nouvelles questions. *Enfance, 53*, 221–225.

Brun, P. (2001b). Psychopathologie de l'émotion chez l'enfant: L'importance des données développementales typiques. *Enfance, 53*, 281–291.

Brun, P., & Nadel, J. (1998). La perception intermodale des émotions: Approche comparative développementale. *L'Encéphale*, 107–109.

Brun, P., Nadel, J., & Mattlinger, M. J. (1998). L'hypothèse émotionnelle dans l'autisme. *Psychologie Française, 43*, 147–156.

Brun, P., & Mellier, D. (2004). Régulation émotionnelle et retard mental: étude chez l'enfant trisomique 21. *Handicap, 101–102*, 19–31.

Buffington, D. M., Krantz, P. J., McClannahan, L. E., & Poulson, C. L. (1998). Procedures for teaching appropriate gestural communication skills to children with autism. *Journal of Autism and Developmental Disorders, 28*, 535–545.

Buitelaar, J. K., & van der Wees, M. (1997). Are deficits in the decoding of affective cues and in mentalizing abilities independent? *Journal of Autism and Developmental Disorders, 27*, 539–556.

Buitelaar, J. K., van der Wees, M., Swaab-Barneveld, H., & van der Gaag, R. J. (1999a). Theory of mind and emotion–recognition in autistic spectrum disorders and in psychiatric control and normal children. *Development and Psychopathology, 11*, 39–58.

Buitelaar, J. K., van der Wees, M., Swaab-Barneveld, H., & van der Gaag, R. J. (1999b). Verbal memory and performance IQ predict theory of mind and emotion recognition ability in children with autistic spectrum disorders and in psychiatric control children. *Journal of Child Psychology and Psychiatry, 40*, 869–881.

Buron, K. D., & Curtis, M. (2004). *The incredible 5-Point Scale: Assisting students with autism spectrum disorders in understanding social interactions and controlling their emotional responses.* Shawnee Mission, KS: Autism Asperger Publishing Company.

Campos, J. J., Campos, R. G., & Barret, K. C. (1989). Emergent themes in the study of emotional development and emotion regulation. *Developmental Psychology, 25*, 394–402.

Capps, L., Kasari, C., Yirmiya, N., & Sigman, M. (1993). Parental perception of emotional expressiveness in children with autism. *Journal of Consulting and Clinical Psychology, 61*, 475–484.

Capps, L., Sigman, M., & Yirmiya, N. (1995). Self-competence and emotional understanding in High-Functioning children with autism. *Development and Psychopathology, 7*, 137–149.

Capps, L., Yirmiya, N., & Sigman, M. (1992). Understanding of simple and complex emotions in non-retarded children with autism. *Journal of Child Psychology and Psychiatry, 33*, 1169–1182.

Cassidy, K. W., Ball, L. V., Rourke, M. T., Werner, R. S., Feeny, N., Chu, J. Y., et al. (1998). Theory of mind concepts in children's literature. *Applied Psycholinguistics, 19*, 463–470.

Castelli, F. (2005). Understanding emotions from standardized facial expressions in autism and normal development. *Autism, 9*, 428–449.

Celani, G., Battacchi, M., & Arcidiacono, L. (1999). The understanding of emotional meaning of facial expressions in people with autism. *Journal of Autism and Developmental Disorders, 29*, 57–66.

Ceschi, G., & Scherer, K. R. (2001). Contrôler l'expression faciale et changer l'émotion: Une approche développementale. *Enfance, 53*, 257–269.

Charlop-Christy, M. H., & Daneshvar, S. (2003). Using video modelling to teach perspective taking to children with autism. *Journal of Positive Behavior Interventions, 5*, 12–21.

Charman, T., Swettenham, J., Baron-Cohen, S., Cox, A., Baird, G., & Drew, A. (1997). Infants with autism: An investigation on empathy, pretend play, joint attention, and imitation. *Developmental Psychology, 33*, 781–789.

Charman, T., Swettenham, J., Baron-Cohen, S., Cox, A., Baird, G., & Drew, A. (1998). An experimental investigation of social cognitive abilities in infants with autism: Clinical implications. *Infant Mental Health Journal, 19*, 260–275.

Chawarska, K., Klin, A., & Volkmar, F. (2003). Automatic attention cueing through eye movement in 2-year-old children with autism. *Child Development, 74*, 1108–1122.

Cole, P. M. (1986). Children's spontaneous control of facial expression. *Child development, 57*, 1309–1321.

Cole, P. M., Martin, S. E., & Dennis, T. A. (2004). Emotion regulation as a scientific construct: Methodological challenges and directions for child development research. *Child Development, 75*, 317–333.

Colvert, E., Custance, D., & Swettenham, J. (2002). Rule-based reasoning and theory of mind in autism: A commentary on the work of Zelazo, Jacques, Burack and Frye. *Infant and Child Development, 11*, 197–200.

Constantino, J. N., & Gruber, C. P. (2005). *Social responsiveness scale.* Los Angeles: Western Psychological Services.

Corbett, B. A., Constantine, L. J., Hendren, R., Rocke, D., & Ozonoff, S. (2009). Examining executive functioning in children with autism spectrum disorder, attention deficit, hyperactivity disorder and typical development. *Psychiatry Research, 166*, 210–222.

Corona, R., Dissanayake, C., Arbelle, S., Wellington, P., & Sigman, M. (1998). Is affect aversive to young children with autism? Behavioral and cardiac responses to experimenter distress. *Child Development, 69*, 1494–1502.

Cotugno, A. J. (2009). Social competences and Social skills training and intervention for children with autism spectrum disorders. *Journal of Autism and Developmental Disorders, 39*, 1268–1277.

Critchley, H. D., Daly, E. M., Bullmore, E. T., Williams, S. C., Van Amelsvoort, T., Robertson, D. M., et al. (2000). The functional neuroanatomy of social behaviour: Changes in cerebral blood flow when people with autistic disorder process facial expressions. *Brain, 123*, 2203–2212.

Cutting, A. L., & Dunn, J. (1999). Theory of mind, emotion understanding, language, and family background: Individual differences and interrelations. *Child Development, 70*, 853–865.

Czapinski, P., & Bryson, S. E. (2003). Reduced facial muscle movements in autism: Evidence for dysfunction in the neuromuscular pathway? *Brain and Cognition, 51*, 177–179.

Da Fonseca, D., Santos, A., Bastard-Rosset, D., Rondan, C., Poinso, F., & Deruelle, C. (2009). Can children with autistic spectrum disorders extract emotions out of contextual cues? *Research in Autism Spectrum Disorders, 3*, 50–56.

Dahlgren, S. O., & Trillingsgaard, A. (1996). Theory of mind in non-retarded children with autism and Asperger's syndrome: A research note. *Journal of Child Psychology and Psychiatry, 37*, 759–763.

Dapretto, M., Davies, M. S., Pfeifer, J. H., Scott, A. A., Sigman, M., Bookheimer, S. Y., et al. (2006). Understanding emotions in others: Mirror neuron dysfunction in children with autism spectrum disorders. *Nature Reviews Neuroscience, 9*, 28–30.

Davies, S., Bishop, D., Manstead, A. S., & Tantam, D. (1994). Face perception in children with autism and Asperger's syndrome. *Journal of Child Psychology and Psychiatry, 35*, 1033–1057.

Dawson, G., & Adams, A. (1984). Imitation and social responsiveness in autistic children. *Journal of Abnormal Child Psychology, 12*, 209–226.

Dawson, G., Carver, L., Meltzoff, A. N., Panagiotides, H., McPartland, J., & Webb, S. J. (2002). Neural correlates of face and object recognition in young children with autism spectrum disorder, developmental delay, and typical development. *Child Development, 73*, 700–717.

Dawson, G., & Galpert, L. (1990a). Mother's use of imitative play for facilitating social responsiveness and toy play on autistic children. *Development and Psychopathology, 2*, 151–162.

Dawson, G., Hill, D., Spencer, A., Galpert, L., & Watson, L. (1990b). Affective exchanges between young autistic children and their mothers. *Journal of Abnormal Child Psychology, 18*, 335–345.

Dawson, G., Webb, S. J., Carver, L., Panagiotides, H., & McPartland, J. (2004). Young children with autism show atypical brain responses to fearful versus neutral facial expressions of emotion. *Developmental Science, 7*, 340–359.

Dawson, G., Webb, S. J., & McPartland, J. (2005). Understanding the nature of face processing impairment in autism: Insights from behavioral and electrophysiological studies. *Developmental Neuropsychology, 27*, 403–424.

de Schonen, S., Mathivet, E., & Deruelle, C. (1989). Hemispheric specialization for face recognition in infancy. In C. von Euler, H. Forssberg, & H. Lagercrantz (Eds.), *Neurobiology of early infant behavior* (pp. 261–271). Houndmills: Macmillan.

de Wit, T. C. J., Falck-Ytter, T., & von Hofsten, C. (2008). Young children with autism spectrum disorder look differently at positive versus negative emotional faces. *Research in Autism Spectrum Disorders, 2*, 651–659.

Decety, J. (2002). Naturaliser l'empathie. *L'Encéphale, 28*, 9–20.

Deneault, J., & Morin, P. (2007). La Théorie de l'Esprit: Ce que l'enfant comprend de l'univers psychologique. In S. Larivée (Ed.), *L'intelligence. Tome 1. Les approches biocognitives, développementales et contemporaines* (pp. 154–162). Montréal: ERPI.

Denham, S. A. (1998). *Emotional development in young children.* New York: Guilford press.

Denham, S. A., Blair, K. A., DeMulder, E., Levitas, J., Sawyer, K., Auerbach-Major, S., et al. (2003). Preschool emotional competence: Pathway to social competence? *Child Development, 74*, 238–256.

Denham, S. A., & Couchoud, E. (1990). Young preschoolers' understanding of emotion. *Child Study Journal, 23*, 171–192.

Denham, S. A., Mason, T., Caverly, S., Schmidt, M., Hackney, R., Caswell, C., et al. (2001). Preschoolers at play: Co-socialisers of emotional and social competence. *International Journal of Behavioral Development, 25*, 290–301.

Denham, S. A., McKinley, M., Couchoud, E. A., & Holt, R. (1990). Emotional and behavioural predictors of peer status in young preschoolers. *Child Development, 61*, 1145–1152.

Dennis, T. A. (2006). Emotional self regulation in preschoolers: The interplay of temperamental approach reactivity and control processes. *Developmental Psychology, 42*, 84–97.

Dennis, T. A., & Kelemen, D. A. (2009). Preschool children's views on emotion regulation: Functional associations and implications for social–emotional adjustment. *International Journal of Behavioral Development, 33*, 243–252.

Dennis, M., Lockyer, L., & Lazenby, A. L. (2000). How high-functioning children with autism understand real and deceptive emotion. *Autism, 4*, 370–381.

Dennis, T. A., Malone, M., & Chen, C. (2009). Emotional face processing and emotion regulation in children: An ERP study. *Developmental Neuropsychology, 34*, 85–102.

Dissanayake, C., Sigman, M., & Kasari, C. (1996). Long-term stability of individual differences in the emotional responsiveness of children with autism. *Journal of Child Psychology and Psychiatry, 37*, 461–467.

Dixon, D. R., Tarbox, J., & Najdowski, A. (2009). Social skills in autism spectrum disorders. In J. L. Matson (Ed.), *Social behavior and skills in children* (pp. 117–140). New York: Springer Sciences.

Dodge, K. A., Pettit, G. S., McClaskey, C. L., & Brown, M. M. (1986). Social competence in children. *Monographs of the Society for Research in Child Development, 51*(2, Serial No. 213), 1–85.

Doussard-Roosevelt, J. A., Joe, C. M., Bazhenova, O. V., & Porges, S. W. (2003). Mother–child interaction in autistic and nonautistic children: Characteristics of maternal approach behaviors and child social responses. *Development and Psychopathology, 15*, 277–295.

Downs, A., & Smith, T. (2004). Emotion understanding, cooperation, and social behavior in high functioning autism. *Journal of Autism and Developmental Disorders, 34*, 625–635.

Draghi-Lorenz, R., Reddy, V., & Costall, A. (2001). Rethinking the development of "nonbasic" emotions: A critical review of existing theories. *Developmental Review, 21*, 263–304.

Dumas, C., & Lebeau, S. (1998). Le changement représentationnel affectif chez les enfants d'âge préscolaire. *Revue canadienne de psychologie expérimentale, 52*, 25–33.

Dumont-Mathieu, T., & Fein, D. (2005). Screening for autism in young children: The modified checklist for autism in toddlers (M-CHAT) and other measures. *Mental Retardation and Developmental Disabilities Research Reviews, 11*, 253–262.

Dunn, J. (1996). The Emanuel Miller Memorial Lecture 1995: Children's relationships: Bridging the divide between cognitive and social development. *Journal of Child Psychology and Psychiatry and Allied Disciplines, 37*, 507–518.

Dunn, W. (1999). *The sensory profile manual.* San Antonio, TX: The Psychological Corporation.

Dunn, J. (2003). Emotional development in early childhood: A social relationship perspective. In R. Davidson, H. H. Goldsmith, & K. Scherer (Eds.), *The handbook of affective science* (pp. 332–346). Oxford: Oxford University Press.

Dyck, M. J., Ferguson, K., & Shochet, I. M. (2001). Do autism spectrum disorders differ from each other and from nonspectrum disorders on emption recognition tests? *European Child and Adolescent Psychiatry, 10*, 105–116.

Dyer, J. R., Shatz, M., & Wellman, H. M. (2000). Young children's storybooks as a source of mental state information. *Cognitive Development, 15*, 17–37.

Eisenberg, N., & Fabes, R. A. (1992). Emotion, regulation, and the development of social competence. In M. S. Clark (Ed.), *Emotion and social behavior* (Vol. 14, pp. 119–150). Newbury Park, CA: Sage.

Eisenberg, N., Fabes, R. A., Guthrie, I. K., & Reiser, M. (2000). Dispositional emotionality and regulation: Their role in predicting quality of social functioning. *Journal of Personality and Social Psychology, 78*, 136–157.

Eisenberg, N., Fabes, R. A., Murphy, B. C., Maszk, P., Smith, M., & Karbon, M. (1995). The role of emotionality and regulation in children's social functioning: A longitudinal study. *Child Development, 66*, 1360–1384.

Eisenberg, N., Fabes, R. A., Shepard, S. A., Murphy, B. C., Guthrie, I. K., Jones, S., et al. (1997a). Contemporaneous and longitudinal prediction of children's social functioning from regulation and emotionality. *Child Development, 68*, 642–664.

Eisenberg, N., Guthrie, I. K., Fabes, R. A., Reiser, M., Murphy, B. C., Holgren, R., et al. (1997b). The relations of regulation and emotionality to resiliency and competent social functioning in elementary school children. *Child Development, 68*, 295–311.

Eisenberg, N., Hofer, C., & Vaughan, J. (2007). Effortful control and its socio-emotional consequences. In J. J. Gross (Ed.), *Handbook emotion regulation* (pp. 287–306). New York: The Guilford Press.

Eisenberg, N., & Spinrad, T. L. (2004). Emotion-related: Sharpening the definition. *Child development, 75*, 331–339.

Eisenberg, N., Zhou, Q., Liew, J. C., Pidada, S., & Champion, C. (2006). Emotion, emotion-related regulation, and social functioning. In X. Chen, D. French, & B. Schneider (Eds.), *Peer relationships in cultural context* (pp. 170–200). Cambridge: Cambridge University Press.

Eisenmajer, R., & Prior, M. (1991). Cognitive linguistic correlates of "theory of mind" ability in autistic children. *British Journal of Developmental Psychology, 9*, 351–364.

Ekman, P. (1992). Are there basic emotions? *Psychological Review, 99*, 550–553.

Ekman, P., & Friesen, W. V. (1975). *Unmasking the face.* Englewood Cliffs, NJ: Prentice Hall.

Ekman, P., & Friesen, W. V. (1977). *Manual for the facial action coding system.* Palo Alto, CA: Consulting Psychologists Press.

Ekman, P., & Friesen, W. V. (1978). *The facial action coding system.* Palo Alto, CA: Consulting Psychologists Press.

Emery, N. J. (2005). The evolution of social cognition. In A. Easton & N. J. Emery (Eds.), *The cognitive neuroscience of social behaviour* (pp. 115–156). New York: Psychology Press.

Fabes, R. A., Eisenberg, N., Jones, S., Smith, M., Guthrie, I., Poulin, R., et al. (1999). Regulation, emotionality, and preschoolers' socially competent peer interactions. *Child Development, 70*, 432–442.

Fein, D., Lucci, D., Braverman, M., & Waterhouse, L. (1992). Comprehension of affect in context in children with pervasive developmental disorders. *Journal of Child Psychology and Psychiatry, 33*, 1157–1167.

Feinman, S. (1982). Social referencing in infancy. *Merrill-Palmer Quarterly, 28*, 445–470.

Feinman, S., Roberts, D., Hsieh, K., Sawyer, D., & Swanson, D. (1992). A critical review of social referencing in infancy. In S. Feinman

(Ed.), *Social referencing and the social construction of reality in infancy* (pp. 15–54). New York: Plenum Press.

Feng, H., Lo, Y., & Tsai, S. (2008). The effects of theory of mind and social skills training on the social competence in a sixth-grade student with autism. *Journal of Positive Behaviour Interventions, 10*, 228–242.

Field, T., Field, T., Sanders, C., & Nadel, J. (2001). Children with autism display more social behaviors after repeated imitation sessions. *Autism, 5*, 317–323.

Field, T. M., & Walden, T. A. (1982). Production and discrimination of facial expressions by preschool children. *Child Development, 53*, 1299–1300.

Fisher, N., & Happé, F. (2006). A training study of theory of mind and executive function in children with autistic spectrum disorders. *Journal of Autism and Developmental Disorders, 35*, 757–771.

Flavell, J. H. (1999). Cognitive development: Children's knowledge about the mind. *Annual Review of Psychology, 50*, 21–45.

Fletcher, P. C., Happé, F., Frith, U., Baker, S. C., Dolan, R. J., Frack-owiak, R. S. J., et al. (1995). Other minds in the brain: A functional imaging study of 'theory of mind' in story comprehension. *Cognition, 57*, 109–128.

Frith, U. (2001). Mind blindness and the brain in autism. *Neuron, 32*, 969–979.

Frith, U. (2003). *Autism: Explaining the enigma* (2nd ed.). Oxford: Blackwell.

Frith, U. (2004). Emanuel Miller lecture: Confusions and controversies about Asperger syndrome. *Journal of Child Psychology and Psychiatry, 45*, 672–686.

Frith, U., & Happé, F. (1994). *Autism: 'Beyond theory of mind'. Cognition, 50*, 115–132.

Frye, D., Zelazo, P. D., & Palfai, T. (1995). Theory of mind and rule-based reasoning. *Cognitive Development, 10*, 483–527.

Gallagher, H. L., & Frith, C. (2003). Functional imaging of 'theory of mind'. *Trends in Cognitive Neurosciences, 7*, 77–83.

Gallese, V., & Goldman, A. (1998). Mirror-neurons and the simulation theory of mind-reading. *Trends in Cognitive Sciences, 2*, 493–501.

Garitte, C. (2003). La reconnaissance des expressions faciales chez des enfants de 8 ans d'âge réel et/ou mental: Processus cognitifs ou sociaux? *Approche Neuropsychologique des Apprentissages chez l'Enfant, 71*, 48–52.

Gattegno, M. P., Ionescu, S., Malvy, J., & Adrien, J. L. (1999). Etude préliminaire de la recherche d'un lien spécifique entre les troubles de l'attention conjointe et de la Théorie de l'Esprit dans l'autisme de l'enfant. *Approche Neuropsychologique des Apprentissages chez l'Enfant, 52*, 42–48.

Gena, A., Krantz, P. J., McClannahan, L. E., & Poulson, C. L. (1996). Training and generalization of affective behaviour displayed by youth with autism. *Journal of Applied Behavior Analysis, 29*, 291–304.

Gepner, B., de Schonen, S., & Buttin, C. (1994). Face processing in young autistic children. *Infant Behavior and Development, 17*, 661.

Gepner, B., Deruelle, C., & Grynfeltt, S. (2004). Motion and emotion: A novel approach to the study of face processing by young autistic children. *Journal of Autism and Developmental Disorders, 31*, 37–45.

Gervais, H., Belin, P., Boddaert, N., Leboyer, M., Coez, A., Sfaello, I., et al. (2004). Abnormal cortical voice processing in autism. *Nature Neuroscience, 7*, 801–802.

Gevers, C., Clifford, P., Mager, M., & Boer, F. (2006). Brief report: A theory of mind based social cognition training program for school-aged children with pervasive developmental disorders: An open study of its effectiveness. *Journal of Autism and Developmental Disorders, 36*, 567–571.

Gewirtz, J. L., & Pelaez-Nogueres, M. (1992). Social referencing as a learned process. In S. Feinman (Ed.), *Social referencing and the social construction of reality in infancy*. New York: Plenum Press.

Gilbert, P. (2004). Evolution, attractiveness, and the emergence of shame and guilt in a self-aware mind: A reflection on Tracy and Robins. *Psychological Inquiry, 15*, 132–135.

Golan, O., & Baron-Cohen, S. (2006b). Systemizing empathy: Teaching adults with Asperger syndrome or high functioning autism to recognize complex emotions using interactive multimedia. *Development and Psychopathology, 18*, 589–615.

Golan, O., Baron-Cohen, S., & Hill, J. (2006a). The Cambridge mindreading (CAM) face-voice battery: Testing complex emotion recognition in adults with and without Asperger syndrome. *Journal of Autism and Developmental Disorders, 36*, 169–183.

Gordon, R. M. (1992). The simulation theory: Objections and misconceptions. *Mind and Language, 7*, 11–34.

Gosselin, P. (1995). Le développement de la reconnaissance des expressions faciales des émotions chez l'enfant. *Revue Canadienne des Sciences du Comportement, 27*, 107–119.

Gosselin, P. (2005). Le décodage de l'expression faciale des émotions au cours de l'enfance. *Psychologie Canadienne, 46*, 126–138.

Gottman, J. M. (1986). The world of coordinated-play: Same and cross-sex friendship in young children. In J. M. Gottman & J. G. Parker (Eds.), *Conversations of friends: Speculations on affective development* (pp. 139–191). Cambridge: Cambridge University Press.

Grandin, T. (1995). *Thinking in pictures*. New York: Vintage Books.

Gray, C. (1994). *Comic strip conversations: Colorful illustrated interactions with students with autism and related disorders*. Jenison, MI: Jenison Public Schools.

Gray, C. (2004). *Social stories 10.0*. Jenison, MI: Jenison Public Schools.

Gray, C., & Garand, J. D. (1993). Social stories: Improving responses of students with autism with accurate social information. *Focus on Autistic Behaviour, 8*, 1–10.

Gresham, F. M., & Elliott, S. N. (1990). *The social skills rating system*. Circle Pines, MN: American Guidance Services.

Gross, J. (1998). The emerging field of emotion regulation: An integrative review. *Review of General Psychology, 2*(3), 271–299.

Gross, T. F. (2004). The perception of four basic emotions in human and nonhuman faces by children with autism and other developmental disabilities. *Journal of Abnormal Child Psychology, 32*, 469–480.

Gross, T. F. (2005). Global-local precedence in the perception of facial age and emotional expression by children with autism and other developmental disabilities. *Journal of Autism and Developmental Disorders, 35*, 773–785.

Gross, J. J., & Thompson, R. A. (2007). Emotion regulation: Conceptual foundations. In J. J. Gross (Ed.), *Handbook of emotion regulation* (pp. 3–24). New York: Guilford Press.

Grossman, J. B., Klin, A., Carter, A. S., & Volkmar, F. R. (2000). Verbal bias in recognition of facial emotions in children with Asperger syndrome. *Journal of Child Psychology and Psychiatry, 41*, 369–379.

Grossman, R. B., & Tager-Flusberg, H. (2008). Reading faces for information about words and emotions in adolescents with autism. *Research in Autism Spectrum Disorders, 2*, 681–695.

Gutstein, S. E. (2000). *Solving the relationship puzzle*. Arlington, TX: Future Horizons.

Hadwin, J., Baron-Cohen, S., Howlin, P., & Hill, K. (1996). Can we teach children with autism to understand emotions, beliefs, or pretence? *Development and Psychopathology, 8*, 345–365.

Hadwin, J., Baron-Cohen, S., Howlin, P., & Hill, K. (1997). Does teaching theory of mind have an effect on the ability to develop conversation in children with autism? *Journal of Autism and Developmental Disorders, 27*, 519–537.

Halberstadt, A. G., Denham, S. A., & Dunsmore, J. C. (2001). Affective social competence. *Social Development, 10*, 79–119.

Hale, C. M., & Tager-Flusberg, H. (2005). Brief report: The relationship between discourse deficits and autism symptomatology. *Journal of Autism and Developmental Disorders, 35*, 519–524.

Happé, F. (1995). The role of age and verbal ability in the theory of mind task performance of subjects with autism. *Child Development, 66*, 843–855.

Happé, F. (1999). Autism: Cognitive deficit or cognitive style? *Trends in Cognitive Sciences, 3*, 216–222.

Happé, F. (2000). Parts and wholes, meanings and minds: Central coherence and its relation to theory of mind. In S. Baron-Cohen, H. Tager-Flusberg, & D. Cohen (Eds.), *Understanding other minds, perspectives from autism and development neuroscience* (2nd ed., pp. 203–221). Oxford: Oxford University Press.

Happé, F., Ronald, A., & Plomin, R. (2006). Time to give up on a single explanation for autism. *Nature Neuroscience, 9*, 1218–1220.

Harris, P. L. (2000). *The work of the imagination*. Oxford: Blackwell.

Harris, P. L., Brown, E., Marriott, C., Whittall, S., & Harmer, S. (1991). Monsters, ghosts and witches – testing the limits of the fantasy reality distinction in young-children. *British Journal of Developmental Psychology, 9*, 105–123.

Harris, P. L., Johnson, C. N., Hutton, D., Andrews, B., & Cooke, T. (1989). Young children's theory of mind and emotion. *Cognition and Emotion, 3*, 379–400.

Hartup, W. W. (1983). Peer relations. In P. Mussen & E. M. Hetherington (Eds.), *Handbook of child psychology, Vol. 4. Socialization, personality, and social development* (4th ed., pp. 103–196). New York: Wiley.

Haxby, J. V., Hoffman, E. A., & Gobbini, M. I. (2000). The distributed neural system for face perception. *Trends in Cognitive Sciences, 4*, 223–233.

Haynie, D. L., & Lamb, M. E. (1995). Positive and negative facial expressiveness in 7-, 10-, 13-month-old infants. *Infant behaviour and Development, 18*(2), 257–259.

Heerey, E. A., Keltner, D., & Capps, L. M. (2003). Making sense of self-conscious emotion: Linking theory of mind and emotion in children with autism. *Emotion, 3*, 394–400.

Heimann, M. (1998). Imitation in neonates, in older infants and in children with autism: Feedback to theory. In S. Bräten (Ed.), *Intersubjective communication and emotion in early ontogeny* (pp. 47–62). Cambridge: Cambridge University Press.

Herbé, D., Tremblay, H., & Mallet, P. (2007). La coopération dyadique entre enfants de 5-6 ans: Effets de la complexité cognitive et de l'activité motrice sollicitées par les situations de résolution de problème. *Enfance, 59*, 393–413.

Hill, E., Berthoz, S., & Frith, U. (2004). Brief report: Cognitive processing of own emotions in individuals with autistic spectrum disorder and in their relatives. *Journal of Autism and Developmental Disorders, 34*, 229–235.

Hillier, A., & Allinson, L. (2002). Understanding embarrassment among those with autism: Breaking down the complex emotion of embarrassment among those with autism. *Journal of Autism and Developmental Disorders, 32*, 583–592.

Hilton, C., Graver, K., & LaVesser, P. (2007). Relationship between social competence and sensory processing in children with high functioning autism spectrum disorders. *Research in Autism Spectrum Disorders, 1*, 164–173.

Hippolyte, L., Barisnikov, K., Van der Linden, M., & Detraux, J. J. (2009). From facial emotional recognition abilities to emotional attribution: A study in Down syndrome. *Research in Developmental Disabilities, 30*, 1007–1022.

Hobson, R. P. (1986a). The autistic child's appraisal of expressions of emotion. *Journal of Child Psychology and Psychiatry, 27*, 321–342.

Hobson, R. P. (1986b). The autistic child's appraisal of expressions of emotion: A further study. *Journal of Child Psychology and Psychiatry, 27*, 671–680.

Hobson, R. P. (1989). Beyond cognition: A theory of autism. In G. Dawson (Ed.), *Autism: New perspectives on diagnosis, nature and treatment* (pp. 22–48). Guilford: New York.

Hobson, R. P. (1991). Methodological issues for experiments on autistic individuals' perception and understanding of emotion. *Journal of Child Psychology and Psychiatry, 32*, 1135–1158.

Hobson, R. P. (1993). *Autism and the development of mind*. Hillsdale, NJ: Erlbaum.

Hobson, R. P., & Lee, A. (1998). Hello and goodbye: A study of social engagement in autism. *Journal of Autism and Developmental Disorders, 28*, 117–127.

Hobson, R. P., Ouston, J., & Lee, A. (1988). Emotion recognition in autism: Co-ordinating faces and voices. *Psychological Medicine, 18*, 911–923.

Hobson, R. P., Ouston, J., & Lee, A. (1989). Naming emotion in faces and voices: Abilities and disabilities in autism and mental retardation. *British Journal of Developmental Psychology, 7*, 237–250.

Howlin, P., Baron-Cohen, S., & Hadwin, J. (1999). *Teaching children with autism to mind-read: A practical guide*. New York: Wiley.

Hudry, K., & Slaughter, V. (2009). Agent familiarity and emotional context influence the everyday empathic responding of young children with autism. *Research in Autism Spectrum Disorders, 3*, 74–85.

Huebner, R. A., & Dunn, W. (2001). Introduction and basic concepts. In R. Huebner (Ed.), *Autism: A sensorimotor approach to management* (pp. 61–99). Gaithersburg, MD: Aspen.

Hugues, C., Soares-Boucaud, I., Hochman, J., & Frith, U. (1997). Social behaviour in pervasive developmental disorders: Effects of informants group and "theory of mind". *European Child and Adolescents Psychiatry, 6*, 191–198.

Hwang, B., & Hughes, C. (2000). Increasing early social-communicative skills of preverbal preschool children with autism through social interactive training. *Journal of the Association for Persons with Severe Handicaps, 25*, 18–28.

Iacobani, M., & Dapretto, M. (2006). The mirror neuron system and the consequences of its dysfunction. *Nature Reviews Neuroscience, 7*, 942–951.

Izard, C. E., & Malatesta, C. Z. (1987). Perspectives on emotional development I: Differential emotions theory of early emotional development. In J. D. Osofsky (Ed.), *Handbook of infant development* (pp. 494–554). New York: Wiley.

Jaedicke, S., Storoschuk, S., & Lord, C. (1994). Subjective experience and causes of affect in high-functioning children and adolescents with autism. *Development and Psychopathology, 6*, 273–284.

Jemel, B., Mottron, L., & Dawson, M. (2006). Impaired face processing in autism: Fact or artifact? *Journal of Autism and Developmental Disorders, 36*, 91–106.

Jones, E. A. (2009). Establishing response and stimulus classes for initiating joint attention in children with autism. *Research in Autism Spectrum Disorders, 3*, 375–389.

Jones, E. A., & Carr, E. G. (2004). Joint attention and autism: Theory and intervention. *Focus on Autism and Developmental Disabilities, 19*, 13–26.

Jones, E. A., Carr, E. G., & Feeley, K. M. (2006). Multiple effects of joint attention intervention for children with autism. *Behavior Modification, 30*, 782–834.

Jones, E. A., & Feeley, K. M. (2007). Parent implemented joint attention intervention for preschoolers with autism. *Journal of Speech-Language Pathology and Applied Behavior Analysis, 2*, 252–268.

Joseph, R. M., Tager-Flusberg, H., & Lord, C. (2002). Cognitive profiles and social–communicative functioning in children with autism spectrum disorder. *Journal of Child Psychology and Psychiatry and Allied Disciplines, 43*(6), 807–821.

Joseph, R. M., & Tanaka, J. (2003). Holistic and part-based face recognition in children with autism. *Journal of Child Psychology and Psychiatry, 44*, 529–542.

Josephs, I. E. (1994). Display rule behavior and understanding in preschool children. *Journal of Nonverbal Behavior, 18*, 301–326.

Kahana-Kalman, R., & Goldman, S. (2008). Intermodal matching of emotional expressions in young children with autism. *Research in Autism Spectrum Disorders, 2*, 301–310.

Kamio, Y., Wolf, J., & Fein, D. (2006). Automatic processing of emotional faces in high-functioning pervasive developmental disorders: An affective priming study. *Journal of Autism and Developmental Disorders, 36*, 155–167.

Karmiloff-Smith, A., Klima, E., Bellugi, U., Grant, J., & Baron-Cohen, S. (1995). Is there a social module? Language, face processing and theory of mind in individuals with Williams Syndrome. *Journal of Cognitive Neuroscience, 7*, 196–208.

Kasari, C., Chamberlain, B., & Bauminger, N. (2001a). In J. Burack, T. Charman, N. Yirmiya, & P. Zelazo (Eds.), *The development of autism: Perspectives from theory and research* (pp. 309–325). Mahwah, NJ: Erlbaum.

Kasari, C., Freeman, S. F. N., & Paparella, T. (2001b). Early intervention in autism: Joint attention and symbolic play. In L. M. Glidden (Ed.), *International review of research in mental retardation*. Autism (Vol. 23, pp. 207–237). San Diego, CA: Academic Press.

Kasari, C., Freeman, S. F. N., & Paparella, T. (2006). Joint attention and symbolic play in young children with autism: A randomized controlled intervention study. *Journal of Clinical Psychology and Psychiatry, 47*, 611–620.

Kasari, C., & Sigman, M. (1996). Expression and understanding of emotion in atypical development: Autism and Down syndrome. In M. Lewis & M. W. Sullivan (Eds.), *Emotional development in atypical children* (pp. 109–130). Mahwah, NJ: Lawrence Erlbaum Associates.

Kasari, C., Sigman, M. D., Baumgartner, P., & Stipek, D. J. (1993b). Pride and mastery in children with autism. *Journal of Child Psychology and Psychiatry, 34*, 353–362.

Kasari, C., Sigman, M., Mundy, P., & Yirmiya, N. (1990). Affective sharing in the context of joint attention interactions of normal, autistic, and mentally retarded children. *Journal of Autism and Developmental Disorders, 20*, 87–100.

Kasari, C., Sigman, M., & Yirmiya, N. (1993a). Focused and social attention of autistic-children in interactions with familiar and unfamiliar adults – A comparison of autistic, mentally-retarded, and normal-children. *Development and Psychopathology, 5*, 403–414.

Kieras, J. E., Tobin, R. M., Graziano, W. G., & Rothbart, M. K. (2005). You can't always get what you want effortful control and children's responses to undesirable gifts. *Psychological Science, 16*, 391–396.

Klin, A. (2000). Attributing social meaning to ambiguous visual stimuli in higher-functioning autism and Asperger syndrome: The social attribution task. *Journal of Child Psychology and Psychiatry and Allied Disciplines, 41*, 831–846.

Klin, A., & Jones, W. (2008). Altered face scanning and impaired recognition of biological motion in a 15-month-old infant with autism. *Developmental Science, 11*, 40–46.

Klin, A., Jones, W., Schultz, R., & Volkmar, F. (2003). The enactive mind, or from actions to cognition: Lessons from autism. *Philosophical transactions of the Royal Society of London series B-Biological Sciences, 358*, 345–360.

Klin, A., Jones, W., Schultz, R., Volkmar, F., & Cohen, D. (2002a). Defining and quantifying the social phenotype in autism. *American Journal of Psychiatry, 159*, 895–908.

Klin, A., Jones, W., Schultz, R., Volkmar, F. R., & Cohen, D. J. (2002b). Visual fixation patterns during viewing of naturalistic social situations as predictors of social competence in individuals with autism. *Archives of General Psychiatry, 59*, 809–816.

Kloo, D., & Perner, J. (2003). Training transfer between card sorting and false belief understanding: Helping children apply conflicting descriptions. *Child Development, 74*, 1823–1839.

Koning, C., & Magill-Evans, J. (2001). Social and language skills in adolescent boys with Asperger syndrome. *Autism, 5*, 23–36.

Konstantareas, M. M., & Stewart, K. (2006). Affect regulation and temperament in children with autism spectrum disorder. *Journal of Autism and Developmental Disorders, 36*, 143–154.

Kusché, C. A., & Greenberg, M. T. (1994). *The PATHS curriculum*. Seattle, WA: Developmental Research and Programs, Inc.

Kylliainen, A., & Hietanen, J. K. (2006). Skin conductance responses to another person's gaze in children with autism. *Journal of Autism and Developmental Disorders, 36*, 517–525.

LaBounty, J., Wellman, H. M., & Olson, S. (2008). Mother's and father's use of internal state talk with their young children. *Social Development, 17*, 757–775.

Lagattuta, K. H. (2005). When you shouldn't do what you want to do: Young children's understanding of desires, rules, and emotions. *Child Development, 76*, 713–733.

Lahaie, A., Mottron, L., Arguin, M., Berthiaume, C., Jemel, B., & Saumier, D. (2006). Face perception in high-functioning autistic adults: Evidence for superior processing of face parts, not for a configural face processing deficit. *Neuropsychology, 20*, 30–41.

Langdell, T. (1978). Recognition of faces: An approach to the study of autism. *Journal of Child Psychology and Psychiatry, 19*, 225–268.

Le Sourn-Bissaoui, S., Caillies, S., Gierski, F., & Motte, J. (2009). Inference processing in adolescents with Asperger syndrome: Relationship with theory of mind abilities. *Research in Autism Spectrum Disorders, 3*, 797–808.

LeBlanc, L. A., Coates, A. M., Daneshvar, S., Charlop-Christy, M. H., Morris, C., & Lancaster, B. M. (2003). Using video modelling and reinforcement to teach perspective-taking skills to children with autism. *Journal of Applied Behavior Analysis, 36*, 253–257.

Leppänen, J. M., & Hietanen, J. K. (2001). Emotion recognition and social adjustment in school-aged girls and boys. *Psychology in the Schools, 42*, 405–417.

Leslie, A. M. (1987). Pretence and representation: The origins of 'theory of mind'. *Psychological Review, 94*, 412–426.

Leslie, A. M. (1991). Theory of mind impairment in autism. In A. Whiten (Ed.), *The emergence of mindreading: The evolution development, and simulation or second-order mental representation* (pp. 63–78). Oxford: Basil Blackwell.

Leslie, A. M. (2000). How to acquire a 'representational theory of mind'. In D. Sperber (Ed.), *Metarepresentation: A multidisciplinary perspective* (pp. 197–223). Oxford: Oxford University Press.

Leslie, A. M., & Roth, D. (2000). What autism teaches us about representation. In S. Baron-Cohen, H. Tager-Flusberg, & D. J. Cohen (Eds.), *Understanding other minds: Perspectives for autism* (pp. 83–111). Oxford: Oxford University Press.

Leslie, A. M., & Thaiss, L. (1992). Domain specificity in conceptual development: Evidence from autism. *Cognition, 43*, 225–251.

Lewis, M., & Sullivan, M. W. (1996). *Emotional development in atypical children*. Mahwah, NJ: Lawrence Erlbaum Associates.

Lewis, M., Sullivan, M. W., Stanger, C., & Weiss, M. (1989). Self development and self-conscious emotions. *Child development, 60*, 146–156.

Lindner, J. L., & Rosen, L. A. (2006). Decoding of emotion through facial expression, prosody and verbal content in children and adolescents with Asperger's syndrome. *Journal of Autism and Developmental Disorders, 36*, 769–777.

Losh, M., & Capps, L. (2006). Understanding of emotional experience in autism: Insights from the personal accounts of high-functioning children with autism. *Developmental Psychology, 42*, 809–818.

Loveland, K. A., & Landry, S. H. (1986). Joint attention and language in autism and developmental language delay. *Journal of Autism and Developmental Disorders, 16*, 335–349.

Loveland, K. A., & Tunali, B. (1991). Social scripts for conversational interactions in autism and Down syndrome. *Journal of Autism and Developmental Disorders, 21*, 177–186.

Loveland, K. A., Tunali-Kotoski, B., Chen, R., Brelsford, K. A., Ortegon, J., & Pearson, D. A. (1995). Intermodal perception of affect in persons with autism or Down syndrome. *Development and Psychopathology, 7*, 409–418.

Loveland, K. A., Tunali-kotoski, B., Pearson, D. A., Brelsford, K. A., Ortegon, J., & Chen, R. (1994). Imitation and expression of facial affect in autism. *Development and Psychopathology, 6*, 433–444.

Luminet, O. (2002). *Psychologie des émotions*. Bruxelles: De Boeck.

Luminet, O., & Lenoir, V. (2006). Alexithymie parentale et capacités émotionnelles des enfants de 3 et 5 ans. *Enfance, 4*, 335–356.

MacDonald, H., Rutter, M., Howlin, P., Rios, P., Le Conteur, A., Evered, C., et al. (1989). Recognition and expression of emotional cues by autistic and normal adults. *Journal of Child Psychology and Psychiatry, 30*, 865–877.

Maestro, S., Muratori, F., Cavallaro, M. C., Pei, F., Stern, D., Golse, B., et al. (2002). Attentional skills during the first 6 months of age in autism spectrum disorder. *Journal of the American Academy of Child and Adolescent Psychiatry, 41*, 1239–1245.

Malatesta, C. Z., & Haviland, J. M. (1982). Learning display rules – the socialization of emotion expression in infancy. *Child Development, 53*, 991–1003.

Malatesta-Magai, C., Leak, S., Tesman, J., & Shepard, B. (1994). Profiles of emotional development: Individual differences in facial and vocal expression of emotion during the second and third years of life. *International Journal of Behavioral Development, 17*, 239–269.

Mann, T. A., & Walker, P. (2003). Autism and a deficit in broadening the spread of visual attention. *Journal of Child Psychology and Psychiatry and Allied Disciplines, 44*(2), 274–284.

Matson, J. L., Rotatori, A. F., & Helsel, W. J. (1983). Development of a rating scale to measure social skills in children: The Matson evaluation of social skills with youngsters (MESSY). *Behaviour Research and Therapy, 21*, 335–340.

McAfee, J. (2001). *Navigating the social world: A curriculum for educating individuals with Asperger's syndrome and high-functioning autism*. Arlington, TX: Future Horizons, Inc.

McGovern, C. W., & Sigman, M. (2005). Continuity and change from early childhood to adolescence in autism. *Journal of Child Psychology and Psychiatry, 46*, 401–408.

McGregor, E., Whiten, A., & Blackburn, P. (1998). Teaching Theory of Mind by highlighting intention and illustrating thoughts: A comparison of their effectiveness with three-year-olds and autistic subjects. *British Journal of Developmental Psychology, 16*, 281–300.

Meltzoff, A. (1999). Origins of theory of mind, cognition and communication. *Journal of Communication Disorders, 32*, 251–269.

Meltzoff, A., & Gopnik, A. (1993). The role of imitation in understanding persons and developing a theory of mind. In S. Baron-Cohen, H. Tager-Flusberg, & D. Cohen (Eds.), *Understanding other minds: Perspectives from Autism* (pp. 335–366). Oxford: Oxford University Press.

Mikolajczak, M., Quoidbach, J., Kotsou, I., & Nélis, D. (2009). *Les compétences émotionnelles*. Paris: Dunod.

Mills, R. S. L. (2005). Taking stock of the developmental literature on shame. *Developmental Review, 25*, 26–63.

Mitchell, P. (1996). *Acquiring a conception of mind: A review of psychological research and theory*. Hove: Psychology Press.

Mottron, L. (2004). *L'autisme: Une autre intelligence*. Liège: Mardaga.

Mottron, L., & Burack, J. (2001). Enhanced perceptual functioning in the development of autism. In J. Burack, T. Charman, N. Yirmiya, & P. D. Zelazo (Eds.), *The development of autism: Perspectives from theory and research* (pp. 131–148). Mahwah, NJ: Erlbaum.

Mottron, L., Dawson, M., Soulieres, I., Hubert, B., & Burack, J. (2006). Enhanced perceptual functioning in autism: An update, and eight principles of autistic perception. *Journal of Autism and Developmental Disorders, 36*, 27–43.

Mundy, P., & Crowson, M. (1997). Joint attention and early social communication: Implications for research on intervention with autism. *Journal of Autism and Developmental Disorder, 27*, 653–676.

Mundy, P., & Gomes, A. (1998). Individual differences in joint attention skill development in the second year. *Infant Behavior and Development, 21*, 469–482.

Mundy, P., Sigman, M., & Kasari, C. (1990). A longitudinal study of joint attention and language development in autistic children. *Journal of Autism and Developmental Disorders, 20*, 115–128.

Nadel, J. (1998a). L'imitation: Son déficit est-il démontré chez l'enfant autiste? *L'Encéphale*, 128–129.

Nadel, J. (1998b). Les habits neufs de l'âge mental. *Enfance, 1*, 111–117.

Nadel, J., Croué, S., Mattlinger, M. J., Canet, P., Hudelot, C., Lécuyer, C., et al. (2000). Do children with autism have expectancies about social behaviour of unfamiliar people? *Autism, 4*, 133–145.

Nadel, J., & Pezé, A. (1993). What makes immediate imitation communicative in toddlers and autistic children. In J. Nadel & L. Camaioni (Eds.), *New perspectives in early communicative development* (pp. 139–156). London: Routledge.

Nader-Grosbois, N. (2007a). L'autorégulation et la dysrégulation chez des jeunes enfants à autisme en situation d'évaluation développementale. *Revue Francophone de la Déficience Intellectuelle, 17*, 34–52.

Nader-Grosbois, N. (2007b). Comment la dysrégulation chez de jeunes enfants autistes et à déficience intellectuelle se manifeste-t-elle en situation d'évaluation développementale? In N. Nader-Grosbois (Ed.), *Régulation, autorégulation et dysrégulation* (pp. 83–100). Wavre: Mardaga.

Nader-Grosbois, N. (2009). *Resilience, regulation and quality of life*. Louvain-la-Neuve: Presses Universitaires de Louvain.

Nader-Grosbois, N. (2011). *Théorie de l'esprit: Entre cognition, émotion et adaptation sociale: chez des personnes typiques et atypiques*. Bruxelles: De Boeck.

Nelson, C. A. (1987). The recognition of facial expressions in the first two years of life: Mechanisms of development. *Child Development, 58*, 889–909.

Noens, I. L. J., & van Berckelaer-Onnes, I. A. (2008). The central coherence account of autism revisited: Evidence from the ComFor study. *Research in Autism Spectrum Disorders, 2*, 209–222.

Oberman, L. M., Hubbard, E. M., McCleery, J. P., Altschuler, E. L., Ramachandran, V. S., & Pineda, J. A. (2005). EEG evidence for mirror neuron dysfunction in autism spectrum disorders. *Cognitive Brain Research, 24*, 190–198.

Ontai, L. L., & Thompson, R. A. (2002). Patterns of attachment and maternal discourse effects on children's emotion understanding from 3 to 5 years of age. *Social Development, 11*(4), 433–450.

Oster, H. (2003). Emotion in the infant's face – insights from the study of infants with facial anomalies. *Annals of the New York Academy of Science, 1000*, 197–204.

Osterling, J. A., Dawson, G., & Munson, J. A. (2002). Early recognition of 1-year-old infants with autism spectrum disorder versus mental retardation. *Development and Psychopathology, 14*, 239–251.

Ozonoff, S., & Miller, J. (1995). Teaching theory of mind: A new approach to social skills training for individuals with autism. *Journal of Autism and Developmental Disorders, 25*(4), 415–433.

Ozonoff, S., Pennington, B. F., & Rogers, S. J. (1990). Are there emotion perception deficits in young autistic children? *Journal of Child Psychology and Psychiatry, 31*, 343–361.

Ozonoff, S., Pennington, B. F., & Rogers, S. J. (1991). Executive function deficits in high functioning autistic children: Relationship to Theory of Mind. *Journal of Child Psychology and Psychiatry, 32*, 1081–1105.

Palomo, R., Belinchon, M., & Ozonoff, S. (2006). Autism and family home movies: A comprehensive review. *Journal of Developmental and Behavioral Pediatrics, 27*, 59–68.

Paris, B. (2000). Characteristics of autism. In C. Murray-Slutsky & B. Paris (Eds.), *Exploring the spectrum of autism and pervasive developmental disorders* (pp. 7–23). Therapy Builder: Harcourt Health Sciences Co.

Parker, J. G., & Asher, S. R. (1987). Peer relations and later personal adjustment: Are low-accepted children at risk? *Psychological Bulletin, 102*(3), 357–389.

Parron, C., Da Fonseca, D., Santos, A., Moore, D. G., Monfardini, E., & Deruelle, C. (2008). Recognition of biological motion in children with autistic spectrum disorders. *Autism, 12*, 261–274.

Parsons, S., & Mitchell, P. (1999). What children with autism understand about thoughts and thought-bubbles. *Autism, 3*, 17–38.

Pellicano, E. (2007). Links between theory of mind and executive function in young children with autism: Clues to developmental primacy. *Development Psychology, 43*, 974–990.

Pellicano, E., Maybery, M., Durkin, K., & Maley, A. (2006). Multiple cognitive capabilities/deficits in children with an autism spectrum disorder: "Weak" central coherence and its relationship to theory of mind and executive control. *Development and Psychopathology, 18*, 77–98.

Pelphrey, K. A., Sasson, N. J., Reznick, J. S., Paul, G., Goldman, B. D., & Piven, J. (2002). Visual scanning of faces in autism. *Journal of Autism and Developmental Disorders, 32*, 249–261.

Perner, J., Frith, U., Leslie, A. M., & Leekam, S. (1989). Exploration of the autistic child's theory of mind: Knowledge, belief, and communication. *Child Development, 60*, 689–700.

Perner, J., Lang, B., & Kloo, D. (2002). Theory of mind and self-control: More than a common problem of inhibition. *Child Development, 73*, 752–767.

Perra, O., Williams, J. H. G., Whiten, A., Fraser, L., Benzie, H., & Perrett, D. I. (2008). Imitation and 'theory of mind' competencies in discrimination of autism from other neurodevelopmental disorders. *Research in Autism Spectrum Disorders, 2*, 456–468.

Perron, M., & Gosselin, P. (2004). Le développement de la simulation des émotions: Une étude de la vraisemblance des expressions faciales produites par les enfants. *Enfance, 2*, 109–125.

Peterson, C. C., & Slaughter, V. (2003). Opening windows into the mind: Mothers' preferences for mental state explanations and children's theory of mind. *Cognitive Development, 18*, 399–429.

Peterson, C. C., & Slaughter, V. (2009). Theory of mind (ToM) in children with autism or typical development: Links between eye-reading and false belief understanding. *Research in Autism Spectrum Disorders, 3*, 462–473.

Peterson, C. C., Wellman, H. M., & Liu, D. (2005). Steps in theory-of-mind development for children with deafness or autism. *Child Development, 76*, 502–517.

Philippot, P. (2007). *Emotions et Psychothérapies*. Wavre: Mardaga.

Phillips, W., Baron-Cohen, S., & Rutter, M. (1992). The role of eye contact in goal detection: Evidence from normal infants and children with autism or mental handicap. *Development and Psychopathology, 4*, 375–383.

Piggot, J., Kwon, H., Mobbs, D., Blasey, C., Lotspeich, L., Menon, V., et al. (2004). Emotional attribution in high-functioning individuals with autistic spectrum disorder: A functional imaging study. *Journal of the American Academy of Child and Adolescent Psychiatry, 43*, 473–480.

Pine, E., Luby, J., Abbacchi, A., & Constantino, J. N. (2006). Quantitative assessment of autistic symptomatology in preschoolers. *Autism, 10*(4), 344–352.

Plaisted, K., Swettenham, J., & Rees, L. (1999). Children with autism show local precedence in a divided attention task and global precedence in a selective attention task. *Journal of Child Psychology and Psychiatry and Allied Disciplines, 40*, 733–742.

Pollak, S., & Sinha, P. (2002). Effects of early experience on children's recognition of facial displays of emotion. *Developmental Psychology, 38*, 784–791.

Prior, M., Dahlstrom, B., & Squires, T. L. (1990). Autistic children's knowledge of thinking and feeling states in other people. *Journal of Child Psychology and Psychiatry, 31*, 587–601.

Rajendran, G., & Mitchell, P. (2007). Cognitive theories of autism. *Developmental Review, 27*, 224–260.

Reddy, V., Williams, E., & Vaughan, A. (2002). Sharing humour and laughter in autism and Down's syndrome. *British Journal of Psychology, 93*, 219–242.

Repacholi, B. M. (1998). Infants' use of attentional cues to identify the referent of another person's emotional expression. *Developmental Psychology, 34*, 1017–1025.

Repacholi, B. M., & Gopnik, A. (1997). Early reasoning about desires: Evidence from 14- and 18-month-olds. *Developmental Psychology, 33*, 12–21.

Rieder, S., Perez, M., Reicherts, M., & Horn, A. (2007). Interpersonal emotion regulation in the family: A review of assessment tools. In A. M. Fontaine & M. Matias (Eds.), *Family, work and parenting: international perspectives* (pp. 17–45). Porto: Legis/livpsic.

Rieffe, C., Meerum Terwogt, M., & Cowan, R. (2005). Children's understanding of mental states as causes of emotions. *Infant and Child Development, 14*, 259–272.

Rieffe, C., Meerum Terwogt, M., & Kotronopoulou, C. (2007). Awareness of single and multiple emotions in high-functioning children with autism. *Journal of Autism and Developmental Disorders, 37*, 455–465.

Rieffe, C., Meerum Terwogt, M., & Stockmann, L. (2000). Understanding atypical emotions among children with autism. *Journal of Autism and Developmental Disorders, 30*, 195–203.

Riggs, N. R., Greenberg, M. T., Kusche, C. A., & Pentz, M. A. (2006). The mediational role of metacognition in the behavioral outcomes of a socio-emotional prevention program in elementary school students: Effects of the PATHS Curriculum. *Prevention Science, 7*, 91–102.

Rimé, B. (2007). Interpersonal emotion regulation. In J. J. Gross (Ed.), *Handbook of emotion regulation* (pp. 466–485). New York: Guilford Press.

Rinehart, N. J., Bradshaw, J. L., Moss, S. A., Brereton, A. V., & Tonge, B. J. (2000). Atypical interference of local detail on global processing in high-functioning autism and Asperger's disorder. *Journal of Child Psychology and Psychiatry and Allied Disciplines, 41*, 769–778.

Robel, L., Ennouri, K., Piana, H. N., Vaivre-Douret, L., Perier, A., Flament, M. F., et al. (2004). Discrimination of face identities and expressions in children with autism: Same or different? *European Child & Adolescent Psychiatry, 13*, 227–233.

Robertson, J. M., Tanguay, P. E., L'Ecuyer, S., Sims, A., & Waltrip, C. (1999). Domains of social communication handicap in autism spectrum disorder. *Journal of American Academy of Child and Adolescent Psychiatry, 38*, 738–745.

Rogers, S. J., & Penington, B. F. (1991). A theoretical approach to the deficits in infantile autism. *Development and Psychopathology, 3*, 137–162.

Russell, J. (1997). How executive disorders can bring about an inadequate 'theory or mind'. In J. Russell (Ed.), *Autism as an executive disorder* (pp. 256–304). Oxford: Oxford University Press.

Russell, J., Hala, S., & Hill, E. (2003). The automated windows task: The performance of preschool children, children with autism, and children with moderate learning difficulties. *Cognitive Development, 18*, 111–137.

Russell, J., & Hill, E. L. (2001). Action-monitoring and intention reporting in children with autism. *Journal of Child Psychology and Psychiatry and Allied Disciplines, 42*, 317–328.

Russell, J., Mauthner, N., Sharpe, S., & Tidswell, T. (1991). The windows task as a measure of strategic deception in preschoolers and autistic subjects. *British Journal of Developmental Psychology, 9*, 331–349.

Rutherford, M. D., Baron-Cohen, S., & Wheelwright, S. (2002). Reading the mind in the voice: A study with normal adults and adults with Asperger syndrome and high functioning autism. *Journal of Autism and Developmental Disorders, 32*, 189–194.

Saarni, C. (1999). *The development of emotional competence*. New York: Guilford Press.

Saarni, C., Mumme, D. L., & Campos, J. J. (1998). Emotional development: Action, communication, and understanding. In W. Damon (Ed.), *Handbook of child psychology, 5th Edition: Social, emotional, and personality development* (pp. 237–309). New York: Wiley.

Salovey, P. (2003). Introduction: Emotion and social processes. In R. Davidson, H. H. Goldsmith, & K. Scherer (Eds.), *The handbook of affective science* (pp. 747–751). Oxford: Oxford University Press.

Salovey, P., Hsee, C. K., & Mayer, J. D. (1993). Emotional intelligence and the self-regulation of affect. In D. M. Wegner & J. W. Pennebaker (Eds.), *Handbook of mental control. Century psychology series*. Upper Saddle River, NJ: Prentice Hall.

Sasson, N. J. (2006). The development of face processing in autism. *Journal of Autism and Developmental Disorders, 36*, 381–394.

Saxe, R., Carey, S., & Kanwisher, N. (2004). Understanding other minds: Linking developmental psychology and functional neuroimaging. *Annual Review of Psychology, 55*, 87–124.

Scambler, D. J., Hepburn, S., Rutherford, M. D., Wehner, E. A., & Rogers, S. J. (2007). Emotional responsivity in children with autism, children with other developmental disabilities, and children with typical development. *Journal of Autism and Developmental Disorders, 37*, 553–563.

Seltzer, M. M., Krauss, M. W., Shattuck, P. T., Orsmond, G., Swe, A., & Lord, C. (2003). The symptoms of autism spectrum disorders in adolescence and adulthood. *Journal of Autism and Developmental Disorders, 33*, 565–581.

Serra, M., Loth, F. L., van Geert, P. L., Hurkens, E., & Minderaa, R. B. (2002). Theory of mind in children with 'lesser variants' of autism: A longitudinal study. *Journal of Child Psychology and Psychiatry, 43*, 885–900.

Seynhaeve, I., & Nader-Grosbois, N. (2008a). Sensorimotor development and dysregulation of activity in young children with autism and with intellectual disabilities. *Research in Autism Spectrum Disorders, 2*(1), 46–59.

Seynhaeve, I., Nader-Grosbois, N., & Dionne, C. (2008b). Functional abilities and neuropsychological dysfunctions in young children with autism and with intellectual disabilities. *Alter, 2*(3), 230–252.

Siegal, M., & Varley, R. (2002). Neural system involved in Theory of mind. *Nature Reviews Neuroscience, 3*, 462–471.

Sigman, M., Arbelle, S., & Dissanayake, C. (1995). Current research findings on childhood autism. *Canadian Journal of Psychiatry, 40*, 289–294.

Sigman, M. D., Kasari, C., Kwon, J. H., & Yirmiya, N. (1992). Responses to the negative emotions of others by autistic, mentally retarded, and normal children. *Child Development, 63*, 796–807.

Silver, M. (2000). *Can people with autistic spectrum disorders be taught emotional understanding? The development and randomised controlled trial of a computer training package*. Unpublished Doctoral Dissertation, Hull University, Kingston-upon-Hull, UK.

Silver, M., & Oakes, P. (2001). Evaluation of a new computer intervention to teach people with autism or Asperger syndrome to recognize and predict emotions in others. *Autism, 5*, 299–316.

Sissons Joshi, M., & McLean, M. (1994). Indian and English children's understanding of the distinction between real and apparent emotion. *Child Development, 65*, 1372–1384.

Smith, I. M., & Bryson, S. E. (1994). Imitation and action in autism: A critical review. *Psychological Bulletin, 116*, 259–273.

Smith, V., Mirenda, P., & Zaidman-Zait, A. (2007). Predictors of expressive vocabulary growth in children with autism. *Journal of Speech, Language, and Hearing Research, 50*, 149–160.

Snow, M. E., Hertzig, M. E., & Shapiro, T. (1987). Expression of emotion in young autistic children. *Journal of the American Academy of Child and Adolescent Psychiatry, 26*, 836–838.

Southam-Gerow, M., & Kendall, P. (2002). Emotion regulation and understanding implication for child and psychopathology and therapy. *Clinical Psychological Review, 22*, 189–222.

Spinrad, T. L., Eisenberg, N., Cumberland, A., Fabes, R. A., Valiente, C., Shepard, S. A., et al. (2006). Relation of emotion-related regulation to children's social competence: A longitudinal study. *Emotion, 6*(3), 498–510.

Steele, S., Joseph, R. M., & Tager-Flusberg, H. (2003). Brief report: Developmental change in theory of mind abilities in children with autism. *Journal of Autism and Developmental Disorders, 33*, 461–467.

Steerneman, P., Jackson, S., Pelzer, H., & Muris, P. (1996). Children with social handicaps: An intervention programme using a Theory of Mind approach. *Clinical Child Psychology and Psychiatry, 1*, 251–263.

Stein, L., Trabasso, T., & Liwag, M. (1993). The representation and organization of emotional experience, unfolding the emotion episode. In M. Lewis & J. M. Haviland (Eds.), *Handbook of emotions* (pp. 279–300). New York: Guilford.

Stewart, C. A., & Singh, N. N. (1995). Enhancing the recognition and production of facial expressions of emotion by children with mental retardation. *Research in Developmental Disabilities, 16*, 365–382.

Swettenham, J. (1996). Can children with autism be taught to understand false belief using computers? *Journal of Child Psychology and Psychiatry, 37*, 157–165.

Swettenham, J., Baron-Cohen, S., Gomez, J.-C., & Walsh, S. (1996). What's inside a person's head? Conceiving of the mind as a camera helps children with autism develop an alternative theory of mind. *Cognitive Neuropsychiatry, 1*, 73–88.

Tanguay, P. (1987). *Early infantile autism: A disorder of affect*. USA: University of Illinois, Department of Psychiatry.

Tantam, D., Monaghan, L., Nicholson, H., & Stirling, J. (1989). Autistic children's ability to interpret faces: A research note. *Journal of Child Psychology and Psychiatry, 30*, 623–630.

Tardif, C., Lainé, F., Rodriguez, M., & Gepner, B. (2007). Slowing down presentation of facial movements and vocal sounds enhances facial expression recognition and induces facial–vocal imitation in children with autism. *Journal of Autism and Developmental Disorders, 37*, 1469–1484.

Teunisse, J. P., Cools, A. R., van Spaendonck, K. P. M., Aerts, F., & Berger, H. J. C. (2001a). Cognitive styles in high-functioning adolescents with autistic disorder. *Journal of Autism and Developmental Disorders, 31*, 55–66.

Teunisse, J. P., & de Gelder, B. (2001b). Impaired categorical perception of facial expressions in high-functioning adolescents with autism. *Child Neuropsychology, 7*, 1–14.

Thirion-Marissiaux, A. F., & Nader-Grosbois, N. (2008a). Theory of Mind "emotion", developmental characteristics and social understanding in children and adolescents with intellectual disability. *Research in developmental Disabilities, 29*, 414–430.

Thirion-Marissiaux, A. F., & Nader-Grosbois, N. (2008b). Theory of Mind "belief," developmental characteristics and social understanding in children and adolescents with intellectual disability. *Research in Developmental Disabilities, 29*, 547–566.

Thirion-Marissiaux, A. F., & Nader-Grosbois, N. (2008c). Theory of mind and socio-affective abilities in disabled children and adolescents. *Alter, 2*, 133–155.

Thompson, R. (1994). Emotion regulation: A theme in search of definition. In N. Fox (Ed.), The development of emotion regulation: Biological and behavioral considerations. *Monographs of the Society for Research in Child Development, 59*(2–3, Serial 240), 25–52.

Toth, K., Munson, J., Meltzoff, A. N., & Dawson, G. (2006). Early predictors of communication development in young children with autism spectrum disorder: Joint attention, imitation, and toy play. *Journal of Autism and Developmental Disabilities, 36*, 993–1005.

Tourrette, C. (1999). Apprentissage du monde, interactions sociales et communication. In J. A. Esperet & E. Esperet (Eds.), *Manuel de psychologie de l'enfant* (pp. 445–478). Sprimont: Mardaga.

Tourrette, C., Recordon, S., Barbe, V., & Soares-Boucaud, I. (2000). Attention conjointe pré-verbale et théorie de l'esprit à 5 ans: La relation supposée entre ces deux capacités peut-elle être démontrée? Etude exploratoire chez des enfants non autistes. In V. Gererdin-Collet & C. Riboni (Eds.), *Autisme: Perspectives actuelles* (pp. 61–75). Paris: L'Harmattan.

Tracy, J. L., Robins, R. W., & Lagattuta, K. H. (2005). Can children recognize pride? *Emotion, 5*, 251–257.

Travis, L. L., & Sigman, M. (1998). Social deficits and interpersonal relationships in autism. *Mental Retardation and Developmental Disabilities Research Reviews, 4*, 65–72.

Travis, L., Sigman, M., & Ruskin, E. (2001). Links between social understanding and social behavior in verbally able children with autism. *Journal of Autism and Developmental Disorders, 31*, 119–130.

Trevarthen, C. (1989). Les relations entre autisme et le développement socioculturel normal: Arguments en faveur d'un trouble primaire de la régulation du développement cognitif par les émotions. In G. Lelord, J. P. Muh, M. Petit, & D. Sauvage (Eds.), *Autismes et troubles du développement global de l'enfant* (pp. 56–80). Paris: Expansion scientifique française.

Turner, M. (1997). Toward an executive dysfunction account of repetitive behavior. In J. Russell (Ed.), *Autism as an executive disorder* (pp. 57–100). Oxford: Oxford University Press.

Valdivia-Salas, S., Luciano, C., Gutierrez-Martinez, O., & Visdomine, C. (2009). Establishing empathy. In R. A. Rehfeldt, Y. Barnes-Holmes, & S. C. Hayes (Eds.), *Derived relational responding: Applications for learners with autism and other developmental disabilities* (pp. 301–311). Oakland, CA: New Harbinger Publications.

van der Geest, J. N., Kemner, C., Verbaten, M. N., & van Engeland, H. (2002). Gaze behavior of children with pervasive developmental disorder toward human faces: A fixation time study. *Journal of Child Psychology and Psychiatry, 43*, 1–11.

van Lang, N. D. J., Bouma, A., Sytema, S., Kraijer, D. W., & Minderaa, R. B. (2006). A comparison of central coherence skills between adolescents with an intellectual disability with and without comorbid autism spectrum disorder. *Research in Developmental Disabilities, 27*, 217–226.

Vaughan, A., Mundy, P., Block, J., Burnette, C., Delgado, C., Gomez, Y., et al. (2003). Child, caregiver, and temperament contributions to infant joint attention. *Infancy, 4*, 603–616.

Völlm, B. A., Taylor, A. N., Richardson, P., Corcoran, R., Stirling, J., McKie, S., et al. (2006). Neuronal correlates of theory of mind and empathy: A functional magnetic resonance imaging study in a nonverbal task. *Neuroimage, 29*, 90–98.

Walden, T. A., & Smith, M. C. (1997). Emotion Regulation. *Motivation and Emotion, 2*, 7–25.

Wang, A. T., Dapretto, M., Hariri, A. R., Sigman, M., & Bookheimer, S. Y. (2004). Neural correlates of facial affect processing in children and adolescents with autism spectrum disorder. *Journal of the American Academy of Child and Adolescent Psychiatry, 43*, 481–490.

Warreyn, P., Roeyers, H., & De Groote, I. (2005). Early social communicative behaviours of preschoolers with autism spectrum disorder during interaction with their mothers. *Autism, 9*, 342–361.

Webster, S., & Potter, D. D. (2008). Eye direction detection improves with development in autism. *Journal of Autism and Developmental Disorders, 38*, 1184–1186.

Wellman, H. M. (1990). *The child's theory of mind*. Cambridge, MA: MIT Press.

Wellman, H. M. (1991). From desires to beliefs: Acquisition of a theory of mind. In A. Whiten (Ed.), *Natural theories of mind* (pp. 19–38). Cambridge, MA: Basil Blackwell.

Wellman, H. M. (2000). Early understanding of mind: The normal case. In S. Baron-Cohen, H. Tager-Flusberg, & D. J. Cohen, *Understanding other minds: Perspectives from autism and developmental neuroscience* (2nd ed., pp. 10–39). Oxford: Oxford University Press.

Wellman, H. M., Caswell, R., Gomez, J. C., Swettenham, J., Toye, E., & Lagattuta, K. (2002). Thought-bubbles help children with autism acquire an alternative to a theory of mind. *Autism, 6*, 343–363.

Wellman, H. M., Harris, P. L., Banerjee, M., & Sinclair, A. (1995). Early understanding of emotion – evidence from natural-language. *Cognition & Emotion, 9*, 117–149.

Wellman, H., Hollander, M., & Schult, C. (1996). Young children's understanding of thought-bubbles and of thoughts. *Child Development, 67*, 768–788.

Wellman, H. M., Phillips, A. T., & Rodriguez, T. (2000). Young children's understanding of perception, desire, and emotion. *Child Development, 71*, 895–912.

Werner, E., Dawson, G., Osterling, J., & Dinno, N. (2000). Brief report: Recognition of autism spectrum disorder before one year of age: A retrospective study based on home videotapes. *Journal of Autism and Developmental Disorders, 30*, 157–162.

Whalen, C., & Schreibman, L. (2003). Joint attention training for children with autism using behavior modification procedures. *Journal of Child Psychology and Psychiatry, 44*, 456–468.

Whalen, C., Schreibman, L., & Ingersoll, B. (2006). The collateral effects of joint attention training on social initiations, positive affect, imitation, and spontaneous speech for young children with autism. *Journal of Autism and Developmental Disabilities, 36*, 655–664.

Whitman, T. (2004). *The development of autism: A self-regulatory perspective*. New York: Jessica Kingsley Publishers.

Widen, S. C., & Russel, J. A. (2002). Gender and preschoolers' perception of emotion. *Merrill-Palmer Quarterly, 48*, 248–262.

Wing, L. (1986). Clarification on Asperger's syndrome. *Journal of Autism and Developmental Disorders, 16*, 513–515.

Yeates, K. O., Bigler, E. D., Dennis, M., Gerhardt, C. A., Rubin, K. H., Stancin, T., et al. (2007). Social outcomes in childhood brain disorder: A heuristic integration of social neuroscience and developmental psychology. *Psychological Bulletin, 133*, 535–556.

Yirmiya, N., Erel, O., Shaked, M., & Solomonica-Levi, D. (1998). Meta-analyses comparing theory of mind abilities of individuals with autism, individuals with mental retardation, and normally developing individuals. *Psychological Bulletin, 124*, 283–307.

Yirmiya, N., Kasari, C., Sigman, M., & Mundy, P. (1989). Facial expressions of affect in autistic, mentally retarded and normal children. *Journal of Child Psychology and Psychiatry, 30*, 725–735.

Yirmiya, N., Pilowsky, T., Solomonica-Levi, D., & Shulman, C. (1999). Brief Report: Gaze behaviour and theory of mind abilities in individuals with autism, Down syndrome, and mental retardation of unknown etiology. *Journal of Autism and Developmental Disorders, 29*(4), 333–341.

Yirmiya, N., Sigman, M. D., Kasari, C., & Mundy, P. (1992). Empathy and cognition in high-functioning children with autism. *Child Development, 63*, 150–160.

Zelazo, P. D., Burack, J. A., Boseovski, J. J., Jacques, S., & Frye, D. (2001). A cognitive complexity and control framework for the study of autism. In J. A. Burack, T. Charman, N. Yirmiya, & P. R. Zelazo (Eds.), *The development of autism: Perspectives from theory and research* (pp. 195–217). Mahwah, NJ: Lawrence Erlbaum Associates.

Zelazo, P. D., & Frye, D. (1997). Cognitive complexity and control: A theory of the development of deliberate reasoning and intentional action. In M. Stamenov (Ed.), *Language structure, discourse, and the access to consciousness*. Amsterdam and Philadelphia: John Benjamins.

Zelazo, P. D., Jacques, S., Burack, J. A., & Frye, D. (2002). The relation between theory of mind and rule use: Evidence from persons with autism-spectrum disorders. *Infant and Child Development, 11*(2), 171–195.

Zeman, J., Cassano, M., Perry-Parrish, C., & Stegall, S. (2006). Emotion regulation in children and adolescents. *Journal of Developmental and Behavioral Pediatrics, 27*, 155–168.

Izard, C. E., Huebner, R. R., Risser, D., McGuinnes, G. C., & Dougherty, L. M. (1980). The young infant's ability to produce discrete emotion expressions. *Developmental psychology, 16*(2), 132–140.

Maestro, S., Muratori, F., Cavallaro, M. C., Pecini, C., Cesari, A., Paziente, A., et al. (2005). How young children treat objects and people? An empirical study of the first year of life in autism. *Child Psychiatry & Human Development, 35*, 383–396.

Developmental Issues and Milestones

Audrey Thurm, Somer Bishop, and Stacy Shumway

Introduction

Autism has been described as a lifelong disorder that emerges in the first year or two of life (Kanner, 1943). Whereas Kanner's longitudinal assessment of his original cohort (Kanner & Eisenberg, 1956) and the few follow-up studies that have been conducted through to adulthood suggest a generally stable diagnosis, recent literature challenges the notion that autism is definitively stable in all individuals diagnosed earlier in life. Prior studies indicate that most individuals diagnosed with autism continue to exhibit symptoms, whether profound or residual, through developmental stages; however, specific information about patterns of symptom change continues to be limited. In part, this is because research focused on examining symptomatology over the life course is inherently impeded by changes in diagnostic methodology, limitations of currently available assessment technology (particularly for older individuals), and other factors that may influence our ability to measure changes in the presentation of autism symptoms over time. This chapter explores the extant literature on symptom presentation across various developmental stages, ranging from onset during infancy, patterns of onset that include developmental regression, preschool through school-age years, and the adolescent/adulthood period. The chapter will focus on autistic disorder, but will consider the fuller spectrum that includes pervasive developmental disorder, not otherwise specified (PDD-NOS) and Asperger syndrome (AS), particularly in the discussion of diagnostic stability. The term autism spectrum disorders (ASD) will be used when collectively referencing this group of disorders.

A striking feature of autism as a disorder (as opposed to delay) is the notion that autism is affected by development at the same time that autism affects development (Lord & Risi, 2000). Autism is affected by development, such that autism symptoms change over time with the influence of various developmental factors. Although information about such changes requires longitudinal study as well as large samples that include a wide age range, prior studies have provided some indications of how developmental factors may influence both core and associated symptoms. Changes that occur with adolescence illustrate this phenomenon of symptoms being affected by development and include initial manifestations of comorbid psychiatric symptoms, such as anxiety and depression (Hutton, Goode, Murphy, Le Couteur, & Rutter, 2008), and increasing risk for seizure onset (Volkmar & Nelson, 1990). As described below, changes in symptom presentation also occur in earlier years. In some areas, such as the emergence of restricted and repetitive behaviors, symptoms may become more pronounced as children develop past age 3 (Cox et al., 1999). In other areas, such as deficits in joint attention, early childhood years may be the peak time of impairment, with gaps closing as children grow older and are explicitly taught or learn these skills.

The ways in which autism affects development are also inherently difficult to investigate. It is thought that the experience of individuals with autism differs from others in such a way that the course of typical development is significantly changed as a result. This notion was recently discussed in terms of the potential for early intervention to be ameliorative, and even preventative, if symptoms are arrested early (Dawson, 2008). Early intervention may provide an "enriching environment" that forces exposure to social stimuli that are often avoided in children with significant social impairments (e.g., lack of social reciprocity and lack of shared enjoyment). In fact, building on the early intervention literature, a recent study found that in very young children, specific intensive therapy can be efficacious in reducing severity of autism symptoms (Dawson et al., 2010). Since it is difficult (and in some ways unethical) to fully control for all aspects of intervention (e.g., intensity/amount/type), information is still quite limited about

A. Thurm (✉)
Pediatrics and Development Neuroscience Branch, National Institute of Mental Health, Bethesda, MD 20892-1255, USA
e-mail: athurm@mail.nih.gov

J.L. Matson, P. Sturmey (eds.), *International Handbook of Autism and Pervasive Developmental Disorders*,
Autism and Child Psychopathology Series, DOI 10.1007/978-1-4419-8065-6_10, © Springer Science+Business Media, LLC 2011

what types of environments, when, and for whom specific enriching experiences most effectively alleviate the specific symptoms of autism (Lord et al., 2005) and shift development toward an optimal trajectory.

Autism also affects development because it *is* a developmental disorder. When compared to other neuropsychiatric disorders, it is one of the earliest developing, oftentimes emerging in infancy, and thus pervasively altering development in its earliest stages. In addition, although other disorders have both "positive" and "negative" symptoms, the "negative" symptoms of autism may actually begin as developmental delays, which later result in deficits when the delays persist. In relation to the symptoms defined as deficits in reciprocal social interaction and communication, for example, it is this delay vs. deficit distinction that is imperative to differentiate in order to make a diagnosis of ASD. Therefore, for the study of how symptoms of autism change over time, one of the main topics of study is not whether overt symptoms abate, but how a lack of skills over a significant amount of time (and possibly over a critical developmental period) affects development in a variety of functional areas.

Stability of Diagnosis

As mentioned above, autism spectrum disorders have traditionally been conceptualized as pervasive, lifelong disorders, and indeed, long-term longitudinal investigations have generally reported high levels of diagnostic stability (Billstedt & Gillberg, 2005; Howlin, Goode, Hutton, & Rutter, 2004; Lord et al., 2006). Stability is lower when the diagnosis is made at very young ages and/or when the initial diagnosis is PDD-NOS as opposed to autism. Recent studies, albeit mostly of children at younger ages, have reported that not even autism diagnoses are 100% stable, with some studies finding the stability of an autism diagnosis range from 68 to 89% (Charman et al., 2005; Chawarska, Klin, Paul, Macari, & Volkmar, 2009; Lord et al., 2006; Turner & Stone, 2007; Turner, Stone, Pozdol, & Coonrod, 2006). These studies have found children moving diagnostically in both directions, such that some children initially diagnosed as more severe (i.e., autism diagnosis) in the early years moved to a less severe diagnosis (i.e., PDD-NOS) or completely off the autism spectrum after a few years, while other children initially diagnosed as non-spectrum were later diagnosed with ASD at follow-up assessment (Chawarska et al., 2009).

Studies of diagnostic stability have typically evaluated children first in the early preschool years (approximately age 2) and followed them to different ages, most often into the early school-age years. Differences in findings across studies likely relate to many factors, such as greater diagnostic instability at the earliest years, particularly under age 3, or varying lengths of time before follow-up and differences in intensity of treatments received across studies. Studies that have monitored children closely over the early preschool through school-age years have also examined *when* change in diagnosis is most likely to occur. Two recent studies followed children from age 2 and found that diagnostic changes are more likely to occur prior to age 5 than after age 5 (Charman et al., 2005; Lord et al., 2006).

It is important to emphasize that although movement across diagnostic categories does occur, longitudinal studies of children with autism typically report that only very small percentages of individuals show such significant improvement that they move to a diagnostic classification that is not on the autism spectrum. Given the small percentages, it has been difficult to track what is different about this small group of individuals with significant improvement. Literature specifically concerning children whose symptoms improve over time, either through specific interventions or as a group who "recover" or "remit," has recently emerged (Helt et al., 2008). These studies propose that some children may lose their autism diagnosis by failing to meet DSM-IV criteria, with only subtle difficulties in pragmatics distinguishing this "recovered" group from typically developing controls on standardized tests. As reports of cases with such improvement are beginning to emerge in the literature (Granpeesheh, Tarbox, Dixon, Carr, & Herbert, 2009), it will be important to explore both the early symptom patterns and the current neurocognitive and psychiatric profiles of these individuals. Recovery does raise questions about whether some individuals may simply "mature" over time – grow out of an autism diagnosis, even with minimal treatment (Turner & Stone, 2007) – or whether individuals are benefitting from specific treatments or combinations of treatments that are proving effective in treating core symptoms of autism. Cross-sectional and retrospective case reports are informative, but are limited in their ability to determine predictors of optimal outcome. Longitudinal studies following children over time are critical in examining early predictors of the most favorable prognoses.

Although to date we do not have enough data on children who fully "recover" to describe this group's functioning or early features, data from larger prospective, longitudinal studies of children with autism have been used to explore predictors of best outcome (see below). Such studies (many of which are ongoing) of larger samples with smaller time intervals between follow-ups may provide information on how the patterns of symptoms in autism change over time and begin to give clues about predictors and different outcomes. However, full interpretation of this extant literature remains difficult, due to varying definitions of best outcome and even weaker rigor used in assessment methods for evaluation.

Developmental Changes in Specific Symptom Areas

In addition to addressing questions related to broad categorical outcomes (e.g., diagnostic stability), researchers are increasingly recognizing the importance of tracking the development and manifestation of specific symptom areas over time. The following sections explore core symptoms of autism, as well as cognition and adaptive behavior, highlighting findings from studies that have assessed these symptoms at various developmental stages. Though separated for the purposes of this discussion, it may be more appropriate for future studies of ASD symptom development to examine the traditionally separate domains of communication and reciprocal social interaction as one grouping of social communication deficits, consistent with findings from recent factor analyses of measures such as the Autism Diagnostic Observation Schedule (Gotham, Risi, Pickles, & Lord, 2007), as well as proposals for revised diagnostic criteria.

Communication

Communication deficits in autism have been studied quite extensively, with literature devoted to detailed descriptions of specific communication deficits seen in ASD compared to other developmental problems, delineation of early markers for predicting outcome, and the study of how communication deficits evolve over time. Although the pattern of communication and language development is quite variable across individuals with autism, early life symptoms in communication (particularly language delay) are very commonly brought to the attention of professionals as a first concern during the child's second year of life (Coonrod & Stone, 2004). There is great variability in the course of communication and language development in autism, though communication impairments are generally present early on, persist into adolescence and beyond, and likely influence development in other areas.

Much of the research on communication impairments in autism has been devoted to the development of spoken language (often defined as functional speech), possibly due to the relative ease with which this can be assessed. Other early delays in nonverbal communication, such as decreased use of gestures (e.g., pointing), basic requesting behaviors, and joint attention skills, have also been studied extensively in young children. Findings from these studies have highlighted the importance of early communication skills as diagnostic markers of ASD and as predictors of communication and language development, particularly in the case of joint attention (Charman et al., 2003; Mundy, Sigman, & Kasari, 1990; Sigman & Ruskin, 1999b). The following sections discuss spoken language in ASD, as well as joint attention and other specific (mostly nonverbal) communicative behaviors in terms of their impact on later autism symptoms.

Spoken Language

The language skills of individuals with ASD vary greatly, ranging from no productive expressive language to verbal fluency. In addition, there appears to be even greater variability in the growth patterns of speech development over time. Early studies of spoken language indicated that approximately half of individuals with autism "were without useful speech" even by adolescence (Rutter, Greenfield, & Lockyer, 1967). "Functional language" has been defined in a variety of ways. Based on a definition that includes use of at least some single words, one recent study found that approximately 80–90% of individuals with autism develop some functional speech by age 9 (Turner et al., 2006). A different longitudinal investigation of children from 2 to 9 years of age reported that by age 9, 28.6% of individuals with autism did not yet spontaneously use words on a consistent basis, 23.8% were speaking with single words but not in spontaneous and meaningful phrases, 23.8% were speaking in phrases/short sentences but were not considered fluent, and 23.8% were verbally fluent (Anderson et al., 2007).

Longitudinal investigations have found that the presence of spoken language skills by age 5 is pivotal in differentiating individuals with more positive outcomes (Billstedt & Gillberg, 2005; Howlin et al., 2004; Szatmari, Bryson, Boyle, Streiner, & Duku, 2003; Venter, Lord, & Schopler, 1992). A recent study of a large sample of children with autism followed from age 2 to 5 indicated that nonverbal cognitive ability at age 2 was the strongest predictor of language at age 5. At age 3, communication scores (from the Vineland Adaptive Behavior Scales) were a stronger predictor of language at 5 years (Thurm, Lord, Lee, & Newschaffer, 2007). A further longitudinal follow-up of the same sample at 9 years of age revealed similar trends. While outcomes in verbal abilities were more variable in children with autism compared to children with PDD-NOS or non-spectrum developmental delays, age 2 variables of nonverbal cognitive ability and joint attention were found to predict language outcome (Anderson et al., 2007).

Type and degree of language impairment itself may vary over time in autism. Some verbal children with ASD show similar skill levels to typically developing children in specific language areas, such as grammar and vocabulary development. On the other hand, there appears to be a group of individuals with autism who have a specific language impairment evident even when language does develop (Kjelgaard & Tager-Flusberg, 2001). Because some children with autism who exhibit early language delays may "catch up" over time, a reliable diagnosis of a separate language disorder may not be possible until the child reaches school age. Studies have shown that among individuals with high-functioning autism and AS, a child's later grammatical language abilities (specific language impairment) between 6 and 8 years may be more predictive of later outcome in adaptive functioning and autism symptoms than early language delay (as measured by retrospective recall of language milestones) or structural language at 4–6 years of age (Bennett et al., 2008). Thus, early variation in language abilities may not become stable impairment until school age, making it difficult to separate out this "specific language impairment" group in preschool years.

Nonverbal Communication and Joint Attention

Deficits in aspects of nonverbal communication, such as gesture use and joint attention, have been identified as early indicators of ASD. In addition to being diagnostic markers, many of these early social communication skills are associated with both concurrent and later language development (Carpenter, Nagell, Tomasello, Butterworth, & Moore, 1998; Charman et al., 2003; Dawson et al., 2004; Mundy et al., 1990; Sigman & McGovern, 2005; Sigman & Ruskin, 1999a).

From a diagnostic perspective, impairments in joint attention are arguably one of the most noticeable areas of deficit in young children with ASD. By the end of the first year of life, typically developing children communicate to express several intentions (Bruner, 1981), ranging from a less social intention of behavior regulation (regulating another person's behavior to obtain a specific result, such as requesting and protesting) to the very social communicative intention of joint attention (directing another's attention to objects and events for the purpose of sharing interest, such as commenting). Joint attention behaviors typically emerge between 9 and 15 months of age (Carpenter et al., 1998; Siller & Sigman, 2008) as infants are becoming intentional communicators. During this time, infants begin to follow the direction of others' gaze (respond to bids for joint attention), alternate gaze between an object and a person, and use communicative means, such as pointing and showing, to draw others' attention to objects and events to share interest. Researchers have long affirmed the theory that joint attention provides for the development of language (Carpenter et al., 1998; Siller & Sigman, 2008).

Children with autism exhibit abnormalities in numerous joint attention behaviors (Tager-Flusberg et al., 2009; Werner & Dawson, 2005). Signs and symptoms of ASD are often becoming apparent around the same time that joint attention skills would be expected to emerge in typical development. Deficits in a variety of joint attention behaviors are often apparent in children later diagnosed with ASD long

before a diagnosis is formally made. For example, deficits in declarative pointing have been observed in children as young as 12 months of age who were later diagnosed with ASD (Werner, Dawson, Munson, & Osterling, 2005). In addition, joint attention abnormalities have been shown to persist over time in children with ASD, with preschool-age and older children showing continued difficulty in this area (Dawson et al., 2004; Mundy, Sigman, & Kasari, 1994; Sigman & Ruskin, 1999a).

As a predictor of communication and language development among children with ASD, results have consistently revealed a strong relationship between joint attention behaviors and both concurrent and later communication and language development (Anderson et al., 2007; Charman et al., 2003; Dawson et al., 2004; Mundy et al., 1990; Wetherby, Prizant, & Hutchinson, 1998). Mundy and colleagues (1990) found that measures of gestural joint attention (e.g., showing, pointing to direct attention) at initial testing significantly predicted language development 1 year later for preschool children with ASD, while nonverbal communication measures, initial language scores, mental age, chronological age, and IQ did not emerge as significant predictors. These findings were further substantiated in a larger follow-up study examining the communicative behaviors and language skills of more than 50 children with ASD between 10 and 13 years of age (Sigman & Ruskin, 1999b). Response to others' bids for joint attention has also been found to be a positive predictor of language development, with preschoolers with autism who responded more frequently showing better language at 9 and 15 years of age (Sigman & McGovern, 2005; Sigman & Ruskin, 1999b). In another study, Charman and colleagues (2003) found that measures of joint attention at 20 months of age predicted language outcomes at 42 months in a sample of 18 children with autism. Overall, findings from these longitudinal studies suggest that whereas the specific nature of joint attention difficulties may change over time, deficits in joint attention manifest early in development in children with ASD, with effects of these deficits evident through adolescence and impacting social communication and language development over time (Mundy et al., 1990; Sigman & Ruskin, 1999b).

In addition to joint attention, other aspects of communication have been found to be important concurrent and predictive correlates of verbal and nonverbal development as well as social impairments of ASD. For instance, rate of communication (acts/bids directed toward another person for a communicative purpose such as requesting or commenting) in children with ASD between 18 and 24 months of age has been shown to be concurrently associated with many other social communication skills (e.g., gestures, shared positive affect, gaze shifts). In these same children, rate of communication was found to predict age 3 nonverbal cognitive level and communication symptoms of autism (Wetherby, Watt,

Morgan, & Shumway, 2007). Furthermore, rate of communication late in the second year was recently found to be the strongest predictor of verbal and nonverbal outcome at 3 years of age in a group of children with ASD (Shumway & Wetherby, 2009). Charman et al. (2005) reported that communicative rate in children with ASD at age 2 was significantly associated with outcome in several domains at age 7. In contrast, scores on standard measures of cognitive and language ability (such as adaptive behavior and functioning as reported on the ADI-R) collected at age 2 did not predict outcome at age 7, though scores on these measures were found to be predictive by age 3 (Charman et al., 2005). Charman and colleagues (2005) concluded that assessing early social communication skills, such as communicative acts, may be just as important, if not more important at very early ages, as measuring IQ and formal language abilities in young children with ASD.

Social Impairment

Despite being the defining feature of ASD, few longitudinal studies have directly addressed how deficits in reciprocal social interaction manifest and change over time. This is likely due to the difficulty the field has in defining and measuring social behavior at different developmental stages. For example, participating in peek-a-boo may be an important measure of social skill in a very young child, but this skill has less relevance for an older school-aged child or adolescent. Thus, limited by a reliance on existing measurements, literature in this area has only described changes in "social symptoms" on a fairly general level and has not provided detailed information about how social impairments evolve over time in individuals with ASD.

Previous longitudinal studies have used scores on parent report measures such as the socialization domain of the Vineland Adaptive Behavior Scales (Sparrow, Balla, & Cicchetti, 1984) or the Autism Diagnostic Interview-Revised (Lord, Rutter, & Le Couteur, 1994) to assess changes in social behavior over time. A recent study followed children from 2 to 13 years of age and found that age 2 nonverbal cognitive ability (along with socialization scores at age 2) was a significant predictor of reports of socialization abilities at age 13 (Anderson, Oti, Lord, & Welch, 2009). However, the study also found wide variability in the growth of socialization abilities, with some children with autism developing socialization abilities at a rate as high as (or higher than) would be expected in typically developing children. In a slightly older sample at the first study time point (age 5), factors such as speech before age 5, gender, and comorbid medical disorder (including epilepsy), as well as cognitive ability, were found to predict social deficits as measured on a parent interview, the Diagnostic Interview for Social and

Communication Disorders (DISCO; Billstedt, Gillberg, & Gillberg, 2007). In a study that followed individuals ranging from 10 to 52 years of age over a 4-year period, parent-reported social symptoms on the ADI-R tended to generally abate over time (Shattuck et al., 2007). Taken together, these findings indicate the potential for varying outcomes in social deficits in children with autism as they grow older and indicate the need to identify more specific predictors (beyond cognitive ability and language) that could be targeted in interventions to improve social functioning.

Because "social impairment" involves different behaviors at different points in development, it has been challenging to identify instruments that provide meaningful, quantitative measures of social abnormality for individuals of varying ages and ability levels. In response to this, a new method for approximating severity of ASD symptoms based on scores on the Autism Diagnostic Observation Schedule (Lord et al., 2000) has recently been developed (Gotham, Pickles, & Lord, 2009). The ADOS, designed as a diagnostic assessment tool, did not originally provide severity ratings. It was not standardized to differentiate between scores above (or below) the determined cutoff scores. In addition, different modules (administered according to an individual's language level) included discrepant numbers and types of items, limiting comparability across individuals. More recently developed algorithms that are standardized by language level and age allow for greater comparability of scores, both above and below cutoffs (Gotham et al., 2007). Individuals with differing language levels can now be compared with respect to a social communication domain. This also allows for longitudinal comparisons within and across individuals, even if language level (and thus module administered) changes over time.

Recent efforts to modify existing assessment tools (Gotham et al., 2009, 2007), as well as to create continuous measures of social behavior that can be administered to individuals across a wide range of ages (Constantino et al., 2004), enhance our ability to conduct longitudinal investigations of social behavior. However, there remains a critical need to develop new tools that will adequately capture the range of social strengths and deficits that are most relevant to individuals at different stages of development. These measures can then be employed as meaningful measures of social outcomes for individuals with ASD.

Restricted Interests and Repetitive Behaviors

Restricted interests and repetitive behaviors (RRBs) are often conceptualized as "positive" symptoms, as opposed to "negative" symptoms characteristic of the social and communication domains. RRBs are, therefore, arguably less difficult to assess, compared to social and communication deficits, because their mere presence can be considered abnormal. However, study of these symptoms over time has been limited by assessment techniques, with challenges in how best to capture these behaviors observationally in a short time period and how to differentiate ASD-specific RRBs from those that occur in non-spectrum disorders and in typically developing young children (Richler, Bishop, Kleinke, & Lord, 2007).

Whereas earlier studies found that RRBs were less apparent than social communication deficits in 2- and 3-year-old children (Cox et al., 1999; Lord, 1995), recent research using more finely tuned observational methods of assessment (as opposed to parent report) has reported the presence of RRBs in children with ASD as young as 12–18 months (Morgan, Wetherby, & Barber, 2008; Zwaigenbaum et al., 2005). In fact, the presence of RRBs between 18 and 24 months of age was found to be predictive of both RRBs and social deficits of autism in the same children at age 3, indicating that early repetitive behaviors may be predictive of more global autism symptoms over time (Morgan et al., 2008). In young children with ASD, repetitive sensory-motor (RSM) behaviors, such as motor mannerisms, repetitive use of objects, and unusual sensory interests, have been found to be more common than insistence on sameness (IS) behaviors, such as compulsions/rituals and resistance to change (Richler et al., 2007). These findings highlight the importance of examining different types of RRBs in investigations of how repetitive behavior emerges and changes over the course of development in individuals with ASD.

Although RSM behaviors appear to be less prevalent in older school-age children with ASD, particularly those with higher cognitive abilities, IS behaviors may actually be more common in these individuals (Bishop, Richler, & Lord, 2006). In one of the only longitudinal studies of RRB trajectories in children with ASD, Richler, Huerta, Bishop, and Lord (2010) used growth curve modeling to show that IS behaviors become more prevalent and severe in children with ASD between the ages of 2 and 9 years. This study also found that nonverbal IQ impacted RSM behaviors over time but not IS behavior. Thus, as with the other core domains, it is important to consider how different aspects of these symptoms may "travel" in different patterns throughout developmental stages and how they may be affected by other symptoms and more general cognitive development.

To examine the presence of RRBs in individuals with ASD beyond the preschool and school-age period, a recent cross-sectional study assessed scores on the Repetitive Behavior Scale-Revised (RBS-R; Lam & Aman, 2007) in a very large sample of children and adults. Results indicated that the mean RBS-R score for children aged 2–9 years was more than twice as high as those aged 51 and older (Esbensen, Seltzer, Lam, & Bodfish, 2009). Clearly, it will be important for future research to more carefully pinpoint the developmental periods during which certain types of RRBs are most

or least prevalent in individuals with ASD and in individuals with other types of developmental disabilities.

Cognition and Adaptive Behavior

Interestingly, relative to the core symptoms of autism, associated problems of cognitive ability and adaptive behavior have generally been studied more extensively over time in individuals with autism, possibly due to more established methods for assessment of these variables. Because of the high prevalence of intellectual disability (typically defined by IQ below 70 with accompanying impairments in adaptive behavior) in autism, researchers have been interested in examining the relationships between cognitive abilities and other features of the ASD phenotype. Epidemiological studies report that approximately 70% of individuals with autism have a comorbid intellectual disability, with level of intellectual disability ranging from mild to profound (Fombonne, 2005). Although IQ is generally held to be a stable trait, there has been considerable interest in examining the stability of IQ scores in children with autism. While studies have varied considerably with respect to tests used, age ranges, and time between reassessments, a recent review of prior studies reported that IQ was quite stable (described by "no change") in 19 out of 23 studies surveyed (Begovac, Begovac, Majic, & Vidovic, 2009).

Several questions emerge when considering how to integrate IQ stability into the broader concept of developmental changes in autism. One question is whether differences in how IQ is measured from preschool to school age may affect IQ scores (in autism and in general) and how these measurement issues may be impacted by both development and autism symptoms (Rapin, 2003). Another question concerns interrelatedness of cognitive and other deficits in autism. Since IQ is often used as a predictor and/or outcome in longitudinal studies, the stability of IQ scores as they relate to core symptom severity is an important avenue for exploration. In other words, do symptoms change differently in individuals with ASD who have significant IQ changes during childhood? Finally, with increased availability of early intervention, it will be important to determine what types/aspects/intensity of intervention increase cognitive abilities and, further, how increases in cognitive abilities affect symptoms of autism and vice versa.

The relationship between cognitive ability and adaptive behavior is also of interest, as adaptive behavior assessment is an important part of the diagnostic evaluation for intellectual disability and therefore important in differential diagnosis and assessment of individuals with ASD (Tomanik, Pearson, Loveland, Lane, & Bryant Shaw, 2007). Findings from a recent cross-sectional study that primarily included a preschool sample suggest that when standard scores are used, adaptive behavior scores tend to decline as young children reach school age (Perry, Flanagan, Dunn Geier, & Freeman, 2009). Whereas age equivalent scores increased with age, the rate of growth was much slower than expected, giving rise to lower standard scores in the older children. In addition, this study found that adaptive behavior scores tended to be lower than cognitive ability in children with higher cognitive abilities, suggesting that even higher functioning children with ASD do not exhibit adaptive skills commensurate with their intellectual abilities.

Studies have also investigated the predictive utility of cognitive factors in determining adaptive behavior outcomes. A recent study included nonverbal cognitive ability and several specific neurocognitive measures, including tasks of learning and reward associations, memory and novelty preference, and spatial working memory in children aged 3–4. Findings suggested that in addition to nonverbal cognitive ability, both learning and reward associations and memory and novelty preference had unique contributions to later growth in socialization (Munson, Faja, Meltzoff, Abbott, & Dawson, 2008). Learning and reward associations also had a unique contribution to communication behavior. These findings underscore the complex neuropsychological deficits in autism and their interplay with core features over time.

Autism Symptom Patterns by Developmental Stages

The first section of this chapter explored how symptoms of autism may change over time within various domains of deficit or across domains as part of a total diagnostic picture. In the next section, we discuss the extant literature as it relates to symptom patterns at different periods of development. We begin with infancy and toddlerhood, with a focus on differentiating key onset patterns of autism compared to other developmental delays. We then focus on the presentation of symptoms during school-age years, adolescence and adulthood, including a discussion of findings from studies that have followed children from early development of autism through these transitions.

Symptom Patterns in Early Life Course

Evidence continues to grow that symptom onset in autism often occurs before age 2 (Coonrod & Stone, 2004; Short & Schopler, 1988), but the age of first diagnosis has not been reduced accordingly. Most recent reports still estimate that the majority of children are diagnosed after 3 years of age (CDC, 2009). Reasons for the difference between reported concern and diagnosis are not completely known.

As indicated by retrospective analyses of home videotapes (Baranek, 1999; Werner, Dawson, Osterling, & Dinno, 2000), as well as more recently by studies of parent report (Ozonoff et al., 2009) and even observational data (Young, Merin, Rogers, & Ozonoff, 2009; Zwaigenbaum et al., 2009, 2005), symptoms of autism are present in some children by the age of 12 months. However, several groups have now confirmed that by looking at both standardized cognitive and language measures, as well as more subtle measures of affect and social reciprocity between both infant and mother, and infant and examiner, no clear differences are apparent between 6 month infants (siblings) who later develop autism and infant siblings who later appear to be developing in a typical trajectory (Ozonoff et al., 2009; Young et al., 2009; Zwaigenbaum et al., 2005). Study of infant siblings of children with autism has been critical in developing this understanding of very early symptom-onset patterns. Overall, research on early identification indicates that given more developmentally appropriate assessment tools, risk, if not diagnosis, can be established before the age of 2 in at least some children. However, it also indicates that at least in terms of behavioral assessment, early detection of symptom onset may not be possible before the age of 12 months.

One reason for lagging diagnosis (as compared to first concern and even observable symptoms) may be the nature of the symptoms in infancy/early toddlerhood. Significant early markers of ASD include language delay (without compensation through other means of communication), as well as deficient skills in joint attention, imitation, and social–emotional reciprocity (e.g., lack of response to name, showing, and sharing enjoyment). Literature on the presence of RRBs indicates that, while not absent in infancy/early toddlerhood, these behaviors may show a more subtle onset and/or emerge later than social communication. Several studies have found that RRB symptoms become more significant closer to the age of 3 years (Lord, 1995; Moore & Goodson, 2003; Stone et al., 1999), though some retrospective analyses of videotapes have shown repetitive behavior/restricted interests to be present in children as young as 12 months (Baranek, 1999; Werner et al., 2005), with prospective observations confirming their presence as young as 18 months (Morgan et al., 2008; Watt, Wetherby, Barber, & Morgan, 2008; Wetherby et al., 2004).

The symptoms of autism that are present in children younger than age 2 are often quite variable and can be difficult to distinguish from variations in typical development. This is especially the case for RRBs. Recent literature in typical development has indicated that certain types of repetitive behaviors are seen in typically developing children around the age of 2 (Leekam et al., 2007; Richler et al., 2007). However, whereas typically developing children appear to "grow out" of these behaviors, RRBs in children with autism may begin to impact functional play skills (and ultimately language), thus differentiating them from the behaviors characteristic of more typical development (Honey, Leekam, Turner, & McConachie, 2007).

Another reason why autism diagnoses may not be possible in all children before the age of 2 relates to the complexity of symptom onset. Presentation of autism onset appears to differ widely across children. Previously, two onset patterns were described: "early onset" of symptoms, in which abnormalities were apparent early in life, and regressive autism, in which a loss of previously acquired skills was observed following a period of typical development (Ozonoff, Williams, & Landa, 2005). This dichotomous conceptualization of onset is outdated, with more recent research suggesting a complex pattern of symptom onset, with the possibility of autism emerging in many ways. For example, four broad groupings have been proposed that include the traditional early onset and regressive autism, but expand the groupings to include the addition of two intermediate-onset groups with mixed features of early onset and regressive autism (Ozonoff, Heung, Byrd, Hansen, & Hertz-Picciotto, 2008). Early onset of symptoms, in which a child shows symptoms somewhere between the first few months of life and the second year of life, with no loss of skills, has been reported to occur in the majority of children with autism.

The frequency of the traditional conceptualization of regressive autism, in which a loss of skills (usually communication or social skills) occurs following a period of typical development, has been difficult to ascertain given the many different methods, instruments, and definitions of skill loss that have been used to study this phenomenon. Studies vary widely in the percentage of children who follow the trajectory of having obtained certain social and/or communication skills and then subsequently lose them, leading to the onset of autism. Prevalence estimates for this pattern of onset range between 15 and 40% of children with autism, with the mean age of loss differing across studies, but most commonly ranging from 16 to 24 months (Davidovitch, Glick, Holtzman, Tirosh, & Safir, 2000; Goldberg et al., 2003; Luyster et al., 2005; Richler et al., 2006).

Variability in the reported prevalence of regression is likely due to differences in the definition of regression across studies. In much of the literature, regression has been conceptualized as a language loss only (see Ozonoff et al., 2008 for a review), without regard to loss of other communication or social skills. More recently, research has indicated that a loss of words alone occurs relatively infrequently, and that most children with a reported spoken language loss also lose other communication and social skills. Thus, recent studies have used an expanded definition of regression that includes loss of both spoken language and other social communication skills. Furthermore, examination of development prior to regression has indicated that even among children who are reported to regress, most show some delays prior to the

loss of skills, suggesting the need to expand a dichotomous categorization of regression/no regression into a more comprehensive conceptualization of symptom-onset patterns. An additional consideration regarding these patterns is the idea that at least some children may not lose skills at all, but instead show a plateau or slowing of progress in some developmental areas (Luyster et al., 2005; Ozonoff et al., 2005). Infant sibling studies have reported drastic reductions in developmental progress, as indicated by standardized measures of developmental level (serving as proxies for cognitive functioning) and language, often beginning to decline at approximately 12 months and continue declining through the second year of life (Rogers, 2009). Thus, young children with ASD may also show a different developmental trajectory compared to children with other delays and typical development, with a broadening developmental delay and a deceleration of cognitive growth observed across the second year (Landa & Garrett-Mayer, 2006). These findings indicate that the second year of life may be a critical time to examine when and how development goes awry in children with ASD.

Infant sibling studies evaluating children in the first and second year of life have also included measures of so-called associated symptoms, including temperament, early signs of other psychopathology, irritability, sensory reactivity, and motor problems. These studies have reported that clinically significant impairments in non-core symptoms are coming online at approximately the same time as the onset of autism-specific symptoms. This more global pattern symptom onset raises questions about whether certain associated features may actually be core aspects of ASD in very young children (Rogers, 2009). Continued follow-up of these infant sibling samples will be necessary to determine if these features that appear to travel with core autism symptoms from the onset of the disorder are stable in the same way as core features or if they vary according to progress made in social communication, repetitive behavior, or other factors such as cognitive ability.

Symptom Patterns in School-Age Children

In the school-age period, symptoms may express themselves at their peak, as the deficits (particularly in communication) become evident as impairments rather than delays and compensatory strategies are often not yet in place. Many cross-sectional studies have included school-age populations to examine specific aspects of autism; however, compared to studies of children with other developmental disorders or typical development, relatively little prospective research has been conducted to longitudinally evaluate developmental course of symptoms or associated problems in school-age children.

More and more studies of young children are showing that significant improvement in symptoms and associated problems occur in some children with ASD, particularly with early intervention. A critical question is whether there can still be improvements in skills during the school-age years. When comparing growth in school-age years to that during later adolescence, findings from one of the longest term longitudinal studies indicate that growth in language is greater during school-age years compared to adolescence, and that cognitive ability remains stable during school age but may decline later in adolescence (Sigman & McGovern, 2005). Another longitudinal investigation examined language and cognitive variables as predictors of adaptive behavior in communication and socialization, as well as more direct measures of autism symptoms, in children with autism or AS (Szatmari et al., 2003). While language and cognitive scores predicted communication, socialization, and autism symptoms, early language and cognitive scores were most predictive of communication and least predictive of the direct measure of autism symptoms. A follow-up examination of the developmental trajectories of children with AS found that although children with AS scored higher on most measures compared to those with autism or PDD-NOS, the *pattern* was the same in both groups for trajectories of communication and socialization scores from age 4–6 through adolescence, such that standard scores increased, but rate of growth slowed down considerably by late adolescence (Szatmari et al., 2009). Taken together, findings from these few longitudinal studies indicate that while growth in skills appears to slow as children move into adolescence, children with ASD may still make considerable progress in at least language and cognitive skills during the school-age years.

As indicated elsewhere in this book, individuals with ASD may present with comorbid psychopathology, including symptoms of affective disorders, hyperactivity, and aggression. Studies investigating comorbidity have generally included the school-age population and upward, although a recent study investigating younger children reported high rates of comorbid psychopathology even in preschoolers (Gadow, DeVincent, Pomeroy, & Azizian, 2004). In school-age children, studies are now beginning to explore whether subgroups of children with ASD are prone to higher rates of comorbidity, with some indication that children with autism (compared to PDD-NOS) have higher rates of several significant comorbid symptoms such as depression and atypical behavior/psychosis (Pearson et al., 2006). Studies are also beginning to explore predictors of associated symptoms during school age. Although the literature is not completely consistent, higher intellectual functioning at earlier ages (defined by higher IQ scores) is generally associated with later internalizing symptoms (e.g., depression, anxiety), whereas lower intellectual functioning at earlier ages is generally associated with externalizing behaviors (e.g., challenging behaviors that affect others, such as aggression, irritability, hyperactivity) (Estes, Dawson, Sterling, & Munson, 2007).

Symptom Patterns in Adolescence/Adulthood

Adolescents and adults with ASD have received relatively little attention in the literature compared to school-age children and, more recently, infants and toddlers. Very few large-scale longitudinal studies have followed children with autism into adulthood (Gillberg & Steffenburg, 1987; Howlin et al., 2004; Sigman & McGovern, 2005) As shown in Table 10.1, while these studies were quite detailed in variables that included cognitive, social and adaptive functioning, they were lacking in quantitative measurements of autism symptom domains. Thus, information is still limited with respect to if and how variability in core features of autism predict or are concurrently associated with various adult outcomes. Studies that include larger samples and more in-depth evaluations of ASD-related features are required to report on how different aspects of the ASD phenotype, as observed at different points in development, are related to outcomes in adolescence and adulthood.

Beyond the many logistical difficulties in conducting long-term outcome studies of individuals with ASD (e.g., the time and expense required to follow children into adulthood), this type of research presents significant challenges related to identifying and measuring meaningful outcomes. As mentioned earlier in this chapter, many longitudinal studies have used ASD diagnostic status as one measure of outcome. However, little attention has been given to best practice guidelines for assessment of adults with suspected ASD. Because ASD is normally diagnosed during childhood, most empirically derived assessment tools have been designed for and validated with samples of children with ASD. Furthermore, DSM-IV criteria for ASD are based on behavioral observations of school-age samples (Volkmar et al., 1994) and therefore may not adequately capture the range or quality of symptoms typical of adolescents and adults with the disorder. Detailed behavioral studies of older individuals with ASD are needed to develop more age-appropriate assessment tools so that researchers and clinicians are not left to rely on extrapolations of diagnostic tools designed for children.

Studies of adults with ASD have also reported on the presence of comorbid medical conditions (e.g., epilepsy) or psychiatric disorders as a dimension of outcome. Billstedt and Gillberg (2005) found that about half of their sample of 120 adults with ASD had a medical problem that required regular medical attention, though it should be noted that a relatively large percentage of this sample had additional diagnoses of severe intellectual disability (ID) and/or genetic syndromes (e.g., Fragile X syndrome and Williams syndrome) that may

Table 10.1 Longitudinal studies of autism: studies that have followed children through puberty

Authors (year)	Study population	Variables studied over time	Main findings	Early predictors of outcome (+/−)
Gillberg and Steffenberg (1987)	$N = 23$ (Infantile autism group) age>16; $N = 23$ (Other childhood psychoses) age = 16–23	IQ, epilepsy, psychiatric symptoms, medication use, social style (Wing, 1983), chromosomal abnormalities	Puberty associated with increase in behavior problems, psychiatric symptoms, and seizures	IQ >50 (+) Communicative speech before age 6 (+) Epilepsy diagnosis (−) "Aloof" social style (−)
Venter, Lord, and Schopler (1992)	$N = 58$, higher functioning individuals (IQ>60) diagnosed with autism during preschool and early school years followed over 8 years (average age at follow-up = 14)	NVIQ, language comprehension, social adaptive behavior, academic achievement	Verbal skills strongest predictor of social-adaptive functioning; positive relationships between IQ and academic success	Higher NVIQ (+) Higher VIQ (+) Speech before 5 years (+) More severe parent-reported RRBs (−)
Howlin et al. (2004)	$N = 69$, individuals diagnosed with autism, seen before age 16 and after age 21, minimum IQ >50	IQ, autism symptoms (ADI), employment, friendships, residential placement	Majority were classified as having "Poor" or "Very Poor outcome"	Combination NVIQ and VIQ >70 (+)
Billstedt, I.C. Gillberg, and C. Gillberg (2005)	$N = 120$, individuals with autism followed from childhood to adulthood	Employment, higher education/vocational training, independent living, and peer relations	4/120 lived independent (isolated) lives	Higher IQ (+) Phrase speech by age 6 (+)
Sigman and McGovern (2005)	$N = 48$, individuals diagnosed with autism during early childhood (mean age at follow-up = 19 years)	Nonverbal communication skills, language, and cognitive abilities	Cognitive and language skills tended to remain stable or decline. Gains in mental age were far less than changes in chronological age	Functional play skills (+) Responsiveness to others' bids for joint attention (+) Frequency of requesting behaviors (+)

have led to an unusually high number of medical problems in this group. Matson and colleagues (2010) found that among 377 adults, those with ASD and comorbid psychopathology exhibited the lowest scores on the Vineland Adaptive Behavior Scales (Sparrow et al., 1984). Esbensen, Bishop, Seltzer, Greenberg, and Taylor (2010) found that over 60% of a community sample of adults with ASD were receiving psychological or psychiatric services compared to only 19% of adults with Down syndrome (DS), and that receipt of psychological and psychiatric services related to overall independence among adults with ASD. Studies of psychiatric comorbidity in adults with ASD have not generally looked closely at early life predictors (besides IQ) of comorbid diagnoses. Particularly with respect to different characteristics of the ASD phenotype (e.g., presence of insistence on sameness behaviors and children who are "aloof" vs. "active but odd"), it is not yet understood whether certain individuals are more likely to develop depression or other psychiatric problems as adolescents and adults.

Similar measurement problems exist when assessing comorbidity as when evaluating ASD in these adults, because many diagnostic tools are not appropriate and/or have not been normed for use in individuals with developmental disabilities. Assessment of adult psychopathology often relies heavily on self-report of symptoms, for example. But given that many adults with ASD have cognitive impairments that impede their ability to comprehend traditional self-report measures, and that lack of insight is one of the characteristics associated with ASD, self-report may not always be the most effective means of assessing the presence or absence of symptoms in this population. More research is needed to determine the most valid methods of collecting information about adults with ASD, both for the purposes of ASD diagnostic assessment and for the identification of comorbid psychopathology. In terms of self-report, adults with ASD have a perspective that is worth considering in assessment and treatment, and for some individuals with ASD, the internal experience of the disorder may be quite different from another person's external perspective. Moving beyond generalizations about ASD and considering that some individuals may have higher levels of social motivation than their behavior would suggest, for example, has implications for how ASD is conceptualized as a disorder. Collecting information directly from individuals who are diagnosed with ASD, rather than relying solely on the ability of professionals to accurately "translate" behaviors, may also inform efforts to identify the underlying causes of certain behaviors.

In addition to diagnostic status of ASD or comorbid psychopathology, traditional measures of outcome include employment, number of close personal relationships, and other factors considered to be markers of adult independence. Howlin et al. (2004) conducted a seminal study of 68 adults who were initially diagnosed with ASD at an average age of 7 years. Based on combined information about the participants' current employment, friendships (as measured by the ADI-R friendship item), and residential placement, 12% were rated as having a "Very Good" overall social outcome (i.e., paid employment, some friends, high level of residential independence), whereas more than half of the participants were rated as having "Poor" or "Very Poor" outcomes. Though higher IQ in childhood (i.e., nonverbal IQ score > 70) was associated with better adult outcomes, verbal and nonverbal IQ scores were not reliable predictors of outcome within the higher functioning individuals. That is, low IQ was found to be more meaningful as a predictor of poor outcome than high IQ predicting a good outcome. Given that more recent studies are following children who were assessed at ages younger than 7 years, it will be interesting to examine whether, and at what ages, verbal or nonverbal abilities in these children become predictive of various aspects of adolescent and adult outcome.

Work by Howlin and others has been influential in identifying certain areas in which many adults with ASD have difficulty. However, measures of "good" or "poor" outcome are defined on the basis of relatively broad and subjective criteria that may be difficult to operationalize or assess for certain individuals. It will be important for future research to move beyond categorical designations to capture the full range of possible outcomes in this population and to identify meaningful constructs that can be more feasibly predicted by factors other than IQ. Certain types of competitive employment or independent living situations may only be realistically attainable by a very small subset of high-functioning adults with ASD, whereas other dimensions of adult success such as friendship/relationship quality, employment satisfaction, or general life satisfaction may exhibit much more variability. Developing continuous measures of life quality for individuals with ASD may prove very useful in identifying new ways of defining outcome that are more predictable and ultimately more susceptible to the effects of intervention and social supports at different points in development.

Some studies have attempted to describe large samples of adolescents and adults with ASD, but they have relied primarily on parent reports of symptoms that may or may not be relevant to individuals past the childhood years. Kobayashi and Murata (2003) used the Child Behavior Checklist (CBCL; Achenbach, 1991; Achenbach & Edelbrock, 1983) to describe the behavioral characteristics of 187 adults with autism and reported a high frequency of obsessive and perfectionist behaviors across adults with varying degrees of language abilities. Seltzer and colleagues have used the ADI-R and other parent report measures to assess the behavioral presentation of 405 individuals with community diagnoses of ASD who were between 10 and 53 years at the initial assessment. These reports have provided important information about the types of symptoms that parents most commonly observe in their adolescent and adult children with ASD (Seltzer, Shattuck, Abbeduto, & Greenberg, 2004) and have been informative about showing that there is a continued trajectory of symptom abatement even after adolescence (Shattuck et al., 2007). However, because of the reliance on the ADI-R, which is a parent report instrument designed to gather information about symptoms that are thought to be most prevalent during the 4- to 5-year-old period, the descriptions do not offer much information about adolescent and adult behavioral phenotypes. What are the behaviors that are most problematic or impairing for adolescents with ASD? How do these older individuals present in face-to-face interactions? Future research in this area must move us beyond surface-level descriptions in order to identify characteristics of adolescents and adults with ASD that can serve as concurrent predictors of outcome or as alternative outcome measures in their own right.

Comparative studies of adults with ASD will also be informative in determining what characteristics are specific to ASD in adulthood and what features are common across developmental disorders. Though these types of studies have been commonly undertaken in children, there is strikingly little comparative work for adults. Esbensen and colleagues (2010) recently conducted a comparison of 70 adults with ASD and intellectual disability and 70 age-matched adults with Down syndrome (DS). Consistent with comparisons of children with ASD vs. children with DS, adults with ASD generally had less good outcomes than those with DS. Only one-third of adults with ASD were rated as having a moderate or high level of independence in adult life, compared to almost two-thirds of adults with DS. Adults with ASD were living in less independent residential settings and had less contact with friends and neighbors compared to adults with DS, though the two groups were comparable on measures of vocational independence. Adults with ASD were also more impaired in their ability to carry out typical tasks of daily living, had poorer literacy skills, exhibited more behavior problems, received fewer services, and had more unmet service needs than adults with DS. The authors suggest that the gap between individuals with ASD and DS persists into adulthood, and that the pattern of behavior problem and symptom abatement observed in adults with ASD (Shattuck et al., 2007) is not so prominent as to overcome existing group differences with adults with DS.

To identify meaningful measures of outcome for adults with ASD, research must delve more deeply into the behavioral characteristics of adults with ASD. We are in need of descriptions that provide more information about what adults with ASD *look* like – not only with reference to childhood diagnostic criteria, but from the perspective of their presentation *as* adults. Just as many researchers who study children with depression or other traditionally "adult disorders" have argued that children with these disorders must be studied and conceptualized differently than their adult counterparts (Kaufman, Martin, King, & Charney, 2001), ASD researchers must make more concerted efforts to consider adolescents and adults with ASD as more than just older, larger versions of children with ASD.

Methodological Limitations of Studies Looking at Symptom Patterns Over Time

Most of the literature summarized in this chapter comes from longitudinal studies of children with ASD. Additional longitudinal studies of autism samples with large heterogeneity in symptomatology are critical for understanding predictors of various outcomes, but they may not provide answers to all questions about the nature of how symptoms change over time. Because specific outcomes of interest, such as "optimal outcomes," are infrequent and not found in large numbers from even mid- to large-sized longitudinal investigations, more targeted studies that recruit specifically for such populations may be necessary.

Prospective, longitudinal studies that start with children as young as possible, preferably in early infancy, will allow for the most comprehensive investigation of symptom onset and progression over time, but large-scale study of pre-clinical to symptom-onset presentation is fraught with issues of feasibility, even in "high-risk" populations such as infant sibling studies. While sibling studies yield a high percentage (possibly up to 20%) of individuals diagnosed with an ASD, these samples, in isolation, are not sufficiently large to produce enough statistical power to study inter-relationships among various symptom domains over time. Thus, different types of studies, some prospective and some retrospective, may be necessary to answer remaining questions about how symptom patterns change over time in ASD.

Other limitations of longitudinal investigations need to be considered in relation to specific hypotheses of developmental trajectory studies in autism. For instance, when considering questions about how the *trajectory* of skill development in a particular area (e.g., language) compares with that of other developmental disorders (or typical development), comparison groups may be necessary, although there may be alternate cross-sectional approaches to determining how age affects very specific skill deficits (Thomas et al., 2009). These types of comparative *trajectory* studies are still necessary, because although much literature now contributes significant understanding to how autism differs from other

developmental problems in specific periods of development, there is much to be learned about how specific deficits change over time and compare with disorders that show similar types of deficits. Do children with autism catch up in communication, cognitive ability, or neuropsychological constructs (e.g., theory of mind) as much as children who start out with similar cognitive abilities and do not have autism?

Finally, when re-considering the reciprocal influences of development affecting autism and autism affecting development, the difficult disentanglement of these mutually influencing factors gives rise to the ultimate methodological challenges of understanding *how* deficits at a certain point in time, especially early in development, impact later outcomes in the same or different domains (Burack et al., 2001).

Conclusions and Future Directions

Although the study of developmental changes in autism has been quite limited thus far, from the literature that exists it is apparent that symptoms of autism do change over time. Patterns differ by symptom and developmental stage, and various patterns are likely to be moderated by individual factors such as early intellectual ability and symptom severity.

Issues that need to be disentangled to truly understand the nature of lifelong stability in autism symptoms include (1) how to interpret findings from prior longitudinal studies to current investigations (e.g., changes in diagnostic criteria, access to accurate early diagnosis, and changes in early intervention and treatment strategies); (2) how variability in treatment affects our understanding of symptom change; (3) the impact of co-occurring psychiatric, neurologic, or other medical problems; and (4) the changing nature of autism symptoms themselves. In addition, tools that are more finely tuned to quantitative delineation of symptom presentations within specific developmental periods will be critical in these investigations.

Finally, as is the growing trend in the study of ASD, autism is currently conceptualized as a heterogeneous spectrum with nomenclature that includes a wide spectrum. As such, future studies should likely continue taking the approach that some have begun utilizing in breaking up samples into meaningful phenotypes (subtypes) and endophenotypes, both by severity and types of core and associated symptoms, as well as by other functional differences. Such phenotypes will be useful in determining if there are different patterns or trajectories in the development of specific symptoms or in profiles of symptom clusters over time.

Acknowledgments The views expressed in this chapter do not necessarily represent the views of the NIMH, NIH, HHS, or the United States Government. This chapter was written as part of the first author's official duties as a Federal Government employee. Therefore, it cannot be copyrighted. Government materials are in the public domain and may be reproduced without permission, even when they appear as part of a publication bearing a general copyright notice. (Reference: U.S. Copyright Law, Title 17 of the U.S. Code, Section 105: "Copyright protection under this title is not available for any work of the United States Government prepared by an officer or employee of the United States Government as part of a person's official duties.")

References

Achenbach, T. (1991). *Manual for the child behavior checklist/4-18 and 1991 profile*. Burlington, VT: Department of Psychiatry of the University of Vermont.

Achenbach, T., & Edelbrock, C. (1983). *Manual for the child behavior checklist and revised child behavior profile*. Burlington, VT: Department of Psychiatry of the University of Vermont.

Anderson, D. K., Lord, C., Risi, S., DiLavore, P. S., Shulman, C., Thurm, A., et al. (2007). Patterns of growth in verbal abilities among children with autism spectrum disorder. *Journal of Consulting and Clinical Psychology, 75*, 594–604.

Anderson, D. K., Oti, R. S., Lord, C., & Welch, K. (2009). Patterns of growth in adaptive social abilities among children with autism spectrum disorders. *Journal of Abnormal Child Psychology, 37*, 1019–1034.

Baranek, G. T. (1999). Autism during infancy: A retrospective video analysis of sensory-motor and social behaviors at 9–12 months of age. *Journal of Autism and Developmental Disorders, 29*, 213–224.

Begovac, I., Begovac, B., Majic, G., & Vidovic, V. (2009). Longitudinal studies of IQ stability in children with childhood autism – Literature survey. *Psychiatr Danub, 21*, 310–319.

Bennett, T., Szatmari, P., Bryson, S., Volden, J., Zwaigenbaum, L., Vaccarella, L., et al. (2008). Differentiating autism and Asperger syndrome on the basis of language delay or impairment. *Journal of Autism and Developmental Disorders, 38*, 616–625.

Billstedt, E., & Gillberg, C. (2005). Autism after adolescence: Population-based 13- to 22-year follow-up study of 120 individuals with autism diagnosed in childhood. *Journal of Autism and Developmental Disorders, 35*, 351–360.

Billstedt, E., Gillberg, I. C., & Gillberg, C. (2005). Autism in adults: Symptom patterns and early childhood predictors. Use of the DISCO in a community sample followed from childhood. *Journal of Child Psychology and Psychiatry and Allied Disciplines, 48*, 1102–1110.

Bishop, S., Richler, J., & Lord, C. (2006). Association between restricted and repetitive behaviors and nonverbal IQ in children with autism spectrum disorders. *Child Neuropsychology (Neuropsychology, Development and Cognition: Section C), 12*(4), 247–267.

Bruner, J. (1981). The social context of language acquisition. *Language and Communication, 1*, 155–178.

Burack, J. A., Pasto, L., Poporino, M., Iarocci, G., Mottron, L., & Bowler, D. (2001). Applying developmental principles to the study of autism. In E. Schopler, N. Yirmiya, C. Shulman, & L. M. Marcus (Eds.), *The research basis for autism intervention* (pp. 25–38). New York: Kluwer Academic.

Carpenter, M., Nagell, K., Tomasello, M., Butterworth, G., & Moore, C. (1998). Social cognition, joint attention, and communicative competence from 9 to 15 months of age. *Monographs of the Society for Research in Child Development, 63*.

CDC (2009). Prevalence of autism spectrum disorders – autism and developmental disabilities monitoring network, United States, 2006. *MMWR, 58*, 1–20.

Charman, T., Baron-Cohen, S., Swettenham, J., Baird, G., Drew, A., & Cox, A. (2003). Predicting language outcome in infants with autism and pervasive developmental disorder. *International Journal of Language and Communication Disorders, 38*, 265–285.

Charman, T., Taylor, E., Drew, A., Cockerill, H., Brown, J. A., & Baird, G. (2005). Outcome at 7 years of children diagnosed with autism at age 2: Predictive validity of assessments conducted at 2 and 3 years of age and pattern of symptom change over time. *Journal of Child Psychology and Psychiatry and Allied Disciplines, 46*, 500–513.

Chawarska, K., Klin, A., Paul, R., Macari, S., & Volkmar, F. (2009). A prospective study of toddlers with ASD: Short-term diagnostic and cognitive outcomes. *Journal of Child Psychology and Psychiatry and Allied Disciplines, 50*, 1235–1245.

Constantino, J. N., Gruber, C. P., Davis, S., Hayes, S., Passanante, N., & Przybeck, T. (2004). The factor structure of autistic traits. *Journal of Child Psychology and Psychiatry and Allied Disciplines, 45*, 719–726.

Coonrod, E. E., & Stone, W. L. (2004). Early concerns of parents of children with autistic and nonautistic disorders. *Infants & Young Children, 17*, 258–268.

Cox, A., Klein, K., Charman, T., Baird, G., Baron-Cohen, S., Swettenham, J., et al. (1999). Autism spectrum disorders at 20 and 42 months of age: Stability of clinical and ADI-R diagnosis. *Journal of Child Psychology and Psychiatry and Allied Disciplines, 40*, 719–732.

Davidovitch, M., Glick, L., Holtzman, G., Tirosh, E., & Safir, M. (2000). Developmental regression in autism: Maternal perception. *Journal of Autism and Developmental Disorders, 30*, 113–119.

Dawson, G. (2008). Early behavioral intervention, brain plasticity, and the prevention of autism spectrum disorder. *Development and Psychopathology, 20*, 775–803.

Dawson, G., Rogers, S., Munson, J., Smith, M., Winter, J., Greenson, J., et al. (2010). Randomized, controlled trial of an intervention for toddlers with autism: The early start Denver model. *Pediatrics, 125*, 17–23.

Dawson, G., Toth, K., Abbott, R., Osterling, J., Munson, J., Estes, A., et al. (2004). Early social attention impairments in autism: Social orienting, joint attention, and attention to distress. *Developmental Psychology, 40*, 271–283.

Esbensen, A., Bishop, S., Seltzer, M., Greenberg, J., & Taylor, J. (2010). Comparisons between individuals with autism spectrum disorders and individuals with down syndrome in adulthood. *Intellectual and Developmental Disabilities, 115*, 277–290.

Esbensen, A. J., Seltzer, M. M., Lam, K. S., & Bodfish, J. W. (2009). Age-related differences in restricted repetitive behaviors in autism spectrum disorders. *Journal of Autism and Developmental Disorders, 39*, 57–66.

Estes, A. M., Dawson, G., Sterling, L., & Munson, J. (2007). Level of intellectual functioning predicts patterns of associated symptoms in school-age children with autism spectrum disorder. [Journal; Peer Reviewed Journal]. *American Journal on Mental Retardation, 112*, 439–449.

Fombonne, E. (2005). Epidemiology of autistic disorder and other pervasive developmental disorders. *Journal of Clinical Psychiatry, 66*(Suppl 10), 3–8.

Gadow, K. D., DeVincent, C. J., Pomeroy, J., & Azizian, A. (2004). Psychiatric symptoms in preschool children with PDD and clinic and comparison samples. *Journal of Autism and Developmental Disorders, 34*, 379–393.

Gillberg, C., & Steffenburg, S. (1987). Outcome and prognostic factors in infantile autism and similar conditions: A population-based study of 46 cases followed through puberty. *Journal of Autism and Developmental Disorders, 17*(2), 273–287.

Goldberg, W., Osann, K., Filipek, P., Laulhere, T., Jarvis, K., Modahl, C., et al. (2003). Language and other regression: Assessment and timing. *Journal of Autism and Developmental Disorders, 33,* 607–616.

Gotham, K., Pickles, A., & Lord, C. (2009). Standardizing ADOS scores for a measure of severity in autism spectrum disorders. *Journal of Autism and Developmental Disorders, 39,* 693–705.

Gotham, K., Risi, S., Pickles, A., & Lord, C. (2007). The autism diagnostic observation schedule: Revised algorithms for improved diagnostic validity. *Journal of Autism and Developmental Disorders, 37,* 613–627.

Granpeesheh, D., Tarbox, J., Dixon, D. R., Carr, E., & Herbert, M. (2009). Retrospective analysis of clinical records in 38 cases of recovery from autism. *Annals of Clinical Psychiatry, 21,* 195–204.

Helt, M., Kelley, E., Kinsbourne, M., Pandey, J., Boorstein, H., Herbert, M., et al. (2008). Can children with autism recover? If so, how? *Neuropsychology Review, 18,* 339–366.

Honey, E., Leekam, S., Turner, M., & McConachie, H. (2007). Repetitive behaviour and play in typically developing children and children with autism spectrum disorders. *Journal of Autism and Developmental Disorders, 37,* 1107–1115.

Howlin, P., Goode, S., Hutton, J., & Rutter, M. (2004). Adult outcome for children with autism. *Journal of Child Psychology and Psychiatry and Allied Disciplines, 45,* 212–229.

Hutton, J., Goode, S., Murphy, M., Le Couteur, A., & Rutter, M. (2008). New-onset psychiatric disorders in individuals with autism. *Autism, 12,* 373–390.

Kanner, L. (1943). Autistic disturbances of affective contact. *Nervous Child, 2,* 217–250.

Kanner, L., Eisenberg, L. (1956). Early infantile autism. *American Journal of Orthopsychiatry, 26,* 55–65.

Kaufman, J., Martin, A., King, R. A., & Charney, D. (2001). Are child-, adolescent-, and adult-onset depression one and the same disorder? *Biological Psychiatry, 49,* 980–1001.

Kjelgaard, M., & Tager-Flusberg, H. (2001). An investigation of language impairment in autism: Implications for genetic subgroups. *Language and Cognitive Processes, 16,* 287.

Kobayashi, R., & Murata, T. (2003). Behavioral characteristics of 187 young adults with autism. *Psychiatry and Clinical Neurosciences, 52,* 383–390.

Lam, K. S., & Aman, M. G. (2007). The repetitive behavior scale-revised: Independent validation in individuals with autism spectrum disorders. *Journal of Autism and Developmental Disorders, 37,* 855–866.

Landa, R., & Garrett-Mayer, E. (2006). Development in infants with autism spectrum disorders: A prospective study. *Journal of Child Psychology and Psychiatry and Allied Disciplines, 47,* 629–638.

Leekam, S., Tandos, J., McConachie, H., Meins, E., Parkinson, K., Wright, C., et al. (2007). Repetitive behaviours in typically developing 2-year-olds. *Journal of Child Psychology and Psychiatry and Allied Disciplines, 48,* 1131–1138.

Lord, C. (1995). Follow-up of two-year-olds referred for possible autism. *Journal of Child Psychology and Psychiatry, 36,* 1365–1382.

Lord, C., & Risi, S. (2000). Diagnosis of autism spectrum disorder in young children. In A. M. Wetherby & B. M. Prizant (Eds.), *Autism spectrum disorders: A transactional developmental perspective* (pp. 11–30). Baltimore: Brookes.

Lord, C., Risi, S., DiLavore, P. S., Shulman, C., Thurm, A., & Pickles, A. (2006). Autism from 2 to 9 years of age. *Archives of General Psychiatry, 63,* 694–701.

Lord, C., Risi, S., Lambrecht, L., Cook, E. H., Jr., Leventhal, B. L., DiLavore, P. C., et al. (2000). The autism diagnostic observation schedule-generic: A standard measure of social and communication deficits associated with the spectrum of autism. *Journal of Autism and Developmental Disorders, 30,* 205–223.

Lord, C., Rutter, M., & Le Couteur, A. (1994). Autism diagnostic interview-revised: A revised version of a diagnostic interview for caregivers of individuals with possible pervasive developmental disorders. *Journal of Autism and Developmental Disorders, 24,* 659–685.

Lord, C., Wagner, A., Rogers, S., Szatmari, P., Aman, M., Charman, T., et al. (2005). Challenges in evaluating psychosocial interventions for autistic spectrum disorders. *Journal of Autism and Developmental Disorders, 35,* 695–708.

Luyster, R., Richler, J., Risi, S., Hsu, W., Dawson, G., Bernier, R., et al. (2005). Early regression in social communication in autism spectrum disorders: A CPEA study. *Developmental Neuropsychology, 27,* 311–336.

Matson, J. L., Hess, J. A., Neal, D., Mahan, S., Fodstad, J. C. (2010). Trend in symptoms in children diagnosed with autistic disorder as measured by the Autism Spectrum Disorders-Diagnostic for Children (ASD-DC). *Journal of Developmental and Physical Disabilities, 22,* 47–56.

Moore, V., & Goodson, S. (2003). How well does early diagnosis of autism stand the test of time? Follow-up study of children assessed for autism at age 2 and development of an early diagnostic service. *Autism, 7,* 47–63.

Morgan, L., Wetherby, A. M., & Barber, A. (2008). Repetitive and stereotyped movements in children with autism spectrum disorders late in the second year of life. *Journal of Child Psychology and Psychiatry and Allied Disciplines, 49,* 826–837.

Mundy, P., Sigman, M., & Kasari, C. (1990). A longitudinal study of joint attention and language development in autistic children. *Journal of Autism and Developmental Disorders, 20,* 115–128.

Mundy, P., Sigman, M., & Kasari, C. (1994). Joint attention, developmental level, and symptom presentation in autism. *Development and Psychopathology, 6,* 389–401.

Munson, J., Faja, S., Meltzoff, A., Abbott, R., & Dawson, G. (2008). Neurocognitive predictors of social and communicative developmental trajectories in preschoolers with autism spectrum disorders. *Journal of the International Neuropsychological Society, 14,* 956–966.

Ozonoff, S., Heung, K., Byrd, R., Hansen, R., & Hertz-Picciotto, I. (2008). The onset of autism: Patterns of symptom emergence in the first years of life. *Autism Research, 1,* 320–328.

Ozonoff, S., Williams, B. J., & Landa, R. (2005). Parental report of the early development of children with regressive autism: The delays-plus-regression phenotype. *Autism, 9,* 461–486.

Ozonoff, S., Young, G., Steinfeld, M., Hill, M., Cook, I., Hutman, T., et al. (2009). How early do parent concerns predict later autism diagnosis? *Journal of Developmental and Behavioral Pediatrics, 30,* 367.

Pearson, D. A., Loveland, K. A., Lachar, D., Lane, D. M., Reddoch, S. L., Mansour, R., et al. (2006). A comparison of behavioral and emotional functioning in children and adolescents with autistic disorder and PDD-NOS. *Child Neuropsychology, 12,* 321–333.

Perry, A., Flanagan, H. E., Dunn Geier, J., & Freeman, N. L. (2009). Brief report: The Vineland Adaptive Behavior scales in young children with autism spectrum disorders at different cognitive levels. *Journal of Autism and Developmental Disorders, 39,* 1066–1078.

Rapin, I. (2003). Value and limitations of preschool cognitive tests, with an emphasis on longitudinal study of children on the autistic spectrum. *Brain and Development, 25,* 546–548.

Richler, J., Bishop, S. L., Kleinke, J. R., & Lord, C. (2007). Restricted and repetitive behaviors in young children with autism spectrum disorders. *Journal of Autism and Developmental Disorders, 37,* 73–85.

Richler, J., Huerta, M., Bishop, S. L., & Lord, C. (2010). Developmental trajectories of restricted and repetitive behaviors and interests in children with autism spectrum disorders. *Developmental Psychopathology, 22*(1), 55–69.

Richler, J., Luyster, R., Risi, S., Hsu, W., Dawson, G., Bernier, R., et al. (2006). Is there a 'regressive phenotype' of autism spectrum disorder associated with the measles-mumps-rubella vaccine? A CPEA study. *Journal of Autism and Developmental Disorders, 36,* 299–316.

Rogers, S. J. (2009). What are infant siblings teaching us about autism in infancy? *Autism Research, 2,* 125–137.

Rutter, M., Greenfield, D., & Lockyer, L. (1967). A five-to-fifteen-year follow-up study of infantile psychosis: II. Social and behavioral outcome. *British Journal of Psychiatry, 113,* 1183–1199.

Seltzer, M., Shattuck, P., Abbeduto, L., & Greenberg, J. (2004). Trajectory of development in adolescents and adults with autism. *Mental Retardation and Developmental Disabilities Research Reviews, 10,* 234–247.

Shattuck, P. T., Seltzer, M. M., Greenberg, J. S., Orsmond, G. I., Bolt, D., Kring, S., et al. (2007). Change in autism symptoms and maladaptive behaviors in adolescents and adults with an autism spectrum disorder. *Journal of Autism and Developmental Disorders, 37,* 1735–1747.

Short, A. B., & Schopler, E. (1988). Factors relating to age of onset in autism. *Journal of Autism and Developmental Disorders, 18,* 207–216.

Shumway, S., & Wetherby, A. M. (2009). Communicative acts of children with autism spectrum disorders in the second year of life. *Journal of Speech, Language, and Hearing Research, 52,* 1139–1156.

Sigman, M., & McGovern, C. (2005). Improvement in cognitive and language skills from preschool to adolescence in autism. *Journal of Autism and Developmental Disorders, 35,* 15–23.

Sigman, M., & Ruskin, E. (1999a). Continuity and change in the social competence of children with autism, Down syndrome and developmental delays. *Monographs of the Society for Research in Child Development, 64,* 1–114.

Sigman, M., & Ruskin, E. (1999b). Social competence in children with autism, Down syndrome and developmental delays: A longitudinal study. *Monographs of the Society for Research in Child Development, 64.*

Siller, M., & Sigman, M. (2008). Modeling longitudinal change in the language abilities of children with autism: Parent behaviors and child characteristics as predictors of change. *Developmental Psychology, 44,* 1691–1704.

Sparrow, S., Balla, D., & Cicchetti, D. V. (1984). *Vineland adaptive behavior scales.* Circle Pines, MN: American Guidance Service, Inc.

Stone, W., Lee, E. B., Ashford, L., Brissie, J., Hepburn, S. L., Coonrod, E. E., et al. (1999). Can autism be diagnosed accurately in children under 3 years? *Journal of Child Psychology and Psychiatry, 40,* 219–226.

Szatmari, P., Bryson, S. E., Boyle, M. H., Streiner, D. L., & Duku, E. (2003). Predictors of outcome among high functioning children with autism and Asperger syndrome. *Journal of Child Psychology and Psychiatry and Allied Disciplines, 44,* 520–528.

Szatmari, P., Bryson, S., Duku, E., Vaccarella, L., Zwaigenbaum, L., Bennett, T., et al. (2009). Similar developmental trajectories in autism and Asperger syndrome: From early childhood to adolescence. *Journal of Child Psychology and Psychiatry and Allied Disciplines, 50,* 1459–1467.

Tager-Flusberg, H., Rogers, S., Cooper, J., Landa, R., Lord, C., Paul, R., et al. (2009). Defining spoken language benchmarks and selecting measures of expressive language development for young children with autism spectrum disorders. *Journal of Speech, Language, and Hearing Research, 52,* 643–652.

Thomas, M. S., Annaz, D., Ansari, D., Scerif, G., Jarrold, C., & Karmiloff-Smith, A. (2009). Using developmental trajectories to understand developmental disorders. *Journal of Speech, Language, and Hearing Research, 52,* 336–358.

Thurm, A., Lord, C., Lee, L. C., & Newschaffer, C. (2007). Predictors of language acquisition in preschool children with autism spectrum disorders. *Journal of Autism and Developmental Disorders, 37,* 1721–1734.

Tomanik, S., Pearson, D., Loveland, K., Lane, D., & Bryant Shaw, J. (2007). Improving the reliability of autism diagnoses: Examining the utility of adaptive behavior. *Journal of Autism and Developmental Disorders, 37,* 921–928.

Turner, L. M., & Stone, W. L. (2007). Variability in outcome for children with an ASD diagnosis at age 2. *Journal of Child Psychology and Psychiatry and Allied Disciplines, 48,* 793–802.

Turner, L. M., Stone, W. L., Pozdol, S. L., & Coonrod, E. E. (2006). Follow-up of children with autism spectrum disorders from age 2 to age 9. *Autism, 10,* 243–265.

Venter, A., Lord, C., & Schopler, E. (1992). A follow-up of high-functioning autistic children. *Journal of Child Psychology and Psychiatry, 33,* 489–507.

Volkmar, F., Klin, A., Siegel, B., Szatmari, P., Lord, C., Campbell, M., et al. (1994). Field trial for autistic disorder in DSM-IV. *American Journal of Psychiatry, 151,* 1361.

Volkmar, F. R., & Nelson, D. S. (1990). Seizure disorders in autism. *Journal of the American Academy of Child and Adolescent Psychiatry, 29,* 127–129.

Watt, N., Wetherby, A. M., Barber, A., & Morgan, L. (2008). Repetitive and stereotyped behaviors in children with autism spectrum disorders in the second year of life. *Journal of Autism and Developmental Disorders, 38,* 1518–1533.

Werner, E., & Dawson, G. (2005). Validation of the phenomenon of autistic regression using home videotapes. *Archives of General Psychiatry, 62,* 889–895.

Werner, E., Dawson, G., Munson, J., & Osterling, J. (2005). Variation in early developmental course in autism and its relation with behavioral outcome at 3–4 years of age. *Journal of Autism and Developmental Disorders, 35,* 337–350.

Werner, E., Dawson, G., Osterling, J., & Dinno, N. (2000). Brief report: Recognition of autism spectrum disorder before one year of age: A retrospective study based on home videotapes. *Journal of Autism and Developmental Disorders, 30,* 157–162.

Wetherby, A., Prizant, B., & Hutchinson, T. (1998). Communicative, social/affective, and symbolic profiles of young children with autism and pervasive developmental disorders. *American Journal of Speech-Language Pathology, 7,* 79.

Wetherby, A. M., Watt, N., Morgan, L., & Shumway, S. (2007). Social communication profiles of children with autism spectrum disorders late in the second year of life. *Journal of Autism and Developmental Disorders, 37,* 960–975.

Wetherby, A. M., Woods, J., Allen, L., Cleary, J., Dickinson, H., & Lord, C. (2004). Early indicators of autism spectrum disorders in the second year of life. *Journal of Autism and Developmental Disorders, 34,* 473–493.

Wing, L. (1983). Social and interpersonal needs. In E. Schopler, & G. B. Mesibov (Eds.), *Autism in adolescents and adults* (pp. 337–354). New York: Plenum Press.

Young, G. S., Merin, N., Rogers, S. J., & Ozonoff, S. (2009). Gaze behavior and affect at 6 months: Predicting clinical outcomes and language development in typically developing infants and infants at risk for autism. *Developmental Science, 12,* 798–814.

Zwaigenbaum, L., Bryson, S., Lord, C., Rogers, S., Carter, A., Carver, L., et al. (2009). Clinical assessment and management of toddlers with suspected autism spectrum disorder: Insights from studies of high-risk infants. *Pediatrics, 123,* 1383–1391.

Zwaigenbaum, L., Bryson, S., Rogers, T., Roberts, W., Brian, J., & Szatmari, P. (2005). Behavioral manifestations of autism in the first year of life. *International Journal of Developmental Neuroscience, 23,* 143–152.

Sensory Processing and Motor Issues in Autism Spectrum Disorders

Claudia List Hilton

Although sensory processing and motor abnormalities are not among the three pathognomonic features of autism spectrum disorders (ASDs; American Psychiatric Association, 2000), many studies have found children with autism to have a higher incidence of both compared to the typically developing population. Atypical sensory processing may limit participation in meaningful activities, such as playing with others or participating in other social activities. Children who have motor impairments also tend to engage in less diversity of activities than do other children, with more frequent participation in quiet recreational activities and less frequent participation in social activities, especially social activities that are spontaneous (Brown & Gordon, 1987; Margalit, 1981; Sillanpää, 1987). Significant differences were seen in participation between children with ASD and typically developing children in the number of activities in which children participate, the numbers of individuals with whom they participate, and the variety of environments in which they participate (Hilton, Crouch, & Israel, 2008). Both sensory processing and motor abnormalities can limit children with ASD from participation in meaningful activities.

Sensory Processing

The sensory systems are the sources for a living being to acquire information about the world and support that being in successfully responding and adapting to environmental demands. Sensory systems in humans provide pathways for the brain to receive information through which it interprets the stimulus and implements a response. Children with an ASD seem to experience atypical patterns of processing sensory input and have difficulty responding to tasks and environmental demands (Dunn, Saiter, & Rinner,

2002). Children who have difficulty integrating the continuous stream of sensory input and responding appropriately may also have difficulty with self-esteem, self-actualization, socialization, and play (Bundy, Lane, & Murray, 2002).

Sensory Processing Disorders

Sensory processing disorders comprise sensory modulation disorders, sensory discrimination disorders, and sensory-based motor disorders (Miller, Anzalone, Lane, Cermak, & Osten, 2007). Sensory modulation disorders occur when a child is unable to respond to sensory information with behavior that is regulated relative to the intensity of the input. Sensory discrimination disorders are present when an individual has difficulty interpreting qualities of sensory stimuli and is unable to perceive similarities and differences among stimuli, such as having a problem with acuity. Sensory discrimination forms the foundation of adequate body scheme because accurate interpretation of sensory stimulation is the basis for planning movement and postural responses. Sensory-based motor disorders consist of postural disorder and dyspraxia. Postural disorder is characterized by inappropriate muscle tension, hypotonic or hypertonic muscle tone, inadequate control of movement, or inadequate muscle contraction to achieve movement against resistance. Dyspraxia is the impaired ability to conceive of, plan, sequence, or execute novel actions, or the impairment of praxis. People with dyspraxia appear to be unsure of where their bodies are in space and have trouble judging their distance from objects or people. They have difficulty grading force during movement and may seem accident prone, frequently breaking toys or objects.

Sensory Modulation Disorders

Three types of sensory modulation disorders have been identified: sensory over-responsiveness occurs when the

C.L. Hilton (✉)
Department of Psychiatry, Washington University School of Medicine, St. Louis, MO 63110, USA
e-mail: hiltonc@psychiatry.wustl.edu

child responds to sensory input more quickly or with increased intensity than typically observed; sensory under-responsiveness occurs when the child does not respond to or disregards sensory input; and sensory seeking behavior occurs when the child actively engages in actions that provide intense sensory input (Miller et al., 2007). Dunn (1997) identifies a fourth category of responding – sensation avoiding. In this category, the person is overly sensitive to certain input but instead of over-responding, avoids the input. A strong relationship has been observed between the degree of atypical sensory responsiveness and the severity of social impairment experienced by children with high-functioning autism spectrum disorders (Hilton, Graver, & LaVesser, 2007).

Atypical patterns of sensory modulation were identified in 69–100% of children with ASD in various studies (Baranek, David, Poe, Stone, & Watson, 2006; Baranek, Foster, & Berkson, 1997; Leekman, Nieto, Libby, Wing, & Gould, 2007; Tomcheck & Dunn, 2007). Although specific results vary, children with ASD present with more sensory difficulties do than children with no diagnosis across studies (Baker, Lane, Angley, & Young, 2008; Ben-Sasson et al., 2007; Dunn, Myles, & Orr, 2002; Kern et al., 2007; 2007; Kientz & Dunn, 1997; Liss, Saulnier, Fein, & Kinsbourne, 2006; Tomcheck & Dunn, 2007; Watling, Deitz, & White, 2001). Ben-Sasson et al. (2007) confirm the early onset of sensory modulation disorders in toddlers with ASD, indicating that this deficit begins to impact child development at an early age. Atypical sensory responsiveness is often one of the first signs that parents notice in their children with ASD (Baker et al., 2008).

Neurological Basis

In typically developing children, two processes naturally occur to help them regulate sensory input in order to actively participate in a variety of activities. The first of these processes, habituation, is the ability of the central nervous system (CNS) to recognize a stimulus as familiar and then decrease transmission of the stimulus since there is no need to respond (Dunn, 1997). If a child has difficulty with habituation, stimuli, such as the feeling of one's clothing, can become overwhelming, limiting the child's ability to attend to anything else. Sensorimotor gating, the ability to dampen responses to repeated stimuli, was found to be significantly impaired in two studies of adult subjects with ASD in quantitative magnetic resonance imaging that compared brain structure with control groups (McAlonon et al., 2002; Perry, Minassian, Lopez, Maron, & Lincoln, 2007). It was also seen in a study of young children with autism and intellectual disabilities, using electroencephalogram analysis (Orekhova

et al., 2008). This slowing of the ability to dampen responses to repeated stimuli may offer some explanation for the hyper-responsiveness in persons who have ASD. To be continually stimulated by non-novel sensory events, which are quickly habituated by others, may place one in a heightened alertness level and may influence their ability to tolerate and their preferences for certain types of activities.

The second process, sensitization, involves the CNS recognizing the stimulus as important and therefore generating a heightened response (Dunn, 1997). We become aware of an insect's light touch by this mechanism, and the quick response to swat it before being stung is important to ensure safety. Without this mechanism working correctly, a child may be more vulnerable to unsafe temperatures, stimuli, and objects. Sensitization and habituation in children with ASD are often disrupted.

Casanova (2007) proposed that autism has a monotopic effect in which a basic abnormality early in brain development results in a cascade of pathological events that are significantly influenced by environmental factors. Microcellular columns in a postmortem examination of the brains of individuals with autism were smaller, more numerous, and more dispersed in their cellular formations than those of matched controls (Casanova, Buxhoeveden, Switala, & Roy, 2002). It is suggested that this pattern leads to over-connected and insufficient neural networks that consequently leave the child hyper-aroused and with impaired selection. Therefore autistic children may use over-selective attention and repetitive behavior to compensate for the hyper-aroused state.

Coskun et al. (2009) used magnetoencephalography to examine the cortical response to passive tactile stimulation of the thumb and index finger of the dominant hand and lip of individuals affected and unaffected with ASD. The distance between cortical representations of the thumb and lip was significantly larger in the group with autism and the typical cortical representation of the thumb being closer to the lip than that of the index finger was not seen in the group with autism. These findings indicate a difference in the cortical organization of the brain in persons with ASD.

Mottron and associates (2006) proposed a model of enhanced perceptual functioning (EPF), which describes over-functioning of brain regions in individuals with ASD, which are typically involved in primary perceptual functioning for the visual and auditory systems. This phenomenon of enhanced functioning was further defined to consist of enhanced detection of patterns and completion of missing information, which seem to explain these superior abilities in the savant syndrome (Mottron, Dawson, & Soulieres, 2009). In a study of gifted children with no ASD diagnosis, their sensitivity to the environment and emotional and behavioral responses were found to be greater than those of children of average intelligence (Gere, Capps, Mitchell, & Grubbs, 2009).

Baron-Cohen and associates (2009) proposed a similar hyper-systemizing theory, which argues that the excellent attention to detail seen in individuals with ASD is a consequence of sensory hypersensitivity and is directed toward detecting law-based pattern recognition ("if p, then q" rules). This systemizing or the identification of rules that govern a system is suggested to be associated with multiple sensory systems and to explain the talent seen in individuals with ASD.

Relationship Between Sensory Modulation and Behaviors Common to ASD

The underlying reason for repetitive stereotypical behaviors or strong aversive responses (also referred to as defensiveness) to commonly occurring sensory experiences in children with ASD has been attributed to either generating or avoiding sensory stimulation or to attempts to achieve homeostasis or to modulate the sensory system (Baker et al., 2008; Ermer & Dunn, 1998; Frick & Lawton-Shirley, 1994; Liss et al., 2006). Children with ASD who have sensory disorders can also experience psychological stress related to the sensory impairment. Wiggins, Robins, Bakeman, and Adamson (2009) found that the consequences associated with these perceptual differences may include anxiety-related behaviors or disorders and may have a detrimental impact on self-concept or social empathy. A strong correlation between sensory defensiveness and anxiety, and a significant relationship between hyposensitivity and symptoms of depression were found in children with Asperger syndrome (Pfeiffer, Kinnealey, Reed, & Herzberg, 2005). In a large population-based young twin study, tactile and auditory defensiveness were found to be moderately correlated with a fearful temperament and anxiety (Goldsmith, Van Hulle, Arneson, Schreiber, & Gernsbacher, 2006).

Sensory modulation difficulties can also lead to difficulties in interacting and relating to people and objects. Bundy, Shia, Qi, and Miller (2007) observed that when autistic children finally master an activity, they often repeat it with little variation, which creates little opportunity for others to engage with these children or for them to encounter new experiences important for development. Ashburner, Ziviani, and Rodger (2008) found auditory responsiveness difficulties, sensory under-responsiveness, and sensory seeking to be associated with academic underachievement in children with ASD. In a study of young children, parents attributed poor sensory modulation abilities as factors impacting their children's social, cognitive, and sensorimotor development (Dickie, Baranek, Schultz, Watson, & McComish, 2009).

Literature Addressing Specific Sensory Systems

Many studies have attempted to determine the sensory modulation deficits by examining the acuity and patterns of responsiveness with individual senses to gain an understanding of which processes are most affected in children with autism. Hans Asperger originally described hypersensitivity, especially touch, smell, and taste, in his first description of children with ASD (Asperger, 1944/1991). A number of studies have provided useful information about sensory discrimination or acuity and atypical responsiveness in the auditory, visual, vestibular, tactile, multisensory, and oral sensory/olfactory senses in typically developing individuals and in individuals with ASD.

Auditory system. Atypical auditory responsiveness has been frequently reported in children with autism (Dahlgren & Gillberg, 1989; Tomcheck & Dunn, 2007). Hyper-responsiveness to particular noises that are not unpleasant to most typical individuals or hyperacusis has been reported in several studies of children with autism (O'Neill & Jones, 1997; Rosenhall, Nordin, Sandstrom, Ahlsen, & Gillberg, 1999), and auditory under-responsivity has been reported in several others (Baranek, 1999b; Osterling & Dawson, 1994). Superior musical pitch processing has been seen in individuals with autism (Heaton, Hemelin, & Pring, 1998). Nieto del Rincon (2008) reports that disturbances found in cognitive-evoked potentials show alterations in auditory processing, auditory identification, attentional processing, and decision making in people with autism. Difficulties in auditory information processing were observed in another study of children with ASD (Tecchio et al., 2003). These difficulties may also lead to inappropriate behaviors if the child is not able to understand the teacher or classmates, or if the child's auditory system becomes easily over stimulated.

Visual system. Visual hyper-responsiveness might be seen in children who prefer to be in the dark or avoid bright lights, while hypo-responsiveness might involve looking intensely or staring at objects or people (Dunn, 1999). Visual motion perception and pursuit eye movement deficits have been reported in individuals with autism (Takarae, Luna, Minshew, & Sweeney, 2008). Increased visual acuity (Ashwin, Ashwin, Rhydderch, Howells, & Baron-Cohen, 2009) and prolonged pupillary light reflex latency, smaller constriction amplitude, and lower constriction velocity (Fan, Miles, Takahashi, & Yao, 2009) have been observed in individuals with ASD in comparison to a control group. Each of these findings could help to explain the atypical visual responsiveness sometimes seen in children with ASD.

Vestibular system. Vestibular hyper-responsiveness might include becoming anxious or distressed when feet leave the ground or avoiding playground equipment or moving toys, while hypo-responsiveness might include inability to sit still or rocking unconsciously (Dunn, 1999). The ability to navigate in the world and make appropriate motor responses is dependent upon the development of accurate internal representations of the body's orientation in space and what happens with movement (Green, Shaikh, & Angelaki, 2005). The otolith organs and the semicircular canals work together to construct this internal model. Kuo (2005) proposed that this model is also dependent on the senses of joint proprioception and vision. Difficulties in vestibular responsiveness, including difficulties in balance and body orientation, are often reported in children with autism (Kern et al., 2007). Symptoms often associated with autism, such as spinning or difficulty in navigating unsteady surfaces, may be related to deficits in vestibular modulation.

Tactile system. Tactile hyper-responsiveness might include expressing distress during grooming, reacting emotionally or aggressively to touch, becoming irritated by wearing shoes or socks, avoiding going barefoot, or having difficulty standing in line close to others (Dunn, 1999). Hypo-responsiveness might include decreased awareness of pain and temperature, not seeming to notice when face or hands are messy, avoiding wearing shoes, or displaying unusual need for touching certain toys, surfaces, or textures. Tactile hyper-responsiveness and hypo-responsiveness have often been reported in children with ASD (Baranek et al., 1997; Blakemore et al., 2006; Cesaroni & Garber, 1991; Tomcheck & Dunn, 2007). In one study, children with tactile hypersensitivity were also more likely to display other autistic behaviors, including inflexible behaviors, repetitive verbalizations, visual stereotypies, and abnormally focused attention (Baranek et al., 1997). In a recent study by Hilton and associates (in press), multiple regression analyses revealed atypical scores from multisensory processing and the proximal senses of oral sensory/olfactory and touch processing as the strongest predictors of greater social impairment in children affected and unaffected with ASD.

Several studies have examined tactile acuity. Increased forearm sensitivity to low-frequency vibration and thermal pain were seen in individuals with autism compared to a control group (Cascio et al., 2008). In another study, tactile stimuli were perceived as more tickly by individuals with ASD than by controls (Blakemore et al., 2006).

Oral sensory and olfactory systems. Children with ASD have narrower food preferences, more feeding problems, and are more resistant to trying new foods than children who do not have ASD (Lockner, Crowe, & Skipper, 2008; Schreck, Williams, & Smith, 2004). Differences have been shown in taste and olfaction identification, but not in detection, in individuals diagnosed with ASD (Bennetto, Kuschner, & Hyman, 2007; Suzuki, Critchley, Rowe, Howlin, & Murphy, 2003). Olfaction plays a critical role not only in selection and enjoyment of food (Nolte, 2007) but also in

controlling and regulating multiple social behaviors in mammals (Halpern, 1987; Nicot, Otto, Brabet, & DiCicco-Bloom, 2004). In addition, current data from animal models show that neuropsychiatric manifestations are intimately associated with smell impairment and autoimmune dysregulation (Moscavitch, Szyper-Kravitz, & Shoenfeld, 2009).

Multisensory systems. Multisensory modulation occurs in activities that involve managing multiple incoming sensations. Tasks invoking multisensory processing include difficulty paying attention, getting lost easily, seeming oblivious in an active environment, or leaving clothing twisted on body (Dunn, 1999). Multisensory processing has been shown to be either enhanced or attenuated, depending upon whether the content of the two modalities is associated (Baier, Kleinschmidt, & Muller, 2006). In multiple regression analyses of sensory responsiveness and autistic traits of children with ASD, multisensory responsiveness, derived as a Sensory Profile subscore (Dunn, 1999), significantly predicted the degree of autistic pathology in the children (Gaines, 2002), as measured by the Child Autism Rating Scale (Schopler, Reichler, & Renner, 2002).

Sensory Assessments

Sensory assessments appropriate for children with ASD are quite varied by age group and psychometric strength. Very few assessments are standardized quantitative observational measures. Table 11.1 provides a list of some of the more commonly used assessments. Physiological measures are also used for determining responsiveness to sensory stimuli which include somatosensory-evoked potential (Parush, Sohmer, Steinberg, & Kaitz, 2007), skin conductance (Miller et al., 1999), event-related potential (ERP; Whitehouse & Bishop, 2008), salivary cortisol (Kimball et al., 2007), MEG procedure (Tecchio et al., 2003), and PET scan to measure regional cerebral blood flow (Boddaert et al., 2004).

Motor Issues

Motor impairment has been frequently reported in studies of children with ASD (Dzuik, Gidley-Larson, Mahone, Denckla, & Mostofsky, 2007; Fuentes, Mostofsky, & Bastian, 2009; Green et al., 2009; Jansiewicz et al., 2006; Ming, Brimacombe, & Wagner, 2007). Assessments of various areas of motor ability have been used to identify these impairments, which include fine manual control/writing, manual dexterity/coordination, ball skills, gait, balance, body coordination, strength and agility, praxis, imitation, postural stability, and speed, and the subtle neurological signs of overflow, dysrhythmia, motor impersistence, and muscle tone. In each study, children with ASD had significantly

Table 11.1   Sensory assessments

Assessment	Age group	Properties
Sensory Behaviour Schedule (Harrison & Hare, 2004)	All ages	Questionnaire. 10 senses, 17 questions (choices of ongoing, in past, no, don't know) No psychometrics
Children's Eating Behavior Inventory (Archer, Rosenbaum, & Streiner, 1991)	Children	40-Item caregiver report for evaluating mealtime behaviors, eating behaviors, and the disruption of feeding problems on family dynamics. Five-point rating scale (1 = never to 5 = always) to measure the frequency of 19 different eating behaviors
Author-developed tactile stimuli response test (Pernon, Pry, & Baghdadli, 2007)	Children	Three-part protocol developed by authors to assess responses to textures, temperature changes, and fluid (air)
Sensory Rating Scale for Infants and Young Children (Provost & Oetter, 1993)	Birth to 3 years	Parent report measure that can be used to identify and quantify sensory responsiveness, including sensory defensive behaviors. Consists of 136 questions with five-point Likert scale responses. Categories are touch, movement/gravity, hearing, vision, taste/smell, and temperature/general sensitivity
Test of Sensory Function for Infants (DeGangi & Greenspan, 1989)	4–18 months	24 items. Provides an overall measure of sensory processing and reactivity, as well as scores on the following subdomains: reactivity to tactile deep pressure, visual tactile integration, adaptive motor function, ocular motor control, and reactivity to vestibular stimulation
Sensory Experiences Questionnaire (Baranek et al., 2006)	5–80 months	15-Min caregiver report that evaluates behavioral responses to common everyday sensory experiences (e.g., child dislikes cuddling), infancy through preschool. Total score and subscales are derived for hyper- and hypo-responsiveness
Sensory Processing Assessment for Young Children (Baranek, 1999a)	Infant–preschool	Play-based observational assessment that measures responsiveness to novel toys and environmental stimuli that present a variety of sensory experiences (e.g., tactile, auditory, and visual). Specifically, the SPA examines patterns of approach avoidance, orientation, and habituation as well as stereotypical behaviors displayed by the child in response to sensory toys and stimuli
Infant/Toddler Sensory Profile (Dunn, 2002)	7 months–3 years	48-Item caregiver questionnaire. Scores have categorical standards (typical, probable difference, and definite difference)
Sensory Defensiveness subscale of the revised Toddler Behavior Assessment Questionnaire (TBAQ; Goldsmith, 1996)	18–36 months	120-Item caregiver report measure that assesses temperamental dimensions (activity level, anger, attention, inhibitory control, interest, object fear, pleasure, sadness, social fear, soothability, and sensory defensiveness). Scale of 1 (never)–7 (always). Sensory Defensiveness subscale comprises two 5-item subscales, Auditory Defensiveness and Tactile Defensiveness
Tactile & Vestibular Questionnaire (Bar-Shalita, Goldstand, Hann-Markowitz, & Parush, 2005)	3–4 years	Author-developed questionnaire, 65 tactile questions and 32 vestibular questions, five-point Likert scale between likes very much and greatly dislikes
The DeGangi-Berk Test of Sensory Integration (DeGangi & Berk, 1983)	3–5 years	36 items measuring overall sensory integration as well as three clinically significant subdomains: postural control, bilateral motor integration, and reflex integration. These vestibular-based functions are essential to the development of motor skills, visual–spatial and language abilities, hand dominance, and motor planning
Sensory Profile (Dunn, 1999)	3–10 years	125-Item questionnaire, five levels of frequency (always, frequently, occasionally, seldom, and never), sensory processing scores, factor scores, quadrant scores. Scores have categorical standards (typical, probable difference, and definite difference), but no t scores, z scores, quotients, etc.
Short Sensory Profile (McIntosh, Miller, Shyu, & Dunn, 1999)	3–10 years	10-Min questionnaire, 38 items, 0–4 scale with higher scores having more impairment. Standardized categorically for entire age group, no differentiation by gender. Done on 1,200 children, reliability was 0.90, discriminant validity was >95% in identifying children with and without sensory modulation dysfunction. Seven factors. Scores have categorical standards (typical, probable difference, and definite difference) but no t scores, z scores, quotients, etc.

Table 11.1 (continued)

Assessment	Age group	Properties
Sensory Profile School Companion (Dunn, 2006)	3–12 years	15-Min, 62-item teacher questionnaire, quadrant scores, factor scores, section scores for auditory, visual, movement, touch, and behavior. Scores have categorical standards (typical, probable difference, and definite difference) but no t scores, z scores, quotients, etc.
Tactile Defensiveness and Discrimination Test – Revised (TDDT-R; Baranek, 1997)	3–12 years	Standardized behavioral assessment measuring tactile processing that has been validated previously for use in children with developmental disabilities between the ages of 3 and 12 years (Baranek & Berkson, 1994; Baranek et al., 1997). Total scores are derived for each of two scales: *externally controlled* tactile experiences (responses to stimuli such as stickers or a finger puppet applied by the examiner) and *internally controlled* tactile experiences (responses during child-initiated exploration of tactile media, such as lotion, dried noodles, or sand)
Sensory Approach–Avoidance Rating (Baranek et al., 2002)	3–12 years	Author-developed assessment, children are presented with nine novel multisensory toys to explore individually
Sensory Over-Responsivity Scales: Assessment & Inventory (Schoen, Miller, & Green, 2008)	3–55 years	SensOR Assessment: Examiner administered, 16 sensory activities, 7 sensory domains, scores 1–4 (startle, elimination, dislike, and negative stop) Inventory: 76-item questionnaire Over-responsivity is the only construct that has been developed. It has only been pilot tested on 125 subjects (65 with over-responsivity and 60 controls)
Sensory Integration and Praxis Test (SIPT) (Ayres, 1989)	4–8 years, 11 months	The SIPT measures visual, tactile, and kinesthetic perception as well as motor performance. It is composed of the following 17 brief tests: 1. Space visualization 2. Figure-ground perception 3. Standing/walking balance 4. Design copying 5. Postural praxis 6. Bilateral motor coordination 7. Praxis on verbal command 8. Constructional praxis 9. Postrotary nystagmus 10. Motor accuracy 11. Sequencing praxis 12. Oral praxis 13. Manual form perception 14. Kinesthesia 15. Finger identification 16. Graphesthesia 17. Localization of tactile stimuli
Sensory Processing Measure – Home Form (Parham & Ecker, 2007)	5–12 years	75-Item questionnaire. Raw scores and T scores for total and seven sensory categories (social participation, vision, hearing, touch, body awareness, balance and motion, and planning and ideas) are derived. Standard scores allow classification into typical, some problems, and definite dysfunction. Norm referenced on over 1,000 children. It is unique in that it is standardized in both the home and the main classroom with all the same students making those environments statistically comparable. It is also unique in that it includes separate environment forms for the art, music, PE, recess, cafeteria, and bus environments
Sensory Processing Measure – School Environments Forms (Kuhaneck, Henry, & Glennon, 2007)	5–12 years	62-Item questionnaire. Raw scores and T scores for total and seven sensory categories (social participation, vision, hearing, touch, body awareness, balance and motion, and planning and ideas). Standard scores allow classification into typical, some problems, and definite dysfunction
Touch Inventory for Elementary School Aged Children (TIE; Royeen & Fortune, 1990)	6–12 years	26-Question screening tool designed for children of elementary school age to screen for tactile defensiveness
Adolescent/Adult Sensory Profile (Brown & Dunn, 2002)	11 years–adult	65-Item questionnaire, five levels of frequency (always, frequently, occasionally, seldom, and never). It produces sensory processing scores, factor scores, and quadrant scores
Adult Sensory Interview (ADULT-SI; Kinnealey, Oliver, & Wilbarger, 1995)	Adults	82-Item semistructured, open-ended questions to elicit information regarding a person's perception and responses to various sensory stimuli. It has a scoring range from 0 to 82 with each question receiving a score of 1 (defensive) or 0 (non-defensive)

Table 11.1 (continued)

Assessment	Age group	Properties
Adult Sensory Questionnaire (ASQ; Kinnealey & Oliver, 2002)	Adults	Self-report screening tool for sensory defensiveness in adults; clients answer yes or no to items that describe behaviors typical of sensory defensiveness. A total score is obtained, and cut-off scores help to determine whether the client indicates sensory defensiveness. Research has established concurrent validity between the ASQ and the Adult Sensory Interview ($r = 0.94$, $p < 0.01$) (Kinnealey et al., 1995) and between the Adolescent/Adult Sensory Profile and the Adult Sensory Interview ($r = 0.81$, $p < 0.01$) (Kinnealey & Smith, 2002)

poorer motor abilities and more frequent subtle neurological signs compared to controls. Studies reveal motor impairment rates that generally converge on 80–90% (Ghazuiddin & Butler, 1998; Ghazuiddin, Butler, Tsai, & Ghazuiddin, 1994; Gillberg, 1989; Green et al., 2002; Manjiviona & Prior, 1995; Miyahara et al., 1997). Minshew, Goldstein, and Siegel (1997) found motor function to be one of the discriminating domains differentiating individuals with ASD from unaffected controls. A recent robust meta-analysis concluded that ASD is associated with significant and widespread alterations in motor performance, suggesting a tentative argument that motor deficits are a potential core feature of ASD (Fournier, Hass, Lodha, & Cauraugh, 2010). In a recent study examining familial patterns of motor impairment, Hilton, Zhang, White, & Constantino (2010) found that motor proficiency exhibited a pathologically shifted, continuous distribution in ASD and that the degree of motor impairment was correlated with the degree of social impairment in ASD but absent among unaffected siblings, suggesting that motor impairment constitutes a core feature of the autistic phenotype.

Motor Skills and Participation in ASD

Motor skill performance was linked to participation in a retrospective chart review of 40 children with Asperger syndrome (Church, Alisanski, & Amanullah, 1999). Motor clumsiness was believed to limit the participation by children between ages 6 and 11 in outdoor sports, with substitution of computer and television activities. Fine motor skill deficits sometimes limited their ability to grasp, write, or use scissors or utensils and 58% received occupational therapy services to address fine motor issues. More than half of the group had histories of being klutzy, clumsy, or awkward and 33% received physical therapy to address large motor movements for such activities as bike riding and climbing. In a separate study, fine motor skills were found to be highly correlated with competence in daily living skills in children with an ASD (Jasmin et al., 2009). In a study of children in Taiwan, the ASD-diagnosed children were found to be less active during recess and lunch time, compared to the typically developing children (Pan, 2008). These findings have implications for overall fitness among children with ASD and

suggest the possibility that lower activity levels may have a relationship with the presence of motor impairment.

Motor Impairment in ASD

Using the Test of Motor Impairment (TOMI-H), the precursor to the Movement Assessment Battery for Children (MABC; Henderson & Sugden, 1992), Stott and colleagues (Stott, Moyes, & Henderson, 1984) found that 7 of their 12 subjects with AS between the ages of 7 and 17 scored below the 15th percentile. Ghazuiddin et al. (1994) used the Bruininks Oseretsky Test of Motor Proficiency (BOT, Bruininks, 1978) to find that 73% of the AS children in their study exhibited abnormally poor performance (at least one standard deviation below the mean) on all three sections of the test (gross motor, fine motor, and upper limb coordination/ball skills). Ghazuiddin and Butler (1998) found that all 12 of their subjects with ASD, aged 8–15, demonstrated motor coordination problems on the BOT.

Another research group (Miyahara et al., 1997) reported that 85% of their 26 Japanese subjects with ASD between the ages of 6 and 15 obtained MABC scores at least two standard deviations below the norm (Henderson & Sugden, 1992). Green et al. (2002) found that all of the 11 children with ASD and aged between 6 years, 5 months and 10 years, 6 months in their study met the criteria for motor impairment, according to the MABC (Henderson & Sugden, 1992). They found that tasks involving aiming and catching of a ball were the most significantly impaired skills.

Jansiewicz et al. (2006) found that the subtle sign of overflow and motor scores for gait, balance, and speed of patterned timed movements were significant predictors of a diagnosis in children with high-functioning autism spectrum disorders but that dysrhythmia in the tasks involving repeated rhythmic movements was not. In an examination of handwriting, Fuentes et al. (2009) found letter formation to be significantly impaired in children with ASD, but no significant differences were seen in ability to write letters with correct size, alignment (placement on the lines), and spacing between the letters. Hilton and associates (2007) found motor impairment and social severity to be strongly correlated in 107 children affected and unaffected with Asperger syndrome.

Gestural Performance

Gestures comprise non-verbal communicative motor actions, skilled motor acts, and the ability to use tools. Gestural performance can involve praxis and may include four types of performances: gestures that are performed from a verbal command, gestures that require another person to imitate the movement, gestures that use objects (e.g., using a scissors, a comb, or a spoon), and gestures that do not use objects (e.g., crossing fingers, waving, snapping fingers, or pretending to hold a scissors, a comb, or a spoon). Numerous studies have examined praxis and gestural performance. Ming et al. (2007) found hypotonia, dyspraxia, toe walking, delayed gross motor milestones, and reduced ankle mobility to be present, but less prevalent in the older ages in a cohort of 154 children with ASD between 2 and 18 years of age. Dewey, Cantell, and Crawford (2007) found that gestural performance was impaired even when the overall level of motor skills was controlled for in children with ASD. Similarly, praxis was shown to be impaired in children with ASD, even after accounting for basic motor skills in two studies (Dzuik, Larson, Apostu, Mahone, Denckla, and Mostofsky, 2007; Mostofsky et al., 2006). Dzuik et al. (2007) also found praxis performance to be a strong predictor of the defining features of autism. Staples and Reid (2009) found that children with ASD had particular difficulty coordinating both sides of their bodies or both arms and legs while performing motor skills, almost like each body segment acting independently of the others. Expanding on this concept, Fabbri-Destro, Cattaneo, Boria, and Rizzolatti (2009) found that the children with ASD in their study were unable to translate their motor intention into an action but would program single motor acts independently, which suggests that they may have a deficit in chaining motor acts into a global action.

Handedness in ASD

Another motor issue discussed in the literature is hand dominance or handedness. Handedness, rather than being a single construct, encompasses both hand preference and hand performance, and frequently refers to the hand one prefers to use during unimanual activities (Cavill & Bryden, 2003; Pederson, Sigmundsson, Whiting, & Ingvaldsen, 2003). Approximately 90% of the general population show a preference for the right hand (Annett, 1985). It is important to examine handedness in children with autism because of its relationship to neuropathology and cerebral organization. Pederson et al. (2003) explain that handedness is caused by lateralization, which is the process that leads to an asymmetrical nervous system. Dawson, Warrenburg, and Fuller (1983) support this idea in their research concerning hemisphere functioning, describing subjects with ASD as

showing a preference for the right hemisphere rather than a general lack of cerebral lateralization. Other theories of atypical handedness patterns in children with ASD suggest the possibility of handedness being related to an overall developmental lag (Annett, 1970; Fein, Humes, Kaplan, Lucci, & Waterhouse, 1984; Satz, Soper, & Orsini, 1988), bilateral brain dysfunction (Fein, Waterhouse, Lucci, Pennington, & Humes, 1985; Soper & Satz, 1984; Tsai, 1983), and poor motor functioning (Bishop, 1990; Cornish & McManus, 1996).

Higher left-handedness. Research conducted on children diagnosed with ASD has frequently indicated higher left-hand preference when compared to typically developing counterparts (Bryson, 1990; Cornish & McManus, 1996; Dane & Balci, 2007; McManus, Murray, Doyle, & Baron-Cohen, 1992; Raja & Azzoni, 2001). Two studies (Escalante-Mead, Minshew, & Sweeney, 2003; Hauck & Dewey, 2001) did not find a greater left-hand preference among the children with autism because they set up higher criteria for determination of handedness, so the children who would have been categorized as left-handed in other studies were categorized as having ambiguous handedness in these studies.

Ambiguous handedness and skill-preference discordance. Ambiguous handedness or mixed hand preference has been a common finding in studies examining children with ASD. Ambiguous handedness is differentiated from ambidextrous handedness because it involves switching hands within a task rather than across tasks (Soper et al., 1986). For example, an ambiguously handed individual would perform tasks such as writing, throwing a ball, or picking up a coin with either hand, while an ambidextrous individual might write with his right hand but throw a ball with his left hand. In a study examining 20 children with autism (mean chronological age, 11.1 years, SD 3.2) who were matched by mental age with 20 typically developing children (mean chronological age, 4.9 years, SD 1.8), and 12 cognitively impaired children (mean chronological age, 12.2 years, SD 1.5), the children with autism had a more ambiguous handedness compared to children from the other two groups (McManus et al., 1992). They compared children with autism and cognitive impairment, and those who are typically developing in the areas of hand skill and hand preference showed that children with autism had higher degrees of ambiguous handedness and skill-preference discordance. Sixty-five percent of children with autism were more skilled with their left hands; however, 50% (10 subjects) chose to use their lesser skilled hand as the preferred hand, so had discordance between skill and preference. In the typical group, only 10% (two subjects) of the typical children and only 8% (one subject) of the children with cognitive impairment were discordant.

In another study comparing 35 cognitively impaired children with autism, 26 with learning disabilities, and 89 who were typically developing, subjects were from two age groups, one from 3 to 5 years and another from 11 to 13 years (Cornish & McManus, 1996). The children with autism or learning disabilities showed more ambiguous handedness than did the typically developing children. Results of the Annett Pegboard Test and 10 unimanual tasks indicated that the degree and consistency of hand preference of those with autism was significantly different from that of typically developing children, showing a higher left-hand preference, especially with the younger subjects.

Handedness in high-functioning autism. Escalante-Mead et al. (2003) studied 47 individuals with high-functioning autism who did not have a history of disordered early language development (mean age, 16.85 years), 22 individuals with high-functioning autism without a history of disordered early language development (mean age, 18.42 years), and 112 typically developing individuals (mean age, 18.82 years), using the Edinburgh Handedness Inventory (Oldfield, 1971), a self-report measure of 23 tasks. In this group of subjects, a criterion of 17 (74%) of the 23 items needing to be performed by one hand was used to determine the presence of a lateral dominance. Both groups of subjects with high-functioning autism had lower rates of right-handedness and higher rates of ambiguous handedness compared to the typically developing group, with the disordered early language development group having significantly greater differences. However, with the high criterion for handedness, an increased left-handedness, which had been seen in many other studies, was not seen with this group. No examination of performance handedness was included in this study, so skill-preference discordance was not examined.

Relationships between handedness and skill performance. Hauck and Dewey (2001) examined the relationship between ambiguous handedness and cognitive, language, and motor skills in a group of young children. They examined three groups of 20 subjects with autism (mean chronological age, 56.60 months; mean mental age, 27.46 months), developmental delay (mean chronological age, 57.35 months; mean mental age, 34.48 months), and typical development (mean chronological age, 33.25 months; mean mental age, 33.53 months). Subjects with developmental delay were matched to those with autism by mental and chronological age and typically developing subjects were matched by mental age. A 90% criterion was used to determine the presence of a lateral dominance or a preferred hand and very few subjects with autism qualified as being left-handed, so increased left-handedness was not found in this group. They found that children with ASD who had an ambiguous handedness performed more poorly on cognitive and language tasks than those who had a preferred hand (Hauck & Dewey, 2001). Children with autism who had not developed a hand preference had significantly lower fine motor skills compared to the children with autism who had a definite hand preference.

A trend toward a significant relationship was seen with gross motor skills in the children with autism. These relationships were not seen in the typical or developmentally delayed groups.

Fein et al. (1985), in a population of 75 cognitively impaired children with autism, found that left-handers did better than right-handers on cognitive tests, while children with ambiguous dominance did the poorest. Tsai (1983) found similarly, in an earlier study, that among 70 children with a wide IQ range, those with a definite handedness tended to function better in intelligence, language, and visuospatial abilities. Lucas, Rosenstein, and Bigler (1989) examined 238 cognitively impaired subjects without autism between ages 11 and 82 and found that left-handedness was associated with poor language in those individuals.

Neurological Explanation for Motor Impairment

Several studies have proposed neurological explanations for motor impairment in children with ASD. Gidley Larson, Bastian, Donchin, Shadmehr, and Mostofsky (2008) echo earlier beliefs of Ayres (1985) that the ability to process and integrate sensation forms the basis for the development of body scheme or internal model. This allows the individual to predict the sensory consequences of motor commands and learn from errors to improve performance on the next attempt and indicates an important role of sensory processing in motor performance.

The cerebellum appears to be one of the key structures involved in forming accurate internal models (Lang & Bastian, 1999; Martin, Keating, Goodkin, Bastian, & Thach, 1996; Maschke, Gomez, Ebner, & Konczak, 2004). Examination of the cerebellum, both in postmortem and imaging studies, suggests an abnormal development of the cerebellum in individual with autism (Bauman & Kemper, 1994; Ritvo et al., 1986; Williams, Hause, Purpura, DeLong, & Swisher, 1980). Mostofsky, Burgess, and Gidley Larson (2007) found that children with autism showed a positive correlation between total motor score and left hemisphere primary motor and premotor white matter volumes such that increased white matter volume predicted poorer motor skill, which directly contrasts with typically developing children. Haswell, Izawa, Dowell, Mostofsky, and Shadmehr (2009) found that greater reliance on proprioception by ASD children was associated with greater social and imitation impairment. Decreased connectivity and cerebellar activity were seen during motor activities in children with ASD (Mostofsky et al., 2009).

Evidence supporting this sensory motor mapping mechanism came from the discovery of mirror neurons that fired when monkeys either performed a given motor act or observed another individual performing the same or similar motor act (Rizzolatti, Fabbri-Destro, & Cattaneo, 2009). Another explanation for motor planning and movement adjustment problems is that poor executive function reduces the ability to plan movements (Booth, Charlton, Hughes, & Happe, 2003).

Motor Assessments

Motor assessments appropriate for children with ASD are varied by age group and psychometric strength. Unlike the sensory assessments, many of the motor assessments are standardized quantitative observational measures. Table 11.2 provides a list of some of the more commonly used assessments.

Sensory and Motor Intervention

Issues with sensory responsiveness and motor impairment are often addressed by occupational or physical therapists. It is important that sensory and motor interventions target changes in the child's ability to participate in meaningful activities or occupations, such as play or leisure, self-care, school, and social activities, and the changes effected by intervention should support that participation. The most common therapeutic approaches used for sensory and motor intervention in children with ASD are sensory integration, other sensory interventions, acquisitional, behavioral, environmental, task expectation, cognitive, and client centered. Descriptions of interventions based on these approaches follow.

Sensory Integration Approach

A sensory integration approach is often appropriate when the child demonstrates difficulties in sensory processing or motor impairment (Schaaf et al., 2010). Ayres (1972) defined sensory integration as "the neurological process that organizes sensation from one's own body and from the environment and makes it possible to use the body effectively within the environment" (p. 11). Based on this frame of reference, certain types of sensory experiences, including deep pressure, proprioception (e.g., muscle resistance, joint traction, and compression), and vestibular input, have been suggested for reducing sensory defensive responses in children (Wilbarger & Wilbarger, 2002). Outcome studies of the impact of sensory integration intervention are limited, but it has been shown to reduce sensory modulation problems in children with autism (Fazlioglu & Baran, 2008). Positive changes were seen in social interaction, purposeful play, and decreased sensitivity in three small studies of children with

autism (Ayres & Tickle, 1980; Case-Smith & Bryan, 1999; Lindermann & Stewart, 1999). It has also been shown to improve fine and gross motor skills, upper limb coordination, and sensory integrative functioning in children with mild cognitive impairment (Wuang, Wang, Huang, & Su, 2009), to improve the child's ability to participate in home, school, and family activities in two small studies of children with poor sensory processing (Miller, Coll, & Schoen, 2007; Schaaf & Nightlinger, 2007), and to improve behavior regulation in a child with sensory modulation disorder (Roberts, King-Thomas, & Boccia, 2007).

To qualify as a sensory integration approach, the intervention must include the following qualities: (1) provide sensory opportunities in more than one sensory modality (tactile, vestibular, and proprioceptive), (2) provide activities that present challenges to the child that are neither too difficult nor too easy, (3) collaborate on activity choice with the child, (4) support and guide the child's self-organization of behavior to make choices and plan own behavior, (5) ensure that the therapy situation is conducive to attaining or sustaining the child's optimal level of arousal, (6) create a context of play by building on the child's intrinsic motivation and enjoyment of activities, (7) maximize the child's success, (8) ensure that the child is physically safe, (9) arrange the room and equipment to motivate the child to choose and engage in an activity, and (10) foster a therapeutic alliance and create a climate of trust and emotional safety with the child (Parham et al., 2007). Sensory activities that do not meet these criteria are not considered under the strict definition of sensory integration.

Other Sensory Intervention Approaches

Other intervention approaches that are sensory based would be classified in the category of sensory intervention but would not be included under the stricter definition of sensory integration intervention (Parham et al., 2007). These might be included in a sensory diet and consist of activities that provide a variety of sensory input.

Sensory activities, sometimes referred to as *sensory strategies or a sensory diet*, can be used to gain and maintain regulation of the child's arousal state. These strategies are carefully designed, personalized activity plan that provides the sensory input a person needs to stay focused and organized throughout the day. They might include various activities that involve tactile, vestibular, and proprioceptive sensory input, such as exercise, slow rhythmic rocking, deep pressure massage, gum chewing, wearing of a weighted vest or a hug vest, or a brushing protocol (Fertel-Daly, Bedell, & Hinojosa, 2001; Hall & Case-Smith, 2007; VandenBerg, 2001). Just as one person may jiggle his or her knee, chew gum to stay awake, or soak in a hot tub to unwind, children

Table 11.2 Motor assessments

Assessment	Age group	Properties
Pediatric Evaluation of Disability Inventory (PEDI; Haley, Coster, Ludlow, Haltiwanger, & Andrellos, 1992)	Birth to school age	Norm- and criterion-referenced assessment of functional ability as reported by caregiver or teacher Includes caregiver assistance score and modifications needed
Peabody Developmental Motor Scales, 2nd Ed. (PDMS2; Folio & Fewell, 2000)	0–5 years, 11 months	Norm- and criterion-referenced scores for gross and fine motor skills. Also provides educational and therapeutic programming
Vineland II Adaptive Behavior Scales (Sparrow, Cicchetti, & Balla, 2005)	Birth to adult	Parent/teacher interview that derives norm-referenced adaptive behavior scores for communication, socialization, daily living skills, and motor skills. Additionally, maladaptive behavior is scored
Bayley Scales of Infant and Toddler Development – III (Bayley III; Bayley, 2006)	1–42 months	Norm-referenced scales for cognitive, language, motor, social–emotional, and adaptive behavior
Toddler and Infant Motor Evaluation (TIME; Miller & Roid, 1994)	2–42 months	Norm- and criterion-referenced observational assessment of quality of movement, specifically mobility, the ability to move the body from one position to another, and stability, the dynamic control of the body within positions or during locomotion
Quality of Upper Extremity Skills Test (QUEST; DeMatteo et al., 1993)	18 months to 8 years	Criterion-referenced observational assessment designed with minimal developmental sequencing so that scoring reflects the severity of the disability rather than age Scores are calculated as percentages with a maximum score of 100
The Miller Function and Participation Scales (M-FUN; Miller, 2006)	2 years, 6 months to 7 years, 11 months	Norm-referenced observational assessment of functional tasks needed to successfully participate in classroom and school activities. Addresses participation, activity, and body function. Scores are derived for fine motor, gross motor, and visual motor scales. Parent and teacher questionnaires are included
Miller Assessment for Preschoolers (MAP; Miller, 1982)	2 years, 9 months to 5 years, 8 months	Norm-referenced observational assessment of school readiness for sensory, motor, and cognitive skills to identify potential learning problems
Test of Gross Motor Development (TGMD) (Ulrich, 1985)	3–10 years	Standardized observational assessment of 12 fundamental movement skill items with 3–4 observable criteria specified for each movement skill. Criteria are based upon typical movement patterns identified from motor development literature and consensus among content experts. Skills are divided into two subtests: locomotion and object control
Movement Assessment Battery for Children (MABC; Henderson & Sugden, 1992)	4–12 years	Norm-referenced observational assessment of impairment of motor function. Categorical scores are derived for manual dexterity, ball skills, and static and dynamic balance. A teacher checklist and remedial activities are included
Bruininks Oseretsky Test of Motor Proficiency, 2nd Ed. (BOT2; Bruininks & Bruininks, 2005)	4–21 years	Individually administered direct assessment that generates gender-specific motor area composite scores, scale scores, standard scores, and percentile ranks for fine manual control, manual coordination, body coordination, and strength and agility, and a full motor composite score
Physical & Neurological Assessment of Subtle Signs (PANESS; Denckla, 1985)	4–21 years	Neurological examination for children used to evaluate subtle neurological signs, which is standardized for age, sex, and handedness. It includes a lateral preference assessment, measures of axial motor skill, and measures of appendicular (limb) motor skill. It also includes scores for balance, speed of repetitive timed movements, speed of patterned timed movements, dysrhythmia, overflow, gaits, and impersistence
Sensory Processing Measure – Home Form (Parham & Ecker, 2007)	5–12 years	75-Item questionnaire. Raw scores and T scores for total and seven sensory categories (social participation, vision, hearing, touch, body awareness, balance and motion, and planning and ideas). Standard scores allow classification into typical, some problems, and definite dysfunction. Norm referenced on over 1,000 children. It is unique in that it was standardized in both the home and the main classroom with all the same students making those environments statistically comparable. And it is also unique in that it includes separate environment forms for the art, music, PE, recess, cafeteria, and bus environments
Sensory Processing Measure – School Environments Forms (Kuhaneck et al., 2007)	5–12 years	62-Item questionnaire. Raw scores and T scores for total and seven sensory categories (social participation, vision, hearing, touch, body awareness, balance and motion, and planning and ideas). Standard scores allow classification into typical, some problems, and definite dysfunction

Table 11.2 (continued)

Assessment	Age group	Properties
Developmental Coordination Disorder Questionnaire 2007 (DCDQ'07; Wilson, Kaplan, Crawford, & Roberts, 2007)	5–15 years	15-Item questionnaire for caregivers who rate the children on particular motor skills on a five-level scale
		Standardized for categorical scoring for control during movement, fine motor/handwriting, and general coordination. Categories are in three age groups and consist of indication or DCD or suspect DCD and probably not DCD
Gesture Test (Cermak, Coster, & Drake, 1980)	9–13 years (in study)	Non-standardized observational assessment contains two components, each comprising 10 items. The first component includes tasks that require the subject to mime the use of specified tools (representational actions). The second requires the imitation of non-meaningful actions (non-representational actions). On both components of the test, actions/gestures are scored on a four-point scale

often need to engage in stabilizing, focusing activities too. Infants, young children, teens, and adults with mild to severe sensory issues can each benefit from a personalized sensory diet. Listening programs may be included in sensory interventions (Hall & Case-Smith, 2007). A small study examining the effect of a sensory diet and therapeutic listening showed significant improvement in visual perception and writing legibility and sensory responsiveness (Hall & Case-Smith, 2007). Use of weighted vests resulted in improved attention to task and reduced self-stimulatory behaviors in two small studies (Fertel-Daly et al., 2001; Hall & Case-Smith, 2007; VandenBerg, 2001). Results from the seven small studies that have been done on the impact of weighted vests, however, are equivocal, so the value of their impact is not clear (Stephenson & Carter, 2009). Use of enhanced proprioceptive input through seating on therapy balls was shown to increase staying in seats and writing legibility for school-age students with attention-deficit hyperactivity disorder (Schilling, Washington, Billingsley, & Deitz, 2003) and ASD (Schilling & Schwartz, 2004).

Acquisitional Approaches

Acquisitional. One of the assumptions of the acquisitional frame of reference is that humans acquire skills through repetition and practice with appropriate reinforcement within a particular environment (Kandel, 2006; Luebben & Royeen, 2010). An approach based on this frame of reference is frequently used with children who have an ASD diagnosis to acquire new skills, such as motor skills. It is important to break the task down into smaller pieces that provide some challenge to the child, but are not unreasonable. Finding a reinforcement that is effective for a child with ASD may be challenging.

Motor skill acquisition. The motor skill acquisition frame of reference defines the continua of function and dysfunction by the performance in the specific skill to be acquired (Kaplan, 2010). It assumes that functional tasks help organize behavior and that motor problems observed are the result

of all systems interacting and compensating for some damage or problem in one or more of those systems. Motor skill acquisition would result from the combination of the child's abilities, the task demands, and the supports and constraints of the environment.

Handwriting. The handwriting frame of reference assumes that functional visual perceptual skills are prerequisite skills for good handwriting and that good posture and good proximal control are necessary for good handwriting (Roston, 2010). It identifies practice as the single most important factor for learning a new skill and that to make the motor skill more accurate, it needs to be practiced in varied conditions with varied sensory input. Handwriting intervention has resulted in improved letter legibility in children with handwriting problems (Case-Smith, 2002; Denton, Cope, & Moser, 2006) and in children at risk for handwriting problems (Marr & Dimeo, 2006), and improved fine motor and graphomotor skills in children who had poor visual–motor scores (Ratzon, Efraim, & Bart, 2007). In other studies of students receiving occupational therapy services, improvement was seen in fine motor skills (Bazyk et al., 2009), and in fine motor skills, self-care, and mobility (Case-Smith, 1996).

Behavioral Approach

As with other areas of deficit for children with ASD, the use of a behavioral approach is very important. Behaviorism, founded by psychologist B. F. Skinner (1976), suggests that all behaviors are a response to an environmental stimulus and that behavior is reinforced by environmental consequences that follow. Behavior modification is a technique of altering an individual's reaction to stimuli through positive reinforcement and the extinction of maladaptive behavior. A measurable system of rewards and punishments needs to be established to focus specifically on behavior. The system encourages using positive reinforcement only, thus lessening the emphasis on negative behavior and is another common model used to promote the development of many skills of children with ASD.

Environment and Task Expectation Approaches

Several occupational therapy models of practice suggest that occupational performance (performance of a meaningful activity) is dependent on environmental demands or expectations (Baum & Christiansen, 2005; Dunn, Brown, & McGuigan, 1994; Law et al., 1996). These models view the environment as a potential enabler or inhibiter to performance. Changes in the environment through modification or adaptation can support the sensory modulation and motor skills in children with an ASD (Rigby & Letts, 2003). For example, the expectation of the task can be adapted with shoes that do not need to be tied or pants with an elastic waist instead of snaps or buttons for children who do not have adequate fine motor skills to perform these tasks. The sensory environment as it relates to light, sound, and touch may also be modified to reduce aversive stimuli for the child. A study using a weighted or hugging vest, along with lighting and auditory adaptations to the environment, found significantly reduced anxiety levels in children with and without disabilities during potentially stress-provoking medical situations (Shapiro, Sgan-Cohen, Parush, & Melmed, 2009).

Cognitive Approaches

Several types of intervention programs use a cognitive approach to help children recognize, quantify, and describe different levels or intensities of their emotions and behaviors that can enable them to modulate their responses to various situations and types of sensory input. These self-regulation tools can help children identify and recognize different degrees of specific behaviors or feelings that they may be experiencing or exhibiting. These tools can address behaviors, such as voice volume or aggressive behaviors, or feelings, such as stress level, anger level, or obsessions or compulsions (how frequently they are thinking about something or engaging in a certain behavior). Increasing the child's awareness of the feeling or behavior is believed to support the child's ability to change it and initial evidence supporting this concept is encouraging (Barnes, Vogel, Beck, Schoenfeld, & Owen, 2008; Berger, Kofman, Livneh, & Henik, 2007). Cognitive approaches can also be used in motor skill acquisition.

Alert Program. The Alert Program (Williams & Shellenberger, 1996) uses the analogy of an automobile engine to identify the child's level of excitability – high, low, or just right. Children use this understanding and various sensory input to work on self-regulation of their own levels of excitability. Use of the Alert Program resulted in improved self-regulation, behavioral adjustments, and sensory processing skills per self-report in a small group of school children diagnosed with emotional disturbance (Barnes et al., 2008).

Thermometers. For the anger or stress thermometer, the therapist gives the child a template for a thermometer with graded levels of anger or stress (McAfee, 2002). It may include 4–10 levels, depending on the understanding of the child. The therapist can list the emotions for the child (e.g., calm, irritated, furious, enraged), and the child can look for pictures of faces in a magazine to match those emotions. The child may code the thermometer with colors, according to the emotion. He or she may also use special interests as themes for the thermometer, such as weather (with "Tornadoes" at the top level and "Calm and breezy" at the bottom) or dinosaurs (with "*Tyrannosaurus rex*" at the top and "Pterodactyl" at the bottom). The therapist and the child can then determine where the child's level of anger fits on the thermometer during a specific situation.

Incredible 5-Point Scale. The Incredible 5-Point Scale (Buron & Curtis, 2003) organizes behaviors, such as voice volume, along a five-point continuum. The scales can be used to help children better understand the social impact of their behaviors, to regulate their responses, and to calm themselves when they over-respond. Like thermometers, the scales should be introduced at a quiet time after an event in which the child had difficulty with regulation. The scale can be used by the therapist to quantify the behavior and to give the child a way to communicate about the behavior in a quantifiable way. For example, if a child has difficulty with being too loud, a voice volume scale can help the child with understanding the need to modulate his or her vocal volume. The therapist can orient the child to the scale and coach him or her by demonstrating the different vocal levels represented on the scale. Then, the scale should be shared with others who will interact with the child, including parents and teachers who can then use the scale and give the child feedback about his or her volume level when it is not appropriate for the situation.

Sensory stories. Sensory stories are stories written to help guide children in coping with their sensory modulation issues. They encourage the children to employ calming strategies (see other sensory interventions) throughout the course of the day that can help them to feel calmer during stressful activities. Stressful activities may include transitions between classes, attendance at a student assembly, or going to the dentist. Results of a small study examining its effect on behavior of children with autism during preschool showed positive results (Marr, Mika, Miraglia, Roerig, & Sinnott, 2007).

CO-OP Program. Cognitive Orientation for daily Occupational Performance (CO-OP) is a client-centered, cognitive approach to acquisition of skills necessary for specific occupations, such as play, writing, or jumping rope. Children are taught a global problem-solving framework and are guided to discover domain-specific strategies to enable mastery of skills that they have chosen (Polatajko, Mandich, & Martini, 2000). Its use was shown to be successful in the acquisition of new motor skills, to overcome organizational and social–emotional difficulties, and for generalization and transfer of skills in two siblings with Asperger syndrome (Rodger, Springfield, & Polatajko, 2007).

Client-Centered Approaches

Client-centered practice is based on developing a partnership with the recipients of the services in determining and carrying out the goals and intervention (Law, Baptiste, & Mills, 1995). For children, this typically involves collaboration with the child and his or her parents in identifying priorities for goals and interventions that are the most practical. In addition to the CO-OP Program (see above for details.), use of a client-centered approach was found to be effective in the improvement of motor and process skills in children with developmental disabilities (Kang et al., 2008).

Conclusion

Sensory processing and motor issues in ASD are very complex and there is a clear need for more in-depth examination of their neurobiological and behavioral bases. Even though neither has been identified as a core characteristic of the autistic syndrome, new evidence suggests that this possibility for each may need to be reconsidered. Assessment of sensory responsiveness is in an early stage and attention to development of a more comprehensive, age-inclusive standardized observational measure would support a higher level of examination and understanding. Unusual sensory responsiveness is often among the first indicators of autism noticed by parents and therefore may be useful to facilitate early diagnosis and intervention (Baker et al., 2008). The earlier a disorder is recognized, the earlier a child is able to receive help, and the more effective outcome can be achieved. In addition, the relationship between sensory processing and other autistic traits seems more important than previously recognized and addressing sensory processing issues in children with ASD may be more critical than previously understood.

Similar to the paucity of evidence illuminating the mechanism for atypical sensory processing issues in ASD, the effects of intervention are not well documented. For example, the value of knowing the sensory predictors of social severity would be increased by knowing how they can be altered and how social severity changes as a result of sensory responsiveness changes. In addition, acuity differences in children with ASD may impact sensory responsiveness and continued investigation across senses may continue to provide implications for further understanding of sensory processing.

References

American Psychiatric Association. (2000). *Diagnostic and statistical manual-text revision.* Chicago: Author.

Annett, M. (1970). The growth of manual preference and speed. *British Journal of Psychology, 61,* 545–588.

Annett, M. (1985). *Left, right, hand and brain: The right shift theory.* Hillsdale, NJ: Erlbaum.

Archer, L. A., Rosenbaum, P. L., & Streiner, D. L. (1991). The children's eating behavior inventory. *Journal of Pediatric Psychology, 16,* 629–642.

Ashburner, J., Ziviani, J., & Rodger, S. (2008). Sensory processing and classroom emotional, behavioral, and educational outcomes in children with autism spectrum disorder. *American Journal of Occupational Therapy, 62,* 564–573.

Ashwin, E., Ashwin, C., Rhydderch, D., Howells, J., & Baron-Cohen, S. (2009). Eagle-eyed visual acuity: An experimental investigation of enhanced perception in autism. *Biological Psychiatry, 65,* 17–21.

Asperger, H. (1944/1991). "Autistic psychopathy" in childhood. (U. Frith, Trans, Annot.). In U. Frith (Ed.), *Autism and Asperger syndrome* (pp. 37–92). New York: Cambridge University Press (Original work published in 1944).

Ayres, A. J. (1972). *Sensory integration and learning disorders.* Los Angeles: Western Psychological Services.

Ayres, A. (1985). *Developmental dyspraxia and adult-onset apraxia.* Torrance, CA: Sensory Integration International.

Ayres, A. J. (1989). *Sensory integration and praxis test (SIPT).* Los Angeles: Western Psychological Services.

Ayres, A. J., & Tickle, L. (1980). Hyperresponsivity to touch and vestibular stimuli as a predictor of positive response to sensory integration procedures in autistic children. *American Journal of Occupational Therapy, 34,* 375–381.

Baier, B., Kleinschmidt, A., & Muller, N. G. (2006). Cross-modal processing in early visual and auditory cortices depends on expected statistical relationship of multisensory information. *The Journal of Neuroscience, 26*(47), 12260–12265.

Baker, A. E. Z., Lane, A., Angley, M. T., & Young, R. L. (2008). The relationship between sensory processing patterns and behavioural responsiveness in autistic disorder: A pilot study. *Journal Autism and Developmental Disorders, 38,* 867–875.

Bar-Shalita, T., Goldstand, S., Hann-Markowitz, J., & Parush, S. (2005). Typical children's responsivity patterns of the tactile and vestibular systems. *American Journal of Occupational Therapy, 59*(2), 148–156.

Baranek, G. T. (1997). *Tactile defensiveness & discrimination test–revised.* Unpublished manuscript, University of North Carolina at Chapel Hill, NC.

Baranek, G. T. (1999a). *Sensory processing assessment for young children (SPA).* Unpublished manuscript, University of North Carolina at Chapel Hill, NC.

Baranek, G. T. (1999b). Autism during infancy: A retrospective video analysis of sensory-motor and social behaviors at 9–12 months of age. *Journal of Autism and Developmental Disorders, 29,* 213–224.

Baranek, G. T., & Berkson, G. (1994). Tacrile defensiveness in children with developmental disabilities: Responsiveness and habiruarion. *Journal of Autism and Developmental Disorders, 24,* 457–471.

Baranek, G. T., Chin, Y. H., Hess, L. M. G., Yankee, J. G., Hatton, D. D., & Hooper, S. R. (2002). Sensory processing correlates of occupational performance in children with fragile X syndrome: Preliminary findings. *American Journal of Occupational Therapy, 56,* 538–546.

Baranek, G., David, F., Poe, M., Stone, W., & Watson, L. (2006). Sensory experiences questionnaire: Discriminating sensory features in young children with autism, developmental delays, and typical development. *Journal of Child Psychology & Psychiatry, 47*(6), 591–601.

Baranek, G., Foster, L. G., & Berkson, G. (1997). Tactile defensiveness and stereotyped behaviors. *American Journal of Occupational Therapy, 51*, 91–95.

Barnes, K. J., Vogel, K. A., Beck, A. J., Schoenfeld, H. B., & Owen, S. V. (2008). Self-regulation strategies of children with emotional disturbance. *Physical and Occupational Therapy in Pediatrics, 28*, 369–387.

Baron-Cohen, S., Ashwin, E., Ashwin, C., Tavassoli, T., & Chakrabarti, B. (2009). Talent in autism: Hyper-systemizing, hyper-attention to detail and sensory hypersensitivity. *Philosophical Transactions of the Royal Society B, 364*, 1377–1383.

Baum, C. M., & Christiansen, C. H. (2005). Person-environment-occupation-performance: An occupation-based framework for practice. In C. Christiansen, C. Baum & J. Bass-Haugen (Eds.), *Occupational therapy: Performance, participation, and well-being* (pp. 242–267). Thorofare, NJ: Slack.

Bauman, M. L., & Kemper, T. L. (1994). *Neuroanatomic observation of the brain in autism*. Baltimore: The Johns Hopkins University Press.

Bayley, N. (2006). *Bayley scales of infant and toddler development* (3rd ed.). San Antonio, TX: Pearson.

Bazyk, S., Michaud, P., Goodman, G., Papp, P., Hawkins, E., & Welch, M. A. (2009). Integrating occupational therapy services in a kindergarten curriculum: A look at the outcomes. *American Journal of Occupational Therapy, 63*, 160–171.

Ben-Sasson, A., Cermak, S. A., Orsmond, G. I., Tager-Flusberg, H., Carter, A. S., Kadlec, M. B., et al. (2007). Extreme sensory modulation behaviors in toddlers with autism spectrum disorders. *The American Journal of Occupational Therapy, 61*(5), 584–592.

Bennetto, L., Kuschner, E. S., & Hyman, S. L. (2007). Olfaction and taste processing in autism. *Biological Psychiatry, 62*, 1015–1021.

Berger, A., Kofman, O., Livneh, U., & Henik, A. (2007). Multidisciplinary perspectives on attention and the development of self-regulation. *Progress in Neurobiology, 82*, 256–286.

Bishop, D. V. M. (1990). *Handedness and developmental disorder*. Oxford: Mac Keith Press.

Blakemore, S. J., Tavassoli, T., Calo, S., Thomas, R., Catmur, C., Frith, U., et al. (2006). Tactile sensitivity in Asperger syndrome. *Brain and Cognition, 61*, 5–13.

Boddaert, N., Chabane, N., Belin, P., Bourgeois, M., Roye, V., Barthelemy, C., et al. (2004). Perception of complex sounds in autism: Abnormal auditory cortical processing in children. *American Journal of Psychiatry, 161*(11), 2117–2120.

Booth, R., Charlton, R., Hughes, C., & Happe, F. (2003). Disentangling weak coherence and executive dysfunction: Planning drawing in autism and attention-deficit/hyperactivity disorder. *Philosophical Transactions of the Royal Society of London B, 358*, 387–392.

Brown, C. E., & Dunn, W. (2002). *Adolescent/adult sensory profile*. San Antonio, TX: The Psychological Corporation.

Brown, M., & Gordon, W. A. (1987). Impact of impairment on activity patterns of children. *Archives of Physical Medicine and Rehabilitation, 68*, 828–832.

Bruininks, R. (1978). *Bruininks Oseretsky test of motor proficiency*. Circle Pines, MN: American Guidance Service.

Bruininks, R. H., & Bruininks, B. D. (2005). *Bruininks-Oseretsky test of motor proficiency* (2nd ed.). Minneapolis, MN: Pearson.

Bryson, S. (1990). Autism and anomalous handedness. *Behavioral Implications and Anomalies, 15*, 441–456.

Bundy, A., Lane, S., & Murray, E. (2002). *Sensory integration: Theory and practice*. Philadelphia: F. A. Davis.

Bundy, A. C., Shia, S., Qi, L., & Miller, L. J. (2007). How sensory processing dysfunction affects play? *The American Journal of Occupational Therapy, 61*, 201–208.

Buron, K. D., & Curtis, M. (2003). *The incredible 5-point scale: Assisting students with autism spectrum disorders in* understanding social interactions and controlling their emotional responses. Shawnee Mission, Kansas: Autism Asperger Publishing Co.

Casanova, M. F. (2007). The neuropathology of autism. *Brian Pathology, 17*, 422–433.

Casanova, M. F., Buxhoeveden, D. P., Switala, A. E., & Roy, E. (2002). Minicolumnar pathology in autism. *Neurology, 58*, 428–432.

Cascio, C., McGlone, F., Folger, S., Tannan, V., Baranek, G., Pelphrey, K., et al. (2008). Tactile perception in adults with autism: A multidimensional psychophysical study. *Journal of Autism and Developmental Disorders, 38*, 127–137.

Case-Smith, J. (1996). Fine motor outcomes in preschool children who receive occupational therapy services. *American Journal of Occupational Therapy., 50*(1), 52–61.

Case-Smith, J. (2002). Effectiveness of school-based occupational therapy intervention on handwriting. *American Journal of Occupational Therapy., 56*, 17–25.

Case-Smith, J., & Bryan, T. (1999). The effects of occupational therapy with sensory integration emphasis on preschool-age children with autism. *American Journal of Occupational Therapy, 53*, 489–497.

Cavill, S., & Bryden, P. (2003). Development of handedness: Comparison of questionnaire and performance-based measures of preference. *Brain and Cognition, 53*, 149–151.

Cermak, S. A., Coster, W., & Drake, C. (1980). Representational and nonrepresentational gestures in boys with learning disabilities. *American Journal of Occupational Therapy, 34*, 19–26.

Cesaroni, L., & Garber, M. (1991). Exploring the experience of autism through firsthand accounts. *Journal of Autism and Developmental Disorders, 21*, 303–313.

Church, C., Alisanski, S., & Amanullah, S. (1999). The social, behavioral, and academic experiences of children with Asperger syndrome. *Focus on Autism and Other Developmental Disabilities, 15*(1), 12–20.

Cornish, K. M., & McManus, I. C. (1996). Hand preference and hand skill in children with autism. *Journal of Autism and Developmental Disorders, 26*(6), 597–609.

Coskun, M. A., Varghese, L., Reddoch, S., Castillo, E. M., Pearson, D. A., Loveland, K. A., et al. (2009). How somatic cortical maps differ in autistic and typical brains. *NeuroReport, 20*, 175–179.

Dahlgren, S. O., & Gillberg, C. (1989). Symptoms in the first two years of life: A preliminary population study of infantile autism. *European Archives of Psychiatry Neurological Sciences, 238*, 169–174.

Dane, S., & Balci, N. (2007). Handedness, eyedness and nasal cycle in children with autism. *International Journal of Developmental Neuroscience, 25*, 223–226.

Dawson, G., Warrenburg, S., & Fuller, P. (1983). Hemisphere functioning and motor imitation in autistic persons. *Brain and Cognition, 2*, 346–354.

DeGangi, G. A., & Berk, R. A. (1983). *DeGangi-Berk test of sensory integration (TSI)*. Los Angeles: Western Psychological.

DeGangi, G. A., & Greenspan, S. (1989). *Test of sensory functions in infants*. Los Angeles: Western Psychological.

DeMatteo, C., Law, M., Russell, D., Pollock, N., Rosenbaum, P., & Walter, S. (1993). The reliability and validity of the quality of upper extremity skills test. *Physical and Occupational Therapy in Pediatrics, 13*, 1–18.

Denckla, M. B. (1985). Revised neurological examination for subtle signs. *Psychopharmacology Bulletin, 21*, 773–800.

Denton, P. L., Cope, S., & Moser, C. (2006). The effects of sensorimotor-based intervention versus therapeutic practice on improving handwriting performance in 6- to 11-year-old children. *American Journal of Occupational Therapy., 60*(1), 16–27.

Dewey, D., Cantell, M., & Crawford, S. G. (2007). Motor and gestural performance in children with autism spectrum disorders, developmental coordination disorder, and/or attention deficit hyperactivity disorder. *Journal of the International Neuropsychological Society*, *13*, 246–256.

Dickie, V. A., Baranek, G. T., Schultz, B., Watson, L. R., & McComish, C. S. (2009). Parent reports of sensory experiences of preschool children with and without autism: A qualitative study. *American Journal of Occupational Therapy, 63*, 172–181.

Dunn, W. (1997). The impact of sensory processing abilities on the daily lives of young children and their families: A conceptual model. *Infants and Young Children, 9*, 23–35.

Dunn, W. (1999). *Sensory profile user's manual*. San Antonio, TX: The Psychological Corporation.

Dunn, W. (2002). *Infant/Toddler sensory profile user's manual*. San Antonio, TX: The Psychological Corporation.

Dunn, W. (2006). *Sensory profile school companion user's manual*. San Antonio, TX: The Psychological Corporation.

Dunn, W., Brown, C., & McGuigan, A. (1994). The ecology of human performance: A framework for considering the effect of context. *American Journal of Occupational Therapy, 48*, 595–607.

Dunn, W., Myles, B. S., & Orr, S. (2002). Sensory processing issues associated with Asperger's syndrome: A preliminary report. *American Journal of Occupational Therapy, 56*(1), 97–102.

Dunn, W., Saiter, J., & Rinner, L. (2002). Asperger Syndrome and Sensory Processing: A conceptual model and guidance for intervention planning. *Focus on Autism and Developmental Disabilities, 17*(3), 172–185.

Dzuik, M. A., Gidley-Larson, J. C., Mahone, E. M., Denckla, M. B., & Mostofsky, S. H. (2007). Dyspraxia in autism: Association with motor, social and communicative deficits. *Developmental Medicine & Child Neurology, 49*, 734–739.

Ermer, J., & Dunn, W. (1998). The Sensory Profile: A discriminant analysis of children with and without disabilities. *American Journal of Occupational Therapy, 52*(4), 283–290.

Escalante-Mead, P. R., Minshew, N. J., & Sweeney, J. A. (2003). Abnormal brain lateralization in high-functioning autism. *Journal of Autism and Developmental Disorders, 33*(5), 539–543.

Fabbri-Destro, M., Cattaneo, L., Boria, S., & Rizzolatti, G. (2009). Planning actions in autism. *Experimental Brain Research, 192*, 521–525.

Fan, X., Miles, J., Takahashi, N., & Yao, G. (2009). Abnormal transient pupillary light reflex in individuals with autism spectrum disorders. *Journal of Autism and Developmental Disorders, 39*(11), 1499–1508.

Fazlioglu, Y., & Baran, G. (2008). A sensory integration therapy program on sensory problems for children with autism. *Perceptual and Motor Skills, 106*, 415–422.

Fein, D., Humes, M., Kaplan, E., Lucci, D., & Waterhouse, L. (1984). The question of left-hemisphere dysfunction in infantile autism. *Psychological Bulletin, 95*, 258–281.

Fein, D., Waterhouse, L., Lucci, D., Pennington, B., & Humes, M. (1985). Handedness and cognitive functions in pervasive developmental disorders. *Journal of Autism and Developmental Disorders, 15*, 77–95.

Fertel-Daly, D., Bedell, G., & Hinojosa, J. (2001). Effects of a weighted vest on attention to task and self-stimulatory behaviors in preschoolers with pervasive developmental disorders. *American Journal of Occupational Therapy, 55*, 629–640.

Folio, M. R., & Fewell, R. R. (2000). *Peabody developmental motor scales: Examiner's manual*. Austin, TX: PROED.

Fournier, K. A., Hass, C. J., Lodha, N., & Cauraugh, J. H. (2010). Motor coordination in autism spectrum disorders: A synthesis and meta-analysis. *Journal of Autism and Developmental Disorders* [e-pub ahead of print]. doi: 10.1007/s10803-010-0981-3.

Frick, S. M., & Lawton-Shirley, N. (1994). Auditory integrative training from a sensory integrative training from a sensory integrative perspective. *Sensory Integration Special Interest Section Newsletter, 17*, 1–3.

Fuentes, C. T., Mostofsky, S. H., & Bastian, A. J. (2009). Children with autism show specific handwriting impairments. *Neurology, 73*, 1532–1537.

Gaines, E. C. (2002). The relationship between sensory processing and play in children with autistic spectrum disorders. *Dissertation Abstracts International: Section B; The Sciences and Engineering, 63*, 2055.

Gere, D. R., Capps, S. C., Mitchell, D. W., & Grubbs, E. (2009). Sensory sensitivities of gifted children. *American Journal of Occupational Therapy, 64*, 288–296.

Ghazuiddin, M., & Butler, E. (1998). Clumsiness in autism & AS: A further report. *Journal of Intellectual Disability Research, 42*(pt.1), 43–48.

Ghazuiddin, M., Butler, E., Tsai, L., & Ghazuiddin, N. (1994). Is clumsiness a marker for AS? *Journal of Intellectual Disability Research, 38*, 519–527.

Gidley Larson, J., Bastian, A., Donchin, O., Shadmehr, R., & Mostofsky, S. (2008). Acquisition of internal models of motor tasks in children with autism. *Brain, 131*, 2894–2903.

Gillberg, C. (1989). Asperger syndrome in 23 Swedish children. *Developmental Medicine & Child Neurology, 31*(4), 520–531.

Goldsmith, H. H. (1996). Studying temperament via construction of the Toddler Behavior Assessment Questionnaire. *Child Development, 67*, 218–235.

Goldsmith, H. H., Van Hulle, C. A., Arneson, C. L., Schreiber, J. E., & Gernsbacher, M. A. (2006). A population-based twin study of parentally reported tactile and auditory defensiveness in young children. *Journal of Abnormal Child Psychology, 34*, 393–407.

Green, D., Baird, G., Barnett, A., Henderson, L., Huber, J., & Henderson, S. (2002). The severity and nature of motor impairment in Asperger syndrome: A comparison with specific developmental disorder of motor function. *Journal of Child Psychology & Psychiatry, 43*(5), 655–668.

Green, D., Charman, T., Pickles, A., Chandler, S., Loucas, T., Simonoff, E., et al. (2009). Impairment in movement skills of children with autistic spectrum disorders. *Developmental Medicine & Child Neurology, 51*, 311–316.

Green, A. M., Shaikh, A. G., & Angelaki, D. E. (2005). Sensory vestibular contributions to constructing internal models of self-motion. *Journal of Neural Engineering, 2*, S164–S179.

Haley, S. M., Coster, W. J., Ludlow, L. H., Haltiwanger, J. T., & Andrellos, P. J. (1992). *Pediatric evaluation of disability inventory: Development, standardization and administration manual*. Boston: Trustees of Boston University.

Hall, L., & Case-Smith, J. (2007). The effect of sound-based intervention on children with sensory processing disorders and visual–motor delays. *American Journal of Occupational Therapy, 61*, 209–215.

Halpern, M. (1987). The organization and function of the vomeronasal system. *Annual Review of Neuroscience, 10*, 325–362.

Harrison, J., & Hare, D. J. (2004). Brief Report: Assessment of Sensory Abnormalities in People with Autistic Spectrum Disorders. *Journal of Autism and Developmental Disorders, 34*(6), 727–730.

Haswell, C. C., Izawa, J., Dowell, L. R., Mostofsky, S. H., & Shadmehr, R. (2009). Representation of internal models of action in the autistic brain. *Nature Neuroscience, 12*, 970–972.

Hauck, J. A., & Dewey, D. (2001). Hand preference and motor functioning in children with autism. *Journal of Autism and Developmental Disorders, 31*(3), 265–277.

Heaton, P., Hemelin, B., & Pring, L. (1998). Autism and pitch processing: A precursor for savant musical ability? *Music Perception, 15*, 291–305.

Henderson, S. E., & Sugden, D. (1992). *The movement assessment battery for children*. London: The Psychological Corporation.

Hilton, C. L., Crouch, M. C., & Israel, H. (2008). Out-of-school participation patterns in children with high functioning autism spectrum disorders. *American Journal of Occupational Therapy, 62*, 554–563.

Hilton, C. L., Graver, K., & LaVesser, P. (2007). Relationship between social competence and sensory processing in children with high functioning autism spectrum disorders. *Research in Autism Spectrum Disorders, 1*(2), 164–173.

Hilton, C. L., Harper, J., Kueker, R., Lang, A., Abbacchi, A., Todorov, A., & LaVesser, P. (2010). Sensory processing as a predictor of social severity in children with high functioning autism spectrum disorders. *Journal of Autism and Developmental Disorders, 40,* 937–945.

Hilton, C. L., Wente, L., LaVesser, P., Ito, M., Reed, C., & Herzberg, G. (2007). Relationship between motor skill impairment and severity in children with Asperger syndrome. *Research in Autism Spectrum Disorders, 1,* 339–349.

Hilton, C. L., Zhang, Y., White, M., & Constantino, J. N. (2010). *Motor impairment in sibling pairs concordant and discordant for autism.* Manuscript submitted for publication.

Jansiewicz, E. M., Goldberg, M. C., Newschaffer, C. J., Denckla, M. B., Landa, R., & Mostofsky, S. H. (2006). Motor signs distinguish children with high functioning autism and Asperger's syndrome from controls. *Journal of Autism and Developmental Disorders, 36,* 613–621.

Jasmin, E., Couture, M., McKinley, P., Reid, G., Fombonne, E., & Gisel, E. (2009). Sensori-motor and daily living skills of preschool children with autism spectrum disorders. *Journal of Autism and Developmental Disorders, 39,* 231–241.

Kandel, E. (2006). *In search of memory: The emergence of a new science of mind.* New York: W. W. Norton.

Kang, D. H., Yoo, E. Y., Chung, B. I., Jung, M. Y., Chang, K. Y., & Jeon, H. S. (2008). The application of client-centered occupational therapy for Korean children with developmental disabilities. *Occupational Therapy International, 15,* 253–268.

Kaplan, M. (2010). A frame of reference for motor skill acquisition. In P. Kramer & J. Hinojosa (Eds.), *Frames of reference for pediatric occupational therapy* (3rd ed., pp. 390–424). Baltimore: Lippincott, Williams & Wilkins.

Kern, J. K., Garver, C. R., Grannemann, B. D., Trivedi, M. H., Carmondy, T., Andrews, A. A., et al. (2007). Response to vestibular sensory events in autism. *Research in Autism Spectrum Disorders, 1,* 67–74.

Kern, J. K., Trivedi, M. H., Garver, C. R., Grannemann, B. D., Andrews, A. A., Savla, J., et al. (2007). Sensory correlations in autism. *Autism, 11*(2), 123–134.

Kientz, M. A., & Dunn, W. (1997). A comparison of the performance of children with and without autism on the Sensory Profile. *American Journal of Occupational Therapy, 51*(7), 530–537.

Kimball, J. G., Lynch, K. M., Stewart, K. C., Williams, N. E., Thomas, M. A., & Atwood, K. D. (2007). Using salivary cortisol to measure the effects of a Wilbarger protocol-based procedure on sympathetic arousal: A pilot study. *American Journal of Occupational Therapy., 61*(4), 406–413.

Kinnealey, M., & Oliver, B. (2002). *Adult sensory questionnaire.* Unpublished raw data, Temple University, College of Allied Health Professionals, Department of Occupational Therapy, Philadelphia.

Kinnealey, M., Oliver, B., & Wilbarger, P. (1995). A phenomenological study of sensory defensiveness in adults. *American Journal of Occupational Therapy, 49*(5), 444–451.

Kinnealey, M., & Smith, S. (2002, June). *Sensory defensive and non-defensive adults: Physiological and behavioral differences.* Poster session presented at the World Federation of Occupational Therapy Conference, Stockholm, Sweden.

Kuhaneck, H. M., Henry, D. A., & Glennon, T. (2007). *Sensory processing measure – School environments form.* Los Angeles: Western Psychological Services.

Kuo, A. D. (2005). An optimal state estimation model of sensory integration in human postural balance. *Journal of Neural Engineering, 2,* S235–S249.

Lang, C. E., & Bastian, A. J. (1999). Cerebellar subjects show impaired adaptation of anticipatory EMG during catching. *Journal of Neurophysiology, 82,* 2108–2119.

Law, M., Baptiste, S., & Mills, J. (1995). Client-centered practice: What does it mean and does it make a difference? *Canadian Journal of Occupational Therapy, 62,* 250–257.

Law, M., Cooper, B., Strong, S., Stewart, D., Rigby, P., & Letts, L. (1996). The person–environment–occupation model: A transactive approach to occupational performance. *Canadian Journal of Occupational Therapy, 63,* 186–192.

Leekman, S. R., Nieto, C., Libby, S. J., Wing, L., & Gould, J. (2007). Describing the sensory abnormalities of children and adults with autism. *Journal of Autism and Developmental Disorders, 37,* 894–910.

Lindermann, T. M., & Stewart, K. B. (1999). Sensory integrative-based occupational therapy and functional outcomes in young children with pervasive developmental disorders: A single subject study. *American Journal of Occupational Therapy, 53,* 207–213.

Liss, M., Saulnier, C., Fein, D., & Kinsbourne, M. (2006). Sensory and attention abnormalities in autistic spectrum disorders. *Autism, 10*(2), 155–172.

Lockner, D. W., Crowe, T. K., & Skipper, B. J. (2008). Dietary intake and parents' perception of mealtime behaviors in preschool-age children with autism spectrum disorder and in typically developing children. *Journal of the American Dietetic Association, 108,* 1360–1363.

Lucas, J. A., Rosenstein, L. D., & Bigler, E. D. (1989). Handedness and language among the mentally retarded: Implications for the model of pathological left-handedness and gender differences in hemispheric specialization. *Neuropsychologia, 27,* 713–723.

Luebben, A. J., & Royeen, C. B. (2010). An acquisitional frame of reference. In P. Kramer & J. Hinojosa (Eds.), *Frames of reference for pediatric occupational therapy* (3rd ed., pp. 461–488). Baltimore: Lippincott, Williams & Wilkins.

Manjiviona, J., & Prior, M. (1995). Comparison of Asperger syndrome and high functioning autistic children on a test of motor impairment. *Journal of Autism and Developmental Disorders, 25*(1), 23–39.

Margalit, M. (1981). Leisure activities of cerebral palsied children. *Israel Journal of Psychiatry and Relational Science, 18*(3), 209–214.

Marr, D., & Dimeo, S. B. (2006). Outcomes associated with a summer handwriting course for elementary students. *American Journal of Occupational Therapy, 60,* 10–15.

Marr, D., Mika, H., Miraglia, J., Roerig, M., & Sinnott, R. (2007). The effect of sensory stories on targeted behaviors in preschool children with autism. *Physical and Occupational Therapy in Pediatrics, 27*(1), 63–79.

Martin, T. A., Keating, J. G., Goodkin, H. P., Bastian, A. J., & Thach, W. T. (1996). Throwing while looking through prisms. I. Focal olivocerebellar lesions impair adaptation. *Brain, 119*(Pt. 4), 230–238.

Maschke, M., Gomez, C., Ebner, T., & Konczak, J. (2004). Hereditary cerebellar ataxia progressively impairs force adaptation during goal-directed arm movements. *Journal of Neurophysiology, 91,* 230–238.

McAfee, J. (2002). *Navigating the social world.* Future Horizons, Inc.: Arlington, TX.

McAlonon, G. M., Daly, E., Kumari, V., Critchley, H. D., van Amelsvoort, T., Suckling, J., et al. (2002). Brain anatomy and sensorimotor gating on Asperger's syndrome. *Brain, 127,* 1594–1606.

McIntosh, D. N., Miller, L. J., Shyu, V., & Dunn, W. (1999). Overview of the Short Sensory Profile (SSP). In W. Dunn (Ed.), *The American Journal of Occupational Therapy,* 237. *The sensory profile: Examiner's manual* (pp. 59–73). San Antonio, TX: Psychological Corporation.

McManus, I. C., Murray, B., Doyle, K., & Baron-Cohen, S. (1992). Handedness in childhood autism shows a dissociation of skill and preference. *Cortex, 28*, 373–381.

Miller, L. J. (1982). *Miller assessment for preschoolers manual* (rev. ed.). San Antonio, TX: Psychological Corporation.

Miller, L. J. (2006). *The miller function and participation scales*. San Antonio, TX: Psychological Corporation.

Miller, L. J., Anzalone, M. E., Lane, S. J., Cermak, S. A., & Osten, E. T. (2007). Concept evolution in sensory integration: A proposed nosology for diagnosis. *American Journal of Occupational Therapy, 61*(2), 135–140.

Miller, L. J., Coll, J. R., & Schoen, S. A. (2007). A randomized controlled pilot study of the effectiveness of occupational therapy for children with sensory modulation disorder. *American Journal of Occupational Therapy, 61*, 228–238.

Miller, L. J., McIntosh, D. N., McGrath, J., Shyu, V., Lampe, M., Taylor, A. K., et al. (1999). Electrodermal responses to sensory stimuli in individuals with fragile X syndrome: A preliminary report. *American Journal of Medical Genetics., 83*(4), 268–279.

Miller, L. J., & Roid, G. H. (1994). *The T.I.M.E., Toddler and infant motor evaluation: A standardized assessment*. Tucson, AZ: Therapy Skill Builders.

Ming, X., Brimacombe, M., & Wagner, G. C. (2007). Prevalence of motor impairment in autism spectrum disorders. *Brain & Development, 29*, 563–570.

Minshew, N. J., Goldstein, G., & Siegel, D. J. (1997). Neuropsychologic functioning in autism: Profile of a complex information processing disorder. *Journal of the International Neuropsychological Society, 3*, 303–316.

Miyahara, M., Tsujii, M., Hori, M., Nakanishi, K., Kageyama, H., & Sugiyama, T. (1997). Brief report: Motor incoordination in children with Asperger syndrome and learning disabilities. *Journal of Autism and Developmental Disorders, 27*(5), 595–603.

Moscavitch, S., Szyper-Kravitz, M., & Shoenfeld, Y. (2009). Autoimmune pathology accounts for common manifestations in a wide range of neuro-psychiatric disorders: The olfactory and immune system interrelationship. *Clinical Immunology, 130*, 235–243.

Mostofsky, S. H., Burgess, M. P., & Gidley Larson, J. C. (2007). Increased motor cortex white matter volume predicts motor impairment in autism. *Brain, 130*, 2117–2122.

Mostofsky, S. H., Dubey, P., Jerath, V., Jansiewicz, E., Goldberg, M., & Denckla, M. (2006). Developmental dyspraxia is not limited to imitation in children with autism spectrum disorders. *Journal of the International Neuropsychological Society, 12*, 314–326.

Mostofsky, S. H., Powell, S. K., Simmonds, D. J., Goldberg, M. C., Caffo, B., & Pekar, J. J. (2009). Decreased connectivity and cerebellar activity in autism during motor task performance. *Brain, 132*, 2413–2425.

Mottron, L., Dawson, M., & Soulieres, I. (2009). Enhanced perception in savant syndrome: Patterns, structure and creativity. *Philosophical Transactions of the Royal Society B, 364*, 1385–1391.

Mottron, L., Dawson, M., Soulieres, I., Hubert, B., & Burack, J. (2006). Enhanced perceptual functioning in autism: An update, and eight principles of autistic perception. *Journal of Autism and Developmental Disorders, 36*, 27–43.

Nicot, A., Otto, T., Brabet, P., & DiCicco-Bloom, E. M. (2004). Altered social behavior in pituitary adenylate cyclase-activating polypeptide type I receptor-deficient mice. *Journal of Neuroscience, 24*, 8786–8795.

Nieto del Rincon, P. L. (2008). Autism: Alteration in auditory perception. *Reviews in Neurosciences, 19*, 61–78.

Nolte, J. (2007). *Elsevier's integrated neuroscience*. Philadelphia: Mosby Elsevier.

Oldfield, R. C. (1971). The assessment and analysis of handedness: The Edinburgh inventory. *Neuropsychologia, 9*, 97–113.

Orekhova, E. V., Stroganova, T. A., Prokofyev, A. O., Nygren, G., Gillberg, C., & Elam, M. (2008). Sensory gating in young children with autism: Relation to age, IQ, and EEG gamma oscillations. *Neuroscience Letters, 434*, 218–223.

Osterling, J., & Dawson, G. (1994). Early recognition of children with autism: A study of first birthday home videotapes. *Journal of Autism and Developmental Disorders, 28*, 25–32.

O'Neill, M., & Jones, R. (1997). Sensory–perceptual abnormalities in autism: A case for more research. *Journal of Autism and Developmental Disorders, 27*, 283–293.

Pan, C. (2008). Objectively measured physical activity between children with autism spectrum disorders and children without disabilities during inclusive recess settings in Taiwan. *Journal of Autism and Developmental Disorders, 38*, 1292–1301.

Parham, L. D., Cohn, E. S., Spitzer, S., Koomar, J. A., Miller, L. J., Burke, J. P., et al. (2007). Fidelity in sensory integration intervention research. *American Journal of Occupational Therapy, 61*, 216–227.

Parham, L. D., & Ecker, C. (2007). *Sensory processing measure – Home form*. Los Angeles: Western Psychological Services.

Parush, S., Sohmer, H., Steinberg, A., & Kaitz, M. (2007). Somatosensory function in boys with ADHD and tactile defensiveness. *Physiology & Behavior, 90*, 553–558.

Pederson, A. V., Sigmundsson, H., Whiting, H. T. A., & Ingvaldsen, R. P. (2003). Sex differences in lateralization of fine manual skills in children. *Experimental Brain Research, 149*, 249–251.

Pernon, E., Pry, R., & Baghdadli, A. (2007). Autism: Perception and emotion. *Journal of Intellectual Disability Research, 51*, 580–587.

Perry, W., Minassian, A., Lopez, B., Maron, L., & Lincoln, A. (2007). Sensorimotor gating deficits in adults with autism. *Biological Psychiatry, 61*, 482–486.

Pfeiffer, B., Kinnealey, M., Reed, C., & Herzberg, G. (2005). Sensory modulation and affective disorders in children and adolescents with Asperger's disorder. *American Journal of Occupational Therapy, 59*(3), 335–345.

Polatajko, H. J., Mandich, A., & Martini, R. (2000). Dynamic performance analysis: A framework for understanding occupational performance. *American Journal of Occupational Therapy, 54*, 65–72.

Provost, B., & Oetter, P. (1993). The Sensory Rating Scale for infants and young children: Development and reliability. *Physical and Occupational Therapy in Pediatrics, 13*(4), 15–35.

Raja, M., & Azzoni, A. (2001). Asperger's disorder in the emergency psychiatric setting. *General Hospital Psychiatry, 23*(5), 285–293.

Ratzon, N. Z., Efraim, D., & Bart, O. (2007). A short-term graphomotor program for improving writing readiness skills of first-grade students. *American Journal of Occupational Therapy, 61*, 339–405.

Rigby, P., & Letts, L. (2003). Environment and occupational performance: Theoretical considerations. In L. Letts, P. Rigby, & S. Stewart (Eds.), *Using environments to enable occupational performance* (pp. 17–32). Thorofare, NJ: Slack.

Ritvo, E. R., Freeman, B. J., Scheibel, A. B., Duong, T., Robinson, H., Guthrie, D., et al. (1986). Lower Purkinje cell counts in the cerebella of four autistic subjects: Initial findings of the UCLA-NSAC autopsy research report. *American Journal of Psychiatry, 143*, 862–866.

Rizzolatti, G., Fabbri-Destro, M., & Cattaneo, L. (2009). Mirror neurons and their clinical relevance. *Nature Clinical Practice. Neurology, 5*, 24–34.

Roberts, H. E., King-Thomas, L., & Boccia, M. L. (2007). Behavioral indexes of the efficacy of sensory integration therapy. *American Journal of Occupational Therapy, 61*, 555–562.

Rodger, S., Springfield, E., & Polatajko, H. J. (2007). Cognitive Orientation for daily Occupational Performance approach for children with Asperger's Syndrome: A case report. *Physical & Occupational Therapy in Pediatrics., 27*(4), 7–22.

Rosenhall, U., Nordin, V., Sandstrom, M., Ahlsen, G., & Gillberg, C. (1999). Autism and hearing loss. *Journal of Autism and Developmental Disorders, 29*, 349–366.

Roston, K. (2010). A frame of reference for the development of handwriting skills. In P. Kramer & J. Hinojosa (Eds.), *Frames of reference for pediatric occupational therapy* (3rd ed., pp. 425–460). Baltimore: Lippincott, Williams & Wilkins.

Royeen, C. B., & Fortune, J. C. (1990). TIE: Tactile inventory for school aged children. *American Journal of Occupational Therapy, 44*, 155–160.

Satz, P., Soper, H. V., & Orsini, D. L. (1988). Human hand preference: Three nondextral subtypes. In D. C. Molfese & S. J. Segalowitz (Eds.), *Brain lateralization in children: Developmental implications* (pp. 281–287). New York: Guilford Press.

Schaaf, R. C., & Nightlinger, K. M. (2007). Occupational therapy using a sensory integrative approach: A case study of effectiveness. *American Journal of Occupational Therapy, 61*, 239–246.

Schaaf, R. C., Schoen, S. A., Smith Roley, S., Lane, S. J., Koomar, J., & May-Benson, T. (2010). A frame of reference for sensory integration. In P. Kramer & J. Hinojosa (Eds.), *Frames of reference for pediatric occupational therapy* (3rd ed., pp. 99–186). Baltimore: Lippincott, Williams & Wilkins.

Schilling, D. L., & Schwartz, I. S. (2004). Alternative seating for young children with autism spectrum disorder: Effects on classroom behavior. *Journal of Autism and Developmental Disorders, 34*, 423–432.

Schilling, D. L., Washington, K., Billingsley, F. F., & Deitz, J. (2003). Classroom seating for children with attention deficit hyperactivity disorder: Therapy balls versus chairs. *American Journal of Occupational Therapy, 57*, 534–541.

Schoen, S., Miller, L., & Green, K. (2008). Pilot study of the sensory over-responsivity scales: Assessment and inventory. *American Journal of Occupational Therapy, 62*, 393–406.

Schopler, E., Reichler, R. J., & Renner, B. R. (2002). *The childhood autism rating scale.* Los Angeles: Western Psychological Services.

Schreck, K. A., Williams, K., & Smith, A. F. (2004). A comparison of eating behaviors between children with and without autism. *Journal of Autism and Developmental Disorders, 34*, 433–438.

Shapiro, M., Sgan-Cohen, H. D., Parush, S., & Melmed, R. N. (2009). Influence of Adapted Environment on the Anxiety of Medically Treated Children with Developmental Disability. *Journal of Pediatrics, 154*(4), 546–550.

Sillanpää, M. (1987). Social adjustment and functioning of chronically ill and impaired children and adolescents. *Acta Paediatrica Scandinavica 340* (Suppl. 340), 1–70.

Skinner, B. F. (1976). *Walden two.* New York: Macmillan.

Soper, H. V., & Satz, P. (1984). Pathological left-handedness and ambiguous handedness: A new explanatory model. *Neuropsychologia, 22*(4), 511–515.

Soper, H. V., Satz, P., Orsini, D. L., Henry, R. R., Zvi, J. D., & Schulman, M. (1986). Handedness patterns in autism suggest subtypes. *Journal of Autism and Developmental Disorders, 16*, 155–167.

Sparrow, S., Cicchetti, D., & Balla, D. (2005). *Vineland-II: Vineland adaptive behavior scales: Survey forms manual* (2nd ed.). Circle Pines, MN: American Guidance Services.

Staples, K. L., & Reid, G. (2009, August). Fundamental movement skills and autism spectrum disorders. *Journal of Autism and Developmental Disorders, 40*(2), 209–217.

Stephenson, J., & Carter, M. (2009). The use of weighted vests with children with autism spectrum disorders and other disabilities. *Journal of Autism and Developmental Disorders, 39*, 105–114.

Stott, D. H., Moyes, F. A., & Henderson, S. E. (1984). *Manual: Test of Motor Impairment* (Henderson Revision). Guelph: Brook International.

Suzuki, Y., Critchley, H. D., Rowe, A., Howlin, P., & Murphy, D. G. (2003). Impaired olfactory identification in Asperger's syndrome. *Journal of Neuropsychiatry and Clinical Neurosciences, 15*, 105–107.

Takarae, Y., Luna, B., Minshew, N. J., & Sweeney, J. A. (2008). Patterns of visual sensory and sensorimotor abnormalities in autism vary in relation to history of early language delay. *Journal of the International Neuropsychological Society, 14*, 980–989.

Tecchio, F., Benassi, F., Zappasodi, F., Gialloreti, L. E., Palermo, M., Seri, S., et al. (2003). Auditory sensory processing in autism: A magnetoencephalographic study. *Society of Biological Psychiatry, 54*, 647–654.

Tomcheck, S. D., & Dunn, W. (2007). Sensory processing in children with and without autism: A comparative study using the short sensory profile. *American Journal of Occupational Therapy, 61*(2), 190–200.

Tsai, L. Y. (1983). The relationship of handedness to the cognitive, language and visuo-spatial skills of autistic patients. *British Journal of Psychiatry, 142*, 156–162.

Ulrich, D. A. (1985). *Test of gross motor development.* Austin, TX: PRO-ED.

VandenBerg, N. L. (2001). The use of a weighted vest to increase on-task behavior in children with attention difficulties. *American Journal of Occupational Therapy, 55*, 621–628.

Watling, R. I., Deitz, J., & White, O. (2001). Comparison of sensory profile scores of young children with and without autism spectrum disorders. *American Journal of Occupational Therapy, 55*, 416–423.

Whitehouse, A., & Bishop, D. (2008). Do children with autism "switch off" to speech sounds? An investigation using event-related potentials. *Developmental Science, 11*(4), 516–524.

Wiggins, L. D., Robins, D. L., Bakeman, R., & Adamson, L. B. (2009). Brief report: Sensory abnormalities as distinguishing symptoms of autism spectrum disorders in young children. *Journal of Autism and Developmental Disorders, 39*, 1087–1091.

Wilbarger, J., & Wilbarger, P. (2002). The Wilbarger approach to treating sensory defensiveness. In A. Bundy, S. Lane, & E. Murray (Eds.), *Sensory integration theory and practice* (2nd ed., pp. 335–338). Philadelphia: F. A. Davis.

Williams, R. S., Hause, S. L., Purpura, D. P., DeLong, G. R., & Swisher, C. N. (1980). Autism and mental retardation: Neuropathologic studies performed in four retarded persons with autistic behavior. *Archives of Neurology, 37*, 749–753.

Williams, M., & Shellenberger, S. (1996). *How does your engine run? A leader's guide to the alert program for self-regulation.* Albuquerque, NM: TherapyWorks.

Wilson, B. N., Kaplan, B. J., Crawford, S. G., & Roberts, G. (2007). *The developmental coordination disorder questionnaire 2007.* Calgary, AB: Alberta Children's Hospital.

Wuang, Y., Wang, C., Huang, M., & Su, C. (2009). Prospective study of the effect of sensory integration, neurodevelopmental treatment, and perceptual–motor therapy on the sensorimotor performance in children with mild mental retardation. *American Journal of Occupational Therapy, 63*, 441–452.

Early Detection of Autism Spectrum Disorders

Dennis R. Dixon, Doreen Granpeesheh, Jonathan Tarbox, and Marlena N. Smith

Early Detection of ASD

The US Centers for Disease Control and Prevention (CDC) now estimates that 1 out of every 110 children aged 8 or below have an autism spectrum disorder (ASD; Autism and Developmental Disabilities Monitoring Network, 2009). The CDC has labeled this increase a significant public health concern and with increased prevalence, the need for effective intervention is greater than ever before. The research on treatment of ASD has revealed that early intensive behavioral intervention (EIBI) is highly effective. Beginning with research in the 1980s (e.g., Lovaas, 1987) and continuing to the present day (e.g., Zachor, Ben-Itzchak, Rabinovich, & Lahat, 2007), studies have consistently demonstrated that EIBI produces substantial gains across domains of functioning (see Granpeesheh, Tarbox, & Dixon, 2009, for a recent review and Eldevik et al., 2009, for a recent meta-analysis). The substantial published research supporting EIBI has led multiple independent bodies to endorse it for the treatment of autism, including the National Academy of Sciences (National Academy of Sciences, 2001), the U.S. Surgeon General (US Department of Health and Human Services, 1999), the New York State Department of Health (New York State Department of Health & Early Intervention Program, 1999), and the American Academy of Pediatrics (Myers & Plauché Johnson, 2007). Public policy changes have also been impacted by research supporting EIBI, such as state-level legislation requiring medical insurance to cover EIBI treatment (e.g., "Steven's Law," Arizona House Bill 2487).

An outcome of the general acceptance of EIBI as an effective treatment for ASD has been an emphasis upon the "early" component of the treatment (Granpeesheh, Dixon, Tarbox, Kaplan, & Wilke, 2009; Matson & Smith, 2008;

Matson, 2007). However, early intervention requires early detection and thus a great deal of effort has been placed upon the development of instruments to screen for ASD (Matson, Wilkins, & González, 2008).

Few studies have specifically addressed the impact of age on EIBI outcomes; however, those that have analyzed this factor have reported that overall earlier is better (Granpeesheh et al., 2009). Intervening early and intensively optimizes long-term outcomes (Lord, 1995; Mays & Gillon, 1993; Prizant & Wetherby, 1988). Likewise, treatment interventions may show diminishing returns as a child's age increases. Recently in our own clinical practice, we found that children between 2 and 5 years performed significantly better than children in the two older age groups (5–7 years and 7–12 years; Granpeesheh et al., 2009). This finding is striking when one considers that children are typically not diagnosed until 5–7 years (Matson, Boisjoli, Hess, & Wilkins, 2010; Fombonne et al., 2004; Oslejsková, Kontrová, Foralová, Dusek, & Némethová, 2007; Siklos & Kerns, 2007). Clearly, the most important years for intervention are being missed for a large portion of children.

Regarding the age of first diagnosis, there has been much discussion as to how early the diagnosis can be made and whether it can remain stable (Matson et al., 2008). It is without debate that ASD can be detected with greater accuracy as a child ages (Landa & Garrett-Mayer, 2006). Further, the diagnosis of autistic disorder is much more stable than PDD-NOS or Asperger's disorder (Cox et al., 1999; Stone et al., 1999; Turner, Stone, Pozdol, & Coonrod, 2006). Overall, results of studies indicate that diagnoses made at 2 years of age are more stable as the severity of ASD increases (i.e., autistic disorder) and less stable as the severity of symptoms decreases (i.e., PDD-NOS).

In a series of publications, Lord (1995) and Lord et al. (2006) examined the long-term stability of diagnoses made at 2 years of age, which were reevaluated at 3 years and again at 9 years. While evaluating the diagnoses from 2 to 3 years, Lord reported good stability when clinical judgment was included; however, when the ADI was used alone, diagnoses

D.R. Dixon (✉)
The Center for Autism and Related Disorders, Tarzana, CA 91356, USA
e-mail: d.dixon@centerforautism.com

J.L. Matson, P. Sturmey (eds.), *International Handbook of Autism and Pervasive Developmental Disorders*,
Autism and Child Psychopathology Series, DOI 10.1007/978-1-4419-8065-6_12, © Springer Science+Business Media, LLC 2011

were less stable. At the follow-up at 9 years of age, Lord et al. (2006) again reported excellent stability as long as clinical judgment was included. Similar results have been found by a number of other researchers (e.g., Chawarska, Klin, Paul, & Volkmar, 2007; Moore & Goodson, 2003; Turner et al., 2006).

Not all studies have found early diagnoses to be stable. For example, Charman et al. (2005) evaluated children diagnosed with autism at 2 years of age and again at 3 and 7 years. They found that standard assessments at 2 years were not stable enough to predict outcomes at 7 years. Likewise, Turner and Stone (2007) found diagnoses, evaluated at 2 and 4 years of age, to be less stable than previously reported. Overall, early diagnoses appear to be stable after 2 years of age if clinical judgment is included and rating scales are not relied upon solely.

Early Signs of ASD

The first step in screening for ASD is identifying what may serve as an early warning sign. Parents of children with ASD typically begin to suspect problems with their child's development before 24 months (Gray, Tonge, & Brereton, 2006) and early research reported that up to 50% may actually suspect problems with their child's development before age 1 (Ornitz, Guthrie, & Farley, 1977). The investigation of home videos has yielded significant information regarding very early symptoms of ASD. These studies typically contrast behavioral observations made on home videos, taken at an early age, of children who later receive an ASD diagnosis and children who do not. For example, Adrien et al. (1993) contrasted ratings of home videos taken of children with ASD and other children with typical development. They reported five specific behaviors that significantly differentiated the two groups. These behaviors fell in the categories of socialization, communication, and motor development.

A number of researchers have found specific variables in infants that predict diagnostic classification. The early signs of ASD appear to be similar to the symptoms upon which the diagnosis is eventually made. Recently, Maestro et al. (2005) found that 87.5% of their sample showed significant signs within the first year of life. As with the study by Adrien et al. (1993), these infants showed a general lack of motor, social, and emotional initiative.

Baranek (1999) found nine items that were able to correctly classify diagnostic group with 93% accuracy among children with developmental disability, ASD, and typical development. Their first factor accounted for 72% of the variance observed. It essentially discriminated the children with ASD from the other two groups based upon mouthing, social touch aversion, orientation to visual stimuli, and response

to name. Again, we see a general pattern of deficits in socialization.

Recently, Landa (2008) discussed a number of symptoms that emerge before 24 months of age. Among these were response to name, faces, joint attention, and motor delays. However, these symptoms were variable in their presentation and some children who eventually received an ASD diagnosis never showed all of these symptoms. They further reported that there appears to be two distinct onset patterns. The first is a pattern of slow development and the second is that of regressive onset.

A particular challenge for the early detection of ASD is that some children exhibit a period of seemingly normal development followed by a rapid loss of skills relating to the core symptoms of ASD (Matson & Kozlowski, 2010; Werner & Dawson, 2005). The regression of skills in children with ASD has been documented in numerous studies. An early report by Hoshino et al. (1987) found that approximately half of their sample showed regression. Further, 56% of their sample reported a specific event associated with the regression onset. Kurita (1985) examined speech loss before 30 months of age. He found that loss of speech occurred from 10 to 30 months of age and most commonly occurred from 15 to 26 months. More recently, Goldberg et al. (2003) extended the ADI-R to gather information regarding regression. They found that skill regression occurred on average between 18 and 21 months. Matson, Wilkins, and Fodstad (2010) found a slightly later mean onset of regression in their group occurring at 27.7 months of age.

Regression may prove to be a specific ASD phenotype (Goldberg et al., 2003; Ozonoff, Williams, & Landa, 2005). Children who experience regression show an overall pattern of much slower development following the regression (Luyster et al., 2005). Further, Matson and Kozlowski (2010) found that regression occurred primarily in communication and social skills.

The etiology of regression is unknown. A large portion of parents of children with ASD report a specific event associated with the regression (e.g., Hoshino et al., 1987). Epilepsy has been reported to potentially play a causal role in the occurrence of regression (Matson & Kozlowski, 2010). For example, Oslejsková et al. (2008) reported that 60% of their sample of children who experienced regression also showed signs of epilepsy. In spite of these reports, no clear antecedent has been identified for all cases of regression in ASD. As with the etiology of ASD, it is likely that no single factor can account for all cases.

Siblings

Siblings of children with ASD have a significantly increased risk of developing ASD, relative to other children (Iverson & Wozniak, 2007). Estimates of recurrence vary but it may be as high as 9% (Szatmari, Jones, Zwaigenbaum, & MacLean,

1998).When contrasted to infants who are not at risk for ASD, siblings showed more delays in sitting, babbling, showing, first word, and posturing (Iverson & Wozniak, 2007). The increased recurrence risk in siblings of children with ASD has made siblings a fruitful population from which to recruit participants for research on early detection (Nadig et al., 2007). In fact, much of what is currently known about early signs has come from studying younger siblings of individuals with autism.

Response to Name

Several studies have documented that lack of response to name in infancy may be predictive of later diagnosis of ASD. Osterling, Dawson, and Munson (2002) investigated whether 1-year-old infants who were later diagnosed with ASD could be distinguished from infants of the same age who had either an intellectual disability or typical development. Videotapes from first year birthday parties were retrospectively rated by blind observers and data were collected on a number of social and verbal measures. The results indicated that children with ASD oriented to their names less frequently and looked at others less frequently than those with ID. Similarly, Baranek (1999) found that response to name was one of several factors that, when combined, accurately distinguished 9- to 12-month-old infants who later were or were not diagnosed with an ASD.

Joint Attention

The role of joint attention (JA) in ASD has been the subject of a significant amount of research. Joint attention is a developmental concept that refers to the process of sharing one's experience with someone else by coordinating one's own attention with the attention of the other person, in response to a third object or event. JA interactions involve active responding on the part of two people. JA is divided into two basic subtypes, defined by the behavior of the person who either initiates the interaction – referred to as initiating joint attention (IJA) – or responds to the initiation – referred to as responding to joint attention (RJA). For example, if a child sees a picture of a preferred event hanging on the wall, he might orient his face toward it, point to it, and say "Look!" while looking at another person, which would constitute an instance of IJA. An RJA in response to such an initiation might consist of the person looking at the child, following his gaze or point, and then looking at the picture to which he was pointing. Researchers have posited that both types of JA are critical parts of early social and language development (Sullivan et al., 2007). In addition, research has shown that deficits in JA can discriminate between children with and without ASD (Dawson et al., 2002, 2004).

A significant amount of research has been done on the role of early JA deficits as predictors of later ASD diagnoses. In an early study, 20-month-old children with autism were found to perform poorly on tests of JA, when compared to typically developing children in the same age group (Charman et al., 1997). These results imply that JA may be a predictor of ASD, if examined at a younger age. More recent research has attempted to do just that. For example, a prospective study on RJA as a predictor of ASD diagnosis found that poor RJA performance (defined as responding to less than 50% of experimenter bids for JA) at both 14 and 24 months of age predicted later ASD diagnosis at 30–36 months (Sullivan et al., 2007). Similarly, Landa, Holman, and Garrett-Mayer (2007) found that children who were diagnosed with an ASD at 14 months of age performed significantly worse than typically developing controls on tests of JA. However, another subset of children who later developed ASD, but did not qualify for ASD diagnosis at 14 months, differed from typically developing controls on only one of several measures of JA. It is possible, then, that two distinct subtypes of ASD exist, one which develops at a very young age and can be detected via JA tests, and another which develops at a slightly older age (e.g., diagnosable by 30–36 months) may not be possible to predict their later diagnosis on the basis of very early JA deficits.

From a behavioral perspective, it is not surprising that JA is important to early social and language development. An analysis of the operant function of JA reveals that it is likely to be an early indicator of the value of social interaction to the developing infant/toddler. This is because the immediate consequence of IJA behavior is clearly to recruit and secure the attention of another person. Given that IJA behavior, by definition, occurs spontaneously (i.e., not in response to the request of another person), it is a direct indication that the social attention of another person is positively reinforcing for the child. In essence, IJA can be conceptualized as a form of requesting or "manding" (Skinner, 1957) for attention. Similarly, the maintaining consequences of RJA likely are the subsequent social responses by the person with whom one is interacting. For example, if an infant's mother says "Look at that train!" (IJA), and the infant responds by looking at the mother and then looking at the train (RJA), the mother very likely will respond to the RJA response with another verbal (e.g., naming the color of the train and describing its properties) or non-verbal (e.g., patting the child on the back or tickling him) social response.

It is entirely possible, then, that poor JA performance in some infants reveals that attention from and interaction with others is not a source of positive reinforcement for them. If attention from others is not positively reinforcing, then delays in the development of social skills and language are not surprising. Engaging in most social behavior results in reactions (attention) from the people with whom one is interacting. Similarly, the function of much language – other than requests to have basic needs met – is to secure attention from others, in one form or another. For example, the consequence of basic vocal imitation ("echoics") of the speech of others is generally positive attention from the caregiver one is imitating, as is the consequence for basic labeling and naming ("tacting") in young children. The development of more advanced language, such as conversational exchanges ("intraverbals"), also likely depends on the natural consequence of such behavior (social interaction with others) being positively reinforcing (Skinner, 1957).

Communication

Some data have also been published which suggest that deficits in communication at very early ages may be predictive of later diagnosis of ASD. For example, Landa et al. (2007) found that children who were diagnosable with ASD at age of 14 months exhibited significantly less vocal and gestural communication behaviors than typically developing children. Children who were not diagnosable at 14 months (but who later were diagnosed with ASD at 30–36 months) did not differ significantly from typically developing controls in communication at 14 months, but did differ significantly from controls on measures of gestural communication at 24 months. Adrien et al. (1993) retrospectively compared home videos of children who were later diagnosed with autism to those who were not. Videos taken before 1 year of age and others taken between 1 and 2 years of age were analyzed. Before 1 year of age, children with ASD engaged in significantly less pre-verbal behaviors such as "social smile" and "appropriate facial expressions." Furthermore, between 1 and 2 years of age, children with ASD displayed significantly less gestures and "expressive postures" than typically developing controls.

Motor and Sensory

Children with ASD show significant impairments in motor skills relative to their typically developing peers (Jansiewicz et al., 2006). This domain also appears to be an area that can be used to screen for ASD at an early age. Adrien et al. (1993) found that children who developed autism were rated as too calm, engaging in unusual posturing, and hypoactive. Further, Baranek (1999) found that unusual posturing of body parts, excessively mouthing objects, aversion to social touch, and stereotyped play with objects were significantly different among their groups of children with developmental disabilities, ASD, and typical development. It is noteworthy that the DD group showed higher stereotypical play than the ASD group.

Early Diagnosis

As noted above, parents of children with ASD typically begin to suspect problems with their child's development before

24 months (Gray et al., 2006). However, there appears to be about a 6-month delay between when a parent first suspects a problem and when they first seek help (De Giacomo & Fombonne, 1998; Howlin & Moore, 1997). The estimate of 6 months may be a lower estimate as a significant portion of the parents in the study by Howlin and Moore (1997) waited as long as 2 years to report problems to a healthcare provider.

Awareness has significantly increased over the past decade since the publication of these studies; however, this increased awareness in the general population may not be leading to earlier diagnoses. Recently, Wiggins, Baio, and Rice (2006) found significant delays (13 months) between when a parent first seeks help and when a formal diagnosis is made. So although the delay between first concern and seeking help may be improving, the delay between reporting the problem and formal diagnosis (and subsequent treatment) is still unacceptably long. Further, Wiggins et al. (2006) found that the mean age at first evaluation was 48 months whereas the actual diagnosis occurred at 61 months. These ages are significantly higher than those that are typically recommended (American Academy of Pediatrics, 2006; Gray et al., 2006).

There are no simple solutions for the task of early detection. While the development of instruments with acceptable psychometric properties is required, the overall task is much broader; consideration of who is responsible for this screening, under what context screening should occur, and at what age is also required.

The American Academy of Pediatrics (AAP) has recently stressed the need for ongoing screening for ASD and recommended initial screening to occur at the 18-month evaluations (American Academy of Pediatrics, 2001, 2006). ASD screening should ideally take place by 18–24 months (Gray et al., 2006). A two-level system has been suggested (Filipek et al., 2000) in which primary care providers perform routine screening on a regular basis (level 1) and refer children identified through this screening process to specialists for more rigorous assessment and diagnosis (level 2). While this is likely the best system, it is difficult to implement. First, physicians are increasingly being asked to complete more tasks with less time. Screening for ASD must be prioritized along with screening for the myriad of other critical disorders. Second, adequate level 1 screening for a disorder still requires some form of training for the physician. Third, pediatricians may have limited access to screening instruments with sufficient psychometric properties that also meet the requirement of brevity.

It should be noted that most research on early detection of ASD has necessarily utilized group designs, which compare groups of children who are later diagnosed with ASD to groups of children who are not. This research methodology has helped identify targets for early detection; however, it has done little to help the clinician or the parent to achieve early detection in the case of a particular child. Essentially, a large list of potential symptoms has been identified yet no single symptom or cluster of symptoms applies to all children who will later receive a diagnosis of ASD. Thus, the consistency of pediatricians' responses to parents' concerns will largely depend upon the individual clinician's experience with other cases of ASD. This highlights the need for an accurate and reliable clinical screening protocol. The next section of this chapter reviews research on attempts to develop such tools.

Screening Methods

Methods for the screening and eventual diagnosis of ASD have almost exclusively relied upon behavioral observation or indirect assessment of behavior. While a general assumption has been made by many researchers that the etiology of ASD is primarily genetic, these assumptions have yet to yield means by which to screen for or diagnose ASD (Matson et al., 2008). It is likely that behavioral assessments will continue to constitute the primary mode of screening for ASD for some time to come.

Over the past decade, the publication of screening tools has proliferated. However, evaluation of the utility of these screening tools, in regard to their psychometric properties, has not kept pace (Matson, 2007). There seems to be a pattern that after an instrument is introduced, development of the tool soon languishes. Only a few research groups continue to evaluate and further develop their tool after it has been introduced (Matson, 2007).

Screening instruments are typically evaluated in regard to sensitivity and specificity. Sensitivity is the degree to which the tool detects a disorder when it is indeed present. Specificity is the degree to which the tool correctly states that the disorder is absent. Both of these are important aspects of a screening instrument. Perfect sensitivity can be obtained simply by stating that the disorder is present in every individual. However, this would be at the cost of specificity, given that a number of individuals would be incorrectly identified as having the disorder. Low specificity wastes time and resources in addition to causing unnecessary heartache. An ideal screening tool would have both high sensitivity and specificity.

Various arguments have been made in regard to whether sensitivity or specificity is more important. For example, Baron-Cohen et al. (2000) argued that sensitivity is less important, stating "The high false-negative rate is not a serious drawback of the test, because the condition is not life-threatening" (p. 524). While ASD does not threaten the viability of an individual to continue living, we disagree with the implication of their statement. In light of the recent findings regarding EIBI outcomes and the importance of providing these services early, failure to detect ASD will result in a significant loss of development that will impact the rest of an individual's life. In such a case, low sensitivity will result in lost opportunities and diminished quality of life, whereas low specificity will waste funding resources and cause families to needlessly worry. Considering both outcomes, we feel that the benefits of early detection far outweigh the costs of false positives.

Screening instruments are also evaluated along two other lines, positive predictive value (PPV) and negative predictive value (NPV). PPV is calculated by dividing the number of true positives by the number of positives reported by the assessment (both true positives and false positives). PPV is an index of the degree to which positive test results reflect true positive classification decisions. Likewise, NPV is an index of the degree to which negative results reflect true negative classification decisions. PPV and NPV interpretation is impacted by the overall prevalence of the disorder being detected. Therefore, changes in the base rate of the disorder will bias PPV and NPV. To address this limitation, study samples should include proportions of the disorder that are equivalent to prevalence estimates within the population; however, this is rarely insured within studies.

Finally, there are additional factors to consider, apart from a purely psychometric evaluation, that impact the utility of a screening tool. These include the test length, format, item readability, who can use the tool, and the training required to both administer and interpret the results. All of these factors affect the degree to which a tool successfully reaches the goal of being routinely used to screen for ASD at an early age.

Assessment Tools

Baby and Infant Screen for Children with Autism Traits

The Baby and Infant Screen for Children with Autism Traits (BISCUIT; Matson, Boisjoli, & Wilkins, 2007) is a recently developed screening tool designed to identify children with ASD. The items that make up the BISCUIT were developed from reviews of pertinent literature, DSM-IV-TR and ICD-10 criteria, and clinical observations. The BISCUIT was created to evaluate the development of 17- to 37-month-old children (Matson et al., 2007).

The BISCUIT contains three sections, which are completed by professionals via caregiver report. Part 1 of the BISCUIT focuses on symptoms of ASD. It contains 62 items and takes approximately 20 min to complete. Items are answered using a point system. The response "0" suggests that a child displays no differences in comparison to typically developing children. Alternatively, "1" implies that a child exhibits slight differences and "2" indicates that a child demonstrates major differences. Children who score 21 points or more in part 1 are regarded as at risk for ASD and should be referred for diagnostic evaluation. Part 2 of the BISCUIT is an evaluation of behavioral symptoms of conditions that frequently co-occur with ASD. These conditions include ADHD, tic disorder, OCD, specific phobia, and eating/feeding difficulties. Part 2 contains 65 items, which are answered using a point system similar to the BISCUIT – part 1. Children who score high in this section should be referred for further evaluation of those particular symptoms. Finally, part 3 of the BISCUIT was created to evaluate problem behaviors that are often seen in children with ASD. These behaviors include aggression, disruption, self-injury, and stereotypies. Part 3 contains 17 items. Children scoring high on part 3 of the BISCUIT should be referred for behavioral evaluation (Matson et al., 2007).

The internal reliability of the BISCUIT was evaluated in Matson et al. (2010). Trained staff used the BISCUIT to evaluate 276 children at risk for developmental delay. All children were between 17 and 37 months of age. Item reliability was evaluated for each part of the BISCUIT and items were removed if they had inadequate endorsement or correlation. Following the removal of inadequate items, the internal reliability coefficient for the remaining 62 items in the BISCUIT – part 1 was 0.97. The BISCUIT – part 2 originally had 84 items, 19 of which were removed. The internal reliability coefficient for the remaining 65 items was 0.96. Finally, the BISCUIT – part 3 initially contained 20 items, 3 of which were removed. The remaining 17 items received an internal reliability coefficient of 0.91. Overall, the BISCUIT shows excellent internal reliability.

The sensitivity and specificity of the BISCUIT – part 1 was evaluated by Matson et al. (2010). In their study, 1,007 children aged 17–37 months, who were receiving services for developmental delay, were screened with the BISCUIT and the M-CHAT. All children in their study went on to receive full diagnostic evaluations. A cutoff score of 17 or more was found to best distinguish children with PDD-NOS from children with abnormal development. Moreover, a cutoff score of 39 or greater was found to best differentiate children with autism from children with PDD-NOS. Using these cutoff scores, the BISCUIT and M-CHAT were compared in their ability to screen for an ASD. More specifically, these contrasts were based on the instrument's ability to differentiate children with ASD from children with abnormal development. The M-CHAT was found to have sensitivity of 74.1%, specificity of 87.5%, and correct classification rate of 83.0%. In contrast, the BISCUIT was found to have sensitivity of 93.4%, specificity of 86.6%, and correct classification rate of 88.8%.

Two studies regarding the factor structure of the BISCUIT – part 1 are presented in Matson, Boisjoli, et al. (2010). In the first study, 270 children with ASD, between 17 and 37 months, were screened with the 62-item BISCUIT – part 1. Exploratory factor analysis identified three factors.

Factor 1, involving socialization and non-verbal communication, showed excellent internal stability (Cronbach's α = 0.93). Factor 2, concerning repetitive behavior and restricted interests, also showed excellent internal stability (Cronbach's α = 0.91). Finally, factor 3, relating to communication, showed satisfactory internal stability (Cronbach's α = 0.82). In the second study, 775 children, between 17 and 37 months old, were screened with the BISCUIT – part 1. Of these children, 270 had ASD diagnoses. The remaining 505 children did not meet diagnostic criteria for ASD; however, these children were receiving state-funded services for developmental delay. In general, the children with ASD received higher scores on all factors than the children without ASD. Additionally, total scores attained for each factor could accurately identify group membership.

Matson, Dempsey, and Fodstad (2009) used the BISCUIT – part 1 to assess stereotypic and repetitive behavior in children with autism, PDD-NOS, and developmental delay. A total of 760 children, between 17 and 37 months old, were screened with the repetitive behavior and restricted interests subscale in the BISCUIT – part 1. Of these children, 140 were found to have autism and 121 were diagnosed with PDD-NOS. The remaining 499 children did not meet diagnostic criteria for ASD; however, they were at risk for other developmental disorders. In general, the children with autism scored higher on the repetitive behavior and restricted interests subscale than the children with PDD-NOS. Furthermore, the children with PDD-NOS attained higher scores than the children without an ASD. The repetitive behavior and restricted interests subscale could accurately identify group membership in this sample.

Fodstad, Matson, Hess, and Neal (2009) used the BISCUIT – part 1 to evaluate social and communication skills in children with autism, PDD-NOS, and developmental delay. They screened 886 children, aged 17–37 months, with the socialization and non-verbal communication subscale, and the communication subscale of the BISCUIT – part 1. Of these children, 161 had ASD and 140 had PDD-NOS. The remaining 585 children did not meet diagnostic criteria for ASD; however, they were recognized by pediatricians as having abnormal development. Overall, children with autism attained higher scores than children with PDD-NOS on both subscales. Likewise, children with PDD-NOS generally received higher scores than children with abnormal development.

Two studies concerning the factor structure of the BISCUIT – part 2 are presented in Matson, Boisjoli, Hess, and Wilkins (2011). In the first study, 270 children with ASD, aged 17–30 months, were screened with the 65-item BISCUIT – part 2. Exploratory factor analysis identified five factors. Factor 1, involving tantrum and conduct behavior, had a Cronbach's α of 0.92. Factor 2, concerning inattention and impulsivity, had a Cronbach's α of 0.88. Furthermore, a

Cronbach's α of 0.83 was found for factor 3, pertaining to avoidance behavior. Factor 4, regarding anxiety and repetitive behavior, had a Cronbach's α of 0.82. Finally, factor 5, involving eating and sleep problems, had a Cronbach's α of 0.75. Eight items, used in the first study, were not included in the second study due to low correlation. In the second study, 775 children, aged 17–37 months, were screened with the BISCUIT – part 2. Two hundred and seventy of these children had ASD. The remaining 505 did not meet diagnostic criteria for ASD; however, these children were receiving state-funded resources for developmental delay. Overall, the children with ASD scored considerably higher than the children without ASD on all five factors. In addition, total scores tallied for each factor could accurately detect group membership.

Matson, Fodstad, Mahan, and Sevin (2009) reported on two studies involving the subscales in the BISCUIT – part 2. In the first study, 309 children with ASD, aged 17–37 months, were screened with the 57-item BISCUIT – part 2. Cutoff scores were determined for both moderate deficits and severe deficits. In the tantrum and conduct behavior subscale, scores between 17 and 24 were considered moderate and higher scores were deemed severe. For the inattention and impulsivity subscale, scores between 16 and 22 were regarded as moderate and higher scores were considered severe. In the avoidance behavior subscale, scores between 7 and 10 were regarded as moderate and higher scores were deemed severe. For the anxiety and repetitive behavior subscale, scores between 7 and 9 were considered moderate and higher scores were regarded as severe. Finally, in the eating and sleep problems subscale, scores of 4 or 5 were deemed moderate and higher scores were considered severe. In the second study, 769 children, aged 17–37 months, were screened with the 57-item BISCUIT – part 2. Of these children, 169 had autism, 140 had PDD-NOS, and 460 had abnormal development. The children with autism were more likely to score high on the BISCUIT – Part 2 and the individual subscales than the children with PDD-NOS. Likewise, the children with PDD-NOS were more likely to score high than the children with abnormal development. Of the children with autism, 29.6% received a severe rating on one or more subscales, compared to 17.9% of the children with PDD-NOS and 0.4% of the children with abnormal development. Matson, Fodstad, and Mahan (2009) further evaluated the subscales of the BISCUIT – part 2. In their study, 651 children, aged 17–37 months, were screened with the BISCUIT – part 2. All children were receiving state-funded services for developmental delay. The frequency and severity of symptoms detected by the BISCUIT – part 2 were measured. Eating and sleep problems were most prevalent with 16.1% of the children attaining moderate to severe scores. Of the children, 13.5% received a severe rating on one or more subscales.

Two studies regarding the factor structure of the BISCUIT – part 3 are presented in Matson, Boisjoli, Rojahn, and Hess (2009). In the first study, 270 children with ASD, aged 17–37 months, were screened with the BISCUIT – part 3. Exploratory factor analysis identified three factors. Factor 1, regarding aggressive and disruptive behavior, had a Cronbach's α of 0.88. Factor 2, involving stereotypic behavior, had a Cronbach's α of 0.72. Finally, factor 3, concerning self-injurious behavior, had a Cronbach's α of 0.51. In the second study, 775 children, between 17 and 37 months old, were screened with the BISCUIT – part 3. Of these children, 270 had ASD diagnoses. The remaining 505 children did not meet diagnostic criteria for ASD; however, these children were receiving state-funded services for developmental delay. Overall, the children with ASD received higher scores than the children without ASD on all factors. Furthermore, scores attained within each factor could accurately detect group membership.

Rojahn et al. (2009) further evaluated the subscales in the BISCUIT – part 3. In their study, 762 children, aged 17–37 months, were screened with the BISCUIT – part 3. Of these children, 172 had autism, 140 had PDD-NOS, and 450 had abnormal development. The children with autism were more likely to receive moderate to severe scores on BISCUIT – part 3 and the individual subscales than the children with PDD-NOS. Likewise, the children with PDD-NOS were more likely to attain moderate to severe scores than the children with abnormal development. Of the children with autism, 29.7% received a severe rating on one or more subscales, compared to 8.6% of the children with PDD-NOS and 1.3% of the children with abnormal development.

Overall, the BISCUIT is a fairly new assessment tool that has received significant evaluation considering the amount of time it has been available. The BISCUIT shows strong psychometric properties. Two strengths of its design really stand out. First, it is designed to screen for symptoms across the autism spectrum and not simply detect the more severe forms of the spectrum (e.g., autistic disorder). Second, by including a comorbidity scale (part 2), and a problem behavior scale (part 3), the clinician is given the option to use these domains in their screening evaluation, or to skip them, if time does not permit. Based upon these factors, the BISCUIT is a promising scale for the screening of ASD.

Checklist for Autism in Toddlers

The Checklist for Autism in Toddlers (CHAT; Baron-Cohen, Allen, & Gillberg, 1992; Baron-Cohen et al., 1996), developed in Great Britain, is a screening instrument for early identification of ASD. More specifically, the CHAT is a rating scale created to evaluate developmental progress in 18-month-old children. The instrument was designed to be administered by trained healthcare professionals and takes approximately 5–10 min to complete (Baron-Cohen et al., 2000). Two subsequent versions of the CHAT have been developed, the Modified CHAT (M-CHAT) and the Quantitative CHAT (Q-CHAT).

The CHAT contains two parts. In section A, a parent is asked questions regarding the child's development. In section B, a healthcare professional describes behaviors observed through direct interaction with the child. Section B was integrated into the CHAT in order to confirm the parental responses provided in section A. The CHAT contains 14 yes/no items, 9 in section A and 5 in section B. These items were derived from behaviors that are either affected or unaffected by ASD. Items intended to assess developmental delay focus on five areas including pretend play, protodeclarative pointing, joint attention, social interest, and social play. The authors regarded pretend play and joint attention as critical components in the detection of ASD. Items concerning behaviors that are unaffected by ASD were derived from areas concerning rough and tumble play, motor development, protoimperative pointing, and functional play. The authors report that these items were integrated into the checklist in order to avoid yes or no favoritism by allowing all parents to answer "yes" to various items (Baron-Cohen et al., 1992).

The CHAT contains five items that are considered critical in determining risk for ASD. These five items involve pretend play and joint attention. Children who receive negative responses on all critical items are regarded as high risk. Those who are not deemed high risk but nevertheless fail both items pertaining to protodeclarative pointing are considered medium risk. All other children are considered low risk (Baron-Cohen et al., 2000). If a child screens positive, another CHAT should be completed within a month. Screening positive a second time is a reason to seek diagnostic evaluation (Blackwell, 2002).

The psychometric properties of the CHAT were first reported by Baron-Cohen et al. (1992). In their study, 91 children, between 17 and 21 months old, were screened using the CHAT. Fifty children were randomly selected from a London medical center and 41 children were younger siblings of children previously diagnosed with ASD (thus at a high risk for ASD). All children from the randomly selected group screened negative on the CHAT. On the other hand, four children, who had older siblings with ASD, screened positive. These four children went on to receive an ASD diagnosis between 24 and 30 months of age. No children from the randomly selected group were found to have ASD. Agreement between parental report and professional observation was measured in the randomly selected group, finding 92% reliability.

In a subsequent study, Baron-Cohen et al. (1996) reported data on 16,000 children who were screened with the CHAT by general practitioners or home health visitors during 18-month checkups. Following the screens, children were divided into three groups. Those who received negative responses on all items regarding protodeclarative pointing, gaze monitoring, and pretend play made up the "risk for ASD" group. The group at risk for developmental delay contained children who passed the item concerning gaze monitoring but failed all items concerning protodeclarative pointing, or protodeclarative pointing and pretend play. All other children fell into the "typical development" group. Children who received two positive screens were referred for diagnostic evaluation. A modification of the ADI-R was used to diagnose children with suspected ASD. The cutoff scores for "reciprocal social interaction" and "communication" were maintained, while the cutoff score for "repetitive behavior" was lowered. The children considered at risk for ASD in this study scored above the original cutoff for "reciprocal social interaction" and "communication" but not "repetitive behavior."

Using the CHAT, Baron-Cohen et al. (1996) detected 12 children at risk for ASD and 44 children at risk for developmental delay. All children in the risk for ASD group and half the children in the risk for developmental delay group received diagnostic evaluations. Ten children in the risk for ASD group were found to have ASD while the remaining two received diagnoses of developmental delay. Furthermore, 15 children in the risk for developmental delay group were diagnosed with developmental delay while the remaining 7 were found to have typical development. Of the children who received diagnostic evaluations, the CHAT accurately identified 83.3% of those with ASD and 68.2% of those with developmental delay. The CHAT had a 16.6% false-positive rate in identifying ASD. Gaze monitoring was found to be a critical item in differentiating children with ASD from children with developmental delay and typical development. Other items found to be significant within the ASD group were interest in other children (failed by 50%) and protoimperative pointing (failed by 90%).

Baird et al. (2000) further report on the psychometric properties of the CHAT. In their study, 16,235 children were screened with the CHAT by healthcare professionals during 18-month checkups. The screens, however, were evaluated with different parameters than those used by Baron-Cohen et al. (1996). Like the 1996 population study, children failing all five items relating to protodeclarative pointing, gaze monitoring, and pretend play were regarded as high risk for developing ASD. In contrast, children who were not considered high risk but who failed both items regarding protodeclarative pointing were deemed medium risk for developing ASD. All other children were considered low risk. After completing an initial CHAT, 38 children were identified as high risk and 369 children were identified as medium risk. All children considered high risk received a second screen while roughly half the children regarded as medium risk were screened again. After the second screen, the CHAT detected 12 children at high risk for ASD and 22 children at medium risk.

Within the sample of 16,235 children, 50 children went on to be diagnosed with autism and 44 children received PDD diagnoses.

Regarding the first screening in Baird et al. (2000), 10 of the 38 children identified as high risk received autism diagnoses. The PPV for detecting autism in the high-risk group was 26.3%, sensitivity was 20.0%, and specificity was 99.8%. One child in the high-risk group was found to have PDD. Therefore, PPV for identifying PDD in this group was 2.6%, sensitivity was 2.3%, and specificity was 99.8%. Of the remaining children in the high-risk group, 7 were diagnosed with other developmental disorders and 20 were found to have typical development. Nine of the 369 children identified as medium risk after the first CHAT were diagnosed with autism, 2 of whom had Asperger's disorder. The PPV for detecting autism in the medium-risk group was 2.4%, sensitivity was 18.0%, and specificity was 97.8%. Thirteen children in the medium-risk group received PDD diagnoses. Here, PPV was 3.5%, sensitivity was 29.5%, and specificity was 97.8%. Of the remaining children in the medium-risk group, 37 had other developmental disorders and 310 were found to have typical development.

Next, Baird et al. (2000) report data concerning the second CHAT screening. Nine of the 12 children identified as high risk after the second CHAT were diagnosed with autism. The PPV for identifying autism in the high-risk group was 75.0%, sensitivity was 18.0%, and specificity was 100%. One child was found to have PDD in this group. Thus, the PPV for detecting PDD in the high-risk group was 8.3%. Furthermore, sensitivity was 2.3% and specificity was 99.9%. Of the remaining children in the high-risk group, one had a language disorder and the other was found to have typical development. One of the 22 children identified as medium risk after the second CHAT received an autism diagnosis. Here, PPV was 4.5%, sensitivity was 2.0%, and specificity was 99.9%. Nine children in the medium-risk group were diagnosed with PDD. Therefore, the PPV for detecting PDD in the medium-risk group was 40.9%, sensitivity was 20.5%, and specificity was 99.9%. Of the remaining children in the medium-risk group, 10 were diagnosed with other developmental disorders and 2 had typical development.

Scambler, Rogers, and Wehner (2001) report on the psychometric properties of the CHAT after applying both standard and modified scoring parameters. Forty-four children between 2 and 3 years old participated in this study. Twenty-six children had ASD and 18 children had other developmental disorders. Diagnoses were confirmed by the ADI-R, ADOS, DSM-IV criteria, and clinical judgment. All children were screened with the CHAT and their scores were evaluated in two ways. First, the parameters used in Baird et al. (2000) were applied. Next, modified parameters (the

Denver criteria) were used. The Denver criteria is a modification of the medium-risk requirements described in Baird et al. (2000). The Denver criteria differ in that a positive screen occurs if a child fails the parental reported items pertaining to either or both protodeclarative pointing and pretend play, in addition to failing the observational item concerning protodeclarative pointing. When the standard parameters were applied, 17 of the 26 children with ASD were identified as either high risk or medium risk. No children with other developmental disorders were detected. The sensitivity for identifying children with ASD as either high or medium risk was 65%. In addition, specificity was 100%, false-positive rate was 0%, and false negative was 35%. When the Denver criteria was used, 22 of the 26 children with ASD were detected. Again, no children with other developmental disorders screened positive. Here, sensitivity was 85% and specificity remained 100%.

In a follow-up study, Scambler, Hepburn, and Rogers (2006) reevaluated children who were screened with the CHAT at 2 and 3 years. Thirty children, 19 with ASD and 11 with other developmental disorders, received follow-up evaluations at 4 and 5 years. The children's diagnoses were reassessed using the ADI-R, ADOS-G, MSEL, VABS, and clinical judgment. Diagnoses were for the most part stable; only two children, who were previously diagnosed with autism, received PDD-NOS diagnoses at reevaluation. When the parameters described by Baird et al. (2000) were applied, 14 of the 19 children with ASD at follow-up were previously detected by the CHAT as either high or medium risk. Here, sensitivity was 74%. When the Denver criteria was used, 17 of the 19 children with ASD at follow-up were formerly detected by the CHAT. Here, sensitivity was 89%. Scambler et al. (2001, 2006) demonstrate that the modified scoring parameters can increase sensitivity without decreasing specificity.

The psychometric properties of the CHAT have also been evaluated by Eaves and Ho (2004). In their study, 49 two-year-old children identified with possible autism by "community professionals" were screened with the CHAT. All children went on to receive diagnostic evaluations and follow-up assessments at 4.5 years. The CHAT maintained a 91% agreement with clinical diagnoses made at 2.5 and 4.5 years.

Recently, VanDenHeuvel, Fitzgerald, Greiner, and Perr (2007) reported the CHAT to be a cost-effective and time-efficient screening tool for the detection of ASD at 18-month developmental checkups. In their study, 156 public health nurses trained to administer the CHAT screened 2,117 children at 18-month developmental evaluations. A screen was considered positive if a child was identified as high risk or medium risk for ASD. Those who screened positive received a second CHAT. Children who received two positive screens were referred for diagnostic evaluation. Twenty-nine children were detected by the first CHAT and seven were identified by the second CHAT. Ten children who screened positive on the first CHAT did not go on to receive a second CHAT. Of the seven children who received two positive screens, three were found to have ASD and one was diagnosed with learning disability. Five children, who did not receive a second CHAT, were given diagnostic evaluations and four were diagnosed with ASD. The prevalence rate for ASD diagnosis was 33.1 per 10,000 in this study.

Overall the CHAT is quick to administer and uses a multimethod assessment approach, which includes direct observation. However, when the original scoring criteria are used, the CHAT's ability to detect ASD is relatively weak. On the other hand, when the scoring procedures used by Scambler et al. (2001, 2006) are implemented, the sensitivity is greatly increased without reducing specificity. Thus, the criteria used by Scambler et al. (2001) are recommended over those used by Baird et al. (2000). One limitation of the CHAT is the use of a dichotomous rating approach. This presents additional concerns in that it gives credit for minimal use of the skill reported which may lead to false negatives along with parent-inaccurate reporting.

Modified Checklist for Autism in Toddlers

The Modified Checklist for Autism in Toddlers (M-CHAT; Robins, Fein, Barton, & Green, 2001) is an extension of the original CHAT. Unlike the CHAT, all items in the M-CHAT are completed via parental response; a healthcare professional is not required to administer this instrument. The authors report that the observational section from the CHAT was not included in the M-CHAT for a couple of reasons. First, since there is no position equivalent to the home health visitor in the United States, eliminating the observational section gives the M-CHAT greater utility abroad. Additionally, they argue that professional observation performed in a single session is actually less accurate than parental response (Robins et al., 2001).

The M-CHAT contains 23 yes/no items that assess sensory and motor function, social interaction, language and communication, and joint attention. Nine items were taken verbatim from the parental response section in the CHAT. Additional items, designed to detect disorders across the broader autism spectrum, were included to replace the omitted observational items. Further alterations were applied to improve the sensitivity of the CHAT. Most importantly, the screening age was increased to 24 months of age. Also, cutoff scores were decreased and structured telephone interviews were employed to confirm parental response in children whose scores elicit concern (Robins et al., 2001).

The psychometric properties of the M-CHAT were first reported by Robins et al. (2001). In their study, 1,122 children recruited from wellness checkups and 171 children recruited from early intervention centers were screened with

the M-CHAT. A screen was considered positive if a child endorsed two key items or any three items. Telephone interviews were conducted to confirm the responses of parents whose children received positive screens. Children considered at risk after the interview process were referred for diagnostic evaluation. One hundred and thirty two children required telephone interviews and 58 children qualified for diagnostic evaluation. Of these children, 39 were diagnosed with ASD and 19 were diagnosed with other developmental delays; no children who received diagnostic evaluations were found to have typical development. Overall, the children who screened negative on the M-CHAT endorsed 0.5 items while the children who did not elicit concern after the interview process endorsed 3.4 items. Furthermore, the children found to have other developmental delays generally endorsed 6.4 items whereas the children found to have ASD endorsed 10.3 items. Internal reliability was found to be satisfactory for the M-CHAT (Cronbach's $\alpha = 0.85$). In addition, six items concerning joint attention, social interest, and communication were found to best detect ASD. Cronbach's α was 0.83 for these key items.

Robins et al. (2001) compared psychometric properties for the two cutoff criteria. A cutoff score of 3 or more items confirmed over the telephone revealed a PPV of 0.68 in detecting ASD. Here, NPV was 0.99, sensitivity was 0.97, and specificity was 0.99. On the other hand, the same cutoff criteria without telephone confirmation reduced PPV to 0.36. NPV stayed the same at 0.99, likewise, sensitivity and specificity stayed relatively the same (0.97 and 0.95, respectively). When a cutoff score of 2 or more key items confirmed over the telephone was evaluated, PPV was 0.79, NPV was 0.99, sensitivity was 0.95, and specificity was 0.99. In contrast, the same cutoff criteria without telephone confirmation yielded a PPV of 0.64, NPV of 0.99, sensitivity of 0.95, and specificity of 0.98. Regardless of which criteria were used, scores improved if the interview process was considered part of the screening procedure.

The sensitivity and specificity of the M-CHAT have also been evaluated by Eaves, Wingert, and Ho (2006) who found significantly lower scores than those reported by Robins et al. (2001). In an evaluation of 84 children aged 17–48 months, they found sensitivity to be 0.77, specificity to be 0.43, and PPV to be 0.65. Similar results were found by Snow and Lecavalier (2008) who evaluated 82 children aged 18–70 months. Snow and Lecavalier (2008) found the optimal sensitivity to be 0.70, specificity to be 0.38, PPV to be 0.81, and NPV to be 0.36.

Kleinman et al. (2008) conducted two studies to evaluate the psychometric properties of the M-CHAT. In their first study, 3,309 children, recruited from wellness checkups, and 484 children, recruited from early intervention centers, were screened with the M-CHAT between 16 and 30 months of age. The cutoff scores and the telephone interview process applied in Robins et al. (2001) were used in this study. A total of 385 children screened positive on the M-CHAT and required telephone interviews. Of these children, 185 qualified for diagnostic evaluation and 137 were diagnosed with ASD. M-CHAT scores confirmed over the telephone yielded a PPV of 0.74. In contrast, scores analyzed without telephone confirmation revealed a PPV of 0.36. Diagnostic evaluations were given to 18 additional children who were not detected by the M-CHAT, however, were deemed at risk according to alternative measures. Only one child in this group was diagnosed with ASD.

In their second study, Kleinman et al. (2008) reassessed children who were previously screened with the M-CHAT either in their first study or the study by Robins et al. (2001). A total of 1,416 children, who did not formerly qualify for diagnostic evaluation, were rescreened and 120 children, who previously required diagnostic evaluation, were reevaluated. Participants in this study were between 42 and 54 months of age. A child was referred for diagnostic evaluation if the telephone interview confirmed a positive screen on the M-CHAT, a professional identified the child with potential ASD sometime after the initial screen, or the child received a diagnostic evaluation in a previous study. One hundred and thirty one children received diagnostic evaluations and 80 children were found to have ASD. The PPV of the initial screen coupled with telephone confirmation was 0.59 at reevaluation. In contrast, initial M-CHAT scores analyzed without telephone confirmation revealed a PPV of 0.38. Seven children, who screened negative on the initial M-CHAT, were found to have ASD at reevaluation.

Robins (2008) provides further data on the M-CHAT. A total of 4,797 children, recruited from wellness checkups, were screened with the M-CHAT between 14 and 26 months of age. Four hundred and sixty-six children screened positive on the M-CHAT; however, only 362 children were available to participate in telephone interviews. After the interview process, 61 children qualified for a diagnostic evaluation; however, only 37 children were able to participate. Of these children, 21 were diagnosed with ASD, 17 were diagnosed with other developmental delays, and 3 were found to have typical development. M-CHAT scores confirmed over the telephone yielded a PPV of 0.57. In contrast, M-CHAT scores analyzed without telephone confirmation revealed a PPV of 0.058. Diagnostic evaluations were given to four additional children who were not detected by the M-CHAT, however, were identified with potential ASD by physicians. No children in this group were found to have ASD.

Recently, Pandey et al. (2008) evaluated the impact of ASD risk and age on the PPV of the M-CHAT. For the younger high-risk children, PPV was 0.79. For the older high-risk children PPV was 0.74. For the younger low-risk children PPV was 0.28 and for the older low-risk children

PPV was 0.61. Thus, we see a significant impact of risk status on the PPV of the M-CHAT.

Screening instruments for ASD have been developed almost exclusively in English for use in the United States or the United Kingdom. However, research groups recently have made efforts to translate the M-CHAT into various languages and evaluate the psychometric properties of the translated version. For example, Wong et al. (2004) translated the M-CHAT items and CHAT observational items into traditional Chinese and evaluated the items for cultural appropriateness. They found that the modified version had sensitivity of 0.93, specificity of 0.77, and PPV of 0.74. The M-CHAT has also been translated into Arabic (Eldin et al., 2008). The authors report sensitivity of 0.86, specificity of 0.80, and PPV of 0.88. Most recently the M-CHAT has been translated and evaluated for use in Sri Lanka with less success (Perera, Wijewardena, & Aluthwelage, 2009). The instrument was translated into the local languages and evaluated for cultural appropriateness. The authors found relatively low sensitivity for the translated version. They report a number of factors that may have influenced the low sensitivity; primary among these were the mother not considering the behaviors to be abnormal and social stigma regarding the child having ASD.

The M-CHAT has several benefits of which the most important is its quick administration. However, psychometric evaluations consistently have found that the follow-up phone interview is more or less required for good PPVs. A second limitation is that the target age was raised from 18 months, for the CHAT, to 24 months for the M-CHAT. While this change certainly increases the sensitivity of the M-CHAT, it also results in screening that is 6 months later. Thus, referral for intervention is delayed. In spite of these limitations, the M-CHAT still remains one of the most frequently recommended screening tools. A definite strength of the M-CHAT is that it has been translated and evaluated for use in various cultures and languages. Since ASD is a global challenge, this development is essential.

Quantitative Checklist for Autism in Toddlers

The Quantitative Checklist for Autism in Toddlers (Q-CHAT; Allison et al., 2008) is the most recent revision of the CHAT. The Q-CHAT is comprised of 25 items that are completed via caregiver report. CHAT items regarding pretend play and joint attention were incorporated into the Q-CHAT. In addition, the Q-CHAT contains supplementary items concerning language development, repetitive behaviors, and social communication. Items are scored using a five-point rating scale with possible answers ranging from 0 to 4. The point scale was applied in order to increase sensitivity. Unlike the CHAT and M-CHAT, which are limited to yes/no responses, the Q-CHAT accounts for the rate at which behaviors occur (Allison et al., 2008).

Allison et al. (2008) present psychometric data concerning the Q-CHAT. A total of 779 typically developing children and 160 children with ASD were screened with the Q-CHAT. The mean total score was 51.8 in the ASD group, compared to 26.7 in the typical development group. Internal reliability was satisfactory (Cronbach's $\alpha = 0.83$) in the ASD group but weaker (0.67) in the typical development group. Finally, test–retest reliability was measured in the typical development group, finding an intraclass correlation coefficient of 0.82. While these initial evaluations of internal stability are encouraging, further psychometric research on the Q-CHAT is needed.

The recent construction of the Q-CHAT provides it with current diagnostic theory, definitions, and psychometrics. Unlike the previous version, it uses a dimensional rating approach which accounts for minimal use of the skill reported. However, more data are required to fully evaluate the utility of the Q-CHAT to screen for ASD.

Early Screening of Autistic Traits Questionnaire

The Early Screening of Autistic Traits Questionnaire (ESAT; Dietz, Swinkels, van Daalen, van Engeland, & Buitelaar, 2006; Swinkels et al., 2006;) is a screening instrument designed to identify children at risk for ASD. This instrument appears in two formats, the 4-item ESAT and the 14-item ESAT. The four-item ESAT is a pre-screening tool in which caregivers answer questions regarding their child's play, emotional expression, and response to stimuli. The pre-screening tool takes only 3 min to administer. A positive prescreen occurs if a child fails one or more of the four items. In contrast, the 14-item ESAT requires that both a child's caregiver and a psychologist answer questions concerning the child's behavior. A positive screen occurs if a child fails 3 or more of the 14 items, as reported by either the parent or the psychologist (Dietz et al., 2006).

Swinkels et al. (2006) report on two studies concerning the development of the ESAT. The initial ESAT consisted of 19 items concerning pretend play, joint attention, interest in others, eye contact, verbal and non-verbal communication, stereotypy, preoccupations, reaction to sensory stimuli, emotional reaction, and social interaction. In the first study, 707 children, aged 8–226 months, were screened with the ESAT. Of these children, 478 were from a non-selected population, 153 had ASD, and 76 had ADHD. Parents of older children were told to retrospectively report on behaviors demonstrated by their child at 14 months. Test–retest reliability for the ASD group was found to be 0.81. Additionally, the first 14 items with a cutoff score of 3 or more failed responses were determined to best detect ASD. This combination identified 0% of the non-selected population, 90.1% of the ASD group, and 19.0% of the ADHD group. Additional evaluation revealed that 94.3% of the ASD group failed one or more

of the first four items compared to only 2.0% of the non-selected population. In the second study, 34 children with ASD, aged 16–48 months, were screened with the 14-item ESAT. Parents were told to retrospectively report on behaviors exhibited by their child at 14 months. Of the children, 94% received positive screens on the 14-item ESAT and 91% failed one or more of the first 4 items. The items "play in varied ways" and "express feelings on expected and appropriate moments" were failed most often by children whose parents reported feeling concerned during their child's first year of life.

Dietz et al. (2006) further discuss the psychometric properties of the ESAT. A total of 31,724 children, aged 14–15 months, were prescreened by physicians trained to administer the four-item ESAT. Children who received positive prescreens were reevaluated by psychologists trained to administer the 14-item ESAT. One hundred children screened positive on the 14-item ESAT. Of these children, 73 were referred for diagnostic evaluation and 18 were diagnosed with ASD. The PPV for the 14-item ESAT was 25%; however, all children who received false-positive screens were found to have other developmental disorders including intellectual disability, language disorder, and ADHD. The items found to be most predictive of ASD were "interest people," "smiles directly," and "reacts when spoken to." Parent and psychologist agreement on the 14-item ESAT was evaluated with a high overall accordance of 82.4%. Conversely, parent and psychologist agreement within the children diagnosed with ASD was only 65.9%. Fifteen of the 18 children diagnosed with ASD would have screened negative based on parental response alone. Children diagnosed with ASD and other developmental disorders were reevaluated at 42 months to determine diagnostic stability. Fourteen of the 16 children with ASD, who were available for reevaluation, maintained their diagnoses. The remaining two children were found to have other developmental disorders. Additionally, two children who were previously diagnosed with other developmental disorders were found to have ASD at reevaluation.

Additional psychometric properties of the ESAT are reported by Oosterling et al. (2009). Two hundred and thirty eight children identified with possible ASD by the 14-item ESAT and clinical judgment participated in this study. In addition to the ESAT, children were screened with the Social Communication Questionnaire (SCQ), Communication and Symbolic Behavior Scales-Developmental Profile (CSBS-DP), and critical items from the CHAT. The children were divided into two age groups. The younger group included 8- to 24-month olds and the older group included 25- to 44-month olds. All children received diagnostic evaluations. The psychometric properties of the ESAT were measured. Within the younger group, the PPV for identifying ASD was 0.75 and the NPV was 0.17. Additionally, sensitivity was 0.86 and specificity was 0.09.

In the older group, the PPV was 0.66 and the NPV was 0.42. Furthermore, sensitivity was 0.89 and specificity was 0.15. For all children combined, PPV was 0.68, NPV was 0.37, sensitivity was 0.88, and specificity was 0.14.

Oosterling et al. (2009) incorporated the ESAT into a two-stage early screening program comprised of training, a specific referral procedure, and a multidisciplinary diagnostic team. A total of 2,793 children between 0 and 11 years participated in this study. The participants were from two geographic regions, the experimental region and the control region. Healthcare professionals, in both regions, were trained to identify early signs of ASD. In addition, children identified with possible ASD from both regions were referred for diagnostic evaluation performed by a multidisciplinary team. Professionals in the experimental region received additional training to administer the ESAT. They were also given a specific referral procedure which required an ESAT to be administered before a child could receive diagnostic evaluation. Data were collected at baseline and for the following 3 years. Professionals in the experimental region referred considerably more children, between 0 and 2 years, for diagnostic evaluation than professionals in the control region. Two-thirds of the children, between 0 and 36 months, who were referred for diagnostic evaluation by professionals in the experimental region, were found to have ASD. The remaining third were diagnosed with other developmental disorders. Only two of these children were found to have typical development. Overall, children in the experimental region were diagnosed with ASD 21 months earlier than children in the control region. The amount of children diagnosed with ASD, between 0 and 36 months old, increased by 22.4% in the experimental region during the 3 years following training. In contrast, the control region saw a 1.7% decrease.

Overall the ESAT shows excellent sensitivity but relatively poor specificity. In spite of the poor specificity, the ESAT has a number of strengths. First, the ESAT is a very brief assessment in its four-item version. Further, the four-item version may be completed by caregivers, thus increasing its availability and utility. On the other hand, these same attributes may also cause the high rate of false positives. The ESAT merits consideration but should certainly be used within the context of a two-tier screening system, in which more specific diagnostic scales are used to catch false positives.

Infant–Toddler Checklist
The Infant–Toddler Checklist (ITC; Wetherby & Prizant, 2002; Wetherby et al., 2004) is a 24-item broadband screening instrument developed to detect communication delays in young children. The ITC, designed to be completed by a parent at a doctor's office or healthcare facility, is a

part of the Communication and Symbolic Behavior Scales-Developmental Profile (CSBS-DP; Wetherby & Prizant, 2002). Wetherby, Brosnan-Maddox, Peace, and Newton (2008) reported on the utility of ITC in screening for ASD. A total of 5,385 children from the general population were screened with the ITC between 6 and 24 months of age. A three-part surveillance procedure was used to detect children with ASD in this sample. Children identified with possible ASD were referred for diagnostic evaluation at 3 years or older. Sixty children attained a "best estimate diagnosis of ASD." Of these children, 56 screened positive on the ITC. Although the ITC demonstrated 93.3% sensitivity in detecting ASD (Wetherby et al., 2008), it is important to keep in mind that the ITC does not differentiate children with ASD from children with other communication delays.

Screening Tool for Autism in Two-Year-Olds
The Screening Tool for Autism in Two-Year-Olds (STAT; Stone, Coonrod, & Ousley, 2000) is a screening tool developed to distinguish children with autism from children with other developmental delays. The STAT is designed to evaluate the development of children between 24 and 35 months. A trained professional is required to administer the STAT, which takes approximately 20 min. Twelve pass/fail items comprise the STAT. These items are completed via direct interaction and assess areas regarding imitation, play, and communication (Stone et al., 2000).

Stone et al. (2000) report on the psychometric properties of the STAT. Two samples of children, between 24 and 35 months, were screened with the STAT. The first sample, containing 7 children with ASD and 33 children with other developmental delays, was used to establish cutoff scores for the STAT. The second sample, consisting of 12 children with ASD and 21 children with other developmental delays, was used to evaluate the validity of the cutoff scores. Scores were calculated in three assessment areas based on the sum of passed items. A cutoff score of less than 2 in any two assessment areas was established. This accurately detected 100% of the children with ASD and 91% of the children with other developmental delays in the first sample. In the second sample, the established cutoff score accurately identified 83% of the children with ASD and 86% of the children with other developmental delays. Here, sensitivity was 0.83, specificity was 0.86, PPV was 0.77, and NPV was 0.90.

Stone, Coonrod, Turner, and Pozdol (2004) report on two studies involving the STAT. In the first study, two samples of children, between 24 and 35 months, were screened with the STAT. Both samples consisted of 13 children with ASD and 13 children with other developmental delays who were matched based on chronological and mental age. The first sample was used to establish cutoff scores and the second sample was used to evaluate validity. A scoring procedure differing from that which was used by Stone et al. (2000)

was applied in this study. Four assessment areas regarding play, requesting, directing attention, and motor imitation were scored with equal weight. Possible scores in each area ranged between 0 and 1 and total scores ranged between 0 and 4. Higher scores illustrated more severe deficits. A total score of 2 or more was found to best detect ASD. Sensitivity was 0.92, specificity was 0.85, PPV was 0.86, and negative predicative value was 0.92.

In the second study, Stone et al. (2004) further investigate the psychometric properties of the STAT. Fifty children with autism, 15 children with PDD-NOS, and 39 children with other developmental delays were administered the STAT and the ADOS-G. Participants were between 24 and 35 months. Interrater agreement on the STAT was measured finding a Cohen's κ of 1.00. Furthermore, test–retest reliability was evaluated revealing a Cohen's κ of 0.90. Agreement between STAT detection and ADOS-G classification was measured in the children classified by the ADOS-G as having autism and children classified as having other developmental delays. Here, Cohen's κ was 0.95. Next, STAT and ADOS-G agreement was reevaluated in children classified with autism and children classified with other developmental delays, who were matched based on mental age. This yielded a Cohen's κ of 0.92. Since the STAT is a screening tool for the detection of autism, the children with PDD-NOS were evaluated independently. Of the children classified by the ADOS-G as having PDD-NOS, 64% attained low-risk scores on the STAT and 36% attained high-risk scores. Mean STAT scores were compared revealing that children with autism attained higher scores than children with PDD-NOS. In addition, children with PDD-NOS were found to score higher than children with other developmental delays. Mean scores were reevaluated in children with autism, children with PDD-NOS, and children with other developmental delays, who were matched based on mental age. Both the children with autism and the children with PDD-NOS showed considerable differences in comparison to the children with other developmental delays; however, no significant differences were identified between the children with autism and the children with PDD-NOS. Agreement between STAT detection and clinical diagnosis was measured in the children with autism and the children with other developmental delays, finding a Cohen's κ of 0.91.

Stone, McMahon, and Henderson (2008) evaluated the utility of the STAT in screening children younger than 24 months old. Seventy-one children, between 12 and 23 months, were screened with the STAT. All children were at risk for ASD. Fifty-nine children had older siblings with ASD and 12 children had been referred for potential ASD. Participants received diagnostic evaluations at the age of 24 months or older. Nineteen children were diagnosed with ASD, 15 children were diagnosed with other developmental delays, and 37 children did not elicit concern. The scoring procedure used in Stone et al. (2004) was applied in this

study; however, a cutoff score of 2.75 was found to best detect ASD in this sample of young children. This cutoff score yielded a sensitivity of 0.95, specificity was 0.73, PPV was 0.56, and NPV was 0.97. Children screened between 12 and 13 months attained the greatest percentage of false positives on the STAT. Moreover, the children who did not elicit concern after diagnostic evaluation attained a smaller percentage of false positives than the children who were diagnosed with other developmental delays.

The STAT appears to be a promising measure for differentiating ASD from other developmental delays. While psychometric evaluations of the STAT have found favorable results, it should be noted that these studies have used relatively small sample sizes. Thus, the STAT's ability to screen for ASD should be evaluated further in larger samples.

Social Communication Questionnaire

The Social Communication Questionnaire (SCQ; Berument, Rutter, Lord, Pickles, & Bailey, 1999), formerly known as the Autism Screening Questionnaire (ASQ), is a screening instrument developed to detect ASD in individuals aged 4 years or older. The SCQ contains 40 items which were derived from the ADI-R. Items assess areas concerning social interaction, language and communication, and repetitive and stereotyped behaviors. The SCQ, designed to be completed by a caregiver, is scored using a point system. The response "1" suggests that an atypical behavior is exhibited. Alternatively, "0" implies that an atypical behavior is not demonstrated. Total possible scores range from 0–39 in individuals with language and 0–34 in individuals without language (Berument et al., 1999).

The psychometric properties of the SCQ were first reported in Berument et al. (1999). Two hundred individuals, between 4 and 40 years, were screened with the SCQ. Of these individuals, 160 had PDD and 40 had other diagnoses. A cutoff score of 15 or more was found to best identify PDD. This cutoff score yielded a sensitivity of 0.85. Additionally, specificity was 0.75, PPV was 0.93, and NPV was 0.55.

Wiggins, Bakeman, Adamson, and Robins (2007) investigated the utility of the SCQ in screening young children. Thirty-seven children, between 17 and 45 months, were screened with the SCQ. Of these children, 19 had ASD and 18 had other developmental disorders. The cutoff score of 15, established in Berument et al. (1999), yielded a sensitivity of 0.47 and a specificity of 0.89; however, a lower cutoff score of 11 was found to best detect ASD in this sample of young children. Here, sensitivity was 0.89 and specificity was 0.89.

Oosterling et al. (2009) further evaluated the use of the SCQ in young children. Two hundred and thirty eight children, between 8 and 44 months, identified as at risk for ASD were screened with the SCQ, ESAT, CSBS-DP, and critical items from the CHAT. All children received diagnostic evaluations. The SCQ with a cutoff score of 15 yielded a PPV of 0.79 and an NPV of 0.48. Additionally, sensitivity was 0.66 and specificity was 0.64. In children aged 8–24 months, a cutoff score of 15 revealed a PPV of 0.84 and an NPV of 0.40. Furthermore, sensitivity was 0.74 and specificity was 0.55. A cutoff score of 11, in this age group, yielded a PPV of 0.79, NPV of 0.43, sensitivity of 0.89, and specificity of 0.27.

Overall, the SCQ shows weak sensitivity to detect ASD when using the procedures reported by Berument et al. (1999). However, scores may be improved significantly when using the procedures reported by Wiggins et al. (2007) and Oosterling et al. (2009). A significant strength of the SCQ is that it has been evaluated for use in very young children (<18 months), thus increasing the utility of the scale for early detection. The inclusion of very young children in the evaluation samples may be partially responsible for why psychometric scores have been somewhat less robust than those reported on other scales.

Conclusion and Future Directions

Early detection is essential for the treatment of ASD. While much research has been conducted over the past 30 years that demonstrates the effectiveness of EIBI programs, these programs can only benefit those who have access to services. The detection of ASD is a necessary first step in diagnosis and subsequent EIBI treatment. The age at which ASD diagnosis is believed to be stable has become increasingly younger, with current estimates showing stability at 18 months of age.

The dramatic increase in development of early screening tools over the past 10 years is encouraging. In this chapter, we have reviewed the most commonly used assessment tools that have some published evaluations on their psychometric properties. While each of these assessment tools merits consideration, there are two assessment tools in particular that stand out from the crowd; these are the M-CHAT in the BISCUIT.

Both the M-CHAT and the BISCUIT have received considerable attention from researchers who have evaluated their psychometric properties. One strength of the BISCUIT is that it has been designed with the entire autism spectrum in mind rather than simply a categorical diagnosis of autistic disorder. This is a significant strength because it allows for mild cases of ASD to be detected. Further, the clinician has access to an evaluation of comorbid disorders as well as problem behaviors. Information from both of these domains may prove to be directly useful to the treating clinician.

The BISCUIT is a relatively new instrument, whereas the M-CHAT is based upon the CHAT, which has a very long history of use. The M-CHAT has improved upon the psychometric properties of the original CHAT considerably. However, the improved psychometric properties are dependent upon the use of the follow-up phone interview. This

significantly increases the amount of time required for the M-CHAT to be administered, thus reducing the benefit of its brevity. Further, the M-CHAT has attained these improved psychometric properties by restricting the range of ages intended for screening from 18 months, in the CHAT, to 24 months in the M-CHAT. The BISCUIT has attained strong psychometric properties while maintaining a screening age of 17 months.

A significant limitation of almost all of the developed screening tools is the reliance upon English versions and cultural considerations. This is one area that the M-CHAT is particularly strong in that it has received considerable attention in non-English-speaking countries. It is clear that ASD is a global problem affecting children in all countries. Thus, developing and evaluating translated versions of these tools should be considered a top priority.

Little has been done to evaluate what training is required to administer the screening instruments. From a review of study descriptions and/or assessment manuals, the majority of assessments are intended to be administered by trained clinicians or in medical settings (BISCUIT, CHAT, 14-item ESAT, ITC, and STAT). However some tools have been developed to be completed by parents/caregivers (four-item ESAT, M-CHAT, Q-CHAT, and SCQ). The development of scales intended to be completed by caregivers is likely to result in a greater overall number of detected ASD cases, which is favorable. However, this may also come at the price of decreased reliability and specificity. More research is needed to evaluate the impact of training and familiarity with ASD on an instrument's ability to effectively screen for the disorder.

A final consideration regarding the early detection of ASD is how do specific responses to test items help in the development of child-specific treatment plans. The entire purpose of early detection is to facilitate early treatment of ASD. EIBI programs have been described (e.g., Hayward, Gale, & Eikeseth, 2009), yet little has been mentioned regarding how clinicians determine the content of their training programs. While, the primary purpose of a screening instrument is to detect likely cases of ASD, an additional benefit would be for these instruments to yield information regarding the particular diagnostic areas that are impaired.

References

Adrien, J. L., Lenoir, P., Martineau, J., Perrot, A., Hameury, L., Larmande, C., et al. (1993). Blind ratings of early symptoms of autism based upon family home movies. *Journal of the American Academy of Child and Adolescent Psychiatry, 32,* 617–626.

Allison, C., Baron-Cohen, S., Wheelwright, S., Charman, T., Richler, J., Pasco, G., et al. (2008). The Q-CHAT (Quantitative CHecklist for Autism in Toddlers): A normally distributed quantitative measure of autistic traits at 18–24 months of age: Preliminary report. *Journal of Autism and Developmental Disorders, 38,* 1414–1425.

212

D.R. Dixon et al.

American Academy of Pediatrics. (2001). Developmental surveillance and screening of infants and young children. *Pediatrics, 108*, 192–196.

American Academy of Pediatrics. (2006). Identifying infants and young children with developmental disorders in the medical home: An algorithm for developmental surveillance and screening. *Pediatrics, 118*, 405–420.

Autism and Developmental Disabilities Monitoring Network. (2009). Prevalence of autism spectrum disorders – Autism and developmental disabilities monitoring network, United States, 2006. *MMWR Surveillance Summaries, 56*, 1–11.

Baird, G., Charman, T., Baron-Cohen, S., Cox, A., Swettenham, J., Wheelwright, S., et al. (2000). A screening instrument for autism at 18 months of age: A 6-year follow-up study. *Journal of the American Academy of Child and Adolescent Psychiatry, 39*, 694–702.

Baranek, G. T. (1999). Autism during infancy: A retrospective video analysis of sensory-motor and social behaviors at 9–12 months of age. *Journal of Autism and Developmental Disorders, 29*, 213–224.

Baron-Cohen, S., Allen, J., & Gillberg, C. (1992). Can autism be detected at 18 months? The needle, the haystack, and the CHAT. *British Journal of Psychiatry, 161*, 839–843.

Baron-Cohen, S., Cox, A., Baird, G., Swettenham, J., Nightingale, N., Morgan, K., et al. (1996). Psychological markers in the detection of autism in infancy in a large population. *British Journal of Psychiatry, 168*, 158–163.

Baron-Cohen, S., Wheelwright, S., Cox, A., Baird, G., Charman, T., Swettenham, J., et al. (2000). Early identification of autism by the CHecklist for Autism in Toddlers (CHAT). *Journal of the Royal Society of Medicine, 93*, 521–525.

Berument, S. K., Rutter, M., Lord, C., Pickles, A., & Bailey, A. (1999). Autism screening questionnaire: Diagnostic validity. *British Journal of Psychiatry, 175*, 444–451.

Blackwell, P. B. (2002). Screening young children for autism and other social-communication disorders. *The Journal of the Kentucky Medical Association, 100*, 390–394.

Charman, T., Swettenham, J., Baron-Cohen, S., Cox, A., Baird, G., & Drew, A. (1997). Infants with autism: An investigation of empathy, pretend play, joint attention, and imitation. *Developmental Psychology, 33*, 781–789.

Charman, T., Taylor, E., Drew, A., Cockerill, H., Brown, J., & Baird, G. (2005). Outcome at 7 years of children diagnosed with autism at age 2: Predictive validity of assessments conducted at 2 and 3 years of age and pattern of symptom change over time. *Journal of Child Psychology and Psychiatry, 46*, 500–513.

Chawarska, K., Klin, A., Paul, R., & Volkmar, F. (2007). Autism spectrum disorder in the second year: Stability and change in syndrome expression. *Journal of Child Psychology and Psychiatry, 48*, 128–138.

Cox, A., Klein, K., Charman, T., Baird, G., Baron-Cohen, S., Swettenham, J., et al. (1999). Autism spectrum disorders at 20 and 42 months of age: Stability of clinical and ADI-R diagnosis. *Journal of Child Psychology and Psychiatry, 40*, 719–732.

Dawson, G., Munson, J., Estes, A., Osterling, J., McPartland, J., Toth, K., et al. (2002). Neurocognitive function and joint attention ability in young children with autism spectrum disorder versus developmental delay. *Child Development, 73*, 345–358.

Dawson, G., Toth, K., Abbott, R., Osterling, J., Munson, J., Estes, A., et al. (2004). Early social attention impairments in autism: Social orienting, joint attention, and attention to distress. *Developmental Psychology, 40*, 271–283.

De Giacomo, A., & Fombonne, E. (1998). Parental recognition of developmental abnormalities in autism. *European Child & Adolescent Psychiatry, 7*, 131–136.

Dietz, C., Swinkels, S., van Daalen, E., van Engeland, H., & Buitelaar, J. K. (2006). Screening for autistic spectrum disorder in children aged 14–15 months. II: Population screening with the Early Screening of Autistic Traits Questionnaire (ESAT). Design and general findings. *Journal of Autism and Developmental Disorders, 36*, 713–722.

Eaves, L. C., & Ho, H. H. (2004). The very early identification of autism: Outcome to age 4½-5. *Journal of Autism and Developmental Disorders, 34*, 367–378.

Eaves, L. C., Wingert, H., & Ho, H. H. (2006). Screening for autism. *Autism, 10*, 229–242.

Eldevik, S., Hastings, R. P., Hughes, C., Jahr, E., Eikeseth, S., & Cross, S. (2009). Meta-analysis of early intensive behavioral intervention for children with autism. *Journal of Clinical Child & Adolescent Psychology, 38*, 439–450.

Eldin, A. S., Habib, D., Noufal, A., Farrag, S., Bazaid, K., Al-Sharbati, M., et al. (2008). Use of the M-CHAT for a multinational screening of young children with autism in the Arab countries. *International Review of Psychiatry, 20*, 281–289.

Filipek, P. A., Accardo, P. J., Ashwal, S., Baranek, G. T., Cook, E. H., Jr., Dawson, G., et al. (2000). Practice parameter: Screening and diagnosis of autism: Report of the quality standards subcommittee of the American academy of neurology and the child neurology society. *Neurology, 55*, 468–479.

Fodstad, J. C., Matson, J. L., Hess, J., & Neal, D. (2009). Social and communication behaviours in infants and toddlers with autism and pervasive developmental disorder-not otherwise specified. *Developmental Neurorehabilitation, 12*, 152–157.

Fombonne, E., Heavey, L., Smeeth, L., Rodrigues, L. C., Cook, C., Smith, P. G., et al. (2004). Validation of the diagnosis of autism in general practitioner records. *BMC Public Health, 4*. doi:10.1186/1471-2458-4-5.

Goldberg, W. A., Osann, K., Filipek, P. A., Laulhere, T., Jarvis, K., Modahl, C., et al. (2003). Language and other regression: Assessment and timing. *Journal of Autism and Developmental Disorders, 33*, 607–616.

Granpeesheh, D., Dixon, D. R., Tarbox, J., Kaplan, A. M., & Wilke, A. E. (2009). The effects of age and treatment intensity on behavioral intervention outcomes for children with autism spectrum disorders. *Research in Autism Spectrum Disorders, 3*, 1014–1022.

Granpeesheh, D., Tarbox, J., & Dixon, D. R. (2009). Applied behavior analytic interventions for children with autism: A description and review of treatment research. *Annals of Clinical Psychiatry, 21*, 162–173.

Gray, K. M., Tonge, B. J., & Brereton, A. V. (2006). Screening for autism in infants, children, and adolescents. *International Review of Research in Mental Retardation, 32*, 197–227.

Hayward, D. W., Gale, C. M., & Eikeseth, S. (2009). Intensive behavioural intervention for young children with autism: A research-based service model. *Research in Autism Spectrum Disorders, 3*, 571–580.

Hoshino, Y., Kaneko, M., Yashima, Y., Kumashiro, H., Volkmar, F. R., & Cohen, D. J. (1987). Clinical features of autistic children with setback course in their infancy. *The Japanese Journal of Psychiatry and Neurology, 41*, 237–246.

Howlin, P., & Moore, A. (1997). Diagnosis in autism: A survey of over 1,200 patients in the UK. *Autism, 1*, 135–162.

Iverson, J. M., & Wozniak, R. H. (2007). Variation in vocal-motor development in infant siblings of children with autism. *Journal of Autism and Developmental Disorder, 37*, 158–170.

Jansiewicz, E. M., Goldberg, M. C., Newschaffer, C. J., Denckla, M. B., Landa, R., & Mostofsky, S. H. (2006). Motor signs distinguish children with high functioning autism and Asperger's syndrome from controls. *Journal of Autism and Developmental Disorders, 36*, 613–621.

Kleinman, J. M., Robins, D. L., Ventola, P. E., Pandey, J., Boorstein, H. C., Esser, E. L., et al. (2008). The modified Checklist for Autism in Toddlers: A follow-up study investigating the early detection of autism spectrum disorders. *Journal of Autism and Developmental Disorders, 38,* 827–839.

Kurita, H. (1985). Infantile autism with speech loss before the age of thirty months. *Journal of the American Academy of Child Psychiatry, 24,* 191–196.

Landa, R. J. (2008). Diagnosis of autism spectrum disorders in the first 3 years of life. *Nature Clinical Practice Neurology, 4,* 138–147.

Landa, R. J., & Garrett-Mayer, E. (2006). Development in infants with autism spectrum disorders: A prospective study. *Journal of Child Psychology and Psychiatry, 47,* 629–638.

Landa, R. J., Holman, K. C., & Garrett-Mayer, E. (2007). Social and communication development in toddlers with early and later diagnosis of autism spectrum disorders. *Archives of General Psychiatry, 64,* 853–864.

Lord, C. (1995). Follow-up of two-year-olds referred for possible autism. *Journal of Child Psychology and Psychiatry, 36,* 1365–1382.

Lord, C., Risi, S., DiLavore, P. S., Shulman, C., Thurm, A., & Pickles, A. (2006). Autism from 2 to 9 years of age. *Archives of General Psychiatry, 63,* 694–701.

Lovaas, O. I. (1987). Behavioral treatment and normal educational and intellectual functioning in young autistic children. *Journal of Consulting and Clinical Psychology, 55,* 3–9.

Luyster, R., Richler, J., Risi, S., Hsu, W., Dawson, G., Bernier, R., et al. (2005). Early regression in social communication in autism spectrum disorders: A CPEA study. *Developmental Neuropsychology, 27,* 311–336.

Maestro, S., Muratori, F., Cesari, A., Cavallaro, M. C., Paziente, A., Pecini, C., et al. (2005). Course of autism signs in the first year of life. *Psychopathology, 38,* 26–31.

Matson, J. L. (2007). Current status of differential diagnosis for children with autism spectrum disorders. *Research in Developmental Disabilities, 28,* 109–118.

Matson, J. L., Boisjoli, J. A., Hess, J., & Wilkins, J. (2010). Factor structure and diagnostic fidelity of the Baby and Infant Screen for Children with aUtIsm Traits – Part 1 (BISCUIT – Part 1). *Developmental Neurorehabilitation, 13,* 72–79.

Matson, J. L., Boisjoli, J. A., Hess, J., & Wilkins, J. (2011). *Comorbid psychopathology factor structure on the baby and infant screen for children with aUtIsm traits – Part 2 (BISCUIT – Part 2). Research in Autism Spectrum Disorders, 5,* 426–432.

Matson, J. L., Boisjoli, J. A., Rojahn, J., & Hess, J. (2009). A factor analysis of challenging behaviors assessed with the Baby and Infant Screen for Children with aUtism Traits (BISCUIT-Part 3). *Research in Autism Spectrum Disorders, 3,* 714–722.

Matson, J. L., Boisjoli, J. A., & Wilkins, J. (2007). *The Baby and Infant Screen for Children with aUtIsm Traits (BISCUIT).* Baton Rouge, LA: Disability Consultants, LLC.

Matson, J. L., Dempsey, T., & Fodstad, J. C. (2009). Stereotypies and repetitive/restrictive behaviours in infants with autism and pervasive developmental disorder. *Developmental Neurorehabilitation, 12,* 122–127.

Matson, J. L., Fodstad, J. C., & Mahan, S. (2009). Cutoffs, norms, and patterns of comorbid difficulties in children with developmental disabilities on the Baby and Infant Screen for Children with aUtIsm Traits (BISCUIT-Part 2). *Research in Developmental Disabilities, 30,* 1221–1228.

Matson, J. L., Fodstad, J. C., Mahan, S., & Sevin, J. A. (2009). Cutoffs, norms, and patterns of comorbid difficulties in children with an ASD on the baby and infant screen for children with aUtIsm traits (BISCUIT-Part 2). *Research in Autism Spectrum Disorders, 3,* 977–988.

Matson, J. L., & Kozlowski, A. M. (2010). Autistic regression. *Research in Autism Spectrum Disorders, 4,* 340–345.

Matson, J. L., & Smith, K. R. M. (2008). Current status of intensive behavioral interventions for young children with autism and PDD-NOS. *Research in Autism Spectrum Disorders, 2,* 60–74.

Matson, J. L., Wilkins, J., & Fodstad, J. C. (2010). Children with autism spectrum disorders: A comparison of those who regress versus those who do not. *Developmental Neurorehabilitation, 13,* 37–45.

Matson, J. L., Wilkins, J., & González, M. (2008). Early identification and diagnosis in autism spectrum disorders in young children and infants: How early is too early? *Research in Autism Spectrum Disorders, 2,* 75–84.

Matson, J. L., Wilkins, J., Sevin, J. A., Knight, C., Boisjoli, J. A., & Sharp, B. (2009). Reliability and item content of the Baby and Infant Screen for Children with aUtIsm Traits (BISCUIT): Parts 1–3. *Research in Autism Spectrum Disorders, 3,* 336–344.

Matson, J. L., Wilkins, J., Sharp, B., Knight, C., Sevin, J. A., & Boisjoli, J. A. (2009). Sensitivity and specificity of the Baby and Infant Screen for Children with aUtIsm Traits (BISCUIT): Validity and cutoff scores for autism and PDD-NOS in toddlers. *Research in Autism Spectrum Disorders, 3,* 924–930.

Mays, R. M., & Gillon, J. E. (1993). Autism in young children: An update. *Journal of Pediatric Health Care, 7,* 17–23.

Moore, V., & Goodson, S. (2003). How well does early diagnosis of autism stand the test of time? *Autism, 7,* 47–63.

Myers, S. M., & Plauché Johnson, C. (2007). Management of children with autism spectrum disorders. *Pediatrics, 120,* 1162–1182.

Nadig, A. S., Ozonoff, S., Young, G. S., Rozga, A., Sigman, M., & Rogers, S. J. (2007). A prospective study of response to name in infants at risk for autism. *Archives of Pediatrics and Adolescent Medicine, 161,* 378–383.

National Academy of Sciences. (2001). *Educating children with autism.* Commission on Behavioral and Social Sciences and Education.

New York State Department of Health, Early Intervention Program. (1999). *Clinical practice guideline: Report of the recommendations: Autism/Pervasive developmental disorders: Assessment and intervention for young children (Age 0–3 years).*

Oosterling, I. J., Swinkels, S. H., van der Gaag, R. J., Visser, J. C., Dietz, C., & Buitelaar, J. K. (2009). Comparative analysis of three screening instruments for autism spectrum disorder in toddlers at high risk. *Journal of Autism and Developmental Disorders, 39,* 897–909.

Oosterling, I. J., Wensing, M., Swinkels, S., van der Gaag, R. J., Visser, J. C., Woudenberg, T., et al. (2009). Advancing early detection of autism spectrum disorder by applying an integrated two-stage screening approach. *The Journal of Child Psychology and Psychiatry.* doi:10.1111/j.1469–7610.2009.02150.x.

Ornitz, E. M., Guthrie, D., & Farley, A. H. (1977). The early development of autistic children. *Journal of Autism and Childhood Schizophrenia, 7,* 207–229.

Oslejsková, H., Dusek, L., Makovská, Z., Pejcochová, J., Autrata, R., & Slapák, I. (2008). Complicated relationship between autism with regression and epilepsy. *Neuroendocrinology Letters, 29,* 558–570.

Oslejsková, H., Kontrová, I., Foralová, R., Dusek, L., & Némethová, D. (2007). The course of diagnosis in autistic patients: The delay between recognition of the first symptoms by parents and correct diagnosis. *Neuroendocrinology Letters, 28,* 895–900.

Osterling, J. A., Dawson, G., & Munson, J. A. (2002). Early recognition of 1-year-old infants with autism spectrum disorder versus mental retardation. *Development and Psychopathology, 14,* 239–251.

Ozonoff, S., Williams, B. J., & Landa, R. (2005). Parental report of the early development of children with regressive autism: The delays-plus-regression phenotype. *Autism, 9,* 461–486.

Pandey, J., Verbalis, A., Robins, D. L., Boorstein, H., Klin, A., Babitz, T., et al. (2008). Screening for autism in older and younger toddlers with the modified Checklist for Autism in Toddlers. *Autism, 12,* 513–535.

Perera, H., Wijewardena, K., & Aluthwelage, R. (2009). Screening of 18–24-month-old children for autism in a semi-urban community in Sri Lanka. *Journal of Tropical Pediatrics, 55*, 402–405.

Prizant, B., & Wetherby, A. (1988). Providing services to children with autism (ages 0 to 2 years) and their families. *Focus on Autistic Behavior, 4*, 1–16.

Robins, D. L. (2008). Screening for autism spectrum disorders in primary care settings. *Autism, 12*, 537–556.

Robins, D. L., Fein, D., Barton, M. L., & Green, J. A. (2001). The modified Checklist for Autism in Toddlers: An initial study investigating the early detection of autism and pervasive developmental disorders. *Journal of Autism and Developmental Disorders, 31*, 131–144.

Rojahn, J., Matson, J. L., Mahan, S., Fodstad, J. C., Knight, C., Sevin, J. A., et al. (2009). Cutoffs, norms, and patterns of problem behaviors in children with an ASD on the Baby and Infant Screen for Children with aUtIsm traits (BISCUIT-Part 3). *Research in Autism Spectrum Disorders, 3*, 989–998.

Scambler, D. J., Hepburn, S. L., & Rogers, S. J. (2006). A two-year follow-up on risk status identified by the Checklist for Autism in Toddlers. *Developmental and Behavioral Pediatrics, 27*, 104–110.

Scambler, D. J., Rogers, S. J., & Wehner, E. A. (2001). Can the Checklist for Autism in Toddlers differentiate young children with autism from those with developmental delays? *Journal of the American Academy of Child and Adolescent Psychiatry, 40*, 1457–1463.

Siklos, S., & Kerns, K. A. (2007). Assessing the diagnostic experiences of a small sample of parents of children with autism spectrum disorders. *Research in Developmental Disabilities, 28*, 9–22.

Skinner, B. F. (1957). *Verbal behavior*. Acton, MA: Copley.

Snow, A. V., & Lecavalier, L. (2008). Sensitivity and specificity of the modified Checklist for Autism in Toddlers and the social communication questionnaire in preschoolers suspected of having pervasive developmental disorders. *Autism, 12*, 627–644.

Stone, W. L., Coonrod, E. E., & Ousley, O. Y. (2000). Brief report: Screening Tool for Autism in Two-Year-Olds (STAT): Development and preliminary data. *Journal of Autism and Developmental Disorders, 30*, 607–612.

Stone, W. L., Coonrod, E. E., Turner, L. M., & Pozdol, S. L. (2004). Psychometric properties of the STAT for early autism screening. *Journal of Autism and Developmental Disorders, 34*, 691–701.

Stone, W. L., Lee, E. B., Ashford, L., Brissie, J., Hepburn, S. L., Coonrod, E. E., et al. (1999). Can autism be diagnosed accurately in children under 3 years? *Journal of Child Psychology and Psychiatry, 40*, 219–226.

Stone, W. L., McMahon, C. R., & Henderson, L. M. (2008). Use of the Screening Tool for Autism in Two-Year-Olds (STAT) for children under 24 months: An exploratory study. *Autism, 12*, 557–573.

Sullivan, M., Finelli, J., Marvin, A., Garrett-Mayer, E., Bauman, M., & Landa, R. (2007). Response to joint attention in toddlers at risk for autism spectrum disorder: A prospective study. *Journal of Autism and Developmental Disorders, 37*, 37–48.

Swinkels, S. H. N., Dietz, C., van Daalen, E., Kerkhof, I. H. G. M., van Engeland, H., & Buitelaar, J. K. (2006). Screening for autistic spectrum in children aged 14 to 15 months. I: The development of the Early Screening of Autistic Traits Questionnaire (ESAT). *Journal of Autism and Developmental Disorders, 36*, 723–732.

Szatmari, P., Jones, M. B., Zwaigenbaum, L., & MacLean, J. E. (1998). Genetics of autism: Overview and new directions. *Journal of Autism and Developmental Disorders, 28*, 351–368.

Turner, L. M., & Stone, W. L. (2007). Variability in outcome for children with an ASD diagnosis at age 2. *Journal of Child Psychology and Psychiatry, 48*, 793–802.

Turner, L. M., Stone, W. L., Pozdol, S. L., & Coonrod, E. E. (2006). Follow-up of children with autism spectrum disorders from age 2 to age 9. *Autism, 10*, 243–265.

US Department of Health and Human Services. (1999). *Mental health: A report of the surgeon general*. Rockville, MD: US Department of Health and Human Services Substance Abuse and Mental Health Services Administration Center for Mental Health Services National Institutes of Health National Institute of Mental Health.

VanDenHeuvel, A., Fitzgerald, M., Greiner, B., & Perr, I. J. (2007). Screening for autism spectrum disorder at the 18-month developmental assessment: A population-based study. *Irish Medical Journal, 100*, 565–567.

Werner, E., & Dawson, G. (2005). Validation of the phenomenon of autistic regression using home videotapes. *Archives of General Psychiatry, 62*, 889–895.

Wetherby, A. M., Brosnan-Maddox, S., Peace, V., & Newton, L. (2008). Validation of the infant-toddler checklist as a broadband screener for autism spectrum disorders from 9 to 24 months of age. *Autism, 12*, 487–511.

Wetherby, A. M., & Prizant, B. (2002). *Communication and symbolic behavior scales developmental profile – first normed edition*. Baltimore: Paul H. Brookes.

Wetherby, A. M., Woods, J., Allen, L., Cleary, J., Dickinson, H., & Lord, C. (2004). Early indicators of autism spectrum disorders in the second year of life. *Journal of Autism and Developmental Disorders, 34*, 473–493.

Wiggins, L. D., Baio, J., & Rice, C. (2006). Examination of the time between first evaluation and first autism spectrum diagnosis in a population-based sample. *Journal of Developmental and Behavioral Pediatrics, 27*, 79–87.

Wiggins, L. D., Bakeman, R., Adamson, L. B., & Robins, D. L. (2007). The utility of the social communication questionnaire in screening for autism in children referred for early intervention. *Focus on Autism and other Developmental Disabilities, 22*, 33–38.

Wong, V., Hui, L. H. S., Lee, W. C., Leung, L. S. J., Ho, P. K. P., Lau, W. L. C., et al. (2004). A modified screening tool for autism (Checklist for Autism in Toddlers [CHAT-23]) for Chinese children. *Pediatrics, 114*, e166–e176.

Zachor, D. A., Ben-Itzchak, E., Rabinovich, A. L., & Lahat, E. (2007). Change in autism core symptoms with intervention. *Research in Autism Spectrum Disorders, 1*, 304–317.

Diagnostic Instruments for the Core Features of ASD

13

Julie A. Worley and Johnny L. Matson

Autism spectrum disorders (ASDs) are a group of lifelong, heterogeneous disorders that share overlapping diagnostic criteria. The broad diagnostic criteria first defined by Kanner (1943) have remained consistent; however, the diagnostic systems classifying these core impairments (i.e., in socialization, communication, and restricted interests/repetitive behavior) have changed over time. Thus, to account for these changes, measures used to assess symptoms of various forms of ASDs have amended and transformed. With the increasing knowledge about the various ASDs, the development of diagnostic measures and screeners that assess for symptoms of ASD continues. Therefore, the focus of this chapter will be on measures specific to ASDs that assist in screening for symptoms and for diagnostic decision making. The standardization of ASD diagnoses remains complicated by research on the symptoms of ASD, differential diagnoses between ASDs, and the promotion of diagnosing ASD in preschoolers (Matson, Nebel-Schwalm, & Matson, 2007). Therefore, measures included in this chapter may cover one or a number of the above (e.g., for younger versus older children, just for autism versus differentiating between ASDs).

This review focuses on three of the five pervasive developmental disorders outlined in the *Diagnostic and Statistical Manual of Mental Disorders, Fourth Edition, Text Revision (DSM-IV-TR*; American Psychiatric Association [APA], 2000). Thus, measures that assess for symptoms of autistic disorder (AD), Asperger's syndrome (AS), and pervasive developmental disorder – not otherwise specified (PDD-NOS) are included in this review. Furthermore, throughout this review, AD is often referred to as autism to keep the "trueness" of the various studies and measures as described by the authors. Due to the rarity of Rett's disorder and childhood disintegrative disorder, they will be excluded

in this chapter. In addition, only measures with known psychometric investigations (i.e., reliability and validity analyses) are included in the review. Prior to the utilization of an assessment measure, psychometric information must be considered. Thus, in order for assessments to be of value, they need to be reliable and demonstrate validity.

Additional variables are important to consider while reviewing this chapter. That is, when assessing the utility of various measures, it is important to take into account the age cohort for which each measure is intended, administration time of the measure, and the measure's ability to discriminate between various ASDs. This review will assist clinicians in choosing the most appropriate measure. Table 13.1 provides an overview of measures with published psychometric analyses found in a literature review for assessing symptoms of ASD. Discussed first are those measures that assess for symptoms of AD, second those that can differentiate between ASDs, and lastly, those that assess for symptoms of AS.

Assessment Tools for ASD

Autism Behavior Checklist (ABC)

The *ABC* is an informant-based checklist designed to be completed independently by a caregiver or teacher and subsequently interpreted by a clinician (Krug, Arick, & Almond, 1980). Primarily, this measure was developed for use in the school systems to assess symptoms of autism and to assist with educational placements and planning. Furthermore, it is one of the five components of the autism screening instrument for educational planning (ASIEP). A total of 57 items comprise this scale which were included in this checklist based on a review of the literature, expert consultation, relevant checklists/measures, and an item analysis. The *ABC* takes approximately 20 min to complete and is intended for use with children aged 3 through school-aged.

The items of the *ABC* comprise five symptom areas: sensory, relating, body and object use, language, and social and

13

J.L. Matson (✉)
Department of Psychology, Louisiana State University, Baton Rouge, LA 70803, USA
e-mail: johnmatson@aol.com

Table 13.1 Assessment measures for autism spectrum disorders

Assessment measures	Age suitability	Administration time	Type of measure
Autism			
Autism Behavior Checklist (ABC)	3 years through school age	20 min	Rating scale
Autism diagnostic interview (ADI)	5 years through early adulthood	2–3 h	Interview
Autism diagnostic interview revised (ADI-R)	Children and adults with a mental age above 2.0 years	1 to 2 h	Interview
Autism diagnostic observation schedule (ADOS)	6 years through adulthood	20–30 min	Observation
Autism Diagnostic Observation Schedule Generic (ADOS-G)	Children with limited or no language Verbally fluent, high-functioning adolescents and adults	20–30 min	Observation
Behavior observation system (BOS)	Children	30 min observations: One per day for 3 days	Observation
Checklist for Autism in Toddlers (CHAT)	18 months	5–10 min	Rating scale
Childhood Autism Rating Scale (CARS)	Childhood through adult	30 min	Rating scale
Developmental dimensional and diagnostic interview (3di)	Not specified	90 or 45 min (short version)	Interview
Diagnostic Interview for Social and Communication Disorders (DISCO)	Children and adults all ages	2–4 h	Interview
Diagnostic Checklist for Behavior-Disturbed Children, Form E2 (E2-DC)	Not specified	Not specified	Rating scale
Gilliam Autism Rating Scale (GARS)	3–22	20 min	Rating scale
Modified Checklist for Autism in Toddlers (M-CHAT)	24 months	5–10 min	Rating scale
Pervasive developmental disorders in mentally retarded persons (PDD-MRS)	2–55 years	15 min	Rating scale
Pervasive Developmental Disorders Rating Scale (PDDRS)	Not specified	20 min	Rating scale
Pre-linguistic Autism Diagnostic Observation Schedule (PL-ADOS)	Under 6 years	30 min	Rating scale
Screening Test for Autism in 2-Year Olds (STAT)	24–35 months	20 min	Rating scale
Autism spectrum disorders			
Autism spectrum disorders diagnosis for adult (ASD-DA)	Adults	10–15 min	Rating scale
Autism spectrum disorders diagnostic for child (ASD-DC)	3–16 years	10–15 min	Rating scale
Baby and Infant Screen for Children with aUtIsm Traits-Part 1	17–37 months	30 min	Rating scale
Behavior function inventory (BFI)	Not specified	2 days	Rating scale
Pervasive developmental disorders behavior Inventory (PDDBI)	1.6–12.5 years	20–30 min Extended form, 45 min	Rating scale
Asperger's syndrome			
Asperger Syndrome Diagnostic Scale (ASDS)	5–18 years	10–15 min	Rating scale
Autism Spectrum Screening Questionnaire (ASSQ)	6–17 years	10 min	Rating scale
Childhood Asperger Syndrome Test (CAST)	4–11 years	10 min	Rating scale
Gilliam Asperger's Disorder Scale (GADS)	3–22 years	5–10 min	Rating scale
Krug Asperger's Disorder Index (KADI)	6–21 years	5–10 min	Rating scale

self-help. However, other researchers have suggested that a three-factor solution better represents the measure (Volkmar et al., 1988; Wadden, Bryson, & Rodgers, 1991). Each item on this measure is provided a weight, and thus the higher the weight of the item, the more frequently it occurs within the ASD population. Krug and colleagues (1980) weighted the item scores, which ranged from 1 to 4, with 4 indicating the highest predictor of ASD. Cutoff scores have been established for this measure; thus up to 53 indicates that the child is unlikely to have autism, a score of 53–67 indicates questionable autism, and a score of 68 and above indicates a high probability of autism (Krug et al., 1980). However, other researchers have suggested that a cutoff of 44 better classifies autism (Wadden et al., 1991). Using 44 as a cutoff, sensitivity was 91.1%, positive predictive power (PPP) was 86.6%, and negative predictive power (NPP) was 96.4%. With the original cutoff scores, only approximately 81% of participants diagnosed with autism fell into the questionable or probably autism range, thus indicating that the original cutoffs may be too high (Volkmar et al., 1988).

Krug and colleagues examined the internal consistency of the *ABC*, which was found to be $\alpha = 0.94$. Interrater reliability was found to be $r = 0.94$, with an agreement score of 95%. However, when comparing the agreement between teachers and parents on this measure, all correlations were low for the subscales and total score (Szatmari, Archer, Fisman, & Streiner, 1994). In regard to validity, the *ABC* is able to discriminate well between those diagnosed with ASD and those without ASD (four comparison groups: severe intellectual disability [ID], deaf–blind, severely emotionally disturbed, and typically developing) (Krug et al., 1980). That is, when compared to control groups, those with ASD scored higher in the five symptoms areas and total score. Further support for the use of this measure came from a comparison of the *ABC* to the *autism diagnostic interview* (*ADI*; LeCouteur et al., 1989). The *ABC* had higher sensitivity than the *ADI*, although the *ADI* demonstrated somewhat higher specificity (Yirmiya, Sigman, & Freeman, 1994). In addition, criterion-related validity was assessed comparing sex, age, living setting, language development, and student–teacher ratio between those with and without an ASD. Almost all analyses were statistically significant. The *ABC* has a large body of published research and is easy to administer; however, it is not designed for use in children under the age of 3.

Autism Diagnostic Interview (ADI)

The *ADI* is a standardized interview designed to be used with a primary caregiver, for those aged five through early adulthood that also have a mental age of at least 2 years (LeCouteur et al., 1989). The *ADI* focuses on social interaction, communication and language, repetitive behaviors and restricted interests, and age of symptom onset. This measure assesses a child's behavior related to the above-mentioned areas during the first 5 years of life and during the 12-month time period leading up to the *ADI* administration. Each item of the *ADI* contains the following: an initial probe, codes with instructions regarding the detail of information required, and supplemental probes. The interviewer must obtain details of the behaviors specific to each item. Thus, skilled interviewers and those familiar with ASD symptoms are essential. Each item in this measure can be scored as a 0 (behavior was not present), 1 (behavior was exhibited, but not severe or frequent enough to warrant a rating of 2), 2 (abnormality is present), 3 (abnormality is present and more severe than a 2), or 7 (some abnormality is present, but not as specified in the coding instructions). This interview takes approximately 2–3 h to complete.

During *ADI* development, a scoring algorithm was created based on ICD-10 (WHO, 1992) diagnostic criteria (LeCouteur et al., 1989). Thus, not all items comprising the ADI factor into the algorithm (i.e., only 14 items from the social interaction area, 12 from the language/communication area, and 6 from the restricted interests and repetitive behavior factor into the algorithm). Deficits related to one of the above-mentioned areas need to be present prior to age 36 months, with at least a score of 10, 8, and 4, on the socialization, verbal communication, and restricted and repetitive interests domains, respectively. Similarly, the same cutoffs are required for nonverbal individuals; however, only a score of 6 is needed in the language/communication area to meet criteria for autism.

In regard to psychometric properties of the *ADI*, there have been studies assessing its reliability and validity (LeCouteur et al., 1989). Item endorsement agreement within each of the three content areas was computed. For items comprising the social interaction content area, $K = 0.66–0.97$. For items comprising the communication/language, restricted interests/repetitive behaviors, and age of onset content areas, $K = 0.64–0.87$, $0.55–0.92$, and $0.76–0.90$, respectively. In addition, intraclass correlation coefficients (ICCs) were above 0.93 for the socialization, communication, and restricted interests/repetitive behaviors content areas.

In regard to diagnostic differentiation between those with autism and those with "mental handicap," abnormalities were more evident in all content areas for those with autism. Thus, all individuals who had a diagnosis of autism met criteria on the algorithm for autism. In addition, specificity was 100%. Although the psychometric properties are stable, a limitation of this measure is that it cannot be used for children below 5 years of age and takes a few hours to complete.

Autism Diagnostic Interview – Revised (ADI-R)

The *ADI-R* is a semistructured interview administered to a parent or guardian by a trained interviewer (Lord, Rutter, & LeCouteur, 1994). It is a modified version of the ADI, which allows for the assessment of symptoms of autism prior to 5 years of age, with a shorter administration time. Some items were taken from the *ADI* with the addition of new items to allow for better differentiation between those with autism and those with "mental handicaps." Items that are asked during the interview focus on actual behaviors and rely on the interviewer's judgment for coding. The coding for the *ADI-R* is the same as for the *ADI*. Items relating to typical development or deficits in these skills are coded for abnormality during the ages of 4–5. There are a total of 93 items over four content areas: 1 (impairments in social interaction), 2 (impairments in communication, either verbal or nonverbal), 3 (restricted and repetitive interests or behaviors), or 4 (age of onset by 36 months of age). Of the 93 items, a total of 37 are included in the diagnostic algorithm, which aligns with the *DSM-IV* (APA, 1994) and ICD-10 (WHO, 1992). In order to meet criteria for AD an individual must meet (i.e., exceed) cutoff in all four areas. Cutoffs for the content areas are as follows: social impairment = 10, restricted and repetitive interests or behaviors = 3, and age of onset = 1. For the communication content area, there are separate cutoffs for verbal and nonverbal participants, which are 8 and 7, respectively.

Using the above-mentioned cutoffs, sensitivity and specificity exceeded 0.90. Initial psychometric analyses by Lord et al. (1994) indicated that the $K_W = 0.64$–0.89 for social interaction, 0.69–0.89 for communication, and 0.63–0.86 for restricted and repetitive behaviors. Furthermore, interrater and test–retest reliabilities were good (K_W ranging from 0.62 to 0.89). In addition, social, restricted and repetitive behaviors, and communication content areas of the ADI-R had internal consistencies of $\alpha = 0.95$ (social), 0.69 (restricted and repetitive behaviors), and 0.84 (communication). The *ADI-R* is able to best differentiate between pervasive (ASD) and specific (language disorders) developmental disorders. That is, on all domains, those with autism scored higher when compared to the scores of those with language disorders (Mildenberger, Sitter, Noterdaeme, & Amorosa, 2001). Psychometric studies conducted by independent researchers have yielded lower, although still acceptable, reliability estimates for the *ADI-R* (Lecavalier et al., 2006). More recently, Charman et al. (2005) showed that the ADI-R at age 2 did not predict a diagnosis of autism age 7, but assessment at age 3 did. Also, the utility of the *ADI-R* total algorithm for distinguishing between autism and other developmental disabilities has been tested with sensitivity estimates ranging from 0.86 to 1.00 and specificity estimates ranging from 0.75 to 0.96 (Lord et al., 1997).

Autism Diagnostic Observation Schedule (ADOS)

The *ADOS* is a standardized observation of behaviors associated with social and communication impairments in autism (Lord et al., 1989). The examiner is considered a participant and observer in the assessment session, supplying contextual and social presses (i.e., preplanned activities that appear to occur naturally). This measure is used for individuals aged 6 through adulthood that are within the normal range of intelligence or only have mild impairments in cognition. The *ADOS* does not examine the presence or absence of social and communication behaviors, but the quality of the behaviors. Items for this measure emerged from diagnostic definitions, research, and reliable and valid descriptions of behaviors. The measure contains eight tasks that can be completed within 20–30 min. Each task contains two options, which vary according to the individual's chronological and developmental level. The eight tasks are construction task, unstructured presentation of toys, drawing game, demonstration task, poster task, book task, conversations, and socioemotional questions. Each of these tasks is rated during the observation as 0 (within normal limits), 1 (infrequent or possible abnormality), 2 (definite abnormality), or 7 (the behavior is abnormal, but not as defined by the other codings). After the commencement of the observation, general ratings are made by the clinician in regard to social interaction, communication and language, stereotyped/restricted behaviors, and abnormal behaviors (nonspecific).

Psychometric properties of the *ADOS* have shown promise (Lord et al., 1989). Thus, weighted kappas for interrater reliability ranged from 0.61 to 0.92 for the tasks and from 0.58 to 0.87 for the general ratings. Weighted kappas for test–retest reliability ranged from 0.57 to 0.84 and from 0.58 to 0.92 for the tasks and general ratings, respectively. To examine the criterion-related validity of the algorithm, items in the *ADOS* matching the diagnostic criteria in the ICD-10 (WHO, 1992) were grouped together: reciprocal social interaction, communication/language, and restricted/stereotyped behaviors. In addition, a total score of the identified items was computed. The above-mentioned algorithm was able to discriminate those diagnosed with autism from those without. That is, significant differences were found between groups for all three content areas in the algorithm. Interrater and test–retest reliabilities ranged from 0.70 to 0.96 (ICCs) for the algorithm content areas and the overall scores. Noterdaeme, Sitter, Mildenberger, and Amorosa (2000) found that the *ADOS* was able to differentiate between children with autism and children diagnosed with an expression/receptive language disorder, especially within the socialization dimension. Their findings indicate that the specificity was at 100%, but sensitivity was low. That is, only 3 of the 11 children diagnosed with autism met criteria for autism on the *ADOS* because of failure to meet the cutoff of the stereotyped behavior domain. A limitation of this scale is that the administration heavily relies on the skills of the assessor and requires great training to complete reliably. Also, it can only be used for those with a mental age greater than 2.

Autism Diagnostic Observation Schedule – Generic (ADOS-G)

The *ADOS-G* is a semistructured assessment, which standardizes observations of behavior (i.e., social and communication behaviors) to assess for symptoms of ASD (Lord et al., 2000). The *ADOS-G* was developed as an extension of the *ADOS* and *PL-ADOS* in order to assess functioning at infant and toddler levels and to extend age and verbal limits for younger and nonverbal children. Thus, the clinician is able to use the module that best matches the language skills (i.e., expressive) of the individual being assessed. Four different modules are included, each reflecting a different developmental/language level. These modules provide a social and communication series using presses to spontaneously observe behaviors in a standardized way. Regarding scoring, notes can be taken throughout the interview, but scoring is not completed until the commencement of the session. Items are rated from 0 (no evidence of abnormality related to autism) to 2 (definite evidence). Although this measure contains 28–31 ratings (depending on the module used), only a subset of these items within each module are used for the diagnostic algorithms. Scores need to exceed thresholds on the social behavior domain, communication domain, and the social communication domain to meet criteria for autism. Restricted interests and repetitive behaviors are not accounted for in the diagnostic algorithms for each module since there is only one observation period.

For psychometric studies, reliability of the *ADOS-G* was examined through interrater and test–retest. Test–retest correlations were found to range from 0.73 to 0.78 for the domains used in the scoring algorithm and interrater reliability was found to be excellent, ranging from 0.84 to 0.93. Cronbach's alpha was utilized to measure the internal consistency of the *ADOS-G*. Collapsing across all modules, $\alpha = 0.74$–0.94 for the social domain, communication domain, and social communication total. Sensitivity of the *ADOS-G* was determined to be 95% and specificity was 92%. In regard to validity, the *ADOS-G* was good at discriminating between those with an ASD and those without, but not between autism and PDD-NOS.

A benefit of this measure is that behavior changes over time can be measured with repeated assessments at the individual level. Limitations of this scale are that assessors have to attend workshops in order to administer this measure reliably. Also, restricted interests and repetitive behaviors are

not used in the algorithm; therefore; this omission may cause individuals falling in the PDD-NOS category (i.e., those who have social deficits, no communication deficits, and restricted and repetitive behaviors) to not meet the cutoff on the measure. In addition, age of symptom onset is not assessed; therefore, there is no way to determine if criterion were met before age 3. Thus, the *ADOS-G* cannot be used in isolation for diagnostic decision making; however, it does give a good current picture of clinical functioning.

Behavior Observation Scale (BOS)

The *BOS* contains objectively defined behaviors, each of which was included after a review of literature and clinicians' reports of behaviors important for diagnostic decisions in autism (Freeman, Ritvo, Guthrie, Schroth, & Ball, 1978). The goals of the *BOS* were stated to be to differentiate typically developing children from those with autism, ID, and other developmental disabilities; to differentiate subgroups of autism; to generate continua of severity in children with autism; and to generate profiles of the course of autism over the years (Freeman & Ritvo, 1981). This scale contains 67 objectively defined items, with each behavior rated on a 3-point Likert scale: 0 (did not occur in the 3 min interval), 1 (occurred rarely, but at least once), 2 (occurred moderately, not continuously), and 3 (engaged in the behavior continuously). Behaviors (items) are coded through an observation of the child through a one-way mirror.

Preliminary analyses were conducted (Freeman, Schroth, Ritvo, Guthrie, & Wake, 1980). The factor solution which best defined the scale was interaction with people, interaction with objects, solitary behaviors, and response to stimuli. Although the authors did not analyze discriminant validity (because of the low sample size), the autistic group was found to be best characterized by behaviors relating to inappropriate interaction with people and objects, when compared to those in the ID group and typically developing group. Freeman and colleagues (1978) examined the interrater reliability of the BOS, with correlation coefficients exceeding 0.84 for all except 12 of the items. Elsewhere, Freeman & Schroth (1984) examined the agreement of the items between raters. Results indicate that on 57 of the 67 items, agreement was 75% or better. In addition, these authors (i.e., Freeman & Schroth, 1984) indicate that a revised version of the BOS should be used. That is, items that occur infrequently or those that did not differentiate between groups were removed.

A major limitation of the *BOS* is that extensive training (i.e., 2 months as in the psychometric studies) is required in order to complete the observations of behaviors, which also includes a need to memorize the coding system.

Checklist for Autism in Toddlers (CHAT)

The *CHAT* serves as an autism screener (Baron-Cohen et al., 2000). This test was developed to assess children at 18 months of age who demonstrate deficits in joint attention and pretend play. Children are assessed to determine if they may be at risk for a diagnosis of autism later in life. This screener is designed to be used in conjunction with a comprehensive diagnostic session and takes approximately 5–10 min to complete. The measure is administered by a professional to the caretaker of the child. A professional refers to primary health-care workers or clinicians. The *CHAT* is comprised of two sections. Section A contains key questions related to the constructs measured in this scale: joint attention and pretend play. Only five items in Section A are key items, the rest are utilized to assist the clinician in differentiating autism from other general developmental delays. A failure on all of the five keys items in Section A indicates a high risk for autism. However, children can be at medium risk for autism if they fail both items for protodeclarative pointing. Section B is comprised of observational items that are directly filled out by the clinician. The authors make a recommendation to administer the *CHAT* twice in order to determine if the failed items remain failed for both administrations.

Effectiveness of the *CHAT* was demonstrated by assessing 91 toddlers, 18 months old, with only 4 of the 91 children failing the five key item questions. These four children were all reassessed at 34 months of age and all were diagnosed with autism (Baron-Cohen et al., 2000). In addition, 16,235 children, 18 months old, were assessed with the *CHAT* with 38 failing the key items. At a 1-month follow-up, 12 of these 38 again failed all five items. A reassessment at 42 months revealed that 10 of 12 who failed all five key items twice had diagnosis of ASD (Baron-Cohen et al., 2000). The sensitivity of the *CHAT* was found to be 18%, specificity was 100%, PPP was 75%, and NPP was 99.7% (for autism). However, for all PDDs, the sensitivity was 21.3%, specificity was 99.9%, and PPV 58.8%. Therefore, the *CHAT* has limited utility due to the inability to identify those with autism who meet criteria (i.e., low sensitivity).

Modified Checklist for Autism in Toddlers (M-CHAT)

The *M-CHAT* is a 23 item, parent report measure that can be used as a screener during pediatric visits (Robins, Fein, Barton, & Green, 2001); therefore it helps to identify symptoms of autism in the primary care setting. This measure relies on parental reports of skills and behaviors exhibited by their child to help with the identification of early signs of autism (i.e., at 24 months of age). The *M-CHAT* assesses for the attainment of developmental milestones and is an

extension of the *CHAT*. The *M-CHAT* symptom checklist was broadened to identify a greater range of PDDs and to make up for not completing an observation (as with the *CHAT*). Items were derived from the *CHAT*, findings from home videos, clinical experience, instruments used for older children, and hypotheses in the literature. Items are answered as "Yes" or "No" about how their child typically functions. Directions for the parents are printed at the top of the page. The screener is brief and can be completed quickly.

Psychometric analyses were conducted on the *M-CHAT* (Robins et al., 2001). First, 6 of the 23 items on this scale (i.e., those measuring communication and social skills) were found to best discriminate between those with and without an ASD (i.e., critical items). Internal reliability was 0.85 for the entire scale and 0.83 for critical items. A discriminant function analysis classified 33 of 38 toddlers correctly as ASD and 1188 of 1196 correctly as without an ASD. Thus, the sensitivity and specificity were 0.87 and 0.99, respectively. In addition, PPP was found to be 0.8 with the NPP being 0.99. Cutoffs were determined; thus, three items in general or two endorsements of the critical items indicate the necessity for follow-up. Using these cutoffs, sensitivity increases from the above mentioned, ranging from 0.87 to 0.97. However, it is just used as a screener and should not be the sole basis for a diagnosis. Thus, observations may be more appropriate in the follow-up assessments when the *M-CHAT* is failed.

Childhood Autism Rating Scale (CARS)

The *CARS* is a behavior rating scale, first developed in 1988 with items originating from Kanner's description of the disorder, characteristics of autism outlined by Creak, and existing assessment scales (Schopler, Reichler, & Renner, 1988). The goal of this scale is to identify symptoms of autism in younger children, as a first step in the diagnostic process. Currently, this scale is comprised of 15 items: relating to people; imitation; emotional response; body use; object use; adaptation to change; visual response; listening response; taste, smell, and touch response and use; fear or nervousness; verbal communication; nonverbal communication; activity level; level and consistency of intellectual response; and general impressions. Each item on this scale can be scored: 1 (within normal limits for a child that age), 2 (mildly abnormal), 3 (moderately abnormal), or 4 (severely abnormal) and all item scores are summed to yield a total score. Midpoints between these values can be used when behaviors fall between two of the aforementioned values. Items are scored by comparing the child's behavior to that of a typically developing child and items are scored after completing the entire observation. The total score can fall into the nonautistic range (below 30), mild to moderate autistic range (score between 30 and 36.5), and moderate to severe autistic range (score between 37 and 60).

The psychometric studies for the *CARS* yielded promising results. That is, the internal consistency of this scale was $\alpha = 0.94$. Reliability analysis has shown that interrater reliability for the items ranged from 0.55 to 0.93, with an average of 0.71 (indicating good agreement). In addition, the test–retest reliability yielded a K_W of 0.64, with a correlation of 0.88. In regard to validating the scale, the criterion-related validity of the measure was assessed. This was determined during diagnostic sessions and through clinical ratings ($r = 0.84$). Since this measure can be filled out from classroom observations, parent interviews, and reports of behavioral history in addition to observations during testing situations, the validity of the CARS was determined for these alternate conditions. The validity for these conditions was as follows: classroom observation ($r = 0.73$), parent interview ($r = 0.82$), and review of behavioral information from history ($r = 0.82$). Discriminant validity was also assessed and showed that the *CARS* can be used to discriminate between those diagnosed with and without autism, as the five symptom areas and the total scores were significantly different between the two groups (Volkmar et al., 1988). As the above-mentioned cutoff for the autistic range is 30, this yielded an agreement rate of 87%, false negative rate of 14.6%, and false positive rate of 10.7%. The authors also note that the *CARS* can be used for adolescents and adults, but a cutoff of 28 instead of 30 is recommended to be sensitive to differences in symptom expression over time. That is, the *CARS* is able discriminate between adolescents with and without autism because the scores were significantly different between the two groups (Garfin, McGallon, & Cox, 1988). Also, convergence of this scale with the *ADI-R* was examined (Saemunden, Magnusson, Smari, & Sigurdardottir, 2003). Saemundsen et al. found that correlations were all significant between the *ADI-R* total and domain scores with the *CARS* total score ($r = 0.60$–0.81). However, diagnostic agreement was only 66.7% between the *CARS* and *ADI-R* when using their respective cutoff scores, with the *CARS* correctly classifying more cases of autism.

Developmental Dimensional and Diagnostic Interview (3di)

The *3di* is a standardized and computerized interview that is most appropriately used to examine and assess symptoms of autism in children without intellectual disabilities (or those diagnosed with Mild ID) (Skuse et al., 2004). The *3di* contains a total of 740 items: 183 examining demographic and background information, 266 related to the symptoms of autism, and 291 relating to mental states indicative of other diagnoses. The computer program generates a structured report including complete symptom profiles. Items are coded following a 3-point Likert type scale: 0 (no such behavior), 1 (minimal evidence of such behavior), or 2 (definite or persistent evidence of such behavior). The full interview takes about 90 min to complete; however, a shorter interview (45 min) can be conducted if questionnaires are completed before the assessment session.

The psychometric properties of the *3di* were assessed by Skuse and colleagues (2004). Reliability (i.e., test–retest and interrater) analyses were conducted for each subscale and all ICCs exceeded 0.86 for both reliabilities, and thus the test–retest and interrater reliabilities were excellent. Criterion validity was examined by combining items into subscales that matched the *ADI-R* algorithm and ICCs ranged from 0.85 to 1.00. Besides having research assessing reliability, there is research examining the validity of the *3di*. Concurrent validity was assessed by comparing clinical diagnoses of ASD and those meeting criteria on the *3di* ($K = 0.74$ for "atypical autism"). Discriminant validity was also examined, indicating that the *3di* is able to differentiate between those diagnosed with ASD from those without. That is, PPP was 0.93 and NPP was 0.91. The kappa value for differentiating ASD from non-ASD was 0.95. Next, criterion validity was assessed by comparing the *3di* subscales to the ADI-R algorithm. The threshold agreement for social interaction was 86%, for repetitive and stereotyped behaviors it was 76%, and for communication it was 100%.

Two benefits of this measure include: training is easily completed through a DVD and illogical questions are automatically eliminated (e.g., if a child is nonverbal, questions relating to verbal language are not asked). Despite the above-mentioned benefits, a limitation is that the *3di* needs to be used in combination with an observation. Additionally, participants assessed for the psychometric analyses more often fit into the "mild" cases of autism and not "classic" autism. As a result, this measure may not be able to accurately assess for the spectrum of autism symptoms.

Diagnostic Interview for Social and Communication Disorders (DISCO)

The *DISCO* is a semistructured interview that is used to make diagnoses of AD and/or psychiatric disorders, to obtain developmental history, and to obtain a current pattern of behavior (Wing, Leekam, Libby, Gould, & Larcombe, 2002). Other uses of the *DISCO* include research, recommendations for education, occupation, leisure, and care. This scale originated prior to 1970 (although under a different name) and has since been revised numerous times (i.e., currently, the *DISCO 9* is described). Items for this scale were derived from diagnostic criteria for ASD, clinical experience, and developmental items from measures of adaptive functioning. This measure records the worst age of observation for untypical behaviors and the age of onset for items related to development. In addition, the *DISCO* covers a large range of developmental domains including self-care, independence, visuospatial, untypical responses to sensory stimuli, motor stereotypies, catatonia, psychiatric disorders, forensic problems, and difficulties related to sexual behavior. Items are coded only if the behavior can be easily remembered by the parent/caregiver. The *DISCO* should be used in conjunction with ratings, observations, psychological assessment, and interviews with multiple informants.

Psychometric analyses for this version of the *DISCO* were conducted by Wing and colleagues (2002). Interrater reliability was examined and the researchers found that all kappa coefficients exceeded 0.75 for 85.2% and 85% of school-age and preschool-age children, respectively. In addition, two algorithms were established, one for the *International Classification of Diseases, Tenth Edition* (ICD-10; World Health Organization, 1992) criteria for autism (i.e., 91 items in the *DISCO*) and the other for Wing and Gould's autism spectrum disorder definition (i.e., 5 items in the *DISCO*). The interrater reliability of the ICD-10 algorithm was ICC = 0.82 and for Wing and Gould's ASD algorithm it was 0.94. Clinical diagnoses and the diagnoses produced by the algorithms were compared to examine discriminant validity. There was a significant relationship between both algorithms and the clinical diagnoses assigned. However, more discrepancies were found for the ICD-10 algorithm (Leekam, Libby, Wing, Gould, & Taylor, 2002). It was not as effective in discriminating between autism and learning and language problems.

A major benefit of the *DISCO* is that it was not developed based on any specific diagnostic systems (i.e., the ICD or DSM) and, therefore, can be adopted under new revisions of these systems over time. However, a limitation of this measure is that at this time, only the ASD algorithm can be used and not the ICD-10 algorithm.

Diagnostic Checklist for Behavior – Disturbed Children, Form E2 (E2-DC)

The *E2-DC* was developed as a diagnostic instrument and is a revised version of the E1 form (same author) (Rimland, 1971). Compared to the E1, the *E2-DC* obtains information regarding the child's behavior and speech before 5 years of age. The measure was originally developed in 1965, with items derived from descriptions of symptoms and from parents' reports of symptoms documented in letters. From the above mentioned, a total of 80 items comprise the *E2-DC* and all items are summed to obtain the total score. If an item is applicable to the individual being assessed, then it is scored as "+1" and if not, then it is scored as "−1." Thus, the total score is the difference between the + (autism) and −

(nonautism) scores. A total score of +20 is indicative of autism. This number is conservative, but represents the best tradeoff between sensitivity and specificity.

Regarding psychometrics (Rimland, 1971), construct validity was assessed by examining those scoring above +20 on the measure and those who were previously diagnosed with autism. Those scoring high on the *E2-DC* had a previous diagnosis of autism. In addition, items comprising the scoring algorithm were able to discriminate between those with and without autism (or those with some autistic like symptoms). Rimland also looked at the agreement with the scores of the *E2-DC* and 30 children Kanner labeled autistic ($n = 22$) or nonautistic ($n = 8$). Those labeled nonautistic scored significantly below those who were labeled as autistic; however, the average score of those labeled as autistic on the *E2-DC* form ($M = 13.23$) was below the conservative cutoff score of +20. Although the *E2-DC* correlated with Kanner's description and diagnoses of children, a limitation is that not all those diagnosed by Kanner met criteria on the *E2-DC* because of the conservative scoring criteria.

Gilliam Autism Rating Scale – Second Edition (GARS-2)

The *GARS-2* is used for screening symptoms indicative of autism, for educational planning, and for research (Gilliam, 2006). It is the second version, with the first published in 1995. The *GARS-2* is useful for those aged 3–22 and distinguishes between those with behavior problems from those with autism. It incorporates observations, parent interviews, and questions completed by the examiner according to their interpretation. The *GARS-2* contains 42 items that load onto three factors: stereotyped behaviors, communication, and social interaction. Items are scored on a 4-point Likert scale: 0 (never observed) to 3 (frequently observed). Also, 11 additional items are included (key questions) that assist the assessor in reaching a diagnosis. Furthermore, a parent interview is included and contains 25 questions that are answered "Yes" or "No." These questions focus on social interaction, language used in social communication, and symbolic or imaginative play (and delays or abnormal functioning in these areas). The assessor should be a trained professional and one that has experience in the administration and interpretation of measures assessing symptoms of autism.

Cronbach's alpha was used to measure internal consistency, with $\alpha = 0.94$ for the entire scale. Additionally, $\alpha = 0.84$, 0.86, and 0.88, for the stereotyped behavior, communication, and social interaction subscales, respectively. In regard to the reliability of the test, test–retest ranged from 0.64 to 0.83 for the subscales and was 0.84 for the Autism Index. Concurrent validity was demonstrated with the comparison of the *GARS-2* to the *ABC*, $r = 0.62$. In addition, discriminant validity was demonstrated by the ability of *GARS-2* to discriminate between those with autism and those with severe behavioral problems. Also, with lower functioning individuals, discriminant validity has been demonstrated. Lastly, the sensitivity of the *GARS-2* ranged from 0.84 to 1, the specificity from 0.84 to 0.87, and PPP from 0.84 to 0.85. One limitation of this measure is that it does not address symptom presentation before 36 months of age, a diagnostic criterion for autism.

Pervasive Developmental Disorders in Mentally Retarded Persons (PDD-MRS)

The *PDD-MRS* was developed to be used for children and adults (i.e., 2–55 years old) diagnosed with ID and to assess for symptoms of ASD (Kraijer, 1997). It contains 12 items related to social interaction, communication, and stereotyped behavior. Items were derived from diagnostic criteria, a review of the literature, and an examination of existing scales. Each item also has a weight assigned to it, ranging from 1 to 3. Thus, the total score can be as high as 19. Providing weights for the items helped with the discriminating power of the scale. The sum of the scores falls into one of the three categories: 6 or less (non-PDD), scores between 7 and 9 (doubtful PDD/non-PDD category), or scores of 10 or greater (PDD category). The assessment period should range from 2 to 6 months.

Interrater reliability ranged from $r = 0.83$ to 0.89 and test–retest ranged from 0.7 to 0.8. The *PDD-MRS* was validated against diagnoses from psychologists and medical experts. Thus, the *PDD-MRS* correctly identified 94.4% of those diagnosed with an ASD and 92.7% of those without ASD. Discriminant validity was also examined and results indicate that the measure is able to discriminate between those with ID and those with ID and ASD. In a more recent study comparing the interrelationship between the *PDD-MRS* and the *ABC*, sensitivity was higher for the *PDD-MRS*; in contrast, specificity was higher for the *ABC* (de Bildt et al., 2003). The same authors demonstrated that the *PDD-MRS* had the highest validity when compared to the *ADOS-G*. That is, those scoring in the PDD category on the *PDD-MRS* had a 4.2 (odds ratio) chance of being classified as the same on the *ADOS-G*. Important to note is that the *PDD-MRS* does not differentiate between various ASDs, but assesses for symptoms of ASD (i.e., AD and PDD-NOS) in general.

Pervasive Developmental Disorders Rating Scale (PDDRS)

The *PDDRS* is a rating scale used to assess symptoms of ASD (Eaves, 1993). The 51 items comprising this scale were derived from a literature review on autism, behavioral symptoms from the DSM-III-R, existing measures, and clinic files of children diagnosed with autism. Each of the 51 items is rated on a 5-point Likert scale, rated according to the degree an individual exhibits the item/behavior. The 51 items of this scale comprise three subscales: arousal, affect, and cognition. In addition, the items can be summed to yield a total score.

In regard to the psychometric properties of the *PDDRS*, the internal consistency of the total scale was $\alpha = 0.92$, with the three subscales ranging from 0.79 to 0.90. Reliability coefficients for the scale ranged from $r = 0.48$ to 0.91 for the total score, from 0.53 to 0.89 for the arousal factor, from 0.40 to 0.87 for the affect factor, and from 0.44 to 0.87 for the cognition factor. Eaves, Campbell, and Chambers (2000) examined the criterion-related validity of the *PDDRS* and found that the *PDDRS* converges with the *ABC*; thus they measure similar constructs. In addition, Eaves and Colleagues found that when using a cutoff of 1 SD below the mean (i.e., for the total and arousal factor scores), the sensitivity, specificity, and correct classification rate was 88%. Furthermore, when examining the scores on the *PDDRS* between those with autism and those with other diagnoses commonly confused with autism, the autism group had a significantly higher mean.

More recently, the reliability of test scores of the *PDDRS* was examined by Williams and Eaves (2002). Results indicated that test–retest reliability for the total score was good ($r = 0.92$). Furthermore, Eaves and Williams (2006) examined the construct validity of the *PDDRS* through an exploratory and confirmatory factor analysis. Results indicated that best solution for *PDDRS* was the three-factor solution as mentioned above. However, for children aged 1 through 6 years, a confirmatory factor analysis indicated a two-factor solution was the best fit for the *PDDRS*.

Pre-linguistic Autism Diagnostic Observation Schedule (PL-ADOS)

The *PL-ADOS* is a semistructured assessment that measures play, interaction, and social communication skills through observation (DiLavore, Lord, & Rutter, 1995). This measure was developed as an alternative to the *ADOS*, as it requires less time on the examiner's part and less structure during the observation (e.g., the child does not have to remain sitting at a table). The observation is conducted during a limited time period with a focus on the child's social and communication behaviors and not just the absence or presence of these behaviors. The observation is intended for children less than 6 years of age, who are suspected of having an ASD; they do not use phrase speech during communication. The diagnoses yielded from the *PL-ADOS* are based on the ICD-10 (WHO,

1992) and DSM-IV-TR (APA, 2000). The observation takes about 30 min to complete and focuses on 12 activities absent in young children with ASD (e.g., joint attention, imitation), which yields 17 separate ratings. The examiner interacts with the child in order to complete the 12 activities: independent use of toys, engagement with parents, repeats own action when imitated, responding to joint attention, anticipates routine with objects, initiates joint attention, anticipates a social routine, requesting, functional/symbolic imitation, turn taking, imitation during play, request during snack, response to name, social smile, response to another's distress, separation from mother, and reunion with mother. Once the observation ends, the clinician generates overall ratings based on the observations of the child's behavior including communication (6 summary ratings), reciprocal social interaction (10 summary ratings), play (2 summary ratings), stereotyped behavior and restricted interests (5 summary ratings), other abnormal behavior (5 summary ratings), and finally an overall autism clinical rating. Observations of behaviors can be scored as 0 (indicating no abnormality), 1 (a response that is not typical but not indicative of an ASD), or 2 (consistent with autism). The overall level of communication is rated on a Likert scale from 0 to 4.

Interrater reliability was assessed and an 80% agreement was achieved with K_W ranging from 0.63 to 0.95 for the activity codes. For the overall summary ratings, $K_W = 0.71$–0.83 for communication, 0.60–0.94 for reciprocal social interaction, 0.78–1.00 for play, 0.60–0.92 for stereotyped behavior and restricted interests, 0.65–0.79 for other abnormal behaviors, and lastly was 0.86 for the overall autism rating (DiLavore et al., 1995). An algorithm was developed based on the ICD-10 and DSM-IV criteria, and using only those items that significantly discriminated between groups. An algorithm score was computed for social interaction/communication (with a cutoff of 12) and for restricted, repetitive behaviors (with a cutoff of 2). The *PL-ADOS* discriminates well between those with nonverbal autism and those with developmental disorders. In contrast, the algorithm is not yet able to differentiate children with ASD who are verbal from those with developmental disorders.

Screening Test for Autism in 2-year Olds: (STAT; Stone & Ousley, 1997)

The *STAT* is a screening tool designed for use with toddlers aged 24–35 months. Twelve items comprise this scale: two play items, four imitation items, four directing attention items, and two requesting items. Items for the *STAT* were derived from measures of play, imitation, and communication and were selected on the basis that they showed a large differentiation between those with autism and developmentally matched controls. All 12 items can be completed within

20 min with the assessment session set up as a play like interaction. Items are scored as "pass" or "fail" and areas scores are obtained by summing "passes" in each area (however, requesting items are not included in the scoring system). An area is considered failed if the score is less than 2 (Stone, Coonrod, & Ousley, 2000) and two of the three areas need to be failed to meet criteria for autism according to this measure. Using this criterion for the validation sample, Stone and colleagues found that the specificity was 86% and sensitivity was 83%. Elsewhere, Stone, Coonrod, Turner, and Pozdol (2004) identified a cutoff score of 2 which yielded a higher sensitivity of 0.92. The specificity with this cutoff was 0.85, PPP was 0.86, and NPP was 0.92. A benefit of this scale is that the items were empirically derived. That is, an existing database was used to identify items that yielded differentiation between developmentally matched controls and those diagnosed with autism. Stone and colleagues (2004) also investigated the interobserver agreement, which was $K = 1.0$ and test–retest reliability was $K = 0.90$. In addition, agreement between the *STAT* and *ADOS-G* was 0.95. A limitation of this scale is that the samples used for the psychometric investigations were small (i.e., $n = 12$).

ASD Measures

Autism Spectrum Disorders – Diagnosis for Adults (ASD-DA)

The *ASD-DA* was developed to assess symptoms of autism in adults diagnosed with ID (Matson, Terlonge, & Gonzalez, 2006). Additionally, this measure can be used to monitor symptom changes over time and for research purposes. A total of 31 items comprise this scale and were generated from a review of the literature, diagnostic guidelines from the DSM-IV-TR (APA, 2000) and ICD-10 (WHO, 1992), from other scales measuring ASD symptoms, and observations of persons with ASD and ID by experts in the field. The assessment is conducted as an interview (by a master's level professional in psychology, social work, etc.) with someone who has known the individual well for at least 6 months. Informants score all items as 0 (not different, no impairment) or 1 (different, some impairment). The instructions are outlined on the top of the protocol and the informants score the items comparing the person they are rating to a same-aged typically developing person. Also, items are rated to the extent they were ever a problem (not a current rating). Once all items are scored, a total score is calculated by summing the endorsements.

The 31 items on this scale load onto three factors (derived during factor analysis): social, communication, and repetitive behaviors/restricted interests. Cutoffs have been established; thus a score of 19 or greater is indicative of an ASD (Matson,

Boisjoli, González, Smith, & Wilkins, 2007). In addition, the scoring algorithm differentiates between PDD-NOS and AD. Thus, a score of 11 or higher on the social factor/subscale and 8 or higher on the repetitive behavior/restricted interests subscale is indicative of AD. In contrast, if these cutoffs are not met, but the total score is greater than 19, then the individual meets criteria for PDD-NOS. The internal consistency as measured by Cronbach's alpha for the subscales was 0.94 (social), 0.90 (communication), and 0.87 (repetitive behaviors/restricted interests). The internal consistency of the entire scale was, $\alpha = 0.94$. Reliability analysis of the *ASD-DA* indicates that the average item interrater reliability was 0.30 and average test–retest reliability for the items was 0.39. Lastly, convergent and divergent validities were examined (Matson, Wilkins, Boisjoli, & Smith, 2008). Thus, convergence was demonstrated through high correlations with a DSM-IV-TR/ICD-10 checklist comprised of symptoms indicative of an ASD diagnosis ($r = 0.60$), with a social skills measures ($r = -0.67$), and with an adaptive measures ($r = -0.42$). Divergence was demonstrated with a measure of psychopathology ($r = 0.12$).

Limitations of this measure are that kappa values for the test–retest and interrater reliabilities are slightly low on average. However, the measure is quick to administer and is able to distinguish between adults with ID alone and adults with ID and ASD and those with ID and PDD-NOS from those with ID and AD. Additionally, it is the only ASD scale available to assess adults with severe ID at this time.

Autism Spectrum Disorder – Diagnosis for Child (ASD-DC)

The *ASD-DC* is an informant-based measure that contains 40 items, which assess for symptoms of ASD in children aged 3–16 years (Matson & González, 2007). The scale was also designed to differentiate between AD, PDD-NOS, and AS, and furthermore, these disorders from typically developing children. The *ASD-DC* is part of a larger battery, the *autism spectrum disorders – child (ASD-C)*, which also assesses for symptoms of comorbid problems and for problem behaviors. Items included in the *ASD-DC* were compiled from a comprehensive research review of the ASD literature, current diagnostic guidelines (i.e., DSM-IV-TR, ICD-10), and clinical psychologist's observations from their experience working with this population. The 40 items on this scale comprise four factors, which were empirically derived: nonverbal communication/socialization, verbal communication, social relationships, and insistence of sameness/restricted interests (Matson, Boisjoli, & Dempsey, 2009). All items are rated on a 3-point Likert scale for severity of items as being either: 0 (not a problem or impairment), 1 (mild problem or impairment), or 2 (severe problem or impairment). Parents

or caregivers rate all 40 items based on how their children compare to other children their age. The total completion time for the *ASD-DC* is approximately 10–15 min.

In regard to psychometric properties of the *ASD-DC*, it has good interrater reliability ($K_W = 0.67$), excellent test–retest reliability ($K_W = 0.77$), and excellent internal consistency ($\alpha = 0.99$; Matson, González, Wilkins, & Rivet, 2008). In addition, cutoff scores have been established for the *ASD-DC* differentiating ASD versus non-ASD (i.e., 33). Just as important, cutoffs have been established to differentiate between AD, AS, and PDD-NOS (Matson, González, & Wilkins, 2009). A cutoff score of 40 or higher was determined to be indicative of a diagnosis of PDD-NOS (differentiating from AS) and a total score of 53 or higher was determined to be the cutoff for AD (differentiating between PDD-NOS). The sensitivity of the *ASD-DC* in correctly identifying cases of ASD as determined by DSM-IV-TR and ICD-10 criteria was 84.3%. The specificity for correctly identifying those without ASD was 98.2%, and the overall rate of correct classification was 91.3%. For autism, sensitivity was 59.8%, specificity was 100%, and the overall rate of correct classification was 83.1%. For PDD-NOS, sensitivity was 0%, specificity was 100%, and the overall rate of correct classification was 95.4%. Lastly, the sensitivity for Asperger's was 0%, the specificity was 100%, and the overall rate of correct classification was 97.3%. It should be noted that only six participants met checklist criteria for Asperger's and 10 met criteria for PDD-NOS, which likely contributed to the lack of sensitivity in identifying cases of these two ASDs.

More recently, convergent validity of the *ASD-DC* was demonstrated with the *CARS* and *ADI-R*. First, the correlation between *ASD-DC* and *CARS* total scores was moderately high ($r = 0.54$). In addition, factors of the *ASD-DC* converged with related items from the *CARS*, ranging from $r = 0.37$ to 0.68. Thus, the *ASD-DC* correctly classified 76.5% of the sample with ASD compared to 58.8% for the *CARS* (Matson, Mahan, Hess, Neal, & Fodstad, 2010). Next, convergence was demonstrated with the *ASD-DC* to the *ADI-R*. Correlations between the factors of the *ASD-DC* and content areas of the *ADI-R* ranged from 48 to 0.61. Correct classification of ASD by the *ASD-DC* was 73% compared to 46% by the *ADI-R* (Matson, Hess, Mahan, & Fodstad, 2010). A major advantage of this scale is that cutoff scores were established for differentiating among the three most common ASDs. In addition, the *ASD-DC* can be completed and scored quickly.

Baby and Infant Screen for Children with aUtIsm Traits-Part 1 (BISCUIT-Part 1)

The *BISCUIT-Part 1* is a 62 item informant-based measure that was designed to assess symptoms of AD and

PDD-NOS in infants and toddlers aged 17–37 months (Matson, Boisjoli, & Wilkins, 2007). Items comprising the *BISCUIT-Part 1* were obtained from a review of research literature, the DSM-IV-TR (APA, 2000), the ICD-10 (WHO, 1992), and a clinical psychologist with expertise with this population. Items are read to the parent or caregiver aloud and they are instructed to rate each item by comparing the child to other children his/her age with the following ratings: 0 (not different; no impairment), 1 (somewhat different; mild impairment), or 2 (very different; severe impairment).

An exploratory factor analysis of the items yielded a three-factor solution: socialization/nonverbal communication, repetitive behavior/restricted interests, and communication (Matson, Boisjoli, Hess, & Wilkins, 2010). The internal consistency of these factors was 0.93, 0.91, and 0.82, respectively. The *BISCUIT-Part 1* had an internal consistency coefficient of 0.97 (Matson, Wilkins, Sevin, et al., 2009). Cutoff scores were determined to differentiate between autistic disorder, PDD-NOS, and no ASD ($n = 1007$; Matson, Wilkins, Sharp, et al., 2009). A score of 17 had the best trade-off between sensitivity and specificity and was chosen as the cutoff for non-ASD and probable ASD/PDD-NOS. A score of 39 was selected to differentiate between autism and PDD-NOS. Overall, the sensitivity and specificity of the *BISCUIT-Part 1* was found to be 93.4 and 86.6%, respectively, with an overall correct classification of 88.8%.

In addition, psychometric analyses were conducted to examine the convergent and divergent validity (with the *Modified Checklist for Autism in Toddlers [M-CHAT*; Robins et al., 2001 and the *Battelle Developmental Inventory-Second Edition [BDI-2*; Newborg, 2005]). The *BISCUIT-Part 1* converged with the *M-CHAT* ($r = 0.80$) and with the personal–social domain of the *BDI-2* ($r = -0.50$). Divergence between the BISCUIT-Part 1 and the adaptive domain from the *BDI-2* was demonstrated ($r = -0.19$) (Matson, Wilkins, & Fodstad, in press).

Test administrators should have at least bachelor-level degrees in health services-related disciplines and experience in early childhood assessment and intervention. Also, this measure should not be used in isolation for a diagnosis, but inform a clinician if further testing and assessment is warranted.

Behavior Function Inventory (BFI)

The *BFI* was developed to provide information on the functional symptomatology of autism (Adrien et al., 2001). It is based on 11 neurophysiological functions: attention, perception, association, intention, motility, imitation, emotion, contact, communication, regulation, and cognition, with five items comprising each of these 11 domains. Authors indicate that the checklist should be completed after a 2 day

observation by professionals experienced with symptoms and assessment of autism. At the completion of the observation, each item on this scale is rated on a 5-point Likert type scale: 1 (behavior never observed), 2 (sometimes observed), 3 (often observed), 4 (very often observed), or 5 (always observed).

Psychometric analyses have been completed on the *BFI* (Adrien et al., 2001). Interrater reliability ranges from $K_W = 0.40$ to 1.0 for the items; however, a total of 37 items had $K_W \geq 0.60$. A factor analysis of the items yielded a six-factor solution: interaction dysfunction, praxis dysfunction, auditory dysfunction, attention dysfunction, islet of ability, and emotional dysfunction. When examining results from an ANOVA between those diagnosed with an AD, PDD-NOS, and ID, those with AD scored higher than the other two groups on all factors, with five of the six being significantly different.

A major limitation of this measure is that the *BFI* would be difficult to use as a clinical instrument during assessment sessions due to the time constraints and the length of time (i.e., 2 days) that it takes to complete the observation for this measure.

Pervasive Developmental Disorders Behavior Inventory (PDDBI)

The *PDDBI* is an informant-based measure that assesses children aged 1.6 through 12.5 years (Cohen & Sudhalter, 1999). This measure was initially designed for use with children diagnosed with ASD to assess treatment outcomes. The *PDDBI* contains two versions: the parent version, containing 176 items, and the teacher version, containing 144 items. All of the items are rated on a Likert scale: 0 (never), 1 (rarely), 2 (sometimes/partially), or 3 (often/typically). Including both versions allows for an examination of agreement between different situations and across informants. The items of the *PDDBI* comprise two broad dimensions of behaviors. First are the approach-withdrawal problems (i.e., maladaptive behaviors), which include nine behavioral domains with only the first four including items typically associated with autism: sensory/perceptual approach behaviors, ritualisms/resistance to change, social pragmatic problems, and semantic/pragmatic problems. The second broad area is receptive/expressive social communication abilities, which contains seven behavioral domains, with only two associated with autism (i.e., the lack of or deficits in skills): social approach behaviors and expressive language. In addition, a total autism composite score can be computed, and thus, higher scores represent a higher severity of autism. The six above-mentioned behavioral domains associated with autism are those included in the calculation of the total score. The *t*-scores sum for social approach behaviors and expressive language are subtracted from the *t*-scores sum of the remaining four behavioral domains.

Psychometric analyses were conducted by Cohen, Schmidt-Lacknew, Romanczyk, and Sudhalter (2003). Internal consistency ranged from $\alpha = 0.73$ to 0.97 for both the teacher and the parent versions. ICCs were computed for parent–teacher and teacher–teacher reliability, ranging from 0.28 to 0.85 and 0.55 to 0.93, respectively. Factor analysis of the items yielded factors consistent with the *PDDBI* subscales, thus demonstrating good construct validity. A cutoff score of 40 yielded a sensitivity of 89–91% and specificity of 80–81% for the parent and teacher scales. Furthermore, a cutoff of 42 discriminates between autism and PDD-NOS, which yielded a sensitivity of 85% and specificity of 50–52%. Although statistics on discriminating between these two groups are provided, the authors suggest that it may be illogical to interpret this score or diagnose this condition until better diagnostic criteria are defined for PDD-NOS (Cohen et al., 2003). Cohen (2003) examined the criterion-related validity. Statistically significant correlations were found between the *PDDBI* and the *CARS* and *ADI-R*. However, they were low. As with most measures, the *PDDBI* should not be used in isolation for a diagnosis.

Asperger's Assessment Measures

Asperger's syndrome (AS) first introduced by Hans Asperger (1944/1991), however, was not popularized until Lorna Wings review (1981; Attwood, 2007), when the term Asperger's syndrome was coined. In addition, AS was not entered into the DSM until the development of the DSM-IV (APA, 1994). Differentially diagnosing between AS and other disorders on the spectrum (e.g., high-functioning autism [HFA]) is often debated. To date, five measures have been developed specifically for the purpose of assessing symptoms indicative of an AS diagnosis.

Asperger Syndrome Diagnostic Scale (ASDS)

The *ASDS* contains 50 items that aid in the diagnosis of AS for children and adolescents, aged 5–18 years (Myles, Bock, & Simpson, 2000). It assesses for the presence or absence of symptoms and in addition to aiding in the diagnosis of AS, the *ASDS* also assists in formulating goals for IEPs, can be used for research purposes and can be used to track behavioral progress. Items for this measure were taken from a review of the literature for AS and from the DSM-IV criteria (APA, 2000), which comprise five domains/subscales: language, social, maladaptive, cognitive, and sensorimotor ($M = 10$, $SD = 3$). In addition, the 50 items on this scale

are utilized to obtain the Asperger syndrome quotient (ASQ; $M = 100$, $SD = 15$). The measure takes approximately 10–15 min to administer and should be administered to an informant who knows the child or adolescent well and who has had sustained contact with them for 2 weeks prior to the administration of this measure.

In regard to the psychometrics of the *ASDS*, the internal consistency of the scale was found to be good for the ASQ ($\alpha = 0.83$). In addition, validity of the *ASDS* was good, with 85% of children across groups (i.e., AD, autism, behavioral disorder, ADHD, and LD) being correctly classified. In regard to construct validity, convergence was demonstrated with the *GADS* and discriminant validity was demonstrated by examining the correlations between the ASQ scores and the age. One limitation of this scale was that participants in the psychometric analyses did not have an assessment of their cognitive functioning, which would be integral to differentiate between AS and AD. In addition, only the total score (ASQ) shows promising reliability and therefore is the only score that should be interpreted.

Autism Spectrum Screening Questionnaire (ASSQ)

The *ASSQ* is a 27 item screening checklist that assesses for symptoms of AS and AD (high functioning) (Ehlers & Gillberg, 1993). Items are rated on a 3-point Likert scale: 0 (indicating abnormality), 1 (some abnormality), or 2 (definite abnormality). Of the 27 items, a total of 11 relate specifically to social interaction, communication, and restricted and repetitive behavior. The remaining 16 items relate to motor clumsiness and motor and vocal tics. It is administered in a brief amount of time (i.e., 10 min) and can be completed by informants without training. All item scores are summed to yield the total score, and it is designed to be a screener to identify children who need a more thorough evaluation.

Psychometric analyses were conducted with two separate samples (Ehlers & Gillberg, 1993; Ehlers, Gillberg, & Wing, 1999). Test–retest reliability was excellent, ranging from $r = 0.90$ to 0.96 and interrater reliability ranged from 0.66 to 0.79 (for the ASSQ total scores). In regard to validation studies, the *ASSQ* is able to differentiate between those with ASD, ADHD/DBD, and LD groups, with the mean scores differing between these groups, demonstrating discriminant validity. In addition, divergent validity was demonstrated by examining the relationships between the mean *ASSQ* scores with the Rutter and Conners' rating scales (Ehlers et al., 1999). Sensitivity and specificity were also examined and ranged from 0.62 to 0.82 and 0.90 to 0.91, respectively. The aforementioned results are found when using a cutoff of 13 for parent scores and 11 for teacher scores (Ehlers & Gillberg, 1993).

The *ASSQ* has promising psychometrics; however, it cannot be used in isolation for a diagnosis. In addition, this measure does identify not only children matching AS criteria, but also children with other ASDs who are in the average range of cognitive functioning (Ehlers & Gillberg, 1993). Therefore, this scale cannot be used for a diagnosis of AS, but to identify symptoms of ASD in children with average cognitive functioning.

Childhood Asperger Syndrome Test (CAST)

The *CAST* is a 37 item parent rating scale that assesses for symptoms of AS and other social and communication disorders (Scott, Baron-Cohen, Bolton, & Brayne, 2002). The overall goals of the *CAST* are to identify children at an early age who are at risk for AS, gain an increased understanding of differences between those diagnosed with AS versus AD, understand the educational/psychological needs of these children, to develop a screening tool for AS, and lastly, to investigate environmental, education, and family factors pertaining to these children. In addition, this scale was designed to assist in the detection of those children and adolescents on the high-functioning end of the spectrum. Items were derived from the ICD-10 (WHO, 1992), DSM-IV (APA, 2000), and a review of items from existing measures designed for AS. This measure screens school-age children aged 4–11 years. A total of 31 of the 37 items on this scale are utilized to determine the overall score. The remaining 6 of the 37 items do not weigh into the overall score, but rather are questions related to overall development. Informants rate each item as "present" or "absent" and a total score of 15 or higher indicates the need for a further evaluation of symptoms related to AS.

This measure was initially piloted with a total of 50 children (13 whom were diagnosed with Asperger's syndrome or autistic disorder). This aforementioned statement leads to a questionable sample in the pilot study (i.e., included children diagnosed with other ASDs aside from AS). To date, no reliability studies have been conducted; however, the sensitivity, specificity, and PPP have been examined in a larger validation study following up the initial pilot study. Results indicated that the sensitivity for ASD was 0.88, with a specificity of 0.98, and PPP of 0.64. As with the *ASSQ*, the *CAST* can only be used to identify those at the high-functioning end of the autism spectrum due to the nature of the sample used in psychometric analyses.

Gilliam Asperger's Disorder Scale (GADS)

The *GADS* is a standardized, norm-referenced measure that can be used to assess the frequency of behaviors associated with a diagnosis of AS for those aged 3–22 years (Gilliam, 2001). Other uses of the *GADS* include the following: to assess progress resulting from interventions, for research, and to develop goals for IEPs. The *GADS* contains 32 items derived from the DSM, ICD, a review of existing instruments, and a review of the literature on AS. Four domains are assessed in the *GADS*: social interaction (items 1–10), restricted patterns of behavior (items 11–18), cognitive patterns (items 19–25), and pragmatic skills (items 26–32). The 32 items are rated by teachers, aids, parents, or psychologists who have had sustained contact with the child or adolescent for at least 2 weeks as 0 (never observed), 1 (seldom observed), 2 (sometimes observed), or 3 (frequently observed). The four subtests scores are summed in order to obtain the Asperger's disorder quotient (ADQ, $M = 100$, $SD = 15$). The *GADS* can be completed in approximately 5–10 min. The *GADS* also includes a parent interview, only for use with parents that have had sustained contact with the child during the first 36 months of life. This interview assists in ensuring that the child or adolescent had no clinical delays in language or cognitive development.

Regarding the psychometric analyses of the *GADS*, the internal consistency was assessed using Cronbach's alpha and found to be 0.87 for the ADQ, with the subscales ranging from $\alpha = 0.70$ to 0.81. An examination of the reliability showed that test–retest ranged from 0.71 to 0.77 for the four subscales, with the test–retest of the ADQ = 0.93. In addition, the interrater reliability was 0.89 for the ADQ and ranged from 0.72 to 0.84 for the four subscales. Validity of the *GADS* was also assessed (i.e., construct and content validity). Construct validity was demonstrated through item and subscale correlations, the lack of correlations between age and GAD scores, and mean difference scores on the *GADS* between those diagnosed with AS, AD, other disabilities, and non-disabled groups. Content validity was demonstrated through item discrimination coefficients. Thus, an item analysis showed that the median coefficients for subscales ranged from 0.56 to 0.68 enabling a correct classification accuracy of 83%. Also, ICCs between the subscales and total score (ADQ) were all significant, and thus they measure the same construct. A notable benefit of this test is that it has the largest standardization sample of the AS scales.

Krug Asperger's Disorder Index (KADI)

The *KADI* is a norm-referenced measure that assesses for symptoms indicative of AS and can be used to develop IEP goals and for research purposes (Krug & Arick, 2003). Two separate forms are included in the *KADI*: the elementary form for those aged 6–11 and the secondary form for those aged 12–21 years. The *KADI* contains 32 items that are rated as "absent" or "present." Eleven of these items are utilized for an initial screen. Only those exceeding a score of 18 complete the remaining items of the *KADI*. All items are summed to obtain a *KADI* total standard score. Higher scores indicate a greater likelihood of AD and each item score can range from 0 to 4. The *KADI* takes about 5–10 min to administer and can be administered to a parent or teacher who have had constant contact with the person for a few weeks. The directions for this assessment are printed at the top of the page.

The *KADI* was initially comprised of 106 items prior to any psychometric investigations. However, 32 items discriminated the best between typical functioning children and adolescents and those diagnosed with AD. Furthermore, the initial 11 screening items discriminate between those diagnosed with AS and AD. The internal consistency of the scale is $\alpha = 0.93$. The interrater and test–retest percent agreement ranged from 90 to 98%. Concurrent validity for the *KADI* was demonstrated by the specificity, sensitivity, and PPP, not only for AS and typically developing children and adolescents but also for AS and high-functioning AD, with a sensitivity of 78%, specificity of 94%, and a PPP of 83%. Results of psychometric studies indicate that the *KADI* is able to accurately differentiate between AS and high-functioning AD. That is, the mean scores between those two groups were significantly different. Evidence for content validity of the *KADI* was conducted through an item analysis (for item discrimination). In addition, the *KADI* produces standardized scores ($M = 100, SD = 15$) and percentile ranks. The authors suggest that the *KADI* should not be used in isolation to arrive at a diagnosis. However, a benefit of the *KADI* is that it has been show to demonstrate the strongest reliability to date (i.e., of the AS measures). A limitation of the scale is that the authors did not assess or report cognitive functioning of their sample used for the psychometric analyses.

Conclusion

The large number of measures available to assess symptoms of ASDs illustrates advancements made over time. Although each measure has its own benefits, a common theme regarding a limitation of all of those mentioned above is that no one measure can be used in isolation to make a diagnosis. Measures designed for the purpose of assisting in diagnostic decisions with strong psychometric properties would be the most reliable and valid way to make a diagnostic decision (Matson et al., 2007). Doss (2005) indicated that to date, best practices include utilizing unstructured assessments in combination with clinical judgment. Elsewhere, Matson, Hess, Mahan, and Fodstad (2010) suggest that clinicians should incorporate multiple methods when assessing symptoms for diagnostic purposes. Specifically, clinicians should include a standardized test for making evidence-based diagnoses. At this point, what may be most beneficial to clinicians would be to utilize a measure that can not only differentiate between those with ASD and those without but also one that can differentiate between the various ASDs (i.e., ASD-DA, ADS-DC, BISCUIT-Part 1, BFI, and PDDBI). Further assessment decisions can then be made after the interpretation of the results from a more comprehensive measure of ASD symptoms.

References

Adrien, J. L., Roux, S., Courutier, G., Malvy, P., Guerin, P., Debuly, S., et al. (2001). Towards a new functional assessment of autistic dysfunction in children with developmental disorders: The Behavior Function Inventory. *Autism, 5*, 249–264.

American Psychiatric Association. (1994). *Diagnostic and statistical manual of mental disorders* (4th ed). Washington, DC: Author.

American Psychiatric Association. (2000). *Diagnostic and statistical manual of mental disorders* (4th Ed., -Text revision). Washington, DC: Author.

Asperger, H. (1991). 'Autistic psychopathology' in childhood. In U. Frith (Ed., Trans.), *Autism and asperger syndrome* (pp. 37–92). New York: Cambridge University Press. (Original work published in 1944)

Attwood, T. (2007). *The complete guide to asperger's syndrome.* London: Jessica Kingsley Publishers.

Baron-Cohen, S., Wheelwright, S., Cox, A., Baird, G., Charman, T., Swettenham, J., et al. (2000). The early identification of autism: The checklist for autism in toddlers (CHAT). *Journal of the Royal Society of Medicine, 93*, 521–525.

Charman, T., Taylor, E., Drew, A., Cockerill, H., Brown, J., & Baird, G. (2005). Outcome at 7 years of children diagnosed with autism at age 2: Predictive validity of assessment conducted at 2 and 3 years of age and pattern of symptom change over time. *Journal of Child Psychology and Psychiatry, 46*, 500–513.

Cohen, I. L. (2003). Criterion-related validity of the PDD Behavior Inventory. *Journal of Autism and Developmental Disorders, 33*, 47–53.

Cohen, I. L., Schmidt-Lackner, S., Romanczyk, R., & Sudhalter, V. (2003). The PDD Behavior Inventory: A rating scale for assessing response to intervention in children with pervasive developmental disorders. *Journal of Autism and Developmental Disorders, 33*, 31–45.

Cohen, I. L., & Sudhalter, V. (1999). *PDD behavior inventory: professional manual.* Lutz, FL: Psychological Assessment Resources.

de Bildt, A., Sytema, S., Ketelaars, C., Kraijer, D., Volkmar, F., & Minderaa, R. (2003). Measuring pervasive developmental disorders in children and adolescents with mental retardation: A comparison of two screening instruments used in a study of the total mentally retarded population from a designated area. *Journal of Autism and Developmental Disorders, 33*, 595–605.

DiLavore, P. C., Lord, C., & Rutter, M. (1995). The pre-linguistic autism diagnostic observation schedule. *Journal of Autism and Developmental Disorders, 25*, 355–379.

Doss, A. J. (2005). Evidence-based diagnosis: Incorporating diagnostic instruments into clinical practice. *Journal of the American Academy of Child & Adolescent Psychiatry, 44*, 947–952.

Eaves, R. C. (1993). *The pervasive developmental disorders rating scale.* Opelika, AL: Small World.

Eaves, R. C., Campbell, H. A., & Chambers, D. (2000). Criterion-related and construct validity of the Pervasive Developmental Disorders Rating Scale and the Autism Behavior Checklist. *Psychology in the Schools, 37,* 311–321.

Eaves, R. C., & Williams, T. O. (2006). Exploratory and confirmatory factor analyses of the pervasive developmental disorders rating scale for young children with autistic disorders. *The Journal of Genetic Psychology, 167,* 65–92.

Ehlers, S., & Gillberg, C. (1993). The epidemiology of Asperger syndrome. A total population study. *Journal of Child Psychology and Psychiatry, 34,* 1327–1350.

Ehlers, S., Gillberg, C., & Wing, L. (1999). A screening questionnaire for Asperger syndrome and other high-functioning autism spectrum disorders in school age children. *Journal of Autism and Developmental Disorders, 29,* 129–141.

Freeman, B. J., & Ritvo, E. R. (1981). The syndrome of autism: A critical review of diagnostic systems and follow-up studies and the theoretical background in Behavior Observation Scale. In J. Gilliam (Ed.), *Autism, diagnosis, instruction, management, and research.* Springfield, IL: Charles C. Thomas.

Freeman, B. J., Ritvo, E. R., Guthrie, D., Schroth, P. C., & Ball, J. (1978). The behavior observation scale for autism: Initial methodology, data analysis, and preliminary findings on 89 children. *The Journal of the American Academy of Child Psychiatry, 17,* 576–588.

Freeman, B. J., & Schroth, P. C. (1984). The development of the Behavioral Observation System (BOS) for autism. *Behavioral Assessment, 6,* 177–187.

Freeman, B. J., Schroth, P. C., Ritvo, E., Guthrie, D., & Wake, L. (1980). The behavior observation scale (BOS) for autism: Initial results of factor analyses. *Journal of Autism and Developmental Disorders, 10,* 343–346.

Garfin, D. G., McGallon, D., & Cox, R. (1988). Validity and reliability of the Childhood Autism Rating Scale with autistic adolescents. *Journal of Autism and Developmental Disorders, 18,* 367–378.

Gilliam, J. E. (2006). *GARS-2: Gilliam autism rating scale-second edition.* Austin, TX: Pro-Ed Inc.

Gilliam, J. E. (2001). *Gilliam asperger's disorder index.* Austin, TX: Pro-Ed Inc.

Kanner, L. (1943). Autistic disturbances of affective contact. *Nervous Child, 2,* 217–250.

Kraijer, D. (1997). *Autism and autistic-like conditions in mental retardation.* Lisse: Swets & Zeitlinger.

Krug, D. A., & Arick, J. R. (2003). *Krug asperger's disorder index.* Austin, TX: Pro-Ed Inc.

Krug, D., Arick, J., & Almond, P. (1980). Behavior checklist for identifying severely handicapped individuals with high levels of autistic behavior. *Journal of Child Psychology and Psychiatry, 21,* 221–229.

Lecavalier, L., Aman, M. G., Scahill, L., McDougle, C. J., McCracken, J. T., Vitiello, B., et al. (2006). Validity of the autism diagnostic interview-revised. *American Journal on Mental Retardation, 111,* 199–215.

LeCouteur, A., Rutter, M., Lord, C., Rios, P., Robertson, S., Holdgrafer, M., et al. (1989). Autistic diagnostic interview: A semi-structured interview for parents and caregivers of autistic persons. *Journal of Autism and Developmental Disorders, 19,* 363–387.

Leekam, S. R., Libby, S. J., Wing, L., Gould, J., & Taylor, C. (2002). The Diagnostic Interview for Social and Communication Disorders: Algorithms for ICD-10 childhood autism and Wing and Gould autistic spectrum disorder. *Journal of Child Psychology and Psychiatry, 43,* 327–342.

Lord, C., Pickles, A., McLennan, J., Rutter, M., Bregman, J., Folstein, S., et al. (1997). Diagnosing autism: Analyses of data from the Autism Diagnostic Interview. *Journal of Autism and Developmental Disorders, 27,* 501–517.

Lord, C., Risi, S., Lambrecht, L., Cook, E. H., Leventhal, B. L., DiLavore, P. C., et al. (2000). The autism diagnostic observation schedule-generic: A standard measure of social and communication deficits associated with the spectrum of autism. *Journal of Autism and Developmental Disorders, 30,* 205–223.

Lord, C., Rutter, M., Goode, S., Heembsbergen, S., Jordon, J., Mawhood, L., et al. (1989). Autism diagnostic observation schedule: A standardized observation of communicative and social behavior. *Journal of Autism and Developmental Disorders, 19,* 185–212.

Lord, C., Rutter, M., & LeCouteur, A. (1994). Autism Diagnostic Interview-Revised: A revised version of a diagnostic interview for caregivers of individuals with possible pervasive developmental disorders. *Journal of Autism and Developmental Disorders, 24,* 659–685.

Matson, J. L., Boisjoli, J. A., & Dempsey, T. (2009). Factor structure of the Autism Spectrum Disorders-Diagnostic for Children (ASD-DC). *Journal of Developmental and Physical Disabilities, 21,* 195–211.

Matson, J. L., Boisjoli, J. A., González, M. L., Smith, K. R., & Wilkins, J. (2007). Norms and cut off scores for the autism spectrum disorders diagnosis for adults (ASD-DA) with intellectual disability. *Research in Autism Spectrum Disorders, 1,* 330–338.

Matson, J. L., Boisjoli, J. A., Hess, J., & Wilkins, J. (2010). Factor structure and diagnostic fidelity of the Baby and Infant Screen for Children with aUtIsm Traits-Part 1 (BISCUIT-Part 1). *Developmental Neurorehabilitation, 13,* 72–79.

Matson, J. L., Boisjoli, J., & Wilkins, J. (2007). *The baby and infant screen for children with autism traits (BISCUIT).* Baton Rouge, LA: Disability Consultants, LLC.

Matson, J. L., & González, M. L. (2007). *Autism spectrum disorders – diagnosis – child version.* Baton Rouge, LA: Disability Consultants, LLC, Translated into Italian, Chinese, Hebrew, and Japanese.

Matson, J. L., González, M., & Wilkins, J. (2009). Validity study of the Autism Spectrum Disorders-Diagnostic for Children (ASD-DC). *Research in Autism Spectrum Disorders, 3,* 196–206.

Matson, J. L., González, M. L., Wilkins, J., & Rivet, T. T. (2008). Reliability of the Autism Spectrum Disorders-Diagnostic for Children (ASD-DC). *Research in Autism Spectrum Disorders, 2,* 696–706.

Matson, J. L., Hess, J. A., Mahan, S., & Fodstad, J. C. (2010). Convergent validity of the Autism Spectrum Disorder Diagnostic for Children (ASD-DC) and Autism Diagnostic Interview-Revised (ADI-R). *Research in Autism Spectrum Disorders, 4,* 741–745.

Matson, J. L., Mahan, S., Hess, J. A., Neal, D., & Fodstad, J. C. (2010). Convergent validity of the autism spectrum disorder diagnostic for children (ASD-C) and childhood autism rating scale (CARS). *Research in Autism Spectrum Disorders, 4,* 633–638.

Matson, J. L., Nebel-Schwalm, M., & Matson, M. L. (2007). A review of methodological issues in the differential diagnosis of autism spectrum disorders in children. *Research in Autism Spectrum Disorders, 1,* 38–54.

Matson, J. L., Terlonge, C., & Gonzalez, M. L. (2006). *Autism spectrum disorders-diagnosis (ASD-D).* Baton Rouge, LA: Disability Consultants, LLC.

Matson, J. L., Wilkins, J., Boisjoli, J. A., & Smith, K. R. (2008). The validity of the autism spectrum disorders-diagnosis for intellectually disabled adults (ASD-DA). *Research in Developmental Disabilities, 29,* 537–546.

Matson, J. K., Wilkins, J., & Fodstad, J. C. (in press). The validity of the baby and infant screen for children with autism Traits (BISCUIT Part 1). *Journal of Autism and Developmental Disorders.*

Matson, J. L., Wilkins, J., Sevin, J. A., Knight, C., Boisjoli, J., & Sharp, B. (2009). Reliability and item content of the baby and infant screen for children with autism traits (BISCUIT): Parts 1, 2, and 3. *Research in Autism Spectrum Disorders, 3,* 336–344.

Matson, J. L., Wilkins, J., Sharp, B., Knight, C., Sevin, J. A., & Boisjoli, J. A. (2009). Sensitivity and specificity of the baby and infant screen for children with autism traits (BISCUIT). Validity and cutoff scores for autism and PDD-NOS in toddlers. *Research in Autism Spectrum Disorders, 3,* 924–930.

Mildenberger, K., Sitter, S., Noterdaeme, M., & Amorosa, H. (2001). The use of the ADI-R as a diagnostic tool in the differential diagnosis of children with infantile autism and children with a receptive language disorder. *European Child and Adolescent Psychiatry, 10*, 248–255.

Myles, B. S., Bock, S. J., & Simpson, R. L. (2000). *Asperger syndrome diagnostic scale*. Austin, TX: Pro-Ed.

Newborg, J. (2005). *Battelle developmental inventory* (2nd ed). Itasca, IL: Riverside.

Noterdaeme, M., Sitter, S., Mildenberger, K., & Amorosa, H. (2000). Diagnostic assessment of communicative and interactive behaviors in children with autism and receptive language disorders. *European Child and Adolescent Psychiatry, 9*, 295–300.

Rimland, B. (1971). The differentiation of childhood psychosis: An analysis for 2218 psychotic children. *Journal of Autism and Childhood Schizophrenia, 1*, 161–174.

Robins, D. L., Fein, D., Barton, M. L., & Green, J. A. (2001). The modified checklist for autism in toddlers: An initial study investigating the early detection of autism and pervasive developmental disorders. *Journal of Autism and Developmental Disorders, 31*, 131–144.

Saemunden, E., Magnusson, P., Smari, J., & Sigurdardottir, S. (2003). Autism Diagnostic Interview-Revised and the Childhood Autism Rating Scale: Convergence and discrepancy in diagnosing autism. *Journal of Autism and Developmental Disorders, 33*, 319–328.

Schopler, E., Reichler, R. J., & Renner, B. R. (1988). *The childhood autism rating scale (CARS)* (Rev.). Los Angeles: Western Psychological Services.

Scott, F. J., Baron-Cohen, S., Bolton, P., & Brayne, C. (2002). The CAST (Childhood Asperger Syndrome Test): Preliminary development of a UK screen for mainstream primary-school age children. *Autism, 6*, 9–31.

Skuse, D., Warrington, R., Bishop, D., Chowdhury, V., Lau, J., Mandy, W., et al. (2004). The Developmental Dimensional and Diagnostic Interview (3di): A novel computerized assessment for autism spectrum disorder. *Journal of the American Academy of Child and Adolescent Psychiatry, 43*, 548–558.

Stone, W. L., Coonrod, E. E., & Ousley, O. Y. (2000). Brief report: Screening Tool for Autism in Two-year-olds (STAT): Development and preliminary data. *Journal of Autism and Developmental Disorders, 30*, 607–612.

Stone, W. L., Coonrod, E. E., Turner, L. M., & Pozdol, S. L. (2004). Psychometric properties of the STAT for early autism screening. *Journal of Autism and Developmental Disorders, 34*, 691–701.

Stone, W. L., & Ousley, O. Y. (1997). *STAT manual: Screening tool for autism in two-year-olds*. Nashville, TN: Vanderbilt University, Unpublished manuscript.

Szatmari, P., Archer, L., Fisman, S., & Streiner, D. L. (1994). Parent and teacher agreement in the assessment of pervasive developmental disorders. *Journal of Autism and Developmental Disorders, 24*, 703–717.

Volkmar, F. R., Cicchetti, D. V., Dykens, E., Sparrow, S. S., Leekman, J. F., & Cohen, D. J. (1988). An evaluation of the autism behavior checklist. *Journal of Autism and Developmental Disorders, 18*, 81–97.

Wadden, N. P. K., Bryson, S. E., & Rodgers, R. S. (1991). A closer look at the Autism Behavior Checklist: Discriminant validity and factor structure. *Journal of Autism and Developmental Disorders, 21*, 529–541.

Williams, T. O., & Eaves, R. C. (2002). The reliability of test scores for the Pervasive Developmental Disorders Rating Scale. *Psychology in the Schools, 39*, 605–611.

Wing, L., Leekam, S. R., Libby, S. J., Gould, J., & Larcombe, M. (2002). The Diagnostic Interview for Social and Communication Disorders: Background inter-rater reliability and clinical use. *Journal of Child Psychology and Psychiatry, 43*, 307–325.

Yirmiya, W., Sigman, M., & Freeman, B. J. (1994). Comparison between diagnostic instruments for identifying high-functioning children with autism. *Journal of Autism and Developmental Disorders, 24*, 281–291.

World Health Organization. (1992). *International classification of diseases* (10th ed.). Geneva, Switzerland: World Health Organization.

Assessment of Rituals and Stereotypy

Olive Healy and Geraldine Leader

Individuals diagnosed with autism spectrum disorder (ASD) present with a "triad of impairments" that negatively affect social interaction and communication abilities and result in the presence of restricted, repetitive, and stereotyped patterns of behavior. Although repetitive stereotyped behavior is one of the three defining features of ASD, compared with the extensive literature published on the other impairments related to this disorder, this class of behaviors continues to be relatively underrepresented in the literature (Lam & Aman, 2007; MacDonald et al., 2007). This actuality becomes clear when one considers the challenges that ritualistic/repetitive or stereotyped behaviors evince for individuals with ASD, their families and service providers (Turner, 1999), and the diagnostic significance of such behaviors (Bodfish, Symons, Parker, & Lewis, 2000).

The term "stereotypy" in autism may be obfuscating given that some clinicians use the term synonymously with self-stimulation, ritualistic, and perseverative behaviors (Cunningham & Schreibman, 2008). It is important, therefore, to clarify what the terms "stereotypy" and "ritualistic behavior" mean. According to the Diagnostic and Statistical Manual of Mental Disorders (DSM-IV-TR; American Psychiatric Association, 2000), individuals with ASD present with "restricted, repetitive, and stereotyped patterns of behavior, interests, and activities" (p. 71). Such restricted, repetitive, and stereotyped behaviors may manifest as inflexible adherence to patterns of behavior or ritualistic movements or mannerisms. In addition, preoccupation with maintaining and/or manipulating specific objects or parts of objects may be observed. This may include unusual attachment to an inanimate object or objects or repetitive manipulation of parts of the object. There may also be a preoccupation with the movement of particular objects such as placement of items at particular angles, repeated turning

on and off switches/opening and closing doors, or sustained attention to revolving objects (e.g., washing machines). Stereotyped body movements related to the hands or whole body (clapping, finger flicking, limb twisting, body rocking, swaying) or abnormalities in posture such as tip-toe walking or unusual hand and body positioning may be present (DSM-IV-TR, 2000, p. 71). In addition, an individual may become very agitated or disturbed if they are prevented from engaging in such stereotyped patterns of behaviors. A wide range of specific topographies of abnormal repetitive behaviors have been identified in ASD. The term "stereotypy" often encompasses rituals, compulsions, obsessions, insistence on sameness, echolalia, stereotyped self-injury, tics, and perseveration (Lewis & Bodfish, 1998). Other related terms include "stereotyped behavior" and "stereotypic behavior" (Rapp & Vollmer, 2005).

Various authors have proposed different definitions of stereotypy and what the term encompasses in relation to topographies of behaviors. Rapp and Vollmer (2005) argue that there may be "dozens if not hundreds of response forms called stereotypy" (p. 527). Lewis and Bodfish (1998) define stereotypy as repetitive body or body part movements or use of body parts to manipulate object movements. Such behavior, they argue, lack purpose for the individual emitting the response forms. Indeed, many authors have argued for the purposeless nature of stereotyped patterns of behavior and ritualistic behaviors and some have adopted their definition of the term stereotypy based on that which persists in the absence of social consequences (e.g., Rapp & Vollmer, 2005). Such a definition points to the automatic reinforcement attained by the individual who emits such behavior and many researchers have provided evidence for this view (e.g., Piazza, Adelinis, Hanley, Goh, & Delia, 2000; Rapp, 2006). Not only can varying stereotyped patterns of behaviors be observed across individuals with ASD but numerous topographies of abnormal stereotypies can occur within the individual themselves. For example, an individual with ASD may present with a single or multiple patterns of stereotyped behaviors at different development levels or chronological

O. Healy (✉)
School of Psychology, National University of Ireland, Galway, Ireland
e-mail: olive.healy@nuigalway.ie

J.L. Matson, P. Sturmey (eds.), *International Handbook of Autism and Pervasive Developmental Disorders,*
Autism and Child Psychopathology Series, DOI 10.1007/978-1-4419-8065-6_14, © Springer Science+Business Media, LLC 2011

ages. As with most of the characteristics of ASD, stereotyped patterns of behavior are idiosyncratic across individuals diagnosed with the condition.

It is clear that the presence of stereotyped patterns of behavior is a diagnostic feature of ASD (ICD-10, World Health Organization, 1990; DSM-IV-TR, American Psychiatric Association, 2000). While the topographies of such patterns of behavior may vary within and across individuals, the function of such behavior is vital to the design and implementation of intervention. There is a wide body of research to suggest that stereotyped behavior may be an operant behavior maintained by sensory stimulation delivered from the particular movement of body parts, whole body, or visual stimulation. In such cases, the behavior may be maintained by automatic positive reinforcement (e.g., Vollmer, Marcus, & LeBlanc, 1994) or automatic negative reinforcement (e.g., Tang, Kennedy, Koppekin, & Caruso, 2002). There are some limited cases evidencing that stereotypy may be mediated by social attention (Kennedy, Meyer, Knowles, & Shukla, 2000) or escape from a demanding situation (Durand & Carr, 1987; Mace & Belfiore, 1990). The issue of function of such behavior will be addressed later in the chapter.

The following section of this chapter will outline the specific behaviors that make up the behavioral cluster of stereotyped patterns of behavior and outline specific studies that have examined topographical forms. The debilitating effects that contribute to the overall disorder of ASD will be provided. In addition, specific methods and considerations in assessment will also be addressed by providing an overview of some assessment instruments for stereotypy and ritualistic behaviors. We have chosen to include the most researched measures by providing descriptions of the instruments and studies that have incorporated them.

Topographies of Behavior Linked by Invariance

Neuringer (2002) has described "variability in responding" as dispersion of responses and unpredictability in responding, but "it can also refer to a continuum ranging from repetitive at one end to stochastic at the other" (p. 672). An individual's behavior can be reinforced, not only for repeating a particular behavior but for distributing responses across a wide array of possibilities in a way that may be quite unpredictable. Much of the early literature on repetitive behavior in ASD tended to focus on stereotyped and ritualistic behaviors as movement repetition and movement invariance (Rapp & Vollmer, 2005). It has been posited that variability is operant behavior that is shaped and maintained by its consequences (Miller & Neuringer, 2000; Neuringer, 2002). Therefore, by delivering reinforcement contingent on variable responding it is possible to increase the variability of an individual's behavior, allowing them to react in more complex ways to

a variety of situations. This is a particularly relevant point when analyzing the lack of variance in behavior that may be displayed by individuals with ASD. According to Miller and Neuringer (2000), normal behavior manifests "differing levels of behavioral variability, which are controlled by discriminative stimuli and reinforcement contingencies" (p. 162), as is the case with the more commonly studied operant behaviors such as response rate.

Miller and Neuringer (2000) determined that direct reinforcement of variable responding could increase variability in individuals with autism. In their study, reinforcement was initially delivered independently of variable responding, next it was contingent on variability, and then it was independent of variability again. Individuals with autism responded less variably overall than adult and child controls. However, all participants demonstrated significantly higher variability when reinforcement was contingent on it, than when it was not. Also, for all groups, variability remained high in the second phase when reinforcement again was delivered independently of response variation. This suggests a maintenance effect for reinforced variability in both ASD and typically developing children and adults.

The lack of response variability across different repertoires evident in ASD may account for the presence of high rates of stereotypy and ritualistic behaviors present in the condition. Connolly and Bruner (1974) report that simple actions are reorganized into more complex behavior patterns in order to develop motor skills. Stability and consistency are valued in the development of such skills as motor skills often have a stable and unchanging goal. In the same way, stereotypy is likely to be influenced by the propensity of an individual with a diagnosis of ASD to develop inflexible behavioral routines (Mason, 1991a, b).

The organism–environment interactions are everchanging and variability in motor actions may be reinforced as a result of the various contingencies encountered. It is possible that individuals with ASD, who commonly show a lack of sensitivity to various reinforcers, experience limited opportunities to acquire reinforcers for behavioral variations which permit alternative behaviors/strategies to be created. This is, of course, true for all repertoires of behavior and is the fundamental advantage of the ability to vary behavior. Carr and Kologinsky (1983) described aspects of language such as spontaneity and flexible conversational skills as difficult to teach to individuals with autism. This may be due to the absence of effective contingencies rather than an inherent inability of this population to vary their verbal behavior (Miller & Neuringer, 2000).

The prevalence of echolalia among children with autism supports the idea of low variability in verbal behavior among this population. Rydell and Prizant (1995) report that 85% of children with ASD who acquire language will emit echolalia. Echolalia is, by definition, restrictive and repetitive. It appears to be non-functional though it is possible that it may serve different purposes for the individual such as auditory feedback/stimulation or escape from demanding situations.

Prevalence of Ritualistic and Stereotyped Behavior

Stereotypy and ritualistic patterns of responding are considered a prevalent behavior and a significant diagnostic feature of children with ASD. A number of authors have suggested that children with ASD engage in unusually and substantially high rates of stereotypy (Baumeister & Forehand, 1973; Lancioni, Smeets, Ceccarani, & Goossens, 1983).

A recent study by Murphy, Healy, and Leader (2009) examining challenging behavior in 157 children with ASD showed that overall, 139 participants (72%) emitted stereotyped patterns of behavior. The main forms of stereotypy shown were engaging in repetitive body movements, repetitive hand movements, and waving or shaking arms. The measure used was the Behavior Problems Inventory (BPI-01; Rojahn, Matson, Lott, Esbensen, & Smalls, 2001).

Lord (1995) has suggested that repetitive behaviors may not be present or fully developed until at least 3 years of age in individuals with ASD. Parent report studies have indicated that stereotyped behaviors in children with ASD generally increase during development from the ages of 2 to 4 (see also Moore & Goodson, 2003).

Certain topographies of stereotyped behaviors are commonly evident in typically developing young infants. These are often presented in the form of repetitive motor movements such as head or body movements. Singer (2009) recently presented a report of repetitive arm and hand movements in a sample of 81 children without diagnoses of intellectual disability or pervasive developmental disorder. The study showed that 56 (69%) participants evinced stereotypy onset at age younger than 24 months, 19 (23%) at age 24–35 months, and 6 (8%) at the age of 36 months or older.

Particular forms of repetitive movements are common to other developmental disorders or psychiatric conditions, e.g., Rett syndrome, Tourette's syndrome, Prader–Willi syndrome, fragile X syndrome, and schizophrenia (Turner, 1999). MacDonald et al. (2007) compared stereotyped patterns of behavior in 30 children with ASD or pervasive developmental disorder – not otherwise specified (PDD-NOS) and 30 typically developing children matched at ages 2, 3, and 4 years old. Each child's performance of several early learning and play skills was assessed using a direct observational assessment protocol developed for children with autism who were entering early intensive behavioral treatment. Duration of episodes of vocal and motor stereotypy was recorded from a videotaped 10 min portion of an assessment of play and basic skill sets. Interestingly, results demonstrated that the 2-year-old children diagnosed with autism or PDD-NOS showed a higher level of stereotypy than their matched

typically developing 2-year-old counterparts during assessment conditions. In addition, the 3- and 4-year-old children diagnosed with autism or PDD-NOS displayed substantially higher levels of stereotypy than their matched same-age peers. This study demonstrates that although stereotypy may be observed in young typically developing children, those diagnosed with a developmental disorder such as ASD or PDD-NOS display higher rates at the same chronological age.

Bodfish et al. (2000) conducted a systematic study of the occurrence of specific topographies of ritualistic behaviors and their severity in individuals with intellectual disability with and without ASD. Both groups had significant patterns of the co-occurrence of stereotypy forms. The presence of each behavior type, other than dyskinesia, was higher in the ASD group. Individuals with ASD emitted a significantly higher number of topographies of stereotypy and compulsions. In addition, participants diagnosed with ASD scored significantly greater severity ratings for compulsions, stereotypy, and self-injury. The severity of ASD predicted the severity of stereotypy. Bodfish et al. (2000) argue that although abnormal ritualistic and repetitive behavior is not specific to the condition of ASD, an elevated pattern of occurrence and severity does seem to characterize the disorder.

Stereotypies and rituals occur at a higher rate and intensity in children and adults with ASD than for any other developmental disorder (Matson, Dempsey, & Fodstad, 2009). Matson et al. (2009) conducted the first large-scale study consisting of an evaluation of the type and extent of stereotyped and ritualistic behavior across 760 young children (age range 17–37 months) with autism, pervasive developmental disorder – not otherwise specified (PDD-NOS), or no diagnosis of ASD but at risk for other delays in development or physical disorders. Findings showed that stereotypies and repetitive/ritualistic behaviors were most common in those with a diagnosis of ASD than those diagnosed with PDD-NOS. Consistent with other literature, individuals without ASD but presenting with other developmental delays were less likely to present with stereotypies or ritualistic patterns of responding. Matson et al. (2009) contend that their findings purport to the possibility of the identification of stereotypies and rituals at very early ages of development (the mean age of infants in this study was 26.63 months). Motor stereotypies can affect development and learning at an early age (see section below) and persist at least through adolescence.

Matson and Dempsey (2008) examined characteristics of stereotypies in adults with ASD (age range of 16–88 years). Stereotypies and ritualistic behaviors were more frequent in individuals diagnosed with ASD than those diagnosed with an intellectual disability. In addition, the authors showed that rates of stereotypic and ritualistic behaviors were highest among adults diagnosed with ASD compared to individuals with a pervasive developmental disorder – not otherwise specified or intellectual disability alone. The severity of stereotypy was much greater in the ASD adult group in the overall analysis.

The next section of this chapter will seek to organize topographies of stereotypy and ritualistic behaviors into topographical forms. Other researchers have sought to identify categories of stereotyped behavior. For example, Berkson (1967) proposed categories of repetitive and non-repetitive movements and subsequently classified stereotypy into five separate criteria: (1) the voluntary nature of the behavior (this rules out tics as non-operant behavior); (2) an absence of response variability (the behavior is manifested in a repetitive manner); (3) endurance of the behavior over a period of time, usually several months; (4) resistance to environmental alterations (implying insensitivity to competing social variables); and (5) the behavior would not be expected given the individual's chronological age (see Berkson, 1983 or Rapp and Vollmer, 2005 for further review). In addition, Turner (1999) classified stereotyped behavior as categories of "lower-level" and "higher-level" behaviors. Lower-level behaviors constitute repetitive movements that Turner describes as "dyskinesias, tics, stereotyped movements, repetitive manipulation of objects, and repetitive forms of self-injurious behaviors" (p. 839). On the other hand, higher-level behaviors include "object attachments, insistence on the maintenance of sameness, repetitive language, and circumscribed interests" (see Turner, 1999, pp. 839–841). In the following section, we organize and discuss topographical forms of this class of problematic behavior under two broad categories consistent with Turner (1999): first, stereotyped behaviors and repetitive movements that are specific to the syndrome of ASD including repetitive or stereotyped motor movements, vocal stereotypy, repetitive manipulation of objects, ritualistic responding, reliance on sameness, and preoccupation with aspects of the environment; and second, classes of ritualistic behavior that may be evinced by individuals with ASD, but that may be related to more nonspecific factors or associated impairments of the condition. These include repetitive self-injurious patterns of behavior, spontaneous dyskinesias/akathisias, and obsessions and compulsions.

Stereotyped Behaviors and Ritualistic Movements That Are Specific to the Syndrome of ASD

Stereotyped Motor Movements

Stereotyped movements observed in individuals with ASD are often described as repetitive patterned motions that are invariant, purposeless, and inappropriate to developmental level. Stereotyped motor movements can be divided into two topological classes: (1) repetitive, including orofacial (e.g., tongue, mouth, and facial movements; sniffing), bodily limbs (e.g., hand, finger, toe, legs), and head and body (e.g., rolling, tilting, or banging of the head; rocking the body) and (2) non-repetitive including limb and/or body posturing. Such stereotyped behavior, it has been argued, does not seem to be advantageous to an individuals' adaptive functioning. Repetitive and non-repetitive stereotypies are commonly referred to as self-stimulatory behavior (SSB) (Cunningham & Schreibman, 2008). The most prominently cited maintaining reinforcement contingency of repetitive and non-repetitive topographies of stereotypy is self-stimulation or automatic reinforcement (Lovaas, Newsom, & Hickman, 1987; Rapp & Vollmer, 2005; Rogers & Ozonoff, 2005; Schreibman, 1988). Such behaviors can manifest as highly characteristic abnormal movements, such as placing a hand with fingers separately outstretched before the eyes and rapidly moving the hand back and forth producing a visual feedback, hand-flapping, rocking, to name some examples.

Symons, Sperry, Dropik, and Bodfish (2005) reviewed 12 studies that provided information on the prevalence, nature, or development of stereotypic and/or self-injurious behavior in children aged 5 years or less and who were identified as at risk for developmental delay. The authors provide a list of discrete forms of stereotypic behaviors examined across the 12 studies. These included tip-toe walking, mouth opening, lip sucking, eyebrow movements, mouth twitching, smell/sniff movements, and covering eyes/ears. Such stereotypies often provide a source of sensory input (e.g., visual, auditory, tactile vestibular, taste, or smell) (Cunningham & Schreibman, 2008). Both typically developing and "at-risk" children displayed the following topographies of stereotypy: body rocking, head rolling/tilting, object manipulation, hand/finger movement, foot kicking, facial grimacing, breathing/puffing noises, tongue wagging, and hand gazing (Symons et al., 2005).

Repetitive Manipulation of Objects

This type of stereotyped behavior is one of the few forms of stereotypy that has been described as being nonspecific to individuals with ASD. Evans et al. (1997) described the development of what they termed "compulsive-like" behavior in typically developing infants. They argue, in line with the developmental theory in explaining the presence of stereotypies, that very young children frequently display ritualistic behavior such as repeated manipulation of objects in a consistent and predictable fashion (see Gesell, 2007 for a review of ritualistic types of behavior in typical development). Thelen (1996) has also described how typically developing infants engage in a broad class of repetitive stereotyped behavioral movements.

Baranek (1999) completed an analysis of early sensory and motor signs of autism using home video recordings and found that early object stereotypies (i.e., mouthing objects) were particularly relevant in discriminating among children with ASD, developmental disabilities, and typically developing children. Symons et al. (2005) demonstrated, in their review of the literature, that typical developing infants presented with repetitive stereotyped patterns of behavior involving object manipulations. However, Ozonoff, Macari, Young, Goldring, Thompson, and Rogers (2008) showed that children with ASD displayed significantly more spinning, rotating, and unusual visual exploration of objects than those who were not diagnosed with or at risk of a developmental delay.

A number of studies have shown that it is possible to replace repetitive manipulation of objects with "matched stimulation" (Rapp, 2007), indicating the sensory feedback that this type of behavior may provide. The concept of "reinforcer substitutability" has been used to decrease repetitive behavior maintained by automatic reinforcement. Piazza et al. (2000) demonstrated, for example, that providing access to items that matched the hypothesized sensory consequences of repetitive behavior may be effective in decreasing and eliminating such problem behavior in ASD.

Repetitive Vocal or Vocal Stereotypy

Some authors have provided a topographical definition of stereotypic behavior that characterizes it as repetitive vocal responses (e.g., Matson, Kiely, & Bamburg,1997; Smith & Van Houten, 1996). Vocal stereotypic behavior has received limited empirical investigation in the behavioral literature (Ahearn, Clark, Macdonald, & Chung, 2000). Such forms of stereotypy may be classed as "immediate echolalia," "delayed echolalia," and repetitive vocal sounds or noises that are not related to the immediate context and do not bear any resemblance to words. Schreibman and Carr (1978) defined immediate echolalia as the "parroting of the speech of others" that were considered contextually inappropriate repetitions or partial repetitions in an immediate manner. These authors focused on the development of replacement vocal statements such as an accurate and correct response to a given question or an accurate and appropriate tact of lack of knowledge to respond to the question. Such communication training significantly reduced repetitive vocal behavior.

Delayed echolalia, as a form of vocal stereotypy, has been described as the repetition of text or components of a narrative heard or read from previously viewed videos or books (Taylor, Hoch, & Weissman, 2005). The delay can be up to a few minutes, hours, days, weeks, months, or even years. It has been described by Charlop, Konarski, and Favell (1992) as "perseverative speech" differentiating it from "parrot speech." Prizant and Rydell (1984) attempted to determine how children with ASD use delayed echolalia in naturalistic interactions with familiar people. Individual differences in functional usage were evident across all three participants. "Delayed echolalia was found to vary along the dimensions of interactiveness, comprehension of the utterance produced, and relevance to linguistic or situational context" (p. 183). Earlier work by Prizant and Duchan (1981) demonstrated that echolalia (immediate and delayed) may not be as purposeless as thought and may, in fact, serve various communicative functions for individuals. Charlop et al. (1992) reported a prevalence rate of 75% among individuals with ASD who are verbal.

Karmali, Greer, Nuzzolo-Gomez, Ross, and Rivera-Valdes (2005) described delayed echolalia using the term "palilalia." The term describes a pathological condition in which a word is rapidly and involuntarily repeated. The authors used a combined multiple baseline and reversal design to investigate the effectiveness of presenting replacement vocal verbal tact operants (labeling objects and actions) as corrections for occurrences of palilalia. The frequency of such vocal stereotypy decreased to low levels and mand (requests) and tact operants increased as a result.

Taylor et al. (2005) have described vocal stereotypy (that is not immediate or delayed echolalia) as "non-contextual vocalizations." Such behavior, they postulate, may consist of vocalizations unrelated to the context such as repeating portions of conversations, videos or books previously heard, and general unintelligible vocalizations. The authors found that providing contingent access to matched stimulation through a negative punishment contingency (i.e., differential reinforcement of other behavior) produced a low level of vocal stereotypy for a child with ASD, but response-independent access to that stimulation was ineffective.

In addition, Ahearn et al. (2000) describe repetitive vocalizations, involving sounds or noises, as that which do not involve immediate or near-immediate repetitions of the vocalizations of others and can vary in comprehensibility, intensity, and bout length (p. 264). A recent study by Falcomata, Roane, Hovanetz, Kettering, and Keeney (2004) determined that an 18-year-old individual with ASD who exhibited repetitive vocalizations chose more appropriate forms of auditory stimulation (music) over self-generated vocalizations (singing), which indicated that these vocalizations may have been maintained by the sensory consequence of auditory stimulation. In such cases the repetitive vocalizations produce auditory stimulation which is viewed as the reinforcer for the behavior. Ahearn et al. (2000) assessed and treated the non-communicative vocalizations of four children with ASD. For all four participants the function of vocal stereotypy was clearly not maintained by social consequences but by automatic reinforcement. Intervention involved the use of response interruption and redirection (RIRD) by delivering vocal demands contingent on the occurrence of vocal stereotypy and a criterion for compliance. For each participant, RIRD substantially decreased levels of vocal stereotypy compared to baseline measures.

High-Level Repetitive Behavior

Turner (1999) used the term "high-level" to refer to more complex stereotyped responding that may manifest as fixation on objects or aspects of one's environment, insistence on sameness, or ritualistic routines, each of which result in restricted, delineated interests in individuals with ASD. Restricted interests and fixation have been described by Turner (1999) as possibly the "highest level" of repetitive or stereotyped behavior in ASD. Such fixation on the environment can manifest as perseverance with models of cars, home appliances, phone numbers, and many more examples. There may also be an extreme and intensive focus on one particular topic, e.g., dinosaurs, cities, and airplanes. Often individuals who present with this type of repetitive behavior are considered "high functioning" on the autism spectrum. High-functioning autism has been defined by the presence of IQ levels that are greater than 70 (Howlin, 2004, p. 6). Howlin (2004) postulates that this type of perseverance is often most evident in both children and adults with Asperger syndrome and that the specific interests are often dysfunctional without any connection to current contexts, while in other cases individuals with ASD can apply "specialist" and focused knowledge to adaptive living.

Ritualistic patterns of behavior and insistence on sameness involve overall habitual movements, repetition in routines, and behavioral inflexibility. Such tendencies are very frequently associated with ASD (Prior & MacMillan, 1973). This kind of invariance and reliance on consistent environments, schedules, and movements can cause serious problem behavior when any kind of inconsistency is encountered. Prior and MacMillan (1973) used the Sameness Questionnaire to assess reliance on sameness across 10 children with ASD and all participants were found to display multiple sameness behaviors. The Sameness Questionnaire includes a 28-item scale measuring different aspects of ritualistic behavior or reliance on routine. The term insistence on sameness has been used by Rutter (1978) to refer to repetitive behaviors, including limited play patterns, intense object attachments, unusual preoccupations, rigid routines, and resistance to change. It is also possible that the lack of behavioral flexibility is overlooked until it manifests itself in significant problem behavior (Green et al., 2006).

Stereotyped or Ritualistic Behavior That May Be Related to More Nonspecific Factors or Associated Impairments of ASD

Repetitive Self-Injurious Behavior

A particularly severe form of stereotypy is self-injurious behavior described as repetitive movements that produce self-inflicted injuries (Baumeister & Rollings, 1976). Self-injury has been described in numerous studies as the following forms: skin picking; self-biting, head punching and slapping; head-to-object and body-to-object banging; body punching and slapping; eye gouging or rectal-poking; lip chewing; hair and nail pulling or removal; and teeth banging. Schroeder, Schroeder, Smith, and Dalldorf (1978) reported that self-injury occurred in 30% of inpatient with ASD. More recent data reported by Bodfish et al. (2000) demonstrated a substantially higher rate of occurrence, with 69% of adults with ASD studied evincing at least one topography of self-injury.

Research by Romanczyk, Lockshin, and O'Connor (1992) suggests that some forms of self-injurious behavior (SIB) may be classed as stereotyped self-injurious behavior (SSIB). Stereotyped self-injurious behavior may be the product of aberrant physiological processes as hypothesized by the organic theory of SIB (Carr, 1977). Romanczyk et al. (1992) postulated an operant-respondent model of SIB, in which SIB is elicited and mediated by physiological arousal and shaped and maintained by environmental events. In this account, the genesis of the behavior is quite different from what subsequently maintains the behavior. Stereotyped self-injurious movements are not included as the archetype of stereotyped movements in the DSM-IV-TR (American Psychiatric Association, 2000). Gal, Dyck, and Passmore (2009) concluded that "self-injurious behavior is a more severe form of stereotyped movements and there is a distinctive pattern of stereotyped movements, including self-injurious behavior, that characterizes children with autism" (p. 342).

Baumeister (1978) classified the theoretical explanations of SSIB as developmental, hemeostatic, organic, psychodynamic, and learned responses which overlap with Turner's (1999) account (see below for an outline). SSIB has been considered to be the most concerning of repetitive behaviors seen in ASD, and it often requires the involvement of expert intervention from experienced practitioners trained in intensive behavioral and/or medical intervention. "Although self-injury is traditionally viewed as a separate category of behavior disorder, its highly stereotyped nature and its frequent co-occurrence with other repetitive, non-injurious movements warrant its inclusion as a repetitive behavior" (Lewis & Bodfish, 1998, p. 82).

Dyskinesia and Akathisia

Owens, Johnstone, and Frith (1982) have described the traditional view of dyskinesia as a "neuroleptic-induced movement disorder" and the more recently developed concept of such repetitive behavior as spontaneous movements occurring mostly in the orofacial areas (lips and tongue) independent of any exposure to neuroleptic medication. Children and adults diagnosed with ASD often evince high rates of orofacial repetitive actions without contacting neuroleptic intervention. However, neuroleptic antipsychotic medications are often used to treat challenging problem behavior in children and adults with ASD (Sheehan, Leader, & Healy, 2009) and such intervention may result in medication-induced movement disorders as a side effect of such intervention. Campbell et al. (1990) demonstrated how difficult it may be to distinguish dyskinesia from abnormal movements or stereotypy in ASD. Results showed no significant predictors of the development of dyskinesias as a side effect of neuroleptic antipsychotic medication. The stereotyped behavior of 224 children with ASD was examined, and stereotypies (mostly in the orofacial areas) were identified in at least mild form in most children studied. Other authors have described the difficulties in differentiating stereotypy and neuroleptic-related dyskinesia in ASD (Meiselas, Spencer, Oberfield, Peselow, Angrist, & Campbell, 1989). The authors argue that repetitive movements in individuals can be misdiagnosed as neuroleptic-related dyskinesias.

Akathisia, on the other hand, refers to repetitive restless movements (e.g., walking/marching on the spot, fidgeting, rocking, pacing repeatedly) and/or the inability to remain motionless whether standing, seated, or lying down (Sachdev, 1995). As with dyskinesia, akathisia is also traditionally conceptualized as neuroleptic-induced but may also occur spontaneously and independent of exposure to neuroleptic medication. Some authors have found significant co-occurrence of stereotypy, dyskinesia, and akathisia (Bodfish, Newell, Sprague, Harper, & Lewis, 1996, 1997; Rutter, 1985).

Obsessions and Compulsions

In the context of ASD, Fischer-Terworth and Probst (2009) describe obsessive and compulsive behaviors as "autism-related obsessive-compulsive phenomena" (AOCP) including all kinds of obsessional, compulsive, ritualistic, stereotyped, and repetitive behaviors. "Compulsions" have been defined as repetitive and intentional behaviors that appear to be governed by particular stringent rules, and "obsessions" have been defined as importunate and repetitive thoughts, impulses, or images (Lewis & Bodfish, 1998). Such behaviors can frequently cause extreme anxiety and distress to the

individual (e.g., Zandt, Prior, & Kyrios, 2008). McDougle et al. (1995) examined obsessive and compulsive behaviors across 50 adults with ASD and compared outcomes to 50 age- and sex-matched individuals diagnosed with OCD. All 50 individuals with autism displayed compulsive behaviors. Interestingly, the authors reported a significant difference between the groups with respect to the forms of compulsive behavior displayed. They found that individuals with ASD evinced topographies involving ordering, hoarding, and touching compulsions but significantly less cleaning, checking, and counting compulsions. The excessive collecting and hoarding of objects like stones, CDs, or books can be characteristic of some individuals with ASD who present with obsessive stereotyped behaviors (Howlin, 2004). More recently, Bodfish et al. (2000) demonstrated that 30 of 32 adults (94%) with ASD studied displayed at least one compulsive behavior. Further research by McDougle et al. (1995) demonstrated that 32 of the 50 participants with ASD studied were found to emit obsessive types of behaviors. However, given the abstract nature of obsessive and compulsive types of responding, these behaviors can be difficult to operationally define and assess.

Contribution of the Presence of Stereotypy to the Disorder of Autism

Given the examples of the various topographies of stereotypy and ritualistic behavior outlined above, and the possibility that such topographies may co-occur, it is not surprising that the presence of such behaviors can impede acquisition of novel and appropriate replacement repertoires. Empirical evidence has related stereotypies with lowered awareness of, or attention to, external environmental contingencies and events. The presence of stereotypies and ritualistic behavior constitutes one of the core features of ASD and their presence immediately sets the individual apart from others and therefore can be highly stigmatizing (Jones, Wint, & Ellis, 1990). Dunlap, Dyer, and Koegel (1983) outlined the possible effects of high-frequency stereotypy as social isolation, exposure to restrictive types of interventions, reduced and limited educational opportunities, and decreased educational programming as a result of over-emphasis on reductive interventions for stereotypy. Although it is behavior that occurs during typical stages of development in infants (Foster, 1998; Troster, 1994), the persistence seen in the repertoires of persons with ASD is thought to interfere with the acquisition of new adaptive skills (e.g., Dunlap et al., 1983; Morrison & Rosales-Ruiz, 1997; Wolery, Kirk, & Gast, 1985) and can have negative social consequences (e.g., Jones et al., 1990; Wolery et al., 1985).

The extent to which repetitive behaviors contribute to the overall severity of ASD has been examined for only a small number of repetitive behaviors. Overall severity of autism has been shown to be significantly positively correlated with severity of stereotypy (Campbell et al., 1990) and with insistence on sameness behaviors (Prior & MacMillan, 1973). Scores for stereotypy, self-injury, compulsions, dyskinesia, and akathisia have significantly predicted higher scores of autism severity using the Autism Behavior Checklist (Bodfish et al., 2000). Repetitive motor stereotypies and insistence on sameness have been associated with a variety of participant characteristics such as IQ or age. Such repetitive and ritualistic behavior has been correlated with impairments in social and communication skills, whereas circumscribed interests appeared to be independent of participant characteristics. Lam, Bodfish, and Piven (2008) have argued that the presence of multiple forms of AOCP in an individual with ASD is associated with more impairment in the social and communication domains, resulting in a greater autism severity rating.

The association between the presence of stereotypy and adaptive functioning has been examined by Cuccaro et al. (2003). For individuals ranging from 3 to 21 years of age ($n = 292$), the authors conducted a component analysis and found that lower-level stereotypic behaviors (e.g., repetitive motor movements, repetitive use of object) were related to poorer adaptive behavior scores with higher-level stereotypies (compulsions, rituals, and abnormal preoccupations) less clearly associated with adaptive functioning. In addition, Bishop, Richler, and Lord (2006) used parent report to provide support for classes of repetitive behaviors in children under the age of 12 years. They reported that the prevalence of most lower-level behaviors was negatively associated with nonverbal IQ, whereas circumscribed and restricted interests showed a positive correlation with nonverbal IQ.

Individuals with ASD frequently present with obsessions and compulsions according to DSM-IV criteria of Obsessive-Compulsive Disorder (OCD), being associated with marked distress and interference with daily life. Symptoms of obsessive-compulsive disorders are time-consuming obsessions and compulsions which can result in elevated distress and significant interference with daily living. Individuals with ASD may experience symptoms of anxiety at a greater level than the general population (Gobrial & Raghavan, 2009; Waller & Furniss, 2004). However, whether the presence of obsessive behavior and/or compulsive types of responding is the underlying factor in relation to the prevalence of anxiety in people with ASD requires more conclusive empirical evidence.

Gabriels, Cuccaro, Hill, Ivers, and Goldson (2005) found that individuals with ASD who had presented with a low nonverbal IQ had a significantly greater number and severity of ritualistic behaviors than a high nonverbal IQ group. They also demonstrated that those participants who presented with higher rates of stereotypy had a lower adaptive behavior score, presented with sleep disturbance, and scored higher on measures of irritability, lethargy, and hyperactivity (measured using the subscales of the *Aberrant Behavior Checklist*). Furthermore, a number of authors have argued that engagement in stereotypy may be a precursor to the development of self-injurious behavior (Morrison & Rosales-Ruiz, 1997; Schroeder, Rojahn, Mulick, & Schroeder, 1990).

"Reinforcement of varied behaviors may facilitate modification of non-functional ritualistic and stereotyped behaviors" (Neuringer, 2002, p. 688). Further research is warranted to determine the relationship between stereotypy, ritualistic behavior, adaptive functioning, and intelligence measures in ASD. This kind of analysis will determine the extent to which the presence of different topographies of stereotypy interferes with adaptive functioning and the possible role that cognitive level can be attributed to this effect.

The remaining sections of this chapter will provide a review of the types of assessment of ritualistic and stereotyped behaviors along with an analysis of the various types of functions that have been posited for such behavior. Some evidence exists to support the view that stereotypy and abnormal repetitive behaviors in ASD may serve a number of functions including sensory stimulation or automatic reinforcement as a result of limited or deficient behavioral repertoires or environments. Some have argued that there is a common assumption that stereotyped behaviors may function as self-stimulation with many practitioners referring to stereotypy as a "self-stim."(Cunningham & Schreibman, 2008). Indeed the literature would suggest that this assumption is a misnomer and that it is imperative to provide an assessment of such behavior in order to design and provide effective intervention. Assessing stereotyped behaviors aids clinicians in the identification of variables maintaining such patterns of responding and provides an analysis of environmental stimuli that both precede and follow them.

Assessment Instruments for Ritualistic and Stereotyped Behaviors

Stereotyped Behavior Scale

The *Stereotyped Behavior Scale* (SBS; Rojahn, Tasse, & Sturmey, 2000) is an empirically developed behavior rating scale for adults and adolescents with developmental delays. Service providers selected 600 clients who displayed stereotypic behaviors, and subsequent refinement resulted in a 26-item scale. These items are scored on a 6-point frequency scale. The scale has an internal consistency alpha of 0.88, test–retest reliability of $p = 0.90$, and interrater reliability of $p = 0.76$ (Rojahn, Tasse, & Sturmey, 1997). It was concluded that internal consistency and test–retest reliability were acceptable to good, but the authors were concerned about the low interrater agreement. Rojahn, Matlock, and Tasse (2000) conducted a study that investigated the test–retest reliability, interrater reliability, and internal consistency of the SBS. In this study 15 participants displayed high rates of stereotyped behaviors, 15 displayed moderate rates while 15 displayed low to 0 rates. Care staff familiar with the participants completed the SBS and the "stereotypy" subscale of the *Aberrant Behavior Checklist Residential* (ABC-R) (Aman, Singh, Stewart, & Field, 1985). Behavior observations were also conducted. After 4 weeks the administration of the instruments was repeated by the same raters. Scores of internal consistency, test–retest reliability, interrater agreement, and criterion validity were found to be good to excellent (Rojahn et al., 2000).

Diagnostic Assessment for the Severely Handicapped-II

The *Diagnostic Assessment for the Severely Handicapped-II* (DASH-II; Matson, Gardner, Coe, & Sovner, 1991) was designed to measure forms of psychopathology which were overlooked by traditional measures of autism for individuals with severe to profound intellectual disability (Matson et al., 1996). There are 13 subscales in this instrument including impulse control, organic problems, anxiety, mood disorders, mania, PDD/autism, schizophrenia, stereotypies, self-injurious behavior, elimination disorders, eating disorders, sleep disorders, and sexual disorders. Several studies have demonstrated the utility of the DASH-II as a measurement of several psychopathology (Matson et al., 1996; Matson, Hamilton, et al., 1997; Sevin, Matson, Williams, & Kirkpatrick-Sanchez, 1995) and demonstrated its reliability and validity. A study by Matson, Hamilton, Duncan, Bamburg, Smiroldo, Anderson, and Baglio (1997) used the Diagnostic and Statistical Manual of Mental Disorders, fourth edition (DSM-IV; American Psychiatric Association, 1994) to validate the stereotypy and self-injury items of the DASH-II. The validity of the DASH-II was confirmed and participants with profound intellectual disability were more likely to evince stereotypies or self-injury compared to severely impaired participants (Matson et al., 1997). Numerous studies have cited the use of the DASH-II in the assessment of stereotypy in ASD.

Repetitive Behavior Scales – Revised

The *Repetitive Behavior Scales – Revised* (RBS-R; Bodfish, Symons, & Lewis, 1999; Bodfish et al., 2000) is an empirically validated rating scale that measures the presence and severity of repetitive behaviors. This scale consists of six subscales (stereotyped behavior, self-injurious behavior, compulsive behavior, routine behavior, sameness behavior, and restricted behavior). Each scale describes topographies of repetitive behaviors which are discrete and observable. Importantly, each scale does not have any item overlap and provides a score which determines the total number of topographies respectively. Researchers have established that the RBS-R has acceptable levels of validity and reliability (Bodfish et al., 1995, 1999; Powell, Bodfish, Parker, Crawford, & Lewis, 1996).

The Aberrant Behavior Checklist

The *Aberrant Behavior Checklist* (ABC; Aman et al., 1985) is a 58-item scale that assesses maladaptive behavior in individuals with developmental disabilities using a 4-point rating scale. The scale ranges from 0 to 3 with behaviors scoring a 3 being most problematic. The ABC provides a score in the areas of irritability, lethargy, stereotypy, hyperactivity, and inappropriate speech. The utility of the ABC in terms of assessing stereotypy is somewhat restricted as it only examines repetitive motor movements. However, several studies have demonstrated the validity and reliability of the ABC (e.g., Aman, Burrow, & Wolford, 1995; Marshburn & Aman, 1992).

The Behavior Problem Inventory

The *Behavior Problem Inventory* (BPI-01; Rojahn, 1986, 1992, 1997; Rojahn et al., 2000) is a 52-item instrument for assessing self-injury, stereotyped behavior, and aggression/destruction in individuals with developmental disabilities. The scale contains 11 self-injury items, 24 stereotypic behavior items, and 11 aggressive/destructive items. Items are scored on two scales: a 5-point frequency scale (0–5) and a 4-point severity scale (0–4). The BPI-01 has undergone several revisions with the original scale (BPI) being developed in German as part of a prevalence study (Rojahn, 1984). The first evaluation of the scale was conducted by Mulick, Dura, Rasnake, and Wisniewski (1988). For stereotyped behavior, this study revealed a mean interrater agreement of 0.98 (0.85–1.0) and a mean test–retest reliability of 0.89 (range 0.80–0.95). Another evaluation was conducted by Rojahn et al. (2001) involving 432 participants. The three-factor solution was confirmed and reliability estimates were termed acceptable. The most recent evaluation of the BPI-01 was conducted by Gonzalez et al. (2009). The internal consistencies of the subscales were reported to be in the good to excellent range. The interrater and test–retest reliabilities of the subscales were found to be adequate with relatively lower reliability reported for the stereotypy subscale.

The Repetitive Behavior Questionnaire

The *Repetitive Behavior Questionnaire* (RBQ; Turner, 1996, Unpublished data) is a parent or teacher behavior interview designed to assess the severity, nature, and frequency of repetitive behaviors. It is a 33-item scale that calculates a score for repetitive language, sameness behavior, and repetitive movements as well as a total repetitive behavior score. To date, information regarding the reliability and validity of this scale has not been published, but this instrument has been frequently incorporated in studies assessing stereotypy in ASD.

The Children's Yale-Brown Obsessive Scale

The Children's Yale-Brown Obsessive Scale (CY-BOSC; Scahill, Riddle, McSwiggin-Hardin, & Ort, 1997) is a measure that is administered by a clinician to both a parent(s) and child and measures the level of obsession and compulsion experience within the previous week. This is a 10-item semi-structured measure of obsession and compulsion. This instrument has most relevance in research pertaining to pediatric obsessive-compulsive disorder and is not suitable for use with individuals with severe/profound mental retardation. Storch Roberti and Roth (2004) evaluated the psychometric properties of the CY-BOSC in a sample of 61 children and adolescents diagnosed with obsessive-compulsive disorder. Findings confirmed that it is a reliable and valid instrument.

As has been documented above, numerous studies have used standardized measurement instruments and rating scales as a methodology to investigate the presence, rate and type of stereotypy, and ritualistic behaviors. However, there is no single instrument that is used for the assessment of these behaviors. Furthermore, there is no evidence to suggest that the use of such instruments permits distinctions between potentially repetitive behaviors (Lewis & Bodfish, 1998).

Rating scales examine the presence of stereotypy and ritualistic behaviors with some examining possible functions of such behavior. These scales are correlational in terms of analyzing the function of stereotypy. This is in contrast to the functional analytic approach adopted by Iwata, Slifer, Bauman, and Richman (1982), where the function of aberrant behavior is identified and analyzed. The goal of functional analysis is to experimentally identify the operant contingencies maintaining behavior in order to design effective treatment interventions. Skinner (1953) suggested that human behavior can be interpreted using a functional analytic approach where the contingencies of reinforcement are used in the analysis and modification of human behavior. From this perspective, stereotypy is operant behavior that is maintained by the consequences that follow the behavior. Functional analytic procedures analyze the extent to which stereotypy is maintained by social positive reinforcement (e.g., attention), social negative reinforcement (e.g., escape from a demand or instruction), or contingent sensory or automatic reinforcement (e.g., self-stimulation). Mace, Browder, and Ying Lin (1987) used functional analytic techniques to analyze the function of stereotypic mouthing in a 6-year-old boy. Researchers showed that stereotypy occurred at high rates during difficult activities (escape) and when stereotypy was allowed to delay instructional demands.

Stereotypy Mediated by Automatic Reinforcement

When a behavior itself provides reinforcement, it is said to be "automatically reinforced" (e.g., Lovaas et al., 1987). In effect, the behavior is reinforced by the sensory stimuli that it produces. The automatic reinforcement hypothesis is supported by studies that demonstrate that stereotypy is resistant to social consequences; the use of matching or alternative forms of stimulation reduces the rate of stereotypy and contingent access to stereotypy functions as reinforcement for other behaviors (Rapp & Vollmer, 2005). A study by Rincover (1979) examined whether automatic reinforcement was maintaining stereotypy in children with a developmental delay. A sensory extinction procedure was implemented where the sensory consequences of the behavior were removed and reintroduced using an ABAB reversal design. When self-stimulation was decreased or eliminated as a result of removing one of the sensory consequences, the functional sensory consequence was designated as a child's preferred sensory reinforcer. The researchers then assessed whether children would play selectively with toys producing the preferred kind of sensory stimulation. When the sensory reinforcer was removed, self-stimulation extinguished. Furthermore, the sensory reinforcers identified for self-stimulatory behavior also served as reinforcers for new, appropriate play. Researchers have also suggested that noncontingent access to stimuli matched in sensory function to the sensory reinforcer may reduce the establishing operation for stereotypy and thus reduce its frequency (Cunningham & Schreibman, 2007). Piazza et al. (2000) conducted a functional analysis which revealed that three behaviors (dangerous climbing, saliva manipulation, and mouthing) were automatically reinforced. Preference assessments were used to identify items that matched and did not match the sensory consequences of the behaviors. The effects of providing noncontingent access to the highly preferred matched and unmatched stimuli relative to a condition in which no stimuli were available were assessed. Providing access to items that matched the sensory consequences of the behaviors was most effective.

Social Positive Reinforcement

Researchers have demonstrated that social positive reinforcement may provide desirable consequences contingent on the occurrence of stereotypy and ritualistic behavior. Goh et al. (1995) conducted a functional analysis of chronic hand mouthing in 12 individuals with ASD. For 10 participants, automatic reinforcement was maintaining the behavior, while social positive reinforcement was responsible for maintaining the behavior of two individuals. Kennedy et al. (2000) studied behavioral functions associated with stereotypy for students with autism. Functional analyses were conducted on the behavior of five participants. For two participants, stereotypy was associated with positive and negative reinforcement and for two additional participants stereotypy occurred across all conditions. For the fifth participant, stereotypy was maintained by negative reinforcement. The results of a second study in this paper showed that similar topographies of stereotypy, based on qualitatively different reinforcers, were reduced only when differential reinforcement contingencies for alternative forms of communication were implemented for specific reinforcer relations. Although research has demonstrated that stereotypy can be maintained by social positive reinforcement, the evidence to date is limited.

Social Negative Reinforcement

A seminal study was conducted by Durand and Carr (1987) which demonstrated that stereotyped behavior increases as a function of difficult task demands and contingent removal of aversive stimuli. In this study, four developmentally disabled children who displayed hand-flapping and body rocking participated in the study. All four children displayed high levels of stereotypy when difficult task demands were introduced (escape from demand). This information was used to develop a functional communication system that consisted of teaching children to request assistance on difficult tasks. This was believed to produce significant reductions of stereotyped behavior. These findings suggest that the social environment of some individuals serves to negatively reinforce stereotypy and ritualistic behaviors.

Ritualistic and stereotyped behaviors are a diagnostic requirement of ASD and are therefore present in the behavioral repertoires of all individuals with this diagnosis. There are numerous topographies of abnormal stereotyped and ritualistic anomalies that can co-occur at high rates in both children and adults diagnosed with ASD. Such individuals present with greater rates of stereotypy than in those with other developmental disorders (Bodfish et al., 2000). No one single topography of ritualistic behavior appears to be specific to ASD. Rather, variations in topographies may be related to the condition itself or the impairments that can be associated with the condition. The idiosyncratic nature of stereotypy in autism can range from simple repetitive movements to complex sequences or patterns. Variations in the co-occurrence of topographies and severity of behavior are also significant in the disorder. There is a clear gap in the literature examining the phenomenology of the full range of ritualistic behaviors seen in ASD using standardized measurement instruments. Much more attention to this issue is needed in future research. In addition, given that the presence of repetitive stereotyped patterns of behavior is evident in the early stages of typical development, the issue of "normal" and "abnormal" movements requires further analysis. Continual research on the long-term assessment of the presence and functions of ritualistic and stereotypic behaviors, along with the overall adverse effects throughout development in persons with ASD, will provide a valuable contribution to behavioral intervention.

References

Ahearn, W. H., Clark, K. M., Macdonald, R. P., & Chung, B. I. (2000). Assessing and treating vocal stereotypy in children with autism. *Journal of Applied Behavior Analysis, 40*, 263–275.

Aman, M. G., Burrow, W. H., & Wolford, P. L. (1995). The aberrant behavior checklist-community: Factor validity and effect of subject variables for adults in group homes. *American Journal of Mental Retardation, 3*, 283–292.

Aman, M. J., Singh, N. N., Stewart, A. W., & Field, C. J. (1985). The aberrant behaviour checklist: A behaviour rating scale for the assessment of treatment effects. *American Journal of Mental Deficiency, 89*, 485–491.

American Psychiatric Association. (1994). *DSM-IV*. Washington, DC: Author.

American Psychiatric Association. (2000). *Diagnostic and statistic manual of mental disorders (DSM-IV)* (4th ed.)., Text Revised (DSM-IV-TR). Washington, DC: APA.

Baranek, G. (1999). Autism during infancy: A retrospective video analysis of sensory-motor and social behaviors at 9–12 months of age. *Journal of Autism and Developmental Disorders, 29*, 213–224.

Baumeister, A. A. (1978). Origins and control of stereotyped movements. In C. E. Meyers (Ed.), *Quality of life in severely and profoundly mentally retarded people: Research foundations for improvement* (Monograph No. 3). Washington, DC: American Association for Mental Deficiency.

Baumeister, A. A., & Forehand, R. (1973). Stereotyped acts. In N. R. Ellis (Ed.), *International review of research in mental retardship* (Vol. 6, pp. 59–96). New York: Academic Press.

Baumeister, A. A., & Rollings, J. P. (1976). Self-injurious behaviour. In N. R. Ellis (Ed.), *International review of research in mental retardation*. New York: Academic Press.

Berkson, G. (1967). Abnormal stereotyped motor acts. In J. Zubin & H. Hunt (Eds.), *Comparative psychology* (pp. 76–94). New York: Grune and Stratton.

Berkson, G. (1983). Repetitive stereotyped behaviors. *American Journal of Mental Deficiency, 88*, 239–246.

Bishop, S. L., Richler, J., & Lord, C. (2006). Association between restricted and repetitive behaviors and nonverbal IQ in children with autism spectrum disorders. *Child Neuropsychology, 12*, 247–267.

Bodfish, J. W., Crawford, T. W., Powell, S. B., Parker, D. E., Golden, R. N., & Lewis, M. H. (1995). Compulsions in adults with mental retardation: Prevalence, phenomenology, and comorbidity with stereotypy and self-injury. *American Journal of Mental Retardation, 100*, 183–192.

Bodfish, J. W., Newell, K. M., Sprague, R. L., Harper, V. N., & Lewis, M. H. (1996). Dyskinetic movement disorder among adults with mental retardation: Phenomenology and co-occurrence with stereotypy. *American Journal of Mental Retardation, 101*, 118–129.

Bodfish, J. W., Newell, K. M., Sprague, R. L., Harper, V. N., & Lewis, M. H. (1997). Akathisia in adults with mental retardation: Development of the Akathisia Ratings of Movement Scale (ARMS). *American Journal of Mental Retardation, 101*, 413–423.

Bodfish, J. W., Symons, F., & Lewis, M. (1999). *The Repetitive Behavior Scale: Test manual*. Morganton: Western Carolina Center Research Reports.

Bodfish, J. W., Symons, F. J., Parker, D. E., & Lewis, M. H. (2000). Varieties of repetitive behavior in autism: Comparisons with mental retardation. *Journal of Autism and Developmental Disorders, 30*, 237–243.

Campbell, M., Locascio, J. J., Choroco, M. C., Spencer, E. K., Malone, R. P., Kafantaris, V., et al. (1990). Stereotypies and tardive dyskinesia: Abnormal movements in autistic children. *Psychopharmacology Bulletin, 26*, 260–266.

Carr, E. G. (1977). The motivation of self-injurious behavior: A review of some hypotheses. *Psychological Bulletin, 84*(4), 800–816.

Carr, E. G., & Kologinsky, E. (1983). Acquisition of sign language by autistic children II. Spontaneity and generalization effects. *Journal of Applied Behavior Analysis, 16*, 297–314.

Charlop, M. H., Konarski, E., & Favell, J. (Eds.) (1992). *Manual for the assessment and treatment of behavior disorders of people with mental retardation* (pp. 1–13). Morganton, NC: WCC Foundation.

Connolly, K. J., & Bruner, J. S. (Eds.) (1974). *The growth of competence*. London, New York: Academic Press.

Cuccaro, M. L., Shao, Y., Grubber, J., Slifer, M., Wolpert, C. M., Donnelly, S. L., et al. (2003). Factor analysis of restricted and repetitive behaviors in autism using the autism diagnostic interview-R. *Child Psychiatry and Human Development, 34*, 3–17.

Cunningham, A. B., & Schreibman, L. (2007). Stereotypy in autism: The importance of function. *Research in Autism Spectrum Disorders, 2*, 469–479.

Cunningham, A. B., & Schreibman, L. (2008). Stereotypy in autism: The importance of function. *Research in Autism Spectrum Disorders, 2*, 469–479.

Dunlap, G., Dyer, K., & Koegel, R. L. (1983). Autistic self-stimulation and intertribal interval duration. *American Journal of Mental Retardation, 88*, 194–202.

Durand, V. M., & Carr, E. G. (1987). Social influences on ''self-stimulatory'' behavior: Analysis and treatment application. *Journal of Applied Behavior Analysis, 20*, 119–132.

Evans, D. M., Leckman, J. F., Carter, A., Reznick, J. S., Henshaw, D., King, R. A., et al. (1997). Ritual, habit and perfectionism: The prevalence and development of compulsive-like behavior in normal young children. *Child Development, 68*(1), 58–68.

Falcomata, T. S., Roane, H. S., Hovanetz, A. N., Kettering, T. L., & Keeney, K. M. (2004). An evaluation of response cost in the treatment of inappropriate vocalizations maintained by automatic reinforcement. *Journal of Applied Behavior Analysis, 37*, 83–87.

Fischer-Terworth, C., & Probst, P. (2009). Obsessive-compulsive phenomena and symptoms in Asperger's disorder and high-functioning autism: An evaluative literature review. *Life Span and Disability, 1*, 5–27.

Foster, L. G. (1998). Nervous habits and stereotyped behaviors in preschool children. *Journal of the American Academy of Child and Adolescent Psychiatry, 37*, 711–717.

Gabriels, R. L., Cuccaro, M. L., Hill, D. E., Ivers, B. J., & Goldsong, E. (2005). Repetitive behaviors in autism: Relationships with associated clinical features. *Research in Developmental Disabilities, 26*, 169–181.

Gal, E., Dyck, M. J., & Passmore, A. (2009). The relationship between stereotyped movements and self-injurious behavior in children with developmental or sensory disabilities. *Research in Developmental Disabilities, 30*, 342–352.

Gesell, A. (2007). *Developmental diagnosis – Normal and abnormal child development – Clinical methods and pediatric applications*. New York: Paul B. Hoeber, Inc.

Gobrial, E., & Raghavan, R. (2009). Unpublished document. Anxiety disorders in children with learning disabilities and autism: a review. Retrieved from: http://www2.warwick.ac.uk/fac/med/staff/bridle/sr/anxiety_in_asd_asp_-_unpublished.doc

Goh, H. L., Iwata, B. A., Shore, B. A., DeLeon, I. G., Lerman, D. C., Ulrich, S. M., et al. (1995). An analysis of the reinforcing properties of hand mouthing. *Journal of Applied Behavior Analysis, 28*, 269–283.

Gonzalez, M. L., Dixon, D. R., Rojahn, J., Esbensen, A. J., Matson, J. L., Terlonge, C., et al. (2009). The behavior problems inventory: Reliability and factor validity in institutionalized adults with intellectual disabilities. *Journal of Applied Research in Intellectual Disabilities, 22*, 223–235.

Green, V. A., Sigafoos, J., Pituch, K. A., Itchon, J., O'Reilly, M., & Lancioni, G. E. (2006). Assessing behavioral flexibility in individuals with developmental disabilities. *Focus on Autism and Other Developmental Disabilities, 21*, 230–236.

Howlin, P. (2004) *Autism and Asperger Syndrome: Preparing for adulthood* (2nd ed). London, New York: Routledge.

Iwata, B. A., Slifer, K. J., Bauman, K. E., & Richman, G. S. (1982). Toward a functional analysis of self-injury. *Journal of Applied Behavior Analysis, 27*, 197–209.

Jones, R. S. P., Wint, D., & Ellis, N. C. (1990). The social effects of stereotyped behavior. *Journal of Mental Deficiency Research, 34*, 261–268.

Karmali, I., Greer, R. D., Nuzzolo-Gomez, R., Ross, D. E., & Rivera-Valdes, C. (2005) Reducing Palilalia by presenting tact corrections to young children with autism. *The Analysis of Verbal Behavior, 21*, 145–154.

Kennedy, C. H., Meyer, K. A., Knowles, T., & Shukla, S. (2000). Analyzing the multiple functions of stereotypical behavior for students with autism: Implications for assessment and treatment. *Journal of Applied Behavior Analysis, 33*, 559–571.

Lam, K. S., & Aman, M. G. (2007). The repetitive behavior scale-revised: Independent validation in individuals with autism spectrum disorders. *Journal of Autism and Developmental Disorders, 37*, 855–866.

Lam, K. S., Bodfish, J. W., & Piven, J. (2008). Evidence for three subtypes of repetitive behavior in autism that differ in familiality and association with other symptoms. *Journal of child psychology and psychiatry, and allied disciplines, 49*(11), 1193–1200.

Lancioni, G. E., Smeets, P. M., Ceccarani, P. S., & Goossens, A. J. (1983). Self-stimulation and task-related responding: The role of sensory reinforcement in maintaining and extending treatment effects. *Journal of Behavior Therapy and Experimental Psychiatry, 14*, 33–41.

Lewis, M. H., & Bodfish, J. W. (1998). Repetitive behavior disorders in autism. *Mental Retardation and Developmental Disabilities Research Reviews, 4*, 80–89.

Lord, C. (1995). Follow-up of 2-year old referred for possible autism. *Journal of Child Psychiatry, 36*, 1365–1382.

Lovaas, O. I., Newsom, C., & Hickman, C. (1987). Self-stimulatory behavior and perceptual reinforcement. *Journal of Applied Behavior Analysis, 20*, 45–68.

MacDonald, R., Green, G., Mansfield, R., Geckeler, A., Gardenier, N., Anderson, J., et al. (2007). Stereotypy in young children with autism and typically developing children. *Research in Developmental Disabilities, 28*, 266–277.

Mace, F. C., & Belfiore, P. (1990). Behavioral momentum in the treatment of escape-motivated stereotypy. *Journal of Applied Behavior Analysis, 23*, 507–514.

Mace, F. C., Browder, D., & Lyn, Y. (1987). Analysis of demand conditions associated with stereotypy. *Journal of Behavior Therapy and Experimental Psychiatry, 18*, 25–31.

Marshburn, E. C., & Aman, M. G. (1992). Factor validity and norms for the Aberrant Behavior Checklist in a community sample of children with mental retardation. *Journal of Autism and Developmental Disorders, 22*, 357–373.

Mason, G. J. (1991a). Stereotypies: A critical review. *Animal Behaviour, 41*, 1015–1037.

Mason, G. J. (1991b). Stereotypies and suffering. *Behavioural Processes, 25*, 103–115.

Matson, J. L., Baglio, C. S., Smiroldo, B. B., Hamilton, M., Packlawskyj, T., Williams, D., et al. (1996). Characteristics of autism as assessed by the diagnostic Assessment for Severely Handicapped-II. *Research in Developmental Disabilities, 17*, 135–143.

Matson, J. L., & Dempsey, T. (2008). Stereotypy in adults with autism spectrum disorders: Relationship and diagnostic fidelity. *Journal of Developmental and Physical Disabilities, 20*, 155–165.

Matson, J. L., Gardner, W. I., Coe, D. A., & Sovner, R. (1991). A scale for evaluating emotional disorders in severely and profoundly retarded persons: Development of the Diagnostic Assessment for the Severely Handicapped (DASH-II). *Research in Developmental Disabilities, 18*, 457–469.

Matson, J. L., Hamilton, M., Duncan, D., Bamburg, J., Smiroldo, B., Anderson, S., et al. (1997). Characteristics of stereotypic movement disorder and self-injurious behaviour assessed with the diagnostic assessment for the severely handicapped (DASH-II). *Research in Developmental Disabilities, 18*, 457–469.

Matson, J. L., Kiely, S. L., & Bamburg, J. W. (1997). The effect of stereotypies on adaptive skills as assessed with the DASH-II and Vineland Adaptive Behavior Scales. *Research in Developmental Disabilities, 18*, 471–476.

Matson, J. L., Smiroldo, B. B., Baglio, C. S., Hamilton, M., Williams, D., & Kirpatrick-Sanchez, S. (1997). Do anxiety disorders exist in individuals with severe and profound mental retardation. *Research in Developmental Disabilities, 18*, 39–44.

Matson, J. M., Dempsey, T., & Fodstad, J. C. (2009). Stereotypies and repetitive/restrictive behaviors in infants with autism and pervasive developmental disorder. *Developmental Neurorehabilitation, 12*, 122–127.

McDougle, C. J., Kresch, L. E., Goodman, W. K., Naylor, S. T., Volkmar, F. R., Cohen, D. J., et al. (1995). A case-controlled study of repetitive thoughts and behavior in adults with autistic disorder and obsessive-compulsive disorder. *American Journal of Psychiatry, 152*, 772–777.

Meiselas, K. D., Spencer, E. K., Oberfield, R., Peselow, E. D., Angrist, B., & Campbell, M. (1989). Differentiation of stereotypies from neuroleptic-related dyskinesias in autistic children. *Journal of Clinical Psychopharmacology, 3*, 207–209.

Miller, N., & Neuringer, A. (2000). Reinforcing operant variability in adolescents with autism. *Journal of Applied Behavior Analysis, 33*, 151–165.

Moore, V., & Goodson, S. (2003). How well does early diagnosis of autism stand the test of time? Follow-up study of children assessed for autism at age 2 and development of an early diagnostic service. *Autism, 7*, 47–63.

Morrison, K., & Rosales-Ruiz, J. (1997). The effect of object preferences on task performance and stereotypy in a child with autism. *Research in Developmental Disabilities, 18*, 127–137.

Mulick, J. A., Dura, J. R., Rasnake, J. K., & Wisniewski, J. (1988). *Self-injurious behavior and stereotypy in nonambulatory children with profound mental retardation.* Poster presented at the 2nd annual North Coast Regional Conference, Society of Pediatric Psychology, May 12–14, Worthington, OH.

Murphy, O., Healy, O., & Leader, G. (2009). *Research in Autism Spectrum Disorders, 3*, 474–482.

Neuringer, A. (2002). Operant variability: Evidence, functions, and theory. *Psychonomic Bulletin & Review, 9*, 672–705.

Owens, D., Johnstone, E., & Frith, C. (1982). Spontaneous involuntary disorders of movement. *Archive of General Psychiatry, 39*, 452–461.

Ozonoff, S., Macari, S., Young, G. S., Goldring, S., Thompson, M., & Rogers, S. J. (2008). Atypical object exploration at 12 Months of age is associated with autism in a prospective sample. *Autism: The International Journal of Research and Practice, 12*, 457–472.

Piazza, C. C., Adelinis, J. D., Hanley, G. P., Goh, H., & Delia, M. D. (2000). An evaluation of the effects of matched stimuli on behaviors maintained by automatic reinforcement. *Journal of Applied Behavior Analysis, 33*, 13–27.

Powell, S., Bodfish, J., Parker, D., Crawford, T. W., & Lewis, M. H. (1996). Self-restraint and self-injury: Occurrence and motivational significant. *American Journal of Mental Retardation, 101*, 41–48.

Prior, M., & MacMillan, M. B. (1973). Maintenance of sameness in children with Kanner's syndrome. *Journal of Autism and Childhood Schizophrenia, 3*(2), 154–167.

Prizant, B., & Duchan, J. (1981). The functions of immediate echolalia in autistic children. *Journal of Speech and Hear Disability, 46*, 241–249.

Prizant, B. M., & Rydell, P. J. (1984). Analysis of functions of delayed echolalia in autistic children. *Journal of Speech and Hearing Research, 27*, 183–192.

Rapp, J. T. (2006). Toward an empirical method for identifying matched stimulation for automatically reinforced behavior: A preliminary investigation. *Journal of Applied Behavior Analysis, 39*, 137–140.

Rapp, J. T. (2007). Further evaluation of methods to identify matched stimulation. *Journal of Applied Behavior Analysis, 40*, 73–88.

Rapp, J. T., & Vollmer, T. R. (2005). Stereotypy. I. A review of behavioural assessment and treatment. *Research in Developmental Disabilities, 26*, 527–547.

Rincover, A. (1979). Sensory extinction: A procedure for eliminating self-injurious behaviors in developmentally disabled children. *Journal of Applied Behavior Analysis, 6*, 299–310.

Rogers, S. J., & Ozonoff, S. (2005). Annotation: What do we know about sensory dysfunction in autism? A critical review of the empirical evidence. *Journal of Child Psychology and Psychiatry, 46*, 1255–1268.

Rojahn, J. (1984). Self-injurious behaviour in institutionalized, severely/profoundly retarded adults: Prevalence and staff agreement. *Journal of Behavioral Assessment, 6*, 13–27.

Rojahn, J. (1986). Self-injurious and stereotypic behaviour of non-institutionalized mentally retarded people: Prevalence and classification. *American Journal of Mental Deficiency, 91*, 268–278.

Rojahn, J. (1992). *Behavior problems inventory: A prospectus.* Unpublished manual. Ohio: The Ohio State University.

Rojahn, J. (1997). Epidemiology and topographic taxonomy of self-injurious behaviour. In T. Thompson (Ed.), *Destructive behaviour in developmental disabilities* (pp. 49–67). Thousand Oaks, CA: Sage.

Rojahn, J., Matlock, S. T., & Tasse, M. J. (2000). The stereotyped behavior scale: Psychometric properties and norms. *Research in Developmental Disabilities, 21*, 437–454.

Rojahn, J., Matson, J. L., Lott, D., Esbensen, A. J., & Smalls, Y. (2001). The Behavior Problems Inventory: An instrument for the assessment of self injury, stereotyped behavior and aggression/destruction in individuals with developmental disabilities. *Journal of Autism and Developmental Disorders, 31*, 577–588.

Rojahn, J., Tasse, M. J., & Sturmey, P. (1997). The stereotyped behavior scale for adolescents and adults with mental retardation. *American Journal of Mental Retardation, 102*, 137–146.

Rojahn, J., Tasse, M. J., & Sturmey, P. (2000). The stereotyped behavior scale for adolescents and adults with mental retardation. *American Journal on Mental Retardation, 102*, 137–146.

Romanczyk, R. G., Lockshin, S., & O'Connor, J. (1992). Psychophysiology and issues of anxiety and arousal. In J. K. Luiselli, J. L. Matson, & N. N. Singh (Eds.), *Self-injurious behavior: Analysis, assessment and treatment* (pp. 93–121). New York: Springer.

Rutter, M. (1978). Diagnosis and definition. In M. Rutter (Ed.), *Autism: A reappraisal of concepts and treatment* (pp. 1–25). New York: Plenum Press.

Rutter, M. (1985). The treatment of autistic children. *Child Psychology and Psychiatry, 26*, 193–214.

Rydell, P., & Prizant, B. (1995). Assessment and intervention strategies for children who use echolalia. In K. A. Quill (Ed.), *Teaching children with autism: Strategies to enhance communication and socialization* (pp. 105–132). Albany, NY: Delmar.

Sachdev, P. (1995). The epidemiology of drug-induced Akathisia: Part II. Chronic, tardive, and withdrawal akathisias. *Schizophrenia Bulletin, 21*, 3451–3461.

Scahill, L., Riddle, M. A., McSwiggin-Hardin, M., & Ort, S. (1997). Children's Yale-Brown obsessive compulsive scale: Reliability and validity. *Journal of the American Academy of Child and Adolescent Psychiatry, 36*, 844–852.

Schreibman, L. (1988). *Autism*. Newbury Park, CA: Sage.

Schreibman, L., & Carr, E. G. (1978). Elimination of echolalic responding to questions through the training of a generalized verbal response. *Journal of Applied Behavior Analysis, 11*, 453–463.

Schroeder, S. R., Rohahn, J., Mulick, J. A., & Schroeder, C. S. (1990). Self-injurious behavior: An analysis of behavior management techniques. In J. L. Matson & J. R. McCartney (Eds.), *Handbook of behavior modification* (2nd ed., pp. 141–180). NewYork: Plenum Press.

Schroeder, S., Schroeder, C., Smith, B., & Dalldorf, J. (1978). Prevalence of self-injurious behavior in a large state facility for the retarded. *Journal of Autism and Child Schizophrenia, 8*, 261–269.

Sevin, J. A., Matson, J. L., Williams, D., & Kirkpatrick-Sanchez, S. (1995). Reliability of emotional problems with the diagnostic assessment for the severely handicapped (DASH). *British Journal of Clinical Psychology, 34*, 93–94.

Sheehan, M., Leader, G., & Healy, O. (2009). *An analysis of the use of psychotropic and psychoactive medication among 135 individuals with an intellectual disability in Ireland*. Unpublished thesis. Galway: National University of Ireland.

Singer, J. (2009). Motor stereotypies. *Seminars in Pediatric Neurology, 16*, 77–81.

Skinner, B. F. (1953). *Science and human behaviour*. New York: McMillan.

Smith, E. A., & Van Houten, R. (1996). A comparison of the characteristics of self-stimulatory behavior in "normal" children and children with developmental disabilities. *Research in Developmental Disabilities, 17*, 253–268.

Storch, E. A., Roberti, J., & Roth, D. (2004). Factor structure, concurrent validity, and internal consistency of the Beck depression inventory-second edition in a sample of college students. *Depression and Anxiety, 19*, 187–189.

Symons, F. J., Sperry, L. A., Dropik, P. L., & Bodfish, J. W. (2005). The early development of stereotypy and self-injury: A review of research methods. *Journal of Intellectual Disability Research, 49*, 144–158.

Tang, J., Kennedy, C. H., Koppekin, A., & Caruso, M. (2002). Functional analysis of stereotypical ear covering in a child with autism. *Journal of Applied Behavior Analysis, 35*, 95–98.

Taylor, B. A., Hoch, H., & Weissman, B. (2005). The analysis and treatment of vocal stereotypy in a child with autism. *Behavioral Interventions, 20*, 239–253.

Thelen, E. (1996). Normal infant stereotypies: A dynamic systems approach. In R. L. Sprague & K. M. Newell (Eds.), *Stereotypies: Brain-behavior relationships* (pp. 139–165). Washington, DC: APA Press.

Troster, H. (1994). Prevalence and functions of stereotyped behaviors in nonhandicapped children in residential care. *Journal of Abnormal Child Psychology, 22*, 79–97.

Turner, M. (1996). *Repetitive behaviour and cognitive functioning in autism*. Unpublished Ph.D. Thesis. Cambridge: University of Cambridge.

Turner, M. (1999). Annotation: Repetitive behaviour in autism: A review of psychological research. *Journal of Child Psychology and Psychiatry and Allied Disciplines, 40*, 839–849.

Vollmer, T. R., Marcus, B. A., & LeBlanc, L. (1994). Treatment of self-injury and hand mouthing following inconclusive functional analyses. *Journal of Applied Behavior Analysis, 27*, 331–344.

Waller, N., & Furniss, F. (2004). Relationship between anxiety and autistic behaviour in persons with severs Learning disabilities. *Journal of Intellectual Disabilities Research, 48*, 320.

World Health Organization. (1990). *International classification of diseases* (10th Rev.). Geneva: Author.

Wolery, M., Kirk, K., & Gast, D. L. (1985). Stereotypic behavior as a reinforcer: Effects and side effects. *Journal of Autism and Developmental Disorders, 15*, 149–161.

Zandt, F., Prior, M., & Kyrios, M. (2008). Similarities and differences between children and adolescents with autism spectrum disorders and those with obsessive compulsive disorder: Executive functioning and repetitive behaviour. *Autism, 12*, 619–633.

Ira L. Cohen, J. Helen Yoo, Matthew S. Goodwin, and Lauren Moskowitz

Challenging behaviors[1] (CBs) are relatively common concerns in persons with intellectual disabilities (ID) and autism spectrum disorders (ASD), have major impacts on the family, and seriously affect the ability of such individuals to reside in more "normalizing" environments. While the term "challenging behavior" covers a wide gamut of problems in people with ID/ASD, the focus of this chapter will be on CBs of most concern to families and professionals: aggression toward others, property destruction, and self-injury; their prevalence; as well as the use of rating scales to assess their frequency or severity. At the end of this section, we will also cover novel autonomic measures that may help in understanding, predicting (and perhaps preventing) their onset. Although we will not cover functional assessment of CBs, as these are discussed elsewhere in the handbook, brief mention of the possible causes of CBs in this population and assessment issues will be mentioned.

Defining Aggression, Property Destruction, and Self-Injury

What do we mean by aggression? In the animal behavioral literature (Miczek & Krsiak, 1979), aggression consists of a number of discrete behavior sequences that take place during a conflict between two individuals and forms part of a group of behaviors categorized as "agonistic behaviors." Agonistic behaviors encompass behaviors such as aggressive displays or pre-attack behaviors, overt attack (e.g., biting), and submission or flight of one of the participants. As discussed below, all rating scales designed to assess aggression in people with ASD and/or ID focus only on display and attack behaviors and not on the submission or

flight components but they probably should do so. Knowing if a person apologized or otherwise tried to "make up" for an aggressive act, complained of an inability to control the behavior, or actually enjoyed the amount of injury caused to the other could be of clinical relevance (Tsiouris, 2010). Property destruction, when it occurs as a form of aggression, may represent an aggressive display, perhaps serving to intimidate others. In data that we show below, physical aggression, verbal threats, and property destruction group together as a single dimension (Cohen et al., 2010b).

Self-injurious behaviors (SIBs) are behaviors that involve overt attack, both initiated and directed toward the same person. Such behaviors include but are not limited to head banging, skin picking, face slapping, eye gouging, rumination and can be quite disturbing to others as well as damaging to the individual. Also of relevance here are self-deprecatory verbalizations such as verbal threats to engage in self-injury or threats of suicide. As we discuss below, our research indicates that SIBs are distinct from other forms of overt aggression and may be related to depressed mood (Cohen et al., 2010b).

Explanations for CBs, Functional Analysis Issues, and ASD

The most common explanations for the maintenance, if not acquisition, of these CBs involve operant models in the form of either positive or negative reinforcement mechanisms (e.g., frustration/arousal reduction (see below); avoidance of demands; attention seeking) (cf. Hanley, Iwata, & McCord, 2003). These models, in turn, are reflected in the use of functional analysis (FA) procedures to identify the variables

I.L. Cohen (✉)
Department of Psychology, New York State Institute for Basic Research in Developmental Disabilities, Staten Island, NY 10314, USA
e-mail: ira.cohen@opwdd.ny.gov

[1]While synonymous, this chapter favors and thus uses the term *challenging behavior* over the term *problem behavior* commonly used in the literature.

maintaining CBs. CBs for which such variables cannot be identified are sometimes said to be maintained by "automatic reinforcement" (Vollmer, 1994). It should be noted, however, that behaviors which persist despite absence of evidence for a reinforcer are quite common in operant studies; e.g., a prolonged period of extinction following an intermittent positive reinforcement schedule or extinction following exposure to a "free-operant" avoidance schedule (e.g., Sidman avoidance; Sidman, 1960). In fact, such avoidance behaviors are notoriously resistant to extinction. In such cases, FA procedures alone may not be successful in identifying the relevant negative reinforcement history.

It is also possible that behaviors presumed to be maintained by automatic reinforcement are actually induced by an adverse reinforcement schedule, i.e., as a form of schedule induced or adjunctive behavior (Falk, 1971; Granger, Porter, & Christoph, 1984; Spiga, Zeichner, & Allen, 1986) in which heightened arousal levels appear to motivate the behaviors. Rumination, for example, would appear to be a behavior readily accounted for as a form of adjunctive behavior. We are not aware of any FA techniques that have been designed to test these alternative hypotheses but autonomic measures might play a role in these and other behaviors in which cues from the autonomic system acquire discriminative and/or reinforcing properties much in the same way that some pharmacological agents can acquire these properties. These issues are described in the last section of this chapter.

Curiously, the known characteristics of ASD that would increase the likelihood of CBs are not part of many FA assessments (but see the *Contextual Assessment Inventory;* CAI; Carr, Ladd, & Schulte, 2008; McAtee, Carr, & Schulte, 2004). These include disruption in routines, change in the physical environment, prevention of an individual from engaging in idiosyncratic rituals, change in the social environment (e.g., new teacher, classmates, or roommates). Based on data we collected as part of a survey of aggression in adults with ID (Cohen et al., 2010b), professional staff reported that a change in schedule or routine provoked aggressive or self-aggressive behaviors in 51% of 1,966 people without an ASD label and in 71% of 255 people with an ASD label ($\chi^2(3) = 61.5$, $p < 0.0001$).

Prevalence of CBs

Several different surveys of the prevalence of CBs in the population of persons with ID have been reported (Crocker et al., 2006; Lowe et al., 2007; Sigafoos, Elkins, Kerr, & Attwood, 1994; Tyrer et al., 2006). However, as noted by Benson and Brooks (2008), they are difficult to compare because each used different methods, populations, and behavioral definitions. These authors concluded, however, that over 50% of this population engages in some type of aggressive behavior

but only a small portion engages in very severe forms of aggression toward self or others. Moreover, some individuals exhibit multiple types of aggression, including physical aggression against others, verbal aggression, and self-injury. Clearly, then, the definition of what constitutes aggression will have a major impact on measures of prevalence as well as on attempts to understand its etiology.

We recently published results of a survey of physical and verbal aggression, property destruction, self-injury, and self-deprecating verbalizations in a large sample ($N > 3,500$) of community-based adults with ID living in New York State (Cohen et al., 2010b). Approximately 9% of this sample had a classification of ASD. We used a version of the Overt Aggression Scale (Yudofsky, Silver, Jackson, Endicott, & Williams, 1986; see below) for data collection which we modified by adding new items and including information on antecedents and consequences of aggressive behaviors, clinical diagnoses, and known etiologies of ID to better define our samples. We named this version the IBR (Institute for Basic Research) Modified Overt Aggression Scale or IBR-MOAS (copies are available from the first author). The four domains (Verbal Aggression Toward Others (VAOTH), Physical Aggression Against Other People (PAOTH), Physical Aggression Against Objects (PAOBJ), and Physical Aggression Against Self (PASLF)) from the original OAS (Yudofsky et al., 1986) were incorporated into the IBR-MOAS form with some modifications in the wording to indicate to the rater that aggressive behaviors toward others and toward objects were being carried out in anger. In addition, a fifth domain (Verbal Aggression Toward Self (VASLF)) consisting of four items that document the occurrence of self-deprecating verbalizations was added. As with the other domains in the OAS, these items varied in severity from showing anger with self by making angry noises to verbal threats of violence toward self. The precise wording of each item is shown in Table 15.1. A Likert measure of the frequency of occurrence of each of the aggression items during the past year was developed as follows: 0 = Never (never happens); 1 = Rarely (averages about once a year to once a month); 2 = Sometimes (averages about several times a month to several times a week); 3 = Often (averages about daily to several times a day); and U (Used to happen but not this past year). For the present analyses, the U rating was coded as equivalent to Never. Unlike the OAS and its modified versions, a weighted scoring system was not used.

Table 15.1 shows the overall distribution of scores for the SURVEY sample ($N = 3,547$). As shown, the distributions were highly positively skewed with the vast majority of people showing relatively little in the way of severe aggression toward self or others, confirming the conclusions of Benson and Brooks (2008). Aggressive incidents that were reported tended to be milder and very severe incidents happened

Table 15.1 Aggressive Behaviors Scale from the IBR-MOAS – percent of total ($n = 3,547$)

	Never	Rarely	Sometimes	Often
Verbal aggression toward others				
1. Makes loud noises, shouts **angrily**, screams at others	33	24	31	12
2. Yells mild personal insults (e.g., "You're stupid!")	63	16	16	4
3. Curses viciously, uses foul language **in anger**, makes moderate threats to others	69	14	14	4
4. Makes clear threats of violence toward others ("I'm going to kill you") or requests help to control self	80	11	7	2
Verbal aggression toward self				
5. Shows frustration and anger with self by making loud noises, screaming, moaning, or whining	50	20	22	9
6. Makes mild personal insults toward self (e.g., "I'm stupid!" "I'm not good!")	85	10	4	1
7. Curses angrily at self, talks more negatively about self ("I'm very bad" "I'm evil")	91	6	2	0
8. Makes clear threats of violence toward self ("I want to die," "I don't want to live," "I want to kill myself")	92	5	3	0
Physical aggression against other people				
9. Makes threatening gestures, swings at people, grabs at clothes	48	24	23	5
10. Strikes, kicks, pushes, pulls others' hair (without injury to them)	56	23	18	3
11. Attacks others, causing mild to moderate physical injury (bruises, sprain, welts)	74	16	9	1
12. Attacks others, causing severe physical injury (broken bones, deep lacerations, internal injury)	94	5	1	0
Physical aggression against objects				
13. Slams door, scatters clothing, makes a mess **in anger**	62	19	15	3
14. Throws objects down, kicks furniture without breaking it, tries to tear clothes, marks the wall **in anger**	67	17	14	2
15. Breaks objects in anger, smashes windows in anger, rips clothes **in anger**	80	11	7	1
16. Sets fires, throws objects dangerously **in anger**	96	3	1	0
Physical aggression against self				
17. Picks or scratches skin, hits self, pulls hair (with no or minor injury only)	67	13	16	5
18. Bangs head, hits fist into objects, throws self onto floor or into objects (hurts self but without serious injury)	77	11	9	2
19. Small cuts or bruises, minor burns as a result of self-injury	83	9	7	1
20. Mutilates self, makes deep cuts, bites that bleed, internal injury, fracture, loss of consciousness, loss of teeth	96	3	1	1

Never = never happens; Rarely = averages about once a year to once a month; Sometimes = averages about several times a month to several times per week; Often = averages about daily to several times a day.
Items added or modified from the OAS are in bold face.
Modified from Cohen et al. (2010b).

relatively infrequently, confirming the ordering of item severity within domains. Such milder forms of verbal or physical aggression toward self or others were actually quite common, appearing in as many as two out of every three cases.

Table 15.2 shows the mean (SD) scores on each of the non-verbal domains as a function of age decade and level of ID (these can be used to develop standardized scores for those who may be interested). Mean scores on each of the non-verbal domains varied significantly (all p values < 0.001) with age decade (ranging from the twenties to over 70 years of age) and with level of ID (ranging from mild to profound) while means on the two verbal domains (Table 15.3)

Table 15.2 Mean (SD) non-verbal domain scores on the IBR-MOAS in community-based adults with ID as a function of ID level and age decade

ID level	Age decade	N	PAOTH	PAOBJ	PASLF
Mild	20_29	114	0.60 (0.65)	0.56 (0.60)	0.23 (0.48)
Mild	30_39	118	0.57 (0.63)	0.54 (0.58)	0.26 (0.49)
Mild	40_49	194	0.48 (0.53)	0.44 (0.54)	0.28 (0.48)
Mild	50_59	150	0.54 (0.61)	0.45 (0.63)	0.25 (0.48)
Mild	60_69	67	0.40 (0.50)	0.25 (0.45)	0.13 (0.33)
Mild	≥70	20	0.33 (0.42)	0.21 (0.52)	0.00 (0.00)
Moderate	20_29	39	0.88 (0.65)	0.74 (0.63)	0.44 (0.64)
Moderate	30_39	62	0.79 (0.61)	0.54 (0.58)	0.24 (0.45)
Moderate	40_49	99	0.57 (0.63)	0.52 (0.61)	0.31 (0.49)
Moderate	50_59	82	0.55 (0.54)	0.43 (0.55)	0.26 (0.44)
Moderate	60_69	53	0.50 (0.61)	0.45 (0.65)	0.23 (0.49)
Moderate	≥70	27	0.41 (0.44)	0.31 (0.44)	0.10 (0.35)
Severe	20_29	18	1.03 (0.74)	0.58 (0.56)	0.39 (0.56)
Severe	30_39	54	0.64 (0.63)	0.46 (0.58)	0.29 (0.35)
Severe	40_49	137	0.64 (0.66)	0.53 (0.64)	0.42 (0.53)
Severe	50_59	147	0.62 (0.63)	0.47 (0.63)	0.38 (0.53)
Severe	60_69	59	0.42 (0.52)	0.28 (0.44)	0.33 (0.56)
Severe	≥70	44	0.48 (0.54)	0.23 (0.34)	0.15 (0.31)
Profound	20_29	26	0.51 (0.67)	0.24 (0.46)	0.37 (0.62)
Profound	30_39	83	0.43 (0.57)	0.28 (0.57)	0.44 (0.57)
Profound	40_49	278	0.46 (0.60)	0.25 (0.46)	0.43 (0.61)
Profound	50_59	299	0.42 (0.56)	0.24 (0.46)	0.39 (0.55)
Profound	60_69	125	0.36 (0.54)	0.19 (0.41)	0.33 (0.47)
Profound	≥70	50	0.29 (0.45)	0.16 (0.36)	0.20 (0.39)

Table 15.3 Mean (SD) verbal domain scores on the IBR-MOAS in community-based adults with ID as a function of ID level

Level of ID	N	VAOTH	VASLF
Mild	663	0.99 (0.80)	0.45 (0.55)
Moderate	362	0.93 (0.76)	0.39 (0.47)
Severe	459	0.73 (0.70)	0.31 (0.36)
Profound	861	0.36 (0.47)	0.24 (0.30)

varied significantly only with ID level with both VAOTH and VASLF decreasing with increasing levels of ID severity (p values <0.001). PAOTH was highest in the youngest groups and declined with age group. It was also highest in the moderate and severe groups. PAOBJ also declined significantly with age and was lowest in the profound ID group. PASLF increased with more severe ID and was highest in the profound groups. There was a drop off in frequency with age starting in the sixth decade which was most obvious in those 70 years of age and older, perhaps due to subject attrition.

As shown in Fig. 15.1, there were significant differences in mean domain scores as a function of an ASD label

($p < 0.044$) and gender ($p < 0.001$) (both levels of ID and age were statistically controlled in this analysis) with people with ASD showing higher levels of PAOTH and PAOBJ. Most striking was the observation that females with ASD were reported to show the highest mean scores for both VASLF and PASLF (all p values <0.001), suggesting that mood disorders may play a role in SIB, especially in this population with these two domains forming an internalizing self-destructive dimension. Both cluster analysis and principal components analysis confirmed that the VASLF and PASLF domains group together and are distinct from VAOTH, PAOTH, and PAOBJ (which also group together as a distinct externalizing aggressive dimension).

Of course, our results may not be quite the same were we to use a different assessment tool (e.g., one that did not include self-deprecating statements), and we do not know the extent to which these subjective ratings correspond to more objective measures. However, they do suggest that self-injury is distinct from other forms of aggression with dysphoric mood perhaps playing a role in its etiology. This indicates the need to assess such mood and arousal problems when measuring aggression and self-injury. In the next section, we review various methods and tools for assessing these CBs. Rating scales that assess psychopathology, although relevant, will not be reviewed here because they are discussed elsewhere in this book.

Assessment Tools

Direct Observational Methods

An essential element of behavioral assessment is collecting observable and quantifiable data to understand and make decisions regarding behaviors targeted for change. This can range from paper-and-pencil or mechanical recordings (handheld counter, video recording) to computer software data collection such as MOOSES (Tapp, Wehby, & Ellis, 1995) or iPhone ABC Data App (Romanczyk & Gillis, 2009). Direct observation methods and analogue conditions relating to functional analysis are discussed elsewhere in this volume. For additional details of this methodology, refer to Cooper, Heron, and Heward (2007).

Various direct recording methods are available depending on the behavioral topography and the availability of time and resources allocated for observation. Examining the reliability and characteristics of different recording methods is still a work in progress (Meany-Daboul, Roscoe, Bourret, & Ahearn, 2007). The first step in direct observation is constructing an "operational definition" of the behavior of interest in order to obtain reliable and valid data (Baer, Wolf, & Risley, 1968). An operational definition requires that a behavior is described in sufficient detail to allow a relatively

Fig. 15.1 This figure shows each of the aggression scale domain means (± sem) for males and females with (AUT) or without (NO-AUT) a diagnosis of autism in the SURVEY sample, controlling for age and level of ID. Persons with autism show greater PAOTH and PAOBJ means than those without autism. Both VASLF and PASLF are highest in females with autism from Cohen et al. (2010b, with permission)

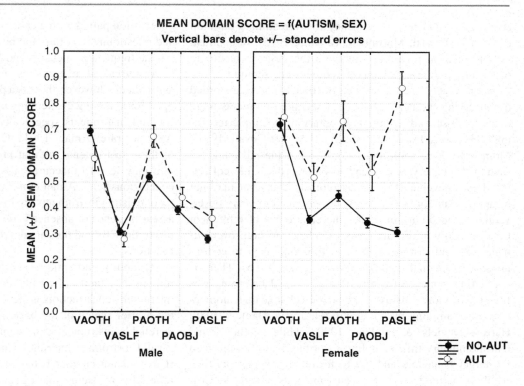

naïve observer who has not seen the target behavior to agree with another observer with minimal disagreement.

Moreover, rather than a general category of behavior (e.g., tantruming), classifying the target behavior into more specific behavioral topographies (e.g., hitting, screaming, throwing) may prove to be more useful in a long run. For example, self-injury for one individual may include head banging and hand biting, each serving a different function. For another individual, head banging alone may serve multiple functions. Therefore, it is advisable to delineate the topography of the CBs during the initial assessment phase and consider combining the behaviors that serve the same function at a later time for data collection purposes (Derby et al., 2000). In addition to operational definitions, the time length of observation; time interval between observations; frequency, and duration of observation sessions; procedures for recording observations; and the level of interaction between the observer and the individual with ASD must be clarified prior to collecting direct observation data.

Antecedent-Behavior-Consequence (ABC) recording is an anecdotal observation method that involves a descriptive *narrative* of the event that immediately preceded the behavior, and the consequence immediately following the behavior (Bijou, Peterson, & Ault, 1968). ABC data collection is widely utilized in functional behavior assessment due to its convenience and minimal training required to collect data.

More sophisticated direct observation methods involve quantifiable collection of data. "Continuous recording" includes simple frequency counts of the CB as well as the duration of each occurrence of such behavior. For

example, the number of self-injurious face slaps may be tallied with a hand-held counter during a fixed observation period. Frequency counts of CBs during a fixed period have an advantage of easily being converted into rate data (frequency/time). A non-discrete behavior such as persistent and inappropriate mouthing is better measured by the total duration of the time engaged in such behavior per observation, usually using a stop watch. Similarly, "latency recording" is useful when observing the time it takes for the individual to start or stop a target behavior (e.g., time between when an instruction or request was given until compliance; e.g., Fjellstedt & Sulzer-Azaroff, 1973; Tiger, Bouxsein, & Fisher, 2007). For behaviors that appear similar in topography yet vary in the magnitude or impact, the intensity of the kinetic force generated by the CB can be measured using a mechanical gauge or sensor (e.g., Fowler, McKerchar, & Zarcone, 2005), but is not typically used in clinical settings.

Where the above methods are not feasible, "interval recording" can be used. It measures occurrence or nonoccurrence of a CB during pre-specified time cycles. Typically, an observation period is divided into multiple 5- to 10-s intervals. For example, during a 5-min observation, there will be thirty 10-s intervals. An automatically resetting timer or stopwatch is useful when conducting observations using interval recordings. There are two types of interval recordings: partial and whole interval. In "partial interval recording," a target behavior is scored if it occurred at *any point* during an interval (even if it occurred only once during that interval). Partial interval observation data are more likely to match those based on frequency data (Meany-Daboul et al., 2007) but have a tendency to overestimate duration of the CB (Powell, Martindale, & Kulp, 1975). In contrast, "whole interval recording" requires the target behavior to occur during the *entire* interval in order to be scored.

Alternatively, the occurrence of the CB can be recorded by observing the behavior only at specified moments (e.g., every tenth second) using "momentary time sample recording" (Harrop & Daniels, 1986; Suen, Ary, & Covalt, 1991). Momentary time sampling recording has the advantage of freeing the observer to attend to other tasks while collecting data (convenient for a classroom teacher) but may not be appropriate for low-rate CBs because a momentary observation would often times miss the occurrence of infrequent CBs. In addition, it may have a tendency to both overestimate and underestimate duration in comparison to continuous observational methods (Powell et al., 1975). There is conflicting evidence for this. Partial interval recording was found to be more sensitive to behavioral change than momentary time sampling by one group (Harrop & Daniels, 1986; Harrop, Daniels, & Foulkes, 1990), while another found that momentary time-sampling recording better represented the target behaviors and led to fewer observer errors than whole or partial interval recording methods (Green, McCoy, Burns, & Smith, 1982).

A "visual product recording" may be used when direct observation is inconvenient or not feasible and the CB almost always results in damage to the same area. For example, a video or a photo of broken skin resulting from self-injurious behavior (SIB), taken weekly, may be used to illustrate the changes made during an intervention. Similarly, a ruler may be useful in quantifying the same injured surface area.

Indirect Rating Scale Measures

Although direct observational methods in combination with analogue FA conditions are likely to be the most accurate and reliable method of understanding the reasons for engaging in the CB, several limitations still remain in practice, including extensive staff training and often prolonged assessment periods to gather sufficient data. While not frequently reported, the physical risk involved with evoking the CB during hypothesis testing and inadvertently introducing non-existing, novel functions through conditioning of trials, sometimes inherent in analogue functional analysis, remain unresolved. In some cases, direct observations are not feasible due to low frequency of CBs or limitations stemming from paucity of expertise and resources. In such cases, subjective rating scales are a quick and convenient way to gather information about the CB.

Due to significant differences between informants, concurrent, multimodal, and multi-informant strategies are recommended to obtain a valid assessment. A detailed direct observation paired with a caregiver interview, record review, and questionnaires offers the best alternative to understanding the frequency, intensity, and function of target behaviors.

A myriad of instruments are available for behavioral assessment. However, there is a paucity of instruments developed for assessing challenging behaviors in individuals with ID, and instruments specifically targeting individuals with ASD are rare (Aman, 1991). Consequently, administration of these instruments without proper psychometric verification may lead to inaccurate assessment results and invalid conclusions (e.g., Aman et al., 2008). Moreover, the majority of existing instruments are informant-based measures that assess presence or absence and/or topographical characteristics of the CBs and thus are not designed to assess behavioral functions.

Reliability and validity are essential elements for determining the quality of an instrument. While an overview of instrument construction is beyond the scope of this chapter, a brief sketch of the basic concepts will be listed here. A reliable instrument consistently measures the CB, while a valid instrument measures what it is intended to measure (CB) and not another behavior (e.g., language). Inter-rater reliability measures the agreement between two or more raters/observers of the same behavior. Test–retest reliability measures the stability of the response over time when the same test is repeated later. Internal consistency measures the homogeneity of an instrument. Validity is often assessed by correlating the newly developed instrument with one or more valid instrument. A coefficient of 0 means no reliability or validity and ± 1.0 means perfect positive/negative reliability or validity.

Maladaptive Behavior Rating Scales

The "Aberrant Behavior Checklist-Community" (ABC-C; Aman, Singh, Stewart, & Field, 1985) is an informant-based 58-item rating scale divided into the following five subcategories: (1) irritability, (2) lethargy, (3) stereotypy, (4) hyperactivity, and (5) inappropriate speech. It is scored on a 4-point Likert scale ($0 = not\ at\ all\ a\ problem$; $3 = the\ problem\ is\ severe\ in\ degree$). The ABC-C was developed for individuals with ID (age 5–54) living in the community in part due to lack of available rating scales targeting treatment effects, especially drug therapies. In particular, the irritability subscale has been widely used in studies evaluating risperidone in children and adolescents with ASD presenting with tantrums, including aggression and SIB (McCracken et al., 2002; McDougle, Stigler, Erickson, & Posey, 2008).

The ABC-C is used most extensively in assessing effects of certain treatments on CBs in individuals with developmental disabilities (see Unwin & Deb, 2008, for number of citations). Internal consistency was 0.92 for the irritability subscale, which contains the majority of the challenging behavior items. Inter-rater reliability ranged from 0.39 to 0.70. Test–retest reliability was 0.98 (Aman et al., 1985). The ABC-C has been shown to measure symptoms of childhood psychopathology in a similar manner as the Child Behavior Checklist (CBCL) (Achenbach, 1991, 1992) and to assess maladaptive behaviors in persons with ID in a similar manner as the American Association on Mental Retardation (AAMD) Adaptive Behavior Scale (Nihira, Foster, Shellhaas, & Leland, 1975).

The "Overt Aggression Scale (OAS)" was developed as an incident reporting system for general psychiatric inpatients with violent aggression (Yudofsky et al., 1986). One of its advantages is that it codes the severity of the four categories of aggressive behavior noted above.

Several modified versions of the OAS are available for use with various populations. The psychometrics associated with these modification indicates adequate reliability and validity (e.g., Alderman, Knight, & Morgan, 1997; Hellings et al., 2005; Kay, Wolkenfield, & Murrill, 1988; Sorgi, Ratey, Knoedler, Markert, & Reichman, 1990). The OAS has been used with children with conduct disorders (e.g., Kruesi et al., 1995) as well as with adolescents and adults with ASD (Hellings et al., 2005; Tsiouris, Cohen, Patti, & Korosh, 2003).

The "IBR Modified Overt Aggression Scale (IBR-MOAS)" described above is an informant-based 107-item scale developed from the OAS. It was modified specifically to study possible biomarkers for aggression and self-injury in individuals with developmental disabilities (Cohen et al., 2010b). The rather large sample ($N = 3,547$) included individuals with ASD who represented 9.4% of the total group. In addition to the aggression scale, level of communication skills, setting events, types of antecedents and consequences used are ranked on a 4-point scale (*never* to *often*). The last section provides items on sensory impairments, medical problems, etiologies of developmental delay, psychiatric diagnoses, and staff estimates of the most effective treatment approach.

Inter-rater ($n = 25$) and test–retest reliabilities ($n = 16$) at 2 weeks were evaluated on the aggression scale. Inter-rater reliability ranged from 0.70 to 0.83. Test–retest reliability ranged from 0.84 to 0.96. Internal consistency ranged from 0.74 to 0.85 in the overall sample and from 0.84 to 0.90 in the smaller ($n = 25$) clinic sample. As noted above, mean domain scores systematically varied with age, level of intellectual disability, and ASD diagnosis (with the autism cases showing more problems), indicating good developmental and diagnostic validity.

The "Repetitive Behavior Scale-Revised (RBS-R)" (Bodfish, Symons, & Lewis, 1999; Bodfish, Symons, Parker, & Lewis, 2000) is a 43-item observer-based rating scale divided into 6 areas: (1) stereotyped behavior, (2) self-injurious behavior, (3) compulsive behavior, (4) ritualistic behavior, (5) sameness behavior, and (6) restricted behavior. It was developed to assess frequently occurring maladaptive behaviors in individuals with various ID and psychiatric disorders (Bodfish et al., 1999). The SIB subscale contains eight items related to hitting, biting, pulling hair or skin, rubbing or scratching, inserting or poking, as well as skin picking. The RBS-R is scored on a 4-point Likert scale (ranging from 0 = *behavior does not occur* to 3 = *behavior occurs and is a severe problem*).

The RBS-R was validated based on data from 307 caregivers of individuals with ASD (aged 3–48 years). Factor analysis produced a five-factor solution. Among them, the mean factor loading was 0.60 for the SIB subscale (Lam & Aman, 2007). Internal consistency was 0.84 for the SIB subscale. Alpha values for the remaining subscales ranged from 0.78 to 0.91. Test–retest reliability conducted with 30 adults with ID was good ($r = 0.71$). The inter-rater reliability varied, with a range of 0.57–0.73 in one sample ($n = 28$) and −0.24 to 0.95 in another ($n = 18$) (Lam & Aman, 2007). The RBS-R has good validity when compared with the Behavior Problems Inventory (BPI) (Bodfish et al., 1999) and has been used in clinical research involving individuals with ASD (Wasserman et al., 2006).

The "Behavior Problems Inventory (BPI-01)" (Rojahn, Matson, Lott, Esbensen, & Smalls, 2001) is a 49-item informant-based rating scale containing 14 SIB items, 24 stereotypy items, and 11 aggression and destruction items scored on a 5-point frequency scale (0 = *never*; 4 = *hourly*) and a 4-point severity scale (0 = *no problem*; 3 = *a severe problem*).

The BPI-01 was normed on 432 individuals with ID (age 14–91), including those diagnosed with PDD and ASD living in a developmental center. Factor loadings were 0.34 for SIB, 0.38 for stereotypy, and 0.54 for aggression/destruction. Full-scale between-interviewer reliability was 0.92 and the test–retest reliability was 0.76. The full-scale internal consistency was 0.83. Moreover, individuals diagnosed with PDD received higher scores on the SIB and aggression/destruction scores than those without (Rojahn et al., 2001). Criterion validity between the BPI and the ABC-C varied between 0.19 and 0.68 (Oliver et al., 2003). Concurrent validity with the autism spectrum disorders–behavior problems for adults (ASD-BPA) has been documented (Matson & Rivet, 2008).

In a more recent finding from 130 adults with ID, 41 of whom were also diagnosed with ASD, inter-rater reliability for the SIB subscale ranged from 0.83 to 0.85 while the aggression/destruction subscale was 0.82. Test–retest reliability after 2 months for the SIB subscale was at 0.91 and ranged from 0.87 to 0.89 for the aggression/destruction subscale. Internal consistency was 0.61 for SIB and 0.79 for aggression/destruction. Concurrent validity with the Inventory for Client and Agency Planning (ICAP) Maladaptive Behavior Items ranged from 0.14 to 0.65 for the SIB subscale and 0.11–0.66 for aggression/destruction (van Ingen, Moore, Haza, & Rojahn, 2010). Concurrent validity with the RBS-R and the ABC-C was good (Bodfish et al., 1999; Rojahn, Aman, Matson, & Mayville, 2003).

The "Challenging Behavior Interview (CBI)" (Oliver et al., 2003) is a standardized clinical interview containing two parts. Part I assesses the topography of the CBs that occurred within the previous month. CBs assessed include SIB, physical and verbal aggression, disruption, property destruction, and stereotypy. Part II assesses the frequency and severity of the CBs and their effects on self and others, as well as intervention strategies used by caregivers (Oliver et al., 2003).

The CBI was standardized on 47 children and 40 adults. Test–retest and inter-rater reliabilities were assessed for 22 adults. Concurrent validity was assessed by correlating child data with the ABC-C. The mean inter-rater and test–retest reliabilities for Part I were 0.67 (range = 0.50–0.80) and 0.86 (range = 0.70–0.91), respectively. The mean inter-rater and test–retest reliabilities for Part II were 0.48 (range = 0.02–0.77) and 0.76 (range = 0.66–0.85), respectively. Correlations with the ABC-C varied between 0.19 and 0.68 (Oliver et al., 2003). Despite this, utilization of the CBI has been limited.

The "Nisonger Child Behavior Rating Form (NCBRF)" (Aman, Tasse, Rojahn, & Hammer, 1996) is a rating scale containing social competence and problem behavior subsections totaling 76 items. The problem behavior subscale, consisting of 60 items, is scored on a 4-point Likert scale (for problem behaviors, 0 = *behavior did not occur or was not a problem*; 3 = *occurred a lot or was a severe problem*). It measures rate and severity of CBs, adapted from the Child Behavior Rating Form (CBRF) (Edelbrock, 1985).

The factor-derived dimensions of behavior included: (1) conduct problems, (2) insecure/anxious, (3) hyperactive, (4) self-injury/stereotypic, (5) self-isolated/ritualistic, and (6) overly sensitive (for parent) or irritable (for teacher).

The NCBRF was standardized on parents of 326 children, aged 3–16 years (Aman et al., 1996). In addition, 260 children, aged 3–16, were rated by teachers. Both parent and teacher ratings were collected for 189 children. Of the total parent and teacher ratings, 19.2% of the children were enrolled in a developmental disabilities classroom and 38.1% were placed in a severe behavior handicap classroom.

The median internal consistency (alpha value) was 0.85 (range = 0.77–0.93) for parent version and 0.88 (range = 0.81–0.91) for the teacher version. Parent–teacher inter-rater reliability for the problem behavior subscales ranged from 0.22 to 0.54 (mean = 0.43). Concurrent validity was assessed with the ABC-C. The median correlation for the ABC-C subscales for the parent version rated on 58

children was 0.72 (range = 0.49–0.80). The median correlation for the teacher version rated on 62 children was 0.69 (range = 0.55–0.85) (Aman et al., 1996).

The construct validity of the NCBRF was confirmed in 330 children and adolescents with ASD (Lecavalier, Aman, Hammer, Stoica, & Mathews, 2004) and has been used to evaluate the effects of psychotropics on CBs (e.g., Aman et al., 2009; Haas, Karcher, & Pandina, 2008; Shea et al., 2004) and other treatment evaluation studies in individuals with ASD (Mudford et al., 2000). Classification and characteristics of CBs in individuals with PDD (Lecavalier, 2006) and normative data based on parent ratings of 485 typically developing children are also available (Aman et al., 2008).

The "Parental Concerns Questionnaire (PCQ)" (McGrew et al., 2007) is a 13-item parent-rated scale developed to quickly identify common developmental and behavioral concerns. It is scored on a 4-point Likert scale (1 = *no problem*; 4 = *severe problems*) reflective of the previous month. Two of the 13 items are specific to challenging behavior: aggression (intentionally hits, bites others) and SIB (bangs head, pinches, bites, hits oneself). Other CBs, such as compulsive behaviors and hyperactivity, are also included.

The PCQ was standardized on 101 children (aged 4–10). Forty-eight of these children were typically developing and served as a control group. Of the 53 in the ASD group, 36 had a diagnosis of autism, 9 with PDD-NOS, and 8 with Asperger syndrome. Children with ASD and comorbid ID were excluded. Therefore, the sample may not be representative of the ASD population.

Test–retest reliability was assessed from 27 parents of the ASD group after a mean of 165 days (range = 22–397 days) and indicated a kappa of 0.60 for SIB while aggression was not reliable over time. Internal consistency was 0.78 for the ASD group and 0.58 for the control group. In regard to external validity, the aggression item was weakly correlated (0.24) with the Child Behavior Checklist (CBCL) aggression score while the self-injury item correlated highly (0.83) with the RBS-R (McGrew et al., 2007). The PCQ is a relatively new instrument and has yet to be widely utilized in the assessment of challenging behaviors in children with ASD.

The "Checklist for Challenging Behaviour (CCB)" (Harris, Humphreys, & Thomson, 1994) is a two-part checklist consisting of aggressive behaviors (14 items) and behaviors that are associated with aggressive behaviors (18 items) in individuals with ID. Items are rated on a 5-point Likert scale on frequency (1 = *has not occurred*; 5 = *occur very often (daily)*), severity of the injury caused (1 = *no injury*; 5 = *very serious injury*) (caused very serious tissue damage such as broken bones, deep lacerations/wounds requiring hospitalization and/or certified absences from work), and the management difficulty that the behavior posed to caregivers (1 = *no problem* (I can usually manage this situation with no difficulty at all); 5 = *extreme problem* (I simply cannot manage this situation without help)) (Harris et al., 1994). Concurrent validity with the PIMRA was 0.35 for the aggressive behaviors portion (Jenkins, Rose, & Jones, 2002). The CCB has been used to evaluate the effects of staff training in the management of aggressive behavior in services in individuals with ASD (McDonnella et al., 2008).

The "Developmental Behavior Checklist (DBC)" (Einfeld & Tonge, 1995) is an informant-based 93-item (teacher) and 96-item (parent) questionnaire containing five subscales: (1) disruptive/antisocial, (2) self-absorbed, (3) communication disturbance, (4) anxiety, and (5) social relating. The disruptive subscale contains items such as "kicks, hits," "throws, breaks," and "hits self." The DBC reflects the major DSM categories. Each item is scored on a 3-point scale from $0 = true$ to $2 = very\ true\ or\ often\ true$ (Einfeld & Tonge, 1992, 2002).

The internal consistency for the disruptive scale was 0.90. Inter-rater reliability for the parent version was 0.78 while the teacher version was 0.68. Test–retest reliability was 0.84. The self-absorbed subscale contains items such as "bangs head" and "throws, breaks." The internal consistency for the disruptive scale was 0.85. Inter-rater reliability for the parent version was 0.79 while the teacher version was 0.74. Test–retest reliability was 0.87. Concurrent validity of the DBC with the Adaptive Behavior Scale was 0.86 and was 0.72 with the scales of independent behavior. Standardization norms are available based on 454 children ascertained from a large survey (Einfeld & Tonge, 1992, 1995).

More recently, a 29-item Developmental Behavior Checklist–Autism Screening Algorithm (DBC–ASA) was developed by using the items from the original DBC. The DBC–ASA was evaluated in 180 children diagnosed with ASD and 180 matched controls. The results indicate adequate validity for children with ASD (Brereton, Tonge, MacKinnon, & Einfeld, 2002).

The "Children's Scale of Hostility and Aggression (C-SHARP)" (Farmer & Aman, 2009) is a recently developed informant-based scale that allows for categorization of the child's behavior as either reactive (impulsive, without clear function) or proactive (function based). The C-SHARP contains 48-items divided into five subscales: (1) verbal aggression, (2) bullying, (3) covert aggression, (4) hostility, and (5) physical aggression (Farmer & Aman, 2009, 2010). The psychometrics of the C-SHARP were examined in individuals (age 3–21 years) with intellectual or developmental disabilities, including 94 children with ASD. Internal consistency ranged from 0.58 to 0.71. Inter-rater reliability ranged from 0.50 to 0.90. Children with ASD were found to have higher scores on bullying, hostility, and physical aggression in comparison to children with other diagnoses (e.g., Down syndrome). An adult version (A-SHARP) is also available (Matlock & Aman, 2011).

Adaptive and Maladaptive Behavior Scales

Several normed adaptive scales also address CBs but only one is specifically targeted to ASD, the "PDD Behavior Inventory (PDDBI)." The PDDBI is a reliable and valid informant-based assessment tool originally designed to monitor treatment outcome in children diagnosed with a pervasive developmental disorder (PDD). The psychometric characteristics of this assessment tool were extensively described in two publications (Cohen, 2003; Cohen, Schmidt-Lackner, Romanczyk, & Sudhalter, 2003b). In 2005, an updated and expanded version was published (with scoring software) and made available to professionals as an assessment tool (Cohen & Sudhalter, 2005). The new PDDBI was standardized on a large, well-diagnosed sample of children, aged 2–12.5 years with PDD (Autism in 86%, PDD-NOS in 12%, and other PDD 2%). Internal consistency measures ranged from 0.80 to 0.98. Unlike other measures, the PDDBI provides age-standardized scoring based on a large, well-diagnosed sample of children with ASD ($n > 300$), which controls for changes in presentation with age. The PDDBI provides for assessment of both maladaptive and adaptive behaviors, permitting assessment of progress or deterioration in both dimensions of behavior. Since the PDDBI measures of social communication correlate highly with IQ, they can also provide an estimate of the functioning level of the child. Separate forms for parents and teachers allow the clinician to assess agreement across informants who see the child in different settings, and tables are provided for assessing the significance of discrepancies between parent and teacher scores.

This instrument consists of 10 domains, comprised of 188 items in the parent version and 180 items in the teacher version. The PDDBI was constructed, a priori, in a hierarchical manner. At the first level, the PDDBI is divided into two behavioral dimensions: (a) approach-withdrawal problems, assessing maladaptive behaviors, and (b) receptive/expressive social communication abilities, assessing social communicative competence. Each of these dimensions is comprised of a number of separate behavioral domains best reflecting that dimension (seven in the first dimension and three in the second dimension). Each domain, in turn, is comprised of behavioral clusters best fitting that domain. Finally, each cluster consists of four or more exemplars, rated on a 4-point Likert scale (never, rarely, sometimes, often) designed to best describe the cluster. The PDDBI generates age-normed T-scores (mean (SD) = 50 (10)) for each domain. An autism composite score is generated based on those domain T-scores most relevant to a diagnosis of ASD. These domain and composite T-scores are normally distributed within the reference sample, enabling complex statistical models to be utilized. Clusters are scored on an ordinal dimension relative to the standardization sample as follows: low (≤33rd percentile), moderate (34th to 74th percentile), high (75th to 94th percentile), and very high (≥95th percentile).

The aggressiveness domain is in the first dimension and consists of aggressive behaviors directed toward self or others as well as the negative mood changes often associated with such behaviors. Coefficient alpha for this domain was 0.89 for the parent version and 0.88 for the teacher version. The criterion-related validity of each domain and the construct validity of the PDDBI have been demonstrated via regression and factor analyses. The aggressiveness domain of the PDDBI correlated 0.47 and 0.52 with the conduct and SIB/stereotypies scales of the NCBRF, respectively.

The PDDBI has been used in the evaluation of music therapy (Kim, Wigram, & Gold, 2008), to evaluate the impact of home and school interventions on the outcome of children with ASD (Crystal, 2008), and in a variety of genetic, familial, and biochemical studies (Chauhan, Chauhan, Brown, & Cohen, 2004; Chauhan, Chauhan, Cohen, Brown, & Sheikh, 2004; Cohen & Tsiouris, 2006; Cohen et al., 2003a; Liu et al., 2009). It is also useful in assisting in ASD diagnosis (Cohen et al., 2010a).

The "Vineland Adaptive Behavior Scales II (VABS-II)" (Sparrow, Cicchetti, & Balla, 2005) is an informant-based standardized interview targeting communication, personal care, social skills, and motor skills in individuals from birth to 90 years of age. There are four different versions: Parent Rating Form, Teacher Rating Form, Survey Interview Form, and the Expanded Interview Form. The optional maladaptive behavior section is included in all but the Teacher Rating Form. The maladaptive behavior section of the Survey Interview Form contains 10 internalizing behaviors, 10 externalizing behaviors, 15 other behavior problems, and 14 critical problems. Among these, four items target overt CBs (i.e., *is physically aggressive; bites fingernails; displays behaviors that cause injury to self; destroys own or another's possessions on purpose*). Maladaptive behaviors are scored on a 3-point frequency scale (0 = *never*; 2 = *often*) and a severity scale (moderate or severe).

The VABS II is widely used in individuals with intellectual and developmental disabilities. Standardization of the VABS II included 77 individuals with ASD. The *Vineland Manual* reports good psychometrics and is readily available (Sparrow et al., 2005).

The "Child Behavior Checklist (CBCL)" (Achenbach & Rescorla, 2000; Achenbach, 1991, 1992) is a parent-based scale for children aged 1½–5 and 6–18 years and for adults 18–59 years of age. It is a widely used norm-referenced instrument. The first section of the CBCL consists of 20 competence items and the second section consists of 120 items on behavior or emotional problems that occurred during the past 6 months. Teacher Report Forms, Youth Self-Reports, and Direct Observation Forms

are also available. Syndromes assessed include aggressive behavior, anxious/depressed, attention problems, delinquent rule-breaking behavior, social problems, somatic complaints, thought problems, and withdrawn, along with externalizing scores, internalizing scores, total problems' scores, and DSM-oriented scales (Achenbach & Rescorla, 2000).

Psychometric characteristics of the CBCL (1½–5 years) were evaluated in 128 preschoolers with ASD (Pandolfi, Magyar, & Dill, 2009). Confirmatory factor analysis indicates that CBCL measures the same constructs in children with and without ASD. The internal consistency for Aggressive Behavior Scale, which contains 19 items, was 0.89.

The AAMR (now the American Association of Intellectual and Developmental Disabilities–AAIDD) Adaptive Behavior Scale (ABS, 2nd Edition, Lambert, Nihira, & Leland, 1993; Nihira, Leland, & Lambert, 1993a, b) is an informant-based scale designed for individuals with ID aged 3–18 years. Two versions are available: ABS School or ABS-S (329 items) and ABS Residential/Community Settings (356 items). The ABS-S is divided into two sections. The first part focuses on personal independence (daily living skills). The second part contains personality/behavior items related to CBs, grouped into seven domains: (1) social behavior, (2) conformity, (3) trustworthiness, (4) stereotyped and hyperactive behavior, (5) self-abusive behavior, (6) social engagement, and (7) disturbing interpersonal behavior.

The ABS-S was normed on 1,254 students without ID and standardized on 2,074 students with ID (Lambert et al., 1993; Watkins, Ravert, & Crosby, 2002). The full-scale test–retest reliability for the ID group ranged from 0.85 to 0.99 (staff) and 0.72 to 0.98 (teacher). Inter-rater reliability between teacher and teacher's aide ranged from 0.49 to 0.80 (Part I) and 0.53 to 0.88 (Part II) (Nihira et al., 1975; 1993a).

The "Scales of Independent Behavior-Revised (SIB-R)" (Bruininks, Woodcock, Weatherman, & Hill, 1996) is a 259-item adaptive behavior interview for individuals with disabilities from birth to 90 years designed to assess their levels of support required. It includes 14 subscales categorized into 4 clusters: motor skills, social interaction and communication skills, personal living skills, and community living skills. There are 24 maladaptive behavior items categorized into 3 domains: internalized (hurts self, repetitive habits, withdrawn or inattentive), asocial (socially offensive, uncooperative), and externalized (hurts others, destructive to property, disruptive). Items are scored on a 4-point Likert scale (0 = *never or rarely performs the task even if asked*; 3 = *does the task very well always or almost always, without being asked*).

The SIB-R was normed on 2,182 individuals stratified to reflect the 1990 US consensus and standardized on 1,681 individuals with intellectual and physical disabilities. Full-scale inter-rater reliability was 0.95 and the test–retest reliability was 0.98. Construct validity was at 0.91 and the criterion validity with other adaptive behavior scales ranged from 0.66 to 0.81 (Bruininks et al., 1996). A modified version for children with visual impairment is also available (Woo & Knowlton, 1992).

Summary

Taken together, the available measures generally have adequate psychometric properties for individuals with developmental disabilities, and the choice of which instrument to use will depend on the needs of the investigator. However, the validity of many of these instruments in individuals with ASD is limited by their content and the small number of individuals who were included in the analysis (Rojahn et al., 2001).

The existing rating scales are useful in attaining an approximate picture of an individual's CBs but most are not designed to assess the types and function of the CBs in individuals with ASD. That is, subjective instruments are helpful in describing the topography and the context rather than causal relations among antecedents and consequences of the CBs. Although higher rates of aggression were reported in people with ASD than those with other types of developmental disability, the majority of existing instruments were not developed specifically for them. Rather, people with ASD continue to be subject to assessments developed for the general developmental disabilities population (Aman, 1991; Farmer & Aman, 2010) with the exception of some instruments such as the PDDBI.

Methodological considerations in refining the assessment instruments for challenging behaviors in individuals with ASD include inclusion of items that delineate the types of CBs frequently observed and that differentiate between clinically significant, extremely high-intensity CBs and frequent but low-impact CBs. Replications of the psychometric properties across independent samples are also urgently needed. Well-thought-out instruments will assist in advancing our knowledge of CBs in individuals with ASD. Such efforts will also facilitate substantive advances in autism research, which in turn may necessitate refinement in these measures accordingly.

These limitations in the use of subjective rating scales in estimating the function of CB and their ability to predict or mitigate them are offset to some extent by their ease of use and unobtrusiveness. Ideally, it would be best to have objective measures that are also unobtrusive, are relatively easy to use, and have the potential to help the investigator predict and understand the functions of CBs. The next section provides some help in this regard by considering the future possibility of assessing autonomic indicators that may both explain and predict some CBs.

Psychophysiological Measures

The following sections focus on the inclusion of psychophysiological measurement to enhance the assessment, understanding, and treatment of CBs in persons with ASD. The first section briefly reviews published theories of CB that incorporate arousal and stress constructs as potential mediating variables. The second section provides an overview of arousal and stress, the autonomic nervous system (ANS), and common forms of autonomic measurement. The third section reviews findings from studies that utilize ANS measures in the assessment of CBs in persons with ASD and severe ID. The fourth section addresses methodological issues associated with these studies and highlights advancements in physiological measurement technology and statistics that can facilitate future assessments of CB. The final section discusses the research and clinical implications of including autonomic measures in the study of CB.

Psychophysiology and Challenging Behavior

A meta-analysis of published literature concluded that behavioral interventions are approximately twice as likely to succeed if they target a CB's underlying function (Carr et al., 1999). While functional analysis is currently the most effective way to identify factors controlling CB, at least 30% of these studies are inconclusive (Derby et al., 1992; Iwata et al., 1994; Vollmer, Marcus, & LeBlanc, 1994). Such findings have motivated a number of researchers and clinicians to consider the possibility that covert physiological factors can serve as setting events or discriminative stimuli that contribute to or maintain CBs, especially when there is a failure to identify any socially mediated functions (Carr & Smith, 1995; Carr, 1977, 1994; Frankel & Simmons, 1976; Harris, 1992; Mace & Mauk, 1999; Newsom, Carr, & Lovaas, 1997; Romancyzk & Goren, 1975; Romancyzk, 1977, 1987; Schroeder & Luiselli, 1992; Vollmer et al., 1994). In this framework, physiological events can be determinants, antecedents, concomitants, and/or consequences of CBs. Moreover, it has been proposed that physiological factors can increase the likelihood of engagement in CBs through a complex interaction of respondent and operant learning (Guess & Carr, 1991; Groden, Cautela, Prince, & Berryman, 1994; Romanczyk, 1992). Romanczyk (1986, 1992) was one of the first to suggest a respondent/operant model of CB that places emphasis on arousal as a central mediating factor. According to this theory, an individual may initially engage in a CB in an attempt to alleviate internal, aversive arousal. Over time, the CB is shaped and maintained by external, environmental events present during the time of high arousal. Romanczyk illustrated this interplay using SIB and restraint-seeking behaviors as examples. In this scenario, SIB produces pain (an unconditioned stimulus), which is followed by arousal (an unconditioned response). In order to reduce pain and arousal, an individual selects a behavior from a hierarchy of strategies that has proven effective in the past (an operant response) at escaping pain and arousal. For an individual with a history of restraint, restraint-seeking behavior may be selected as an effective method of reducing arousal associated with SIB. The restraint and corresponding arousal reduction thereby increases the probability that this form of escape behavior will be selected in the presence of arousal in the future i.e., negative reinforcement.

Guess and Carr (1991) posited a three-level model of CB wherein a wide variety of exogenous (reinforcement consequences, stimulus impoverishment, situational stress, etc.) and endogenous (developmental level and maturation, biological abnormalities, sensory and motor impairments, etc.) variables can interact in dynamic ways to produce and maintain CBs. In the first level, underlying patterns that form the basis for emerging CBs are biologically determined and internally regulated. In the second level, these behaviors are compensatory and employed adaptively to modulate arousal and achieve homeostatic regulation. For instance, an individual may engage in CB to increase arousal in the absence of environmental stimulation or to decrease arousal in a highly stimulating environment. In the third level, CBs are learned through conditioned positive reinforcement (e.g., communication and attention) and/or conditioned negative reinforcement (e.g., escape and avoidance) and actively employed to influence the behavior of other people. While the second level (homeostatic regulation) serves as a transitional stage between the first (internally regulated) and third levels (control the behavior of others), and the second level sets the stage for the third level, the authors note that these levels need not be mutually exclusive nor that the transitions between them hierarchical. That is, a given individual may operate in multiple levels simultaneously or transition between levels in the presence of abrupt, nonlinear exogenous and/or endogenous events or conditions.

Finally, Groden and colleagues suggested that social, cognitive, behavioral, and sensory characteristics of ASD can exacerbate the experience of stress and that CBs may be maladaptive strategies for coping with arousal in this population (Groden, Baron, & Groden, 2006; Groden et al., 1994). According to this model, CBs are employed in the absence of adaptive coping strategies and reinforced through escaping or avoiding aversive stimuli. Moreover, when maladaptive behaviors such as aggression, SIB, and tantrums are reinforced, the opportunity to learn and use adaptive coping strategies lessens. If these behaviors are punished, as they frequently are, they can lead to increases in arousal that exacerbate and perpetuate a loop of accumulating stress, anxiety, and CBs.

Taken together, these models suggest a link between CB, stress, and physiological arousal in persons with ASD such that engagement in CBs is shaped and reinforced by their arousal regulating properties. Before turning to studies that document physiological reactivity before, during, and after engagement in CBs in persons with ASD, the following section reviews arousal and stress constructs, the ANS, and common forms of physiological measurement.

Arousal, Stress, and the Autonomic Nervous System

Arousal is a physiological and psychological state of wakefulness that results in sensory alertness, mobility, and readiness to respond. Arousal is important in regulating consciousness, attention, emotion, and information processing and is closely related to concepts of motivation, stress, and anxiety. It has long been suggested that arousal and stress are useful organizing constructs for understanding motivational aspects of human behavior (Canon, 1932; McEwen & Lasley, 2002; Sapolsky, 1998; Selye, 1982). Bernard (Gross, 1998) was the first to describe the ability to *maintain the constancy of the internal milieu* despite changes in the surrounding environment as a characteristic feature of all living organisms. Cannon (1929) subsequently referred to this power of maintaining consonance *homeostasis*, the ability to remain the same or static. Homeostasis was introduced as a construct to describe and emphasize the dynamic process by which living systems maintain internal states within a functional range. Nearly 25 years later, Selye (1956) observed that many medical conditions share common elements even when they present with unique symptoms. Studying illnesses, he defined stress as the nonspecific or common result of any demand placed upon the body, whether the effect be mental or physical. Selye also highlighted that stress can have both positive (*eustress*) and negative (*distress*) effects.

Any stimulus or circumstance that compromises physical or psychological well-being and that requires an individual to make an adjustment is referred to as a *stressor* (Lazarus & Folkman, 1984). The consequence of stressors for individuals is known as *the stress response*, of which there are emotional, cognitive, behavioral, and physiological correlates. Many variables have been found to moderate the severity of psychological and physiological responses to stressors. Among them are a stressor's severity (amount of impact a stressor will have), temporal factor (length of time before a stressor occurs), event probability (likelihood of the stressor occurring), novelty (prior experience with the stressor), duration (how long the stressor will last), ambiguity (relating to prediction of a stressor's severity, temporal factor, event probability, novelty, and duration), and whether one's responses can affect an outcome (Paterson &

Neufeld, 1989; Turner, 1994). The latter factor, anticipation that an individual's response to a stressor will be successful at reducing perturbation, is especially important as it represents the ability to learn from previous experience. Whenever chronic or specific stressors affect an individual, these conditions are superimposed upon a pre-existing repertoire of behavior wherein the pre-potent reaction (i.e., engagement or disengagement) depends largely on the individual's prior experiences and outcomes in similar situations (Spence, 1956).

Widespread changes in the cardiovascular system, the immune system, the endocrine glands, and brain regions involved in emotion and memory are activated in the presence of a stressor (McEwen & Lasley, 2002; Sapolsky, 1998). These physiological actions are controlled primarily by the ANS and enable an individual to respond adaptively by preparing the body to fight or flee. The peripheral part of the nervous system, the ANS, includes both sympathetic and parasympathetic branches that affect the heart rate, respiration rate, perspiration, salivation, digestion, and diameter of the pupils, among other body organ responses. In general, the sympathetic division is a *catabolic* system associated with arousal and energy generation (*fight or flight*) and the parasympathetic, an *anabolic* system associated with vegetative processes (*rest and digest*). The sympathetic and parasympathetic divisions of the ANS work in compensatory ways to maintain homeostasis: a dynamic equilibrium in which continuous changes occur; yet relatively uniform conditions prevail (Fox, 1996).

Cardiovascular and electrodermal activities are two of the most commonly employed ANS indices of human arousal since they can be measured by electrodes placed directly on the surface of the skin (Stern, Ray, & Quigley, 2001). Cardiovascular and electrodermal responses are typically analyzed in terms of tonic, phasic, and spontaneous activities. Tonic activity refers to the baseline or resting level of an individual (i.e., the absence of a spontaneous response or discrete response to a known stimulus). Phasic activity is a discrete, evoked response to a *specific stimulus* resulting in frequency or amplitude changes relative to tonic activity. Spontaneous responses relate to changes in physiological activity that occurs in the absence of *any known stimuli*.

Significant interactions of heart action occur with somatic (muscle) and central (brain) activities (Andreassi, 2000). Cardiovascular activity is controlled by both sympathetic and parasympathetic branches of the ANS via the vagus nerve and is affected by physical, psychological, or psychosocial stimuli that put demands on the heart's output of blood. The most robust measures of cardiovascular activity in response to conditions of stress are heart rate (HR) and heart rate variability (HRV) (Andreassi, 1995). Heart rate constitutes the number of heartbeats per unit time and is typically expressed as beats per minute (bpm). While HR is a robust measure

of general physiological arousal, it is influenced by both sympathetic and parasympathetic nervous system activities. Heart rate variability, on the other hand, is a measure of the variation in the beat-to-beat interval rather than the variation in instantaneous HR, and thus permits more fine-grained analyses of stress on cardiovascular arousal, including the assessment of vasovagal tone. Physiological research supports the notion that HR patterns are predominantly mediated via the vagus nerve (Levy, 1984). Measures of vagal reactivity to sensory, visceral, or cognitive challenges indicate the adaptive functioning of the nervous system. As such, measures of HRV can provide an important window into the central control of autonomic processes and by inference, the central processes necessary for organized behavior.

Electrodermal activity (EDA) (often used synonymously with skin conductance) reflects autonomic innervation of sweat glands and provides a sensitive and convenient measure for assessing alterations in arousal associated with emotion, cognition, and attention (Critchley, 2002). Sweat secretion from the skin is modulated by postganglionic sympathetic fibers surrounding eccrine sweat glands (Sato, Kang, Saga, & Sato, 1989). Since eccrine sweat glands receive only excitatory sympathetic nerve impulses, EDA constitutes a purely sympathetic response (Boucsein, 1992).

Autonomic Measures and Challenging Behaviors

Many individuals with ASD and severe ID have difficulties identifying and describing internal states through self-report (Allen & Rapin, 1980, 1992; Hill, Berthoz, & Frith, 2004; Landa, 2007). As a result, traditional assessments of arousal and stress that utilize verbal communication (e.g., interviews, paper/pencil tests) have limited use in these populations. In the present context, researchers have attempted to overcome unreliable self-reports and measure autonomic arousal by focusing on physiological reactivity before, during, and after engagement in CBs.

The notion that persons with ASD engage in CBs to achieve homeostatic regulation has been around at least since the 1960s (e.g., Hutt & Hutt, 1965; Hutt & Hutt, 1968; Hutt & Hutt, 1970). However, the first study to directly test this hypothesis using autonomic measures appears to be by Sroufe, Struecher, and Strutzer (1973). They examined the covariation between body rocking, HR, and behavioral indices of stress (e.g., muscular tension, facial expression) in a 6-year-old boy with autism and found a significant correlation between HR accelerations and episodes of body rocking. Hutt, Forrest, and Richer (1975) replicated and extended this study and found that the autistic group ($n = 9$) had higher tonic HR compared to an age-matched and younger group of typically developing children. Furthermore, the group with autism showed a decrease in mean HR 5 s following engagement in repetitive motor movements. The authors interpreted these results as both evidence for heightened general arousal in ASD and engagement in CBs led to decrease in arousal. They further speculated that the mechanisms enabling arousal reduction are the monotony induced by repetitive motor movements and the corresponding blockage of novel sensory input.

Lewis et al. (1989) correlated body rocking with autonomic activity in 17 individuals with severe to profound ID living in institutions. They found increases in mean HR and HRV during periods of stereotypical behavior, but unlike Sroufe et al. (1973), no significant positive correlation was found between HR and body rocking. HRV and body rocking, on the other hand, did correlate highly. The investigators interpreted the results as evidence for cardiac–somatic coupling (Obrist, Webb, Sutterer, & Howard, 1970), whereby an under-aroused individual increases motor movement to maintain efficient metabolic functioning.

Willemsen-Swinkels, Buitellar, Dekker, and van Engeland (1998) investigated 26 children with PDD, attention deficit disorder (ADD), attention deficit hyperactivity disorder (ADHD), developmental expressive language disorder (or a developmentally receptive language disorder), and typically developed children. They measured HR around the onset of stereotypical behaviors associated with distress, elation, and composure. Results revealed a positive correlation between HR increases and stereotypical behaviors associated with distress just before the onset of the behavior. The authors interpreted the finding that individuals with PDD engage in stereotypical behavior while distressed as a functional response for decreasing arousal.

Freeman, Horner, and Reichle (1999) collected naturalistic data on the rate and covariation of CBs (SIB, aggression, property destruction), HR, and environmental activities in two men with severe ID. Using 15-s interval recording during periods of CB and no CB, both men were found to have significant HR increases 15 s *following* engagement in CB. No significant HR increases were found in the 15-s *preceding* CBs, suggesting an absence of autonomic–CB behavior antecedent relations. However, as the authors note, 15-s intervals may not have been a sensitive enough time scale to identify physiological *precursors* of CBs. As a follow-up test of this hypothesis, Freeman, Grzymala-Busse, Riffel, and Schroeder (2001) further analyzed data obtained from one of the participants in the Freeman et al. (1999) study at longer time scales and found that SIB *was* more likely to occur in the presence of high HR 30 s before and during engagement in SIB.

Hirstein, Iversen, and Ramachandran (2001) videotaped and recorded EDA in 37 children with ASD for 35 min as they sat quietly, interacted with their parents, immersed their hands in dry beans, and engaged in a favorite self-stimulating activity (e.g., watching a favorite video, arranging books or toys, flipping through pages of a book). Results suggested two distinguishable groups of responders, whom the authors dubbed "type A" and "type B." The type A group comprised 26 of the 37 children and was characterized by abnormally high tonic and highly variable phasic EDA. The type B group comprised 4 of the 37 children and was characterized by low and flat tonic and phasic EDA. Interestingly, type A responders showed *reduced* EDA when they engaged in apparently calming activities (e.g., immersing their hands in dry beans, sucking on sweets, being wrapped in a heavy blanket, deep pressure massage), while type B responders showed *increased* EDA only during "extreme behaviors" (e.g., SIB). The authors interpreted these findings as evidence for two classes of autonomic responders (hyper-responsive and hypo-responsive) within the diagnostic classification of ASD and suggested that both of these groups actively engage in behaviors and activities to help regulate their arousal. For the hyper-responsive type A group, repetitive and self-stimulatory behaviors and activities appeared to reduce sympathetic activity. For the hypo-responsive type B group, SIB and other high-intensity behavior appeared to increase sympathetic activity.

Finally, Barrera, Violo, and Graver (2007) exposed three adults with PDD who engaged in severe, chronic SIB to multi-element analogue functional analysis conditions while recording HR. Results demonstrated a reliable and consistent HR pattern across all participants for all conditions (attention, demand, alone, and control) wherein increases in HR immediately before SIB and a temporary drop in HR during or after SIB were evident irrespective of SIB topographies, SIB durations, body positioning, movement, respiratory action, or baseline HR activity. The finding that the SIB–HR patterns were consistent across participants and conditions suggested that internal or endogenous mechanisms of SIB were functioning in these participants independent of external consequences (i.e., were not determined by external operant contingency effects). The authors interpreted their results as evidence for SIB as a negative reinforcement mechanism that terminates, reduces, or allows escape from arousal.

Taken together, this small but suggestive literature indicates that a variety of CBs are associated with autonomic arousal in persons with ID and/or ASD and that these individuals may actively engage in CBs to either increase or decrease arousal in an attempt to achieve psychological and metabolic homeostatic regulation. There are, however, several methodological issues associated with this body of research that make it difficult to interpret and generalize the results generated. The following section briefly reviews these shortcomings and highlights a number of methodological, statistical, and measurement issues that if adequately addressed could clarify and enhance the systematic study of autonomic arousal and CBs in persons with ASD.

Methodological, Statistical, and Measurement Issues

Although the findings reviewed above suggest relationships between arousal and CBs in persons with ASD, there are several methodological shortcomings that call into question the reliability, validity, and specificity of the results. For instance, few of these studies reported on or controlled for background factors that can affect arousal responses, including comorbid psychological or medical conditions, participants' use of pharmaceuticals, general physical fitness, affective state, and amount of physical activity during the assessment period. Nearly all of the studies were conducted in laboratory settings unfamiliar to the participants, potentially increasing their arousal responses artificially (i.e., the testing environment was driving arousal, not experimental stimuli or observed behavior) thereby under- or over-representing responses seen in the natural environment. Most of these studies were undertaken only once and included a sole autonomic measure, making it impossible to determine the replicability and specificity of the tonic and phasic responses observed. The majority of these studies averaged arousal responses and CB rates across participants, potentially obscuring important individual differences. Finally, the physiological equipment used in the majority of these investigations was antiquated, likely contributing to participant discomfort, movement artifact, and equipment failures (e.g., questionable instrument calibration) that resulted in a loss of data. Establishing the following methodological protocols and utilizing advancements in technological and statistical tools can overcome many of these limitations.

Thorough screening and documentation of psychological and medical conditions, pharmaceutical use, and level of physical fitness would help determine what influences these background factors have on arousal responses and better clarify the relationships between autonomic activity and CBs. Similarly, measuring concomitant motor movements and postural changes, and conducting subjective ratings of affective state (e.g., positive, negative, or neutral facial expressions), would be useful to decouple autonomic reactivity associated with metabolic demands from affective and cognitive processes.

Conducting assessments in artificial settings can increase reactivity to measurement where the measurement process itself produces change, not the experimental stimuli, activities, or behavioral responses under observation (Campbell & Stanley, 1966; Cook & Campbell, 1979; Shadish, Cook, & Campbell, 2002). Given the potential confound of measurement reactivity when recording autonomic arousal, procedures to help participants acclimate to the measurement process seem especially important. Useful pre-observation activities could include familiarizing participants with the evaluator, providing measurement rationales appropriate to

participants' cognitive levels, and introducing participants to the observation setting and measurement apparatus using modeling, desensitization, and direct instruction as needed. To accommodate for difficulties with changes in daily routines, participants with ASD may also benefit from having autonomic assessments included in their weekly classroom schedules. Finally, all participants should be adequately praised throughout the assessment and rewarded (edible, game, or activity) at the end of their assessments to increase future participation and cooperation.

To increase ecological validity (cf. Bronfenbrenner, 1977, 1979; Brunswik, 1947; Neisser, 1976; Schmuckler, 2001), assessments should strive to measure CBs and autonomic arousal under naturalistic conditions. This includes conducting assessments in settings which a person occupies on a regular basis, observing temporally and spatially relevant variables that reliably produce the behaviors of interest, and focusing on behavior that is both most relevant for investigation and indicative of a person's behavioral repertoire.

Repeating measurements over various time scales (hours, days, weeks) would permit researchers to gather data on autonomic and CB reliability and minimize false-positive and false-negative correlations. Such intensive longitudinal designs (cf. Walls & Schafer, 2006) also have the potential to detect underlying natural behavior processes (e.g., diurnal rhythms or other cyclical or periodic fluctuations in autonomic and behavioral responses), characterize patterns of change over time, and evaluate the effects of either planned or unplanned interventions. Intensive longitudinal studies utilizing repeated measurements can also establish temporal precedence between variables and help in the determination of cause–effect relations. Increasing the number of observations also increases the power of the obtained longitudinal data.

Temporal and response directions of various ANS indices are not always uniform, a concept referred to as *directional fractionation* (Lacey, 1967). Therefore, when possible, multiple measures of ANS reactivity (e.g., EDA, HR) should be obtained simultaneously to clarify the extent and specificity of autonomic responses associated with CBs.

Inductive assessment strategies that employ a combination of single-subject and group designs would appear to be a useful method for studying autonomic activity and CB in persons with ASD given the differences in arousal and CB relations observed across previous studies, the heterogeneous nature of ASD, and the unlikely event that researchers know a priori which potential subgroups are likely to respond in idiosyncratic ways. In this framework, assessments could begin with an idiographic approach (cf. Molenaar, 2004) that focuses on autonomic and behavioral variation over time within a single individual. After studying processes at the individual level, direct and systematic replication (Barlow & Hersen, 1984; Horner et al., 2005) could be undertaken to determine if there are similarities or differences in the processes between individuals. Such an approach has the potential to yield identification of subgroup responders that can then be tested prospectively in larger studies.

Lazarus (2000) argued for such combined within-persons (*ipsitive*) and across-persons (*normative*) research, in both the short-term and the long-term, to study stress and coping. This combined approach may be especially important when including physiological measures, since his early research (Lazarus, Speisman, & Mordkoff, 1963) found almost no correlation between HR and EDA under stress and non-stress conditions across persons, but a nearly 0.50 correlation when a within-subjects method was used. Furthermore, when averaging responses across individuals, one cannot readily extrapolate the findings to any one person (cf. Epstein, 1983). The errors that result from drawing individual-level conclusions from aggregate-level data have been labeled *ecological fallacy* (Dooley, 1995). The fallacy assumes that all members of a group exhibit characteristics of the group at large. However, as Sidman (1960) thoroughly noted, there is no *average* person. As a result, such group-average findings may not be readily translatable or generalizable to any one person (Chassan, 1967, 1979). It may also be the case that differences found in between-group designs are due to a small number of outliers and not representative of the majority of people who make up the group. Finally, as the Hirstein et al. (2001) study nicely illustrated, there may be distinct subtypes of responders within a sample (e.g., hyper-aroused and hypo-aroused) that if averaged together would "wash out" and obscure important individual differences.

It should be noted when considering the above designs that conducting repeated measurements over time on a single subject creates serial dependency that violates the statistical assumption that errors in the data are independent across observations. Analytical approaches that can calculate an autocorrelation between adjacent observations will be needed in these designs to transform serially dependent data to be independent before any further analyses can be carried out. There are a growing number of statistical methods capable of handling the vast number of observations and dependency inherent in intensive longitudinal data and that can model within- and between-person observations simultaneously (for extended reviews of these methods, see Singer & Willett, 2003; Walls & Schafer, 2006; Walls, Höppner, & Goodwin, 2007). Some especially promising approaches are discussed below. They include time series analysis, multilevel modeling, survival analysis and point process modeling, and pattern-based methods, such as cluster analysis and growth mixture models.

Time series analysis (Box & Jenkins, 1976; Chatfield, 1996; Glass, Wilson, & Gottman, 1975; Peña, Tiao, & Tsay, 2001; Velicer & Fava, 2003) can be used to uncover the autoregressive structure of data, examine temporal regularities (i.e., lawfulness) or response variations over time, and assess the effects of either a planned or an unplanned intervention. Techniques capable of visually displaying, quantifying, and analyzing two or more synchronized time series at either the variable level (e.g., HR and EDA) or the person level are also emerging (Höppner, Goodwin, Velicer, & Heltshe, 2008; Lamey, Hollenstein, Lewis, & Granic, 2004). Multilevel models or hierarchical linear models that conceptualize interindividual heterogeneity in intraindividual change as variability around a common trajectory are useful if one wishes to simultaneously examine and explain heterogeneity in data sets containing both within- and across-person observations. Survival analysis (Kalbfleisch & Prentice, 2002; Lawless, 2002; Lee & Wang, 2003) and point process models (Blossfeld & Rohwer, 2002; Diggle, 1998; Lindsey, 1999) could be used to characterize the distribution of time-to-event data, determine the likelihood of an event occurring, test for differences between groups of individuals, and model the influences covariates have on duration data. Lastly, if the existence of subgroups is hypothesized but not known a priori, pattern-based methods, such as cluster analysis and growth mixture models, may be used to classify individuals into more homogenous groups on the basis of similar or dissimilar trajectories (Bauer & Curran, 2003; Bergman & Magnusson, 1997; Dumenci & Windle, 2001; Muthen, 2001; Nagin, 1999).

Finally, with respect to physiological equipment available for autonomic measurement, the extreme process of miniaturization in both electronic circuits and processors are enabling passive (i.e., do not require conscious input from the wearer), on-body perception systems to be sewn into articles of clothing and embedded into wearable accessories, such as shoes, gloves, and jewelry (e.g., Asada, Shaltis, Reisner, Rhee, & Hutchinson, 2003; Poli, 2003; Starner, 2002). For example, a wide variety of small, wireless physiological sensors have recently been developed to unobtrusively record cardiovascular, respiratory, skin conductivity, and muscle activity in freely moving people (for reviews, see Achten & Jeukendrup, 2003; Goodwin, Velicer, & Intille, 2008; Healey, 2000). These passive telemetric sampling devices can store an unprecedented amount of longitudinal autonomic data appropriate for idiographic analyses. Discrete, wireless sensors worn on the body also have the potential to decrease measurement reactivity and increase ecological validity by recording information about a freely moving person's physiological states comfortably, continuously, and passively. A variety of these autonomic sensors are now commercially available, including but not limited to, *FlexComp* (www.thoughttechnology. com), *SenseWear* (www.bodymedia.com), *Vitaport* (www. temec.com), *Alive* (www.alivetec.com), and *Actiheart* (www. bio-lynx.com). Academic researchers such as those in the Massachusetts Institute of Technology (MIT) Media Lab are also developing unobtrusive, wireless, wearable autonomic sensors (see Fig. 15.2) designed specifically for children and persons with special needs to be low-cost, light-weight, comfortable, and easy to use (Fletcher et al., 2010). Finally, open-source data visualization and analysis

software such as *ANSLAB* (www.psycho.unibas.ch/anslab/helpprofessional/index.html) are beginning to emerge.

To illustrate autonomic–CB relations, Fig. 15.3 contains simulated HR, motor movement, and CB data based on actual data obtained through our work at MIT from individuals with ASD who engaged in SIB and stereotypical motor movements while wearing the *Lifeshirt*. The *LifeShirt* (Vivometrics, Inc.) is a noninvasive telemetric recording device that continuously stores electrocardiograph (ECG), respiratory, and movement data (for description, see Wilhelm, Roth, & Sackner, 2003). Motor movements and changes in posture positions are recorded using a dual-axis accelerometer positioned on the anterior surface of the rib cage. The graph illustrates how CB can facilitate homeostatic regulation through its interaction with antecedent and consequent arousal increases and decreases. Relative to the first baseline phase, an increase in autonomic arousal (i.e., high arousal antecedent) precedes engagement in CB that results in a decrease in autonomic arousal (i.e., low arousal consequence) and return to baseline. Relative to the second baseline phase, a decrease in autonomic arousal (i.e., low arousal antecedent) precedes engagement in CB that results

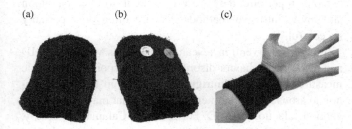

Fig. 15.2 MIT Media Lab wearable autonomic sensor. The wireless autonomic recording system captures EDA, temperature, and motor movement and posture changes through three-axis accelerometry. The three-axis accelerometer and temperature sensors provide information about a person's activity and account for the influence of motion and environmental temperature on EDA signals. (**a**) Sensor is inside elastic-breathable wristband. (**b**) Disposable Ag/AgCl electrodes attach to the underside of the wristband. (**c**) The wristband can be worn comfortably for long periods of time

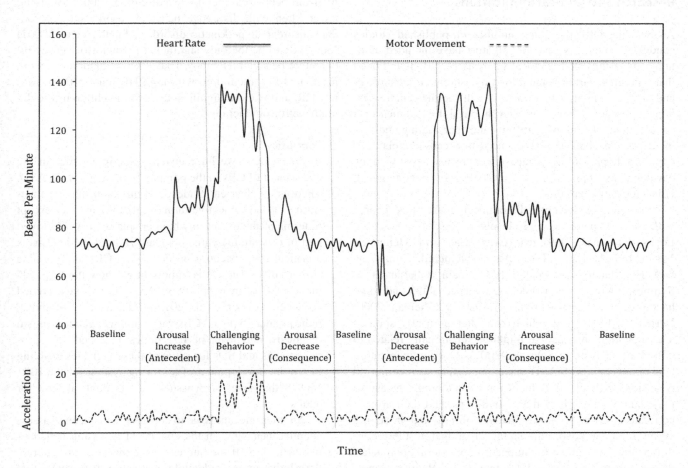

Fig. 15.3 Heart rate, motor movement, and CB homeostatic relations. The graph illustrates how CB can facilitate homeostatic regulation through its interaction with antecedent and consequent arousal increases and decreases (see text)

in an increase in autonomic arousal (i.e., high arousal consequence) and return to baseline. Measurement of motor movement activity confirms that observed arousal increases and decreases are related to the calming and stimulating functions of CB, not metabolic demand associated with increased physical activity.

In sum, establishing careful protocols and study designs, utilizing unobtrusive autonomic measures and sophisticated statistical approaches, repeating assessments, and conducting observations in a variety of settings can enhance the study of autonomic arousal and CBs in persons with ASD. Concomitant use of direct observation and physiological measures could enable a rich, multi-level description of an individual's behavior and arousal profile. Repeated observation of an individual's autonomic reactivity allows for establishing baseline range and an analysis of change or development over time. Finally, conducting assessments across various settings leads to an appreciation of the differential impacts that environmental conditions can have on a CB's frequency, duration, and severity.

Research and Clinical Implications

As evidenced by the small number of published studies conducted, relatively few investigators have included autonomic measures in functional analysis of CB. It is hoped that emerging wireless autonomic measurement technology and advances in statistical models will facilitate more systematic research of this kind. Psychophysiological measures could potentially aid in identifying and appreciating underlying arousal mechanisms associated with or causally related to CBs. Psychophysiological measures may also assist with the development, application, and evaluation of more targeted, efficacious interventions.

An emerging scientific literature suggests that people with ASD experience high levels of anxiety (MacNeil, Lopes, & Minnes, 2009), fear (Evans, Canavera, Kleinpeter, Maccubbin, & Taga, 2005), panic (Steingard, Zimnitzky, DeMaso, Bauman, & Bucci, 1997), pain (Oberlander & Symons, 2006), sleep disorders (Richdale, 1999), and some have other medical conditions (Gillberg & Coleman, 2000; Herbert, 2005), all of which can alter arousal responses and regulation abilities that might be functionally related to CBs (Carr & Owen-DeSchryver, 2007). Poor communication skills in persons with ASD make diagnosing such comorbid conditions difficult; thus inclusion of autonomic measures may help elucidate how these conditions, and their arousal correlates, serve as discriminative stimuli and/or setting events for CBs. Also, eliminating or mitigating these conditions may strengthen the impact of behavioral approaches whose effectiveness can be impeded by their presence. Further, if the display of CB was determined to be casually

related to arousal, then stress reduction (Cautela & Baron, 1973; Cautela & Groden, 1978; Groden & Baron, 1991), functional communication, and other replacement behavior could be taught early on to enhance arousal regulation and prevent CBs from developing into environmentally controlled, learned behaviors. Once CBs are entrenched in a person's repertoire, they are very difficult to intervene upon and invite intrusive methods that are often only partially successful.

Finally, intervention research in persons with severe ID and disruptive behavior disorders that incorporate autonomic measures suggest an intriguing relationship between autonomic arousal and treatment responses that may guide intervention selection in ASD. For instance, Calamari, McNally, Benson, and Babington (1990) observed a positive relationship between high tonic HR and engagement in SIB and aggressive behavior in a 23-year-old woman with severe ID. Administration of propranolol, a non-selective beta-blocker used in the treatment of hypertension, was found to reduce tonic HR and lower the rate and severity of CBs. In addition to pharmacological approaches, autonomic arousal appears to impact the extent to which an individual benefits from behavioral therapy (Stadler et al., 2007). Studying 23 children with disruptive behavior disorders (e.g., conduct disorder, hyperkinetic disorder), Stadler et al. (2007) found HR to be the only significant predictor of successful cognitive-behavioral therapy. That is, CB reduction was more prominent in the children with high HR than in those with low HR, and HR was significantly lower in children who did not benefit from therapy.

Conclusion

In this review, we have covered multiple issues in the assessment of CBs in the population of people with ASD. There is no clear-cut evidence at this point for the superiority of one subjective rating scale over another except in terms of the extent to which people with ASD formed part of or were the entire standardization sample. This is a critical issue because in identifying CBs and possible comorbidity issues, it is important to know the "typical" range of CBs in people with ASD, as we have argued elsewhere (Cohen et al., 2010a). Our data, cited above, indicate that "typical" CBs vary with age, gender, autism diagnosis, and level of ID. Tables 15.2 and 15.3 provide means and SDs for some of these variables enabling the future development of a scoring system for the IBR-MOAS that takes such issues into account, at least for adults.

Another relevant issue to consider is the need to assess adaptive behaviors in the context of assessing maladaptive behaviors. If the interest of the investigator is purely descriptive in an epidemiological sense, then scales that assess only maladaptive behaviors may be sufficient. But if one of the goals of the investigator is to assess treatment efficacy, then we would suggest that inclusion of adaptive skills assessment is critical because of the need to ensure that treatments which suppress maladaptive behaviors do not also suppress adaptive ones.

Autism spectrum disorders are an etiologically and behaviorally heterogeneous group of conditions, and there is some evidence that different etiologies or associated medical conditions will also prove to be important additional sources of information in understanding these challenging behaviors in the future. For example, there is evidence that a functional polymorphism in the promoter region of the X-linked gene responsible for monoamine oxidase-A, influences level of adaptive skills and stereotyped behaviors and arousal in young males with autism (Cohen et al., 2003a), is associated with CBs in adult males with ID (May et al., 2009), and also predicts aggressive behaviors in "typical" males following provocation (McDermott, Tingley, Cowden, Frazzetto, & Johnson, 2008). Sokol et al. (2006) also noted high levels of Alzheimer beta-amyloid precursor protein in severely aggressive individuals with autism.

Therefore, it may be the case that an adequate assessment of CBs in this population will eventually require a complex but systematic decision-making system involving behavior analytic, developmental rating scale, psychopathological, autonomic, and biochemical and/or genetic approaches so as to both understand and treat severe maladaptive behaviors. To this end, future research studies will help to decide the extent to which some or all of these assessments are both necessary and sufficient.

Acknowledgments We would like to acknowledge the late Dr. Edward (Ted) Carr for his pioneering work in the field of functional behavior assessment, biological setting events for self-injury, and intervention for challenging behaviors in individuals with ASD and other developmental disabilities. The research performed at the Institute for Basic Research in Developmental Disabilities was supported by funds from the New York State Office of Mental Retardation and Developmental Disabilities. Research at the MIT Media Lab cited in this chapter is supported by grants from the Nancy Lurie Marks Family Foundation and Autism Speaks. The first author would also like to thank Dr. Paul Starker and his team at Overlook Hospital whose kindness, sensitivity, skills, and expertise enabled this chapter to have been written.

References

Achenbach, T. M. (1991). *Manual for child behavior checklist/4–18 and 1991 profile.* Burlington, VT: University of Vermont, Department of Psychiatry.

Achenbach, T. M. (1992). *Manual for child behavior checklist/2–3 and 1992 profile.* Burlington, VT: University of Vermont, Department of Psychiatry.

Achenbach, T. M., & Rescorla, L. A. (2000). *Manual for the ASEBA preschool forms & profiles.* Burlington, VT: University of Vermont, Research Center for Children, Youth, and Families.

Achten, J., & Jeukendrup, A. E. (2003). Heart rate monitoring: Applications and limitations. *Sports Medicine, 33,* 517–538.

Alderman, N., Knight, C., & Morgan, C. (1997). Use of a modified version of the Overt Aggression Scale in the measurement and assessment of aggressive behaviours following brain injury. *Brain Injury, 11*(7), 503–523.

Allen, D. A., & Rapin, I. (1980). Language disorders in preschool children: Predictors of outcome – a preliminary report. *Brain & Development, 2,* 73–80.

Allen, D. A., & Rapin, I. (1992). Autistic children are also dysphasic. In H. Naruse & E. M. Ornitz (Eds.), *Neurobiology of infantile autism* (pp. 157–163). Amsterdam: Elsevier.

Aman, M. G. (1991). *Assessing psychopathology and behavior problems in person with mental retardation: A review of available instruments.* Rockville, MD: US Department of Health and Human Services.

Aman, M. G., Hollway, J. A., Leone, S., Masty, J., Lindsay, R., Nash, P., et al. (2009). Effects of risperidone on cognitive-motor performance and motor movements in chronically medicated children. *Research in Developmental Disabilities, 30,* 386–396.

Aman, M. G., Singh, N. N., Stewart, A. W., & Field, C. J. (1985). The Aberrant Behavior Checklist: A behavior rating scale for the assessment of treatment effects. *American Journal of Mental Deficiency, 89,* 485–491.

Aman, M. G., Tasse, M. J., Rojahn, J., & Hammer, D. (1996). The Nisonger CBRF: A child behavior rating form for children with developmental disabilities. *Research in Developmental Disabilities, 17,* 41–57.

Aman, M., Leone, S., Lecavalier, L., Park, L., Buican, B., & Coury, D. (2008). Nisonger child behavior rating form: Typical IQ version. *International Clinical Psychopharmacology, 23,* 232–242.

Andreassi, J. L. (1995). Heart activity and behavior: Developmental factors, motor and mental activities, perception, attention, and orienting responses. *Psychophysiology: Human behavior and physiological response* (3rd ed., pp. 218–239). Mahwah, NJ: Erlbaum.

Andreassi, J. L. (2000). *Psychophysiology: Human behavior and physiological response.* Mahwah, NJ: Erlbaum.

Asada, H. H., Shaltis, P., Reisner, A., Rhee, S., & Hutchinson, R. C. (2003). Mobile monitoring with wearable photoplethysmographic biosensors. *IEEE Engineering in Medicine and Biology Magazine, 22,* 28–40.

Baer, D. M., Wolf, M. M., & Risley, T. R. (1968). Some current dimensions of applied behavior analysis. *Journal of Applied Behavior Analysis, 1,* 91–97.

Barlow, D. H., & Hersen, M. (1984). *Single case experimental designs: Strategies for studying behavior change* (2nd ed.). New York: Pergamon Press.

Barrera, F. J., Violo, E. E., & Graver, F. B. (2007). On the form and function of severe self-injurious behavior. *Behavioral Interventions, 22,* 5–33.

Bauer, D. J., & Curran, P. J. (2003). Distributional assumptions of growth mixture models: Implications for overextraction of latent trajectory classes. *Psychological Methods, 8,* 338–363.

Benson, B. A., & Brooks, W. T. (2008). Aggressive challenging behaviour and intellectual disability. *Current Opinion in Psychiatry, 21,* 454–458.

Bergman, L. R., & Magnusson, D. (1997). A person-oriented approach in research on developmental psychopathology. *Development and Psychopathology, 9,* 291–319.

Bijou, S. W., Peterson, R. F., & Ault, M. H. (1968). A method to integrate descriptive and experimental field studies at the level of data and empirical concepts. *Journal of Applied Behavior Analysis, 1,* 175–191.

Blossfeld, H. P., & Rohwer, G. (2002). *Techniques of event history modeling: New approaches to causal analysis* (2nd ed.). Mahwah, NJ: Lawrence Erlbaum.

Bodfish, J. W., Symons, F. J., & Lewis, M. H. (1999). *Repetitive behavior scales*. New York: Western Carolina Center Research Reports.

Bodfish, J. W., Symons, F. J., Parker, D. E., & Lewis, M. H. (2000). Varieties of repetitive behavior in autism: Comparisons to mental retardation. *Journal of Autism and Developmental Disorders, 30*, 237–243.

Boucsein, W. (1992). *Electrodermal activity*. New York: Plenum Press.

Box, G. E. P., & Jenkins, G. M. (1976). *Time series analysis, forecasting, and control*. San Francisco: Holden-Day.

Brereton, A. V., Tonge, B. J., MacKinnon, A. J., & Einfeld, S. T. (2002). Screening young people for autism with the developmental behavior checklist. *Journal of the American Academy of Child and Adolescent Psychiatry, 41*, 1369–1375.

Bronfenbrenner, U. (1977). Toward an experimental ecological of human development. *American Psychologist, 32*, 513–531.

Bronfenbrenner, U. (1979). *The ecology of human development: Experiments by nature and design*. Cambridge, MA: Harvard University Press.

Bruininks, R. H., Woodcock, R. W., Weatherman, R. F., & Hill, B. K. (1996). *Scales of independent behavior—revised*. Chicago: Riverside.

Brunswik, E. (1947). *Systematic and representative design of psychological experiments. With results in physical and social perception*. Berkeley: University of California Press.

Calamari, J. E., McNally, R. J., Benson, D. S., & Babington, C. M. (1990). Case study: Use of propranolol to reduce aggressive behavior in a woman who is mentally retarded. *Behavioral Residential Treatment, 5*, 287–296.

Campbell, D. T., & Stanley, J. C. (1966). *Experimental and quasi-experimental designs for research*. Chicago: Rand McNally.

Cannon, W. B. (1929). Organization for physiological homeostasis. *Physiological Reviews, 9*, 399–431.

Canon, W. B. (1932). *The wisdom of the body*. New York: Norton.

Carr, E. G. (1977). The motivation of self-injurious behavior: A review of some hypotheses. *Psychological Bulletin, 84*, 800–816.

Carr, E. G. (1994). Emerging themes in the functional analysis of problem behavior. *Journal of Applied Behavior Analysis, 27*, 393–399.

Carr, E. G., Horner, R. H., Turnbull, A. P., Marquis, J. G., Magito-McLaughlin, D., McAtee, M., et al. (1999). *Positive behavior support for people with developmental disabilities: A research synthesis*. Washington, DC: American Association on Mental Retardation.

Carr, E. G., Ladd, M. V., & Schulte, C. (2008). Validation of the contextual assessment inventory (CAI) for problem behavior. *Journal of Positive Behavior Interventions, 10*, 91–104.

Carr, E. G., & Owen-DeSchryver, J. S. (2007). Physical illness, pain, and problem behavior in minimally verbal people with developmental disabilities. *Journal of Autism and Developmental Disorders, 37*, 413–424.

Carr, E. G., & Smith, C. E. (1995). Biological setting events for self-injury. *Mental Retardation and Developmental Disabilities Research Reviews, 1*, 94–98.

Cautela, J., & Groden, J. (1978). *Relaxation: A comprehensive manual for adults, children and children with special needs*. Champaign, IL: Research Press.

Cautela, J. P., & Baron, M. G. (1973). Multifaceted behavior therapy of self-injurious behavior. *Journal of Behavior Therapy and Experimental Psychiatry, 4*, 125–131.

Chassan, J. B. (1967, *1979*). *Research designs in clinical psychology and psychiatry* (2nd ed.). New York: Irvington Press.

Chatfield, C. (1996). *The analysis of time series: An introduction* (6th ed.). Boca Raton, FL: CRC Press.

Chauhan, A., Chauhan, V., Brown, W. T., & Cohen, I. L. (2004). Oxidative stress in autism: Increased lipid peroxidation and reduced serum levels of ceruloplasmin and transferrin – the antioxidant proteins. *Life Sciences, 75*, 2539–2549.

Chauhan, V., Chauhan, A., Cohen, I. L., Brown, W. T., & Sheikh, A. (2004). Alteration in amino-glycerophospholipids levels in the plasma of children with autism: A potential biochemical diagnostic marker. *Life Sciences, 74*, 1635–1643.

Cohen, I. L. (2003). Criterion-related validity of the PDD behavior inventory. *Journal of Autism and Developmental Disorders, 33*, 47–53.

Cohen, I. L., Gomez, T. R., Gonzalez, M. G., Lennon, E. M., Karmel, B. Z., & Gardner, J. M. (2010a). Parent PDD Behavior Inventory profiles of young children classified according to autism diagnostic observation schedule-generic and autism diagnostic interview-revised criteria. *Journal of Autism and Developmental Disorders, 40*, 246–254.

Cohen, I. L., Liu, X., Schutz, C., White, B. N., Jenkins, E. C., Brown, W. T., et al. (2003a). Association of autism severity with a monoamine oxidase a functional polymorphism. *Clinical Genetics, 64*, 190–197.

Cohen, I. L., Schmidt-Lackner, S., Romanczyk, R., & Sudhalter, V. (2003b). The PDD behavior inventory: A rating scale for assessing response to intervention in children with PDD. *Journal of Autism and Developmental Disorders, 33*, 31–45.

Cohen, I. L., & Sudhalter, V. (2005). *The PDD behavior inventory*. Lutz, FL: Psychological Assessment Resources, Inc.

Cohen, I. L., & Tsiouris, J. (2006). Maternal recurrent mood disorders and high-functioning autism. *Journal of Autism and Developmental Disorders, 36*, 1077–1078.

Cohen, I. L., Tsiouris, J. A., Flory, M. J., Kim, S. Y., Freedland, R., Heaney, G., et al. (2010b). A large scale study of the psychometric characteristics of the IBR modified overt aggression scale: Findings and evidence for increased self-destructive behaviors in adult females with Autism Spectrum Disorder. *Journal of Autism and Developmental Disorders, 40*, 599–609.

Cook, T. D., & Campbell, D. T. (1979). *Quasi-experimentation*. Chicago: Rand-McNally.

Cooper, J. O., Heron, T. E., & Heward, W. L. (2007). *Applied behavior analysis* (2nd ed.). *Upper. Saddle River, NJ: Merrill/Prentice Hall*.

Critchley, H. D. (2002). *Electrodermal responses: What happens in the brain. Neuroscientist, 8*, 132–142.

Crocker, A. G., Mercier, C., Lachapelle, Y., Brunet, A., Morin, D., & Roy, M. E. (2006). Prevalence and types of aggressive behaviour among adults with intellectual disabilities. *Journal of Intellectual Disability Research, 50*, 652–661.

Crystal, G. (2008). *The impact of home and school interventions on the adjustment of children with autism spectrum disorders*. Unpublished doctoral dissertation. Pullman, WA: Washington State University.

Derby, K. M., Hagopian, L., Fisher, W. W., Richman, D., Augustine, M., Fahs, A., et al. (2000). Functional analysis of aberrant behavior through measurement of separate response topographies. *Journal of Applied Behavior Analysis, 33*, 113–117.

Derby, K. M., Wacker, D. P., Sasso, G., Steege, M., Northrup, J., Cigrand, K., et al. (1992). Brief functional assessment techniques to evaluate aberrant behavior in an outpatient clinic: A summary of 79 cases. *Journal of Applied Behavior Analysis, 25*, 713–721.

Diggle, P. J. (1998). An approach to the analysis of repeated measurements. *Biometrics, 44*, 959–971.

Dooley, D. (1995). *Social research methods* (3rd ed.). Upper Saddle River, NJ: Prentice Hall.

Dumenci, L., & Windle, M. (2001). Cluster analysis as a method of recovering types of intraindividual growth trajectories: A Monte Carlo study. *Multivariate Behavioral Research, 36*, 501–522.

Edelbrock, C. S. (1985). Child behavior rating form. *Psychopharmacological Bulletin, 21*, 835–837.

Einfeld, S. L., & Tonge, B. J. (1992). *Manual for the Developmental Behaviour Checklist*. Clayton, Malbourne, and Sydney: Monash University Center for Developmental Psychiatry and School of Psychiatry, University of New South Wales.

Einfeld, S. L., & Tonge, B. J. (1995). The developmental behavior checklist: The development and validation of an instrument to assess behavioral and emotional disturbance in children and adolescents with mental retardation. *Journal of Autism and Developmental Disorders, 25*, 81–104.

Einfeld, S. L., & Tonge, B. J. (2002). *Manual for the Developmental Behaviour Checklist: Primary Carer Version (DBC-P) & Teacher Version (DBC-T)* (2nd. ed.). Clayton, Melbourne: Monash University Centre for Developmental Psychiatry and Psychology.

Epstein, S. (1983). Aggregation and beyond: Some basic issues on the prediction of behavior. *Journal of Personality, 51*, 360–392.

Evans, D. W., Canavera, K., Kleinpeter, F. L., Maccubbin, E., & Taga, K. (2005). The fears, phobias and anxieties of children with autism spectrum disorders and down syndrome: Comparisons with developmentally and chronologically age matched children. *Child Psychiatry and Human Development, 36*, 3–26.

Falk, J. L. (1971). The nature and determinants of adjunctive behavior. *Physiology and Behavior, 6*, 577–588.

Farmer, C. A., & Aman, M. G. (2009). Development of the children's scale of hostility and aggression: reactive/proactive (C-SHARP). *Research in Developmental Disabilities, 30*, 1155–1167.

Farmer, C. A., & Aman, M. G. (2010). Psychometric properties of the children's scale of hostility and aggression: reactive/proactive (C-SHARP). *Research in Developmental Disabilities, 31*, 270–280.

Fjellstedt, N., & Sulzer-Azaroff, B. (1973). Reducing the latency of child's responding to instructions by means of a token system. *Journal of Applied Behavior Analysis, 6*, 125–130.

Fletcher, R., Dobson, K., Goodwin, M. S., Eydgahi, H., Wilder-Smith, O., Fernholz, D., et al. (2010). iCalm: Wearable sensor and network architecture for wirelessly communicating and logging autonomic activity. *IEEE Transactions on Information Technology in Biomedicine, 14*, 215–223.

Fowler, S. C., McKerchar, T. L., & Zarcone, T. J. (2005). Response dynamics: Measurement of the force and rhythm of motor responses in laboratory animals. In M. Ledoux (Ed.), *Animal models of movement disorders* (pp. 73–100). San Diego, CA: Academic Press.

Fox, S. (1996). *Human physiology* (5th ed.). Dubuque, IA: W. C. Brown.

Frankel, F., & Simmons, J. Q. (1976). Self-injurious behavior in schizophrenic and retarded children. *American Journal of Mental Deficiency, 80*, 512–522.

Freeman, R., Horner, R., & Reichle, J. (1999). Relation between heart rate and problem behaviors. *American Journal of Mental Retardation, 104*, 330–345.

Freeman, R. L., Grzymala-Busse, J. W., Riffel, L. A., & Schroeder, S. R. (2001). Analyzing the relation between heart rate, problem behavior, and environmental events using data mining system LERS. *Computer-Based Medical Systems, CBMS proceedings. 14th IEEE symposium.*

Gillberg, C., & Coleman, M. (2000). *The Biology of the Autistic Syndromes*. London: Mac Keith Press.

Glass, G. V., Wilson, V. L., & Gottman, J. M. (1975). *Design and analysis of time series experiments*. Boulder: Colorado Associate University Press.

Goodwin, M. S., Velicer, W. F., & Intille, S. S. (2008). Telemetric monitoring in the behavior sciences. *Behavioral Research Methods, 40*, 328–341.

Granger, R. G., Porter, J. H., & Christoph, N. L. (1984). Schedule-induced behavior in children as a function of interreinforcement interval length. *Physiology and Behavior, 33*, 153–157.

Green, S. B., McCoy, J. F., Burns, K. P., & Smith, A. C. (1982). Accuracy of observational data with whole interval, partial interval, and momentary time-sampling recording techniques. *Journal of Psychopathology and Behavioral Assessment, 4*, 103–117.

G. Groden & M. G. Baron (Eds.). (1991). *Autism: Strategies for change*. New York: Gardner Press.

Groden, J., Baron, M. G., & Groden, G. (2006). Stress and autism: Assessment and coping strategies. In M. G. Baron, J. Groden, G. Groden, & L. P. Lipsitt (Eds.), *Stress & coping in autism* (pp. 15–51). New York: Oxford University Press.

Groden, J., Cautela, J., Prince, S., & Berryman, J. (1994). The impact of stress and anxiety on individuals with autism and developmental disabilities. In E. Schopler & G. Mesibov (Eds.), *Behavioral issues in autism* (pp. 178–190). New York: Plenum Press.

Gross, C. G. (1998). Claude bernard and the constancy of the internal environment. *The Neuroscientist, 4*, 380–385.

Guess, D., & Carr, E. G. (1991). Emergence and maintenance of stereotypy and self-injury. *American Journal of Mental Retardation, 96*, 335–344.

Haas, M., Karcher, K., & Pandina, G. J. (2008). Treating disruptive behavior disorders with risperidone: A 1-year, open-label safety study in children and adolescents. *Journal of Child and Adolescent Psychopharmacology, 18*, 337–345.

Hanley, G. P., Iwata, B. A., & McCord, B. E. (2003). Functional analysis of problem behavior: A review. *Journal of Applied Behavior Analysis, 36*, 147–185.

Harris, J. C. (1992). Neurobiological factors in self-injurious behavior. In J. K. Luiselli, J. L. Matson, & N. N. Singh (Eds.), *Self-injurious behavior: Analysis, assessment, and treatment* (pp. 93–121). New York: Springer-Verlag.

Harris, P., Humphreys, J., & Thomson, G. (1994). A checklist of challenging behavior. The development of a survey instrument. *Mental Handicap Research, 7*, 118–133.

Harrop, A., & Daniels, M. (1986). Methods of time sampling: A reappraisal of momentary time sampling and partial interval recording. *Journal of Applied Behavior Analysis, 19*, 73–77.

Harrop, A., Daniels, M., & Foulkes, C. (1990). The use of momentary time sampling and partial interval recording in behavioural research. *Behavioural Psychotherapy, 18*, 121–127.

Healey, J. (2000). Future possibilities in electronic monitoring of physical activity. *Research Quarterly for Exercise and Sport, 71*, 137–145.

Hellings, J. A., Nickel, E. J., Weckbaugh, M., McCarter, K., Mosier, M., & Schroeder, S. R. (2005). The overt aggression scale for rating aggression in outpatient youth with autistic disorder: Preliminary findings. *Journal of Neuropsychiatry and Clinical Neurosciences, 17*, 29–35.

Herbert, M. R. (2005). Autism: A brain disorder, or a disorder that affects the brain? *Clinical Neuropsychiatry, 2*, 354–379.

Hill, E., Berthoz, S., & Frith, U. (2004). Brief report: Cognitive processing of own emotions in individuals with autistic spectrum disorder and in their relatives. *Journal of Autism and Developmental Disorders, 34*, 229–235.

Hirstein, W., Iversen, P., & Ramachandran, V. S. (2001). Autonomic responses of autistic children to people and objects. *Proceedings of Biological Sciences, 268*, 1883–1888.

Horner, R., Carr, E., Halle, J., McGee, G., Odom, S., & Wolery, M. (2005). The use of single subject research to identify evidence-based practice in special education. *Exceptional Children, 71*, 165–179.

Hutt, C., Forrest, S., & Richer, J. (1975). Cardiac arrhythmia and behaviour in autistic children. *Acta Psychiatrica Scandinavica, 51*, 361–372.

Hutt, C., & Hutt, S. J. (1965). Effects of environmental complexity on stereotyped behaviours of children. *Animal Behaviour, 13*, 1–4.

Hutt, C., & Hutt, S. J. (1970). Stereotypies and their relation to arousal: A study of autistic children. In S. Hutt & C. Hutt (Eds.), *Behaviour studies in psychiatry* (pp. 175–204). Oxford: Pergamon Press.

Hutt, S. J., & Hutt, C. (1968). Stereotypy, arousal and autism. *Human Development, 11*, 277–286.

Höppner, B. B., Goodwin, M. S., Velicer, W. F., & Heltshe, J. (2008). An applied example of pooled time series analysis: Cardiovascular reactivity to stressors in children with autism. *Multivariate Behavioral Research, 42*, 707–727.

Iwata, B. A., Pace, G. M., Dorsey, M. F., Zarcone, J. R., Vollmer, T. R., Smith, R. G., et al. (1994). The functions of self-injurious behavior: An experimental-epidemiological analysis. *Journal of Applied Behavior Analysis, 27*, 215–240.

Jenkins, R., Rose, J., & Jones, T. (2002). The checklist of challenging behaviour and its relationship with the psychopathology inventory for mentally retarded adults. *Journal of Intellectual Disability Research, 42*, 273 – 278.

Kalbfleisch, J. D., & Prentice, R. L. (2002). *The statistical analysis of failure time data* (2nd ed.). New York: Wiley.

Kay, S. R., Wolkenfield, F., & Murrill, L. M. (1988). *Profiles of aggression among psychiatric patients: II. Covariates and predictors. Journal of Nervous and Mental Disorders, 176*, 547–557.

Kim, J., Wigram, T., & Gold, C. (2008). The effects of improvisational music therapy on joint attention behaviors in autistic children: A randomized controlled study. *Journal of Autism and Developmental Disorders, 38*, 1758–1776.

Kruesi, M. J. P., Hibbs, E. D., Hamburger, S. D., Rapoport, J. L., Keysor, C. S., & Elia, J. (1995). *Measurement of aggression in children with disruptive behaviour disorders. Journal of Offender Rehabilitation, 21*, 159–172.

Lacey, J. I. (1967). Somatic response patterning and stress: Some revisions of activation theory. In M. H. Appley & R. Trumball (Eds.), *Psychological stress: Issues in research*. New York: Appleton-Century-Crofts.

Lam, K. S., & Aman, M. G. (2007). The repetitive behavior scale-revised: independent validation in individuals with autism spectrum disorders. *Journal of Autism and Developmental Disorders, 37*, 855–866.

Lambert, N., Nihira, K., & Leland, H. (1993). *AAMR adaptive behavior scale-school* (2nd ed.). *Austin, TX: Pro-ed.*

Lamey, A., Hollenstein, T., Lewis, M. D., & Granic, I. (2004). GridWare (Version 1.1). [Computer software]. http://www.statespacegrids.org

Landa, R. (2007). Early communication development and intervention for children with autism. *Mental Retardation and Developmental Disabilities, 13*, 16–25.

Lawless, J. F. (2002). *Statistical models and methods for lifetime data* (2nd ed.). New York: Wiley.

Lazarus, R. S. (2000). Toward better research on stress and coping. *American Psychologist, 55*, 665–673.

Lazarus, R. S., & Folkman, S. (1984). Stress, appraisal, and coping. New York: Springer.

Lazarus, R. S., Speisman, J. C., & Mordkoff, A. M. (1963). The relationships between autonomic indicators of psychological stress: Heart rate and skin conductance. *Psychosomatic Medicine, 25*, 19–21.

Lecavalier, L. (2006). Behavioral and emotional problems in young people with pervasive developmental disorders: Relative prevalence, effects of subject characteristics, and empirical classification. *Journal of Autism and Developmental Disorders, 36*, 1101–1114.

Lecavalier, L., Aman, M. G., Hammer, D., Stoica, W., & Mathews, G. L. (2004). Factor analysis of the nisonger child behavior rating form in children with autism spectrum disorders. *Journal of Autism and Developmental Disorders, 34*, 709–721.

Lee, E. T., & Wang, J. W. (2003). *Statistical methods for survival data analysis* (3rd ed.). New York: Wiley.

Levy, M. N. (1984). Cardiac sympathetic-parasympathetic interactions. *Federation Proceedings, 43*, 2598–2602.

Lewis, M., MacLean, W. E., Bryson-Brockmann, W., Arendt, R., Beck, B., Fidler, P. S., et al. (1989). Time-series analysis of stereotyped movements: Relationship of body-rocking to cardiac activity. *American Journal of Mental Deficiency, 89*, 287–294.

Lindsey, J. K. (1999). *Models for repeated measurements* (2nd ed.). New York: Oxford University Press.

Liu, X., Novosedik, N., Wang, A., Hudson, M., Cohen, I., Chudley, A. E., et al. (2009). The DLX1 and DLX2 genes and susceptibility to autism spectrum disorders. *European Journal of Human Genetics, 17*, 228–235.

Lowe, K., Allen, D., Jones, E., Brophy, S., Moore, K., & James, W. (2007). Challenging behaviours: Prevalence and topographies. *Journal of Intellectual Disability Research, 51*, 625–636.

MacNeil, B. M., Lopes, V. A., & Minnes, P. M. (2009). Anxiety in children and adolescents with autism spectrum disorders. *Research in Autism Spectrum Disorders, 3*, 1–21.

Mace, F. C., & Mauk, J. E. (1999). Bio-behavioral diagnosis and treatment of self-injury. In A. C. Repp & R. H. Horner (Eds.), *Functional analysis of problem behaviors: From effective assessment to effective support* (pp. 78–97). Pacific Grove, CA: Brooks/Cole.

Matlock, S. T., & Aman, M. G. (2011). Development of the adult scale of hostility and aggression: Reactive-proactive (A-SHARP). *American Journal on Intellectual and Developmental Disabilities, 116*, 130–141.

Matson, J. L., & Rivet, T. T. (2008). A validity study of the autism spectrum disorders—behavior problems for adults (asd-bpa) scale. *Journal of Developmental and Physical Disabilities, 19*, 557–564.

May, M. E., Srour, A., Hedges, L. K., Lightfoot, D. A., Phillips, J. A., Blakely, R. D., et al. (2009). Monoamine oxidase a promoter gene associated with problem behavior in adults with intellectual/developmental disabilities. *American Journal of Intellectual and Developmental Disabilities, 114*, 269–273.

McAtee, M. L., Carr, E. G., & Schulte, C. (2004). A contextual assessment inventory for problem behavior: Initial development. *Journal of Positive Behavior Interventions, 6*, 148–165.

McCracken, J. T., McGough, J., Shah, B., Cronin, P., Hong, D., Aman, M. G., et al. (2002). Research units on pediatric psychopharmacology autism network. risperidone in children with autism and serious behavioral problems. *New England Journal of Medicine, 347*, 314–321.

McDermott, R., Tingley, D., Cowden, J., Frazzetto, G., & Johnson, D. D. P. (2008). Monoamine oxidase a gene (MAOA) predicts behavioral aggression following provocation. *Proceedings of the National Academy of Sciences Early Edition.*

McDonnella, A., Sturmey, P., Oliver, C., Cunninghama, J., Hayesd, S., Galvind, M., et al. (2008). The effects of staff training on staff confidence and challenging behavior in services for people with autism spectrum disorders. *Research in Autism Spectrum Disorders, 2*, 311–319.

McDougle, C. J., Stigler, K. A., Erickson, C. A., & Posey, D. J. (2008). Atypical antipsychotics in children and adolescents with autistic and other pervasive developmental disorders. *Journal of Clinical Psychiatry, 69*(Suppl 4), 15–20.

McEwen, B., & Lasley, E. (2002). *The end of stress as we know it.* Washington, DC: Joseph Henry Press.

McGrew, S., Malow, B. A., Henderson, L., Wang, L., Song, Y., & Stone, W. (2007). Developmental and behavioral questionnaire for autism spectrum disorders. *Pediatric Neurology, 37*, 108–116.

Meany-Daboul, M. G., Roscoe, E. M., Bourret, J. C., & Ahearn, W. H. (2007). A comparison of momentary time sampling and partial-interval recording for evaluating functional relations. *Journal of Applied Behavior Analysis, 40*, 501–514.

Miczek, K. A., & Krsiak, M. (1979). Drug effects on agonistic behavior. In T. Thompson, P. B. Dews, & W. A. Mckim (Eds.), *Advances in behavioral pharmacology* (Vol. 2, pp. 87–161). New York: Academic Press.

Molenaar, P. C. M. (2004). A manifesto on psychology as idiographic science: Bringing the person back into scientific psychology, this time forever. *Measurement: Interdisciplinary Research and Perspectives, 2*, 201–218.

Mudford, O. C., Cross, B. A., Breen, S., Cullen, C., Reeves, D., Gould, J., et al. (2000). Auditory integration training for children with autism: No behavioral benefits detected. *American Journal on Mental Retardation, 105,* 118–129.

Muthen, B. O. (2001). Second-generation structural equation modeling with a combination of categorical and continuous latent variables: New opportunities for latent class/latent growth modeling. In A. Sayer & L. Collins (Eds.), *New methods for the analysis of change* (pp. 291–322). Washington, DC: American Psychological Association.

Nagin, D. (1999). Analyzing developmental trajectories: A semiparametric, group-based approach. *Psychological Methods, 4,* 139–157.

Neisser, U. (1976). *Cognition and reality.* San Francisco: Freeman.

Newsom, C. D., Carr, E. G., & Lovaas, O. I. (1997). The experimental analysis and modification of autistic behavior. In R. S. Davidson (Ed.), *Modification of pathological behavior* (pp. 109–187). Thousand Oaks, CA: Sage.

Nihira, K., Foster, R., Shellhaas, M., & Leland, H. (1975). *AAMD adaptive behavior scale (rev).* Washington, DC: American Association on Mental Deficiency.

Nihira, K., Leland, H., & Lambert, N. (1993a). *AAMR adaptive behavior scale school edition.* Lutz, FL: Psychological Assessment Resources.

Nihira, K., Leland, H., & Lambert, N. (1993b). *AAMR adaptive behavior scale-residential and community (Second edition): Examiner's manual.* Austin, TX: PRO-ED.

Oberlander, T. F., & Symons, F. (2006). *Pain in children and adults with developmental disabilities.* Baltimore: Brookes.

Obrist, P. A., Webb, R. A., Sutterer, J. A., & Howard, J. L. (1970). The cardiac-somatic relationship: Some reformulations. *Psychophysiology, 6,* 569–587.

Oliver, C., McClintock, K., Hall, S., Smith, M., Dagnan, D., & Stenfert-Kroese, B. (2003). Assessing the severity of challenging behaviour: Psychometric properties of the challenging behavior interview. *Journal of Applied Research in Intellectual Disabilities, 16,* 53–61.

Pandolfi, V., Magyar, C. I., & Dill, C. A. (2009). Confirmatory factor analysis of the child behavior checklist 1.5–5 in a sample of children with autism spectrum disorders. *Journal of Autism and Developmental Disorders, 39,* 986–995.

Paterson, R. J., & Neufeld, R. W. J. (1989). The stress response and parameters of stressful situations. In R. Neufeld & R. Paterson (Eds.), *Advances in the investigation of psychological stress* (pp. 7–42). Oxford: Wiley.

Peña, D., Tiao, G. C., & Tsay, R. S. (2001). *A course in time series analysis.* New York: Wiley.

Poli, A. (2003). The equipped body: Wearable computers and intelligent fabrics. In L. Fortunati, J. E. Katz, & R. Riccini (Eds.), *Mediating the human body: Technology, communication, and fashion* (pp. 169–173). Mahway, NJ: Lawrence Erlbaum & Associates.

Powell, J., Martindale, A., & Kulp, S. (1975). An evaluation of time-sample measures of behavior. *Journal of Applied Behavior Analysis, 8,* 463–469.

Richdale, A. L. (1999). Sleep problems in autism: Prevalence, cause, and intervention. *Developmental Medicine and Child Neurology, 41,* 60–66.

Rojahn, J., Aman, M. G., Matson, J. L., & Mayville, E. (2003). The aberrant behavior checklist and the behavior problems inventory: Convergent and divergent validity. *Research in Developmental Disabilities, 24,* 391–404.

Rojahn, J., Matson, J. L., Lott, D., Esbensen, A., & Smalls, Y. (2001). The behavior problems inventory: An instrument for the assessment of self-injury, stereotyped behavior and aggression/destruction in individuals with developmental disabilities. *Journal of Autism and Developmental Disorders, 31,* 577–588.

Romancyzk, R. G. (1977, October). *Treatment of self-injurious behavior and self-stimulatory behavior: The contrast between treatment*

and follow-up. Paper presented at the 24th annual meeting of the American Association on Mental Deficiency, Pittsfield, MA.

Romancyzk, R. G. (1987, October). *Aversive conditioning as a component of comprehensive treatment: The impact of etiological factors on clinical decision making.* Paper presented at Rutgers Symposium on Applied Psychology, New Brunswick, NJ.

Romancyzk, R. G., & Goren, E. R. (1975). Severe self-injurious behavior: The problem of clinical control. *Journal of Consulting and Clinical Psychology, 43,* 730–739.

Romanczyk, R. G. (1986). Self-injurious behavior: Conceptualization, assessment and treatment. In K. D. Gadow (Ed.), *Advances in learning and behavioral disabilities* (Vol. 5). Greenwich, CT: JAI Press, Inc.

Romanczyk, R. G. (1992, June). *The role of arousal and anxiety in self-injurious behavior: Implications for treatment.* Paper presented at the third international Fragile X Conference, Snowmass, CO.

Romanczyk, R. G., & Gillis, J. M. (2009). An iTunes app for behavior analysts–ABC data just released. *ABPA Newsletter,* Vol. 8. (www.apbahome.net)

Sapolsky, R. (1998). *Why zebras don't get ulcers.* New York: Freeman.

Sato, K., Kang, W. H., Saga, K., & Sato, K. T. (1989). Biology of sweat glands and their disorders. I. Normal sweat gland function. *Journal of the American Academy of Dermatology, 20,* 537–563.

Schmuckler, M. A. (2001). What is ecological validity? A dimensional analysis. *Infancy, 2,* 419–436.

Schroeder, S. R., & Luiselli, J. K. (1992). Self-restraint. In J. K. Luiselli, J. L. Matson, & N. N. Singh (Eds.), *Self-injurious behavior: Analysis, assessment, and treatment* (pp. 293–306). New York: Springer.

Selye, H. (1956). *The stress of life.* New York: McGraw-Hill.

Selye, H. (1982). Foreword. In R. W. J. Neufeld (Ed.), *Psychological stress and psychopathology.* (pp. v–vii). New York: McGraw Hill.

Shadish, W. R., Cook, T. D., & Campbell, D. T. (2002). *Experimental and quasi-experimental designs for generalized causal inference.* Boston: Houghton-Mifflin.

Shea, S., Turgay, A., Carroll, A., Schulz, M., Orlik, H., Smith, I., et al. (2004). Risperidone in the treatment of disruptive behavioral symptoms in children with autistic and other pervasive developmental disorders. *Pediatrics, 114,* 634–641.

Sidman, M. (1960). Tactics of scientific research: Evaluating experimental data in psychology. Boston: Authors Cooperative, Inc.

Sigafoos, J., Elkins, J., Kerr, M., & Attwood, T. (1994). A survey of aggressive behaviour among a population of persons with intellectual disability in Queensland. *Journal of Intellectual Disability Research, 38,* 369–381.

Singer, J. D., & Willett, J. (2003). *Applied longitudinal data analysis.* New York: Oxford University Press.

Sokol, D. K., Chen, D., Farlow, M. R., Dunn, D. W., Maloney, B., Zimmer, J. A., et al. (2006). High levels of Alzheimer beta-amyloid precursor protein (APP) in children with severely autistic behavior and aggression. *Journal of Child Neurology, 21,* 444–449.

Sorgi, P., Ratey, J. M., Knoedler, D. W., Markert, R. J., & Reichman, M. (1990). Rating aggression in the clinical setting: A retrospective adaptation of the overt aggression scale: preliminary results. *Journal of Neuropsychiatry and Clinical Neurosciences, 3,* 52–56.

Sparrow, S. S., Cicchetti, D. V., & Balla, D. A. (2005). *Vineland adaptive behavior scales: Second edition (Vineland II), survey interview form/caregiver rating form.* Livonia, MN: Pearson Assessments.

Spence, K. W. (1956). *Behavior theory and conditioning.* New Haven: Yale University Press.

Spiga, R., Zeichner, A., & Allen, J. D. (1986). Human schedule-induced cardiovascular response. *Physiology and Behavior, 36,* 133–140.

Sroufe, L. A., Struecher, H. U., & Strutzer, W. (1973). The functional significance of autistic behaviors for the psychotic child. *Journal of Abnormal Child Psychology, 1,* 225–240.

Stadler, C., Grasmann, D., Fegert, J. M., Holtmann, M., Poustka, F., & Schmeck, K. (2007). Heart rate and treatment effect in children with disruptive behavior disorders. *Child Psychiatry and Human Development, 39*, 299–309.

Starner, T. E. (2002). Wearable computers: No longer science fiction. In *IEEE Pervasive Computing, 1*, 86–88.

Steingard, R. J., Zimnitzky, B., DeMaso, D. R., Bauman, M. L., & Bucci, J. P. (1997). Sertraline treatment of transition-associated anxiety and agitation in children with autistic disorder. *Journal of Child and Adolescent Psychopharmacology, 7*, 9–15.

Stern, R. M., Ray, W. M., & Quigley, K. S. (2001). *Psychophysiological recording* (2nd ed.). Oxford: Oxford University Press.

Suen, H. K., Ary, D., & Covalt, W. (1991). Reappraisal of momentary time sampling and partial interval recording. *Journal of Applied Behavior Analysis, 24*, 803–804.

Tapp, J. T., Wehby, J. H., & Ellis, D. (1995). MOOSES: A Multi-option observation system for experimental studies. *Behavior Research Methods, Instruments, & Computers, 27*, 25–31.

Tiger, J. H., Bouxsein, K. J., & Fisher, W. W. (2007). Treating excessively slow responding of a young man with asperger syndrome using differential reinforcement of short response latencies. *Journal of Applied Behavior Analysis, 40*, 559–563.

Tsiouris, J. A. (2010). Pharmacotherapy for aggressive behaviours in persons with intellectual disabilities: Treatment or mistreatment? *Journal of Intellectual Disability Research, 54*, 1–16.

Tsiouris, J. A., Cohen, I. L., Patti, P. J., & Korosh, W. M. (2003). Treatment of previously undiagnosed psychiatric disorders in persons with developmental disabilities decreased or eliminated self-injurious behavior. *Journal of Clinical Psychiatry, 64*, 1081–1090.

Turner, J. R. (1994). *Cardiovascular reactivity and stress: Patterns of physiological response*. New York: Plenum Press.

Tyrer, F., McGrother, C. W., Thorp, C. F., Donaldson, M., Bhaumik, S., Watson, J. M., et al. (2006). Physical aggression towards others in adults with learning disabilities: Prevalence and associated factors. *Journal of Intellectual Disability Research, 50*, 295–304.

Unwin, G., & Deb, S. (2008). Psychiatric and behavioural assessment scales for adults with learning disabilities. *Advances in Mental Health and Learning Disabilities, 2*, 37–45.

van Ingen, D. J., Moore, L. L., Haza, R. H., & Rojahn, J. (2010). The Behavior Problems Inventory (BPI-01) in community-based adults with intellectual disabilities: Reliability and concurrent validity vis-à-vis the Inventory for client and agency planning (ICAP). *Research in Developmental Disabilities, 31*, 97–107.

Velicer, W. F., & Fava, J. (2003). Time series analysis. In J. A. Schinka & W. F. Velicer (Eds.), *Handbook of psychology: Research methods in psychology* (Vol. 2, pp. 581–606). New York: Wiley.

Vollmer, T. R. (1994). The concept of automatic reinforcement: Implications for behavioral research in developmental disabilities. *Research in Developmental Disabilities, 15*, 187–207.

Vollmer, T. R., Marcus, B. A., & LeBlanc, L. (1994). Treatment of self-injury and handmouthing following inconclusive functional analyses. *Journal of Applied Behavior Analysis, 27*, 331–344.

Walls, T. A., & Schafer, J. L. (2006). *Models for intensive longitudinal data*. New York: Oxford University Press.

Walls, T. A., Höppner, B. B., & Goodwin, M. S. (2007). Statistical issues in intensive longitudinal data analysis. In A. Stone, S. Shiffman, A. Atienza, & L. Nebelling (Eds.), *The science of real-time data capture* (pp. 338–360). New York: Oxford University Press.

Wasserman, S., Iyengar, R., Chaplin, W. F., Watner, D., Waldoks, S. E., Anagnostou, E., et al. (2006). Levetiracetam versus placebo in childhood and adolescent autism: A double-blind placebo-controlled study. *International Clinical Psychopharmacology, 21*, 363–367.

Watkins, M. W., Ravert, C. M., & Crosby, E. G. (2002). Normative factor structure of the AAMR adaptive behavior scale-school, second edition. *Journal of Psychoeducational Assessment, 20*, 337–345.

Wilhelm, F. H., Roth, W. T., & Sackner, M. A. (2003). The LifeShirt: An advanced system for ambulatory measurement of respiratory and cardiac function. *Behavior Modification, 27*, 671–691.

Willemsen-Swinkels, S., Buitellar, J., Dekker, M., & van Engeland, H. (1998). Subtyping stereotypic behavior in children: The association between stereotypic behavior, mood, and heart rate. *Journal of Autism and Developmental Disorders, 28*, 547–557.

Woo, I., & Knowlton, M. (1992). Developing a version of the Scales of independent behavior, adapted for students with visual impairments. *RE:view, 24*, 72–83.

Yudofsky, S. C., Silver, J. M., Jackson, W., Endicott, J., & Williams, D. (1986). The overt aggression scale for the objective rating of verbal and physical aggression. *American Journal of Psychiatry, 143*, 35–39.

Functional Behavioral Assessment and Analysis

16

John Ward-Horner, Laura J. Seiverling, and Peter Sturmey

Practitioners and caregivers face the important question of what treatment will be most effective for a particular person's presenting problem (Sturmey, 2009a). Information from randomized controlled trials (RCTs) may be helpful in general terms; however, the relevant question is not whether this treatment works for the average person, but whether it works for this specific person here and now. Group experimental designs arose in the field of agriculture where the average weight of the average corn cob was indeed important to the farmer; however, the outcomes for the hypothetical average person are of little use to specific people if these outcomes do not apply to the person of interest. For example, within a RCT with clinically significant results will be participants whose problem changed to a clinically significant degree, participants whose problem changed to a moderate, but unimportant extent, participants who did not change at all, and participants who become significantly worse *because of the treatment*. Thus, even if a RCT based on diagnostic categories produced significant results, these results may be of little help in guiding treatment for individual people. Additionally, RCTs tend to focus on symptom reduction, rather than positive changes in the person's behavior; thus, RCTs may sometimes identify treatments that effectively reduce problematic behavior, but leave the person with few relevant skills and a poor quality of life. Therefore, predicting the most effective treatment for an individual's specific problem is an applied question of paramount importance, but RCTs provide imperfect answers to this question.

Traditional approaches to predicting a person's response to treatment focus on enduring, intra-personal qualities of the person, such as psychiatric diagnosis, hypothetical personality traits, and alleged psychodynamic processes to guide treatment (Sturmey, Ward-Horner, Marroquin, & Doran,

2007). These structural approaches attempt to divide the presence of some underlying trait, illness, or alleged biological cause that summarizes the constellation of presenting behavior, its underlying cause, and the treatment based on that cause. Although such models have been quite effective for some acute physical illnesses, their status for chronic medical problems and psychological and psychiatric problems is less clear. For example, DSM-IV characterized pervasive developmental disorders (PDDs) as disorders having qualitative impairments in the three domains that include social interaction; communication; and restrictive, repetitive, and stereotyped patterns of behavior. The DSM-IV further categorizes clients into five disorders: autistic disorder, pervasive developmental disorder not otherwise specified (PDD-NOS), Asperger's syndrome, Rett disorder, and childhood disintegrative disorder. This classification provides a gross distinction between groups of people with mild and severe disabilities and between people with disabilities in some or all of the three domains and, to the extent that these disorders reflect severity of PDD, may also predict speed of response to early intensive applied behavior analysis (ABA) treatment (Sallows & Graupner, 2005). Nevertheless, research has not shown that these classifications are helpful in predicting treatment of problem behavior in specific people. For example, we are unaware of different treatments for aggression for people with PDD-NOS, as opposed to Asperger's syndrome. Indeed, as subsequent sections will show, people with autistic disorder who act aggressively may require radically different interventions, even though they share the same diagnosis.

In contrast, functional approaches, especially those associated with ABA, focus on identifying independent variables that can be manipulated and that have a large impact on the problem behavior of interest for each specific person, resulting in idiosyncratic assessments and formulations for each individual (Haynes & O'Brien, 2000; Sturmey, 2009b). Thus, Skinner (1953) defined functional analysis as follows: "The external variables of which behavior is a function provide for what may be called a causal or functional analysis...

J. Ward-Horner (✉)
Department of Psychology, Queens College and The Graduate Center, City University of New York, Flushing, NY 11367, USA
e-mail: wardhornerj@yahoo.com

J.L. Matson, P. Sturmey (eds.), *International Handbook of Autism and Pervasive Developmental Disorders*, Autism and Child Psychopathology Series, DOI 10.1007/978-1-4419-8065-6_16, © Springer Science+Business Media, LLC 2011

271

[behavior] is our 'dependent variable'... Our 'independent variables'... are the external conditions of which behavior is a function... [which] must be defined in physical terms..." (pp. 35–36). Baer, Wolf, and Risley (1968) put it like this: "An experimenter has achieved an analysis of behavior when he can exercise control over it... an ability of an experimenter to turn the behavior on and off" (p. 94).

Since the mid-1950s these ideas, derived from basic behavior analytic research, were gradually translated into a technology of functional assessment and analysis and ABA interventions. For example, Ted Carr's (1977) classic review, *The Motivation of Self-Injurious Behavior*, identified two operant functions of self-injury: positive social reinforcement and negative social reinforcement, and subsequent empirical studies supported, refined, and extended these hypotheses to a very wide range of problems (e.g., Iwata, Doresy, Slifer, Bauman, & Richman, 1982/1994; Sturmey, 2008; Sturmey et al., 2007) including aggression in people with PDDs (see below).

There are now many good reasons to conduct functional assessments and analyses of challenging behavior in children with PDDs. Most importantly, there is robust evidence from several meta-analyses that behavioral interventions based on functional assessments and analyses are superior to other behavioral interventions and other non-behavioral interventions (Didden, Duker, & Korzilius, 1997), including people with mild intellectual disabilities (Didden, Korzilius, van Oorsouw, & Sturmey, 2006; Scotti, Evans, Meyer, & Walker, 1991) and people with autism (Campbell, 2003). Further, Federal laws, such as Individuals with Disabilities Improvement Education Act (2004), state laws, and professional standards (US Department of Justice, 2009; Van Houten et al., 1988) all mandate the use of functional assessments prior to behavioral intervention. This chapter provides an overview of the variety of functional assessment and analysis methods that are available for conducting functional assessments and analyses and provides case examples of the application of functional methods for assessing behavior in individuals with PDD.

Assessment Versus Analysis

A functional assessment/functional behavioral assessment refers to the general process of collecting information regarding antecedent and consequent events that are related to the occurrence of challenging behavior (Cooper, Heron, & Heward, 2007; Smith, Vollmer, & St. Peter Pipkin, 2007). There are three categories of functional assessments. These include indirect/anecdotal assessments, descriptive/direct assessments, and functional/experimental analyses. As the name implies, indirect assessment consists of those procedures that do not involve the direct observation and

measurement of the target behavior. For instance, rating scales, questionnaires, and interviews are all considered indirect assessments. Descriptive assessments consist of directly observing challenging behavior and recording environmental events that the observer believes to be correlated with behavior. The data from scatter plots and antecedent behavior consequence (ABC) observations are examples of descriptive assessment methods. In contrast to descriptive assessments, functional analyses are those methods that involve the experimental manipulation of variables that the clinician believes to be causally related to the target behavior. Although each method shares the common goal of attempting to identify the variables occasioning and maintaining instances of a problem behavior, the methods differ in terms of the strength of the conclusions about functional relations. Information obtained through functional analyses is regarded to provide the best/most accurate information, followed by direct and indirect assessment methods, respectively.

It is important to note that the terms used to refer to the various functional assessment methods have been used loosely in practice and in the literature (Cone, 1997; Dunlap & Kincaid, 2001; Kates-McElrath, Agnew, Axelrod, & Bloh, 2007). For instance, some authors have used the term "descriptive assessment" to refer to both indirect and direct assessment methods (Arndorfer & Miltenberger, 1994; Miltenberger, 2008), while others only use the term in reference to direct observations (Iwata, Vollmer, Zarcone, & Rodgers, 1993; Smith et al., 2007). Of greater concern, however, is the lack of consistency when distinguishing between correlation and causal functional assessment methods. For instance, authors have used the terms "functional assessment" and "functional analysis" inconsistently in manuals describing functional approaches to challenging behavior (Dunlap & Kincaid, 2001) and in the educational literature (Kates-McElrath et al., 2007). Nevertheless, the word "analysis" has a long history of being used only when there is an experimental manipulation of variables (Baer et al., 1968). In keeping with this definition of analysis, this chapter will use the term functional analysis to refer to only those methods that experimentally manipulate variables to identify functional relations.

Variables Maintaining Challenging Behavior

As previously noted, the purpose of any functional assessment is to identify the antecedent and consequent variables that occasion and maintain the occurrence of the target behavior. Challenging behavior may be maintained by either positive or negative reinforcement. The type of positive and negative reinforcers maintaining challenging behavior can be further categorized by whether the consequence was socially mediated or was a product of the behavior itself. Accordingly, there are four types of consequences that may maintain challenging behavior (Iwata et al., 1993; Miltenberger, 2008; Smith et al., 2007). These consequences include social positive reinforcement, social negative reinforcement, automatic positive reinforcement, and automatic negative reinforcement. Social positive reinforcement occurs when people deliver or increase the intensity of an event contingently on the occurrence of the target behavior. Examples of social positive reinforcement may include the presentation of attention, such as disapproving statements, or access to tangible items, such as toys, snacks, or drinks. Social negative reinforcement is a consequence that occurs when other people terminate or reduce the intensity of an aversive event or interaction contingently on the occurrence of the target behavior. Examples of social negative reinforcement include the removal of demands, such as academic or work tasks, and/or the removal of a particular aspect of the environment, such as changing the radio station. Automatic positive reinforcement is a consequence that the target behavior itself produces and, thus, does not require the presence of another person. With automatic positive reinforcement, a person's own behavior produces changes in the environment that result in the presentation or increase in intensity of a reinforcing consequence. Examples of automatic positive reinforcement may include the stimulation that skin picking, eye poking, and object mouthing produce, providing that these responses produce some sort of sensory stimulation that functions as a positive reinforce. In contrast to automatic positive reinforcement, automatic negative reinforcement occurs when a person's behavior results in the removal or reduction in intensity of an aversive/unpleasant event. Examples of automatic negative reinforcement may include the attenuation or removal of aversive stimulation, such as repetitive scratching to relieve an itch or ear covering to attenuate certain sounds.

Functional Analysis

A functional analysis is an experimental manipulation of antecedent and consequent events to identify the function of behavior. Iwata and colleagues (1982/1994) developed one method for experimentally investigating the variables maintaining challenging behavior, which many researchers and practitioners use, and as such, the method developed by Iwata et al. is the focus of this section. The functional analysis methodology developed by Iwata et al. consists of three or four test conditions and one control condition. Each test condition has a different arrangement of antecedent and consequent stimuli to evaluate the environmental events that occasion and maintain behavior. The test conditions are designed to simulate a particular situation in the natural environment that could occasion and maintain challenging

behavior. The analog conditions are generally presented in a block-randomized order in the context of a multi-element design (Iwata et al., 1982/1994); however, other researchers have also used reversal (Carr & Durand, 1985) and sequential test control designs (Iwata et al., 1994). The logic of a functional analysis is that the analog condition that produces greatest amounts of the target behavior likely represents the contingency maintaining the behavior in the natural environment.

The typical test conditions included in a functional analysis are the alone, attention (or social disapproval), demand, and tangible conditions. In the alone condition, the client remains alone in a room that does not contain any leisure items. Thus, the alone condition simulates an environment that is deprived of leisure items and social interactions. The purpose of the alone condition is to test whether challenging behavior is maintained by automatic reinforcement.

In contrast to the alone condition, the attention and demand conditions evaluate challenging behavior in a social environment. In the attention condition, an experimenter provides attention in the form of disproving statements contingently on each occurrence of the problem behavior. The attention condition usually begins with the experimenter directing the client to play with some leisure items. Once the client is engaged with the leisure items, the experimenter removes attention by moving away from the client and by pretending to do some work. Thus, the experimenter ignores the client throughout the session, unless the client engages in the target response. Contingently upon each target response, the experimenter briefly interacts with the client by interrupting the target behavior and by presenting statements of disapproval. Therefore, the attention condition evaluates whether the target behavior is maintained by social positive reinforcement because contingent attention is provided for each instance of the target behavior.

The purpose of the demand condition is to test whether the target behavior is maintained by social negative reinforcement. In this condition, the experimenter presents instructional demands on a fixed time schedule, usually every 30 s. Each instructional trial begins with the experimenter verbally instructing the client to complete a task. If the client does not complete the task within a specified amount of time, which is usually 5 s, the experimenter repeats the verbal instruction and provides a prompt, a gesture to or a model of the correct response, to help the client engage in the task. If the client does not respond to the second verbal instruction, the experimenter once again repeats the verbal instruction and physically guides the client to complete the task. If at any point during the instructional trial the client engages in the target behavior, the experimenter terminates the trial, removes the teaching materials, and waits 30 s after the termination of the target behavior before beginning the next instructional trial.

The tangible condition is similar to the attention condition with the exception that the experimenter provides access to a preferred item with each occurrence of the target behavior. Prior to beginning a tangible condition, the client is permitted to engage with preferred items for a few minutes. At the start of the session, the experimenter removes the items and offers the client less preferred items. If the target behavior occurs during the session, the experimenter provides access to the preferred item for 30 s. Therefore, the purpose of this condition is to test whether the challenging behavior is maintained by social positive reinforcement in the form of access to preferred items.

The purpose of the play condition is to serve as a control or comparison condition for the attention, demand, and alone conditions. The play condition begins with the experimenter directing the student to play with the leisure items by verbally instructing the client to play and/or handing the client a leisure item. This condition is similar to the attention condition in that the client is allowed to play freely with the leisure items. In contrast to the attention condition, however, the experimenter provides praise to the client on a fixed time schedule, usually every 30 s, providing that the client is not engaged in the target response. Therefore, the play condition requires that the experimenter ignore all instances of the challenging behavior.

Considerations

When conducting functional analyses, there may not always be a clear pattern of responding across conditions (Hagopian, Bruzek, Bowman, & Jennett, 2007; Hausman, Kahng, Farrell, & Mongeon, 2009; Kuhn, DeLeon, Fisher, & Wilke, 1999; Tarbox, Wallace, Tarbox, Landaburu, & Williams, 2004). In some cases the results are said to be undifferentiated or inconclusive because the rate of challenging behavior is similar across functional analysis conditions. One explanation for this outcome is that the challenging behavior is maintained by automatic reinforcement (Smith et al., 2007). When challenging behavior is maintained by automatic reinforcement, the functional analysis may be undifferentiated because the behavior occurs independently of social consequences. For instance, Kuhn et al. (1999) conducted a functional analysis to examine the function of self-injurious behavior (SIB) in a 35-year-old man with autism, obsessive-compulsive disorder, and severe mental retardation. The functional analysis indicated that escape, sensory reinforcement, or both maintained the self-injurious behavior of face hitting and head banging. To further analyze and clarify the function of SIB, the researchers compared escape extinction, sensory extinction, and a combination of both treatments. While escape extinction alone failed to decrease SIB, sensory extinction alone greatly reduced SIB, indicating that

sensory extinction was sufficient in reducing SIB. The failure of escape extinction and the success of sensory extinction also clarified that the function of the response was most likely due to sensory reinforcement and not both sensory reinforcement and escape. Thus, the evaluation of different treatments may be helpful in clarifying the outcome of an ambiguous functional analysis.

In other cases, functional analyses have been inconclusive when dealing with low-rate problem behavior (Hausman et al., 2009; Tarbox et al., 2004). For instance, Hausman et al. (2009) first conducted a traditional functional analysis (Iwata et al., 1982/1994) to examine problem behavior (i.e., property destruction, SIB) and communication in a 9-year-old girl with autism, mental retardation, and cerebral palsy. The researchers concluded that, due to low rates of problem behavior across all conditions, the results of the analysis were uninterpretable; however, reports from parents and anecdotal observations suggested that the participant engaged in intense bursts of problem behavior when blocked from engaging in ritualistic behavior (i.e., changing the position of doors in close proximity). In such cases, someone would open or close doors in the presence of the participant. Thus, Hausman et al. conducted a second functional analysis of problem behavior in which the participant had access to open and closed doors for 2 min followed by a test condition in which a therapist manipulated the position of the door every 30 s (e.g., if the door was open, the therapist would close it). During the test condition, the experimenter permitted the participant to engage in ritualistic behavior such as opening the door or propping the door open contingent on problem behavior. The analysis showed that problem behavior was maintained by access to the ritualistic behavior of manipulating door position. Thus, treatment involved functional communication training in which the participant learned to request access to ritualistic behavior by handing the therapist a communication card and saying "my way, please" and extinction, namely, the therapist did not provide access to the door contingent upon disruptive behavior.

Another explanation for undifferentiated responding in a functional analysis is that the client might not discriminate the different contingencies in the analog conditions (Iwata et al., 1982/1994; Iwata, Duncan, Zarcone, Lerman, & Shore, 1994). That is, the rapidly changing conditions in the multi-element design might make it difficult for the participant to discriminate when the contingency has changed from social positive reinforcement in the attention or tangible conditions to social negative reinforcement in the demand condition. One solution to this problem is to use a sequential test control design (Iwata et al., 1994), which combines multi-element and reversal designs, and it consists of alternating one test condition with the control condition within each experimental phase. For instance, during the first experimental phase, the play (control condition) might be alternated with the attention condition, and in the second experimental phase, the play condition could be alternated with the demand condition. Iwata et al. demonstrated that this design could clarify the results of undifferentiated responding.

In addition to experimental designs issues, it is also important for clinicians to take into account the idiosyncratic variables that might be responsible for the occurrence of the challenging behavior (Carr, Yarbrough, & Langdon, 1997, Iwata et al., 1982/1994; Kodak, Northup, & Kelley, 2007; O'Reilly, Lancioni, King, Lally, & Dhomhnaill, 2000). Carr et al. (1997) conducted a functional analysis with three individuals with autism that displayed aggression, disruption, or SIB. These researchers identified that idiosyncratic stimuli, such as the presence or absence of magazines, puzzles, and small objects, influenced the frequency of challenging behavior, rather than the contingency embedded within the different analog conditions. For instance, the authors compared the results of the social attention condition with and without the presence of magazines for one participant and found that challenging behavior was much more frequent in the presence of magazines. Finally, research has also demonstrated that the idiosyncratic events that immediately precede a functional analysis can impact the outcome of the analysis. For instance, pre-session attention and prior social context both have been demonstrated to impact behavior during functional analyses (O'Reilly, 1999; O'Reilly, Lancioni, & Emerson, 1999).

Another point to consider is that different consequences may maintain different topographies of challenging behavior within one person (Sigafoos & Tucker, 2000; Thompson, Fisher, Piazza, & Kuhn, 1998). For example, Thompson et al. (1998) conducted a functional analysis of the aggressive behavior of a boy with pervasive developmental disorder (PDD) and intellectual disabilities. Aggressive behavior consisted of kicking, hitting, scratching, pinching, and chin grinding. Chin grinding behavior consisted of firmly pressing his chin against caregivers to the point that it caused pain and bruising. The results of the first functional analysis were undifferentiated, such that aggression occurred at similar rates across all conditions. Based on hypotheses developed during direct observation, the authors conducted a second functional analysis where they recorded chin grinding independently of the other aggressive behavior. The outcome of the second analysis indicated that automatic positive reinforcement maintained chin grinding whereas attention maintained other aggressive responses. Thus, treatment involved two interventions. Treatment of chin grinding involved response blocking and frequent access to an alternate form of chin stimulation in the form of a padded object that did not result in injury to the chin. Treatment of other aggressive responses involved functional communication training to hand over a card to request attention and attention extinction in the form of ignoring.

In addition to the possibility of different topographies serving different operant functions, a single topography can serve multiple functions (Hagopian, Wilson, & Wilder, 2001; Ingvarsson, Kahng, & Hausman, 2008; Kennedy, Meyer, Knowles, & Shukla, 2000; LaBelle & Charlop-Christy, 2002; McKerchar, Kahng, Casioppo, & Wilson, 2001; Shirley, Iwata, & Kahng, 1999). For instance, Hagopian et al. (2001) conducted a functional analysis of the challenging behavior of a boy with autism and intellectual disabilities. During the initial functional analysis, challenging behavior occurred most frequently in the play condition and at lower but similar levels for the other two conditions. Results of the functional analysis were inconclusive because the challenging behavior occurred most often in the control condition. Based on direct observations, the authors conducted a modified functional analysis to evaluate the hypothesis that escape from attention and access to tangibles maintained challenging behavior. The second functional analysis confirmed the authors' hypothesis, and they successfully treated the challenging behavior with a treatment package consisting of functional communication training and non-contingent reinforcement.

Limitations of FA and Modifications

Although functional analyses provide an excellent test of the variables maintaining challenging behavior, there are several limitations that clinicians should take into consideration. One of the main disadvantages of conducting a functional analysis is that they require a substantial amount of time to conduct. For instance, Iwata et al.'s (1982/1994) functional analysis of self-injury required an average of 30 functional analysis conditions spread out over an average of 8 days, and each functional analysis condition took 15 min to complete. Another concern is that a functional analysis requires the intentional reinforcement of challenging behavior, which is problematic for two reasons. First, reinforcing challenging behavior, such as SIB or aggression, poses a risk for the client and potentially the therapist since directly reinforcing the behavior may produce a greater frequency or intensity of the behavior that may cause severe tissue damage to the participant. A second concern is that the behavior may develop new and/or multiple functions from exposure to the contingencies in the analog conditions (Shirley et al., 1999). For instance, a behavior initially maintained by escape might also function to obtain attention following exposure to the attention condition.

One way to reconcile some of the limitations of conducting a traditional functional analysis is to conduct a brief functional analysis. A brief functional analysis is a modified version of the standard functional analysis that generally consists of the same analog conditions as the extended functional analyses (Northup et al., 1991); however, the experimenter presents each condition only once, and the conditions are 10 rather than 15 min in duration. A common element of a brief functional analysis is to include a contingency reversal phase following the presentation of analog conditions (Derby et al., 1992; Northup et al., 1991; Tincani, Castrogiavanni, & Axelrod, 1999). In the contingency reversal phase, the client is exposed to the analog condition that produced the highest rate of challenging behavior; however, the experimenter places the client's challenging behavior on extinction while reinforcing a more appropriate behavior. Although brief analyses generally include a single presentation of each condition and a contingency reversal phase, there have been several modifications that have included a replication of conditions (Luiselli et al., 2004; Tincani et al., 1999) and reversal designs (Sigafoos & Tucker, 2000).

The advantage of a brief functional analysis is that (a) the procedure only takes 90 min or less and (b) the contingency reversal phase allows for the assessment of a replacement behavior for the challenging behavior. Brief analyses, however, do not have the experimental rigor of extended functional analyses as brief functional analyses take place in a single day and typically do not contain replications of analog conditions. Furthermore, brief analyses may be too short in duration to capture behavior that occurs infrequently (Derby et al., 1992).

A functional analysis of precursor behavior – behavior that reliably precedes the target behavior – is another modification to the traditional functional analysis that is a viable option when it is too dangerous or unacceptable to reinforce the target behavior for even brief periods of time (Borrero & Borrero, 2008; Langdon & Carr, 2008; Smith & Churchill, 2002). This approach assumes that precursor and target responses serve the same function, and if intervention is applied to the precursor behavior, then problem behavior will also reduce; this may be true if, for example, the precursor behavior is an earlier member or a response chain and the target behavior is the terminal behavior in the same response chain. For instance, in one study examining precursor behavior, Borrero and Borrero (2008) used both descriptive and experimental analyses to assess precursors to problem behavior in a 12-year-old boy with autism who engaged in aggression and SIB and an 11-year-old boy with autism who engaged in aggression, SIB, and property destruction. The precursor response for both participants was vocalization that occurred at a louder volume than normal conversation. During a series of 60-min descriptive assessments, the observers used a computerized data collection system to record potential reinforcers, such as instruction termination, access to tangible items, and attention. The observers also recorded possible establishing operations, such as instructional demands, restricted access to tangible or edible items, and periods of low attention, in addition to recording the individual problem behavior and precursor responses for each participant. The researchers analyzed descriptive data by calculating conditional probabilities of a precursor given the problem behavior, the problem behavior given a precursor, and the unconditional probability of problem and precursor behavior. They found that the probability of the potential precursor was greater when problem behavior occurred compared to the unconditional probability of the precursor. Further, a lag-sequential analysis indicated that the probability of the precursor behavior occurred most frequently during the 1-s interval prior to the onset of the problem behavior. Borrero and Borrero (2008) then conducted separate functional analyses for problem and precursor behaviors and found that, for both participants, problem behavior and precursor behavior served the same function. For one participant, both precursor and problem behavior occurred most frequently in the tangible condition whereas for the other participant, precursor and problem behavior were elevated during both tangible and escape conditions. Thus, assessing precursor responses that immediately and reliably precede the problem behavior has value when assessing and treating challenging behavior.

Descriptive Methods

Although experimental analyses provide the most convincing demonstration of functional relations, it may not always be possible to use experimental methods due to practical issues related to time constraints and/or ethical issues related to reinforcing dangerous behavior such as SIB. When such issues are a concern, clinicians may use descriptive methods. Descriptive methods consist of measuring target behavior in the presence of antecedent and consequent events in the context of the natural environment (Bijou, Peterson, & Ault, 1968). Thus, descriptive methods do not consist of the systematic manipulation of environmental variables to identify causal relation between behavior and the environment; rather, descriptive methods consist of observing behavior to identify correlations between behavior and environmental events. When descriptive methods identify such correlations, clinicians may develop hypotheses regarding functional relations, and providing that the assessment leads to a strong hypothesis, descriptive assessments may be sufficient for developing a treatment plan (Miltenberger, 2008; O'Neill, Horner, Albin, Sprague, & Newton, 1997). There are three main types of descriptive methods: ABC observation (Bijou et al., 1968), continuous recording (Lerman & Iwata, 1993), and scatter plots (Touchette, MacDonald, & Langer, 1985). In the following sections, we present a description of each descriptive assessment in addition to a discussion of the advantages and disadvantages of each assessment.

ABC Observation

ABC observation refers to recording the antecedent, behavior, and consequences in the natural environment (Bijou et al., 1968) during which clinicians record the antecedent and consequent events that occur in close temporal proximity to the target behavior. The logic of ABC observations is that if there is a clear pattern of antecedent and consequent events that regularly precede and follow the target behavior, then clinicians may develop hypotheses regarding maintaining variables.

There are two ABC observation methods: structured and narrative/open-ended ABC observations (Smith et al., 2007). With structured ABC observations, a number of antecedent and consequent events are pre-defined and observers simply place a mark in the appropriate antecedent and consequent categories each time the target behavior occurs (O'Neill et al., 1997). With narrative ABC observations, the observer provides a brief written description of the activities or events that immediately preceded and followed the target behavior. There are advantages to each type of observation. Structured ABC observations require less effort and data may be easier to interpret than narrative accounts. In contrast, narrative ABC observations provide idiosyncratic information regarding antecedent and consequent stimuli, such as access to specific tangible item following problem behavior; however, this observation system is more cumbersome than structured observations and it may be more difficult to identify patterns of events associated with the target behavior.

Several researchers have demonstrated the utility of ABC observation for formulating hypotheses regarding functional relations (Arndorfer & Miltenberger, 1994; Cunningham & O'Neill, 2000; Sasso et al., 1992). For instance, Sasso et al. (1992) compared the results of ABC data recorded under conditions similar to analog conditions to the results of standard functional analyses. Outcomes for each method were similar and thus ABC observations can be helpful in formulating hypotheses about functional relations. Cunningham and O'Neill (2000) compared indirect assessments and ABC observations with experimental analysis for three children with autism. They also reported that the results of the ABC observations were very similar as those of the experimental analyses. Arndorfer and Miltenberger (1994) used a variety of indirect and direct assessments to develop hypothesis regarding maintaining variables for five children, one of who had autism. Based on the outcome of indirect data and ABC data, the authors conducted brief functional analyses to test the hypothesized functions suggested by the indirect and ABC data. For all children, the brief functional analysis confirmed the results of the ABC observations and indirect assessment. Finally, for two children, the authors validated the outcome of the functional assessments by demonstrating that functional communication training effectively replaced aberrant behavior with a more appropriate behavior.

Although previous research has demonstrated the utility of ABC data, clinicians should cautiously interpret the results because (a) the studies were based on small sample sizes and (b) other studies comparing descriptive and experimental methods found disagreement between descriptive and experimental methods (Lerman & Iwata, 1993; Pence, Roscoe, Bourret, & Ahearn, 2009). Furthermore, one major limitation of ABC observations is that it might produce spurious results because data are recorded only when the target behavior occurs (Cooper et al., 2007). For instance, ABC data might suggest a high correlation between a particular antecedent and/or consequent and the target response. Nevertheless, because ABC data do not indicate how often environmental events occur in the absence of the target behavior, it is difficult determine for certain whether there truly is a correlation between aspects of the environment and the target behavior. Finally, another limitation of ABC data is that it does not take into consideration environmental events that are more distant in time from the target behavior (e.g., O'Reilly, 1995).

Continuous Recording

Continuous recording is very similar to ABC observations in that data are collected on the occurrence of antecedents and consequences in relation to the target behavior. Unlike ABC observations, however, continuous recording consists of observers recording the presence of environmental events in the absence of the target behavior. To score the occurrences and non-occurrences of environmental events, in addition to the target behavior, observation periods are generally divided into intervals and observers record the presence or absence of behavior and environmental events that occur within each interval. For instance, a 15-min observation period may be divided into ninety 10 s intervals and observers record events within each of the intervals. Depending on the interval recording method, observers may record an event only if the event occurred throughout the interval (whole interval recording) or observers may record an event if it happened at all during the interval (partial interval recording). Further, a scoring guide may be created before the assessment to record pre-specified environmental events in the presence or absence of the target response (Mace & Lalli, 1991).

When evaluating data from continuous observation, clinicians and researchers can extract information from antecedent and consequent events that occur in both close and distant in temporal relation to the target behavior. They may also evaluate the relation between target behavior and environmental events by calculating conditional probabilities (Galiatsatos & Graff, 2003; Lerman & Iwata, 1993). Continuous observation data provide a fine-grain analysis of challenging behavior than ABC observations; however, Lerman and Iwata (1993) reported that conclusions from continuous observation data were inconsistent with the outcomes of functional analyses, thereby questioning the utility of continuous observations. Nevertheless, other studies have indicated the utility of descriptive methods for developing better test of hypotheses when conducting functional analyses (Mace & Lalli, 1991) and to help clarify the outcome of ambiguous functional analyses (Galiatsatos & Graff, 2003).

Structured Descriptive Assessments

A structured descriptive assessment (SDA) is one method that researchers have used to improve continuous recording techniques (Anderson & Long, 2002; Freeman, Anderson, & Scotti, 2000). Unlike traditional descriptive methods, SDA involves the manipulation of antecedent events in the natural environment; however, unlike functional analyses, SDA does not involve the manipulation of any consequent events. Thus, a SDA occupies a middle ground between experimental methods that manipulate antecedent and consequences systematically and descriptive methods that do not manipulate independent variables. In conducting an SDA, a clinician identifies situations in the natural environment that are similar to the analog conditions of a functional analysis. For instance, in a school setting, an attention condition may be established by identifying an activity that is neutral in preference and that the teacher requires the student to complete independently. Other situations are identified to represent the antecedents of the tangible, demand, and control conditions of a standard functional analysis. The clinician then provides instructions to the teacher/therapist regarding the appropriate implementation of antecedents, but the clinician instructs the teacher to respond to the student's behavior as usual. Within each observation session, experimenters collect data on the percentage of intervals containing instances of the problem behavior. Finally, to develop hypotheses regarding the function of the behavior, experimenters compare the percentage of interval containing the problem behavior across the different observation conditions.

Scatter Plot

A scatter plot is a grid that is designed to capture the temporal pattern of behavior within and across days (Touchette et al., 1985). The rows of the grid represent different time intervals during a day, and each column of the grid represents a different day. The size of the time intervals on the grid may be created to best suit the goal of the observation, although 15 or 30 min intervals are standard. Observers track behavior by placing a mark in a cell of the grid that corresponds to the interval in which the challenging behavior occurred. Further, observers may use different markings to indicate the frequency of the challenging behavior, such as a completely shaded cell, a cell with a slash, and an empty cell indicating high, low, and zero frequency of behavior, respectively. The purpose of the scatter plot is to identify events that have stimulus control over challenging behavior. Thus, if a client has a set schedule and challenging behavior occurs regularly at the same time of day, researchers can use the information to develop hypotheses about antecedent events that set the occasion for challenging behavior. Therefore, a scatter plot relies on a strong correlation between regularly scheduled events and time of day.

Touchette et al. (1985) used scatter plot data to identify the antecedent events that occasioned instances of challenging behavior in three individuals with autism. For one participant, the challenging behavior consisted of aggression in the form of kicking, hitting, head butting, and object throwing. Scatter plot data were recorded on the aggression in half hour intervals, such that a filled symbol indicated several instances of aggression, open symbols indicated a single instance, and empty cells indicated zero instances. The scatter plot indicated that aggression occurred almost exclusively between 1 and 4 o'clock, which was when the participant was engaged in classroom activity. Given the correlation between aggression and classroom activity, the authors rearranged the participants' schedule to eliminate classroom instruction and to fill that time with activities that did not occasion aggression. The change in schedule virtually eliminated aggression, and after several successful days with low aggression, the authors began to systematically increase the activities that previously produced aggression. Touchette et al. concluded that scatter plot data might be useful for identifying global environmental events that control behavior without necessarily requiring the identification of specific stimuli that are functionally related to the behavior.

There are several limitations to scatter plot data. First, although a scatter plot might indentify global events associated with behavior, the data do not provide information regarding the specific stimuli. This is problematic because it may not be possible or practical to rearrange or eliminate activities that are correlated with the occurrence of challenging behavior. Second, scatter plot data only identify antecedents that are associated with challenging behavior; it does not identify the reinforcing consequence maintaining the occurrence of the behavior. Third, the utility of scatter plots relies on a consistent daily schedule, such that activities occur in the same order and at the same time each day. Without a consistent schedule, it may be challenging to identify patterns of behavior. Finally, although Touchette et al. (1985) identified patterns in two out of three participants, the extent to which such patterns are likely to be identified with other clients and in other situations is questionable (Kahng et al., 1998). For instance Kahng et al. (1998) had 8 behavior analysts visually inspect the scatter plot data for

15 participants, and in each case, the panel was unable to identify patterns of responding. Nevertheless, the authors reported that statistical analysis identified patterns in 12 out of the 15 scatter plots. Given that clinical utility is often touted as an advantage of scatter plots, the value of scatter plot data in the absence of other functional assessments is questionable if it requires statistical analyses to identify temporal patterns in behavior.

Indirect Assessments

Indirect assessments are those assessment methods in which the therapist does not directly observe behavior and its environment, but rather uses third party reports, such as interviews, questionnaires, and rating scales, to identify potential target and replacement behaviors and the functions of target behaviors. Practitioners and researchers commonly use these indirect methods of functional assessment. Although ABA sometimes minimizes the role of indirect assessments, clinicians often use them before conducting descriptive assessments and functional analyses (Cooper et al., 2007). Hence, research on indirect methods of functional assessments may make an important contribution to both practice and research on functional approaches to aggression in people with PDDs.

Interviews

Practitioners and researchers use interviews to identify target responses, identify priorities and clinical goals, develop hypotheses concerning the functions of target behavior(s), and assess the capacity of the service to provide effective interventions (Cooper et al., 2007). For example, Cipani and Schock (2007) proposed several screening questions to use during the preliminary stages of functional assessment to determine the seriousness of the problem and its impact on the client and others (p. 19). It is common to distinguish three types of clinical interviews: unstructured, structured, and semi-structured interviews. Unstructured interviews have no predetermined questions; the interviewer simply follows the client's lead and provides relatively little direction. Hypothesis-driven interviews is also classified as an unstructured interview because there are no predetermined set of questions, but the interviewer has a predetermined theoretical framework and likely a set of hypotheses that s/he uses to drive the interview and to guide the sequence of questions (Wolpe & Turkat, 1985). In contrast, structured interviews use predetermined questions that the interviewer uses with no or relatively little modification. Semi-structured interviews occupy the middle ground in which there are predetermined questions and topics, but the order in which the interviewer presents the questions and the precise wording of the questions is flexible.

Miltenberger and Fuqua (1985) described one of the few studies to teach semi-structured behavioral interviewing skills. They defined interviewing skills operationally to include the following ten topics: asks for a general description of the problem; asks for other problems; sets priorities; specified problem behaviors; asks about onset; asks about frequency, duration, magnitude, and latency; asks about antecedents; asks about consequences; asks about verbal behavior, such as thoughts; and asks about goals. This study provided operational and reliable measures of interviewer behavior. For example, they defined "sets priorities" as "summarizes the problems listed by the client and uses an open-ended question to ask which is the most important and should be addressed first" (p. 324). Almost all of these interviewer target behavior required the use of open rather than closed questions.

Miltenberger and Fuqua (1985) described generic behavioral interviewing strategies that are applicable to any behavior problem; however, some authors have developed specific interview protocols to assess challenging behavior in people with developmental disabilities. For example, O'Neill et al. (1997) developed the *Functional Assessment Interview Form* (FAIF), a structured interview to identify the target and replacement behaviors, antecedents and consequences, ecological variables, such as time of day and diet, client communication skills, client reinforcers, and treatment history. Similar interview schedules include the *Behavioral Diagnosis and Treatment Information Form* (Bailey & Pyles, 1989).

Questionnaires and Rating Scale

Questionnaire measures of function offer a potentially attractive alternative to interviews and direct assessments as they may be easy to administer and many people can provide the necessary information. One of the earliest questionnaire measures of function was the *Motivation Assessment Scale* (MAS; Durand & Crimmins, 1988). The MAS has 16 items that assess 4 functions: sensory, escape, attention, and tangible. Informants rate each item on a 7-point frequency scale. Scores from each of the four items that correspond to each of the four functions are summed to obtain a profile. In the original study, Durand and Crimmins assessed the functions of SIB in 50 people with developmental disabilities using the MAS. They assessed the inter-rater and test–retest reliabilities of the MAS and compared MAS ratings with the results of functional analyses. They found high inter-rater and test-retest reliabilities and very good agreement between the MAS and experimental analyses in terms of identifying the functions of SIB. Subsequent research has applied the MAS to a wide range of problem behavior, including aggression. The MAS was also influential in the development of other questionnaire measures of function, such as the *Questions about Behavioral Function* (QABF; Matson & Vollmer, 1995), the *Functional Assessment for Multiple Causality* (FACT; Matson et al., 2003; www.disabilityconsultants.org), and the *Functional Analysis Screening Tool* (FAST; Iwata & DeLeon, 1995). Although Durand and Crimmins (1988) initially reported impressive psychometric properties and validity data, not all subsequent studies have corroborated this initial report (Duker, Sigafoos, Barron, & Coleman, 1998; Newton & Sturmey, 1992). Thus, the status of the MAS remains in question at this time.

One of the most extensively researched psychometric measures of function is the QABF (Matson & Vollmer, 1995). The *QABF* (Matson & Vollmer, 1995) has 25 items to assess 5 functions: *attention, escape, tangible, non-social* (self-stimulation), and *physical* (physical discomfort reduction). The informant rates the frequency of the behavior on a 4-point Likert scale. Both the authors and independent researchers have evaluated the QABF's psychometric properties (Freeman, Walker, & Kaufman, 2007; Nicholson, Konstantinidi, & Furniss, 2006; Paclawskyj, Matson, Rush, Smalls, & Vollmer, 2000; Paclawskyj, Matson, Rush, Smalls, & Vollmer, 2001; Shogren & Rojahn, 2003). One of the most interesting studies of the QABF went beyond issues of reliability and compared the effectiveness of behavioral interventions based on hypotheses derived from the QABF (Matson, Bamburg, Cherry, & Paclawskyj, 1999). This study compared the effectiveness of behavior programs for 180 adults with intellectual and other developmental disabilities. There were three groups of individuals who had behavior programs for self-injury, aggression, and stereotypes. Within each group, half of the participants did not have interventions based on functional assessments and the other half of the participants had interventions based on behavior plans using the QABF. For all three groups, behavior reductions were statistically significantly greater for the groups whose programs were based on the QABF.

Whereas the previous questionnaires focused on consequence functions, fewer questionnaires have focused on antecedent functions. Examples of checklists that have addressed antecedent stimuli include the *Setting Events Checklist* (Gardner, Cole, Davidson, & Karan, 1986) and the *Contextual Assessment Inventory* (CAI) (Carr, Ladd, & Schulte, 2008). There has been relatively little research on these measures; however, Carr et al. (2008) systematically evaluated the CAI. In this study, 17 adults with severe or profound intellectual disability participated. Clinicians had diagnosed 15 participants with autism and 10 of the 15 participants displayed aggression. The CAI has 80 items in 4 domains: socio-cultural, task/activity, physical, and biological. Informants rated each item on a 5-point Likert scale on frequency. Carr et al. found good convergence between CAI ratings and incidents recorded in logs. For example, approximately 73% of log entries corresponded to frequently rated CAI items, but only 0.1% of log entries corresponded to frequency of CAI ratings. There was also good agreement between CAI ratings and direct observation of challenging behavior in contexts identified in CAI ratings.

Conclusions

Both practitioners and researchers commonly use indirect assessments such as interviews and questionnaires. The literature has now moved beyond the most basic question of evaluating whether or not a particular interview protocol or questionnaire has minimally adequate reliability – at least in some circumstances – and has begun to address other issues. For example, some studies have compared different indirect measures with each other and indirect measures with functional assessment and analyses. For example, Durand and Crimmins (1988) found convergence between the results of the MAS and functional analyses of self-injury. In contrast, Paclawskyj et al. (2001) found that the MAS and QABF correlated strongly with each other; however, they failed to find convergence between the results of two psychometric measures and functional analyses. In some cases, Paclawskyj et al. (2001) were unable to determine the function of challenging behavior during the functional analyses because of the low rate of the target behavior, although questionnaire measures did identify functions in these cases. The discrepancy between Durand and Crimmins (1988) and Paclawskyj et al. (2001) is puzzling. It is unclear whether these different findings reflect differences in the measures used, the target behavior, participants, characteristics of the people completing the ratings, or other factors.

Fifteen years ago the literature on the reliability and validity of questionnaire measures of function was relatively modest and could be readily reviewed (Sturmey, 1994). During the intervening years the number of instruments and papers has greatly increased. Hence, any definitive statement based on a comprehensive review on the relative merits of the different instruments is beyond the scope of this chapter.

One aspect of conducing functional assessments that the literature has failed to address rigorously has been training of observers and informants. Some questionnaires suggest that the person administering the test should have at least a master's degree and that informants should have a certain amount of experience, such as 6 months, working with the client. These suggestions may appear to be judicious, but they fail to specify what skills test administrators and informants should have to result in an accurate assessment of function. For example, reading the question and accurately transcribing an informant's responses are elementary skills; however, obtaining an operational definition of the target behavior and resolving conflicting results from different informants are more complex skills for test administrators. Likewise, informants answering questions, such as what establishing operations and discriminative stimuli occur before a target behavior, sometimes require relatively subtle discrimination skills. Perhaps training on prototypical cases prior to test administration for both test administrators and informants might increase the reliability of the results of indirect measures of function.

Future research should also address two further issues. First, interview protocols have usually assessed both antecedent and consequence functions; however, questionnaire measures have focused on only one of these functions. Future research on questionnaires should develop questionnaires that assess both antecedent and consequential variables. Second, several authors have suggested that hierarchical approaches to identifying the functions of aggression might be efficient. For example, one might start with indirect measures. If these do not result in effective programming one might then proceed to descriptive assessments. Finally, if these methods do not result in effective treatment, one might proceed to experimental analyses of behavior. This approach might be cost-effective and use limited service resources more efficiently. This appears to be a promising approach; however, to date the exact details of such a protocol have not yet been operationalized and evaluated.

Combining Methods

Occasionally, experimenters and clinicians may combine descriptive and experimental methods when assessing problem behavior. It is common for descriptive techniques to be used at first to develop hypotheses about controlling variables, to identify when a behavior occurs, and to determine antecedents and consequences correlated with behavior. In addition, if preliminary descriptive analyses are inconclusive then clinicians can implement experimental analyses. For instance, Tang, Kennedy, Koppekin, and Caruso (2002) first used a descriptive analysis to determine the function of stereotypical ear covering in a 5-year-old boy with autism. During the descriptive analysis, the experimenters made forty three 30-min observations across 4 days using a 30-s partial interval recording to measure ear covering and correlated environmental events such as snacks and instruction. The experimenters found that no antecedent or social consequence consistently correlated with ear covering except for the presence of a classmate's scream. Consequently, when the experimenters conducted a functional analysis in which they exposed the child to the alone, attention, control, and demand conditions, they also manipulated the conditions so that the classmate's scream occurred during each condition. During the functional analysis, ear

covering occurred most often when the classmate's scream was added to the alone, attention, and demand conditions. Thus, the authors concluded that negative automatic reinforcement through noise attenuation maintained ear covering. This study nicely linked descriptive and functional analyses in identifying maintaining variables for problematic behavior particularly when idiosyncratic events (i.e., another student's scream) were involved in the maintenance of a response. This study also shows how descriptive assessments may facilitate hypothesis testing in subsequent functional analyses.

English and Anderson (2004) also combined descriptive and experimental techniques when examining problem behavior in four children with developmental delays. These researchers were particularly interested in differences in problem behavior depending on whether caregivers or unfamiliar therapists conducted the functional analyses. Prior to the functional analyses, they conducted interviews with caregivers using the FAIF to help operationally define the problem behavior and to identify the situations that occasioned the problem behavior and preferred items to use during the functional analysis. In addition, they asked parents to fill out a scatter plot for a 1-week period to record the frequency of recording within 30-min intervals between 6:00 a.m. and 11:00 p.m. Thus, in this study, information from the indirect and descriptive assessments assisted in defining responses as well as identifying potential reinforcers. Interestingly, three of four children exhibited different patterns of responding when caregivers rather than experimenters conducted the functional analysis.

In summary, it might often be necessary and beneficial to combine assessment techniques to identify the variables maintaining challenging behavior, especially in those cases in which the results of one assessment are ambiguous. Although functional analyses provide the most convincing demonstration of the relation between a particular problem behavior and environmental variables, these analyses are conducted in contrived settings and would require clinicians to have at least some information regarding the idiosyncratic variables, if any, that may be correlated with behavior in the natural environment. Clinicians and researchers should use formal and informal interviews and descriptive observations to increase the probability that functional analysis conditions closely approximate the natural environment. This may reduce the probability of obtaining inconclusive results and increase the validity of experimental analyses. Nevertheless, in cases where a functional analysis is ambiguous, further descriptive observation and interview information may assist in clarifying ambiguous results by allowing for a more thorough evaluation of idiosyncratic stimuli associated with challenging behavior and a more comprehensive and clearer definition of the challenging behavior in the natural environment.

Inconclusive Assessments

Sometimes extensive functional assessments and analyses fail to identify the functions of target responses (Sturmey, 1995) or services require treatments that may be effective while clinicians conduct extensive functional assessments and analyses. In either circumstance, it may be necessary to implement interventions that are not based on functions. For example, Ingvarsson et al. (2008) conducted an experimental functional analysis and found that escape from demand and access to edible item maintained the aggressive, disruptive, and SIB of an 8-year-old girl with autism, cerebral palsy, moderate mental retardation, and obsessive-compulsive disorder. Despite the functional analysis revealing multiple functions of the response, researchers implemented noncontingent delivery of an edible item to increase compliance and reduce problem behavior without having to implement escape extinction in a demand context. Thus, while some treatments may be based specifically on the function of the response, sometimes treatment may be successful, even if it does not specifically address the function or all functions of the response identified in a functional assessment.

Case Examples

This section provides some examples of the use of functional assessment and analyses for individuals with Asperger's disorder, Autistic disorder, and PDD-NOS. Several studies have examined various assessment methods in those with Asperger's syndrome (Arvans & LeBlanc, 2009; Clarke, Dunlap, & Vaughn, 1999; Lang et al., 2009). In a recent study, Arvans and LeBlanc conducted a functional assessment prior to implementing an intervention to treat a 14-year-old boy with Asperger's syndrome, Eric, who frequently reported migraines and missed school because of these migraines. The experimenter interviewed both Eric and his mother using the functional assessment interview (FAI), and Eric's mother also filled out the functional assessment screening tool (FAST) checklist. Arvans and LeBlanc compared the participant's FAI responses to those of his mother and found that their responses were fairly consistent with 7 out of 10 responses indicating an escape function. Eric's mother also endorsed all items on the escape subscale of the FAST. Thus, the FAI, as well as the FAST completed by Eric's mother, indicated that the migraine complaints were escape maintained. Consequently, the intervention chosen involved a token economy to reinforce task completion and escape extinction. Eric's parents reinforced his task completion and pro-social behavior using the token economy, and they prompted task completion, such as taking medication and completing academic work, so that he could not escape these situations by reporting a migraine.

This intervention was highly effective in reducing both the number of migraines per week and the number of missed school days.

Studies have also assessed maladaptive responses in people with PDD-NOS (Dawson, Matson, & Cherry, 1998; Galiatsatos & Graff, 2003). For example, Galiatsatos and Graff combined descriptive and functional analyses to assess and treat screaming in a 13-year-old boy with autism and PDD-NOS. In this case, the experimenters conducted a functional analysis prior to the use of a descriptive assessment. During the functional analysis, the authors presented attention, demand, play, alone, tangible-toy, and tangible-edible conditions in a multi-element design. Following the functional analysis, the authors also conducted a series of descriptive assessments that entailed naturalistic observations in the participant's classroom during which another student and teacher were present. Experimenters also used a structured ABC sheet to collect data using a partial interval recording procedure during 10-min sessions. The ABC sheet listed potential activities and antecedent conditions that may have been present when screaming occurred (e.g., demand placed on the student) as well as potential consequences that may follow the screaming.

Galiatsatos and Graff (2003) reported that the child's screaming occurred most frequently during the tangible-toy and tangible-edible conditions of the functional analysis; however, the descriptive assessment revealed that the most highly correlated antecedent condition associated with screaming was when the other student in the classroom received attention. Further, the student was much less likely to scream when interacting with the teacher.

Therefore, according to the descriptive assessment, teacher attention may have maintained screaming. Galiastsatos and Graff further analyzed the descriptive assessments by combining specific events into four general classes: whether the student interacted with the teacher or did not interact with the teacher while screaming and whether materials were present or not present when screaming occurred. They then calculated conditional probabilities for these events and found that screaming did indeed appear to be, in part, socially mediated. Thus, the authors concluded that descriptive assessment did not support the results of the functional analysis and claimed that the functional analysis may have produced a false-positive outcome. Despite these conflicting results during the initial assessment and analysis, a differential reinforcement of other behavior (DRO) procedure with tokens delivered for the absence of screaming and response cost for removal of tokens contingent on screaming led to a 50% reduction in screaming within 4 weeks.

Several studies have examined the use of various assessment procedures prior to implementing interventions to evaluate the problem behavior of adults with ASD (Baker, Valenzuela, & Wieseler, 2005; Chapman, Fisher, Piazza,

& Kurtz, 1993; Wong, Floyd, & Innocent, Woolsey, 1991; Jensen, McConnachie, & Pierson, 2001; Kuhn, DeLeon, Fisher, & Wilke, 1999; Piazza et al., 1998; Piazza, Hanley, & Fisher, 1996; Rehfeldt & Chambers, 2003; Richman, Wacker, Asmus, & Casey, 1998). One example comes from Richman et al. (1998) who conducted a functional analysis of different behavior problems in a 27-year-old woman with profound intellectual disabilities and autism. Disruptive responses included pushing task items away, pulling her hands back from tasks, screaming, and throwing items. The authors also included finger picking in the functional assessment, which produced lacerations on her fingers. Researchers observed the client through video monitoring during two separate 2-week admissions and used a 6-s partial interval recording system to calculate the percentage of intervals in which the responses occurred during 5-min assessments. Researchers then implemented a brief functional analysis that included a free-play condition, contingent attention condition, demand condition, and alone condition. Finger picking occurred continuously and thus, contingencies were not provided contingent on finger picking. Disruptive behavior appeared to be maintained by escape from demands while finger picking appeared to be maintained by automatic reinforcement. The authors then implemented two forms of escape extinction based on the brief functional analysis. Escape extinction led to a reduction in disruptive behavior with no reduction in finger picking while sensory extinction plus a differential reinforcement procedure led to a suppression of finger picking.

Summary and Conclusions

Since the work of Carr (1977) and Iwata et al. (1982/1994), there have been great advancements in the use of functional assessment and analysis methods for identifying variables maintaining challenging behavior in people with ASD. Thirty years ago researchers and clinicians had limited options when deciding on methods for evaluating challenging behavior, such that the alternatives were mainly restricted to the selection of different functional analysis methods that were labor intensive and time consuming, and as a result, they were primarily used for research purposes. Presently there are a wide variety of indirect assessments that allow for a rapid and systematic approach for developing hypotheses regarding functional relations. There also have been substantial developments to improve descriptive methods, such as ABC recording, by incorporating new measurement procedures, such as interval recording procedures and the calculation of conditional probabilities. In addition, ABA has been active in developing and evaluating alternatives to Iwata et al.'s (1982/1994) experimental methods for indentifying functional relations, which has been the bedrock from which

other functional assessment methodologies are based. These modifications to experimental analyses have included the development of new functional analysis conditions designed to evaluate how complex social interactions might occasion and maintain challenging behavior, brief functional analyses, and structured descriptive assessments, which allow for a middle ground between true experimental analysis and descriptive assessments.

The use of functional assessment and analysis methods has led to improvements in intervention by allowing clinicians to tailor the least intrusive, most socially acceptable, and most effective treatments to the individual. Indeed, interventions based on outcomes of functional assessments and analyses stand in stark contrast to the interventions of the past. In the past, clinicians used a structural approach to treat challenging behavior, which consisted of selecting interventions based on topography rather than function. In some of these cases the intervention was effective, but in other cases, the intervention was ineffective or even harmful. With the use of functional assessments and analyses, the selection of interventions is less of a guessing game and more of a task of tailoring the intervention to fit the outcome of the assessment.

The evaluation of challenging behavior through functional assessment/analysis methods is now widespread, which is evident by the plethora of new assessment techniques and functional assessment/analysis manuals that are continually being developed by Federal, state, and professional mandates requiring practitioners to conduct functional assessments prior to behavioral intervention. Future research is now needed to further refine the current functional assessment/analysis methods, to develop a standard protocol for conducting functional assessments/analyses, and to develop the most effective and efficient training procedures to ensure the quality of assessments in school and clinical environments.

References

Anderson, C. M., & Long, E. S. (2002). Use of structured and descriptive assessment methodology to identify variables affecting problem behavior. *Journal of Applied Behavior Analysis, 35*, 137–154.

Arndorfer, R. E., & Miltenberger, R. G. (1994). Home-based descriptive and experimental analysis of problem behaviors in children. *Topics in Early Childhood Special Education, 14*, 64–87.

Arvans, R. K., & LeBlanc, L. A. (2009). Functional assessment and treatment of migraine reports and school absences in an adolescent with Asperger's Disorder. *Education and Treatment of Children, 32*, 151–166.

Baer, D. M., Wolf, M. M., & Risley, T. R. (1968). Some current dimensions of applied behavior analysis. *Journal of Applied Behavior Analysis, 1*, 91–97.

Bailey, J. S., & Pyles, D. A. M. (1989). Behavioral diagnostics. *Monographs of the American Association on Mental Retardation, 12*, 401–409.

Baker, D. J., Valenzuela, S., & Wieseler, N. A. (2005). Naturalistic inquiry and treatment of coprophagia in one individual. *Journal of Developmental and Physical Disabilities, 17*, 361–367.

Bijou, S. W., Peterson, R. F., & Ault, M. H. (1968). A method to integrate descriptive and experimental field studies at the level of data and empirical concepts. *Journal of Applied Behavior Analysis, 1*, 175–191.

Borrero, C. S. W., & Borrero, J. C. (2008). Descriptive and experimental analyses of potential precursors to problem behavior. *Journal of Applied Behavior Analysis, 41*, 83–96.

Campbell, J. M. (2003). Efficacy of behavioral interventions for reducing problem behavior in persons with autism: A quantitative synthesis of single-subject research. *Research in Developmental Disabilities, 24*, 120–138.

Carr, E. G. (1977). The motivation of self-injurious behavior: A review of some hypotheses. *Psychological Bulletin, 84*, 800–816.

Carr, E. G., & Durand, V. M. (1985). Reducing behavior problems through functional communication training. *Journal of Applied Behavior Analysis, 18*, 111–126.

Carr, E. G., Ladd, M. V., & Schulte, C. F. (2008). Validation for the Context Inventory for Problem Behavior. *Journal of Positive Behavioral Support, 10*, 91–104.

Carr, E. G., Yarbrough, S. C., & Langdon, N. A. (1997). Effects of idiosyncratic stimulus variables on functional analysis outcomes. *Journal of Applied Behavior Analysis, 30*, 673–686.

Chapman, S., Fisher, W., Piazza, C. C., & Kurtz, P. F. (1993). Functional assessment and treatment of life-threatening drug ingestion in a dually diagnosed youth. *Journal of Applied Behavior Analysis, 26*, 255–256.

Cipani, E., & Schock, K. M. (2007). *Functional behavioral assessment, diagnosis and treatment. A complete system for education and mental health settings.* New York: Springer.

Clarke, S., Dunlap, G., & Vaughn, B. (1999). Family-centered, assessment-based intervention to improve behavior during an early morning routine. *Journal of Positive Behavior Interventions, 1*, 235–241.

Cone, J. D. (1997). Issues in functional analysis in behavioral assessment. *Behavioral Research and Therapy, 35*, 259–275.

Cooper, J. O., Heron, T. E., & Heward, W. L. (2007) *Applied behavior analysis* (2nd ed.). Upper Saddle River, NJ: Pearson.

Cunningham, E., & O'Neill, R. E. (2000). Comparison of results of functional assessment and analysis methods with young children with autism. *Education and Training in Mental Retardation and Developmental Disabilities, 35*, 406–414.

Dawson, J. E., Matson, J. L., & Cherry, K. E. (1998). An analysis of maladaptive behaviors in persons with autism, PDD-NOS, and mental retardation. *Research in Developmental Disabilities, 19*, 439–448.

Derby, K. M., Wacker, D. P., Sasso, G., Steege, M., Northup, J., Cigrand, K., et al. (1992). Brief functional assessment techniques to evaluate aberrant behavior in an outpatient setting: A summary of 79 cases. *Journal of Applied Behavior Analysis, 25*, 713–721.

Didden, R., Duker, P., & Korzilius, H. (1997). Meta-analytic study of treatment effectiveness for problem behaviors with individuals who have mental retardation. *American Journal on Mental Retardation, 101*, 387–399.

Didden, R., Korzilius, H., van Oorsouw, W., & Sturmey, P. (2006). Behavioral treatment of problem behaviors in individuals with mild mental retardation: A meta-analysis of single-subject research. *American Journal on Mental Retardation, 111*, 290–298.

Duker, P. C., Sigafoos, J., Barron, J., & Coleman, F. (1998). The Motivation Assessment Scale: Reliability and construct validity across three topographies of behavior. *Research in Developmental Disabilities, 19*, 131–141.

Dunlap, G., & Kincaid, D. (2001). The widening world of functional assessment: Comments on four manuals and beyond. *Journal of Applied Behavior Analysis, 34*, 365–377.

Durand, V. M., & Crimmins, D. B. (1988). Identifying the variables maintaining self-injurious behavior. *Journal of Autism and Developmental Disabilities, 18*, 99–117.

English, C. L., & Anderson, C. M. (2004). Effects of familiar versus unfamiliar therapists on responding in the analog functional analysis. *Research in Developmental Disabilities, 25*, 39–55.

Freeman, K. A., Anderson, C. M., & Scotti, J. R. (2000). A structured descriptive methodology: Increasing agreement between descriptive and experimental analyses. *Education and Training in Mental Retardation and Developmental Disabilities, 35*, 55–66.

Freeman, K., Walker, K., & Kaufman, J. (2007). Psychometric properties of the Questions About Behavioral Function scale in a child sample. *American Journal on Mental Retardation, 112*, 122–129.

Galiatsatos, G. T., & Graff, R. B. (2003). Combining descriptive and functional analyses to assess and treat screaming. *Behavioral Interventions, 18*, 123–138.

Gardner, W. I., Cole, C. L., Davidson, D. P., & Karan, O. C. (1986). Reducing aggression in individuals with developmental disabilities: An expanded stimulus control, assessment, and intervention model. *Education and Training in Mental Retardation, 21*, 3–12.

Hagopian, L. P., Bruzek, J. L., Bowman, L. G., & Jennett, H. K. (2007). Assessment and treatment of problem behavior occasioned by interruption of free-operant behavior. *Journal of Applied Behavior Analysis, 40*, 89–103.

Hagopian, L. P., Wilson, D. M., & Wilder, D. A. (2001). Assessment and treatment of problem behavior maintained by escape from attention and access to tangible items. *Journal of Applied Behavior Analysis, 34*, 229–232.

Hausman, N., Kahng, S., Farrell, E., & Mongeon, C. (2009). Idiosyncratic functions: Severe problem behavior maintained by access to ritualistic behaviors. *Education and Treatment of Children, 32*, 77–87.

Haynes, S., & O'Brien, W. (2000). *Principles and practice of behavioral assessment.* Dordrecht, The Netherlands: Kluwer Academic Publishers.

Individuals with Disabilities Education Act of 2004. Pub. L. No. 108-446, 118 Stat. 2647 (2004).

Ingvarsson, E. T., Kahng, S., & Hausman, N. L. (2008). Some effects of noncontingent positive reinforcement on multiply controlled problem behavior and compliance in a demand context. *Journal of Applied Behavior Analysis, 41*, 435–440.

Iwata, B. A., & DeLeon, I. G. (1995). *The functional analysis screening tool (FAST).* Unpublished manuscript. Gainesville, FL: University of Florida.

Iwata, B. A., Dorsey, M. F., Slifer, K. J., Bauman, K. E., & Richman, G. A. (1994). Toward a functional analysis of self-injury. *Journal of Applied Behavior Analysis, 27*, 197–209. (Reprinted from Analysis and Intervention in Developmental Disabilities, 2(3–20), 1982).

Iwata, B. A., Duncan, B. A., Zarcone, J. R., Lerman, D. C., & Shore, B. A. (1994). A sequential, test-control methodology for conducting functional analyses of self-injurious behavior. *Behavior Modification, 18*, 289–306.

Iwata, B. A., Vollmer, T. R., Zarcone, J. R., & Rodgers, T. A. (1993). Treatment classification and selection based on behavioral function. In R. Van Houten & S. Axelrod (Eds.), *Behavior Analysis and Treatment* (pp. 101–125). New York: Plenum.

Jensen, C. C., McConnachie, G., & Pierson, T. (2001). Long-term multicomponent intervention to reduce severe problem behavior: A 63-month evaluation. *Journal of Positive Behavior Interventions, 3*, 225–236.

Kahng, S., Iwata, B. A., Fischer, S. M., Page, T. J., Tredwell, K. R. H., Williams, D. E., et al. (1998). Temporal distributions of problem behavior based on scatter plot analysis. *Journal of Applied Behavior Analysis, 13*, 593–604.

Kates-McElrath, K., Agnew, M., Axelrod, S., & Bloh, C. L. (2007). Identification of behavioral function in public schools and a clarification of terms. *Behavioral Intervention, 22,* 47–56.

Kennedy, C. H., Meyer, K. A., Knowles, T., & Shukla, S. (2000). Analyzing the multiple functions of stereotypical behavior for students with autism: Implications for assessment and treatment. *Journal of Applied Behavior Analysis, 33,* 559–571.

Kodak, T., Northup, J., & Kelley, M. E. (2007). An evaluation of the types of attention that maintain problem behavior. *Journal of Applied Behavior Analysis, 40,* 167–171.

Kuhn, D. E., DeLeon, I. G., Fisher, W. W., & Wilke, A. E. (1999). Clarifying an ambiguous functional analysis with matched and mismatched extinction procedures. *Journal of Applied Behavior Analysis, 32,* 99–102.

LaBelle, C. A., & Charlop-Christy, M. H. (2002). Individualizing functional analysis to assess multiple and changing functions of severe behavior problems in children with autism. *Journal of Positive Behavior Interventions, 4,* 231–241.

Lang, R., Didden, R., Sigafoos, J., Rispoli, M., Regester, A., & Lancioni, G. E. (2009). Treatment of chronic skin-picking in an adolescent with asperger syndrome and borderline intellectual disability. *Clinical Case Studies, 8,* 317–325.

Langdon, N. A., & Carr, E. G. (2008). Functional analysis of precursors for serious problem behavior and related intervention. *Behavior Modification, 32,* 804–827.

Lerman, D. C., & Iwata, B. A. (1993). Descriptive and experimental analyses of variables maintaining self-injurious behavior. *Journal of Applied Behavior Analysis, 26,* 293–319.

Luiselli, J. K., Ricciardi, J. N., Schmidt, S., & Tarr, M. (2004). Brief functional analysis and intervention evaluation for treatment of saliva-play. *Child and Family Therapy, 26,* 53–61.

Mace, F. C., & Lalli, J. S. (1991). Linking descriptive and experimental analyses in the treatment of bizarre speech. *Journal of Applied Behavior Analysis, 24,* 553–562.

Matson, J. L., Bamburg, J. W., Cherry, K. E., & Paclawskyj, T. R. (1999). A validity study on the questions about behavioral function (QABF) scale: Predicting treatment success for self-injury, aggression, and stereotypies. *Research in Developmental Disabilities, 20,* 163–175.

Matson, J. L., Kuhn, D. E., Dixon, D. R., Mayville, S. B., Laud, R. B., Cooper, C. L., et al. (2003). The development and factor structure of the Functional Assessment for multiple causality (FACT). *Research in Developmental Disabilities, 24,* 485–495.

Matson, J. L., & Vollmer, T. R. (1995). *User's guide. Questions about behavioral function (QABF).* Baton Rouge: Scientific Publishers.

McKerchar, T. L., Kahng, S., Casioppo, E., & Wilson, D. (2001). Functional analysis of self-injury maintained by automatic reinforcement: Exposing masked social functions. *Behavioral Interventions, 16,* 59–63.

Miltenberger, R. G. (2008) *Behavior modification. Principles and procedures* (4th ed.). Belmont, CA: Thomson Wadsworth.

Miltenberger, R. G., & Fuqua, R. W. (1985). Evaluation of a training manual for the acquisition of behavioral assessment interviewing skills. *Journal of Applied Behavior Analysis, 18,* 323–328.

Newton, T. J., & Sturmey, P. (1992). The Motivation Assessment Scale: Inter-rater reliability and internal consistency. *Journal of Mental Deficiency Research, 35,* 472–474.

Nicholson, J., Konstantinidi, E., & Furniss, F. (2006). On some psychometric properties of the Questions about Behavior Function Scale. *Research in Developmental Disabilities, 27,* 337–352.

Northup, J., Wacker, D., Sasso, G., Steege, M., Cigrand, K., Cook, J., et al. (1991). A brief functional analysis of aggressive and alternative behavior in an outclinic setting. *Journal of Applied Behavior Analysis, 24,* 509–522.

O'Neill, R. E., Horner, R. H., Albin, R. W., Sprague, J. R., & Newton, J. S. (1997) *Functional assessment and program development for problem behavior. A practical handbook* (2nd ed.). New York: Brooks/Cole.

O'Reilly, M. E., Lancioni, G. E., King, L., Lally, G., & Dhomhnaill, O. N. (2000). Using brief assessments to evaluate aberrant behavior maintained by attention. *Journal of Applied Behavior Analysis, 33,* 109–112.

O'Reilly, M. F. (1995). Functional analysis and treatment of escape-maintained aggression correlated with sleep deprivation. *Journal of Applied Behavior Analysis, 28,* 225–226.

O'Reilly, M. F. (1999). Effects of presession attention on the frequency of attention-maintained behavior. *Journal of Applied Behavior Analysis, 32,* 371–374.

O'Reilly, M. F., Lancioni, G. E., & Emerson, E. (1999). A systematic analysis of the influence of prior social context on aggression and self-injury within analogue analysis assessments. *Behavior Modification, 23,* 578–596.

Paclawskyj, T. R., Matson, J. L., Rush, K. S., Smalls, Y., & Vollmer, T. R. (2000). Questions about behavioral function: A behavioral checklist for functional assessment of aberrant behavior. *Research in Developmental Disabilities, 21,* 223–229.

Paclawskyj, T. R., Matson, J. L., Rush, K. S., Smalls, Y., & Vollmer, T. R. (2001). Assessment of the convergent validity of the Questions About Behavioral Function scale with analogue functional analysis and the Motivation Assessment Scale. *Journal of Intellectual Disability Research, 45,* 484–494.

Pence, S. T., Roscoe, E. M., Bourret, J. C., & Ahearn, W. H. (2009). Relative contributions of three descriptive methods: Implications for behavioral assessment. *Journal of Applied Behavior Analysis, 42,* 425–446.

Piazza, C. C., Fisher, W. W., Hanley, G. P., LeBlanc, L. A., Worsdell, A. S., Lindauer, S. E., et al. (1998). Treatment of pica through multiple analyses of its reinforcing functions. *Journal of Applied Behavior Analysis, 31,* 165–189.

Piazza, C. C., Hanley, G. P., & Fisher, W. W. (1996). Functional analysis and treatment of cigarette pica. *Journal of Applied Behavior Analysis, 29,* 437–450.

Rehfeldt, R. A., & Chambers, M. R. (2003). Functional analysis and treatment of verbal perseverations displayed by an adult with autism. *Journal of Applied Behavior Analysis, 36,* 259–261.

Richman, D. M., Wacker, D. P., Asmus, J. M., & Casey, S. D. (1998). Functional analysis and extinction of different behavior problems exhibited by the same individual. *Journal of Applied Behavior Analysis, 31,* 475–478.

Sallows, G. O., & Graupner, T. D. (2005). Intensive behavioral treatment for children with autism: Four-year outcome and predictors. *American Journal on Mental Retardation, 110,* 417–438.

Sasso, G. M., Reimers, T. H., Cooper, L. J., Wacker, D., Berg, W., Steege, M., et al. (1992). Use of descriptive and experimental analyses to identify the functional properties of aberrant behavior in school setting. *Journal of Applied Behavior Analysis, 25,* 809–821.

Scotti, J. R., Evans, I. M., Meyer, L. H., & Walker, P. (1991). A meta-analysis of intervention research with problem behavior: Treatment validity and standards of practice. *American Journal on Mental Retardation, 96,* 233–256.

Shirley, M. J., Iwata, B. A., & Kahng, S. (1999). False-positive maintenance of self-injurious behavior by access to tangible reinforcers. *Journal of Applied Behavior Analysis, 32,* 201–204.

Shogren, K. A., & Rojahn, J. (2003). Convergent reliability and validity of the Questions About Behavioral Function and the Motivation Assessment Scale: A replication study. *Journal of Developmental and Physical Disabilities, 15,* 367–375.

Sigafoos, J., & Tucker, M. (2000). Brief assessment and treatment of multiple challenging behaviors. *Behavioral Interventions, 15,* 53–70.

Skinner, B. F. (1953). *Science and human behavior.* New York: The Free Press.

Smith, R. G., & Churchill, R. M. (2002). Identification of environmental determinants of behavior disorders through functional analysis of precursor behavior. *Journal of Applied Behavior Analysis, 35*, 125–136.

Smith, R. G., Vollmer, T. R., & St. Peter Pipkin, C. (2007). Functional approaches to assessment and treatment of problem behavior in persons with autism and related disabilities. In P. Sturmey & A. Fitzer (Eds.), *Research in autism spectrum disorders* (pp. 187–234). Austin, TX: PRO-ED.

Sturmey, P. (1994). Assessing the functions of aberrant behaviors: A review of psychometric instruments. *Journal of Autism and Developmental Disorders, 24*, 293–304.

Sturmey, P. (1995). Assessing the functions of self-injurious behavior: A case of assessment failure. *Journal of Behavior Therapy and Experimental Psychiatry, 25*, 331–336.

Sturmey, P. (2008). *Behavioral case formulation and intervention. A functional analytic approach.* Chichester: Wiley-Blackwell.

Sturmey, P. (2009a). *Varieties of case formulation.* Chichester: Wiley.

Sturmey, P. (2009b). Case formulation: A review and overview of this volume. In P. Sturmey (Ed.), *Varieties of case formulation* (pp. 3–30). Chichester: Wiley.

Sturmey, P., Ward-Horner, J., Marroquin, M., & Doran, E. (2007). Structural and functional approaches to psychopathology and case formulation. In P. Sturmey (Ed.), *Functional analysis and clinical treatment* (pp. 1–22). New York: Elsevier.

Tang, J. C., Kennedy, C. H., Koppekin, A., & Caruso, M. (2002). Functional analysis of stereotypical ear covering in a child with autism. *Journal of Applied Behavior Analysis, 35*, 95–98.

Tarbox, J. T., Wallace, M. D., Tarbox, R. S. F., Landaburu, H. J., & Williams, W. L. (2004). Functional analysis and treatment of low rate problem behavior in individuals with developmental disabilities. *Behavioral Interventions, 19*, 187–204.

Thompson, R. H., Fisher, W. W., Piazza, C. C., & Kuhn, D. E. (1998). The evaluation and treatment of aggression maintained by attention and automatic reinforcement. *Journal of Applied Behavior Analysis, 31*, 103–116.

Tincani, M. J., Castrogiavanni, A., & Axelrod, S. (1999). A comparison of the effectiveness of brief versus traditional functional analyses. *Research in Developmental Disabilities, 20*, 327–338.

Touchette, P. E., MacDonald, R. F., & Langer, S. N. (1985). A scatter plot for identifying stimulus control of problem behavior. *Journal of Applied Behavior Analysis, 18*, 343–351.

US Department of Justice. (2009). *CRIPA*, US Department of Justice Civil Rights Division. http://www.justice.gov/crt/split/cripa.php, Downloaded December, 29, 2009.

Van Houten, R., Axelrod, S., Bailey, J. S., Favell, J. E., Foxx, R. M., Iwata, B. A., et al. (1988). Right to effective behavioral treatment. *Journal of Applied Behavior Analysis, 21*, 381–384.

Wolpe, K., & Turkat, I. D. (1985). Behavioral formulation of clinical cases. In I. D. Turkat (Ed.), *Behavioral case formulation* (pp. 1–35). New York: Plenum.

Wong, S. E., Floyd, J., Innocent, A. J., & Woolsey, J. E. (1991). Applying a DRO schedule and compliance training to reduce aggressive and self-injurious behavior in an autistic man: A case report. *Journal of Behavior Therapy and Experimental Psychiatry, 22*, 299–304.

Lisa Underwood, Jane McCarthy, and Elias Tsakanikos

People with autism spectrum disorders (ASD) may also have other conditions such as intellectual disability (ID) and mental health disorders (see Chapters 6 and 7, respectively). The relationships between these conditions are complex and remain under-researched (Matson & Shoemaker, 2009; McCarthy et al., 2009). Recognizing and assessing comorbid psychopathology in individuals with ASD is challenging (Tsakanikos et al., 2006; Tsakanikos, Costello, Holt, Sturmey, & Bouras, 2007b). There is considerable overlap between the characteristics of ASD and some symptoms of comorbid psychopathology, e.g., obsessive-compulsive disorder, which may make it difficult for clinicians to determine whether a specific problem reflects features of ASD or an additional mental health problem (Helvershou, Bakken, & Martinsen, 2009; LoVullo & Matson, 2009). This diagnostic overshadowing can result in symptoms of psychopathology going unrecognized (Xenitidis, Paliokosta, Maltezos, & Pappas, 2007). There is also growing evidence that the presentation of psychopathology in people with ASD is atypical compared with the general population (Hutton, Goode, Murphy, Le Couteur, & Rutter, 2008). In addition, people with ASD often have difficulty understanding and expressing their own thoughts and feelings, and their ability to grasp the meaning of questions about their symptoms may also be impaired (Kannabiran & McCarthy, 2009; Leyfer et al., 2006; MacNeil, Lopes, & Minnes, 2009).

These issues have been further compounded by a number of other factors: reluctance to accept that mental illness can co-occur with ASD and ID; lack of research on psychopathology in people with ASD; a lack of professionals with sufficient training and skills in recognizing and diagnosing psychiatric disorder in people with ASD; and a lack of tools available to aid clinicians in the assessment process

(Ghaziuddin, 2005). In the last 5 years substantial progress has been made in each of these areas. This chapter will cover the specific scales and related methods designed to help arrive at a diagnosis of psychopathology in children and adults with ASD.

Methods of Assessing Psychopathology

The most common method of assessing psychiatric symptomatology is clinical judgment, whereby a health-care professional formulates a diagnosis based on information collected from a variety of sources such as an interview with the person themselves or an informant who knows them well. The disadvantages of this approach are that the technique used may vary between clinicians and across time, leading to different conclusions. The next step up is the use of operationalized criteria which form the basis of classification systems such as the Diagnostic and Statistical Manual of Mental Disorders (DSM-IV; American Psychiatric Association, 1994) and the International Classification of Diseases (ICD-10; World Health Organization, 1992). Additionally, there are diagnostic systems that have been developed for specific groups such as those with ID, for example, the Diagnostic Manual – Intellectual Disability Diagnostic Criteria (DM-ID; Fletcher, Loschen, Stavrakaki, & First, 2007) and the Diagnostic Criteria for Psychiatric Disorders for Use with Adults with Learning Disabilities/Mental Retardation (DC-LD; Royal College of Psychiatrists, 2001). The application of these criteria for assessing psychopathology in people with ASD is covered in Chapter 7. Finally, there is the use of standardized tools which systematically assess the presence/absence of specific symptoms and their severity. The symptoms themselves and the way of measuring their severity are explicitly defined, as is the method of administration.

These standardized assessment tools come in many forms, from in-depth structured interviews to checklists and brief rating scales. Some measures are designed to be administered

E. Tsakanikos (✉)
Department of Psychology, Roehampton University, London, UK
e-mail: elias.tsakanikos@kcl.ac.uk

J.L. Matson, P. Sturmey (eds.), *International Handbook of Autism and Pervasive Developmental Disorders*,
Autism and Child Psychopathology Series, DOI 10.1007/978-1-4419-8065-6_17, © Springer Science+Business Media, LLC 2011

by a specially trained clinician or researcher, while others can be completed by the individual themselves as a self-report measure or by an informant who knows them well such as a family or paid carer. Some tools rely on responses to specific questions but others might be completed by observing the person in a particular setting.

Many instruments have algorithms or cutoff scores that can be used to determine whether an individual meets the "caseness" criteria for a specific psychiatric disorder. Others include scales that cluster symptoms into specific categories. Some measures just record a person's position on a scale at a given point in time and are used to record change or compare scores across individuals.

Psychometric Properties of Assessment Methods

When choosing a specific tool, a careful review of its main characteristics and psychometric properties is required. Depending on the objectives of the assessment, careful consideration should be given to the following aspects:

- Purpose of the tool (screening, diagnosis, or measurement of symptoms)
- Content (behavioral manifestations or clinical symptoms related to the disorder under investigation)
- Population it was developed for and has been tested on (children or adults; ASD with or without LD)
- The level of measurement required for the purpose of the assessment (a number on a scale, a binary outcome, or a measure of change)

Once these factors have been established, it is important to assess the quality of the instrument by examining its psychometric properties, i.e., its reliability and validity.

Inter-rater, intra-rater, and test–retest reliability are assessed by calculating a coefficient, such as Cohen's kappa (κ) coefficient, between two sets of responses. A kappa (κ) coefficient greater than 0.5 indicates acceptable reliability (Streiner & Norman, 2008). The internal consistency of a scale is usually obtained by calculating Cronbach's alpha (α), with a coefficient in the range of 0.6–0.8 indicating acceptable-to-good reliability (Cronbach & Shavelson, 2004). Higher reliability is not necessarily desirable given that the items of an instrument, apart from having a substantial amount of shared variance, are also expected to provide some unique information.

Face and content validity may be addressed by the factors that help to determine how appropriate the tool is. Establishing criterion validity can be difficult in the absence of a "gold standard" measure; however, it is acceptable to test instruments against other criteria such as clinical expert or a similar scale. The suggested acceptable correlation between different scales is between 0.4 and 0.8 (Streiner & Norman,

2008). Concurrent validity looks at how well an instrument can distinguish between groups that it is designed to be able to distinguish between, for example, whether a screening tool for depression can successfully differentiate people with and without a clinical diagnosis of depression. When a measure has a binary outcome, it is also important to consider the sensitivity (proportion of true positives) and specificity (proportion of true negatives) of the instrument. High sensitivity (detecting a large number of potential cases at the expense of including some false positives) may be acceptable for a screening tool, whereas high specificity would be required for a diagnostic tool. A feature to consider when choosing a continuous measure is its responsiveness to change.

Other factors to take into account include the acceptability of the items of a tool to patients, their carers, and those administering it. Practical concerns need to be addressed such as whether the rater needs specific training; whether the person is able to complete a self-rating tool or whether they have a reliable informant; whether the tool will take a long time to complete; and whether its administration requires any special equipment. Furthermore, there are issues around the availability of both published and unpublished instruments, including whether there are costs involved in obtaining or administering them and whether they are available in the appropriate language.

Tools for Assessing Psychopathology

A variety of tools have been developed for assessing psychopathology in the general population, for example, the Structured Clinical Interview for DSM Disorders (SCID; Spitzer, Williams, Gibbon, & First, 1990), Schedules for Clinical Assessment in Neuropsychiatry (SCAN; Wing et al., 1990), and Brief Symptoms Inventory (BSI; Derogatis & Melisaratos, 1983). There are also tools that focus on single disorders, such as the Beck Depression Inventory (BDI; Beck, Ward, Mendelson, Mock, & Erbaugh, 1961) and the Yale-Brown Obsessive Compulsive Scale (Y-BOCS; Goodman et al., 1989). The APA *Handbook of Psychiatric Measures* (American Psychiatric Association, 2000) lists many such tools, and a review of instruments designed specifically for children can be found in Matson, Andrasik, and Matson's (2008) book *Assessing Childhood Psychopathology and Developmental Disabilities*.

Assessment of Comorbid Psychopathology in People with ASD

Evidence on the use of measures designed for the general population and their use in those with ASD is scarce

(MacNeil et al., 2009). For reasons discussed earlier it may be difficult to use these tools with people who have ASD, particularly if they have lower functioning (Stewart, Barnard, Pearson, Hasan, & O'Brien, 2006). Research on the comorbidity of psychopathology and ASD has relied on a variety of techniques for diagnosing both ASD and comorbid psychopathology (Kanne, Abbacchi, & Constantino, 2009). Most often the method is clinical diagnosis (Melville et al., 2008). Much previous research has relied on the assessment of behavioral rather than psychiatric symptoms. While there is evidence to suggest that people with ASD are more likely to exhibit more behavioral problems than those without ASD (Murphy et al., 2005; Tsakanikos, Costello, Holt, Sturmey, & Bouras, 2007a), there is a debate over the extent to which problem behaviors are associated with psychiatric disorders (McCarthy et al., 2009). Specific methods to evaluate challenging behavior in people with ASD are covered in Chapter 17. In a recent review of research on anxiety symptoms in children and adolescents with ASD that identified 40 studies that had used around 20 different methods of assessment, none were specifically for individuals with ASD (White, Oswald, Ollendick, & Scahill, 2009). Another review observed similar findings and also found that only 2 out of the 13 studies they identified reported that the instruments they used had comparative data in ASD populations – these were the Child Symptom Inventory-4 (CSI-4; Gadow & Sprafkin, 2002) and the Personality Inventory for Children – Revised (PIC-R; Wirt, Lachar, Klinedinst, & Seat, 1984) (MacNeil et al., 2009). Information on whether either of these tools had been normed for children with ASD was not provided. In a systematic review of research on depression in autism and Asperger syndrome, 15 studies used 7 different methods of assessing depression; as with the reviews described earlier none of the studies used instruments that were specifically designed for people with ASD (Davis, Atezaz Saeed, & Antonacci, 2008). It is widely acknowledged that there is a great need for more information on the psychometric properties of generic assessment tools when they are used in ASD populations and for instruments developed specifically for people with ASD (Davis et al., 2008; Leyfer et al., 2006; Matson & Boisjoli, 2008; Melville et al., 2008; Stewart et al., 2006; White et al., 2009).

In response to the call for specially designed tools, a range of measures have been developed from brief rating scales to structured, in-depth, diagnostic interviews. Literature on five such instruments has been published; all were developed within the last 15 years, with two emerging recently. These measures vary in approach, design, and purpose; a summary of each tool is provided in Table 17.1 and evidence for their effectiveness is discussed below.

Tools for Children and Adolescents with ASD

Two instruments have been designed specifically for children and adolescents with ASD: the Autism Comorbidity Interview – Present and Lifetime Version (ACI-PL; Leyfer et al., 2006) and the Autism Spectrum Disorder – Comorbid for Children scale (ASD-CC; Matson, LoVullo, Rivet, & Boisjoli, 2009). Two further instruments have been used with both children and adults: the Schedule for the Assessment of Psychiatric Problems Associated with Autism (and Other Developmental Disorders) (SAPPA; Bolton & Rutter, 1994) and the Stress Survey Schedule for Persons with Autism and Other Developmental Disabilities (Groden et al., 2001).

The ACI-PL and SAPPA are both semi-structured diagnostic schedules to be used by trained clinicians in interviews with an informant. The ACI-PL was developed in the USA, especially for children with ASD, from the Kiddie Schedule for Affective Disorders and Schizophrenia (KSADS; Chambers et al., 1985). It has been tested on children aged 5–17 years with high-functioning ASD diagnosed by ADI-R (Lord, Rutter, & Le Couteur, 1994) and ADOS assessment (Lord et al., 1989) with data reported on the reliability and validity of three specific diagnoses (see Table 17.1; Leyfer et al., 2006). Although criterion validity was established by looking at whether participants had received treatment for a psychiatric disorder in the past, the sample did not undergo any other assessment of psychopathology. The authors state that they did not attempt to distinguish some of the behavioral symptoms of ASD from those of comorbid disorders and acknowledge that further testing is needed across the range of disorders, ages, IQ, and verbal ability (Leyfer et al., 2006).

The SAPPA, developed in the UK, has items derived from the Research Diagnostic Criteria (Spitzer, Endicott, & Robins, 1978). The SAPPA has been used in a study of adolescents aged 14–20 years with ID and ASD diagnosed using the ADI-R (Bradley & Bolton, 2006); a follow-up study of adults aged 21–57 years who had been diagnosed with ASD in childhood (using the ADI-R and ADOS) (Hutton et al., 2008); and a study of psychopathology in adults with tuberous sclerosis (Raznahan, Joinson, O'Callaghan, Osborne, & Bolton, 2006). None of these studies report the reliability or validity of the SAPPA. The studies of people with ASD looked at the prevalence of psychiatric disorders in their samples according to the SAPPA; however, no other assessments of psychopathology were carried out to establish the validity of SAPPA.

In contrast to the diagnostic approach of the ACI-PL and SAPPA, the Stress Survey Schedule (SSS) is a rating scale designed to measure the intensity of symptoms related to stress (Groden et al., 2001), and the ASD-CC is a rating scale designed to measure symptoms of emotional difficulties (Matson et al., 2009). The SSS was developed in

Table 17.1 Assessment tools developed specifically for people with autism spectrum disorders (ASD)

	Type of tool	Outcome	Corresponding diagnostic criteria	Population	Psychometric properties
ACI-PL	Diagnostic tool (semi-structured interview between trained professional and informant)	Coding allows determination of whether an individual meets criteria for DSM psychiatric disorders	DSM-IV-TR (items are based on KSADS)	Children with ASD	Leyfer et al., 2006: 109 high-functioning children, reliability tested for major depression, ADHD and OCD sections – IRR (κ) range was 0.7–0.8, TRR (κ) range was 0.61–0.75. Criterion validity: sensitivity was 100%, range of specificity across diagnoses was 83–94%
ASD-CA	Screening checklist (face-to-face interview between trained professional and informant, 37 items rated 0 or 1)	Five subscales: anxiety/repetitive behaviors, conduct problems, irritability/behavioral excesses, attention/hyperactivity/impulsivity, depression. Subscale scores calculated by summing item scores. Cutoffs for "those more likely to have comorbid psychopathology" vary for each subscale	DSM-IV-R and ICD-10 (plus items from the DASH-II and literature review)	Adults with severe or profound ID and ASD	Matson & Boisjoli, 2008: 169 adults, IRR (κ): mean = 0.43 (range, 0.30–0.77), TRR (κ): mean = 0.59 (range, 0.35–0.92). IC: overall KR-20 was 0.91; for subscales, KR-20 ranged from 0.44 to 0.85; for individual item scale, coefficients ranged from 0.35 to 0.92. LoVullo & Matson, 2009: 120 adults with ID and ASD compared with two other groups: ID alone ($N = 151$) and ID and ASD and psychopathology ($N = 42$). No significant differences on mean subscale scores between two ASD groups. On four subscales, mean ASD and ID scores were higher than mean ASD and ID and psychopathology scores
ASD-CC	Rating scale (informant-completed, 49 items rated 0–2)	Measures severity of symptoms of emotional difficulties (seven factors: tantrum behavior, repetitive behavior, worry/depressed, avoidant behavior, under-eating, conduct, over-eating)	DSM-IV-R and ICD-10	Children with ASD	Matson & Wilkins, 2008: 113 children, IRR (κ): mean = 0.46 (range, 0.3–0.64), TRR (κ): mean = 0.51 (range, 0.3–0.85), IC (α) = 0.91. Matson et al., 2009: 177 children, range of intercorrelations between factors was –0.02 to 0.48; between factors and ASD-CC composite the range was 0.23–0.82. Scores on ASD-CC were compared with BASC-2 scores, correlation between ASD-CC composite score and BASC-2 subscales (r) = 0.66. Range of intercorrelations between ASD-CC factors and BASC-2 subscales was –0.22 to 0.68
PAC	Screening checklist (informant-completed, 42 items rated 1–4)	Severity of symptoms on five subscales: psychosis, depression, anxiety, OCD, and general adjustment problems. Subscale scores calculated by taking average item scores. Cutoffs vary for each subscale	DSM-IV and ICD-10	Adults with severe or profound ID and ASD	Helvershou et al., 2009: 35 adults with and without identified psychiatric disorder. Range of IRR (κ) across five subscales was 0.51–0.67, IC (α) ranged from 0.78 to 0.89. Average score subscales were higher for those with psychiatric disorder ($N = 26$) than for those with autism only ($N = 9$)
SAPPA	Diagnostic tool (semi-structured interview between trained professional and informant)	Psychiatric disorder identified as being absent, possible, probable, or definite	Research diagnostic criteria	Children and adults with ID and/or ASD	Bradley & Bolton, 2006: 36 teenagers with ID and ASD compared to a matched group with ID. Hutton et al., 2008: 135 adults with ASD. Both studies used the SAPPA to assess prevalence of psychiatric disorder. No published reports of psychometric properties
Stress Survey Schedule	Rating scale (self- or informant-completed, 49 items, rated 1–5)	Severity of stress (intensity of symptoms on eight subscales)	None	Children and adults with ASD or other developmental disability	Groden et al., 2001: data on 129 adults and children used to identify subscales. Goodwin et al., 2007: 180 adults and children, IC (α) across subscales ranged from 0.57 to 0.89

DSM = Diagnostic and Statistical Manual of Mental Disorders, KSADS = Kiddie Schedule for Affective Disorders and Schizophrenia, ADHD = attention-deficit hyperactivity disorder, OCD = obsessive-compulsive disorder; IRR = inter-rater reliability, κ = Cohen's kappa, TRR = test-retest reliability, ICD-10 = International Statistical Classification of Diseases and Related Health Problems 10th Revision, DASH-II = Diagnostic Assessment for the Severely Handicapped – Revised, ID = intellectual disability, IC = internal consistency, KR-20 = Kuder-Richardson-20, α = Cronbach's alpha, BASC-2 = Behavioral Assessment for Children version 2, r = correlation coefficient.

the USA through a consultation process using open-ended questionnaires and was not designed to map on to any operationalized diagnostic criteria. In the first test of the scale it was administered to children and adults (aged 3–40 years) with autism and other developmental disabilities to establish content validity (Groden et al., 2001). A later study focused on individuals aged 3–41 years with autism diagnosed by psychologists according to DSM-IV criteria and looked at the internal consistency of the SSS (Goodwin, Groden, Velicer, & Diller, 2007). No other tests of reliability or validity were carried out and there were no other measures of stress (or other psychopathology) against which the SSS was compared. It is unclear whether the SSS is equally appropriate for use with children and adults.

Developed in the USA, the ASD-CC items are based on symptoms from the DSM-IV-TR and ICD-10. The aim of the scale is to differentiate symptoms which are usual for children with ASD from those that constitute a comorbid "emotional disturbance" (Matson & Wilkins, 2008). Factor analysis of the ASD-CC identified seven subscales (see Table 17.1); these do not match specific mental disorders and the focus is on certain behaviors rather than clinical symptoms (Matson et al., 2009). Matson and Wilkins (2008) refined the ASD-CC items and tested its reliability in a study of children aged 2–16 years with ASD diagnosed using a checklist of DSM-IV-TR and ICD-10 symptoms. A further study carried out factor analyses and looked at the internal consistency of the ASD-CC in a sample of children (aged 2–17 years) with ASD (Matson et al., 2009). The Behavioral Assessment for Children, version 2 (BASC-2; Reynolds & Kamphaus, 2004) was also administered. In these studies inter-rater and test–retest reliabilities were found to be moderate, while internal consistency was high. When compared with the BASC-2, the range of correlations between the subscales of the two instruments varied widely (see Table 17.1).

Tools for Adults with ASD

Two screening tools have been developed for identifying psychopathology in adults with severe or profound ID and ASD: the Autism Spectrum Disorders – Comorbidity for Adults (ASD-CA; Matson & Boisjoli, 2008) scale from the USA and more recently in Norway, the Psychopathology in Autism Checklist (PAC; Helvershou et al., 2009). Both were developed according to the DSM-IV-R and ICD-10; however, neither tool has subscales that map directly onto the range of clinical diagnoses used in these diagnostic systems (see Table 17.1). The ASD-CA is completed by a trained clinician in an interview with an informant and the PAC is completed by the informant themselves.

Two reports have been published on the ASD-CA so far. In the first study, informants for a sample of adults with severe/profound ID and ASD diagnosed by two raters using DSM-IV-TR and ICD-10 criteria completed a longer version of the ASD-CA (Matson & Boisjoli, 2008). Data from this sample were used in factor and item analyses to further refine the tool, establish subscales, and test for reliability (see Table 17.1). In the second study, a group with ID and ASD (diagnosed using a checklist based on DSM-IV-TR and ICD-10 criteria) was used to establish cutoff scores for the ASD-CA subscales and then compared with a group who had ID, ASD, and psychopathology (diagnosed by consensus of a psychiatrist and a psychologist) and another group with ID alone (LoVullo & Matson, 2009). The reliability and validity of each subscale of the ASD-CA varied widely, and it was unable to distinguish between the group with ASD and psychopathology and the group with ASD alone, although the authors admit that ASD-CA was mainly intended to detect a large number of individuals with potential comorbid psychopathology at the expense of false positives.

One pilot study has been published so far on the PAC; participants were adults with severe/profound ID and ASD (diagnosis confirmed by clinicians using DSM-IV criteria). The sample included those with and without previously identified psychiatric disorders (Helvershou et al., 2009). In this study the PAC was found to have good reliability and those diagnosed with a psychiatric disorder scored significantly higher on all subscales than those without. However, many participants scored highly on a number of the subscales so it did not appear to be able to distinguish between specific psychiatric disorders. Neither the ASD-CA nor the PAC has been tested against other screening tools for psychopathology such as those developed for adults with ID.

The development of tools for assessing psychopathology in children and adults with ASD is in its infancy. The evidence base is currently small but expanding; more data on the tools described in this chapter may soon emerge. Currently, research is at too early a stage to recommend any tool as a "gold standard" against which other instruments should be measured. An alternative approach is to use tools developed for people with other types of developmental disorder or disability which are commonly comorbid in people with ASD. For example, there are several tools for people with ID which may be suitable for use with those with ASD who also have ID. These include the Reiss Screen (Reiss, 1988); the Psychopathology Instrument for Mentally Retarded Adults (PIMRA; Matson, Senatorve, & Kazdin, 1984); the Diagnostic Assessment for the Severely Handicapped-II (DASH-II; Matson, 1995); the Present Psychiatric State for Adults with LD (PPS-LD; Cooper, 1997); and the Psychiatric Assessment Schedule for Adults with Developmental Disabilities (PAS-ADD; Moss, Prosser, Costello, Simpson, & Patel, 1998). There are also tools that assess symptom severity and are condition specific rather than general measures of psychopathology such as the Glasgow Depression Scale for people with ID (Cuthill, Espie, & Cooper, 2003). Other instruments focus on a specific aspect of mental ill-health, such as behavior problems, for example, the Aberrant Behavior Checklist (ABC; Aman & Singh, 1994), or health and social functioning, for example, the Health of the Nation Outcome Scales for People with Learning Disabilities (HoNOS-LD; Roy, Matthews, Clifford, Fowler, & Martin, 2002). For a comprehensive review of tools for people with ID and their psychometric properties, see Mohr and Costello (2007). Currently tools designed for the general population and those tools developed for people with ID have little evidence on their reliability and validity for use with people with ASD (Leyfer et al., 2006; LoVullo & Matson, 2009).

People with ASD do not form a homogenous group for whom one tool will be applicable. Instruments need to take into account critical variables such as age, developmental level, communication skills, and intellectual functioning (LoVullo & Matson, 2009; Matson & Boisjoli, 2008). The standardized assessment of psychopathology in adults and children with ASD is a work in progress as tools need to be further developed and tested. There appears to be a particular lack of tools developed specifically for adults with higher functioning ASD. Existing and future tools must be developed to standards such as those set out by the American Psychiatric Association (1999). It is important that the psychometric properties and results of tests carried out on these instruments are comprehensively reported.

References

Aman, M. G., & Singh, N. N. (1994). *Aberrant behavior checklist-community: Supplementary manual*. East Aurora, NY: Slosson Educational Publications, Inc.

American Psychiatric Association. (1994). *The diagnostic and statistical manual of mental disorders* (4th Ed). Washington, DC: Author.

American Psychiatric Association. (1999). *Standards for educational and psychological testing*. Washington, DC: Author.

American Psychiatric Association. (2000). *Handbook of psychiatric measures*. Washington, DC: Author.

Beck, A. T., Ward, C. H., Mendelson, M., Mock, J., & Erbaugh, J. (1961). An inventory for measuring depression. *Archives of General Psychiatry, 4*, 561–571.

Bolton, P. F., & Rutter, M. (1994). *Schedule for Assessment of Psychiatric Problems Associated with Autism (and Other Developmental Disorders) (SAPPA): Informant version*. Cambridge: University of Cambridge; and London: Institute of Psychiatry.

Bradley, E., & Bolton, P. (2006). Episodic psychiatric disorders in teenagers with learning disabilities with and without autism. *British Journal of Psychiatry, 189*, 361–366.

Chambers, W. J., Puig-Antich, J., Hirsch, M., Paez, P., Ambrosini, P. J., Tabrizi, M. A., et al. (1985). The assessment of affective disorders in children and adolescents by semistructured interview. Test–retest

reliability of the schedule for affective disorders and schizophrenia for school-age children, present episode version. *Archives of General Psychiatry, 42*, 696–702.

Cooper, S. A. (1997). Epidemiology of psychiatric disorders in elderly compared with younger adults with learning disabilities. *British Journal of Psychiatry, 170*, 375–380.

Cronbach, L. J., & Shavelson, R. J. (2004). My current thoughts on coefficient alpha and successor procedures. *Educational and Psychological Measurement, 64*, 391–418.

Cuthill, F. M., Espie, C. A., & Cooper, S. A. (2003). Development and psychometric properties of the Glasgow Depression Scale for people with a Learning Disability: Individual and carer supplement versions. *British Journal of Psychiatry, 182*, 347–353.

Davis, E., Atezaz Saeed, S., & Antonacci, D. J. (2008). Anxiety Disorders in Persons with Developmental Disabilities: Empirically Informed Diagnosis and Treatment. *Psychiatric Quarterly, 79*, 249–263.

Derogatis, L. R., & Melisaratos, N. (1983). The Brief Symptom Inventory: An introductory report. *Psychological Medicine, 13*, 595–605.

Fletcher, R., Loschen, E., Stavrakaki, C., & First, M. (2007). *Diagnostic manual-intellectual disability: A clinical guide for diagnosis of mental disorders in persons with intellectual disability*. Kingston, NY: NADD Press.

Gadow, K. D., & Sprafkin, J. (2002). *Child symptom inventory-4 screening and norms manual*. Stony Brook, NY: Checkmate Plus.

Ghaziuddin, M. (2005). *Mental health aspects of autism and Asperger syndrome*. London: Jessica Kingsley Publishers.

Goodman, W. K., Price, L. H., Rasmussen, S. A., Mazure, C., Fleischmann, R. L., Hill, C. L., et al. (1989). The Yale–Brown Obsessive Compulsive Scale, I: Development, use, and reliability. *Archives of General Psychiatry, 46*, 1006–1011.

Goodwin, M. S., Groden, J., Velicer, W. F., & Diller, A. (2007). Brief report: Validating the Stress Survey Schedule for Persons with Autism and Other Development Disabilities. *Focus on Autism and Other Developmental Disabilities, 22*, 183–189.

Groden, J., Diller, A., Bausman, M., Velicer, W., Norman, G., & Cautela, J. (2001). The development of a Stress Survey Schedule for Persons with Autism and Other Development Disabilities. *Journal of Autism and Developmental Disorders, 31*, 207–217.

Helvershou, S. B., Bakken, T. L., & Martinsen, H. (2009). The Psychopathology in Autism (PAC): A pilot study. *Research in Autism Spectrum Disorders, 3*, 179–195.

Hutton, J., Goode, S., Murphy, M., Le Couteur, A., & Rutter, M. (2008). New-onset psychiatric disorders in individuals with autism. *Autism, 12*, 373–390.

Kannabiran, M., & McCarthy, J. (2009). The mental health needs of people with autism spectrum disorders. *Psychiatry, 8*, 398–401.

Kanne, S. M., Abbacchi, A. M., & Constantino, J. N. (2009). Multi-informant ratings of psychiatric symptom severity in children with autism spectrum disorders: The importance of environmental context. *Journal of Autism and Developmental Disorders, 39*, 856–864.

Leyfer, O. T., Folstein, S. E., Bacalman, S., Davis, N. O., Dinh, E., Morgan, J., et al. (2006). Comorbid psychiatric disorders in children with autism: Interview development and rates of disorders. *Journal of Autism and Developmental Disorders, 36*, 849–861.

LoVullo, S. V., & Matson, J. L. (2009). Comorbid psychopathology in adults with Autism Spectrum Disorders and intellectual disabilities. *Research in Developmental Disabilities, 30*, 1288–1296.

Lord, C., Rutter, M., Goode, S., Heemsbergen, J., Jordan, H., Mawhood, L., et al. (1989). Autism diagnostic observation schedule: A standardized observation of communicative and social behavior. *Journal of Autism and Developmental Disorders, 19*, 185–212.

Lord, C., Rutter, M., & Le Couteur, A. (1994). Autism Diagnostic Interview-Revised – A revised version of a diagnostic interview for caregivers of individuals with possible pervasive developmental disorders. *Journal of Autism and Developmental Disorders, 24,* 659–685.

MacNeil, B. M., Lopes, V. A., & Minnes, P. M. (2009). Anxiety in children and adolescents with Autism Spectrum Disorders. *Research in Autism Spectrum Disorders, 3,* 1–21.

J. L. Matson, F. Andrasik, & M. L. Matson (Eds.) (2008). *Assessing childhood psychopathology and developmental disabilities.* New York: Springer.

Matson, J. L. (1995). *The Diagnostic Assessment for the Severely Handicapped – Revised (DASH-II).* Baton Rouge, LA: Disability Consultants, LLC. www.disabilityconsultants.org

Matson, J. L., & Boisjoli, J. A. (2008). Autism spectrum disorders in adults with intellectual disability and comorbid psychopathology: Scale development and reliability of the ASD-CA. *Research in Autism Spectrum Disorders, 2,* 276–287.

Matson, J. L., LoVullo, S. V., Rivet, T. T., & Boisjoli, J. A. (2009). Validity of the Autism Spectrum Disorder-Comorbid for Children (ASD-CC). *Research in Autism Spectrum Disorders, 3,* 345–357.

Matson, J. L., Senatorve, V., & Kazdin, A. E. (1984). Psychometric properties of the Psychopathology Instrument for Mentally Retarded Adults. *Applied Research in Mental Retardation, 5,* 81–89.

Matson, J. L., & Shoemaker, M. (2009). Intellectual disability and its relationship to autism spectrum disorders. *Research in Developmental Disorders, 30,* 1107–1114.

Matson, J. L., & Wilkins, J. (2008). Reliability of the Autism Spectrum Disorders – Comorbid for Children (ASD-CC). *Journal of Developmental and Physical Disabilities, 20,* 327–336.

McCarthy, J., Hemmings, C., Kravariti., E., Dworsynski, K., Holt, G., Bouras, N., et al. (2009). Challenging behavior and co-morbid psychopathology in adults with intellectual disability and autism spectrum disorders. *Research in Developmental Disabilities.* (Advance online publication: doi:10.1016/j.ridd.2009.10.009)

Melville, C. A., Cooper, S. A., Morrison, J., Smiley, E., Allan, L., Jackson, A., et al. (2008). The prevalence and incidence of mental ill-health in adults with autism and intellectual disabilities. *Journal of Autism and Developmental Disorders, 38,* 1676–1688.

Mohr, C., & Costello, H. (2007). Mental health assessment and monitoring tools for people with intellectual disabilities. In N. Bouras & G. Holt (Eds.), *Psychiatric and behavioural disorders in developmental and intellectual disabilities* (2nd ed., pp. 24–41). Cambridge: Cambridge University Press.

Moss, S., Prosser, H., Costello, H., Simpson, N., & Patel, P. (1998). Reliability and validity of the PAS-ADD Checklist for detecting psychiatric disorders in adults with intellectual disability. *Journal of Intellectual Disability Research, 42,* 173–183.

Murphy, G., Beadle-Brown, J., Wing, L., Gould, J., Shah, A., & Holmes, N. (2005). Chronicity of challenging behaviors in people with severe intellectual disabilities and/or autism: A total population sample. *Journal of Autism and Developmental Disorders, 35,* 405–418.

Raznahan, A., Joinson, C., O'Callaghan, F., Osborne, J. P., & Bolton, P. F. (2006). Psychopathology in tuberous sclerosis: An overview and findings in a population based sample of adults with tuberous sclerosis. *Journal of Intellectual Disability Research, 50,* 561–569.

Reiss, S. (1988). *Test manual for the Reiss Screen for maladaptive behavior.* Worthington, OH: IDS.

Reynolds, C. R., & Kamphaus, R. W. (2004). *Manual: Behavior assessment system for children-Second Edition.* Circle Pines, MN: American Guidance Service.

Roy, A., Matthews, H., Clifford, P., Fowler, V., & Martin, D. M. (2002). Health of the Nation Outcome Scales for people with learning disabilities (HoNOS-LD). *British Journal of Psychiatry, 180,* 16–66.

Royal College of Psychiatrists. (2001). *OP48. DC-LD: Diagnostic criteria for psychiatric disorders for use with adults with learning disabilities/mental retardation.* London: Gaskell.

Spitzer, R. L., Endicott, J., & Robins, E. (1978). Research diagnostic criteria: Rationale and reliability. *Archives of General Psychiatry, 35,* 773–782.

Spitzer, R. L., Williams, J. B. W., Gibbon, M., & First, M. B. (1990). *Structured Clinician Interview for DSM-III-R Axis II Disorders (SCID-II).* Washington, DC: American Psychiatric Press.

Stewart, M. E., Barnard, L., Pearson, J., Hasan, R., & O'Brien, G. (2006). Presentation of depression in autism and Asperger syndrome. *Autism, 10,* 103–116.

Streiner, D. L., & Norman, G. R. (2008). *Health measurement scales. A practical guide to their development and use* (4th ed.). Oxford: Oxford University Press.

Tsakanikos, E., Costello, H., Holt, G., Bouras, N., Sturmey, P., & Newton, T. (2006). Psychopathology in Adults with Autism and Intellectual Disability. *Journal of Autism and Developmental Disorders, 36,* 1123–1129.

Tsakanikos, E., Costello, H., Holt, G., Sturmey, P., & Bouras, N. (2007a). Behaviour management problems as predictors of psychotropic medication and use of psychiatric services in adults with autism. *Journal of Autism and Developmental Disorders, 35,* 1080–1085.

Tsakanikos, E., Sturmey, P., Costello, H., Holt, G., & Bouras, N. (2007b). Referral trends in mental health services for adults with intellectual disability and autism spectrum disorders. *Autism, 11,* 9–17.

White, S. W., Oswald, D., Ollendick, T., & Scahill, L. (2009). Anxiety in children and adolescents with autism spectrum disorders. *Clinical Psychology Review, 29,* 216–229.

Wing, J. K., Babor, T., Brugha, T., Burke, J., Cooper, J. E., Giel, R., et al. (1990). SCAN: Schedules for Clinical Assessment in Neuropsychiatry. *Archives of General Psychiatry, 47,* 589–593.

Wirt, R. D., Lachar, D., Klinedinst, J. K., & Seat, P. D. (1984). *Multidimensional description of child personality: A manual for the Personality Inventory for Children* (Rev., ed.). Los Angeles: Western Psychological Services.

World Health Organization. (1992). *The ICD-10 classification of mental and behavioural disorders: Clinical descriptions and diagnostic guidelines.* Geneva: Author.

Xenitidis, K., Paliokosta, E., Maltezos, S., & Pappas, V. (2007). Assessment of mental health problems in people with autism. *Advances in Mental Health and Learning Disabilities, 1,* 15–22.

Identifying Moderators of Treatment Outcome for Children with Autism

18

Laura Schreibman, Sarah Dufek, and Allison B. Cunningham

The identification of variables that affect treatment outcomes and the development of individualized treatment protocols for children with autism have become a research priority for both researchers and funding agencies. Research indicates the inadequacy of one single treatment approach for all areas of learning for children with autism (National Research Council, 2001; Schreibman, 2000). Indeed, there is now a consensus that there is no "one-size-fits-all" treatment for autism. Despite the benefits for many children, differential response to treatment is common for any behavioral approach, in that up to 50% of children fail to show substantial positive responses. While several different treatment models have been developed and separately empirically validated, little research has addressed *when* and *for whom* each intervention is most appropriate. Very little is known about how to individualize treatment protocols or how to best determine a priori which intervention is most likely to benefit individual children (Schreibman, 2000; Sherer & Schreibman, 2005; Yoder & Comptom, 2004). Individualization research requires an understanding of the pre-treatment characteristics associated with differential outcomes in treatment, including child, family, and practitioner variables. The ultimate goal of this line of research is to enable practitioners to prospectively tailor treatments to specific children and increase the overall rate of positive outcomes for children with autism.

This chapter begins with a review of child, family, and practitioner variables that have been associated with child treatment outcomes. It then continues with a discussion of existing individualization research that has been conducted to date. It concludes with a discussion of where the treatment individualization field is going and recommends future directions.

L. Schreibman (✉)
Department of Psychology, University of California, San Diego, CA 92093-0109, USA
e-mail: lschreibman@ucsd.edu

Child Variables Associated with Outcome

Given the wide heterogeneity of outcomes in children with autism, a number of studies have identified child characteristics associated with positive developmental and treatment outcomes. Developmental studies have used cross-sectional and longitudinal study designs to identify early child variables associated with later child outcomes in general. Although these variables were not evaluated in relation to response to a specific treatment per se, these data have been important in helping researchers and practitioners identify important child features to consider when tailoring interventions to unique child needs. In particular, treatment individualization is likely to be more important for those children least likely to demonstrate positive developmental outcomes.

Early language ability and cognitive ability have emerged as the most robust predictors of overall prognosis for autism during childhood, adolescence, and adulthood (Howlin, Goode, Hutton, & Rutter, 2004; Sigman & Ruskin, 1999; Ventner, Lord, & Schopler, 1992). Without the acquisition of some functional speech by the age of 5, individuals with autism are unlikely to demonstrate advanced long-term gains in communication, social, adaptive, or academic domains (Howlin, 2005; Lotter, 1974). Perhaps because of the importance of early language and cognitive abilities in later prognoses, several studies have looked further at the relationship between early language ability, later language, and overall outcomes. Standardized communication scores from children as young as 3 years old predict later language acquisition (Thurm, Lord, Lee, & Newschaffer, 2006). Early measures of non-verbal IQ also correlate with concurrent and later language ability (Stevens et al., 2000; Tager-Flusberg, Paul, & Lord, 2005; Thurm et al., 2006) but not always before the age of 3 (Charman, Taylor, Drew, Cockerill, Brown, & Baird, 2005). Specifically, Charman et al. (2005) found that while diagnostic and non-verbal cognitive abilities at age 3 were predictive of outcome in children with autism at age 7, similar measures at age 2 were not.

Prelinguistic and early social behaviors, including joint attention, motor imitation, and toy play, have also been identified as variables related to outcomes in children with autism. These features have also been suggested as possible underlying and causal features of other autism deficits (Dawson, Toth, Abbott, Osterling, Munson, Estes et al., 2004; Sigman, Spence, & Wang, 2000). In both typical infant and toddler development, research indicates that early responsivity to social stimuli is important for later social and communicative development (Van Hecke, Mundy, Acra, Block, Delgado, Parlade et al., 2007). Studies of children with autism have found certain socially oriented behaviors (e.g., joint attention, imitation, gesture use) to be strong concurrent and future predictors of development in several areas central to autism, including language and play (Anderson, Lord, Risi, DiLavore, Shulman, Thurm et al., 2007; Bono, Daley, & Sigman, 2004; Charman, Baron-Cohen, Swettenham, Baird, Drew, & Cox, 2003; Luyster, Kadlec, Carter, & Tager-Flusberg, 2008; Rutherford, Young, Hepburn, & Rogers, 2007; Sigman & Ruskin, 1999; Thurm, Lord, Lee, & Newschaffer, 2006; Toth, Munson, Meltzoff, & Dawson, 2006).

One study found that joint attention skills, along with motor imitation, were significantly more impaired in young children with autism who failed to develop language by the age of 5 in comparison to those who became verbal (Thurm et al., 2006). An even larger body of literature confirms that early emerging joint attention skills continue to predict language production and communication skills across the life span (Charman et al., 2003, 2005; Sigman & McGovern, 2005; Toth et al., 2006). Motor imitation has been associated with later development by several investigators (Charman et al., 2003; McDuffie, Yoder, & Stone, 2005; Stone, Ousley, & Littleford, 1997; Sutera et al., 2007; Thurm et al., 2006; Toth et al., 2006). Vocal imitation skills, although less often examined, have also been implicated (Thurm et al., 2006). Lastly, early functional and symbolic play behaviors have been associated with later language, play, and social abilities in this population (Charman et al., 2005; Mundy, Sigman, Ungerer, & Sherman, 1987; Sigman & McGovern, 2005; Toth et al., 2006).

Another important line of research has been the identification of child characteristics that may moderate treatment effects. It is well established that there is a wide variability in treatment responsivity for children receiving early intervention services. A growing body of literature confirms that substantial gains may be achieved for a large minority of children when behavioral intervention is provided at an early age (Ben-Itzchak & Zachor, 2007; Cohen, Amerine-Dickens, & Smith, 2006; Eikeseth & Jahr, 2001; Harris & Handleman, 2000; Ingersoll, Schreibman, & Stahmer, 2001;

McEachin, Smith, & Lovaas, 1993; Sallows & Graupner, 2005; Sheinkopf & Siegel, 1998; Dawson et al., 2009; Sherer & Schreibman, 2005; Smith, 1999; Smith, Eikeseth, Klevstrand, & Lovaas, 1997; Smith, Groen, & Wynn, 2000; Weiss, 1999). Some children show rapid and considerable gains, while others respond minimally or not at all. Mean data representing treatment outcomes should be interpreted with caution. For any behavioral approach, up to 50% of children fail to make substantial gains.

It is this heterogeneity in treatment response that has made individualization research such a priority. These studies have sought to identify those variables related to differences in child treatment outcomes and have begun to search for variables that differentially predict success in varied treatment models. Optimal treatment outcomes in comprehensive early and intensive behavioral interventions have been related to age at the start of treatment, initial learning rate, non-verbal IQ, imitation ability, and autism severity (Ben-Itzchak & Zachor, 2007; Dawson et al., 2009; Harris & Handleman, 2000; Sallows & Graupner, 2005; Smith et al., 1997; Weiss, 1999).

More recently, investigators have begun to look for variables that may be differentially predictive of child response to treatment. While studies identifying predictors of treatment response continue to be important, they are only able to identify child variables associated with response to *one* specific treatment. This is problematic, as there is no consensus on the specific treatment model of choice for children with autism (NRC, 2001; Schreibman, 2005). Several different treatment models have been developed and separately empirically validated, but without information about *when* and *for whom* each intervention is most appropriate. Some single-subject and group comparison designs have argued for the superiority of one treatment over the other (Delprato, 2001; Smith et al., 2000). However, few investigators have examined the possibility that different treatments may be most appropriate for different children and at different points in the treatment process. Indeed, given the heterogeneity of autism presentation and prognosis, it is unlikely that there is a one-size-fits-all best practice intervention (NRC, 2001; Schreibman, 2005). Improved understanding of child variables associated with differential treatment outcomes may enable researchers and practitioners to prospectively tailor treatments to specific children. In turn, this may increase the overall rate of treatment effectiveness across children with autism (Schreibman, Stahmer, Cestone-Bartlet, & Dufek, 2009). This research is becoming even more important as treatment approaches integrating non-behavioral components are gaining support and other treatment options become available (Dawson et al., 2009).

Only a handful of studies, which are discussed later in this chapter, have moved beyond exploring simple main effects to explore possible treatment-by-child interactions. While some theoretical papers suggest that different treatments may be appropriate for different children, very little is known about how to individualize treatment protocols or how to best determine a priori which intervention is most likely to benefit individual children (Schreibman, 2000; Yoder & Comptom, 2004). This type of individualization research has a good deal of promise for the field, but it is in its infancy.

Individualizing Interventions Using Practitioner and Parent Variables

In addition to identifying child variables, researchers are currently examining other variables that affect intervention outcomes such as practitioner (e.g., special education teachers, autism service providers, speech therapists, psychologists) and parent variables. The effectiveness of individualized treatment protocols for children with autism can be further maximized if researchers and practitioners take into account *all* variables affecting these children. Autism experts agree that delivering behavioral intervention during early development is crucial to maximizing outcomes (Anderson & Romanczyk, 1999; Bristol, Cohen, Costello, Denckla, Eckberg, & Kallen, 1996; Guralnick, 1998; Ramey & Ramey, 1998; Schreibman, 2005). During this critical period, practitioners and parents are often faced with difficult decisions about which interventions should be included in a child's early intervention program and how the interventions should be implemented. Unfortunately, since individualizing treatment protocols based on child characteristics is still in its infancy, practitioners and parents are often more heavily influenced by other factors when making intervention program decisions. Providing guidelines for individualizing interventions based on factors outside of child characteristics can also be a valuable way to maximize the effectiveness of those interventions.

Practitioner Variables

Practitioner variables that influence intervention choice usually consist of practitioner knowledge of and training to implement interventions available and practitioner attitudes toward those interventions. Most evidence-based practices (EBPs) available for children with autism are from the field of applied behavior analysis, although other intervention approaches are accumulating evidence to support their use (ABA; e.g., Dawson et al., 2009; National Research Council, 2001; Schreibman, 1988, 1996; Schreibman, 2005; Smith & Magyar, 2003). EBPs are practices (e.g., interventions, assessments, program management systems) that are supported by the current best research evidence available (Sackett, Richardson, Rosenberg, Haynes, & Strauss, 1997).

There is some evidence that practitioners are having difficulty adopting EBP interventions for children with autism in community practice settings, much less individualizing these interventions. Stahmer, Collings, and Palinkas (2005) asked focus groups made up of practitioners to discuss the use of EBP interventions in their programs. Practitioners reported utilizing EBP interventions in addition to other practices that are not evidence based. The practitioners were admittedly unsure as to which interventions were evidence based. They would often report a technique was an EBP intervention if they attended workshops or lectures to learn to use a technique or if a technique was being used in their program.

These findings demonstrate that just disseminating best practice guidelines alone is not an effective technique; often there are other factors influencing best practice guidelines adoption by practitioners. Some researchers suggest individualizing best practice guidelines by *categorizing* these guidelines to help practitioners specify application of EBP. Best practice guidelines can be categorized by level of research evidence support, patient or practitioner characteristics, or implementation setting characteristics (Biglan, Mrazek, Carnine, & Flay, 2003; Hawley & Weisz, 2002; Onion, Dutton, Walley, & Turnbull, 1996). When developing interventions for children with autism, researchers should individualize the interventions to the needs of the practitioners who will be utilizing those interventions, in order to make sure they are adopted and used properly. For example, some of the phases of the Picture Exchange Communication System (PECS; Bondy & Frost, 2001) require an additional person to act as a physical prompter during intervention. Adding the requirement of an additional staff member in a classroom setting, where there is already a high student to teacher ratio, may create a situation where correct implementation of PECS as intended by researchers is unlikely.

In order to develop more individualized interventions, researchers have suggested development of "local" guidelines to address the relevancy of research findings in practice (Antony, 2005; Arthur & Blitz, 2000; Onion et al., 1996; Southam-Gerow, 2004). Arthur and Blitz suggest increasing local ownership of interventions by encouraging practitioners to take responsibility for the development and implementation of interventions in their own communities. They state that local practitioners have the greatest ability to help themselves when it comes to use of interventions. Instead of a "one-size-fits-all approach," interventions themselves should be matched to specific community settings and those settings should inform others about what works and what does not. To improve individualization of intervention for children with autism, autism researchers need to considerably increase the amount of time they spend working directly with practitioners in real-world settings. In addition, more research examining usual care for children with autism (practices that are currently provided in applied settings by practitioners) is needed to determine what information is necessary or desired for practitioners.

Unfortunately, the limited resources available to practitioners often determine the interventions they use. Autism interventions need to be individualized by the resources available to the practitioners who will be utilizing them. However, there are very few efforts put forth to examine *how* these interventions are implemented in the real world. The limited research that has been conducted indicates that practitioners are not implementing interventions developed as intended by researchers. For example, Stahmer and colleagues (2005) found that the practitioners reported using modified versions of interventions, often combining elements of multiple practices or applying adaptations to those practices based on child and/or program characteristics. They caution that combining or changing interventions is problematic because these practices were developed in isolation and researchers have no evidence about their effectiveness when used in combined or modified forms. Practitioners are likely recognizing that interventions designed by researchers in research settings have to be individualized for use in applied settings. However, practitioners are not adapting these interventions in a systematic way and there has been minimal research about how those modifications are influencing child outcome.

Other child mental health researchers have noted practitioner inconsistency of implementation of interventions (Walrath, Sheehan, Holden, Hernandez, & Blau, 2006; Weisz, Donenberg, Han, & Weiss, 1995; Weisz, Weiss, & Donenberg, 1992). Two common themes in the literature relating to what affects correct implementation of interventions are (1) usability of the practice and (2) limited practitioner time and training. Interventions developed for children with autism need to be tailored to address intervention usability and limited practitioner time and training in order to be most effective. Southam-Gerow (2004) urges researchers to reconsider the significance of external variables that influence usability of interventions in applied settings. He reminds researchers that practices developed in a laboratory are usually developed to improve upon client *symptom* patterns. However, in applied settings, often *non-symptom* client variables and/or provider and agency variables are the most responsible for failure of an intervention (e.g., health insurance only pays for half the sessions needed for an intervention, parents are unable to read all materials required for training).

While laboratory work in a controlled setting is critical, research should also be conducted outside of the laboratory to examine possible real-world variables that may interfere with good outcome (Bauman, Stein, & Ireys, 1991; Weisz & Jensen, 2001). Southam-Gerow (2004) suggests the best way to examine the effects of real-world variables is to determine how these variables influence outcome in a laboratory setting (e.g., enroll participants in research projects who present

with comorbid disorders, such that the participants in the research study are more like clients practitioners see in the real world). Research findings from studies conducted in the real world can also allow researchers to obtain more understanding as to the role of subjective "clinical judgment" (Brown, Reeves, Glynn, Majid, & Kothari, 2007). There is little consensus in the literature about what exactly defines clinical judgment. Clinical judgment is defined by Schalock and Luckasson (2005) as "a special type of judgment rooted in a high level of clinical expertise and experience and based on extensive data ... some refer to this ancillary thing as intuition, some as one's better judgment, some as blind faith, and some as professional license" (p. 5). Despite uncertain practitioner understanding of the role of clinical judgment, use of clinical judgment is important to practitioners. However, there is no research to determine if clinical judgment used by practitioners helps or harms positive outcome in clients with autism. Researchers should examine the nature and influence of practitioners' clinical judgment on child outcome. Researchers would then be able to inform practitioners about when (or if) they should rely on clinical judgment when making decisions about a child's intervention program.

Another potentially helpful way to individualize interventions is to clarify what resources are required for successful implementation of those interventions. Biglan and colleagues suggest assigning interventions "grade levels." Grade levels could be determined based on amount of staff, hours of training, and/or level of staff monitoring required for effective implementation of an intervention. Gonzales, Ringeisen, and Chambers (2002) also emphasize the importance of clarifying resources required by applying "implementation feasibility criteria" to interventions and encourage researchers to determine these criteria in the research and development phase of practice creation, testing practices in various settings to determine what resources are needed. The criteria determined should then be part of intervention designations. This technique would allow a more local application of intervention, and practitioners could more easily determine if an intervention is usable given their resources available. For example, an administrator may be given a choice to train the practitioners in her program in two possible interventions. One intervention may be more appropriate for a classroom environment (e.g., classroom has teacher's aides to assist during implementation) and one intervention may be more appropriate for a one-on-one environment (e.g., implementation requires only one therapist). If the interventions in question are rated, the administrator can refer to the grade levels or implementation feasibility criteria to determine which training would be most appropriate for the administrator's practitioners.

One common training tool that *discourages* individualization of interventions is the training manual. Intervention training manuals are often the primary training technique used and usually consist of highly specific guidelines about how to implement an intervention. The specificity is normally required so that researchers can achieve fidelity of implementation when studying the manualized intervention. Fidelity of implementation is a measure of the accuracy with which a practitioner is implementing a practice and is used to ensure the integrity of the independent variable in a study. However, in real-world settings, it may be impractical to implement an intervention with this highly technical level of accuracy. Accordingly, researchers propose some adjustments to training manuals that may be beneficial. Chorpita (2002) criticizes the use of manuals as a primary training technique for two main reasons: practitioners in the real world are usually not highly trained graduate students or laboratory staff, and practitioners' clients are usually more diverse than is typically seen in research settings. He suggests targeting these two issues in the laboratory during manual development (Chorpita & Daleiden, 2004; Chorpita & Nakamura, 2004; Chorpita, 2001, 2002). Kendall and Beidas (2007) propose a "flexibility within fidelity" approach, where manuals provide not only the basic structure, organization, sequence, and duration of a treatment but also flexible alternatives within the text. These alternatives would provide practitioners with some "wiggle room" within the context of good fidelity of implementation. Kendall and Beidas emphasize that since we already know practitioners are modifying interventions to pick and choose components they feel are most useful, researchers have a responsibility to examine modifications to determine if the practice is still effective. Determining allowable flexibility within fidelity is especially relevant to intervention for children with autism, given that researchers know practitioners often adjust interventions for use in their intervention programs. Including any acceptable adjustments may aid practitioners in individualizing interventions without fear of making the implementation ineffective.

Parent Characteristics

Although most intervention options for children with autism are implemented in school settings, an increasing number are becoming available in parent training formats, which are very effective for this population (Breiner & Beck, 1984; Ingersoll & Dvortcsak, 2006; National Research Council, 2001; Singh et al., 2006). Some research findings suggest that parents also benefit from specific training. Bristol, Gallagher, and Holt (1993) found that parent training reduced maternal depression in mothers of children with autism or related disorders compared to mothers who did not participate in parent training. They suggest that parent training increases parent understanding of the disorder and improves parental teaching techniques and management strategies of

child behavior. These help to alleviate maternal depression without direct treatment of the depression. These data suggest that as active parent involvement in children's intervention programs increases, intervention programs should be individualized based on not only child and practitioner characteristics but also parent characteristics. Indeed, even when individualization of intervention programs based on child and practitioner characteristics is happening at an optimal rate, researchers indicate that practitioners still come up against compliance issues during parent training efforts that may interfere with intervention outcome. DiMatteo and Haskard (2006) remind researchers and practitioners that interventions require many resources to be designed and implemented correctly, but emphasize that all intervention utilization efforts will be useless if issues of compliance are ignored. Individualizing interventions for children with autism based on parent variables can ensure that parents will also find those interventions usable and in turn improve child outcome.

Forehand and Kotchick (2002) suggest techniques that can be used to individualize intervention programs based on parent needs and characteristics. Thus, practitioners should provide parents with very detailed information about the interventions they are learning. Parents will likely be more agreeable to an intervention if they know there is research to support that the intervention works, especially when individualized for the specific set of difficulties at hand. Greater issues that can affect compliance may also be present, such as low SES, already present legal issues, or single parenthood. Many parents may have minimal support from the community and will have difficulty traveling away from the community to seek outside help (DiMatteo, 2004). It would be ideal if practitioners could provide some of the real-world benefits of social support, such as child care during treatment sessions, legal help, financial help, making themselves available by phone, or even holding the therapy sessions at neighborhood community centers or churches to reduce commute time and help parents feel more comfortable.

There are some data to suggest that lack of social support is a pertinent problem for parents of children with autism. Parents interviewed by Ruef and colleagues (1999) reported they frequently felt physically and emotionally drained from lack of social support by their community. Stahmer and Gist (2001) found that adding just a 1 h per week parent education support group to a 12-week accelerated training program for parents of children with autism increased parent mastery of training techniques and, in turn, increased child gains. Ingersoll and Dvortcsak (2006) also suggest that providing social support such as child care during sessions, reducing parent time commitment, and offering home visits as an alternative to clinic visits would increase parent compliance. They also stress the need for practitioners to be realistic about whether parents' needs or wants can be accommodated. Parents' needs should be balanced with practitioners' capabilities.

Another possible variable that is a candidate for individualization by parent characteristics is parent gender. Typically, mothers are the primary trainee in parent education programs, although researchers have found involving fathers in parent training programs can benefit children with problem behaviors (Horton, 1984; Webster-Stratton, 1985). Importantly, research indicates that parent training programs may require modifications in order to increase father involvement. Winter (2006) examined factors that contribute to increased father participation in a parent training program for children with autism. She found that modifying an existing parent training program by (1) offering flexible days and times for training, (2) altering location of training by including home visits, and (3) adding a recreational component all influenced father participation. In light of Winter's findings, autism researchers and practitioners need to consider parent gender when individualizing parent training programs. Further research in this area would also be beneficial.

Another technique to individualize intervention for parents is to pre-test parents about variables that may influence parent compliance before implementing parent training (Dush & Stacy, 1987). Dush and Stacy trained practitioners to improve parenting skills of low SES parents by increasing parent management of the needs of their children who were at-risk for various developmental disabilities, mental health, and/or behavior problems. Practitioners were also trained to pre-test one group of parents about variables such as parenting skills, resources available to parents, and parent education to determine how to individualize the parent intervention. Pre-testing of parents consisted of a home observation and some questionnaires about child and parent behavior. These researchers found that pre-testing parents in this manner reduced missed appointments and premature terminations compared to parents who were not pre-tested. Dush and Stacy suggest that pre-testing gives participants more information about what to expect during treatment, made the parents feel more valued, and helped to develop rapport between practitioner and parent. Jahng, Martin, Golin, and DiMatteo (2005) also found benefits from pre-testing patients in a medical setting. They found that when patients and doctors were pre-tested about their beliefs about treatment participation and were subsequently matched on these beliefs, patient outcomes tended to be more positive as measured by self-reported satisfaction with medical care received, adherence to medical regimens, and patient perception of their general health. Interestingly, highest patient satisfaction with medical care received was found in cases where both patients and physicians desired more patient involvement, indicating that physicians' willingness to incorporate their patients' expectations when determining course of treatment may be a key factor.

In addition, collaboration between practitioners and parents is important for individualization of intervention for parents. Brookman-Frazee (2004) found that when parents and practitioners collaborate on identifying target behaviors and method of treatment implementation for children with problem behaviors, parents demonstrated reduced stress and increased confidence compared to parents who did not collaborate. The children also showed more improvement in the collaboration group. The children were more engaged with the parents, responded at higher rates, and had more positive affect during sessions. Forehand and Kotchick (2002) provide guidelines to assess individual family variables that may influence compliance before training to help practitioners determine what level of intervention parents may (or may not) be able to handle: (Level 1) Family discord is not severe: no need to target family variables directly, parent training by itself can sometimes help resolve any problems. (Level 2) Family discord is present and may interfere with treatment: modification of original parent training plan may be helpful to directly target family issues. (Level 3) Family discord is moderate: parent training for the child can be concurrent with family services provided elsewhere. (Level 4) Family discord is severe and will definitely impede any immediate parent training efforts: encourage parents to resolve issues *before* beginning a parent training plan.

Breiner and Beck (1984) reviewed the literature on individualizing interventions for parents of children with developmental disabilities. They found parental characteristics do influence training efficacy, such as family SES (parents of lower SES are more likely to be non-compliant than parents of middle and upper SES), parental adjustment (parental depression, marital distress, stress concerning extended family and social agencies), and parental commands (parents often give children delayed and interrupted commands). Breiner and Beck make recommendations of parenting skills to target in parents of children with developmental disabilities: (1) Parent use of the principles of differential and contingent reinforcement to increase target child behaviors, (2) parent use of time out and extinction to decrease disruptive child behavior, and (3) decrease parents' tendency to use unclear and interrupted commands without having their child's attention. Suggested parent training techniques are (1) practitioner modeling of behavior techniques, (2) parent behavioral rehearsal, (3) practitioner feedback to parents, (4) booster parent training sessions, (5) parent use of self-reinforcement strategies outside the clinic, and (6) practitioner evaluation and (if necessary) correction of therapy expectations of parents (e.g., Is the parent realistic about the benefits of therapy and the projected timeline for change?). Forehand and Kotchick (2002) also discuss the importance of parent expectations about child behavior and the therapy process and how parent expectations can influence compliance.

They emphasize the practitioner's need to assess, validate, and if necessary change parents' expectations.

Unfortunately, many parents have educated themselves incorrectly about what interventions will (or will not) be beneficial for children with autism. For example, many parents incorrectly assume that if their child is mentally challenged, the parent will be unable to change any problem behavior. Often parents have tried many ineffective ways of changing the child's behavior and have failed by the time the parents enter a treatment program. Educating parents about the effectiveness of behavior treatment with children with developmental disabilities can give them hope and motivate them to implement treatment. The practitioner can help a parent to have more positive expectations about what the *parent* can do to increase child outcome, which can increase their feelings of self-efficacy. Assessing parents' expectations will assist practitioners to know what behavior to expect from parents. Practitioners can use information about parent expectations to individualize interventions for parents that are appropriate for the parents' personalities and lifestyle.

Existing Research on Treatment Individualization

Child Behavioral Characteristics

Two prospective studies have examined child variables associated with differential responsivity to one specific naturalistic behavioral intervention, pivotal response training (PRT). One of these studies found that 3- to 5-year-old children demonstrating high levels of non-verbal stereotypy and avoidance, as well as low levels of verbal stereotypy, toy play, and approach behaviors, were less likely to respond to PRT than those exhibiting the opposite behavioral profile prior to treatment (Sherer & Schreibman, 2005). A follow-up study suggested that this predictive profile was specific to PRT and that it was not predictive of response to other behavioral interventions, such as discrete trial training (Schreibman et al., 2009). Additionally, a related study found that level of peer social avoidance influenced the extent to which children with autism benefited from an inclusive school setting (Ingersoll et al., 2001). Collectively, these initial studies provide evidence that specific behavioral profiles may be useful in identifying which children are likely to respond to particular treatments and in making treatment decisions.

Another study evaluated the differential effectiveness of two communication training strategies commonly used to teach early communication skills to nonverbal and minimally verbal young children with autism (Cunningham, Schreibman, Stahmer, Koegel, & Koegel, 2008). Specifically, this randomized comparison study addressed the differential effects of a language-based approach (PRT) and a visually based approach (the picture exchange communication system, PECS; Bondy & Frost, 2001) on the communication, social, and cognitive functioning of very young (i.e. 2–4 years old) children with autism. Thirty-four children who at intake had 10 or fewer functional words were matched and randomly assigned to a PRT or PECS treatment condition. Both programs resulted in substantial spoken language gains for approximately 50% of the children. While early word use was highly predictive of verbal gains in both treatment conditions, it was not predictive of augmentative communication gains. Children with *some* words (i.e. 1–10 words at intake) were equally likely to develop verbal communication skills in PECS or PRT. However, children entering treatment with *no verbal language* were unlikely to develop spoken language. But, over 80% of the PECS participants developed substantial augmentative communication skills. These preliminary results suggest that word use at intake may be an important and parsimonious child variable to consider when deciding between verbal and augmentative communication programs for very young children with autism. In addition, these data suggested that the PRT predictive profile (Sherer & Schreibman, 2005) was not predictive of responsivity in a younger aged sample. The data indicated that the behaviors composing the PRT predictive profile did not discriminate PRT responders from PRT nonresponders in younger children, suggesting that the profile may require adaptations in order to be appropriate for addressing treatment responsivity in younger children with autism.

There has been one other systematic comparison of the differential effects of verbally and visually based communication training programs for young children with autism. Yoder and Stone (2006a, b) conducted a randomized experiment comparing a vocally based naturalistic intervention, responsive education and prelinguistic milieu teaching (RPMT), to PECS in order to examine how the relative treatment effects varied as a function of child variables. The investigators found that while both PECS and RPMT resulted in an increase in initiating joint attention across treatment, RPMT resulted in more initiating joint attention compared to PECS for those children who had at least some joint attention skills prior to intervention. Also, RPMT resulted in more object exchange turns than did PECS. Alternatively, PECS resulted in more requests in comparison to RPMT and greater gains in initiating joint attention bids for those children with little joint attention skill at intake. In a different report based on the same experiment, the authors found that pre-treatment levels of object exploration moderated growth rates in a number of nonimitative words in PECS versus RPMT. Children who began treatment with low object exploration benefited more from RPMT, while children who began treatment with higher levels of object exploration benefited more from PECS. These researchers reasoned that while both PECS and RPMT involve objects as rewards for communicative attempts, only RPMT involves specifically teaching children how to play with objects. Therefore, children with low object exploration at pre-treatment were more likely to benefit from intervention after learning to play with objects. The PECS treatment was superior for children with high object exploration at pre-treatment. Both the PECS versus PRT (Cunningham et al., 2008) and the Yoder and Stone (2006a, b) studies provide information about the differential effects of visually and vocally based interventions and illustrate how detailed information about very specific behavioral effects may be identified.

Collectively, these studies serve as the foundation for research aimed at matching treatment approaches to the individual treatment needs of different children with autism. They begin to suggest methods of tailoring interventions to specific child needs. For example, it may be that PECS may be more appropriate as a first-line treatment approach for children with fewer prerequisite abilities, including early word use and joint attention initiation skills. Alternatively, verbally based programs, such as RPMT and PRT, may be appropriate for children who enter treatment with some early communication skills. Importantly, these data also suggest that treatment providers or family members may select their preferred intervention with little effect on outcome in certain cases. This is a particularly promising finding given the importance of individualizing treatment based on practitioner and family variables. It is important to emphasize that these findings must be replicated and may only apply to early communication treatment. The relative benefits of these interventions for older children or longer term treatment programs, as well as on other areas of development, are yet to be addressed.

Conclusions and Future Directions

The focus on variables affecting the treatment of children with autism, while in its relative infancy, has already produced important findings relating to how we might provide more tailored interventions for individual children. Taking into account important child, treatment practitioner, and family characteristics, autism researchers have already identified significant factors that impact treatment responsiveness. While we are off to a good start, future directions in this line of research will undoubtedly substantially improve our ability to develop tailored treatment protocols.

Child Neurobiological Characteristics

Our ability to measure and evaluate brain structure and brain functioning in young children with autism opens an entirely new and potentially enormous opportunity to design treatments based upon individual brain development. An example of one study in progress will serve to illustrate this potential. The UCSD Autism Center of Excellence (ACE, NIH, Eric Courchesne, PI) focuses on employing a variety of neurophysiological and genetic evaluations of at-risk babies (scanned and evaluated longitudinally at 12, 24, and 36 months of age). These investigators are looking for features of the brain that may differentiate autism from normal brain development during the first 3 years of life. Specifically, our involvement in this research (ACE Treatment Core, Schreibman and Stahmer, Directors) is responsible for the treatment portion of the center and is providing intensive state-of-the-art behavioral treatment to very young (i.e., 18–36 months) children with a provisional diagnosis of autism. The treatment portion ensures a standardized model of intensive treatment to all study participants. The behavioral treatment package employed consists of several empirically validated behavioral treatment components (e.g., PRT, DTT, PECS); we hope to be able to further relate aspects of brain functioning to specific treatment protocols. It is predicted that differential treatment outcomes may subsequently be related to specific features of brain structure and functioning. If this is the case, as we expect, this might allow us to base treatment component decisions on the brain features of these babies and toddlers. Taking this area even further, it may be the case that ultimately in the future we may be able to provide intervention that will help the developing brain develop to exhibit the characteristics of a brain that is associated with the most positive treatment outcome. We view the potential for this line of investigation to be particularly promising and hopeful.

Empirically Based Treatment Combinations

Evidence suggests that treatment providers working in community settings do not select just one intervention. Instead, they report using a combination of highly structured (e.g., discrete trial training; DTT) and naturalistic (e.g., pivotal response training; PRT) interventions (Stahmer et al., 2005). It has been hypothesized that incorporating multiple treatment methods into a comprehensive program and customizing it in terms of the individual needs of specific children should increase overall treatment effectiveness (Hurth, Shaw, Izeman, Whaley, & Rogers, 1999; Iovannone, Dunlap, Huber, & Kincaid, 2003; Rogers, 1996; Schreibman, 2000). Unfortunately, very little data are available to inform specific methods of combining such interventions. Currently, combination treatments are determined by what intervention the teachers are familiar with, what the school district provides, or other factors not based on empirical research. No controlled studies have addressed the relative efficacy of structured and naturalistic interventions when used in combination with each other or suggested empirically tested methods of integrating them into comprehensive programs.

In our laboratory we are currently focusing on evaluating the relative benefits of combining structured and naturalistic behavioral treatment strategies as compared to the use of each treatment approach alone. Although structured and naturalistic models have often been compared, no studies have systematically addressed their effectiveness when used in combination with each other or suggested empirically tested methods for integrating them into comprehensive treatment programs. It has been hypothesized that incorporating multiple treatment methods in a comprehensive program and customizing it in terms of individual needs should increase overall treatment effectiveness, but very little data are available to inform specific methods for integrating approaches. Some treatment outcome studies have included eclectic models, which incorporate a variety of empirically based methods (Eikeseth, Smith, Jahr, & Eldevik, 2002; Howard, Sparkman, Cohen, Green, & Stanislaw, 2005). However, these studies do not identify the specific components making up the model and may represent a lack of strong methodology for combining techniques.

In particular, it is not well understood how DTT and PRT may be differentially effective at targeting different skill areas. It may be that naturalistic and structured teaching procedures accomplish different goals and are mutually beneficial. We are presently conducting a study to identify (1) specific developmental areas or skill domains that may be best addressed using DTT or PRT and (2) child variables that may influence whether specific children are more likely to benefit from DTT or PRT. These data will be used for the subsequent development and evaluation of a treatment model that integrates these approaches into comprehensive treatment programs that address the diverse developmental needs of individual children with autism.

The above are but a few projects underway that will likely have a significant impact on the development of an individualized treatment capability. Of course we still need to continue focusing on the relationship between treatment outcome and child, family, and practitioner variables since there are many more yet to study. However, we feel very confident that the continued pursuit of an understanding of the relationship between outcome and a variety of potentially important treatment effect mediators will greatly enhance our ability to provide for a brighter future for children with autism and their families.

References

Anderson, D. K., Lord, C., Risi, S., DiLavore, P. S., Shulman, C., Thurm, A., et al. (2007). Patterns of growth in verbal abilities among children with autism spectrum disorder. *Journal of Consulting and Clinical Psychology, 75,* 594–604.

Anderson, S. R., & Romanczyk, R. G. (1999). Early intervention for young children with autism: Continuum-based behavioral models. *Journal of the Association for Persons with Severe Handicaps, 24,* 162–173.

Antony, M. M. (2005). Five strategies for bridging the gap between research and clinical practice. *The Behavior Therapist, 28,* 162–163.

Arthur, M. W., & Blitz, C. (2000). Bridging the gap between science and practice in drug abuse prevention through needs assessment and strategic community planning. *Journal of Community Psychology. Special Issue: Bridging the Gap Between Research and Practice in Community-Based Substance Abuse Prevention, 28,* 241–255.

Bauman, L. J., Stein, R. E., & Ireys, H. T. (1991). Reinventing fidelity: The transfer of social technology among settings. *American Journal of Community Psychology. Special Issue: Preventive Intervention Research Centers, 19,* 619–639.

Ben-Itzchak, E., & Zachor, D. A. (2007). The effects of intellectual functioning and autism severity on outcome of early behavioral intervention for children with autism. *Research in Developmental Disabilities, 28,* 287–303.

Biglan, A., Mrazek, P. J., Carnine, D., & Flay, B. R. (2003). The integration of research and practice in the prevention of youth problem behaviors. *American Psychologist. Special Issue: Prevention that Works for Children and Youth, 58,* 433–440.

Bondy, A., & Frost, L. (2001). The picture exchange communication system. *Behavior Modification, 25,* 725–744.

Bono, M. A., Daley, T., & Sigman, M. (2004). Relations among joint attention, amount of intervention and language gain in autism. *Journal of Autism and Developmental Disorders, 34,* 495–505.

Breiner, J., & Beck, S. (1984). Parents as change agents in the management of their developmentally delayed children's noncompliant behaviors: A critical review. *Applied Research in Mental Retardation, 5,* 259–278.

Bristol, M. M., Cohen, D. J., Costello, E. J., Denckla, M., Eckberg, T. J., & Kallen, H. C. (1996). State of the science in autism: Report to the national institutes of health. *Journal of Autism and Developmental Disorders, 26,* 121–155.

Bristol, M. M., Gallagher, J. J., & Holt, K. D. (1993). Maternal depressive symptoms in autism: Response to psychoeducational intervention. *Rehabilitation Psychology, 38,* 3–10.

Brookman-Frazee, L. (2004). Using parent/clinician partnerships in parent education programs for children with autism. *Journal of Positive Behavior Interventions, 6,* 195–213.

Brown, M., Reeves, M., Glynn, T., Majid, A., & Kothari, R. (2007). Implementation of an emergency department-based transient ischemic attack clinical pathway: A pilot study in knowledge translation. *Academic Emergency Medicine,* 1–6.

Charman, T., Baron-Cohen, S., Swettenham, J., Baird, G., Drew, A., & Cox, A. (2003). Predicting language outcomes in infants with autism and pervasive developmental disorder. *International Journal of Language and Communication Disorders, 38,* 265–285.

Charman, T., Taylor, E., Drew, A., Cockerill, J., Brown, J., & Baird, G. (2005). Outcome at 7 years of children diagnosed with autism at age 2: Predictive validity of assessments conducted at 2 and 3 years of age and pattern of symptom change over time. *Journal of Child Psychology and Psychiatry, 46,* 500–513.

Chorpita, B. (2002). Treatment manuals for the real world: Where do we build them? *Clinical Psychology: Science and Practice, 9,* 431–433.

Chorpita, B. F. (2001). Reflections on clinical significance: What do our best treatments accomplish and how can we best find out? *Clinical Psychology: Science and Practice, 8,* 451–454.

Chorpita, B. F., & Daleiden, E. L. (2004). Designs for instruction, designs for change: Distributing knowledge of evidence-based practice. *Clinical Psychology: Science and Practice, 11,* 332–335.

Chorpita, B. F., & Nakamura, B. J. (2004). Four considerations for dissemination of intervention innovations. *Clinical Psychology: Science and Practice, 11*, 364–367.

Cohen, J., Amerine-Dickens, M., & Smith, T. (2006). Early intensive behavioral treatment: Replication of the UCLA model in a community setting. *Developmental and Behavioral Pediatrics, 27*, 145–155.

Cunningham, A. B., Schreibman, L., Stahmer, A. C., Koegel, R. L., & Koegel, L. K. (2008). Individualization of treatment for young children with autism: A randomized comparison of verbal and pictorial communication training strategies. Paper presented at 7th Annual International Meeting for Autism Research. London.

Dawson, G., Rogers, S., Munson, J., Smith, M., Winter, J., Greenson, J., et al. (2009). Randomized, controlled trial of an intervention for toddlers with autism: The early start denver model. *Pediatrics, 125*, e17–e23.

Dawson, G., Toth, K., Abbott, R., Osterling, J., Munson, J., Estes, A., et al. (2004). Early social attention impairments in autism: Social orienting, joint attention, and attention to distress. *Developmental Psychology, 40*, 271–283.

Delprato, D. J. (2001). Comparisons of discrete-trial and normalized behavioral language intervention for young children with autism. *Journal of Autism and Developmental Disorders, 31*, 315–325.

DiMatteo, M. R. (2004). Social support and patient adherence to medical treatment: A meta-analysis. *Health Psychology, 23*, 207–218.

DiMatteo, M. R., & Haskard, K. B. (2006). Further challenges in adherence research: Measurements, methodologies, and mental health care. *Medical Care, 44*, 297–299.

Dush, D. M., & Stacy, E. W. (1987). Pretesting enhancement of parent compliance in a prevention program for high-risk children. *Evaluation & The Health Professions, 10*, 201–205.

Eikeseth, S., & Jahr, E. (2001). The UCLA reading and writing program: An evaluation of the beginning stages. *Research in Developmental Disabilities, 22*, 289–307.

Eikeseth, S., Smith, T., Jahr, E., & Eldevik, S. (2002). Intensive behavioral treatment at school for 4- to 7-year-old children with autism: A 1-year comparison controlled study. *Behavior Modification. Special Issue: Autism, Part, 2*(26), 49–68.

Forehand, R., & Kotchick, B. A. (2002). Behavioral parent training: Current challenges and potential solutions. *Journal of Child and Family Studies, 11*, 377–384.

Gonzales, J. J., Ringeisen, H. L., & Chambers, D. A. (2002). The tangled and thorny path of science to practice: Tensions in interpreting and applying "evidence." *Clinical Psychology: Science and Practice, 9*, 204–209.

Guralnick, M. J. (1998). Effectiveness of early intervention for vulnerable children: A developmental perspective. *American Journal on Mental Retardation, 102*, 319–345.

Harris, S. L., & Handleman, J. S. (2000). Age and IQ at intake as predictors of placement for young children with autism: A four- to six-year follow-up. *Journal of Autism and Developmental Disorders, 30*, 137–142.

Hawley, K. M., & Weisz, J. R. (2002). Increasing the relevance of evidence-based treatment review to practitioners and consumers. *Clinical Psychology: Science and Practice, 9*, 225–230.

Horton, L. (1984). The father's role in behavioral parent training: A review. *Journal of Clinical Child Psychology, 13*, 274–279.

Howard, J. S., Sparkman, C. R., Cohen, H. G., Green, G., & Stanislaw, H. (2005). A comparison of intensive behavior analytic and eclectic treatments for young children with autism. *Research in Developmental Disabilities, 26*, 359–383.

Howlin, P. (2005). Outcomes in autism spectrum disorders. In D. Cohen & F. Volkmar (Eds.), *Handbook of autism and pervasive developmental disorders* (3rd ed., vol. 1, pp. 201–222). New Jersey: Wiley.

Howlin, P., Goode, S., Hutton, J., & Rutter, M. (2004). Adult outcome for children with autism. *Journal of Child Psychology and Psychiatry, 45*, 212–229.

Hurth, J., Shaw, E., Izeman, S., Whaley, K., & Rogers, S. (1999). Areas of agreement about effective practices serving young children with autism spectrum disorders. *Infants and Young Children, 12*, 17–26.

Ingersoll, B., & Dvortcsak, A. (2006). Including parent training in the early childhood special education curriculum for children with autism spectrum disorders. *Journal of Positive Behavior Interventions, 8*, 79–87.

Ingersoll, B., Schreibman, L., & Stahmer, A. (2001). Brief report: Differential treatment outcomes for children with autistic spectrum disorder based on level of peer social avoidance. *Journal of Autism and Developmental Disorders, 31*, 343–349.

Iovannone, R., Dunlap, G., Huber, H., & Kincaid, D. (2003). Effective educational practices for students with autism spectrum disorders. *Focus on Autism and Other Developmental Disabilities, 18*, 150–166.

Jahng, K. H., Martin, L. R., Golin, C. E., & DiMatteo, M. R. (2005). Preferences for medical collaboration: Patient-physician congruence and patient outcomes. *Patient Education and Counseling, 57*, 308–314.

Kendall, P. C., & Beidas, R. S. (2007). Smoothing the trail for dissemination of evidence-based practices for youth: Flexibility within fidelity. *Professional Psychology: Research and Practice, 38*, 13–20.

Lotter, V. (1974). Factors related to outcome in autistic children. *Journal of Autism and Childhood Schizophrenia, 4*, 263–277.

Luyster, R. J., Kadlec, M. B., Carter, A., & Tager-Flusberg, H. (2008). Language assessment and development in toddlers with autism spectrum disorders. *Journal of Autism and Developmental Disorders, 38*, 1426–1438.

McDuffie, A., Yoder, P., & Stone, W. (2005). Prelinguistic predictors of vocabulary in young children with autism spectrum disorders. *Journal of Speech, Language, and Hearing Research, 48*, 1080–1097.

McEachin, J. J., Smith, T., & Lovaas, O. I. (1993). Long-term outcome for children who received early intensive behavioral treatment. *American Journal on Mental Retardation, 97*, 359–372.

Mundy, P., Sigman, M., Ungerer, J., & Sherman, T. (1987). Nonverbal communication and play correlates of language development in autistic children. *Journal of Autism and Developmental Disorders, 17*, 349–364.

National Research Council. (2001). *Educating children with autism. Committee on Educational Interventions for Children with Autism. Division of Behavioral and Social Sciences and Education.* Washington, DC: National Academy Press.

Onion, C. W. R., Dutton, C. E., Walley, T., & Turnbull, C. J. (1996). Local clinical guidelines: Description and evaluation of a participative method for their development and implementation. *Family Practice, 13*, 28–34.

Ramey, C. T., & Ramey, S. L. (1998). Early intervention and early experience. *American Psychologist, 53*, 109–120.

Rogers, S. (1996). Brief report: Early intervention in autism. *Journal of Autism and Developmental Disorders, 26*, 207–214.

Ruef, M. B., Turnbull, A. P., Turnbull, H. R., & Poston, D. (1999). Perspectives of five stakeholder groups: Challenging behavior of individuals with mental retardation and/or autism. *Journal of Positive Behavior Interventions, 1*, 43–58.

Rutherford, M. D., Young, G. S., Hepburn, S., & Rogers, S. J. (2007). A longitudinal study of pretend play in autism. *Journal of Autism and Developmental Disorders, 37*, 1024–1039.

Sackett, D., Richardson, W. S., Rosenberg, W., Haynes, R., & Strauss, S. (1997). *Evidence-based medicine: How to practice and teach EBM*. New York: Churchill Livingstone.

Sallows, G. O., & Graupner, T. D. (2005). Intensive behavioral treatment for children autism: Four-year outcome and predictors. *American Journal on Mental Retardation, 2005*, 417–438.

Schalock, R. L., & Luckasson, R. (2005). *Clinical judgment.* Washington, DC: American Association on Mental Retardation.

Schreibman, L. (1988). *Autism.* Newbury Park: SAGE publications.

Schreibman, L. (1996). Brief report: The case for social and behavioral intervention research. *Journal of Autism and Developmetal Disorders, 26*, 247–251.

Schreibman, L. (2000). Intensive behavioral/psychoeducational treatment for autism: Research needs and future directions. *Journal of Autism and Developmental Disorders, 30*, 373–378.

Schreibman, L. (2005). *The science and fiction of autism.* Cambridge, MA: Harvard University Press.

Schreibman, L., Stahmer, A. C., Cestone-Bartlet, V., & Dufek, S. (2009). Brief report: Toward refinement of a predictive behavioral profile for treatment outcome in children with autism. *Research in Autism Spectrum Disorders, 3*, 163–172.

Sheinkophf, S. J., & Siegel, B. (1998). Home-base behavioral treatment of young children with autism. *Journal of Autism and Developmental Disorders, 28*, 15–23.

Sherer, M. R., & Schreibman, L. (2005). Individual behavioral profiles and predictors of treatment effectiveness for children with autism. *Journal of Consulting and Clinical Psychology, 73*, 525–538.

Sigman, M., & McGovern, C. W. (2005). Improvement in cognitive and language skills from preschool to adolescence in autism. *Journal of Autism and Developmental Disorders, 35*, 15–23.

Sigman, M., & Ruskin, E. (1999). Continuity and change in the social competence of children with autism, Down syndrome, and developmental delays. *Monographs of the Society for Research in Child Development, 64*, 1–10.

Sigman, M., Spence, S. J., & Wang, A. T. (2000). Autism from developmental and neuropsychological perspectives. *Annual Review of Clinical Psychology, 2*, 327–355.

Singh, N. N., Lancioni, G. E., Winton, A. S. W., Fisher, B. C., Wahler, R. G., & McAleavey, K. (2006). Mindful parenting decreases aggression, noncompliance, and self-injury in children with autism. *Journal of Emotional and Behavioral Disorders, 14*, 169–177.

Smith, T. (1999). Outcome of early intervention for children with autism. *Clinical Psychology: Science, and Practice, 6*, 33–48.

Smith, T., Eikeseth, S., Klevstrand, M., & Lovaas, O. I. (1997). Intensive behavioral treatment for preschoolers with severe mental retardation and pervasive developmental disorder. *American Journal on Mental Retardation, 102*, 238–249.

Smith, T., Groen, A. D., & Wynn, J. W. (2000). Randomized trial of intensive early intervention for children with pervasive developmental disorder. *American Journal of Mental Retardation, 105*, 269–285.

Smith, T., & Magyar, C. (2003). Behavioral assessment and treatment. In E. Hollander (Ed.), *Autism Spectrum Disorders* (pp. 369–382). Basel, NY: Marcel Dekker, Inc.

Southam-Gerow, M. A. (2004). Some reasons that mental health treatments are not technologies: Toward treatment development and adaptation outside labs. *Clinical Psychology: Science and Practice, 11*, 186–189.

Stahmer, A. C., Collings, N. M., & Palinkas, L. A. (2005). Early intervention practices for children with autism: Descriptions from community providers. *Focus on Autism and Other Developmental Disabilities, 20*, 66–79.

Stahmer, A. C., & Gist, K. (2001). The effects of an accelerated parent education program on technique mastery and child outcome. *Journal of Positive Behavior Interventions, 3*, 75–82.

Stevens, M. C., Fein, D. A., Dunn, M., Allen, D., Waterhouse, L. H., Feinstein, C., et al. (2000). Subgroups of children with autism by cluster analysis: A longitudinal examination. *Journal of the American Academy of Child and Adolescent Psychiatry, 39*, 346–352.

Stone, W. L., Ousley, O. Y., & Littleford, C. D. (1997). Motor imitation in young children with autism: What's the object? *Journal of Abnormal Child Psychology, 25*, 475–485.

Sutera, S., Pandey, J., Esser, E. E., Rosenthal, M. A., Wislon, L. B., Barton, M., et al. (2007). Predictors of optimal outcome in toddlers diagnosed with autism spectrum disorders. *Journal of Autism and Developmental Disorders, 37*, 98–107.

Tager-Flusberg, H., Paul, R., & Lord, C. (2005). Language and communication in autism. In D. Cohen & F. Volkmar (Eds.), *Handbook of autism and pervasive developmental disorders* (3rd ed., vol. 1, pp. 335–364). New Jersey: Wiley.

Thurm, A., Lord, C., Lee, L., & Newschaffer, C. (2007). Predictors of language acquisition in preschool children with autism spectrum disorders. *Journal of Autism and Developmental Disorders, 37*, 1721–1734.

Toth, K., Munson, J., Meltzoff, A. N., & Dawson, G. (2006). Early predictors of communication development in young children with autism spectrum disorder: Joint attention, imitation, and toy play. *Journal of Autism and Developmental Disorders, 36*, 993–1005.

Van Hecke, A. V., Mundy, P. C., Acra, C. F., Block, J. J., Delgado, C. E. F., Parlade, M. V., et al. (2007). Infant joint attention, temperament, and social competence in preschool children. *Child Development, 78*, 53–65.

Ventner, A., Lord, C., & Schopler, E. (1992). A follow-up study of high-functioning autistic children. *Journal of Child Psychology and Psychiatry, 33*, 489–507.

Walrath, C. M., Sheehan, A. K., Holden, E. W., Hernandez, M., & Blau, G. M. (2006). Evidence-based treatments in the field: A brief report on provider knowledge, implementation, and practice. *Journal of Behavioral Health Services & Research, 33*, 244–253.

Webster-Stratton, C. (1985). The effects of father involvement in parent training for conduct problem children. *Journal of Child Psychology and Psychiatry, 26*, 801–810.

Weiss, M. J. (1999). Differential rates of skill acquisition and outcomes of early intensive behavioral intervention for autism. *Behavioral Interventions, 14*, 3–22.

Weisz, J. R., Donenberg, G. R., Han, S. S., & Weiss, B. (1995). Bridging the gap between laboratory and clinic in child and adolescent psychotherapy. *Journal of Consulting and Clinical Psychology, 63*, 688–701.

Weisz, J. R., & Jensen, A. L. (2001). Child and adolescent psychotherapy in research and practice contexts: Review of the evidence and suggestions for improving the field. *European Child & Adolescent Psychiatry, 10*, 112–118.

Weisz, J. R., Weiss, B., & Donenberg, G. R. (1992). The lab versus the clinic: Effects of child and adolescent psychotherapy. *American Psychologist, 47*, 1578–1585.

Winter, J. (2006). Father involvement in parent training interventions for children with autism: Effects of tailoring treatment to meet the unique needs of fathers. *Dissertation Abstracts International, 67*(03), 1751B.

Yoder, P., & Comptom, D. (2004). Identifying predictors of treatment response. *Mental Retardation and Developmental Disabilities Research Reviews, 10*, 162–168.

Yoder, P., & Stone, W. L. (2006a). A randomized comparison of the effect of two prelinguistic communication intervention on the acquisition of spoken communication in preschoolers with ASD. *Journal of Speech, Language, and Hearing Research, 49*, 698–711.

Yoder, P., & Stone, W. L. (2006b). Randomized comparison of two communication interventions for preschoolers with autism spectrum disorders. *Journal of Consulting and Clinical Psychology, 74*, 426–435.

Identifying Fad Therapies for Autism Spectrum Disorders and Promoting Effective Treatment

Jenny E. Tuzikow and Steve Holburn

The prevalence of autism continues to rise every year. Recently, the results of a 2006 surveillance survey conducted by the Autism and Developmental Disabilities Monitoring Network were released by the Center for Disease Control (CDC, 2009). It was estimated that 1 in 70 boys and 1 in 315 girls in the United States are diagnosed with an ASD (CDC, 2009). The increase in the prevalence of autism is astounding, as is the responsibility placed on parents and professionals to identify effective treatments for individuals with autism. Although the increasing rates of autism are staggering, the desperation of families to find the right treatment for their children can be overwhelming. This sense of urgency can increase parents' susceptibility to embracing fad treatments.

The intent of this chapter is to refine the reader's understanding of fads and the implications of adhering to them. Throughout this chapter we refer to a fad as a popular, but usually short-lived, practice in a given culture. We consider a fad in the treatment of autism and pervasive developmental disorders to be a technique or an approach that is over-promoted in relation to its credibility. The credibility of the approach refers to the extent to which the approach has been confirmed to be therapeutically effective using traditional scientific research methodology. Unproven methods are not necessarily fads, particularly if they are consistent with contemporary concepts and theory, but the determination of their validity rests on the measurability of their outcomes and the replicability of their procedures.

Ethical Considerations

Although there is controversy with regard to what constitutes a fad and what does not, one similarity between fads and evidence-based treatments is that the providers of both claim to be competent in their specialty areas and claim to provide effective treatments. Every fad included in this chapter was developed by professionals who have obtained certification or licensure requirements to practice in the United States. Although the professionals have met the requirements to practice, it is critical to note that the licensing agencies only designate that they are qualified. The licensing boards do not always dictate which types of therapy the practitioners are permitted to conduct.

Competent Practitioners

This brings us to the issue of competence. In order to practice in an ethical manner, one must be competent. Ghezzi and Rehfeldt (1994) addressed the issue of competence and indicated that competence is a judgment of a person's abilities and these judgments of competence are relative. In addition, the concept of competence depends on the advancements in the profession and cultural beliefs about the expectations of the profession (Ghezzi & Rehfeldt, 1994). Therefore, although licensing boards have established criteria for competence, public opinion is an integral part of attributing competence to a service provider. It is unrealistic to expect the public to assess the competence of professionals using fair and systematic criteria, yet it is this lack of a gold standard that enables providers of fads to profit and to continue to promote unsubstantiated theories and treatments.

Effective Treatments

In addition to considering the provider's level of competence when a treatment is selected, the effectiveness of that

J.E. Tuzikow (✉)
Institute for Basic Research in Developmental Disabilities, Staten Island, NY 10314, USA
e-mail: jtuzikow@gmail.com

The views expressed in this chapter do not necessarily reflect the policies of the supporting organizations.

J.L. Matson, P. Sturmey (eds.), *International Handbook of Autism and Pervasive Developmental Disorders*, Autism and Child Psychopathology Series, DOI 10.1007/978-1-4419-8065-6_19, © Springer Science+Business Media, LLC 2011

treatment is also taken into account. Van Houten discussed the rights of clients when receiving behavior analysis services and stated that "the client has the right to the most effective behavior treatment available" (Van Houten, 1994, p. 115). In his review, Van Houten (1994) described the criteria that behavior analysts must meet to determine if a prescribed intervention is the most effective intervention. Although Van Houten's (1994) discussion primarily pertains to behavior analysis, he emphasized the concept of efficacy. While advocating for the effective treatment of individuals through behavior analysis, he encouraged the reader to consider the lack of evidence of other treatment modalities and to demand to see evidence that other treatments are also effective prior to supporting them (Van Houten, 1994).

Concerns about identifying effective treatments apply to all theoretical perspectives and are not solely a concern of behavior analysts. For example, advocates of sensory integration therapy (Schaaf & Miller, 2005) shared this view and indicated that it is the occupational therapists' responsibility to "assure that therapy is helping the child become more functional in their daily life activities" (p. 144). Although different treatments may have the same goals, it is critical that parents select efficacious therapies so that their children will actually meet the goals that they are working toward. This occurs when parents select evidence-based treatments.

Identifying Fad Treatments

Unwitting Promoters of Fad Interventions

An accurate determination of the veracity of a treatment for ASD is a scientific undertaking, which does not always necessitate a complex analysis. Implementation of the treatment rests on the professional credentials of the implementer, which in turn are based on a demonstration of competence and ethical guidelines, and the efficacy of the modality, as discussed earlier. Accordingly, parents of individuals with ASD are less able to make an accurate determination of treatment veracity, unless they understand the empirical principles on which an accurate determination of a treatment rests. Thus, it is the parents and other family members of an individual who tend to be the most vulnerable to fad remedies and misinformation. In a discussion of effective interventions for autism, G. Green (1996) cautioned, "Despite the evidence, families with young autistic children are often told incorrectly that all treatments are equally effective or, even more inaccurately, that behavioral intervention is ineffective or harmful" (p. 29). A discussion of parent susceptibility to fad interventions was provided by Metz, Mulick and Butter (2005), who posit reasons such as desperation, guilt, lack of knowledge, and excessive sources of information.

Another group, whose members are likely to misidentify a fad as a valid treatment, is that of semi-professional practitioners who lack the knowledge and skills to appropriately comprehend research methodology (Greenspan, 2005; Metz et al., 2005). Such practitioners might be inclined to make clinical decisions based on information from workshops, how-to resources, and collegial discussion, rather than on relevant research findings (Blanton, 2000).

We would add that many practitioners incorrectly assume that the effectiveness of a given therapy depends principally on the extent of adherence to the stated procedures of the therapy, rather than the research supporting that therapy. In this case, a practitioner might be susceptible to the faulty reasoning that a fad therapy did not work because it was not conducted properly.

This is not to say that treatment integrity is unimportant; indeed, it is critical to faithfully implement a method that has been demonstrated to be effective. Any legitimate treatment, including applied behavior analysis, can be misapplied. Indeed, there are plenty of practitioners who claim to be conducting behavior analysis in individuals with ASD but in fact are not applying the methods correctly (Sturmey, 2005a). Dawson (2001) contends that there are many unqualified therapists marketing themselves as applied behavior analysts, many of whom do not even grasp basic behavior analytic methods, and when the therapy fails, the parents or the child is blamed.

A third group of individuals that can be at risk of unwittingly promoting an unverified treatment for ASD is medical practitioners. Most medical practitioners are not experts in ASD, and outside of the use of Abilify and Risperdal [Food and Drug Administration (FDA), 2009], there are no verified health-based treatments for ASD; although some have questioned whether it is possible to conduct double-blind trials of a medication with characteristic side effects that might easily break the blind (Singh, Matson, Cooper, Dixon, & Sturmey, 2005). Nonetheless, parents and semi-professional practitioners often defer to these professionals with respect to ASD because of their stature in the health field and their early contact with the child with an ASD. Medical practitioners often employ a multiple-intervention approach to a health problem such that diet, medication, and other physically oriented therapies may be prescribed together as a broad-based approach. This shotgun approach is intuitively attractive and consistent with the notion that "It can't hurt to try everything" and "What do you have to lose?" (G. Green, 1996; Holburn, 2007). According to the Web site, Interactive Autism Network (2008), individuals with ASD are experiencing 400 different treatments; however, for ASD, the try-everything approach is detrimental because it can lure victims away from effective treatment. Multiple simultaneous interventions to treat ASD have both empirical and therapeutic shortcomings in that they can mask or dilute the effects of a valid therapy (Holburn, 2008).

We are not suggesting here that all parents, semi-professional practitioners, and physicians unknowingly promote ineffective treatments for ASD; rather, we believe that individuals in these groups can be subject to influences that might overpower the empirical principles that guide accurate determination of a treatment effectiveness and faithful implementation of a given therapeutic approach. There are countless other therapists, consultants, parents, and media personalities who unwittingly promote illegitimate remedies. Thus, a great deal of misinformation is spread by unsuspecting victims who believe in the approaches and share them with others, although most people believe that such remedies are promoted by charlatans who intentionally exploit others (Barrett, 2009).

Hallmarks of a Credible Intervention

There are many ways to spot a fad treatment designed to remedy or ameliorate autism spectrum disorder. One general approach is to compare the approach with the hallmarks of what is traditionally considered to be a credible therapeutic procedure. In other words, with today's myriad of available therapies and other interventions purporting to treat autism, how can one identify a legitimate one? Three considerations noted here are (a) the qualifications of the therapist, (b) the research history of the approach, and (c) the nature of the treatment plan. First, a valid procedure is carried out by a practitioner with professionally recognized credentials and training experience. Many fad providers claim that they have experience in a particular area or specialty; however their training was actually not specialized or with a different population.

With respect to the treatment itself, the validity or the effectiveness of the intervention will have been determined through rigorous standards of scientific practice. Thus, the approach will have a history of analysis and replication that can be found in peer-reviewed journals. In addition, the assumptions and methods of the intervention are theoretically plausible; they tend to be consistent with and build upon other bodies of knowledge. In short, the approach is evidence based and contributes to an existing foundation of knowledge about successful treatment for a given condition.

The last consideration, the treatment plan for a credible approach, can be distinguished in a number of ways. For one, the plan should directly address the symptoms of ASD, including any deficits in social interaction, repetitive behavior, and communication. It does not attempt to remedy a hypothesized internal cause of the disorder (Holburn, 2005), such as malfunctioning neural pathways in the brain (McGee, 1987). In addition, intensive early intervention and

parent training are considered critical (Kabot, Masi, & Segal, 2003), as is the convergence of services and supports to assist the child in a manner consistent with the characteristics of a credible treatment plan.

Insufficient Empirical Support

Perhaps the most distinctive characteristic of a fad for ASD is the absence of scientific validation of the procedure. Unfortunately, while this shortcoming is obvious to many readers of this volume, it may not be so clear to the many practitioners, family members, and policy makers whose perspectives are swayed by more seductive arguments, some of which are blatantly antiscientific. For example, Newsome and Hovenitz (2005) point to postmodernist philosophies as having threatened the scientific tenets undergirding progress in developmental services today. Here, where science is portrayed as an oppressive and hopeless quest; where realities are socially constructed and multiple voices are weighed equally, a variety of colorful and interesting solutions to ASD can be proffered. Of course, fad victims need not understand postmodernism to be persuaded by a fad. News of sudden breakthroughs, accidental discoveries, and heartwarming cures can eclipse the persuasions of applied science.

Fad therapies for ASD have little or no well-conducted experimental support. Research, if conducted at all, tends to use subjective, qualitative assessment such as field notes, testimonials, interviews, anecdotes, and stories. Empirical therapeutic research, on the other hand, relies on quantifiable outcomes based on observation, observer agreement, and sound experimental design. Fad therapy research investigations also suffer from poor treatment integrity. The procedures are usually too vague to be reproduced and therefore unverifiable as effective treatments. In contrast, empirical research procedures are carefully described so that they can be replicated and failures are studied closely. Failures of a fad tend to be concealed or explained away. Thus, there is no call for outcome measurement precision or accuracy of treatment implementation with fads.

Strategically, technical information about fads is aimed toward the general public rather than the professional or scientific community. The popularity of the fad grows by advertising, Internet sites, and word of mouth. Advances in scientific knowledge are communicated through professional journals and conferences, and they are ponderous by comparison. In this respect, science is at a disadvantage. The healthy skepticism of the scientist cannot compete with the optimistic appeal of the fad promoter. While the scientist is calling for more research, the fad promoter is touting the benefits of the fad, and the latter is often more appealing to the public. When pressed for data, the fad promoter may claim that studies are underway and that preliminary results look promising, even though the technique is so obviously ineffective that further study is really not necessary.

Common Characteristics of a Fad for ASD

To a researcher, the principal identifier of a fad in ASD is insufficient empirical support with the telltale signs of anecdotes, stories, and testimonials as evidence for outcomes; however, the most salient characteristic of a fad remedy for ASD is that it is an unusual or a non-traditional approach. While this characteristic might be another red flag for a knowledgeable professional, it matters little to a parent desperate for a solution. Thus, the fad can represent a breakthrough or cure that was not discovered through science and this can be said to make the fad immune from scientific analysis. Instead, the fad can be based on an ideology or a belief system. For an ideologically based fad, non-believers are said to disrupt the therapeutic process. For example, during the facilitated communication (FC) craze in the early 1990s, the second author was unable to evoke facilitated typing from individuals with no known communication abilities, but several other staff members were finding that these same individuals were able to type complex sentences and even poetry using this technique. The successful staff members were said to be believers who were able to bond with the person and understand his or her true capacities and worth. Those who were unsuccessful were often accused of not accepting the person as an equal, a disparity that was easily detected by the individual, who in turn could not trust the unsuccessful ones and simply failed to cooperate. Some who were unsuccessful were accused of not appreciating the full potential of the person, and in some instances, they were accused of abusing the person.

The operative ideological position in the case of FC seemed to be that if one believed that individuals with intellectual disabilities had the same capacity and value as others in society, then one would likely be successful at FC. Closely related to the common requirement to be a true believer is the need to think positively about the veracity of the treatment and the benefit that should accrue. Sometimes mind over matter is said to be necessary for a fad treatment to be successful. In any case, when the fad fails to produce the desired outcome of an ideologically driven fad intervention, the culpability is shifted from the failed treatment to the failure of the implementer to hold the proper complementary ideological position.

Some fad treatments are characterized as remedies that are natural and safe, including "... dietary interventions, detoxification and supplement therapies...," and that describe "safe chelation and detoxification for children" (Nichols, 2009, p. 1); however, so-called safe therapies such as chelation have been found to be dangerous, even resulting in death

(see Tsouderos & Callahan, 2009). Herbal and homeopathic remedies, including highly diluted mineral products such as "biochemic tissue salt combinations," are used as natural treatments for autism (Native Remedies, 2009). Nutritional supplements and special diets are commonly prescribed for individuals with ASD. In a survey study by V. A. Green et al. (2006), 27% of parents were implementing special diets and 43% were using vitamin supplements. One particularly unusual herbal remedy for people with ASD is called "tantrum tamer." This herb "dissolves easily in the mouth" and "can greatly reduce or eliminate distressing and hard to handle tantrums" (Native Remedies, 2009).

Natural and safe treatments are often termed alternative treatments which often claim to treat the whole person and are not generally accepted by the scientific community whose conventional treatments rarely treat the whole person (Barrett & Hebert, 2007). In the Autism Speaks (2009) Internet Web site, four alternative therapies are described, which, to our knowledge, have no empirical support: facilitated communication, holding therapy, auditory integration therapy, and the Doman/Delacato method. In addition to highlighting environmental toxins as culpable elements, natural and alternative methods also commonly implicate standard treatments as dangerous, including many over-the-counter remedies, fluoridation, food additives, and vaccines such as the MMRI vaccination. In short, the general public can be led to feel that they are slowly being poisoned and that natural or alternative treatments can reverse the damage and restore the individual to a healthier state.

Another characteristic of fads is that they can appeal to the sense of immediacy for improvement that parents and practitioners may experience. As testified by the medical coordinator for the Autism Research Institute, "We feel some urgency that we can't wait for 10 or 20 years" (Tsouderos & Callahan, 2009, p. 2). This urgency is probably intensified with the growing reports of increased incidence of autism, and it potentiates interest in treatments for autism that promise the possibility of quick, dramatic results; however, such results typically occur when a source of a problem or an illness is known or detected and then eliminated or ameliorated. Thus, a method to treat ASD that offers rapid improvement will likely claim to attack the cause of the disorder, but for autism, the cause(s) is not yet known. The hope for rapid improvement is bolstered by enthusiastic testimony. For example, one parent described her surprise at the immediate and powerful effects of detoxifying clay baths:

What a change! Our almost 5 year old son who is on the spectrum is now doing great. After just the first bath, my husband and I saw results! He'll turn to look at us (in the eyes) after calling his name only once! He's using the right words to communicate, and in sentences!! And best of all, he's smiling and laughing, and just seems happier! (Parent Feedback, 2009)

Unfortunately, although such testimony inspires hope for rapid success and even a cure for autism, such quick fixes have not been demonstrated empirically to date. Alternatively, fad remedy promoters sometimes claim that even small effects can be greatly beneficial and that even minor effects can make a big difference in the life of the person with an ASD and the family. These effects might strain the limit of empirical detection, but they are held as justification for the fad therapy, and even small changes might reduce the feeling of desperation and urgency experienced by the parent.

Popular and Controversial Fads

In this section, we present the reader with an introduction to several fads that have gained popularity in recent years, despite having limited or no evidence-based research supporting their use for individuals with autism. Therefore, most studies that lacked experimental control or were not peer reviewed are excluded from this discussion; however, some may be mentioned simply to illustrate the point that there are several non-evidence-based treatments in use today.

Supplements and Allergies

In general, dietary interventions are believed to improve the symptoms of ASD caused by allergies or insufficient consumption of vitamins and minerals. Many individuals with autism tend to be very selective eaters and prefer to consume foods that are of a particular color, texture, or taste, and refuse to consume other foods. An example of this selective behavior is the beige diet, a preference noted in many individuals with an ASD who choose to eat only beige-colored foods such as cookies, crackers, and chicken. As a result, individuals adhering to this diet or similar diets will not meet the recommended daily intake levels of vitamins and minerals. At other times, allergies to particular foods may be an explanation for inadequate consumption of vitamins and minerals.

Herndon, DiGuiseppi, Johnson, Leiferman, and Reynolds (2009) compared the diets of children with ASD and children with typical development. Significant differences in the consumption of vitamins (B6 and E), dairy, non-dairy protein, and calcium were reported. Typically developing children consumed significantly more calcium and dairy products and less non-dairy and vitamins (B6 and E) than did children with ASD. Despite these differences indicating that the diets of children with an ASD significantly differ from the diets of typically developing children, a more suggestive finding reported was that many of the children in both groups failed to consume the daily recommended requirements of vitamins and minerals (Herndon et al., 2009).

This research addresses the need for individuals to meet their daily requirements of vitamins and minerals, regardless of whether they are typically developing or have an ASD. Vitamins and minerals may improve an individual's health, thereby improving any aspect of their overall functioning.

At this time, however, there is limited to no evidence to suggest that the administration of vitamin and mineral supplements beyond the daily recommended requirements will improve the symptoms of individuals with ASD. In fact, attempts to do so could lead to toxicity and result in adverse and potentially dangerous effects.

Gluten-Free, Casein-Free Diets

Gluten-free and casein-free (GFCF) diets have gained a great deal of popularity, especially in recent years. GFCF diets rest on the assumption that individuals with an ASD process gluten and casein proteins differently than do other individuals. Gluten is a type of protein that is found in wheat, rye, and barley; casein is a protein found in lactose and dairy products.

Based on a suspected unique processing of these proteins in the brains of individuals with ASD, it is assumed that an opiate-like influence develops within the brain, which is responsible for the behavioral symptoms of autism. It is believed that this opiate-like influence on the brain can be prevented by removing these proteins from an individual's diet.

We identified two recent comprehensive reviews pertaining to the efficacy of GFCF diets for children with ASD. One study, Millward, Ferriter, Calver, and Connell-Jones (2008), reviewed eight major databases to identify studies that examined the efficacy of gluten-free and casein-free diets. After a thorough review, they concluded that the available evidence for the effectiveness of GFCF diets was lacking and continued studies were needed to gain a better understanding of the impact that GFCF diets have on individuals with ASD (Millward et al., 2008).

Elder et al. (2006) performed a double-blind repeated measure crossover design assessing the efficacy of the GFCF diet in 15 children. Their results showed that GFCF diets were not effective in ameliorating the symptoms of autism. A surprising additional finding was that over half of the parents decided to continue their children on the diet after being informed that there was no evidence that the diet improved their children's behaviors (Elder et al., 2006).

More recently, Buie et al. (2010) released a consensus report based on the research and recommendations of 28 experts in the medical and mental health fields pertaining to issues related to gastrointestinal disorders in individuals with

ASD. The panel reviewed available evidence-based research and concluded that "available research data do not support the use of a casein-free diet, a gluten-free diet, or combined gluten-free, casein-free (GFCF) diet as a primary treatment for individuals with ASD" (Buie et al., 2010, p. 10). Buie et al. (2010) commented that additional research is needed to determine if restrictive diets may be beneficial in improving the behavioral symptoms of individuals with ASD. The authors suggested that if restrictive diets are beneficial, they may be beneficial only to a particular subgroup of individuals with ASD (Buie et al., 2010).

It is also important to note that it is critical that all individuals on GFCF diets be monitored by medical professionals to ensure that their nutritional needs are being met. Eliminating wheat and dairy from an individual's diet may not only result in the deprivation of preferred foods and the obligation to take supplements but also an inadequate intake of the vitamins and minerals that are necessary for healthy development. For example, Hediger et al. (2008) found that boys with an ASD who adhered to a casein-free diet between the ages of 4 and 8 years of age may be more susceptible to reduced rates of appositional bone growth. It is necessary to consider if these potential side effects are worth implementing an unvalidated treatment.

Secretin

Secretin is a hormone produced by the intestine that aids in digestion. It has been believed to effectively treat the gastrointestinal and behavioral problems of individuals with autism. Levy and Hyman (2005) reported that the initial wave of excitement pertaining to secretin as a potentially effective treatment occurred in 1998 after Horvath et al. presented clinical observations of secretin successfully being used to treat gastrointestinal and behavioral symptoms of three children with autism. Parents and professionals were eager to learn of the possibility that secretin could be the missing clue in the mystery of autism and began to advocate for additional research studying the use of secretin for children with autism. Many secretin studies followed.

In 1999, Sandler et al. examined the effects of synthetic human secretin and failed to identify significant improvements in ASD symptoms. The same conclusion was reached by Owley et al. (2001) and Handon and Hofkosh (2005) when they assessed the efficacy of porcine secretin. Despite this evidence, parents continued to question the efficacy of secretin. In 2005, Handon and Hofkosh reported that their motivation for conducting the study was partially due to the pressure that they received from families to respond to questions regarding the effectiveness of secretin. During the same year, Sturmey (2005b) conducted a comprehensive review of 15 double-blind randomized controlled trials examining the

effectiveness of secretin in reducing symptoms of ASD and reconfirmed that secretin was ineffective in treating autism. An independent review of the same studies also reached the same conclusions (Esch & Carr, 2004).

The use of secretin in the treatment of ASD presents several significant concerns. Marie Bristol-Power, the National Institute of Child Health and Human Development (NICHD) special assistant for autism programs, reported that the use of secretin from swine could result in an allergic reaction (NICHD, 1999). While the FDA has approved the use of secretin for the purposes of identifying gastrointestinal problems, it has not approved secretin as an effective treatment for autism. Furthermore, it has not been thoroughly tested on the pediatric population for potential harmful side effects.

Facilitated Communication

FC is a technique that was developed by Crossley (Crossley & McDonald, 1980) and often associated with Biklen (1990). It is used to teach individuals with limited communication skills to communicate with the assistance of a facilitator, a person who physically assists the individual to type or write for the purpose of communicating with others. The facilitator guides the individual's arm, hand, or finger to type on a device to communicate with others. The facilitator's goal is to eventually fade their support, thereby allowing the individual to communicate independently. A major concern with this approach is that the facilitators appear to be communicating instead of the individual (Jacobson, Mulick, & Schwartz, 1995). In 2001, Mostert conducted a review of 29 published studies on FC and found a negative correlation between the degree of experimental control procedures and the effectiveness of FC reported. Hence, the higher the levels of experimental control employed, the less the FC concluded to be effective.

Mostert (2001) recommended that future studies examining the effectiveness of FC include these methodological characteristics: larger sample sizes, control groups, severity of the participants' disorders, examination of the intensity of support provided and influence of the facilitator, and an evaluation of the maintenance of communication skills. Following Mostert's (2001) recommendations, researchers attempting to conduct experimentally sound studies continued to have difficulty showing that FC was effective for individuals with autism. Four years later, Jacobson, Foxx, and Mulick (2005) reviewed additional FC studies and it was again concluded that the facilitators, not the communicators, were responsible for the communication that occurred during FC in practically all experimentally controlled studies.

The rationale behind FC is intriguing and appealing to parents because it enables them to believe that their children may have the opportunity to communicate their wants and needs. It may be the first time a parent is told that their child will be able to share their thoughts and feelings with their family and therefore parents may begin to believe that FC will work for their child. Unfortunately, the experimentally controlled studies available suggest that FC is an ineffective strategy for teaching communication to individuals with autism, and it is critical that parents and educators devote their time and energy to other communication strategies that have evidence-based support. Jacobson et al. (2005) address the nature and appeal of FC by stating:

> FC could be viewed as an important phenomenon because of how the movement to support FC resists disconfirmation of any nature, from any source, at any time, and exemplifies the enormous waste of time, money, and human resources that such fad and bogus treatments and interventions represent (p. 379).

Jacobson et al. (2005) provide an accurate assessment of the nature of FC and it is essential that potential consumers of FC begin to question its efficacy and practitioners voice their concerns. As recently as 2009, a bill was introduced to the Massachusetts legislature requesting that teachers be mandated to receive training in FC. It also reported that FC is a legitimate treatment for students with disabilities (S. 223, 2009). Despite the preponderance of research suggesting otherwise, an unfortunate number of consumers and providers believe FC is effective and continue to promote this fad.

Sensory Integration Therapy

Sensory integration therapy (SIT) was formulated based on the theory proposed by Ayres (1972). Schaaf and Miller (2005) reported that the tenets of this theory rest on the understanding that disorganized neural processing of sensory input results in difficulties in performing adaptive behaviors. The three sensory systems targeted for intervention include the vestibular, tactile, and proprioceptive systems. The vestibular system integrates sensory input from the vestibular organs, eyes, and muscles, and allows a person to maintain balance and understand where they are in space. The tactile system coordinates sensory input through the sense of touch and disintegration of the tactile system is sometimes evidenced as tactile defensiveness. The proprioceptive system integrates sensory input received through muscles and joints. It is believed that sensory difficulties are due to a dysfunction in one or all three of these systems. Sensory integration therapy involves creating sensory experiences that are designed to meet an individual's needs and to then continue to challenge his or her needs to develop more advanced neural processing. Examples of these experiences include carrying heavy objects, swinging, playing with different textured materials, and using a vibrating massager.

Green (1996) discusses concerns related to how some of the activities used in SIT are inherently enjoyable. Since many SIT activities are enjoyable, evaluators need to recognize that an individual may appear to enjoy an activity simply because the activity is fun. In reality, that activity may have no impact on an individual's symptoms of ASD. In addition, Smith, Mruzek, and Mozingo (2005) reviewed studies assessing the efficacy of SIT (Dura, Mulick, & Hammer, 1988; Mason & Iwata, 1990). Smith et al. (2005) concluded that the available studies failed to show that SIT was effective in reducing the symptoms of ASD. A recent review of the effectiveness of weighted vests for reducing the symptoms of ASD was conducted by Stephenson and Carter (2009). They concluded that although additional research may be warranted, the results of the review indicated that weighted vests were not effective in reducing the symptoms of ASD (Stephenson & Carter, 2009).

While advocates of SIT do acknowledge that there are limitations to the approach, they report that this is the result of the limited research available, due to a "lack of funding, paucity of doctorate trained clinicians and researchers in occupational therapy, and the inherent heterogeneity of the population of children affected by sensory integrative dysfunction" (Schaaf & Miller, 2005, p. 143); however, at this time, based on the above noted research studies, it appears that the actual limitation to the approach is the lack of proven effectiveness, not funding.

Auditory Integration Training

Auditory integration training (AIT) was developed by Berard, an ear, nose, and throat doctor in the early 1990s (Berard, 2006). Similar to SIT, AIT also posits disorganization of an individual's ability to process information; however, instead of focusing on neural processing, AIT focuses on auditory processing. The belief is that when individuals organize their auditory processing abilities, they will become more receptive to other therapies (AIT Institute, 2010). AIT is an intensive procedure that involves listening to particular frequencies to ostensibly retrain the acoustical reflex muscle (AIT Institute, 2010). Then, once hearing is retrained, individuals with ASD will become less sensitive to particular sounds in their environment and a reduction in sound distortion will be evident. In order to achieve these goals, the individuals must adhere to a protocol that requires them to listen to 30 min of music or sounds at specified frequencies and volumes twice daily over the course of 10 days. Despite these requirements, AIT evidences several perceived advantages over other fads. The parent is permitted to remain with the child during the treatment sessions, the child is not required to take medications or supplements, and it has a clear time commitment. These treatment characteristics can be appealing to parents; however, another factor should discourage parents, the lack of conclusive evidence supporting AIT.

Although several studies have suggested beneficial results (Edelson et al., 1999; Rimland & Edelson, 1995, 1994), the methodological and statistical procedures employed in these studies have been reported to be highly controversial and flawed. As a result, the positive findings have not been widely accepted by the scientific community (Goldstein, 2000; Mudford & Cullen, 2005). Mudford and Cullen (2005) reviewed three additional studies evaluating the efficacy of AIT. The outcomes indicated that either AIT was ineffective in improving the behaviors of individuals with ASD or the reported behavior changes were due to the influence of repeated behavior rating scales, not AIT (Bettison, 1996; Mudford et al., 2000; Zollweg, Palm, & Vance, 1997). Mudford and Cullen (2005) suggest that parents who are considering utilizing AIT to improve their children's behaviors should reconsider in light of the lack of valid evidence supporting AIT.

Hyperbaric Oxygen Treatment

Hyperbaric oxygen therapy (HBOT) is "a specialized therapy that uses an increase in atmospheric pressure to allow the body to incorporate more oxygen into blood cells, blood plasma, cerebral-spinal fluid, and other body fluids" [The International Hyperbarics Association (IHA), 2004, para. 3]. It is believed that this release of oxygen assists in healing injured tissues (IHA, 2004). Hyperbaric oxygen therapy is used for numerous illnesses and injuries, and the number and the duration of treatment sessions are individualized for each patient based on their doctor's recommendations (IHA, 2004).

Unfortunately, there is a paucity of controlled studies that assess the effectiveness of HBOT in children with autism (Granpeesheh et al., 2009; Rossignol et al., 2009). Granpeesheh et al. (2009) performed a double-blind, placebo-controlled trial designed to assess the efficacy of HBOT for treating children with ASD. HBOT failed to produce significant differences in the behaviors of children when delivered at 24% oxygen and 1.3 atmospheric pressure (Granpeesheh et al., 2009). Rossignol et al. (2009) also delivered 24% oxygen at 1.3 atmospheric pressure. Again, no significant differences in changes in behaviors between the control and treatment groups were found (Rossignol et al., 2009). Results from this study indicated that all children appeared to improve simply through inclusion in the study (Rossignol et al., 2009). At the present time, conclusive evidence supporting the use of hyperbaric oxygen treatment for individuals with ASD does not exist.

Chelation Therapy

Of all of the aforementioned fads, chelation therapy possesses the most harmful side effects. Chelation therapy involves the removal of metals in the body by administering a medication that binds to the metals, allowing them to be eliminated through urine and stools. Chelation has been shown to be effective in reducing excess iron in the body due to chronic transfusion therapy or lead poisoning [Center for Disease Control (CDC), 2006]. Proponents of chelation believe that the cause of autism is excess mercury and other heavy metals in the fetus. A concern with this logic is that studies have not shown that mercury causes autism, yet proponents of this belief are subjecting individuals to potentially harmful unsubstantiated treatment for ASD. Reported side effects of chelation include neutropenia, kidney damage, and liver damage, and in some cases, chelation therapy resulted in the loss of excess calcium that led to hypocalcemia and then cardiac arrest. The CDC (2006) reported three deaths that occurred due to hypocalcemia that resulted in the cardiac arrest of a 2-, a 5-, and a 53-year old. The 5-year old was being treated for autism.

The Promotion of Fads

Reviewing the aforementioned information may cause one to question why fads continue despite the contradictory evidence, potentially harmful side effects, and limited or non-existent support of the efficacy of a fad. In the following section, we discuss why fads not only continue in the face of adversity but also occasionally gain momentum.

The ASD Fad Promoter

Perhaps the greatest factor responsible for the success of a fad is the promoter's enthusiasm and self-confidence about the benefits of the fad. In short, the fad promoter can sell. In doing so, some fad promoters appear authoritative and use the language of science to sell their product (Shermer, 1997). To bolster the credibility of the method, the fad promoter often invents terms that ostensibly represent new phenomena that are central to the fad technique. Highly technical terminology that obfuscates the victim or technical apparatus that amazes the victim appears to add intelligence to authority. The resulting combination of good salesmanship and pseudoscientific procedures and evidence can persuade parents and semi-professionals to support the method and share it with others with zeal. The following excerpt exemplifies this phenomenon by blending technical language with a promise of a longed-for future:

We believe we've discovered the most innovative, unique, and superior treatment available. Our IV Lipid Membrane Therapies restore cell membrane integrity... [and]... it allows a child to, once again, become a whole person. The same becomes true of a once fragmented family, who no longer have to deal with the difficult issues they were facing. (Becker Hilton Medical Institute, n.d., p. 1)

When confronted with opposition about the lack of real research, the fad promoter has many possible counters. One is that of indignation, as demonstrated by a physician when the merits of chelation were being challenged: "I am deeply troubled by any suggestion that the medical profession should not treat the medical problems these children clearly face" (Tsouderos & Callahan, 2009, p. 8). More cerebrally, the promoter is likely to have prepared rebuttals for various challenges to the fad because he or she is likely to have heard the concerns before. The promoter might discredit research findings that do not support the fad, claiming the research is politically motivated or technically flawed. With a breakthrough, the approach might be too new to have been formally evaluated, though sometimes studies are said to be underway, or the entire scientific experimental approach may be challenged if the breakthrough turns on a new and complex theoretical construct or phenomenon that escapes the purview of scientific analysis.

Another approach is to attack conventional treatments that are promoted by "stuffy, old academics" ensconced in "stifling orthodoxy" (Aaronovitch, 2009). More appealing are the newer, out-of-the-box ideas that will counter the corrupt elitists that have acted to oppress many good methods. Here, scientific facts and conventional wisdom are not to be trusted. Applied behavior analysis is a common target because of its status as the principle validated treatment for autism. Smith (2005) pointed out how detractors claim that gains do not generalize outside of the treatment setting, but it is probably more common to hear allegations that children are bribed and punished, and that behavior analysts stifle creativity and teach children to be mindless robots.

Instead of merely trying to convince someone that a fad treatment is effective, some fad promoters will try to convert the victim. In this case, faith trumps facts. Even if a cure requires a miracle, there is hope because *miracles do happen*. When a fad is couched in a quasi-religious framework, the proclamation that science does not have all the answers can become a mantra, even though scientists do not refute that statement. The problem with faith as the operative element in a treatment is that failures can be attributed to insufficient faith, rather than an insufficient intervention. Sometimes spiritual matters blend with the paranormal in the search for unusual abilities of people with ASD. In reviewing the book *The Soul of Autism*, Rudy (2008) recommends the book to anyone who has seen a person with autism demonstrate any of the following: knowledge of existence

before birth, precognition or premonition, telepathy, animal communication, connection with a loved one in Spirit (that is, a dead loved one), apparitions (ghosts), and communion with angels. Parents and practitioners who have witnessed such phenomena in people with ASD are likely to be more persuaded by a faith-based intervention than a scientific one.

The Genesis and Promotion of a Fad Therapy for Autism

Below we have presented a scenario that depicts 10 signs of a fad as they might be presented to a parent by a fictional fad promoter. A few points are exaggerated to exemplify the signs. In the scenario, a fad practitioner discovers by chance a promising treatment and soon it is being promoted by a doctor at an institute. Note the doctor's rebuttals to a wary parent who is looking for an effective treatment for her son:

Practitioner: I tested Billy in my office last month, but this month he did much better and he seemed happier. He even looked better after he left the session.

Friend: What happened?

Practitioner: During the recent session, I think he was able to hear the building air circulation fan that is behind the wall. Can you hear it?

Friend: No

Practitioner: Neither can I. It has a very low frequency, beyond the normal human hearing range, but Billy's autism might have enabled him to detect it, and that frequency or the vibration could have altered something in his neurological system that is connected to his hearing.

Friend: Wow! You need to try this with different people with the fan on and off.

Practitioner: I think it is clear about what happened here... this could be a breakthrough, and I want to talk with his parents about this!

Two months later, a phone rings:

Dr. Charlton: Hello, this is Dr. Charlton, at the Autism Frequency Kinetic Energy (AFAKE) Institute. Can I help you?

Parent: My son has autism, and I want to know how AFAKE works and the research behind it.

Dr. Charlton: It's highly technical, but I think your son could benefit if he can hear. You see, many people with autism have a hypersensitive cochlear system that permits low frequency sound waves to transfer sound energy particles that vibrate and stimulate dormant brain cells – basically, it wakes up the real person inside. Many of my patients have been transformed through AFAKE. Can your son hear? If so we can try to remodulate his glia cell system.

Parent: Yes... I mean wait... What will this do to my son?

Dr. Charlton: That depends a lot on you. You have to commit to the process and follow AFAKE procedures. He will need to start with our 15 Hz low-modulation fan system. Almost immediately, your son can begin to show signs of higher confidence, esteem, and enjoyment. You will feel better too because you will know that you are doing everything you can for him, no matter what cost.

Parent: Of course I want to do all I can for my son. How do I know this will work? Can you show me the research on AFAKE?

Dr. Charlton: Ma'am, if we followed the usual mechanistic research route, we never would have discovered this method. Obviously, those highly researched methods don't work or you wouldn't be here. Personally, I have devoted my own life to helping children with autism. I know when something works and I don't have to quantify the benefit. Your son's life cannot be reduced to a number and I refuse to subject these kids to needless research. Many others feel the same way, including the president of the American Association of Natural Alternative Systems for Autism.

Parent: OK, so if I use the 15 Hz low-modulation fan to remodulate my son's glia cell system, how do you know when his cell system has changed? Do you look at those cells?

Dr. Charlton: You will automatically know when your son's cells wake up because his behavior will change. But you must be adept at detecting the changes because they can be subtle. We can move forward with the 10 Hz lower-modulation fan when you feel comfortable. We call this the organic shift because you and your son decide when to shift. If you trust this method, your son will sense your trust, and this will expedite his recovery. You have to be open to it. If you use this long enough it will work.

Parent: I read a research review of your method, and it concluded that there was no benefit to AFAKE.

Dr. Charlton: Of course! Those researchers' careers reflect the hierarchical, scientific dogma that constrains our sensing of other forms of knowledge. I read the same review, and the researchers had no way to measure the benefits experienced by our patients. Their research methods are based on old theories; our methods reflect new theoretical constructs.

Parent: But the researchers found that your fans did not change behavior in any way; some participants got worse.

Dr. Charlton: Of course! The researchers used the old oppressive prediction and control paradigm. People with autism are sensitive and sometimes reject experimental manipulation. In fact, that research proves my point that you need a great degree of openness and trust for AFAKE to work.

Clearly, in the scenario above, the doctor exemplified many of the tactics used by fad promoters to convince parents to partake in the fad treatment. But the point here is not to convince the reader that faddists use various tactics; rather, it is meant to exemplify the power of the conversational context in which persuasion occurs and the pressure that can be applied to a reasonable parent who might valiantly resist the appeals. Specifically, the intervention had no empirical validity, so the promoter resorted to persuasion with pseudoscientific vernacular and reference to an unsanctioned authoritative organization. There was also emotional pressure, the bandwagon ploy, and an appeal to the parent's hope for a cure. The intervention itself constituted a new and rapidly effective approach that was above scientific review. Ironically, the onus of the treatment was on the parent, who needed to believe in the intervention. In reality, a fad promoter would not likely need to use all of these ploys, but a combination of several ploys is common, as even a brief review of Internet sites for ASD demonstrates.

Why Do ASD Fads Continue?

Fad treatments for autism are profitable. The Web site Quackwatch (2009) lists 10 questionable organizations for autism, all of which are said to promote invalidated treatments. Why would so many organizations be promoting fad remedies for autism? Hundreds of Internet sites also describe a variety of unorthodox solutions to ASD. True, profit would seem to be the main motive behind the never-ending stream of colorful and creative fads for ASD, but why would victims (parents and practitioners) continue to support remedies that do not work? The contagious enthusiasm and self-confidence of the promoter that was initially inspiring cannot, by itself, maintain ineffective therapies for ASD.

Fad treatments in ASD appear to persist for a number of reasons. For one, if a treatment fails, the parent may simply try another. Indeed many parents of children with ASD subject their children to a variety of treatments for ASD, but ultimately they may give up altogether because none of the treatments were effective as promised (Holburn, 2007). These parents may be unaware of effective treatments such as ABA or lack access to it, and those who *have* heard of ABA and *do* have access might be less inclined to participate in the long-term, labor-intensive enterprise that ABA entails, especially when enticed by the myriad of available treatments offering new and rapid recovery or improvement. Another occasion in which unvalidated treatments are maintained is when the original diagnosis or prognosis may have been incorrect. In this case, the individual might have shed his ASD, not because of the treatment but because he or she was wrongly diagnosed as having ASD.

More systemically, professionals may persist in continuing to administer insufficient treatment if the standard of success has diminished. This phenomenon is consistent with Heward and Silvestri's (2005) contention that the field of special education has moved from amelioration to accommodation. When applied to individuals with ASD, this conceptual shift might entail less emphasis on teaching the skills of communication and social interaction and greater emphasis on social support, acceptance, and inclusion; however, the viability of the latter two aspirations, while critically important, *requires* the prerequisite skills of communication and social interaction, which appear to have been replaced in importance by efforts to accommodate the individual with ASD.

Obviously, a main factor governing the continuing treatments is the parent's perception on how well the treatment is working. Counterintuitively, the duration of the treatment for autism may influence the parent's view on whether or not it is effective. This finding was reported by Green (2007), who noted that the longer the parents invested their time and money into the treatment, the more favorable their impression of the effectiveness. In other words, longer term doses of treatments, whether they were effective or not, resulted in positive assessments of the treatment effectiveness. We suspect that cognitive dissonance is operating here, which gives rise to tautological-like speculation that a factor in continuing a fad therapy is the length of time the parent commits to that therapy.

A final reason why ineffective treatments continue to flourish is that not enough professionals speak out about them. According to Greenspan (2005), intelligent professionals are simply not using critical judgment or they are reluctant to share their concerns and alienate families. Given the potential profiting for fad treatments in ASD and the psychological factors maintaining parents' interest in them, we need to find ways to hold practitioners who continue to implement ineffective treatments to a higher standard of proof. This standard, while limiting wasted time and money, is the basis for continuing to improve our existing treatments that have been empirically validated. Although parents are the identified consumers and monetary providers that partially enable fad providers, the professionals are responsible for debunking these fads and informing the consumers of the potential risks and benefits associated with these fads. If parents are not adequately informed, how can the professional community question their decisions? Offit (2008) included the following excerpt from the physicist Robert Park in his book *Autism's False Prophets*:

> While forever bemoaning general scientific literacy, scientists suddenly turn shy when given an opportunity to help educate the public by exposing some preposterous claim. If they comment at all, their words are often so burdened with qualifiers that it appears that nothing can ever be known for sure.

We believe that this excerpt is a testimony to the need for more scientists to vocalize their concerns about unvalidated treatments. It is essential that treatments are based on scientific evidence and not on anecdotal reports, preliminary results, or unsubstantiated findings.

Conclusion

In this chapter we have discussed the role that fads play in our society and why they continue to gain support from parents and professionals despite the preponderance of unsubstantiated claims associated with them. Fads are not confined to the territory of wacky antiscience zealots on the periphery of the culture. Instead, fads are endorsed by a growing army of politicians, media personalities, and sports figures, many of whom have the respect of mainstream society. Fortunately, the US federal government intervened in 1991 by creating the Office of Alternative Medicine, which later became the National Center for Complementary and Alternative Medicine (NCCAM, 2009). NCCAM (2009) researches interventions that involve unconventional approaches and disseminates their findings to the public for the purposes of protecting the public from ineffective or even potentially harmful treatments (NCCAM, 2009). The NCCAM has debunked some unvalidated treatments and even warned of their dangers (Offit, 2008). It is the work of NCCAM and similar organizations that ensures that individuals with ASD are only subjected to treatments that have proven to be safe and effective, and it is our responsibility to uphold the standards that they set forth.

Acknowledgments This work was supported by the New York State Office of Mental Retardation and Developmental Disabilities, Albany, NY, and its Institute for Basic Research in Developmental Disabilities, Staten Island, NY.

References

AIT Institute. (2010). *What is AIT: Berard auditory integration training (Berard AIT)?* Retrieved from http://www.aitinstitute.org/what_is_auditory_integration_training.htm. Accessed 7 February 2010.

Aaronovitch, D. (19 December 2009). A conspiracy-theory theory. *The Wall Street Journal*. Retrieved from http://online.wsj.com/homepage. Accessed 7 February 2010.

Autism Speaks. (2009). Alternative treatments. Retrieved from http://www.autismspeaks.org/whattodo/treatments_non_standard.php. Accessed 5 January 2010.

Ayres, A. J. (1972). *Sensory integration and learning disorders*. Los Angeles: Western Psychological Services.

Barrett, S. (2009). *Quackery: How should it be defined?* Retrieved from http://quackwatch.com/01QuackeryRelatedTopics/quackdef.html. Accessed 5 January 2010.

Barrett, S., & Herbert, V. (2007). *More ploys that can fool you.* Retrieved from http://www.quackwatch.com/01QuackeryRelatedTopics/ploys.html. Accessed 6 January 2010.

Becker Hilton Medical Institute. (n.d.). *Autism therapy in the new decade*. Retrieved from http://www.beckerhilton.com/index.php?page=AutismTherapy&gclid=CPKao8qXiZ8CFQk75Qod-3f7dQ. Accessed 18 December 2009.

Berard, G. (2006). *Understanding the difference between Berard AIT and the Tomatis method: Guy Berard*. Retrieved from http://www.drguyberard.com/tomatis.html. Accessed 4 January 2010.

Bettison, S. (1996). The long-term effects of auditory training on children with autism. *Journal of Autism and Developmental Disorders, 26*, 361–374.

Biklen, D. (1990). Communication unbound: Autism and praxis. *Harvard Educational Review, 60*, 291–315.

Blanton, S. J. (2000). Why consultants don't apply psychological research. *Consulting Psychology Journal: Practice and Research, 52*, 235–247.

Buie, T., Campbell, D. B., Fuchs, G. J., III, Furuta, G. T., Levy, J., VandeWater, J., et al. (2010). Evaluation, diagnosis, and treatment of gastrointestinal disorders in individuals with ASDs: A consensus report. *Pediatrics, 125*, S1–S18. doi: 10.1542/peds.2009-1878CCDC.

Center for Disease Control [CDC]. (2006). Deaths associated with hypocalcemia from chelation therapy – Texas, Pennsylvania, and Oregon, 2003–2005. *Morbidity and Mortality Weekly Report, 2006, 55*(8), 204–207.

Center for Disease Control [CDC]. (2009). Prevalence of autism spectrum disorders – Autism and developmental disabilities monitoring network, United States, 2006. *Surveillance Summaries, December 18, 2009. Morbidity and Mortality Weekly Report 2009, 58*(SS10), 1–20.

Crossley, R., & McDonald, A. (1980). *Annie's coming out*. New York: Penguin.

Dawson, P. F. (2001). The search for effective autism treatment: Options or insanity? In C. Maurice, G. Green, & R. M. Foxx (Eds.), *Making a difference: Behavioral intervention for autism* (pp. 11–22). Austin, TX: PRO-ED.

Dura, J. R., Mulick, J. A., & Hammer, D. (1988). Rapid clinical evaluation of sensory integrative therapy for self-injurious behavior. *Mental Retardation, 26*, 83–87.

Edelson, S. M., Arin, D., Bauman, M., Lukas, S. E., Rudy, J. H., Sholar, M., et al. (1999). Auditory integration training: A double-blind study of behavioral, electrophysiological, and audiometric effects in autistic subjects. *Focus on Autism and Other Developmental Disabilities, 14*, 73–81.

Elder, J. H., Shankar, M., Shuster, J., Theriaque, D., Burns, S., & Sherrill, L. (2006). The gluten-free, casein-free diet in autism. Results of a preliminary double blind clinical trial. *Journal of Autism and Developmental Disorders, 36*, 413–420. doi: 10.1007/s10803-006-0079-0.

Esch, B. E., & Carr, J. E. (2004). Secretin as a treatment for Autism: A review of the evidence. *Journal of Autism and Developmental Disorders, 34*, 543–556.

Food and Drug Administration [FDA]. (2009). Drugs@FDA. Retrieved from http://www.accessdata.fda.gov/Scripts/cder/DrugsatFDA/index.cfm. Accessed 21 December 2009.

Ghezzi, P. M., & Rehfeldt, R. A. (1994). Competence. In L. J. Hayes, G. J. Hayes, S. C. Moore, & P. M. Ghezzi (Eds.), *Ethical issues in developmental disabilities* (pp. 81–88). Reno, NV: Context Press.

Goldstein, H. (2000). Commentary: Interventions to facilitate auditory, visual, and motor integration. "Show me the data." *Journal of Autism and Developmental Disorders, 30*, 423–425.

Granpeesheh, D., Tarbox, J., Dixon, D. R., Wilke, A. E., Allen, M. S., & Bradstreet, J. J. (2009). Randomized trial of hyperbaric oxygen therapy for children with autism. *Research in Autism Spectrum Disorders, 4*, 268–275. doi: 10.1016/j.rasd.2009.09.014.

Green, G. (1996). Evaluating claims about treatment for autism. In C. Maurice, G. Green, & S. Luce (Eds.), *Behavioral intervention for young children with autism: A manual for parents and professionals* (pp. 15–28). Austin, TX: PRO-ED.

Green, V. A. (2007). Parental experience with treatments for autism. *Journal of Developmental Disabilities, 19*, 91–101.

Green, V. A., Pituch, K. A., Itchon, J., Choi, A., O'Reilly, M., & Sigafoos, J. (2006). Internet survey of treatments used by parents of children with autism. *Research in Developmental Disabilities, 27*, 70–84.

Greenspan, S. (2005). Credulity and gullibility among service providers: An attempt to understand why snake oil sells. In J. W. Jacobson, R. M. Foxx, & J. A. Mulick (Eds.), *Controversial therapies for developmental disabilities: Fad, fashion, and science in professional practice* (pp. 129–138). Mahwah, NJ: Lawrence Erlbaum.

Handon, B. L., & Hofkosh, D. (2005). Secretin in children with autistic disorder: A double-blind, placebo-controlled trial. *Journal of Developmental and Physical Disabilities, 17*, 95–106. doi: 10.1007/s10882-005-3682-7.

Hediger, M. L., England, L. J., Molloy, C. A., Yu, K. F., Manning-Courtney, P., & Mills, J. L. (2008). Reduced bone cortical thickness in boys with autism or autism spectrum disorder. *Journal of Autism and Developmental Disorders, 38*, 848–856. doi: 10.1007/s10803-007-0453-6.

Herndon, A. C., DiGuiseppi, C., Johnson, S. L., Leiferman, J., & Reynolds, A. (2009). Does nutritional intake differ between children with autism spectrum disorders and children with typical development? *Journal of Autism and Developmental Disorders, 39*, 212–222. doi: 10.1007/s10803-008-0606-2.

Heward, W. L., & Silvestri, S. M. (2005). The neutralization of special education. In J. W. Jacobson, R. M. Foxx, & J. A. Mulick (Eds.), *Controversial therapies for developmental disabilities: Fad, fashion, and science in professional practice* (pp. 193–214). Mahwah, NJ: Lawrence Erlbaum.

Holburn, S. (2005). Severe aggressive and self-destructive behavior: Mentalistic attribution. In J. W. Jacobson, R. M. Foxx, & J. A. Mulick (Eds.), *Controversial therapies for developmental disabilities: Fad, fashion, and science in professional practice* (pp. 279–293). Mahwah, NJ: Lawrence Erlbaum.

Holburn, S. (2007). Counter the mistreatments for autism with professional integrity. *Intellectual and Developmental Disabilities, 45*, 136–137.

Holburn, S. (2008). Detrimental effects of overestimating the occurrence of autism. *Intellectual and Developmental Disabilities, 46*, 243–246.

Horvath, K., Stefanatos, G., Sokolski, K. N., Wachtel, R., Nabors, L., & Tildon, J. T. (1998). Improved social and language skills after secretin administration in patients with autistic spectrum disorders. *Journal of the Association for Academic Minority Physicians, 9*, 10–15.

Interactive Autism Network. (2008). *IAN State Stats*. Retrieved from http://www.iancommunity.org/cs/for_researchers/ian_statestats. Accessed 15 December 2009.

International Hyperbarics Association, Inc. (2004). *Welcome to the amazing world of hyperbaric medicine*. Retrieved from http://www.ihausa.org. Accessed 18 December 2009.

Jacobson, J. W., Foxx, R. M., & Mulick, J. A. (2005). Facilitated communication: The ultimate fad treatment. In J. W. Jacobson, R. M. Foxx, & J. A. Mulick (Eds.), *Controversial therapies for developmental disabilities: Fad, fashion, and science in professional practice* (pp. 363–384). Mahwah, NJ: Lawrence Erlbaum.

Jacobson, J. W., Mulick, J. A., & Schwartz, A. A. (1995). A history of facilitated communication: Science, pseudoscience, and antiscience. *American Psychologist, 50*, 750–765.

Kabot, S., Masi, W., & Segal, M. (2003). Advances in the diagnosis and treatment of autism spectrum disorders. *Professional Psychology: Research and Practice, 34*, 26–33.

Levy, S. E., & Hyman, S. L. (2005). Novel treatments for autistic spectrum disorders. *Mental Retardation and Developmental Disabilities Research Reviews, 11,* 131–142.

Mason, S. A., & Iwata, B. A. (1990). Artifactual effects of sensory–integrative therapy on self-injurious behavior. *Journal of Applied Behavior Analysis, 23,* 361–370.

McGee, M. (1987). The motor aspects of behavior disorders in mentally retarded individuals: A neuro-developmental approach. In J. A. Mulick & R. Antonak (Eds.), *Transitions in mental retardation: Vol. 2. Issues in therapeutic intervention* (pp. 179–188). Norwood, NJ: Ablex Publishing.

Metz, B., Mulick, J. A., & Butter, E. M. (2005). A late-20th-century fad magnet. In J. W. Jacobson, R. M. Foxx, & J. A. Mulick (Eds.), *Controversial therapies for developmental disabilities: Fad, fashion, and science in professional practice* (pp. 237–263). Mahwah, NJ: Lawrence Erlbaum.

Millward, C., Ferriter, M., Calver, S. J., & Connell-Jones, G. G. (2008). Gluten- and casein-free diets for autistic spectrum disorder. *Cochrane Database of Systematic Reviews, 2.* Art. No.: CD003498. doi: 10.1002/14651858.CD003498.pub3

Mostert, M. P. (2001). Facilitated communication since 1995: A review of published studies. *Journal of Autism and Developmental Disorders, 31,* 287–313.

Mudford, O. C., Cross, B. A., Breen, S., Cullen, C., Reeves, D., Gould, J., et al. (2000). Auditory integration training for children with autism: No behavioral benefits detected. *American Journal on Mental Retardation, 105,* 118–129.

Mudford, O. C., & Cullen, C. (2005). Auditory integration training: A critical review. In J. W. Jacobson, R. M. Foxx, & J. A. Mulick (Eds.), *Controversial therapies for developmental disabilities: Fad, fashion, and science in professional practice* (pp. 351–362). Mahwah, NJ: Lawrence Erlbaum.

National Center for Complementary and Alternative Medicine [NCCAM]. (2009). Retrieved from http://nccam.nih.gov/about. Accessed 5 January 2010.

National Institute of Child Health and Human Development [NICHD]. (1999). *Study shows secretin fails to benefit children with autism.* Retrieved from http://www.nichd.nih.gov/news/releases/secretin1299.cfm?renderforprint=1. Accessed 10 January 2010.

Native Remedies. (2009). *Natural remedies, the natural choice: Approaches to autism treatment.* Retrieved from http://www.nativeremedies.com/ailment/autism-symptoms-info.html. Accessed 7 February 2010.

Newsome, C., & Hovenitz, C. A. (2005). The nature and value of empirically validated interventions. In J. W. Jacobson, R. M. Fox, & J. A. Mulick (Eds.), *Controversial therapies for developmental disabilities: Fad, fashion, and science in professional practice* (pp. 31–44). Mahwah, NJ: Lawrence Erlbaum.

Nichols, A. (2009). *Even better now: Help your behaviorally or developmentally challenged child reach his or her full potential using safe chelation, detoxification and supplement therapies.* Retrieved from http://www.evenbetternow.com/autism.asp?s=gaw5&gclid=CM_QyeDuhp8CFWkN5Qo\djQxj7w. Accessed 20 December 2009.

Offit, P. A. (2008). *Autism's false prophets: Bad science, risky medicine, and the search for a cure.* Chichester, NY: Columbia University Press.

Owley, T., McMahon, W., Cook, E. H., Jr., Laulhere, T., South, M., Mays, L. Z., et al. (2001). A multi-site, placebo-controlled, double-blind study of porcine secretin in the treatment of autistic disorder. *Journal of the American Academy of Child and Adolescent Psychiatry, 40,* 1293–1299.

Parent Feedback. (2009). *Even better now: Parent feedback using Kids Clear^TM Detoxifying Clay Baths.* Retrieved from http://www.evenbetternow.com/autism.asp?s=gaw5&gclid=CM_QyeDuhp8CFWkN5QodjQxj7w. Accessed 15 January 2010.

Quackwatch. (2009). Retrieved from http://www.quackwatch.org/index.html. Accessed 15 January 2010.

Rimland, B., & Edelson, S. M. (1994). The effects of auditory integration training in autism. *American Journal of Speech and Language Pathology, 5,* 16–24.

Rimland, B., & Edelson, S. M. (1995). Auditory integration training: A pilot study. *Journal of Autism and Developmental Disorders, 25,* 61–70.

Rossignol, D. A., Rossignol, L. W., Smith, S., Schneider, C., Logerquist, S., Usman, A., et al. (2009). Hyperbaric treatment for children with autism: A multicenter randomized, double-blind, controlled trial. *BioMed Central Pediatrics, 9,* 21. doi: 10.1186/1471-2431-9-21.

Rudy, L. J. (2008, April 14). *Review of The Soul of Autism,* by William Stillman. Retrieved from http://autism.about.com/od/booksaboutautism. Accessed 7 February 2010.

S. 223. (2009). *An Act to improve augmentative and alternative communication opportunities for children with disabilities.* The Commonwealth of Massachusetts. Retrieved from http://www.mass.gov/legis/bills/senate/186/st00pdf/st00223.pdf. Accessed 20 January 2010.

Sandler, A. D., Sutton, K. A., Deweese, J., Girardi, M. A., Sheppard, V., & Bodfish, J. W. (1999). Lack of benefit of synthetic human secretin in the treatment of autism and pervasive developmental disabilities. *The New England Journal of Medicine, 341,* 1801–1806.

Schaaf, R. C., & Miller, L. J. (2005). Occupational therapy using a sensory integrative approach for children with developmental disabilities. *Mental Retardation and Developmental Disabilities Research Reviews, 11,* 143–148.

Shermer, M. (1997). *Why people believe weird things: Pseudoscience, superstition, and other confusions of our time.* New York: Henry Holt and Company, LLC.

Singh, A. N., Matson, J. L., Cooper, C. L., Dixon, D., & Sturmey, P. (2005). The use of Risperidone among individuals with mental retardation: Clinically supported or not? *Research in Developmental Disabilities, 26,* 203–218.

Smith, T. (2005). The appeal of unvalidated treatments. In J. W. Jacobson, R. M. Foxx, & J. A. Mulick (Eds.), *Controversial therapies for developmental disabilities: Fad, fashion, and science in professional practice* (pp. 45–57). Mahwah, NJ: Lawrence Erlbaum.

Smith, T., Mruzek, D. W., & Mozingo, D. (2005). Sensory integrative therapy. In J. W. Jacobson, R. M. Foxx, & J. A. Mulick (Eds.), *Controversial therapies for developmental disabilities: Fad, fashion, and science in professional practice* (pp. 331–350). Mahwah, NJ: Lawrence Erlbaum.

Stephenson, J., & Carter, M. (2009). The use of weighted vests with children with autism spectrum disorders and other disabilities. *Journal of Autism and Developmental Disorders, 39,* 105–114.

Sturmey, P. (2005a). Ethical dilemmas and the most effective therapies. In J. W. Jacobson, R. M. Foxx, & J. A. Mulick (Eds.), *Controversial therapies for developmental disabilities: Fad, fashion, and science in professional practice* (pp. 435–449). Mahwah, NJ: Lawrence Erlbaum.

Sturmey, P. (2005b). Secretin is an ineffective treatment for pervasive developmental disabilities: A review of 15 double-blind randomized controlled trials. *Research in Developmental Disabilities: A Multidisciplinary Journal, 26,* 87–97.

Tsouderos, T., & Callahan, P. (2009, December 7). *Autism treatments: Risky alternative therapies have little basis in science.* Retrieved from http://www.chicagotribune.com/health/la-he-autism-main7-2009dec07,0,6189104.story. Accessed 7 February 2010.

Van Houten, R. (1994). The right to effective behavioral treatment. In L. J. Hayes, G. J. Hayes, S. C. Moore, & P. M. Ghezzi (Eds.), *Ethical issues in developmental disabilities.* Reno, NV: Context Press.

Zollweg, W., Palm, D., & Vance, V. (1997). The efficacy of auditory integration training: A double blind study. *American Journal of Audiology, 6,* 39–47.

Intensive Early Intervention

20

Svein Eikeseth

Autism: Definition, Prevalence, and Cause

Autism is a pervasive developmental disorder (PDD) characterized by severe impairment in social interaction and communication along with high rates of ritualistic and stereotyped behavior (American Psychiatric Association, 1994). It is one of the most common developmental disorders. The prevalence rate for all forms of PDD is estimated to be around 3–11 per 1,000, and childhood autism is estimated to have a prevalence of approximately 1–4 per 1,000 (Baird et al., 2006; Fombonne, 2003). Researchers have shown that 50–80% of children with autism have intellectual disabilities (Baird et al., 2006; Fombonne, 1999) and that the majority will require professional care throughout their lives (Billstedt, Gillberg, & Gillberg, 2005).

Although specific biological causes of the condition have not yet been identified, researchers have suggested that genetic, epigenetic, and biological–environmental factors are involved (Bailey et al., 1995; Freitag, 2007; Muller, 2007; Volkmar, Lord, Bailey, Schultz, & Klin, 2004). Currently, researchers are searching for medical and biomedical treatments that are effective, safe, and generally accepted (Pangborn & Baker, 2005); however, the only drug approved for autism by the US Food and Drug Administration (FDA) is risperidone (FDA, October 6, 2006). Risperidone may be used to treat aggression, self-injury, and temper tantrums, but it does not address the core deficits of the autistic disorder, that is, the deficits in social interaction, communication, and stereotyped behaviors. Hence, medical treatments are not a substitute for comprehensive early intervention, which currently is the standard intervention for autism (Filipek, Steinberg-Epstein, & Book, 2006; Howlin, 2005).

In this chapter, the term "comprehensive intervention" for children with autism will be defined. Next those comprehensive interventions that have been evaluated in outcome research will be described and reviewed to establish which interventions, if any, are considered evidence based, and hence, recommended as appropriate treatment for children with autism. What constitutes meaningful treatment effect, including effect size and meta-analysis, will also be discussed, as will factors that may moderate or mediate treatment gains. Finally, the chapter provides a review of outcome of interventions for school-aged children as well as research on outcome for children with other types of neurodevelopmental disorders.

What Defines Comprehensive Early Intervention

Comprehensive early interventions are distinguished from those interventions addressing specific deficits exhibited by children with autism, such as communication difficulties or sensory problems. Comprehensive interventions must, at the very least, address all three core deficits defining autism: (i) social skills and social interests, (ii) all aspects of communication, and (iii) ritualistic and/or stereotyped behaviors; however, children with autism may also exhibit other behavioral *excesses* and *deficits*. Examples of these are aggression and self-injurious behavior, attention deficits, learning difficulties, eating problems, and difficulties with motor development and self-help skills. Hence, comprehensive interventions should include procedures to address these types of difficulties in addition to addressing the three core deficits defining autism.

S. Eikeseth (✉)
Faculty of Behavioral Science, Akershus University College, N-2001 Lillestrøm, Norway
e-mail: svein.eikeseth@hiak.no

This chapter is dedicated to the memory of O. Ivar Lovaas, who died at the age of 83 on August 2, 2010. Being one of those who had the privilege of working closely with Dr. Lovaas, I will carry not only his scientific legacy for life but also the memory of a charismatic, passionate, breathtaking, and brilliant man.

J.L. Matson, P. Sturmey (eds.), *International Handbook of Autism and Pervasive Developmental Disorders*,
Autism and Child Psychopathology Series, DOI 10.1007/978-1-4419-8065-6_20, © Springer Science+Business Media, LLC 2011

Some well-researched examples of *noncomprehensive* intervention are picture exchange communication system (PECS; Yoder & Lieberman, 2010), parent-delivered pragmatic language interventions (Aldred, Green, & Adams, 2004; Drew et al., 2002), functional analysis to determine causes of aberrant behaviors (Iwata et al., 1994), noncontingent reinforcement to reduce aberrant behaviors (Carr, Severtson, & Lepper, 2009), and eating interventions (Matson & Fodstad, 2008), among others. Noncomprehensive procedures may well be components of a comprehensive early intervention program. For example, eating interventions, functional analysis, noncontingent reinforcement, and PECS are often components of interventions based on applied behavior analysis (ABA).

Comprehensive Early Intervention Programs

Since the 1970s and until today, a large number of intervention programs for children with autism have been developed, but unfortunately, only a minority of these programs have been evaluated in outcome research (Howlin, 2005; Smith & Wick, 2008). Eikeseth (2009) examined comprehensive intervention for children with autism and found that only three programs had been subjected to outcome research. These included interventions based on (i) treatment and education of autistic and communication-handicapped children (TEACCH), (ii) the Denver model, and (iii) ABA. The next section provides a brief description of these three programs followed by an assessment of the extent to which they are evidence based.

Treatment and Education of Autistic and Related Communication-Handicapped Children

TEACCH was founded at the University of North Carolina in 1966 by Eric Schopler (Schopler & Reichler, 1971). TEACCH is the most influential special education program for children with autism and is used worldwide. The program aims to address multiple problems such as communication, cognition, perception, imitation, social skills, and motor skills. It emphasizes teaching in multiple settings with the involvement of several teachers. TEACCH was traditionally used in segregated self-contained classrooms for children with autism, but recently, focus has been shifting toward exposing children with autism to inclusive settings with typically developing children (Lord & Schopler, 1994). In addition, increased emphasis has been placed on home programming using parents as co-therapists (Ozonoff & Cathcart, 1998). The TEACCH approach, as described in numerous manuals and books (Mesibov, Shea, & Schopler, 2005; Schopler & Mesibov, 1995), typically contains the following five components: (1) focus on structural teaching. Specifically, a teacher and a teacher's assistant share the responsibility of teaching five children with autism. Focus is placed on teaching children independent work skills. (2) Strategies to enhance visual processing are emphasized, including (a) the physical (ecological) structure of the classroom, (b) the use of a visual activity schedule to help children anticipate future events, (c) a visual organization of the work materials to teach the learning tasks and their sequences, and (d) a visual system to teach complicated skills such as language and imitation. (3) The teaching of a communication system based on gesture, pictures, signs, or printed words. (4) The teaching of pre-academic skills (colors, numbers, shapes, drawing, writing, and assembly). (5) Encouragement for parents to work as co-therapists with their child in the home using the same techniques and materials as employed during the TEACCH clinic sessions.

The Denver Model

The Denver model was developed by Sally Rogers and colleagues in the 1980s (Rogers, Hall, Osaki, Reaven, & Herbison, 2001; Rogers, Hayden, Hepburn, Charlifue-Smith, Hall, & Hayes, 2006). The program provides more than 20 h per week of systematic instruction to children from 2 to 5 years. The Denver model is a developmental play-based approach and is based on Piaget's theory of cognitive development, Mahler's psychoanalytic theory of interpersonal development, and the INREAL pragmatic-based communication program (Rogers & DiLalla, 1991). Piaget focused on how children explore their environments to construct schemas about how the world works and how to reason about it. Mahler's theory of interpersonal development centers on how children establish a sense of identity. It also focuses on how children establish an understanding of others through interactions with adults. The Colorado Health Science Program also utilizes the INREAL pragmatic-based communication program (Weiss, 1981), which aims to enhance functional communication in the context of naturally occurring activities. Finally, the program uses behavior analytic techniques to reduce aberrant or undesirable behaviors. The Denver model is offered as a comprehensive, eclectic "best practice" approach with a broad theoretical underpinning.

The Early Start Denver Model (ESDM)

Recently, the Denver model has been labeled the early start Denver model (ESDM). The ESDM has increased its emphasis on behavioral analytics principles. Dawson et al. (2010) described the ESDM as a "comprehensive early behavioral intervention for infant to preschool-aged children with ASD that integrates applied behavior analysis with developmental and relationship-based approaches" (p. 18). Moreover, the principles used for teaching "... are consistent with the principles of ABA" (p. 20). Hence, the contemporary Denver model, the ESDM, employs behavior analytic principles not only for reducing inappropriate behaviors but also to establish appropriate skills such as communication and social skills.

Interventions Based on ABA

Interventions for children with autism based on ABA were pioneered by Ivar Lovaas and colleagues in the 1960s (Ferster & DeMyer, 1961; Lovaas & Simmons, 1969; Wolf, Risley, & Mees, 1964) and rest on several hundred small numbers of experimental and clinical studies published in peer-reviewed journals (Cunningham & Schreibman, 2008; Matson & LoVullo, 2008; Matson, Matson, & Rivet, 2007; Matson & Smith, 2008). Building on this body of knowledge, several empirically supported treatment manuals have been published to guide practitioners in designing effective programs for children with autism (Leaf & McEachin, 1999; Lovaas, 1977, 2003; Lovaas et al., 1981; Maurice, Green, & Foxx, 2001; Maurice, Green, & Luce, 1996). ABA focuses on remediating the children's delays in communication, social, and emotional skills and emphasizes the integration of these children with typical peers in mainstream settings. ABA uses principles derived from laboratory and applied research on learning psychology (Catania, 1998; Cooper, Heron, & Heward, 2007) to teach developmentally appropriate and functional skills. One working hypothesis is that children with autism have a biologically based learning/developmental deficit and that modern principles derived from learning psychology may be used to help the children to develop skills exhibited by typical children and to reduce aberrant behaviors. Moreover, it is hypothesized that some children may overcome their learning deficit, enabling them to acquire age-appropriate behaviors and eventually learn from typical (non-behavioral) education (Lovaas, 2003). Interventions based on ABA will be defined and further described later in this chapter.

Evidence-Based Interventions

Evidence-based interventions are interventions that have been evaluated scientifically in outcome research and found to benefit children with autism. Globally, governmental agencies, including the United States (National Research Council, 2001), have set up national review groups to review research on treatment for autism to establish which types of interventions may be considered evidence based and could thus be recommended as appropriate interventions for children with

autism. In an attempt to do so, Rogers and Vismara (2008) reviewed comprehensive intervention programs using the criteria for "well-established" or "probably efficacious" from Chambliss and Hollon (1998) and Chambliss et al. (1996). "Well-established" interventions required that (a) the treatment was described in treatment manuals, (b) participant groups were clearly specified, and (c) either (i) two independent well-designed group studies showing the treatment to be better than placebo or alternative treatment or equivalent to an established effective treatment, or (ii) nine or more single subject design studies using a strong research design and a comparison to an alternative treatment were available.

To achieve status as a "probably efficacious" intervention, requirements included (a) clearly specified subject groups and (b) either (i) two studies showing better outcomes than a no-treatment control group; or (ii) two strong group studies by the same investigator showing the treatment outperformed placebo or alternative treatment, or treatment was equivalent to an established treatment; or (iii) three or more single subject design studies that have a strong design and compare the intervention to another type of treatment.

Based on these criteria, Rogers and Vismara (2008) concluded that interventions based on ABA ("Lovaas method") could be considered "well established." Moreover, *no* other interventions were either "well established" or "probably efficacious."

Eldevik, Hastings, Hughes, Jahr, and Eikeseth (2010) and Eikeseth (2009) reached similar conclusions based on slightly different criteria. Eikeseth (2009) graded outcome studies according to their scientific merit and the magnitude of treatment effect documented in the studies. For scientific merit, studies were graded into four levels. Eikeseth found that one study received level 1 scientific merit (the highest possible rating) and four studies received level 2 scientific merit, with each of these five studies having evaluated ABA treatment. Eleven outcome studies received level 3 evidence support, representing a relatively low scientific merit. Nine of the 11 studies evaluated interventions based on ABA and 2 studies evaluated TEACCH. Finally, nine outcome studies were classified as having insufficient scientific value. Of these nine studies one evaluated TEACCH, two evaluated the Colorado Health Science Program, and six evaluated ABA.

Based on an evaluation of the magnitude of treatment effects, four ABA studies received level 1 rating (the highest rating), demonstrating that children receiving ABA made significantly more gains than control group children on standardized measures of IQ, language and adaptive functioning. Three studies received level 2 rating, demonstrating that ABA-treated children made significantly more gains than the comparison group on one standardized measure of IQ or adaptive functioning. Finally, five ABA studies and two TEACCH studies received level 3 rating (the lowest treatment effect), requiring significant group differences on developmental (or mental) age, or significant group differences on assessment instruments that are not fully standardized (Eikeseth, 2009). This review shows that treatment based on ABA is more thoroughly researched and has produced better outcome as compared to other comprehensive interventions for children with autism.

Eldevik, Jahr, Eikeseth, Hastings, and Hughes (2010) compared outcome studies with the criteria developed by the Oxford Centre for Evidence Based Medicine (2009) and concluded that the evidence for ABA for young children with autism is at level 1b. This level requires evidence from at least one well-designed randomized controlled study and evidence from systematic reviews. Level 1a (the highest level of evidence) would require a systematic review of several randomized controlled trials showing homogeneity in results. Similarly, Eldevik et al. (2010) argued that the evidence for interventions based on ABA meets the criteria for evidence-based practices in special education, as proposed by Gersten et al. (2005).

Because interventions based on ABA are the only comprehensive early intervention programs that are evidence based to date, the remainder of this chapter will address this type of treatment, currently labeled *early and intensive behavioral intervention (EIBI)*.

What Defines EIBI

EIBI has been described by Green, Brennan, and Fein (2002) as having the following characteristics: (a) individualized and comprehensive treatment, addressing all skill domains; (b) normal developmental sequences (i.e., data from developmental psychology) guide the selection of intervention goals and short-term objectives; (c) several behavior analytic procedures used to teach new skills and to reduce interfering behavior (e.g., differential reinforcement, prompting, discrete trial teaching, natural environment teaching, activity-embedded trials, and task analysis); (d) one or more professionals with advanced training in applied behavior analysis and advanced training in EIBI with young children with autism direct and supervise the intervention; (e) parents serve as active co-therapists for their children; (f) intervention is initially delivered one to one, with gradual transitions to small-group and large-group formats when warranted; (g) intervention typically begins in the home and is carried over into other environments (e.g., community settings), with gradual, systematic transitions to preschool, kindergarten, and elementary school classrooms when children develop the skills required to learn in those settings; (h) intensive, year-round teaching, including 20–40 h of structured sessions per week plus informal instruction and practice throughout most of the children's other waking hours; (i) two or more years of intervention, in most cases; and (j) most children start intervention in the preschool years.

To accurately use the term EIBI to describe a particular intervention, all of the defining characteristics described above must be present. Also, these defining characteristics must be in place in order to achieve maximum clinical gains from an EIBI program.

Treatment

The treatment has been detailed in a number of treatment manuals and is based on a number of principles and procedures from behavior analysis.

Principles

Reinforcement and motivational operations are key treatment principles, as are stimulus control technology and generalization techniques. Reinforcers are environmental events produced by certain behaviors. For example, an infant's cry (i.e., the behavior) results in he/she being comforted, changed, and/or fed by the caretaker (i.e., the environmental events). Hand flapping and gazing by a child with autism (i.e., the behavior) produces visual and kinesthetic feedback (i.e., the environmental event), or a smile to a friend (i.e., the behavior) results in some social gestures in return (i.e., the environmental events). For such environmental events to be classified as reinforcers, however, they must strengthen the behaviors for which they occur as a consequence. In the example above, the infant's cry is strengthened by the caretaker's comfort, hand flapping and gazing is strengthened by sensory feedback, and the smile to a friend is strengthened by the social responses received.

In autism treatment, the principle of reinforcement is used to strengthen behaviors such as communication, play, and social skills in order to remediate core deficits in autism. Reinforcers can also be used to motivate the child for learning by, for example, putting a favorite item out of the child's reach so that the child has to communicate in some way to access it.

Stimulus control concerns how environmental events occasion behaviors. For example, the sight of a cookie (i.e., the environmental event) may evoke saying "I want cookie" (i.e., the behavior) to obtain the cookie (i.e., the reinforcer). Getting the cookie after saying "I want cookie" is the reinforcer which will strengthen the behavior for which it is a consequence. A toy car may be an environmental event for driving the car or perhaps spinning the wheels of the car. A green traffic light serves as the stimulus that signal driving, while a red traffic light tells us to stop driving.

Generalization concerns the extent to which the effects of teaching spread to other situations or responses. For example, if the preschool teacher has taught the child to play lotto in a one-to-one setting in a therapy room, generalization occurs if the child, without further training, plays lotto also with other children, plays lotto in other rooms, and/or plays lotto at home with his/her parents. For a more detailed description of these (and other) learning principles, see Cooper et al. (2007).

Teaching Methods

Teaching includes identifying skills to be taught, performing task analyses, objectively defining target behaviors, identifying materials to be used during teaching (e.g., objects from the child's daily routine such as a toothbrush), identifying reinforcers and performing operations to motivate the child for learning, and planning a specific prompt (how to help the child to perform the target behavior) and prompt fading strategy (how to remove the help after the child starts to correctly perform the target behavior).

Discrete trial teaching is a specific teaching procedure used to maximize learning. It is used to establish a number of important skills, including cognitive skills, communication, play, social, and self-help skills (Lovaas et al., 1981). The teaching strategy involves (a) breaking skills into small steps, (b) teaching each step of the skill individually until mastered, (c) providing repetitions of teaching steps, (d) prompting the correct skill and fading (removing) the prompts whenever possible, and (e) using reinforcement and stimulus control procedures.

Natural environment teaching is another important method used. It focuses on teaching behaviors in the situations they naturally occur. During mealtime, for example, the child is reinforced for sitting nicely or instructed how to use a knife and fork appropriately. Whenever possible the reinforcer used in natural environment teaching is the consequence that naturally follows the target behavior such as going outside to perform a desired activity after practicing tying shoes.

Many skills, however, such as tying shoes may be difficult to learn from natural environment teaching because the skill is very complex and/or because few learning opportunities occur naturally over the course of the day. Consequently, natural environment teaching is often combined with discrete trial teaching, where a particular skill (e.g., shoe tying) can be broken down into smaller components and practiced repeatedly until mastered.

Task analyses and chaining are used to break down complex behaviors (e.g., toy play and language) into smaller units that can be reliably measured and more easily taught. For example when teaching a child to play with a train set, the behavioral components identified as a result of the task analysis could be (1) attaching two pieces of track together; (2) adding subsequent pieces of track one by one; (3) placing the train on the track; (4) pushing the train around the track; (5) saying "choo choo." For teaching language, the behavioral components are identified and teaching begins with the most basic components such as vocal imitation of sounds. These individual behaviors would then be systematically taught and chained together to make one complex behavior, using backward or forward chaining techniques.

Curriculum

Behavioral principles are necessary for optimal learning, but must be combined with an appropriate and comprehensive curriculum for the child to make maximum gains. The content of the curriculum is comprehensive and addresses all areas of deficit and must be individually tailored for each child's needs. The key components of the curriculum are described elsewhere (Leaf & McEachin, 1999; Lovaas, 1977, 2003; Lovaas et al., 1981; Maurice et al., 1996, 2001) and are only summarized below.

Beginning Curriculum
Each child's curriculum is individualized and comprehensive, teaching skills in all areas of development. Beginning skills included prerequisites in the areas of attention, communication, social initiations, and play. Examples include sitting on a chair, responding to simple instructions such as "come here" and "wave bye-bye", requesting favorite items, pointing, joint attention, matching identical objects, imitating gross motor actions or imitating actions with objects, imitating sounds and words, identifying and naming objects, playing independently with toys, and basic interactive skills such as rolling a ball to and from an adult.

Intermediate Curriculum
Intermediate skills included further language training such as identification and naming of abstract concepts, parallel play, turn taking, imitating sentences, early academic skills such as identifying letters and numbers, drawing imitation and tracing, and self-help skills such as dressing and undressing, toilet training, drinking from an open cup, and increasing the range of foods and drink taken.

Advanced Curriculum
Once these skills are acquired, more advanced skills are addressed, such as conversation and asking questions, advanced pretend play and cooperative play, social–emotional skills such as theory of mind, advanced academic skills, observational learning, and learning in the classroom environment.

School Integration

School integration begins once a range of skills have been acquired that enable the child to access materials, follow the curriculum, and interact with peers in the nursery or school environment. It is preferable for a child to gain as many language, play, and social skills as possible before entering nursery or elementary school, in order to optimize generalization and functional use of skills in the classroom. The aim is for a child to learn increasingly from peers, the class teacher, and the school curriculum. A tutor shadows the child at school, ensuring that the child benefits from every learning opportunity, including social situations as well as the academic curriculum. Consistent interventions are used to ensure inappropriate behaviors are minimized and therefore do not interfere with the child's attention skills or ability to be compliant. Once the child can follow segments of activities, whole activities, or parts of the full school day, the therapist will then use shaping and stimulus control procedures to improve the child's ability to learn new information and new skills directly from the school environment, and not specifically from the ABA program. For a child who progressively learns more from the school environment, hence becoming an independent learner, the tutor systematically reduces interventions such as prompting and reinforcement, until the child attends all or part of the school day independently. For a child who does not learn sufficiently from the classroom environment, the therapist will continue to shadow on a long-term basis and concentrate on integrating the child for activities in which he/she can be successful. Time is also allocated to ongoing one-to-one teaching, both at home and school, during which individual learning goals, including independent living skills, can be addressed more efficiently than in the classroom. The primary aim for every child is to become as independent as possible at school, and therefore shadowing is reduced, for each child, on a task-specific basis, or for periods of the school day.

Record of Treatment

Each child has a log book with sections for each current program or intervention (Lovaas, 2003). Within each section, there is a page outlining the name of the program, the instruction that should be used, the materials that are required, and the response the child is learning, as well as further information about prompting, shaping, and chaining procedures. There is also a list of target behaviors for the child to learn, with columns to mark when each one is introduced and mastered. Finally, there is a note section in which each tutor should note the following points at the end of a session: tutor's initials, date, am/pm session, target, progress, and next stage to be taught. When necessary, information on progress within a program includes analysis of trial-by-trial data and data to establish the function of behavioral excesses and deficits and also to monitor progress of interventions used.

Before treatment starts, the child should receive a comprehensive psychological assessment. This assessment should be repeated annually thereafter. The assessment battery should include measures of developmental/intellectual behavior, adaptive skills, and autism symptoms. The purpose of the assessment is to monitor the child's progress, to evaluate the child's treatment, and to aid in program planning.

Outcome Studies: Evidence for EIBI

The first outcome study evaluating effects of ABA for children with autism was conducted by Lovaas and colleagues and published in 1973 (Lovaas, Koegel, Simmons, & Long, 1973). Twenty children with autism participated. Pretreatment and outcome data were recorded in a free-play setting, different from the treatment setting, and included personnel that had not been involved the children's treatment. Following 12–14 months of treatment, stereotyped behaviors including echolalia decreased, appropriate speech, appropriate play, and social non-verbal behaviors increased as compared to the pretreatment baseline measures. Moreover, intelligence quotient (IQ) and social quotient improved during treatment for some of the children. Following treatment, some of the children were discharged to a state hospital while some children remained with their parents, who had received parent training. Follow-up assessments 1–4 years after the end of treatment showed that those children whose parents were trained to carry out the behavioral treatment continued to improve, while children who were institutionalized regressed. After a brief reinstatement of the behavioral treatment, however, some of the original therapeutic gains made by the children who had been institutionalized were recovered.

The 1973 Treatment Study occasioned what has been labeled the 1987 Early Intervention Project (Lovaas, 1987), which today is considered the seminal outcome study examining effects of EIBI for children with autism. Six important observations made during the 1973 Treatment Study played a major role in the design of the 1987 study (Lovaas, 1993). First, Lovaas and his colleagues found that the youngest children in the 1973 study made the greatest gains and hence the 1987 study focused on younger children. Second, they learned that treatment effects were situation specific, and as a result, treatment was moved away from a hospital or clinic setting and into the children's home and everyday environment. Third, they found limited evidence for response generalization (e.g., becoming more social after learning language), and in the 1987 study, treatment was designed to target most or all of the children's excess and deficit behaviors. Fourth, they learned that the parents could become skilled teachers of their children, and they were the best allies in helping to accelerate and maintain treatment gains. Fifth, they offered treatment for most of the child's waking hours, for 2 or more years, and focused on teaching the children to develop friendships with typical peers. This therapeutic arrangement resembled, according to Lovaas, more closely the type of learning environment available to typical children, who learn from their environment from the time they wake up in the morning and until they go to sleep, 365 days per year (Lovaas, 1993).

Number of participants in the 1987 study was larger than in previous studies and many subsequent studies. In addition, normed and standardized measures were used to evaluate progress and participants were diagnosed and assessed by independent agencies. Also, the 1987 study was the first ABA outcome study for children with autism that included control groups. Previous studies and many of the subsequent studies used one-group pretest–posttest design and a small sample size. The inclusion of control groups greatly improved the validity of the findings.

More specifically, Lovaas (1987) studied 19 children who received 40 h per week of one-to-one ABA treatment for a minimum of 2 years. A comparison group of 19 children received 10 h or less per week one-to-one ABA treatment. A second comparison group ($N = 21$) came from the same agency that diagnosed the majority of the other participants and had received services generally available for children with autism in the area. The diagnosis for all participants was set by an independent agency and based on the most current *Diagnostic and Statistical Manual of Mental Disorders* used at the time of the study. Mean intake was age was 33.3 months. Intake measures included IQ and behavioral observations. When reevaluated at a mean age of 7 years, children in the experimental group had gained an average of 20 IQ points to a mean of 83, and they had made major advances in educational placement. Forty-seven percent of the participants achieved IQ scores of 85 or above, and regular educational placement without assistance. In contrast, the control group that had received 10 h or less of behavioral treatment obtained an average IQ score of 52, and the group who had received services as usual obtained a mean follow-up IQ score of 58. Gains were maintained by eight of the nine best outcome children at a second follow-up conducted when the children averaged 13 years of age (McEachin, Smith, & Lovaas, 1993). Although creating a great deal of controversy (Eikeseth, 2001; Gresham & MacMillan, 1997; Lovaas, Smith, & McEachin, 1989; Schopler, 1987; Schopler, Short, & Mesibov, 1989) Lovaas' seminal study provided hope for parents and professionals and opened up a whole new line of research.

The second outcome study evaluating effects of ABA for children with autism appeared prior to the Lovaas, 1987 study and evaluated an ABA-based preschool intervention program called the learning experiences and alternate programs (LEAP) curriculum model (Hoyson, Jamieson, & Strain, 1984). The LEAP curriculum model is a multi-faceted

program using peer-mediated instruction in preschool classes of typically developing children, though part of the intervention was conducted in a one-to-one format. Intervention procedures included incidental learning, self-management training, prompting strategies, and systematic parent training. Intervention was provided for 15 h per week for 9 months. The study design was a pre–post design, and participants were six children with autism with a mean chronological age of 40 months. On average, the participants had improved their LAP scores with 17 points.

The next outcome study appeared the same year as the 1987 study. A research group from the May Institute (Anderson, Avery, DiPietro, Edwards, & Christian, 1987) examined effects of ABA-based early intervention program for children with autism. Participants received 15 h of one-to-one instruction per week for a period of 2 years. In addition, parents were required to provide 10 h per week of intervention. Mean intake age was 43 months. The diagnosis was set by an independent agency and based on the DSM-III (1980) criteria. Fourteen children participated in the study. A one-group pretest–posttest design was used. In addition a multiple baseline design across behaviors was used to demonstrate the relationship between treatment effect and program intervention. Measures included IQ, language functioning, adaptive functioning, school placement, and parent's skills in behavioral techniques. Assessments of IQ, language functioning, and adaptive functioning were carried out independently. Results indicated a significant change between intake and follow-up in mental age, developmental language functioning, and developmental adaptive functioning; however, significant improvements in standard scores on the tests employed were not found. Results also showed that integrated school placement increased, and parents improved their skills in using behavioral techniques.

In 1990 and 1991, Harris, Handleman, and colleagues published three studies evaluating effects of the Douglass preschool program (Handleman, Harris, Celbiberti, Lilleheht, & Tomchek, 1991; Harris, Handleman, Gordon, Kristoff, & Fuentes, 1991; Harris, Handleman, Kristoff, Bass, & Gordon, 1990). All three studies examined the effects of 11 months of 25 h per week of intervention in either self-contained classes or integrated classrooms. In the integrated classrooms, the number of children with autism was approximately the same as the number of typical developing children. Intervention focused on targeting language and social skills, and intervention procedures emphasized incidental teaching, discrete trial teaching, and parent training. Harris et al. (1990) examined outcome of five children with autism participating in the self-contained classes compared to the outcome of five children with autism participating in integrated classrooms. Mean chronological intake age was 57 months, and mean intake IQ and language quotient were 66 and 70, respectively. Children were assigned to the integrated or self-contained classes based on an assessment of which type of service was most appropriate for each individual child. Harris et al. (1990) found that children who participated in the integrated classes made more progress compared to the children in the self-contained class on a measure of language development. Harris and colleagues (1991) and Handleman et al. (1991) replicated these findings using other outcome measures including IQ.

The first attempt to replicate the Lovaas (1987) study was carried out at Murdoch University in Australia. Birnbrauer and Leach (1993) examined effects of 18 h per week of one-to-one ABA treatment for 2 years for nine children with autism. Mean intake age was 39 months. The diagnosis was set by an independent agency and based on the DSM criteria. A one-group pretest–posttest design was used. In addition, a multiple baseline design across behaviors was used to help demonstrate the relationship between treatment effect and program intervention. Measures included IQ, language functioning, adaptive functioning, school placement, and parents' skills in behavioral techniques. Assessments of IQ, language functioning, and adaptive functioning were carried out independently. Results indicated a significant change between intake and follow-up in mental age, developmental language functioning, and developmental adaptive functioning. In addition, integrated school placement increased, and parents improved their skills in using behavioral techniques; however, as a group participants did not achieve significant improvement in standard scores but only in mental or developmental scores. Hence, the results were much more modest than those of Lovaas (1987).

A second attempt to replicate Lovaas (1987) came from Stanford University, and the results of this study were more consistent with Lovaas (1987) than those reported by the Murdoch group. In this study, Sheinkopf and Siegel (1998) examined effects of ABA treatment for children with autism and children with PDD-NOS. Mean intake age was 34 months. The diagnosis was made by consensus from two or more independent clinic staff and was based on the DSM-III criteria. Study design was retrospective. Participants were matched on pretreatment CA, mental age, interval between pre- and post-assessments, diagnosis, and sex. Eleven children (10 with autism) received ABA treatment and 11 children (10 with autism) received services available in the child's local community. Participants in ABA group received a mean of 19.5 h per week of one-to-one ABA treatment for an average of 15.7 months. Measures included IQ and autism symptoms. Assessments may be considered blind since the study was archival and not planned at the time of diagnosis and assessment. There were no significant differences at intake on any of the measures. At follow-up, the ABA treatment group scored significantly higher on both measures. The ABA treatment group gained an average of 27 IQ points. By comparison, the comparison group gained two IQ points.

Another attempt to replicate Lovaas (1987) was conducted at UCLA by Smith and colleagues and published in 2000. Smith, Groen, and Wynn (2000) conducted a randomized, controlled trial to examine effects of EIBI for children with autism and children with PDD-NOS. Mean intake age was 36 months. The diagnosis was set by an independent agency and based on the DSM-III criteria. Participants were matched on pretreatment IQ and randomly assigned by an independent statistician to either EIBI ($N = 15$) group or to a parent training group ($N = 13$). Participants in the EIBI group (seven with autism and eight with PDD-NOS) received a mean of 24.5 h per week of one-to-one ABA treatment during the first year of intervention with a gradual reduction of treatment hours over the next 2 years. Participants in the control group (seven with autism and six with PDD-NOS) received 3–9 months of parent training for several hours per week. Measures included IQ, visual–spatial IQ, language functioning, adaptive functioning, socio-emotional functioning, academic achievement, class placement progress in treatment, and parent evaluation. Tests were carried out by independent assessors. There were no significant differences at intake on any of the measures. At follow-up the EIBI treatment group scored significantly higher as compared to the parent training group on IQ, visual–spatial skills, language (assessed the by score combining comprehension and expression), school placement, and academics, though not adaptive functioning and socio-emotional functioning. The ABA treatment group gained an average of 16 IQ points. By comparison, the parent training group lost one IQ point. Children with PDD-NOS gained more than those with autism. Twenty-seven percent of the children in the EIBI group achieved average post-treatment scores and were succeeding in regular education classrooms.

The Multi-site Young Autism Project

In 1995, Lovaas was awarded funding from the National Institute of Mental Health to coordinate a more comprehensive replication of the Lovaas, 1987 study. The first study from the Multi-site Young Autism Project was published by a Norwegian research group in 2002. In Norway, at the time of the study, most referrals were older than 42 months, which was above the intake cut-off age for the multi-site replication study; however, since no studies had examined outcome for this group of children, and because the data could possibly extend the validity of the EIBI treatment for older children with autism, an outcome study for this group of children was conducted (Eikeseth, Smith, Jahr, & Eldevik, 2002, 2007). Also, in Norway, children with autism are integrated into regular preschools and kindergartens. Hence, the study could possibly extend the intervention setting from a home program to a school-based program.

Eikeseth et al. (2002, 2007) compared effects of EIBI and eclectic, special education treatment for children with autism who were 5.5 years old at intake. The diagnosis was set by an independent agency and based on the ICD-10 diagnostic criteria and confirmed by the ADI-R diagnostic instrument. Group assignment to either an EIBI treatment group ($N = 13$) or to an eclectic treatment group ($N = 12$) was based on availability of supervisors and performed by a person who was independent of the study. Participants in the EIBI treatment group received 28 h per week of one-to-one treatment during the first year of intervention with a gradual reduction of treatment hours over the next 2 years. Participants in the eclectic group received 29 h per week of one-to-one eclectic, special education treatment with a gradual reduction of treatment hours over the next 2 years. Measures included IQ, language functioning, adaptive functioning, maladaptive behavior, and socio-emotional functioning. Tests were carried out by independent assessors. There were no significant differences at intake on any of the measures. Follow-up assessment – conducted approximately 3 years after the treatment begun – showed that the EIBI treatment group scored significantly higher as compared to the eclectic treatment group on intelligence, language, adaptive functioning, maladaptive functioning, and on two of the subscales on the socio-emotional assessment (social and aggression). The EIBI treatment group gained an average of 25 IQ points and 12 points in adaptive functioning. By comparison, the eclectic treatment group obtained an average change of +7 points in IQ and –10 points in adaptive functioning. Seven of 13 children in the ABA group who scored within the range of intellectual disabilities (mental retardation) at intake scored within the average range (> 85) on both IQ and verbal IQ at follow-up, compared to 2 of 12 children in the eclectic treatment group.

The next replication study was published by Sallows and Graupner in 2005, and the participants in this study met the intake criteria set out in the multi-site replication study. Sallows and Graupner examined effects of clinic-based ABA treatment and parent-managed ABA treatment for children with an independent diagnosis of autism, with a mean intake age of 36 months. The diagnosis was set by an independent agency, based on the DSM-IV criteria and confirmed by the ADI-R. Participants were matched on pretreatment IQ and randomly assigned by an independent statistician to either an ABA treatment ($N = 13$) group or to parent-managed ABA treatment ($N = 10$). Participants in ABA group received a mean of 37.6 h per week of one-to-one treatment for 2 years. Participants in the parent-managed ABA control group received a mean of 31.3 h per week of one-to-one treatment for 2 years. It is unclear whether this difference in treatment intensity is statistically significant. Number of one-to-one hours decreased over the next 2 years as the children entered school. Measures included

IQ, visual–spatial IQ, language functioning, adaptive functioning, socio-emotional functioning, and autism symptoms as measured by the ADI-R. Pretests were carried out by the second author prior to group assignment. Posttests were conducted independently. There were no significant differences at intake on any of the measures. At follow-up, there were no significant differences between groups at pre- or posttest. Combining children in both groups, pretest to posttest gains were significant for IQ, language comprehension, and ADI-R Social Skills and ADI-R Communication, but not on visual–spatial IQ, expressive language, adaptive behavior, socio-emotional functioning, and ADI-R rituals. All children in both groups gained an average of 25 IQ points. Forty-eight percent of all children in both groups showed rapid learning, achieved average post-treatment scores, and were succeeding in regular education classrooms.

The next replication study was published by Cohen, Amarine-Dickens, and Smith (2006) and compared effects of EIBI with special education provided at local public schools for children with autism or PDD-NOS. Participants' mean age when the treatment begun was unspecified, but the mean age at diagnosis was 31.2 months (range 18–48 months) and all participants were less than 48 months by the onset of treatment. The diagnosis was set by an independent agency, based on the DSM-IV criteria and confirmed by the ADI-R. Group assignment to either an ABA treatment group ($N = 21$, 20 with autism and 1 with PDD-NOS) or an eclectic treatment group ($N = 21$, 14 with autism and 7 with PDD-NOS) was based on parental preference. Participants in the ABA treatment group received 35–40 h per week of one-to-one EIBI treatment provided in a community setting. Participants in the comparison group received public community services. The child/teacher ratios varied from one-to-one to three-to-one. Classes operated for 3–5 days per week, for up to 5 h per day. Speech, occupational, and behavioral therapies varied from 0 to 5 h per week. Three of the children spent brief sessions (up to 45 min per day) mainstreamed in regular education. Measures included IQ, visual IQ, language functioning, and adaptive functioning. Assessments were carried out by independent assessors. There were no significant differences at intake on any of the measures, though the groups differed on some of the demographic variables. Most notably, the EIBI group had significantly more children with autism (and less with PDD-NOS) as compared to the comparison group. Follow-up assessment – conducted approximately 3 years after the treatment begun – showed that the ABA treatment group scored significantly higher as compared to the two comparison groups on IQ and adaptive functioning, though not on visual IQ and language (language comprehension was marginally significant with $p = 0.06$). The ABA treatment group gained an average of 25 IQ points and 10 points in adaptive functioning. By comparison, the eclectic treatment group obtained average change of 14 points in IQ and −3 points in adaptive functioning. Six of the 21 ABA-treated children were fully included into regular education without assistance and 11 others were included with support.

Eldevik, Eikeseth, Jahr, and Smith (2006) compared effects of low-intensity EIBI and low-intensity eclectic treatment for children with autism. Despite recommendation of 30–40 h per week of one-to-one treatment, low intensive EIBI programs may occur due to circumstances such as costs, availability of trained professionals, and concerns by some that 30–40 h per week of one-to-one treatment might put too much stress on the child or the family. Mean intake age was 51 months. The diagnosis was based on the ICD-10 criteria. Study design was retrospective. An examination of each child's treatment record and a questionnaire completed by case supervisors determined group assignment. Children who had received treatment based only on ABA constituted the EIBI group ($N = 13$). Children who had received a combination of two or more types of treatment comprised an eclectic group ($N = 15$). Group assignment was blind. Participants in the ABA treatment group received 12.5 h per week of one-to-one ABA treatment for 20 months. Participants in the eclectic group received 12 h per week of one-to-one eclectic treatment for 21 months. When not receiving one-to-one treatment, participants in both groups were mainstreamed with typical peers in regular preschool classes. Measures included IQ, non-verbal intelligence, language functioning, adaptive functioning, and psychopathology (no words, affectionate, toy play, peer play, stereotypes, temper tantrums, toilet trained, and sum pathology). Diagnosis and assessment were not provided independently, but may be considered blind since the study was archival and hence not planned at the time of diagnosis and assessment. There were no significant differences at intake on any of the measures. Follow-up assessment showed that the ABA treatment group scored significantly higher as compared to the eclectic treatment group on intelligence and language, but not on adaptive functioning. On the pathology scale, the ABA group scored higher than the eclectic group on affection, toy play, peer play, toilet training, and sum pathology, but not on no words, temper tantrums, or stereotypy. The ABA treatment group gained an average of 8.2 IQ points. By comparison, the eclectic treatment group lost an average of 2.9 IQ points. The degree of intellectual disabilities was reduced for 38% of the children in the ABA group, as compared to 7% in the eclectic group. Results suggest that low-intensity EIBI may be more effective than low-intensity eclectic special education treatment; however, gains in IQ and language skills made in the behavioral treatment group were more modest than those reported in studies employing intensive behavioral treatment. Finally, replacing the one-to-one behavioral treatment with time in mainstream kindergarten was not successful in improving participant's adaptive and social skills.

The most recent outcome study from the multi-site replication group comes from the UK. Hayward, Eikeseth, Gale, and Morgan (2009) examined progress after 1 year of treatment for children with autism who received a mean of 36 h per week one-to-one EIBI. Similar to Sallows and Graupner (2005), two types of service provision were compared: an intensive clinic-based treatment model with all treatment personnel ($N = 23$) and an intensive parent-managed treatment model with intensive supervision only ($N = 21$). A non-concurrent multiple baseline design across participants ($N = 13$) examined whether progress was associated with EIBI or confounds. At intake, there were no significance between group differences on any of the intake measures. Between intake and follow-up, children in both groups improved significantly on IQ, visual–spatial IQ, language comprehension, expressive language, social skills, motor skills, and adaptive behavior. There were no significant differences between the two groups on any of the measures at follow-up, indicating that both services were equally effective. Mean IQ for participants in both groups increased by 16 points between intake and follow-up. The parent-managed service model required the parents to recruit and manage their own tutors in addition to managing their child's program. Hayward et al. (2009) argued that parents may find it difficult, stressful, or too much of a burden to run a parent-managed program, and they questioned whether parents should be expected to administer and be responsible for their child's psycho-educational provision. On the other hand, this service model has increased access to this treatment and was offered because it was a demand-led outreach service.

Recent Outcome Studies Not Part of the Multi-site Young Autism Project

The first outcome study from researchers not involved in the Multi-site Young Autism Replication Project was published by Howard, Sparkman, Cohen, Green, and Stanislaw in 2005. The study compared effects of three treatment approaches for children with autism or PDD-NOS. Twenty-nine children received 25–40 h per week one-to-one EIBI. A comparison group ($N = 16$) received 30 h per week of one-to-one or two-to-one eclectic intervention in public special education classrooms. A second comparison group ($N = 16$) received 15 h per week of public early intervention in small groups. Mean intake age was 36 months. The diagnosis was set by an independent agency and based on the DSM-IV criteria. Measures included IQ, language functioning, and adaptive functioning. Tests were carried out by independent assessors. There were no significant differences at intake on any of the measures. Follow-up assessment – conducted approximately 14 months after the treatment begun – showed that the EIBI treatment group scored significantly higher as compared to the two comparison groups on all measures. There were no statistically significant differences between the mean scores of the two comparison groups. The EIBI group gained an average of 31 IQ points and 11 points in adaptive functioning. The comparison groups obtained an average change of +9 points in IQ and –2 points in adaptive functioning. Learning rates at follow-up were also substantially higher for children in the ABA group than for participants in either of the other two comparison groups.

A persistent question about EIBI has been whether children's gains are due to the specific behavioral techniques used (e.g., discrete trial teaching, systematic use of reinforcement, shaping, and chaining) or to nonspecific or placebo factors such as providing many hours of service and setting treatment goals that address diverse areas of functioning (Dawson & Osterling, 1997; Jordan, Jones, & Murray, 1998). If it is merely the intensity of treatment that is responsible for the positive outcome reported, then similar outcomes should be achieved if other forms of treatment are applied with the same intensity. Both Howard, Sparkman, Cohen, Green, and Stanislaw (2005) and Eikeseth et al. (2002, 2007) compared EIBI with eclectic special education, when both treatments were delivered with a similar intensity. Both studies clearly demonstrated that the children given EIBI made significantly more progress as compared to the children who received eclectic treatment of similar intensity, showing that gains are due to the specific behavioral intervention rather than to nonspecific factors.

Remington et al. (2007) compared effects of EIBI with standard treatment for children with autism. Mean intake age was 37 months. The diagnosis was set by an independent agency and based on the ICD-10 criteria and confirmed by the ADI-R. Group assignment to either an ABA treatment group ($N = 23$) or a treatment as usual group ($N = 21$) was based on parental choice. Participants in the EIBI treatment group received 25.6 h per week of one-to-one EIBI for 2 years. Participants in the comparison group received standard provision from the local education authorities. The number of one-to-one treatment hours in the treatment as usual group was unspecified. Measures included IQ, language functioning, adaptive functioning, rating scales and observation measures for child behavior, and a self-report measure of parent well-being. Tests were carried out by one of the authors of the study, but the assessor was not informed regarding which group the participants belonged to. There were no significant differences at intake on any of the measures. Follow-up assessment showed that the EIBI treatment group scored significantly higher as compared to the comparison group on intelligence, but not on language functioning or adaptive behavior (as measured by standard scores). The EIBI treatment group gained an average of 12 IQ points, whereas children in the comparison group lost, on average, 2 IQ points. Children in the EIBI group showed an advantage over the comparison group in language functioning at follow-up, as more children in the EIBI group reached basal on the Reynell comprehension and expression scales post-treatment. The EIBI group demonstrated significantly better scores on responding to joint attention as compared to the comparison group, but not in initiating joint attention. No other significant changes were reported in child outcome. On parental outcome, no significant group differences were found except that fathers of children in the EIBI group showed a higher degree of depression at follow-up.

Remington et al. used Jacobson and Truax's (1991) RCI statistic as a criterion for assessing "best outcome." Previous studies had typically reported the number of children scoring within the normal range as criterion for "best outcome." Using the RCI statistic, Remington et al. found that 26% of children receiving early intensive behavioral intervention achieved IQ change that was statistically reliable and none showed a correspondingly reliable regression in IQ. In the comparison group, 14% improved reliably, but a further 14% regressed reliably.

By the early 1990s, EIBI had been suggested as beneficial for many children with autism, and as a result, the demand for EIBI accelerated. As there were often no EIBI services available for children with autism, families set up and managed their own EIBI program in order to secure services for their own child. Mudford, Martin, Eikeseth, and Bibby (2001) compared this type of program to the recommendations of the Multi-site Young Autism Project to assess whether parent-managed programs in the UK adhered to the UCLA protocol. They found that most children (57%) started after they were $3\frac{1}{2}$ years old (later than is considered preferable in the UCLA protocol) and 16% did not exceed the minimum IQ criterion. Children experienced fewer hours of treatment (mean of 32 h) and their programs received relatively infrequent supervision. Twenty-one percent of the programs received supervision from individuals identified as competent to supervise EIBI treatment. No child received the full UCLA protocol (starting prior to $3\frac{1}{2}$ years, receiving 40 h per week, and having weekly supervision from qualified personnel).

Subsequently, Bibby, Eikeseth, Martin, Mudford, and Reeves, (2001) analyzed data for 66 children who had participated in the Mudford et al. (2001) study. They found that mental age and Vineland adaptive behavior increased significantly for a subgroup of the participants, but failed to find significant changes in IQ. None of the participants obtained best outcome status, that is, performed within the normal range on IQ tests and achieved unassisted mainstream school placement. Thus, the results were disappointing.

A similar outcome was reported by Magiati, Charman, and Howlin (2007) who also studied UK parent-managed

EIBI treatment compared to autism-specific nursery provision for preschool children with autism spectrum disorders. Forty-four 23- to 53-month-old children with autism participated. Twenty-eight were in EIBI home-based programs and 16 were in autism-specific nurseries. Cognitive ability, language, play, adaptive behavior skills, and severity of autism were assessed at intake and 2 years later. At follow-up, neither group showed improvements in standard scores, nor were there any significant group differences in IQ, language, play, or severity of autism.

Ben-Itzchak and Zachor (2007) examined progress after 1 year of EIBI for 25 children with autism, who received 35 h or more of one-to-one intervention. They found significant improvements in IQ, imitation, receptive language, expressive language, play skills, non-verbal skills, and stereotyped behavior, as well as a rise in IQ scores by a margin of 17.3 points, from an average of 70.67 points pretreatment to 87.9 points after 1 year of intervention.

Perry et al. (2009) reported on the outcomes of 332 children, aged 2- to 7-years, enrolled in a large, community-based, publicly funded EIBI program in Ontario, Canada. The study was an *effectiveness* study, which examines the extent to which the intervention is effective when applied in "real-life" clinical settings. Children were given between 20 and 40 h of one-to-one EIBI. After an average intervention length of 18 months (range 4–47 months), participants showed a statistically significant reduction in autism severity (–5 points as measured by the Childhood Autism Rating Scale), a significant IQ gain of 12 points, and a significant adaptive behavior gain of 1.5 points.

Finally, Dawson et al. (2010) conducted a randomized, controlled trial to evaluate the efficacy of the early start Denver model (ESDM). Forty-eight children between 18 and 30 months of age were randomly assigned to either ESDM intervention or treatment as usual. Children in the ESDM group received 20 h of one-to-one treatment for 2 years, and participants in the treatment as usual group received 9.1 h of one-to-one intervention for 2 years. The ESDM is a comprehensive intervention for toddlers with autism based on developmental and applied behavioral analytic principles delivered by trained therapists. Children who received ESDM showed significant improvements in IQ, adaptive behavior, and autism diagnosis as compared to children in the control group. Two years after entering intervention, the ESDM group on average improved their standard scores on intellectual functioning by 17.6 points as compared to a gain of 7 points for the children in the control group. The ESDM group did not improve their standard scores in adaptive behavior; however, children who received ESDM were more likely to experience a change in diagnosis from autism to pervasive developmental disorder, not otherwise specified, than the control group.

Conclusions

In sum, there are many outcome studies demonstrating that EIBI may facilitate clinically and socially valid gains in intellectual, social, emotional, and adaptive functioning in preschool-aged children with autism. Research also shows that there is variability in outcome across studies. There may be at least two reasons for this. First, child characteristics such as severity in autism symptoms and intellectual and adaptive functioning may have varied across studies. Second, and perhaps more importantly, the quality and quantity in the intervention may have varied across studies, which in turn, may have affected outcome. An adequate EIBI program involves, at minimum, the following elements: (a) the program is individualized and comprehensive, (b) targets guided by normal development, (c) parents serve as active co-therapists, (d) one-to-one intervention is provided initially, (e) the intervention is intensive and lasts for a minimum of 2 years, (f) several behavior analytic procedures are used, (h) the intervention quality is high quality, and finally (j) the program is supervised regularly by a qualified supervisor. Whenever one or more of these conditions are not met, less than optimal outcomes may be expected. For example, Eikeseth, Hayward, Gale, Gitlesen, and Eldevik (2009) found that intensity of supervision was associated with outcome in preschool-aged children with autism receiving EIBI. In this study, supervision intensity ranged from 2.9 to 7.8 h per month per child. Results showed a significant correlation between intensity of supervision and change in IQ scores between intake and follow-up, suggesting that intensity of supervision was reliably associated with skill acquisition. Hence, variables such as insufficient intensity of supervision may explain, in part, the limited gains observed after the UK parent-managed EIBI treatment, as reported by Bibby et al. (2001) and Magiati et al. (2007). In both studies, supervision was provided, on average, every 3 months, as compared to other studies which have reported weekly or bi-weekly supervision (Eikeseth et al., 2002; Lovaas, 1987; Sallows & Graupner, 2005; Smith et al., 2000).

Meta-analysis and Effect Size

Although many of the controlled studies just described have reported statistically significant group differences in favor of EIBI, a statistical method called meta-analysis can be used to analyze the combined results of several studies to allow for a more thorough analysis of intervention effects, often being referred to as effect size. Often effect size is calculated by expressing the difference between the means of the experiment and control groups in terms of the standard deviation of the control group's scores. Reichow and Wolery (2009) performed a meta-analysis based on 12 EIBI outcome studies and reported a mean effect size of 0.69 for IQ change. An effect size of 0.69 is considered, by convention, moderate in terms of clinical effect, and Reichow and Wolery concluded that EIBI is an effective treatment, on average, for children with autism.

Another recent meta-analysis was conducted by Eldevik and colleagues (2009) and replicated and extended the meta-analysis by Reichow and Wolery. In contrast to Reichow and Wolery, Eldevik et al. included only those studies containing comparison or control groups and based the analysis on individual participant's data (obtained from the authors) rather than group average data, as reported in the original studies. Results showed an effect size of 1.10 for IQ change and 0.66 for change in adaptive behavior. The effect size of 1.10 for IQ change is considered, by conventions, large and was larger than the moderate effect size reported by Reichow and Wolery (2009). There may be at least two explanations for this difference. First, Eldevik et al. used the more methodologically rigorous standardized mean difference effect size, whereas Reichow and Wolery computed their mean effect size based on the change within the EIBI group only. The mean change effect size is computed without comparison or control group data and is limited by threats to validity such as maturation. Second, Eldevik et al. applied a more precise yet inclusive definition of EIBI, introduced by Green et al. (2002), that is more in line with how other professionals define EIBI (e.g., Eikeseth, 2009). The effect size for adaptive functioning obtained by Eldevik et al. is considered moderate. Reichow and Wolery (2009) did not include effect size on adaptive behavior in their analysis.

Spreckley and Boyd (2009) performed a meta-analysis of four EIBI studies for children with autism and concluded, in contrast to the two meta-analyses just described, that EIBI did not significantly improve outcomes. Unfortunately, the meta-analysis by Spreckley and Boyd is flawed. Smith, Eikeseth, Sallows, and Graupner (2009) showed that it yielded null findings because of an error made in the handling of the study by Sallows and Graupner (2005). As noted above, this study compared two models of EIBI (clinic based and parent managed). Spreckley and Boyd classified the clinic-based group as EIBI, but the parent-managed group was erroneously misrepresented as a "standard care" control. Smith et al. (2009) noted that simply removing the Sallows and Graupner (2005) study from the meta-analysis, or correctly classifying both models as EIBI, yields significant findings in favor of EIBI.

Finally, two more recent meta-analysis have reported results supporting the efficacy of EIBI (Makrygianni & Reed, 2010; Peters-Scheffer, Didden, Korzilius, & Sturmey, 2011). Makrygianni and Reed (2010) reported a moderate mean change effect size for IQ and a moderate to high effect size for adaptive functioning. The meta-analysis was based on 14 studies, but the studies selected for the analysis were somewhat different from those included in the previously mentioned meta-analysis. Peters-Scheffer et al. (2011) included 11 studies in their meta-analysis and reported that EIBI outperformed the control groups on IQ, non-verbal IQ, expressive and receptive language, and adaptive behavior. Differences between the EIBI and control groups were 11.26–15.70 points on standardized tests. The results of these meta-analysis support the assertion that EIBI may facilitate clinically and socially valid gains in intellectual, social, language, and adaptive functioning in preschool-aged children with autism.

Best Outcome and Meaningful Change

Given that outcomes for individual children vary, an important step in the examination of the effects of EIBI for children with autism is to determine what constitutes "best outcome" or meaningful change for individual children. To date, the method for assessing "best outcome" and meaningful change has varied. Lovaas (1987) defined "best outcome" as IQ scores within the normal range and successful first-grade performance in public schools. Using this definition of best outcome, Lovaas found that 47% of children in the experimental group could be classified as "best outcome," Smith et al. (2000) found that 27% of participants in the experimental group achieved "best outcome," Sallows and Graupner (2005) found that 48% of children could be classified as "best outcome," and finally, Cohen et al. (2006) reported that 29% of children in the EIBI group achieved "best outcome."

Remington et al. (2007) used the RCI (Jacobson & Truax, 1991) to examine meaningful change. The Reliable Change Index (RCI), a statistical analysis borrowed from psychotherapy outcome research, is the amount by which an outcome measure needs to change before one can be 95% certain that the change cannot be accounted for by the variability of scores in the sample and/or measurement error. Remington et al. (2007) found that 26% of the experimental children achieved reliable change on IQ. To achieve reliable change, an IQ gain of 24 or more was required.

Eldevik et al. (2010) calculated the RCI for individual participant data from 309 children from 16 EIBI outcome studies. To achieve reliable change in IQ, a gain of 27 points (almost 2 standard deviations) between intake and follow-up was required. Eldevik et al. found that 30% of children achieved reliable change in IQ. Eldevik et al. also calculated reliable change in adaptive behavior. They found that to achieve reliable change, a gain of 21 points in adaptive behavior was required. Twenty-one percent of the participants achieved reliable change in adaptive functioning.

Eldevik et al. (2010) also argued for the need to identify a dichotomous outcome variable for change at the level of individual participants to supply simple ways to communicate information about intervention efficacy to policy makers and consumers and suggested using number needed to treat (NNT) to do so. The NNT represents the number of children who would need to be treated with a specific intervention to obtain one additional success over the success rate in a comparison intervention (Straus & Sackett, 2005). For example, NNT = 5 means that for every five children who are treated with a particular intervention, one additional child will respond to this intervention who would not have responded to a comparison intervention. The larger the NNT, the less effective the treatment relative to the comparison (Kraemer et al., 2003).

Using this statistic, Eldevik et al. (2010) found that NNT for IQ was 5 and NNT for adaptive behavior was 7. In comparison, NNT for other disorders such as major depression is between 3 and 5, obsessive compulsive disorders is between 4 and 5, and bulimia nervosa is 9 (Pinson & Gray, 2003).

School-Aged Children

Although the diagnosis of autism may now be occurring at younger ages than in the past, and although access to services may have improved, many children with autism do not access EIBI until after they are 4 years of age. To date, only one study has examined outcome of EIBI for older children: As described above, Eikeseth et al., 2002, 2007) examined outcomes for children with autism who were between 4 and 7 years of age at the onset of treatment (mean age = 5.5 years) and demonstrated that EIBI can be effective for children who are up to 7 years of age at intake. Interestingly, Eikeseth et al. (2007) found that age at intake predicted neither treatment outcome nor gains in treatment for children in the EIBI group, suggesting that this variable may not be as important for outcome as previously thought. The same conclusion was reached by Eldevik et al. (2010) when analyzing individual participant data from 309 children receiving behavioral interventions.

Although EIBI is also promising for children who start intervention later, more research is needed before it can be concluded that EIBI for school-aged children is evidence based (Eikeseth, 2009). Hence, research on the efficacy of EIBI for school-aged children should be a priority.

EIBI for Children with Other Diagnosis

EIBI is specifically designed to target the behavioral excesses and deficits exhibited by individual children, and interventions are tailored to replace such deficit and excess behaviors with functional and adaptive skills that are maintained by the child's natural environment. Hence, EIBI is not designed to address "autism" per se or the "cause of autism" (Lovaas,

2003). For those and other reasons, it can be hypothesized that EIBI may be effective for other types of neurodevelopmental conditions.

To date, only two outcome studies have examined the effects of EIBI for non-autistic populations, both addressing intellectual disabilities. Smith, Eikeseth, Klevstrand, and Lovaas (1997) evaluated the effects of EIBI provided to 11 children with severe intellectual disabilities. A comparison group of 10 children received minimal treatment. Groups were similar on all measures at intake, with a mean age at intake of 3.08 years and mean intake IQ of 28. Mean IQ gain for the EIBI group after a minimum of 24 months of intervention was 8 points while the comparison group, on average, lost 3 IQ points over the same period. Moreover, children in the EIBI group acquired more expressive language than children in the comparison group. Hence, EIBI may result in meaningful gains for preschool-aged children with severe intellectual disabilities, although the children in the study remained significantly developmentally delayed.

Recently, Eldevik et al. (2010) evaluated effects of EIBI for children with mild to moderate intellectual disabilities. Eleven children received 10 h per week of one-to-one EIBI. Mean intake age for this group was 54 months and mean intake IQ was 56. Fourteen children with a mean intake age of 46 months and a mean intake IQ of 50 received treatment as usual and constituted the comparison group. After 1 year of intervention, changes in intelligence and adaptive behavior scores were statistically significant in favor of the EIBI group (effect sizes of 1.13 for IQ change and 0.95 for change in adaptive behavior composite). Children in the EIBI group gained an average of 16 IQ points and 3 points in adaptive behavior. Sixty-four percent of the children in the EIBI group met criteria for reliable change in IQ, as compared to 14% of the comparison group.

The results from these two studies give some support for the notion that EIBI may be effective for populations other than children with autism. Additional research, however, is needed to further examine this possibility.

Moderators and Mediators of Treatment Outcome

Several studies have examined relations between intake variables and outcome measures. Positive correlates with outcome include initial skill acquisition (Hayward et al., 2009; Sallows & Graupner, 2005; Weiss, 1999), age at intake (Harris & Handleman, 2000), IQ at intake (Ben-Itzchak & Zachor, 2007; Harris & Handleman, 2000), initial social skills (Eikeseth et al., 2007), toy play, socially avoidant behavior at intake (Sherer & Schreibman, 2005), and autism subtype (Beglinger & Smith, 2005). Other studies, however, have found no relations between age or IQ at intake and outcome (Eikeseth et al., 2007; Hayward et al., 2009; Lovaas & Smith, 1988; Sallows & Graupner, 2005). Hence, conflicting results have been reported.

Ben-Itzchak and Zachor (2007) assessed the relation between pre-intervention variables (cognition, socialization, and communication) and outcome of EIBI for young children with autism. Twenty-five children with autism (20–32 months) were divided into groups based on their IQ scores and on the severity of their social interaction and communication deficits. Six developmental–behavioral domains including imitation, receptive language, expressive language, non-verbal communication skills, play skills, and stereotyped behaviors were assessed at pre- and post-intervention. Significant progress was noted in all six developmental–behavioral domains after 1 year of intervention. Children with higher initial cognitive levels and children with fewer measured early social interaction deficits showed better acquisition of skills in three developmental areas: receptive language, expressive language, and play skills. Both groups showed improvement in receptive language skills. Improvement in expressive language was associated with the child's social abilities, while more significant progress in play skills was related to pre-intervention cognitive level.

Eldevik et al. (2010) examined individual participant data from 16 group design studies of behavioral intervention for children with autism. Three hundred and nine children received behavioral intervention, 39 received comparison interventions, and 105 were in a control group. This large sample size allowed for an analysis of main effects as well as for interactions between key variables (e.g., age at intake combined with IQ at intake) as potential predictors. Such analyses were not possible in previous research because participant numbers were too small. Eldevik et al. found that intervention intensity was the only variable that independently positively predicted both IQ and adaptive behavior gain. In addition, intake adaptive behavior and intake IQ predicted gains in adaptive behavior. Those children with lower adaptive behavior scores at intake had larger adaptive behavior change over 2 years, whereas higher IQ at intake predicted larger adaptive behavior gains.

Despite the considerable sample size, Eldevik et al. (2010) found that no interactions between variables predicted outcome; however, it is important to continue to explore interactions between predictors of outcome in future research where sample size permits because such interactions may provide important information regarding ideal conditions for positive outcomes for EIBI. Eldevik and Hastings et al.'s results are limited by the lack of available data on correlates of outcome, and their results were based on studies where moderator effects were not built into the design of the studies.

Future Research

Clearly, there is a need for additional outcome research. The fact that only three comprehensive intervention programs have been subjected to outcome research illustrates this issue. Also, there is a need to identify effective treatment parameters and mechanisms responsible for change (Kazdin & Nock, 2003). Future research should continue to explore variables that may interact with outcome. Variables interacting with outcome could be system variables (e.g., family variables, socio-economic status, staff characteristics), behavioral variables (e.g., intake functioning including "autistic symptoms"), and/or biological/medical variables. Future research should also aim to improve treatment efficacy in general and specifically to improve treatment efficacy for those children who respond less favorably. Research should follow children who have received EIBI in their preschool years into adulthood to examine how well they function and the extent to which they have maintained their gains. Research should also continue to examine the efficacy of EIBI with older children and adults and for children with other neurodevelopmental disorders. Finally, research should be conducted to examine the long-term cost-effectiveness and cost–benefits of EIBI.

Conclusions

Comprehensive interventions are those addressing, at minimum, all three core deficits that define autism. Unfortunately, only three comprehensive interventions have been subjected to outcome research and the only intervention which is evidence based is intervention based on ABA. This intervention has been labeled early and intensive behavioral interventions (EIBI). Currently there are many outcome studies and several meta-analyses demonstrating that EIBI may facilitate clinically significant gains in intellectual, social, emotional, and adaptive functioning in preschool-aged children with autism.

Acknowledgments The author thanks Tristram Smith, Sigmund Eldevik, Madison Pilato, and Lisa Shull for their valuable comments.

References

Aldred, C., Green, J., & Adams, C. (2004). A new social communication intervention for children with autism: Pilot randomised controlled treatment study suggesting effectiveness. *Journal of Child Psychology and Psychiatry, 45*, 1420–1430.

American Psychiatric Association. (1980). *Diagnostic and statistical manual of mental disorders* (3rd ed.). Washington, DC: American Psychiatric Association.

American Psychiatric Association. (1994). *Diagnostic and statistical manual of mental disorders* (4th ed.). Washington, DC: American Psychiatric Association.

Anderson, S. R., Avery, D. L., DiPietro, E. K., Edwards, G. L., & Christian, W. P. (1987). Intensive home-based intervention with autistic children. *Education and Treatment of Children, 10,* 352–366.

Bailey, A., Le Couteur, A., Gottesman, I., Bolton, P., Simonoff, E., Yuzda, E., & Rutter, M. (1995). Autism as a strongly genetic disorder: Evidence from a British twin study. *Psychological Medicine, 25,* 63–77.

Baird, G., Simonoff, E., Pickles, A., Chandler, S., Loucas, T., Meldrum, D., mfl (2006). Prevalence of disorders of the autism spectrum in a population cohort of children in South Thames: The Special Needs and Autism Project (SNAP). *The Lancet, 368,* 210–215.

Beglinger, L., & Smith, T. (2005). Concurrent validity of social subtype and IQ after early Intensive Behavioral Intervention in children with autism: A preliminary investigation. *Journal of Autism and Developmental Disorders, 35,* 295–303.

Ben-Itzchak, E., & Zachor, D. A. (2007). The effects of intellectual functioning and autism severity on outcome of early behavioral intervention for children with autism. *Research in Developmental Disabilities, 28,* 287–303.

Bibby, P., Eikeseth, S., Martin, N. T., Mudford, O., Reeves, D. (2001). Progress and outcomes for children with autism receiving parent-managed intensive intervention. *Research in Developmental Disabilities, 22,* 425–447.

Billstedt, E., Gillberg, C., & Gillberg, C. (2005). Autism after adolescence: Population-based 13- to 22-year follow-up study of 120 individuals with autism diagnosed in childhood. *Journal of Autism and Developmental Disorders, 35,* 351–360.

Birnbrauer, J. S., & Leach, D. J. (1993). The Murdoch Early Intervention Program after 2 years. *Behavior Change, 10,* 63–74.

Carr, J. E., Severtson, J. M., & Lepper, T. L. (2009). Noncontingent reinforcement is an empirically supported treatment for problem behavior exhibited by individuals with developmental disabilities. *Research in Developmental Disabilities., 30,* 44–57.

Catania, A. C. (1998). *Learning* (4th ed.). Englewood Cliffs, NJ: Prentice Hall.

Chambliss, D. L., & Hollon, S. D. (1998). Defining empirically supported therapies. *Journal of Consulting and Clinical Psychology, 66,* 7–18.

Chambless, D. L., Sanderson, W. C., Shoham, V., Bennett Johnson, S., Pope, K. S., Crits-Christoph, P., et al. (1996). An update on empirically validated therapies. *The Clinical Psychologist, 49,* 5–18.

Cohen, H., Amarine-Dickens, M., & Smith, T. (2006). Early intensive behavioral treatment: Replication of the UCLA model in a community setting. *Developmental and Behavioral Paediatrics, 27,* 145–155.

Cooper, J. O., Heron, T. E., & Heward, W. L. (2007). *Applied behavior analysis* (2nd ed.). Prentice Hall: New Jersey.

Cunningham, A. B., & Schreibman, L. (2008). Stereotypy in autism: The importance of function. *Research in Autism Spectrum Disorders, 2,* 469–479.

Dawson, G., & Osterling, J. (1997). Early intervention in autism. In M. Guralnick (Ed.), *The effectiveness of early intervention.* Baltimore: Brookes.

Dawson, G., Rogers, S., Munson, J., Smith, M., Winter, J., Greenson, J., Donaldson, A., Varley, J. (2010). Randomized, controlled trial of an intervention for toddlers with autism: The Early Start Denver Model. *Pediatrics, 125,* e17–e23.

Drew, A., Baird, G., Baron-Cohen, S., Cox, A., Slonims, V., Wheelwright, S., et al. (2002). A pilot randomized control trial of a parent training intervention for pre-school children with autism: Preliminary findings and methodological challenges. *European Child and Adolescent Psychiatry, 11,* 266–272.

Eikeseth, S. (2001). Recent critiques of the UCLA young autism project. *Behavioral Interventions, 16,* 249–264.

Eikeseth, S. (2009). Outcome of comprehensive psycho-educational interventions for young children with autism. *Research in Developmental Disabilities, 30,* 158–178.

Eikeseth, S., Hayward, D., Gale, C., Gitlesen, J.-P., Eldevik, S. (2009). Intensity of supervision and outcome for preschool aged children receiving early and intensive behavioral interventions: A preliminary study. *Research in Autism Spectrum Disorders, 3,* 67–73.

Eikeseth, S., Smith, T., Jahr, E., & Eldevik, S. (2002). Intensive behavioral treatment at school for 4- to 7-year-old children with autism. A 1-year comparison controlled study. *Behavior Modification, 26,* 49–68.

Eikeseth, S., Smith, T., Jahr, E., & Eldevik, S. (2007). Outcome for children with autism who began intensive behavioral treatment between ages 4 and 7: A comparison controlled study. *Behavior Modification, 31,* 264–278.

Eldevik, S., Eikeseth, S., Jahr, E., & Smith, T. (2006). Effects of low-intensity behavioral treatment for children with autism and mental retardation. *Journal of Autism & Developmental Disorders, 36,* 211–224.

Eldevik, S., Hastings, R. P., Hughes, J. C., Jahr, E., Eikeseth, S., & Cross, S. (2009). Meta-analysis of early intensive behavioral intervention for children with autism. *Journal of Clinical Child and Adolescent Psychology, 38,* 439–450.

Eldevik, S., Hastings, R. P., Hughes, J. K., Jahr, E., Eikeseth, S., & Cross. S. (2010). Analyzing outcome for children with autism receiving early intensive behavioral intervention: Secondary analysis of data from 457 children. *The American Journal on Intellectual and Developmental Disabilities, 34,* 16–34.

Eldevik, S., Jahr, E., Eikeseth, S., Hastings, R. P., & Hughes C. J. (2010). Cognitive and adaptive behavior outcomes of behavioral Intervention for young children with intellectual disability. *Behavior Modification, 34,* 16–34.

FDA. (October 2, 2006). *FDA Approves the First Drug to Treat Irritability Associated with Autism, Risperdal.* Press release. Retrieved on 2006-10-02.

Ferster, C. B., & DeMyer, M. K. (1961). The development of performances in autistic children in an automatically controlled environment. *Journal of Chronic Disease, 13,* 312–345.

Filipek, P. A., Steinberg-Epstein, R., Book, T. M. (2006). Intervention for autistic spectrum disorders. *NeuroRx, 3,* 207–216.

Fombonne, E. (1999). The epidemiology of autism: A review. *Psychological Medicine, 29,* 769–786.

Fombonne, E. (2003). Epidemiological surveys of autism and other pervasive developmental disorders: An update. *Journal of Autism and Developmental Disorders, 33,* 365–382.

Freitag, C. M. (2007). The genetics of autistic disorder and its clinical relevance: A review of the literature. *Molecular Psychiatry, 12,* 2–22.

Gersten, R., Fuchs, L. S., Compton, D., Coyne, M., Greenwood, C., & Innocenti, M. S. (2005). Quality indicators for group experimental and quasi-experimental research in special education. *Exceptional Children, 71,* 149–164.

Green, G., Brennan, L. C., & Fein, D. (2002). Intensive behavioral treatment for a toddler at high risk for autism. *Behavior Modification, 26,* 69–102.

Gresham, F. M., & MacMillan, D. L. (1997). Autistic recovery? An analysis and critique of the empirical evidence on the Early Intervention Project. *Behavioral Disorders, 22,* 185–201.

Handleman, J. S., Harris, S. L., Celbiberti, D., Lilleheht, E., & Tomchek, S. (1991). Developmental changes in preschool children with autism and normally developing peers. *Infant Toddler Intervention, 1,* 137–143.

Harris, S. L., & Handleman, J. S. (2000). Age and IQ at intake as predictors of placement for young children with autism: A four- to six-year follow-up. *Journal of Autism and Developmental Disorders, 30,* 137–142.

Harris, S. L., Handleman, J. S., Gordon, R., Kristoff, B., & Fuentes, F. (1991). Changes in cognitive and language functioning of preschool children with autism. *Journal of Autism and Developmental Disorders, 21*, 281–290.

Harris, S. L., Handleman, J. S., Kristoff, B., Bass, L., & Gordon, R. (1990). Changes in language development among autistic and peer children in segregated and integrated preschool settings. *Journal of Autism and Developmental Disorders, 20*, 23–31.

Hayward, D. W., Eikeseth, S., Gale, C., & Morgan, S. (2009). Assessing progress during treatment for young children with autism receiving intensive behavioural interventions. *Autism, 13*, 613–633.

Howard, J. S., Sparkman, C. R., Cohen, H. G., Green, G., & Stanislaw, H. (2005). A comparison of intensive behavior analytic and eclectic treatments for young children with autism. *Research in Developmental Disabilities, 26*, 359–383.

Howlin, P. (2005). The effectiveness of interventions for children with autism. *Journal of Neural Transmission, 69* (Supplementum), 101–119.

Hoyson, M., Jamieson, B., & Strain, P. S. (1984). Individualized group instruction of normally developing and autistic-like children: A description and evaluation of the LEAP curriculum model. *Journal of the Division of Early Childhood, 8*, 157–181.

Iwata, B. A., Pace, G. M., Dorsey, M. F., Zarcone, J. R., Vollmer, T. R., Smith, R. G. et al. (1994). The functions of self-injurious behavior: An experimental-epidemiological analysis. *Journal of Applied Behavior Analysis, 27*, 215–240.

Jacobson, N. S., & Truax, P. (1991). Clinical significance: A statistical approach to defining meaningful change in psychotherapy research. *Journal of Consulting and Clinical Psychology, 59*, 12–19.

Jordan, R., Jones, G., & Murray, D. (1998). *Educational interventions for children with autism: A literature review of recent and current research*. Birmingham: School of Education, University of Birmingham.

Kazdin, A. E., & Nock, M. K. (2003). Delineating mechanisms of change in child and adolescent therapy: Methodological issues and research recommendations. *Journal of Child Psychology and Psychiatry, 44*, 1116–1129.

Kraemer, H. C., Morgan, G. A., Leech, N. L., Gliner, J. A., Vaske, J. J., & Harmon, R. J. (2003). Measures of clinical significance. *Journal of the American Academy of Child and Adolescent Psychiatry, 42*, 1524–1529.

Leaf, R., & McEachin, J. (1999). *A work in progress: Behavior management strategies and a curriculum for intensive behavioral treatment of autism*. New York: DRL Books, L. L. C.

Lord, C., & Schopler, E. (1994). TEACCH services for preschool children. In S. Harris & J. Handleman (Eds.), *Preschool education programs for children with autism* (pp. 87–106). Austin, TX: PRO-ED.

Lovaas, O. I. (1977). *The autistic child: Language development through behaviour modification*. New York: Irvington Publishers.

Lovaas, O. I. (1987). Behavioral treatment and normal intellectual and educational functioning in autistic children. *Journal of Consulting and Clinical Psychology, 55*, 3–9.

Lovaas, O. I. (1993). The development of a treatment-research project for developmentally disabled and autistic children. *Journal of Applied Behavior Analysis, 26*, 617–630.

Lovaas, O. I. (2003). *Opplæring av mennesker med forsinket utvikling: Grunnleggende prinsipper og prosedyrer*. Oslo: Gyldendal Akademisk.

Lovaas, O. I., Ackerman, A., Alexander, D., Firestone, P., Perkins, M., & Young, D. B. (1981). *Teaching developmentally disabled children: The ME Book*. Austin, TX: PRO-ED.

Lovaas, O. I., Koegel, R. L., Simmons, J. W., & Long, J. S. (1973). Some generalization and follow-up measures on autistic children in behavior therapy. *Journal of Applied Behavior Analysis, 6*, 131–161.

Lovaas, O. I., & Simmons, J. Q. (1969). Manipulation of self-destruction in three retarded children. *Journal of Applied Behaviour Analysis, 2*, 143–157.

Lovaas, O. I., & Smith, T. (1988). Intensive behavioral treatment for young autistic children. Advances in clinical child psychology. In B. B. Lahey & A. E. Kazdin (Eds.), *Advances in clinical child psychology* (Vol. II, pp. 285–323). New York: Plenum.

Lovaas, O. I., Smith, T., & McEachin, J. J. (1989). Clarifying comments on the young autism study: Reply to Schopler, Short, and Mesibov. *Journal of Consulting and Clinical Psychology, 57*, 165–167.

Magiati, I., Charman, T., & Howlin, P. (2007). A two-year prospective follow-up study of community-based early intensive behavioural intervention and specialist nursery provision for children with autism spectrum disorders. *Journal of Child Psychology and Psychiatry, 48*, 803–812.

Makrygianni, M. K., & Reed, P. (2010). A meta-analytic review of the effectiveness of behavioural early intervention programs for children with Autistic Spectrum *Disorders. Research in Autism Spectrum Disorders, 4*, 577–593.

Matson, J. L., & Fodstad, J. J. C. (2008). The treatment of food selectivity and other feeding problems in children with autism spectrum disorders. *Research in Autism Spectrum Disorders, 3*, 455–461.

Matson, J. L., & LoVullo, S. V. (2008). A review of behavioral treatments for self-injurious behaviors of persons with autism spectrum disorders. *Behavior Modification, 32*, 61–76.

Matson, J. L., Matson, M. L., & Rivet, T. T. (2007). Social-skills treatments for children with autism spectrum disorders: An overview. *Behavior Modification, 32*, 61–76.

Matson, J. L., & Smith, K. R. (2008). Current status of intensive behavioral interventions for young children with autism and PDD-NOS. *Research in Autism Spectrum Disorders, 2*, 60–74.

Maurice, C., Green, G., & Foxx, R. M. (Eds.). (2001). *Making a difference: Behavioral intervention for autism*. Austin, TX: PRO-ED.

Maurice, C. (Ed.), Green, G., & Luce, S. (Co-Eds.). (1996). *Behavioral intervention for young children with autism: A manual for parents and professionals*. Austin, TX: PRO-ED.

McEachin, J. J., Smith, T., & Lovaas, O. I. (1993). Long-term outcome for children with autism who received early intensive behavioral treatment. *American Journal of Mental Retardation, 97*, 359–372.

Mesibov, G. B., Shea, V., & Schopler, E. (2005). *The TEACCH approach to autism spectrum disorders*. New York: Springer Publishers.

Mudford O. C., Martin, N., Eikeseth, S., & Bibby, P. (2001). Parent-managed behavioral treatment for pre-school children with autism: Some Characteristics of UK Programs. *Research in Developmental Disabilities, 22*, 173–182.

Muller, R. A. (2007). The study of Autism as a distributed disorder. *Mental Retardation and Developmental Disabilities Research Reviews, 13*, 85–95.

National Research Council, Division of Behavioral and Social Sciences Education. (2001). *Educating children with autism*. Washington, DC: National Academy Press.

Oxford Centre for Evidence Based Medicine. (2009). *Levels of evidence*. Retrieved July 1st, 2009, from http://www.cebm.net/index.aspx?o=1025

Ozonoff, S., & Cathcart, K. (1998). Effectiveness of home program intervention for young children with autism. *Journal of Autism and Developmental Disabilities, 28*, 25–32.

Pangborn, J., & Baker, S. M. (2005). *Autism: Effective biomedical treatments*. San Diego: Autism Research Institute.

Perry, A., Cummings, A., Geier, J. D., Freeman, N. L. Hughes, S., LaRose, L., et al. (2009). Effectiveness of Intensive Behavioral Intervention in a large, community-based program. *Research in Autism Spectrum Disorders, 2*, 621–642.

Peters-Scheffer, N., Didden, R., Korzilius, H., & Sturmey, P. (2011). A meta-analytic study on the effectiveness of comprehensive ABA-based early intervention programs for children with Autism Spectrum Disorders. *Research in Autism Spectrum Disorders, 5,* 60–69.

Pinson, L., & Gray, G. E. (2003). Number needed to treat: An underused measure of treatment effect. *Psychiatric Services, 54,* 145–146.

Reichow, B., & Wolery, M. (2009). Comprehensive synthesis of early intensive behavioral interventions for young children with autism based on the UCLA young autism project model. *Journal of Autism and Developmental Disorders, 39,* 23–41.

Remington, B., Hastings, R. P., Kovshoff, H., Espinosa, F., Jahr, E., Brown, T., et al. (2007). Early intensive behavioral intervention: Outcomes for children with autism and their parents after two years. *American Journal on Mental Retardation, 112,* 418–438.

Rogers, S., Hall, T., Osaki, D., Reaven, J., & Herbison, J. (2001). The Denver model: A comprehensive, integrated educational approach to young children with autism and their families. In J. Handleman & S. Harris (Eds.), *Preschool education programs for children with autism.* Austin, TX: PRO-ED.

Rogers, S. J., & DiLalla, D. L. (1991). A comparative study of the effects of developmentally based instructional model on young children with autism and young children with other disorders of behavior and development. *Topics in Early Childhood Special Education, 11,* 29–47.

Rogers, S. J., Hayden, D., Hepburn, S., Charlifue-Smith, R., Hall, T., & Hayes, A. (2006). Teaching young nonverbal children with autism useful speech: A pilot study of the Denver Model and PROMPT interventions. *Journal of Autism and Developmental Disorders, 36,* 1007–1024.

Rogers, S. J., & Vismara, L. A. (2008). Evidence-based comprehensive treatments for early autism. *Journal of Clinical Child and Adolescent Psychology, 37,* 8–38.

Sallows, G. O., & Graupner, T. D. (2005). Intensive Behavioral Treatment for children with autism: Four-year outcome and predictors. *American Journal on Mental Retardation, 110,* 417–438.

Schopler, E. (1987). Specific and nonspecific factors in the effectiveness of a treatment system. *American Psychologist, 42,* 376–383.

Schopler, E., & Mesibov, G. B. (Eds.). (1995). *Learning and cognition in autism.* New York: Plenum Press.

Schopler, E., & Reichler, R. J. (1971). Parents as cotherapists in the treatment of psychotic children. *Journal of Autism and Childhood Schizophrenia, 1,* 87–102.

Schopler, E., Short, A., & Mesibov, G. (1989). Relation of behavioral treatment to «normal functioning»: Comment on Lovaas. *Journal of Consulting and Clinical Psychology, 57,* 162–164.

Sheinkopf, S. J., & Siegel, B. (1998). Home-based behavioral treatment of young children with autism. *Journal of Autism and Developmental Disorders, 28,* 15–23.

Sherer, M. R., & Schreibman, L. (2005). Individual behavioral profiles and predictors of treatment effectiveness for children with autism. *Journal of Consulting and Clinical Psychology, 73,* 525–538.

Smith, T., Eikeseth, S., Klevstrand, M., & Lovaas, O. I. (1997). Intensive behavioral treatment for preschoolers with severe mental retardation and pervasive developmental disorder. *American Journal on Mental Retardation, 102,* 238–249.

Smith, T., Eikeseth, S., Sallows, G. O., & Graupner, T. D. (2009). Efficacy of applied behavior analysis in autism. *The Journal of Paediatrics, 155,* 151–152.

Smith, T., Groen, A. D., & Wynn, J. W. (2000). Randomized trial of intensive early intervention for children with pervasive developmental disorder. *American Journal on Mental Retardation, 105,* 269–285.

Smith, T., & Wick, J. (2008). Controversial treatments. In K. Chawarska, A. Klin, & F. R. Volkmar (Eds.), *Autism spectrum disorders in infants and toddlers* (pp. 243–273). New York: Guilford Press.

Spreckley, M., & Boyd R. (2009). Efficacy of applied behavioral intervention in preschool children with autism for improving cognitive, language, and adaptive behavior: A systematic review and meta-analysis. *The Journal of Paediatrics, 154,* 338–344.

Straus, S. E., & Sackett, D. L. (2005). *Evidence-based medicine: How to practice and teach EBM.* Edinburgh: Elsevier Churchill Livingstone.

Volkmar, F., Lord, C., Bailey, A., Schultz, R. T., & Klin, A. (2004). Autism and pervasive developmental disorders. *Journal of Child Psychology and Psychiatry, 45,* 135–170.

Weiss, M. J. (1999). Differential rates of skill acquisition and outcomes of early intensive behavioral intervention for autism. *Behavioral Interventions, 14,* 3–22.

Weiss, R. (1981). INREAL intervention for language handicapped and bilingual children. *Journal of the Division of Early Childhood, 4,* 40–51.

Wolf, M. M., Risley, T., & Mees, H. (1964). Application of operant conditioning procedures to the behavior problems of an autistic child. *Behaviour, Research and Therapy, 1,* 305–312.

Yoder, P. J., & Lieberman, R. G. (2010). Brief report: Randomized test of the efficacy of Picture Exchange Communication System on highly generalized picture exchanges in children with ASD. *Journal of Autism Developmental Disorders, 40,* 629–632.

Teaching Adaptive and Social Skills to Individuals with Autism Spectrum Disorders

Kendra Thomson, Kerri Walters, Garry L. Martin, and C.T. Yu

The purpose of this chapter is to review intervention strategies that have been researched for teaching adaptive and social skills to children with autism spectrum disorders (ASDs). We hope that the chapter will be useful for practitioners and that it will also stimulate further research. Before beginning our review, we briefly describe ASDs (a more thorough discussion of the characteristics of ASDs can be found in Chapter 1 of this volume).

The Diagnostic and Statistical Manual of Mental Disorders, Fourth Edition, Text Revision (DSM-IV-TR, American Psychiatric Association, 2000) classifies autistic disorder, Asperger disorder, and pervasive developmental disorders-not otherwise specified (PDD-NOS) under the umbrella of pervasive developmental disorders (PDDs). Autistic disorder is characterized by abnormal language development, qualitative impairments in communication skills and social interactions, and rigid, repetitive behaviors and interests. Asperger syndrome has similar features as autism, although it has less severe symptoms and it is typically not accompanied by language delay. If a child has symptoms of autistic disorder or Asperger syndrome, but does not meet the specific criteria for either, a diagnosis of PDD-NOS is given. The term autism spectrum disorders typically refers to these three disorders, although two other very rare, but severe disorders, Rett syndrome and childhood disintegrative disorder, are also included under PDDs.

Adaptive Skills Interventions

The American Association on Intellectual and Developmental Disabilities defines adaptive skill development as "the ability to apply basic information learned in school to naturally accruing activities in the school, home or community" (Drew & Hardman, 2007, p. 231). A number of different life skills comprise the category of adaptive behaviors, including (a) domestic skills (e.g., chores, meal preparation); (b) self-care (e.g., tooth brushing, toilet training, and dressing); and (c) community skills (e.g., recognition of danger and street crossing). Many of these skills can be found throughout the literature, particularly for teaching individuals with developmental disabilities. For the purposes of this chapter, we will focus solely on domestic, self-care, community, and toileting skills. Among the central concerns experienced by parents of children with ASD is whether their child will lead a productive and independent life (Shipley-Benamou, Lutzker, & Taubman, 2002). Individuals who achieve independence in performing adaptive behaviors at an early age have a better chance of thriving in vocational and domestic settings (Pierce & Schreibman, 1994). Failure to teach daily living skills to individuals with ASD can negatively impact their autonomy, independence, and quality of life (Hayden, 1997). Although there has been a focus on teaching individuals with intellectual disabilities to perform domestic and daily living tasks and although approximately 70% of individuals with autism spectrum disorders also have intellectual disabilities, the application of these interventions with individuals with autism remains limited (Shipley-Benamou et al., 2002). Recently, researchers have begun addressing this dearth in the literature by examining the efficacy of a number of teaching strategies to target adaptive behaviors among individuals with ASD.

Inclusion Criteria

The literature review method used to identify published empirical articles on teaching self-help skills to individuals with ASD involved an electronic search on PsychINFO. Descriptors used in the electronic search included "showering," "hair brushing," "face washing," "shaving," "tooth

G.L. Martin (✉)
Department of Psychology, Rm. 129, St. Paul's College, University of Manitoba, Winnipeg, MB, Canada
e-mail: gmartin@cc.umanitoba.ca

J.L. Matson, P. Sturmey (eds.), *International Handbook of Autism and Pervasive Developmental Disorders*, Autism and Child Psychopathology Series, DOI 10.1007/978-1-4419-8065-6_21, © Springer Science+Business Media, LLC 2011

brushing," "flossing," "oral hygiene," "meal preparation,"
"cooking," "baking," "food preparation," "table setting,"
"sweeping," "cleaning," "chores," "dishwashing," "dusting,"
"housekeeping," "laundry," "bed making," "table clearing,"
"dressing," "street crossing," "community skills," "bus riding," "safety skills," "purchasing skills," "fork use," "utensil
use," "knife use," "spoon use," "straw use," "eating skills,"
and "toilet training." These key terms were used in conjunction with terms such as "PDD," "ASD," "autism," and
"autistic." Relevant references were also identified within
articles generated via the electronic literature search. The
review was refined to studies that met the following criteria:
(a) an intervention was carried out in a controlled experimental design; (b) participants included at least one individual
with a diagnosis of ASD; (c) target behavior comprised one
of the subcategories identified for adaptive skills in this chapter; and (d) the research was published in a peer-reviewed
journal. The intervention strategies and recommendations for
future research described in previous review papers were
summarized in this chapter. Articles published between the
date of the last article included in previous review papers and
October 2009 were reviewed in this chapter. In all, 23 papers
were included and organized into three broad skill areas
(domestic, self-care, and community) and with subareas,
where appropriate.

Domestic Skills

Independent performance of domestic skills can lead to
opportunities to contribute meaningfully during day-to-day
activities for individuals with ASD. A growing body of
research has provided evidence of effective strategies that not
only facilitate learning but also produce generalized, independent skill performance across various domestic tasks over
time. Of the 10 articles reviewed that evaluated interventions
for teaching domestic skills, all produced improved performance on the targeted domestic skill, 3 provided evidence
of generalization following training, and 5 demonstrated
maintenance during follow-up sessions. A variety of teaching procedures were employed across the studies including
(listed according to the frequency of their application in
the literature) (a) task analysis (eight articles); (b) video
prompting (six articles); (c) positive reinforcement and/or
praise (six articles); (d) verbal, gestural, or physical prompting (five articles); (e) picture prompting (four articles); (f)
error correction (four articles); (g) chaining (three articles);
(h) instructor modeling (three articles); (i) video modeling (two articles); (j) prompt fading (two articles); and (k)
generalization programming (two articles).

Successful applications of verbal, gestural, and physical
prompting procedures, along with instructor modeling, were
demonstrated by Datlow Smith and Belcher (1985), who

taught cooking and cleaning skills to individuals with autism
using an AB non-experimental design replicated across five
participants. Instructors in this study provided as much assistance as needed to perform each behavior involved in the
target training tasks. That is, they began by giving the individuals an opportunity to independently perform the task and
provided an increased level of assistance when necessary.
A second demonstration of the efficacy of these prompting
techniques is evidenced in Bock's (1999) training of laundry
sorting to five children with autism using a multiple baseline
across participants research design. Using modeling, verbal, and physical prompts; backward chaining; and positive
reinforcement, Bock successfully taught laundry sorting and
produced generalization to a public laundry facility. All participants maintained their performance for at least 4 months
following training, as demonstrated in a follow-up probe,
and four children displayed their laundry sorting skills under
naturalistic conditions.

Another prompting strategy, picture prompting, involves
presenting pictures to cue learners to respond correctly. A
number of variations on picture prompting procedures were
used across a series of studies investigating teaching domestic tasks to individuals with ASD. These ranged from simple
photograph sequences (Pierce & Schreibman, 1994) to elaborate personal digital assistant (PDA) devices, consisting of
digital still and video images to prompt individuals through a
complex domestic task sequence (Mechling, Gast, & Seid,
2009). Pierce and Schreibman taught three children with
autism self-management picture prompting sequences for
table setting, meal preparation, laundry, and bed making.
With little additional training, generalization emerged across
untrained tasks in novel settings. These findings are consistent with prior research, which suggests that picture prompts
are successful in producing generalization across settings and
tasks (Wacker & Berg, 1983). Advantages to using these systems are that they are small, readily transported to novel
settings as a means for producing generalization, and can be
easily faded if necessary (Pierce & Schreibman, 1994).

Video modeling and video prompting have been used to
teach a variety of skills to individuals with developmental disabilities and ASD. Video modeling involves making
a videotape of a person performing a behavior or completing a task (Sigafoos et al., 2007). The individual views the
entire video without interruption, after which they are given
the opportunity to perform the target behavior depicted in
the video (Charlop & Milstein, 1989; Charlop-Christy &
Daneshvar, 2003). Video prompting is a variation on video
modeling, in which a participant is shown one step of a
task, after which they are given the chance to perform the
modeled step before proceeding to the next step in the
sequence. Video prompting has been demonstrated as effective in teaching table setting in a multiple baseline across
participants with an ABAC within participants research

design (Goodson, Sigafoos, O'Reilly, Cannella, & Lancioni, 2007), meal and snack preparation routines using a multiple probe across behaviors research design (Mechling et al., 2009), putting away groceries using a multiple probe across subjects with alternative treatment within subject research design (Cannella-Malone, Sigafoos, O'Reilly, de la Cruz, Edrisinha, & Lancioni, 2006), and dishwashing using a multiple baseline across participants research design (Sigafoos et al., 2007) among individuals with ASD. One of two perspectives is typically presented in video models or prompts: (a) a first person perspective (i.e., from the view of the person performing the skill) and (b) a third person perspective (from the view of someone watching another person perform a skill). A comparison of perspectives of video models was carried out by Ayres and Langone (2007) while teaching four elementary school-aged students with autism to put away groceries using an adapted alternating treatments design. Although their results demonstrated improved performance in the context of computerized training and produced generalization to some natural conditions for some of the participants, it remains unclear as to which perspective, first or third person, was more efficient in teaching this skill to the children who participated in the study. Further research is needed to identify, and refine, effective and efficient procedures for teaching skills to children with ASD using video modeling and video prompting.

Picture prompting, video modeling, and video prompting have all been demonstrated as effective in teaching a number of adaptive self-help skills to individuals with ASD. Little research, however, has systematically examined the relative effectiveness and efficiency of these three teaching systems. When compared with static picture prompts using an adapted alternating treatments design, video prompts were superior in producing independent cooking skills among five adolescents and one adult diagnosed with autism (Mechling & Gustafson, 2008). The authors recommended extending the findings of their study to teaching daily living skills or vocational tasks consisting of an extended sequence of behaviors, as opposed to the discrete skills taught in the context of their cooking tasks. A more systematic comparison between these visual prompting systems, in conjunction with measures of generalization and maintenance, would serve as a useful contribution to this scarce body of research.

Lovaas (2003) indicated that it is important to work toward eliminating the need for continued prompting so as to promote greater independence and prevent prompt dependence. To address this, Sigafoos et al. (2007) investigated an innovative strategy for fading out the use of video prompts. The fading procedure they developed – video chunking – involved gradually compressing the video prompts into one video segment, by systematically merging the independent steps into the full sequence (i.e., video modeling). Although the researchers successfully removed all of the video prompts

for two of the three participants by the end of the fading procedure, performance for all three participants was variable at a 3-month follow-up. After having the participants review the video model, their performances returned to levels comparable to the final training stage, suggesting that a brief booster session was sufficient in re-establishing the skill.

Although absolute independence is the ultimate goal when teaching individuals with ASD, the use of self-managed prompting strategies, such as those described in this section, may result in reliance on books, pictures, videos, or PDAs in executing complex domestic tasks. If the individual independently retrieves the prompting device and subsequently manipulates the device in a way that facilitates self-management of the behavior, the objective is still being achieved, in that the presence of a caregiver to aid in performing the task has been removed. Considering that we often rely on cookbooks, assembly instruction manuals, and global positioning systems as aids in performing complicated sequences, it is conceivable that similar prompting devices can remain present as strategies to maintain and facilitate otherwise independent behavior among individuals with ASD.

Self-Care Skills

Teaching self-care skills, such as grooming, dressing, tooth brushing, and appropriate mealtime behaviors, can result in improved independence for individuals with ASD. A significant amount of caregiver time is devoted to assisting individuals with ASD to complete their daily living routines. By establishing effective interventions that promote independence, staff and caregiver assistance can be reduced. Not only is it important to identify effective teaching strategies, but consideration must be given to maintenance and generalization. Although limited evidence exists of empirically validated procedures for teaching self-care behaviors to individuals with ASD, researchers have attempted to address these key issues in their investigations. Across the eight articles reviewed on teaching self-care skills, the following procedures were identified (listed according to the frequency of their application in the literature): (a) verbal, gestural, or physical prompting (six articles); (b) task analysis (five articles); (c) positive reinforcement and/or praise (four articles); (d) instructor modeling (four articles); (e) chaining (three articles); (f) generalization programming (three articles); (g) error correction (one article); (h) picture prompting (one article); (i) prompt fading (one article); and (j) negative reinforcement (one article).

Grooming

Matson, Taras, Sevin, Love, and Fridley (1990) taught tooth brushing and hair combing to three children with autism using a multiple baseline across behaviors research design. Each teaching session consisted of the instructor first modeling and verbally describing the steps, physically and verbally assisting the children in completing each step, and finally providing the children an opportunity to independently perform this skill. This strategy was successful in increasing two grooming behaviors across all three children. Datlow Smith and Belcher (1985) applied a least to most prompting system to teach tooth brushing, hair combing, and face washing to three adults with autism using an AB non-experimental design. Because the number of sessions per week varied across participants and weeks, the average number of steps performed independently for all training sessions per week was reported. One individual learned to perform all of the steps identified in the tooth brushing sequence after 34 weeks of training, a second learned to perform all five hair combing steps within 39 weeks of training, while the third child learned to independently perform 11 of 17 steps of a face washing sequence within 19 weeks. Further research on the maintenance and generalization of these skills is needed to determine the long-term impact of training on improved independent grooming skills.

Dressing

Like grooming skills, dressing behaviors often involve lengthy, complex sequences which require the chaining of multiple discrete behaviors. Pierce and Schreibman (1994) applied a picture prompting self-management training procedure to teach dressing skills to one 6-year-old boy with autism using a multiple baseline with probes across behaviors research design. Although he learned to use a picture prompting book to correctly complete the dressing sequence, he did not maintain the skill at the level of independence produced during training. Further, in the absence of the book, he did not perform any of the dressing skills. Matson et al. (1990) taught four dressing skills to children with autism using a multiple baseline across behaviors research design. Two participants improved their shoe-tying skills, although only one maintained the skill at a 7-month follow-up. A third participant learned three dressing skills (i.e., putting on a shirt, pants, and socks) to 100% accuracy during training. Unfortunately, he did not complete the follow-up sessions because he had moved to another city; however, his mother reported that he continued to perform these skills independently. Finally, using a multiple probe across behaviors research design, Sewell, Collins, Hemmeter, and Schuster (1998) successfully taught a 2-year-old girl with a diagnosis of PDD to put on her shirt and shoes using a simultaneous prompting procedure and activity-based instruction. Simultaneous prompting involves delivering a prompt at the same time as the target stimulus is presented (e.g., at the same time as the instruction "Put on your shirt" is issued, the instructor would begin physically guiding the student

to complete the entire task). Activity-based instruction is a strategy used to teach functional skills within the context of child-initiated, planned, or routine scenarios and is designed to incorporate naturally occurring antecedent and consequence events (Bricker & Cripe, 1992). Learners in Sewell et al.'s (1998) study were taught dressing sequences within the context of activities that incorporated the target dressing behaviors. For example, when teaching the child to put on a shirt, instructors arranged a scenario such as painting or water play which began with the child putting on a shirt and then engaging in the selected activity.

The studies described thus far on teaching dressing skills have focused on producing independent performance of the sequences discussed. Using an ABAB withdrawal with baseline probes research design, one study by Fantuzzo and Smith (1983) was designed to remedy a situation where a 12-year-old boy with autism was taking up to an hour to complete his morning dressing routine. With the introduction of a token reinforcement system combined with a back-up reinforcer (chocolate milk with his breakfast) to reinforce appropriate dressing behavior which involved putting on his clothing within the allotted time period, he learned to perform the sequence independently in under 9 min both in a community residential setting and at his mother's home. This case study demonstrates that in addition to the discrete-trial interventions and chaining procedures typically applied to self-care skills, issues such as length of time required to perform a task can impact independent functioning and, therefore, still require careful consideration.

Eating

Two main approaches have been adopted to teach self-feeding skills to individuals with developmental disabilities and ASD: (a) promoting skill acquisition (e.g., basic utensil use) and (b) eliminating inappropriate mealtime behaviors (e.g., reducing sloppiness and spills). Using a multiple baseline across behaviors research design, Sisson and Dixon (1986) applied a group training procedure combined with modeling, verbal, gestural, or physical prompts and tokens following the occurrence of appropriate behaviors to teach a group of children, one of which had a diagnosis of autism, appropriate utensil use, napkin use, to chew with a closed mouth, and to display good posture during mealtimes. When tested under naturalistic conditions, however, performance of these skills was variable. The authors noted that special consideration must be given to generalization programming for mealtime behaviors because food reinforcement is accessible regardless of appropriate mealtime behaviors (i.e., whether your mouth is open or you are slouching, once the food is in your mouth reinforcement will occur despite the presence of undesirable behaviors).

Toilet Training

Independent toileting can improve a number of quality of life factors for individuals with developmental disabilities and ASD including, but not limited to, improved hygiene, self-confidence, and daily activities as well as reduced stigmatism and physical discomfort (Cicero & Pfadt, 2002; Hyams, McCoull, Smith, & Tyrer, 1992; McCartney, 1990). Competent toileting can influence socialization opportunities as well as educational and vocational placements (Kroeger & Sorensen-Burnworth, 2009).

In 1971, Azrin and Foxx introduced their rapid toilet training (RTT) procedure which consisted of (a) positive reinforcement for successful in-toilet urinations; (b) positive punishment, involving an overcorrection and positive practice component following out-of-toilet urinations; (c) increased fluid intake to promote urination; and (d) scheduled sittings to ensure frequent toilet sittings and to promote independence. For almost 40 years this method of toilet training, and variations of it, has produced increased in-toilet urinations and reduced out-of-toilet urinations among individuals with developmental disabilities (Azrin, Bugle, & O'Brien, 1971; Sadler & Merkert, 1977; Smith, 1979). Since its inception, researchers continue to refine the procedures originally outlined by Azrin and Foxx. In doing so, a number of variations have been explored with varying levels of success.

In 2009, a comprehensive review of the toilet training literature for individuals with developmental disabilities and autism was conducted by Kroeger and Sorensen-Burnworth. The authors identified the following common behavioral components in toilet training procedures: (a) graduated guidance (i.e., providing the necessary amount of assistance required to perform the toileting skill); (b) reinforcement-based training (i.e., providing a preferred activity, item, or event following performance of the skill); (c) scheduled sittings to increase opportunities for successful in-toilet eliminations; (d) identification of elimination schedules prior to beginning toilet training, in order to identify the naturally occurring elimination times for each individual; (e) punishment procedures to consequate out-of-toilet eliminations; (f) increased fluid intake to promote eliminations; and (g) stimulus control manipulations (i.e., identifying the conditions under which out-of-toilet eliminations occurred and manipulating the environment in a way that results in transferring those eliminations to the toilet). The intervention strategies and recommendations for future research described in Kroeger and Sorensen-Burnworth were summarized in this chapter and articles published between the date of the last article included in their review and October 2009 were included in this chapter.

Keen, Brannigan, and Cuskelly (2007) provided evidence that video modeling may be an effective tool in toilet training when combined with operant procedures described by Azrin and Foxx (1971). Further investigation of video modeling is needed to determine its efficacy in treating incontinence, as well as other toileting behaviors (e.g., self-initiation) among children with ASD. A second avenue of investigation focuses on the elimination of positive punishment practices (Cicero & Pfadt, 2002), such as overcorrection and positive practice (e.g., having the individual walk from the spot of the accident to the toilet a specific number of times following an accident). Although the application of these procedures has demonstrated effective components of toilet training packages for individuals with autism (e.g., Ando, 1977), others have reported them counterproductive, particularly among some individuals exhibiting challenging behaviors (Cicero & Pfadt, 2002).

One area in need of detailed investigation is the components included in a toileting sequence. Although many behaviors are involved in the sequence (e.g., undressing, eliminating in the toilet, wiping, dressing, and hand washing), little evidence exists detailing empirically based interventions for teaching these component skills. Stokes, Cameron, Dorsey, and Fleming (2004) taught two adult males, one of whom had a diagnosis of autism, to wipe themselves independently following bowel movements using an AB non-experimental design. A task analysis was conducted to identify 10 steps for carrying out self-hygiene practices following bowel movements. The participant was taught to follow a complex chain by providing prompts when needed to ensure proper completion of the sequence. Correspondence training, in which the individual examined a wet wipe at the seventh step of the sequence, after which he was required to report to the instructor whether the wipe was clean, and if so, he could finish up and leave the washroom. If the wipe was discolored, he was instructed to repeat the wiping procedure until the wipe was clean. This step served as a strategy for self-feedback on their cleanliness, a prompt that could be carried out in the absence of a caregiver. Following training, the participant performed the entire task with 100% independence, and his cleanliness improved substantially following 22 training sessions. The authors further extended the toileting sequence by varying four environmental stimuli in order to promote generalization to non-training settings and conditions. Accuracy and independence were maintained at 100% during generalization probes and maintenance sessions at 1- and 9-month follow-up sessions.

Most recently, Ozcan and Cavkaytar (2009) examined the effectiveness of a parent training program designed to teach toileting skills to two children diagnosed with autism using a multiple-probe design with probe sessions across participants. The parent training procedures demonstrated that following intervention, both children carried out 100% of the skills independently and maintained performance during follow-up sessions. The results of this study extended previous toilet training research by demonstrating the effectiveness of parent instruction in producing independent toileting skills among two children with autism.

There are many protocols available in the literature for toilet training individuals with an ASD or with a developmental disability. The majority appear to be modifications of Azrin and Foxx's (1971) original toilet training protocol. The direction of the research and application has been to abbreviate and refine the steps involved in training and to minimize the cost of involving professional training and supervision (e.g., parent training models). In conclusion, Kroeger and Sorensen-Burnworth (2009) recommended the following considerations for future research directions: (a) teaching communication, self-initiation, and bowel movement training; (b) evaluation and investigation of the age and functioning limits based on the positive results of prior research on toilet training; and (c) identification of the prerequisite skills for toilet training individuals within these populations. Finally, refining the toileting procedures and generating cost-effective intervention approaches for addressing toileting among individuals with ASD are needed if parents and caregivers, already busy with other responsibilities in caring for an individual with ASD, are expected to carry out toilet training procedures that can be maintained and generalized across natural settings.

Community Skills

Any curriculum for individuals with developmental disabilities, including autism, should emphasize the inclusion of skills that are both functional and relevant over time (Morse & Schuster, 2000). Deciding which skills to target can be difficult given the adeptness required to independently perform complex behaviors in community settings. With a lack of empirical data to guide these decisions, caregivers and practitioners are left to decide where to start and how to train adaptive community skills. This section describes research on teaching community living skills – including shopping and safety – to individuals with ASD. Across the six articles reviewed the following intervention approaches were identified (listed according to the frequency of their application in the literature): (a) verbal, gestural, or physical prompting (five articles); (b) positive reinforcement and/or praise (five articles); (c) task analysis (three articles); (d) error correction (three articles); (e) prompt fading (three articles); (f) instructor modeling (two articles); (g) picture prompting (two articles); (h) video modeling (two articles); (i) generalization programming (two articles); and (j) virtual reality (VR) (one article). Additional research on applying these intervention procedures in the context of controlled experimental designs is needed to establish evidence-based strategies for teaching community skills to individuals with ASD.

Shopping

Morse and Schuster (2000) examined the efficacy of an intervention to teach shopping skills using in vivo training, prompting according to a predetermined time delay, and a pictorial storyboard using a multiple baseline across participants research design. Eight children, one with a diagnosis of autism, participated. After 20 training sessions, the individual with autism learned to perform the two shopping tasks, generalized those skills to a grocery store not before seen during training, and maintained her performance at 100% accuracy at 2- and 6-week follow-up sessions. A limitation of this intervention was the cost associated with training (e.g., transportation and actual purchases made at the store). Although some research examining generalization to naturalistic versus simulated settings has found training to be superior in simulated settings (van den Pol et al., 1981), others have suggested just the opposite (Marchetti, McCartney, Drain, Hooper, & Dix, 1983).

Haring, Kennedy, Adams, and Pitts-Conway (1987) taught children with autism to make simple purchases in a school cafeteria and at a convenience store. Alcantara (1994) extended these findings by teaching purchasing skills to three children with autism using a multiple baseline across settings research design. First, video modeling training was carried out in isolation, after which all participants showed improvement in their purchasing performance in naturalistic settings. Because none of the students achieved 100% accuracy during training, a second phase was introduced. During this phase, in addition to viewing video models, prompting and reinforcement were provided while participants were shopping at a local convenience store. The introduction of this second training phase produced further improvement for all participants. All three children maintained their purchasing skills with between 94 and 97% independence at a 2-week follow-up. Further, shopping session time decreased from an average of 8 min and 27 s during baseline to 2 min and 48 s during follow-up, indicating that not only did training improve independent purchasing, it also improved the speed with which the skills were performed.

Shopping skills are valuable skills for independent living. Not only can they facilitate opportunities to make meaningful purchases, but other important life skills can be embedded within the shopping sequence (e.g., transportation to and from the store, money management, money use, and preparation of a grocery list to replenish their food supplies). Further investigation of cost-effective shopping skills and strategies for incorporating other useful independent living skills into shopping routines for individuals within this population are needed.

Helping Others

Although helping others is an important social skill, it is also a functional community skill. Harris, Handleman, and

Alessandri (1990) successfully taught three adolescents diagnosed with autism to provide assistance to adults struggling with adaptive and community activities (i.e., putting a key into a lock and putting a letter in an envelope) using a multiple baseline across participants and multiple baseline across tasks within participants research design. Some participants showed evidence of generalization across people and environments; however, generalization to untrained tasks was limited. To extend these findings, Reeve, Reeve, Buffington Townsend, and Poulson (2007) taught four individuals with autism to offer assistance in the context of various community and domestic activities (e.g., cleaning, replacing broken materials, picking up objects, locating objects, carrying objects, and putting items away) using a multiple baseline across participants research design. Training procedures consisted of video modeling, verbal, and physical or gestural prompting, in conjunction with tokens and verbal praise following helping behaviors. Not only was there an increase in the execution of these skills, performance was maintained for up to 2 months following training. Further, all participants offered assistance in the presence of novel stimuli, in an untrained setting, and when presented by a new instructor. These two studies offer evidence of effective interventions for producing increased helping behaviors, which can be maintained over time, and generalized across a variety of contexts. Further research designed to reduce the complexity of this multi-component intervention and to identify the essential training components for teaching helping skills will assist in the development of user-friendly training procedures to increase these behaviors in individuals within this population (Reeve et al., 2007).

Safety Skills

When in community settings, individuals with developmental disabilities and ASD encounter various scenarios that can pose threats to their safety. Some situations can be remedied through teaching visual discrimination (e.g., sign reading), auditory comprehension (e.g., following instructions issued over intercom systems), and personal safety skills (e.g., appropriate street crossing). Until recently, despite ongoing research addressing this topic among individuals with developmental disabilities, little evidence exists to guide clinicians and practitioners supporting children, adolescents, and adults with ASD. In recent years, researchers have only started to extend these findings to this population. Given the restrictions that a lack of safety skills can impose on individuals with ASD, and the dangerous situations that can result from failure to teach safety skills, effective interventions are of the essence.

While offering assistance (Harris et al., 1990; Reeve et al., 2007) is a useful self-help skill that may also facilitate appropriate social interactions, the ability to seek out assistance when separated from a caregiver presents a serious safety concern for individuals with ASD. Using a multiple-baseline probe design across participants, Taylor, Hughes, Richard, Hoch, and Rodriquez Coello (2004) examined whether three adolescents with autism could be taught to request assistance from an adult in community settings when their teacher or parent were not in sight. A vibrating paging device was given to each participant and was activated by a teacher when the individual was no longer in their view. A card with the child's name, a statement that he/she was lost, and an instruction to call or page their parent or teacher was placed in each participant's pocket. Upon sensing vibration of the paging device, students were taught to solicit assistance by handing the communication card to an adult in the community. All three individuals showed success by seeking out an adult to request their help. As evidence of generalization, they all performed the behavior when in the community with a parent. The authors noted that future research is needed to improve the social validity of the procedures used in this study by teaching participants to approach specific community helpers, such as cashiers or sales clerks, so as to minimize the danger of communicating information of being alone and lost to a potentially dangerous person. Overall, however, the results of this study demonstrate the usefulness of advances in technology in teaching community safety skills to individuals with ASD.

A second demonstration of the impact of rapidly evolving technology can be seen in Strickland, McAllister, Coles, and Osborne's (2007) successful teaching of fire safety skills to individuals with ASD using headset and PC-based VR systems using a changing-criterion research design. VR technology is a method used to create the illusion of actually performing an event in a computer-generated environment (Strickland et al., 2007). Self, Scudder, Weheba, and Crumrine (2007) later compared VR with an *integrated visual learning model* consisting of a variety of commonly used teaching strategies for individuals with ASD (e.g., social stories, picture cards, role-play/rehearsal, vide modeling) using a group research design. Both instructional methods were reported as successful in teaching fire safety and tornado safety skills to children with ASD in the context of the VR training conditions; however, controlled studies are still required to determine the efficacy of these interventions for individuals with ASD. An important finding with respect to establishing cost-effective and efficient interventions is that the amount of training time required using the VR approach was half that of the integrated visual learning model.

With rapid advances in technology, it is not surprising that case studies applying innovative techniques, such as those described in this chapter, are emerging in the literature. Empirical investigation of their efficacy in rapid teaching, generalization production, and maintenance of adaptive life skills is still needed to demonstrate their applicability among this population. Further investigation is needed to determine how technology can be used to reduce training time and produce rapid skill acquisition that can be generalized across environments and maintained over time. The use of PDAs and VR computer configurations should be considered a launching point for research investigating the role of advanced technology in teaching individuals with ASD.

Social Skills Interventions

Social impairment is one of the main areas of deficits for individuals with ASDs. With the most recent autism prevalence report of 1 in 110 live births (Centers for Disease Control and Prevention, 2009) and with social skill deficits being one of the most debilitating areas of dysfunction for children diagnosed with ASD (Kanner, 1943; Rogers, 2000), there is an urgent need for empirical validation of effective social interventions for children with ASD (Kransny, Williams, Provencal, & Ozonoff, 2003; Paul, 2003).

There are a large number of social skills training intervention strategies for children with ASDs reported in the literature. These studies can be categorized in many ways including (a) delivery (e.g., teacher-directed, peer-mediated instruction; direct instruction; incidental teaching); (b) theoretical orientation (e.g., behavioral, cognitive-behavioral); (c) setting (e.g., school, clinic); (d) teaching methods (e.g., social stories, video self-modeling, social scripts); and (f) age of participants (preschool, middle school) (Ruble, Willis, & McLaughlin Crabtree 2008; Scattone, 2007).

The majority of the social skills intervention studies to date have employed direct observation in small N research designs and have implemented modeling of target behaviors and reinforcement procedures (Matson, Matson, & Rivet, 2007); however, increasing varieties of intervention approaches continue to develop at a very fast pace. Although this development is very encouraging, the rapid growth in this area has led to lack of consensus in the literature on definitions of social skills and assessment techniques (Matson & Wilkins, 2007). Although further investigations involving behavioral intervention strategies and single-case research are very important, statistical analyses of larger scale intervention studies are lacking, an approach that could help to identify which specific interventions are most effective (Kroeger, Schultz, & Newsom, 2007; Matson et al., 2007).

Given the growth of intervention studies in the literature, a number of comprehensive reviews involving social skills intervention strategies exist, which have garnered important recommendations for future research. Some key issues addressed in these reviews include the (a) need for clarification of variations in diagnostic procedures for ASD and understanding subtypes of ASD to more efficiently individualize and implement treatments (Rao, Beidel, & Murray,

2008; Reynhout & Carter, 2006; Stichter, Randolph, Gage, & Schmidt, 2007); (b) need for assessment of the effectiveness of various intervention strategies through comparative analyses (DiSalvo & Oswald, 2002; Matson et al., 2007); (c) need for increased use of generalization and long-term assessments (Bellini, Peters, Benner, & Hopf, 2007; Goldstein, Schneider, & Thiemann, 2007; Hwang & Hughes, 2000); and (d) need for manualized curricula for public dissemination (Rogers, 2000; Williams White, Keonig, & Scahill, 2007). More recent studies will be reviewed in the context of the recommendations highlighted within those reviews.

Inclusion Criteria

The articles included in this review met the following criteria: (a) an intervention was carried out in a controlled experimental design, (b) participants included at least one individual with a diagnosis of a PDD or ASD, (c) the target behavior comprised one of the subcategories identified for the social skills in this chapter, and (d) the study was published in a peer-reviewed journal.

The literature review procedure used to identify the published empirical articles on social skills interventions included an electronic search of PsychINFO. The search terms, "social skills," were used in conjunction with the terms "PDD," "ASD," "autism," and "autistic." The results of this search resulted in over 1,500 peer-reviewed articles. To refine the search, "social skills training" and "social skills intervention" were used in conjunction with the terms "PDD," "ASD," "autism," and "autistic." Next, even more specific search terms such as "sharing," "turn-taking," "social initiations," "reciprocal interaction," "appropriate display of affection," and "compliment giving" were used in conjunction with the terms "pervasive development disorder (PDD)," "autism spectrum disorder (ASD)," "autism," and "autistic." Any additional references were identified within the articles found in the electronic literature search. For the purposes of this review, the following subcategories of social skills will be discussed: (a) compliment giving/greetings; (b) social initiations/reciprocal interactions; and (c) sharing/turn-taking.

If the search terms generated results for studies involving topics such as play skills (e.g., Bass & Mulick, 2007; Stahmer, Ingersoll, & Carter, 2003), emotion recognition (e.g., Solomon, Goodlin-Jones, & Anders, 2004), theory of mind (e.g., Prelock & Hutchins, 2008), or language skills, they were excluded on the basis that they were encompassed by topics to be covered in other chapters. A number of review papers concerning social skills will be cited in this chapter; however, studies that were included in previous reviews will not be described in detail, with two exceptions (Apple, Billingsley, & Schwartz, 2005; Thiemann &

Goldstein, 2004). A total of 17 articles that met the inclusion criteria are reviewed here and organized into the three broad categories mentioned previously; 5 articles on greetings/compliment giving, 7 on social initiations/reciprocal interactions, and 5 articles on sharing/turn-taking.

Giving Compliments and Greetings

Deficits in social skills obstruct children with ASDs' ability to establish meaningful relationships, which often leads to withdrawal and social isolation (Weiss & Harris, 2001). Therefore such skills are critical to successful social, emotional, and cognitive development. A conceivable way to strengthen relationships maybe by offering compliments and greetings during interactions with others. Three of the five articles reviewed included compliment-giving target behaviors and two included greetings. In all but two of the studies, the target behaviors were assessed in combination with other social skill behaviors. The most common intervention strategies included some form of direct instruction (e.g., written text training, video modeling with reinforcement, direct adult instruction) (three articles). Other interventions included the use of *Social Stories*™ (one article) and a form of music therapy combined with prompting procedures (one article). Although all of the studies resulted in improved performance of the target skills, only two studies included maintenance assessments and only one reported evidence of generalization.

Giving Compliments

Giving compliments to others provides children with ASDs a way to express their approval for, or curiosity about, issues of interest to others (Apple et al., 2005). Apple et al. addressed compliment giving in isolation from other social skills. Although this study was included in Matson et al. (2007), it warrants brief mention here as the literature on compliment giving is very sparse. In a multiple-baseline design across participants, direct instruction in the form of video modeling with explicit rules and tangible reinforcement produced and maintained "response"-type compliments (i.e., when participants used compliment statements such as "neat" in response to another individual's initiation such as "Look at my_____.") When a self-management component was added to the video modeling procedure, compliment-giving behaviors were initiated (i.e., compliment statements made more than 15 s after another persons' initiation statement) and maintained, offering evidence of a successful approach to teaching both reciprocal and self-initiated exchanges. Generalization to other social settings and to naturally occurring social rather than tangible contingencies was not assessed. Evidence of the generality of these findings would strengthen the efficacy of this intervention, in

that the applicability of these techniques to real-life scenarios and settings would increase opportunities for socialization among individuals in this population.

Further support for direct instructional intervention strategies is evidenced in Thiemann and Goldstein (2004). In a multiple-baseline design across behaviors and five participants with PDD, the effectiveness of two intervention strategies for increasing the frequency of five social skills (including compliment giving) was assessed. The two intervention strategies, peer training and direct adult instruction using written text cues (i.e., phrases appropriate to the activity), were assessed consecutively in order to attempt to differentiate the effects of both interventions on children's social initiations (i.e., compliments). Peer training alone was insufficient to increase children's rate of compliment use; however, when written text instruction was introduced, compliment giving increased. Therefore, the combined effects of the intervention strategies lead to favorable results. Maintenance of the skills was also observed; however, generalization of the behaviors outside of the structured classroom environment (e.g., recess) requires further investigation.

Another intervention technique that has been shown to be effective in increasing compliment-giving behavior is the use of *Social Stories*™, which are designed to instruct children with ASD to identify and respond appropriately to social cues across situations and environments (Gray, 2000). In a multiple-baseline design across behaviors with two children diagnosed with PDD-NOS, Dodd, Hupp, Jewell, and Krohn (2008) examined the effectiveness of *Social Stories*™ for decreasing a problem social skill (i.e., excessive directions) and increasing a prosocial skill (i.e., compliment giving). Trained observers recorded frequencies of directions and compliments. Results indicated a 19.5% increase in compliments from baseline demonstrating that *Social Stories*™ were effective at increasing rates of compliment giving for children with PDD. Social validity evaluations of the intervention were positive; however, there were no long-term follow-up assessments or evaluation of generalization to other contexts.

Although *Social Stories*™ have gained increased clinical popularity in teaching social skills to children with ASD for reasons such as ease of implementation, they are not without limitation. A recent review of 16 social stories experiments by Reynhout and Carter (2006) revealed that (a) social story interventions are often combined with empirically validated methods such as prompting and reinforcement which confounded the results; (b) variability in the construction and implementation of social story research exists; and (c) maintenance and generalization are generally not addressed. The authors caution that this type of intervention may be more effective for individuals with mild to moderate functioning levels and for individuals with some basic language abilities.

Greetings

Greetings are a part of daily interactions for children with ASD in inclusive classroom environments; however, these children often do not have the necessary social skills to execute this type of interaction. Given that greetings typically involve peers, it seems plausible that a peer training intervention involving modeling and reinforcement would be a preferred method, as it is for training other social skills (Kamps et al., 2002); however, peer tutoring procedures may be difficult to implement because typically developing preschool children may have difficulty grasping the concepts involved in peer training. Instead, research has focused on other training strategies. For example, Gena (2006) assessed the effectiveness of social reinforcement in combination with prompting procedures in a multiple-baseline design across four participants with autism to increase five categories of social initiations (including greetings). Prompting (verbal, manual guidance) was provided by a skilled teacher and social reinforcement (verbal praise, physical contact) was delivered contingent on target behaviors. The procedures were effective in increasing the social initiations (including compliment giving) as well as appropriate responding to peers' initiations during social interactions. Two of the participants' initiations also generalized to a novel teacher. However, further research on long-term follow-up is needed.

A unique strategy for training greetings involved a "music therapy" procedure in conjunction with standard prompting methods. In a single-subject withdrawal design, Kern, Wolery, and Aldridge (2007) assessed the effects of individualized songs on the behaviors of two children with autism during morning greeting/classroom entry routines in an inclusive classroom setting. The songs included five steps of the greeting routine which were taught to the participants' teachers. The teachers sang the song during the morning routine, in conjunction with a least prompting (verbal and physical) method. Independently executed steps of the greeting routine increased from baseline for Participant 1 and a modified song procedure produced an increase in independently performed steps for Participant 2; however, no follow-up or generalization data were presented. Also, the same limitations that were raised by Reynhout and Carter (2006) in the *Social Stories*[TM] literature should be considered in this case. That is, because the songs were used in conjunction with previously validated prompt-fading procedure, the contribution of "music therapy" is unclear.

Social Initiations and Reciprocal Interactions

Reciprocal social interactions are necessary for social functioning and involve both an initiation and a response. It is well documented in the literature that children with ASD lack social initiation skills (Kern Koegel, 2000). Therefore,

it is not surprising that studies involving social initiation and interaction training are more represented in the literature than other target social skills reviewed in this chapter (e.g., compliment giving). Of the seven recent studies reviewed, the most common intervention strategies focused mainly on direct training methods based in behavior-analytic principles. Among the studies reviewed, six contained some measure of generalization or follow-up. For the purpose of this section, the articles reviewed are organized by intervention method: (a) visual procedures (four articles); (b) standard reinforcement (one article); and (c) peer mediated (two articles).

Visual Intervention

Although children with ASD have delayed language ability, they often possess strong visual ability (Bondy & Frost, 2001). Therefore, it is not surprising that social skills intervention strategies that employ some form of visual intervention have yielded favorable results. Within a multi-experiment study, Buggey (2005) employed a multiple-baseline design across two participants with ASD to assess the effectiveness of videotaped self-modeling (VSM) for increasing social initiations with peers. Social initiations were defined as "unsolicited verbalizations (not preceded by peer or staff prompts for a period of 10 s) addressed to peers (other than their counterpart in the study) or staff" (p. 55). The participants were videotaped participating in social initiations across settings (e.g., walking up to a group of classmates). The videos were modified in that classmates of the participants were given scripts to accompany the videos showing the participants engaging in the desirable behavior. The participants then viewed themselves in the situations where they were performing at a higher functioning level than usual. Results indicated significant increases in social initiations across both participants, and the increased initiations were maintained. The VSM intervention technique was also shown to be effective across other participants and behaviors (e.g., decreasing tantrums). Nikopoulos and Keenan (2007) also demonstrated the effectiveness of video modeling to teach complex social skills (including social initiations) to children with autism. Results indicated increased social initiation behaviors and decreased latency to perform social initiations after the video modeling procedure. Social initiations also generalized to novel peers and were maintained at 1- and 2-month follow-ups. Further support for intervention techniques involving visual cues for increasing social initiations is evident in Laushey, Heflin, Shippen, Alberto, and Fredrick (2009). Laushey and colleagues created visual diagrams using the "Concept Mastery Routine" (see Bulgren, Schumaker, & Deshler, 1988) in combination with direct instruction in small group settings with typical peers. A concept diagram is created interactively by an instructor and student and includes necessary elements to promote student understanding, such as definitions and examples of an idea. A multiple-baseline design across behaviors (including social initiations) revealed that the intervention technique was successful in increasing initiations across four children with high-functioning autism (HFA). Increases in the target behaviors generalized from the small group settings to an inclusive classroom setting; however, further research on generalization effects to a wider population of children with ASD is needed. Follow-up data revealed that the effects were maintained 3 weeks following cessation of the intervention, although more long-term assessment is needed.

Another visual intervention strategy combined the use of computer-presented *Social Stories*™ and visual models. Sansosti and Powell-Smith (2008) assessed the effectiveness of this intervention package for increasing social initiations and reciprocal interactions in a multiple-baseline design across three children with Asperger syndrome (AS) and HFA. Target behaviors were observed during unstructured, naturalistic settings (e.g., recess) and increased significantly after the intervention package was implemented. Maintenance of the effects was also observed at a 2-week follow-up but only one participant demonstrated generalization of the skills. An important consideration is that the intervention package was modified to allow for social reinforcement for two of the participants. Given the combined nature of the intervention strategy and the additional modifications, it is difficult to conclude what specific strategy may have contributed most to the observed effect, especially given vast empirical validation for reinforcement as a powerful tool to increase behavior.

Motivating Antecedent Variables

Another technique that has been shown to be effective for increasing social initiations is use of a motivating antecedent variable, as evidenced in Boyd, Conroy, Mancil, Nakao, and Alter (2007). The authors used a single-subject alternating treatments design to compare the effects of circumscribed interests (CI) and less preferred (LP) tangible stimuli for increasing social behaviors (including social initiations and interactions) of three children with ASD. CIs were defined as the interests or preoccupations of individuals with ASD that are unusual in intensity and focus (Boyd et al., 2007). In this study the CIs were items and, along with the LP stimuli, were identified using a multiple stimulus preference assessment. When children's CIs and LPs were embedded in a play session (i.e., a peer held the respective items), results indicated that CI sessions led to increased and longer durations of the target behaviors compared to the LP sessions. That is, participants were more likely to initiate to peers when the peers had the participant's CI in hand. In addition, it took participant less time to initiate to peers when CIs were present. These results have important implications in that CIs are potentially

powerful reinforcers and when embedded in social situations with peers can serve as motivating antecedent variable to increase the social behavior. Future research should examine whether other appropriate stimuli that are more reinforcing than CIs could be used. Also generalization to other contexts and long-term follow-up assessments are needed.

Peer- and Adult-Mediated Approaches

Both peer-mediated and adult-mediated approaches to intervention strategies have effectively helped to establish social skills in children with autism (Bellini et al., 2007; McConnell, 2002). Owen-DeSchryver, Carr, Cale, and Blakeley-Smith (2008) evaluated the impact of a peer training intervention on social interactions in a multiple-baseline design across three children with ASD. Peers participated in training sessions that targeted increasing social interactions (e.g., initiations) and data were collected in unstructured settings (e.g., recess). Peer training intervention, delivered by trained peers and other children with ASD, was effective in increasing initiations. Another interesting finding was that untrained peers also showed increased initiations. This finding has important implications for classroom-based interventions in which teachers have many responsibilities and peers are readily available. Future research should also address long-term follow-up of the effects.

Another example of favorable collateral effects from social skills training that focused on increasing social initiations is that the training can also lead to decreased problematic behavioral excesses (e.g., repetitive motor behaviors) in children with autism. In a multiple-baseline design across participants, Loftin, Odom, and Lantz (2008) assessed the effectiveness of a multi-component (peer training, direct social initiation training, and self-monitoring) intervention strategy for decreasing repetitive motor behavior of three children with autism. Direct instruction was used to teach participants social initiations, which were defined as, "the participant starting an interaction with a peer(s) with whom there has not been an interaction during the previous 5 s" (p. 1126). Participants were also taught to self-monitor instances of initiations using a wrist counter. Social initiations increased with direct social initiation training, and social interactions continued when self-monitoring was introduced. Further, participants' repetitive motor behavior was significantly reduced and this effect was maintained more than 1 month after the intervention ended. Future research examining the generalizability of these findings across untrained conditions is needed.

As indicated by previous reviews of social skills training and the studies described thus far in this chapter, the majority of intervention strategies to date have involved traditional behavioral methods, and these methods have demonstrated that children with autism can indeed learn to perform discrete social behaviors. Assessments of the efficacy of these strategies indicate that generalization of these skills is lacking (Bellini et al., 2007; Williams White et al., 2007). Another recommendation highlighted in previous reviews is that intervention techniques should be selected based on the individual language and cognitive abilities of children with ASD (Stichter et al., 2007).

Sharing and Turn-Taking

Cooperative skills, including sharing and turn-taking, are necessary for forming positive peer relationships, including accessing opportunities to obtain positive reinforcement through social exchanges; however, research in this area is lacking. For example, of the five articles reviewed here, only two studies (DeQuinzio, Townsend, & Poulson, 2008; Sawyer, Luiselli, Ricciardi, & Gower, 2005) targeted cooperative skills (including sharing and turn-taking); specifically, the remaining three studies assessed cooperative behaviors in conjunction with other social skills (e.g., play). Four of the five articles included some form of direct instruction, such as Pivotal Response Training (PRT), video modeling, priming with prompting and reinforcement, and one article assessed a novel social–behavioral intervention strategy called "SODA" (Stop, Observe, Deliberate, and Act) (Bock, 2001). One of the five studies also involved peer-mediated delivery of this strategy (Harper, Symon, & Frea, 2008). Effectiveness in increasing cooperative skills was demonstrated across all five studies, and all but one study reported some measure of generalization or maintenance (Kroeger, Schultz, & Newsom, 2007).

Sharing
The majority of the research devoted to increasing prosocial behaviors (e.g., sharing) has applied behavior-analytic techniques such as modeling, prompting, and reinforcement (e.g., Kamps et al., 1992). Sawyer et al. (2005) demonstrated the effectiveness of behavioral interventions for increasing sharing skills with children with ASD. In an ABCB single-case design, Sawyer et al. assessed the effectiveness of a multi-component package for increasing instances of physical sharing (e.g., handing an item to another individual) and verbal sharing (e.g., requesting an item from another individual) with one child with autism. Two interventions were employed. The first intervention procedure consisted of priming, prompting, and reinforcement. Priming of sharing behaviors occurred before a play session in which the instructor described the importance of sharing to the participant and then modeled a few examples of both verbal and physical sharing behaviors with one of the participant's peers. The instructor then guided the participant to perform sharing behaviors with the peer while provided prompts and reinforcement. The participant's sharing skills

were then measured in the inclusive classroom. The second intervention procedure was the same except that priming was not included. The combination of priming, prompting, and reinforcement was needed to increase and maintain improvements in sharing behavior. This study was conducted in an inclusive preschool classroom and implemented by the teacher who had other ongoing responsibilities, which has important social validity implications. Maintenance data were also collected 40 and 60 days after the study had ended and showed positive results. Methodological issues include lack of generalization, the use of a non-experimental case study, and some baseline data points increased in the absence of intervention. Therefore, although the results of this study should be interpreted with caution, since sharing skills are rarely targeted in isolation in the literature, it provides preliminary evidence of successful strategies requiring further investigation under controlled experimental conditions.

More recently, in a multiple-baseline design across four participants with autism, DeQuinzio et al. (2008) found that a behavioral intervention package (manual guidance, auditory prompts, and contingent reinforcement) was successful in teaching all four children a sharing response chain. Further, the sharing behaviors generalized to non-trained (non-reinforced) toys, individuals (i.e., peers), and settings. The generalization measures were based on pre- and post-test data, however; so they should be interpreted with caution. Information pertaining to the maintenance of these skills was not reported.

Turn-Taking
In a controlled group design with 25 children with autism, Kroeger et al. (2007) assessed the effectiveness of a direct-teaching strategy (video modeling with prompting and edible reinforcement) compared to an unstructured play activities group for teaching turn-taking skills to children with ASD. Pre-post assessments on videotaped behavior data revealed that children in both groups made prosocial behavioral gains, including increased turn-taking, and, most importantly, the direct-teaching group showed greater success. Long-term follow-up and generalization were not assessed.

Another effective, albeit time-consuming strategy involving direct-teaching strategies for promoting positive social interaction (e.g., social initiations) between children with ASD and peers, is peer-mediated PRT (Pierce & Schreibman, 1995, 1997a, 1997b). PRT is based on principles of applied behavior analysis and incorporates motivational procedures to improve responding. Peer-mediated PRT can assist in increasing generalization of skills to others, although it is yet to be assessed for a wide range of social skills (Pierce & Schreibman, 1997a). More recently, PRT has been demonstrated as effective in increasing cooperative behavior in children with ASD. In a concurrent multiple-baseline design across two children with autism, Harper et al. (2008)

assessed improvements in social skills, including turn-taking, during recess, using peer-mediated PRT. Results indicated increased and maintained turn-taking behaviors in both participants; however, the authors noted that advanced language and cognitive abilities of one participant might have contributed to his prominent improvement. Hence, assessment of the effectiveness of the intervention across a wider range of functioning levels is needed. The majority of research on social skills training to date focuses on children in the higher functioning range (Harper et al., 2008; Hwang & Hughes, 2000; Rogers, 2000). This limitation also speaks to the recommendation that social skills programs for children with ASD require modification to meet the specific needs of subgroups of children within the diagnostic category (Rao et al., 2008).

Bock (2001) developed a social–behavioral learning strategy for children and adolescents with Asperger syndrome: "SODA" (stop, observe, deliberate, and act) which provides a set of rules to help children with AS attend to relevant social cues and select specific social skills that they will use in novel social settings (generalization). The first three steps (S, O, and D) include self-talk questions or statements. The final step (A) assists with development of what they will say and do in novel social settings. A recent evaluation of the SODA strategy revealed its effectiveness for increasing cooperative learning skills of children with Asperger syndrome (Bock, 2007). In a multiple-baseline design across natural settings with four children with Asperger syndrome, participant's cooperation skills increased considerably from baseline in the presence of the SODA intervention. Further, participants' cooperative skill performance was maintained for 5 months after the intervention was terminated and actually increased to levels comparable to their typically developing peers. In addition, the participants demonstrated long-term memory (e.g., recalling SODA components in follow-up interviews) of SODA 1 month after the termination of maintenance assessments. As indicated previously, training methods may require tweaking based on the specific functioning level of the children involved, providing further support for the need for accurate assessment and diagnosis of ASDs (Matson & Wilkins, 2007).

Future Research

We reviewed 23 studies grouped in three adaptive skills domains (domestic, self-care, and community skills), and 17 studies grouped in three social skills domains (compliments and greetings, social initiation and interaction, and sharing and turn-taking). Of the 40 articles, only 15 specified the types of scales that were used to diagnose participants, and only 2 of the 40 studies included independent confirmation of the diagnoses. In order to allow for adequate comparison

of effectiveness of treatments across specific diagnostic categories of ASDs, future research should describe the tools used for diagnoses and include confirmation of diagnoses.

Across articles the intervention strategies were based predominantly on behavior-analytic techniques. The most common strategies included standard prompting and reinforcement procedures, task analysis, and modeling. The majority of articles employed single-subject research designs and demonstrated internal validity of the treatment strategies; however, only 30% of the studies actively programmed for generalization. The independent performance of the various adaptive and social skills under naturalistic conditions requires further research.

Of the 40 articles, only 53% reported some measure of social validity (Kazdin, 1977; Wolf, 1978). Given that caregivers of children with ASDs are often involved in the implementation of treatment programs, measures of social validity are important in developing user-friendly treatment programs for addressing adaptive and social skill needs and future research should include them routinely.

References

Alcantara, P. R. (1994). Effects of videotape instructional package on purchasing skills of children with autism. *Exceptional Children, 61*, 40–55.

American Psychiatric Association. (2000). *Diagnostic and statistical manual of mental disorders* (4th ed, Text Revision). Washington, DC: Author.

Ando, H. (1977). Training autistic children to urinate in the toilet through operant conditioning techniques. *Journal of Autism and Childhood Schizophrenia, 7*, 151–163.

Apple, A. L., Billingsley, F., & Schwartz, I. S. (2005). Effects of video modeling alone and with self-management on compliment-giving behaviors of children with high-functioning ASD. *Journal of Positive Behavior Interventions, 7*, 33–46.

Ayres, K. M., & Langone, J. (2007). A comparison of video modeling perspectives for students with autism. *Journal of Special Education Technology, 22*, 15–30.

Azrin, N. H., Bugle, C., & O'Brien, F. (1971). Behavioral engineering: Two apparatuses for toilet training retarded children. *Journal of Applied Behavior Analysis, 4*, 249–252.

Azrin, N. H., & Foxx, R. M. (1971). A rapid method of toilet training the institutionalized retarded. *Journal of Applied Behavior Analysis, 4*, 89–99.

Bass, J. D., & Mulick, J. A. (2007). Social play skill enhancement of children with autism using peers and siblings as therapists. *Psychology in the Schools. Special Issue: Autism Spectrum Disorders, 44*, 727–735.

Bellini, S., Peters, J. K., Benner, L., & Hopf, A. (2007). A meta-analysis of school-based social skills interventions for children with autism spectrum disorders. *Remedial and Special Education, 28*, 153–162.

Bock, M. A. (1999). Sorting laundry: Categorization strategy application to an authentic learning activity by children with autism. *Focus on Autism and Other Developmental Disabilities, 14*, 220–230.

Bock, M. A. (2001). SODA Strategy: Enhancing the social interaction skills of youngsters with asperger syndrome. *Intervention in School and Clinic, 36*, 272–278.

Bock, M. A. (2007). The impact of social-behavioral learning strategy training on the social interaction skills of four students with asperger syndrome. *Focus on Autism and Other Developmental Disabilities, 22*, 88–95.

Bondy, A., & Frost, L. (2001). The picture exchange communication system. *Behavior Modification. Special Issue: Autism, Part 1, 25*, 725–744.

Boyd, B. A., Conroy, M. A., Mancil, G. R., Nakao, T., & Alter, P. J. (2007). Effects of circumscribed interests on the social behaviors of children with autism spectrum disorders. *Journal of Autism and Developmental Disorders, 37*, 1550–1561.

Bricker, D., & Cripe, J. (1992). *An activity-based approach to early intervention*. Baltimore: Brookes Publishing Company.

Buggey, T. (2005). Video self-modeling applications with students with autism spectrum disorder in a small private school setting. *Focus on Autism and Other Developmental Disabilities, 20*, 52–63.

Bulgren, J., Schumaker, J. B., & Deshler, D. D. (1988). Effectiveness of a concept teaching routine in enhancing the performance of LD students in secondary-level mainstream classes. *Learning Disability Quarterly, 11*, 3–17.

Cannella-Malone, H., Sigafoos, J., O'Reilly, M., de la Cruz, M., Edrisinha, C., & Lancioni, G. E. (2006). Comparing video prompting to video modeling for teaching daily living skills to six adults with developmental disabilities. *Education and Training in Developmental Disabilities, 41*, 344–356.

Centers for Disease Control and Prevention. (2009). *Counting Autism*. Retrieved November 30, from http://www.cdc.gov/ncbddd/features/counting-autism.html

Charlop-Christy, M. H., & Daneshvar, S. (2003). Using video modeling to teach perspective taking to children with autism. *Journal of Positive Behavior Interventions, 5*, 12–21.

Charlop, M. H., & Milstein, J. P. (1989). Teaching autistic children conversational speech using video modeling. *Journal of Applied Behavior Analysis, 22*, 275–285.

Cicero, F. R., & Pfadt, A. (2002). Investigation of a reinforcement-based toilet training procedure for children with autism. *Research in Developmental Disabilities, 23*, 319–331.

Datlow Smith, M., & Belcher, R. (1985). Teaching life skills to adults disabled by autism. *Journal of Autism and Developmental Disorders, 15*, 163–175.

DeQuinzio, J. A., Townsend, D. B., & Poulson, C. L. (2008). The effects of forward chaining and contingent social interaction on the acquisition of complex sharing responses by children with autism. *Research in Autism Spectrum Disorders, 2*, 264–275.

DiSalvo, C. A., & Oswald, D. P. (2002). Peer-mediated interventions to increase the social interaction of children with autism: Consideration of peer expectancies. *Focus on Autism and Other Developmental Disabilities, 17*, 198–207.

Dodd, S., Hupp, S. D. A., Jewell, J. D., & Krohn, E. (2008). Using parents and siblings during a social story intervention for two children diagnosed with PDD-NOS. *Journal of Developmental and Physical Disabilities, 20*, 217–229.

Drew, C. J., & Hardman, M. L. (2007). *Intellectual disabilities across the lifespan* (9th ed.). Upper Saddle River, NJ: Merrill-Prentice Hall.

Fantuzzo, J. W., & Smith, C. S. (1983). Programmed generalization of dress efficiency across settings for a severely disturbed, autistic child. *Psychological Reports, 53*, 871–879.

Gena, A. (2006). The effects of prompting and social reinforcement on establishing social interactions with peers during the inclusion of four children with autism in preschool. *International Journal of Psychology, 41*, 541–554.

Goldstein, H., Schneider, N., & Thiemann, K. (2007). Peer-mediated social communication intervention: When clinical expertise informs treatment development and evaluation. *Topics in Language Disorders, 27*, 182–199.

Goodson, J., Sigafoos, J., O'Reilly, M., Cannella, H., & Lancioni, G. E. (2007). Evaluation of a video-based error correction procedure for teaching a domestic skill to individuals with developmental disabilities. *Research in Developmental Disabilities, 28*, 458–467.

Gray, K. (2000). Review of *children with autism and Asperger syndrome: A guide for practitioners and carers*. *Australian and New Zealand Journal of Psychiatry, 34*, 181–182.

Haring, T. G., Kennedy, C. H., Adams, M. J., & Pitts-Conway, V. (1987). Teaching generalization of purchasing skills across community settings to autistic youth using videotape modeling. *Journal of Applied Behavior Analysis, 20*, 89–96.

Harper, C. B., Symon, J. B. G., & Frea, W. D. (2008). Recess is time-in: Using peers to improve social skills of children with autism. *Journal of Autism and Developmental Disorders, 38*, 815–826.

Harris, S. L., Handleman, J. S., & Alessandri, M. (1990). Teaching youths with autism to offer assistance. *Journal of Applied Behavior Analysis, 23*, 297–305.

Hayden, M. F. (1997). Class-action, civil rights litigation for institutionalized persons with mental retardation and other developmental disabilities: A review. *Mental & Physical Disability Law Reporter, 21*, 411–423.

Hwang, B., & Hughes, C. (2000). The effects of social interactive training on early social communicative skills of children with autism. *Journal of Autism and Developmental Disorders, 30*, 331–343.

Hyams, G., McCoull, K., Smith, P. S., & Tyrer, S. P. (1992). Behavioural continence training in mental handicap: A 10-year follow-up study. *Journal of Intellectual Disability Research, 36*, 551–558.

Kamps, D. M., Leonard, B. R., Vernon, S., Dugan, E. P., & Delquadri, J. C., Gershon, B., Wade, L., & Folk, L. (1992). Teaching social skills to students with autism to increase peer interactions in an integrated first-grade classroom. *Journal of Applied Behavior Analysis, 25*, 281–288.

Kamps, D., Royer, J., Dugan, E., Kravits, T., Gonzalez-Lopez, A., Garcia, J., et al. (2002). Peer training to facilitate social interaction for elementary students with autism and their peers. *Exceptional Children, 68*, 173–187.

Kanner, L. (1943). Autistic disturbances of affective contact. *Nervous Child, 2*, 217–250.

Kazdin, A. E. (1977). Assessing the clinical or applied importance of behavior change through social validation. *Behavior Modification, 1*, 427–452.

Keen, D., Brannigan, K. L., & Cuskelly, M. (2007). Toilet training for children with autism: The effects of video modeling. *Journal of Developmental and Physical Disabilities, 19*, 291–303.

Kern Koegel, L. (2000). Interventions to facilitate communication in autism. *Journal of Autism and Developmental Disorders. Special Issue: Treatments for People with Autism and Other Pervasive Developmental Disorders: Research Perspectives, 30*, 383–391.

Kern, P., Wolery, M., & Aldridge, D. (2007). Use of songs to promote independence in morning greeting routines for young children with autism. *Journal of Autism and Developmental Disorders, 37*, 1264–1271.

Kransny, L., Williams, B. J., Provencal, S., & Ozonoff, S. (2003). Social skills interventions for the autism spectrum: Essential ingredients and a model curriculum. *Child and Adolescent Psychiatric Clinics of North America, 12*, 107–122.

Kroeger, K. A., Schultz, J. R., & Newsom, C. (2007). A comparison of two group-delivered social skills programs for young children with autism. *Journal of Autism and Developmental Disorders, 37*, 808–817.

Kroeger, K. A., & Sorensen-Burnworth, R. (2009). Toilet training individuals with autism and other developmental disabilities: A critical review. *Research in Autism Spectrum Disorders, 3*, 607–618.

Laushey, K. M., Heflin, L. J., Shippen, M., Alberto, P. A., & Fredrick, L. (2009). Concept mastery routines to teach social skills to elementary children with high functioning autism. *Journal of Autism and Developmental Disorders, 39*, 1435–1448.

Loftin, R. L., Odom, S. L., & Lantz, J. F. (2008). Social interaction and repetitive motor behaviors. *Journal of Autism and Developmental Disorders, 38*, 1124–1135.

Lovaas, O. I. (2003). *Teaching individuals with developmental delays: Basic intervention techniques*. Austin, TX: PRO-ED.

Marchetti, A. G., McCartney, J. R., Drain, S., Hooper, M., & Dix, J. (1983). Pedestrian skills training for mentally retarded adults: Comparison of training in two settings. *Mental Retardation, 21*, 107–110.

Matson, J. L., Matson, M. L., & Rivet, T. T. (2007). Social-skills treatments for children with autism spectrum disorders: An overview. *Behavior Modification, 31*, 682–707.

Matson, J. L., Taras, M. E., Sevin, J. A., Love, S. R., & Fridley, D. (1990). Teaching self-help skills to autistic and mentally retarded children. *Research in Developmental Disabilities, 11*, 361–378.

Matson, J. L., & Wilkins, J. (2007). A critical review of assessment targets and methods for social skills excesses and deficits for children with autism spectrum disorders. *Research in Autism Spectrum Disorders, 1*, 28–37.

McCartney, J. R. (1990). Toilet training. In J. L. Matson (Ed.), *Handbook of behavior modification with the mentally retarded* (pp. 255–271). New York: Plenum Press.

McConnell, S. R. (2002). Interventions to facilitate social interaction for young children with autism: Review of available research and recommendations for educational intervention and future research. *Journal of Autism and Developmental Disorders, 32*, 351–372.

Mechling, L. C., Gast, D. L., & Seid, N. H. (2009). Using a personal digital assistant to increase independent task completion by students with autism spectrum disorder. *Journal of Autism and Developmental Disorders, 39*, 1420–1434.

Mechling, L. C., & Gustafson, M. R. (2008). Comparison of static picture and video prompting on the performance of cooking-related tasks by students with autism. *Journal of Special Education Technology, 23*, 31–45.

Morse, T. E., & Schuster, J. W. (2000). Teaching elementary students with moderate intellectual disabilities how to shop for groceries. *Exceptional Children, 66*, 273–288.

Nikopoulos, C. K., & Keenan, M. (2007). Using video modeling to teach complex social sequences to children with autism. *Journal of Autism and Developmental Disorders, 37*, 678–693.

Owen-DeSchryver, J. S., Carr, E. G., Cale, S. I., & Blakeley-Smith, A. (2008). Promoting social interactions between students with autism spectrum disorders and their peers in inclusive school settings. *Focus on Autism and Other Developmental Disabilities, 23*, 15–28.

Ozcan, N., & Cavkaytar, A. (2009). Parents as teachers: Teaching parents how to teach toilet skills to their children with autism and mental retardation. *Education and Training in Developmental Disabilities, 44*, 237–243.

Paul, R. (2003). Promoting social communication in high functioning individuals with autistic spectrum disorders. *Child and Adolescent Psychiatric Clinics of North America, 12*, 87–106.

Pierce, K. L., & Schreibman, L. (1994). Teaching daily living skills to children with autism in unsupervised settings through pictorial self-management. *Journal of Applied Behavior Analysis, 27*, 471–481.

Pierce, K., & Schreibman, L. (1997a). Multiple peer use of pivotal response training social behaviors of classmates with autism: Results from trained and untrained peers. *Journal of Applied Behavior Analysis, 30*, 157–160.

Pierce, K., & Schreibman, L. (1995). Increasing complex social behaviors in children with autism: Effects of peer-implemented pivotal response training. *Journal of Applied Behavior Analysis, 28*, 285–295.

Pierce, K., & Schreibman, L. (1997b). Using peer trainers to promote social behavior in autism: Are they effective at enhancing multiple social modalities? *Focus on Autism and Other Developmental Disabilities, 12*, 207–218.

Prelock, P. A., & Hutchins, T. L. (2008). The role of family-centered care in research: Supporting the social communication of children with autism spectrum disorder. *Topics in Language Disorders, 28*, 323–339.

Rao, P. A., Beidel, D. C., & Murray, M. J. (2008). Social skills interventions for children with Asperger's syndrome or high-functioning autism: A review and recommendations. *Journal of Autism and Developmental Disorders, 38*, 353–361.

Reeve, S. A., Reeve, K. F., Buffington Townsend, D., & Poulson, C. L. (2007). Establishing a generalized repertoire of helping behavior in children with autism. *Journal of Applied Behavior Analysis, 40*, 123–136.

Reynhout, G., & Carter, M. (2006). Social stories™ for children with disabilities. *Journal of Autism and Developmental Disabilities, 36*, 445–469.

Rogers, S. J. (2000). Interventions that facilitate socialization in children with autism. *Journal of Autism and Developmental Disorders. Special Issue: Treatments for People with Autism and Other Pervasive Developmental Disorders: Research Perspectives, 30*, 399–409.

Ruble, L., Willis, H., & Crabtree, V. M. (2008). Social skills group therapy for autism spectrum disorders. *Clinical Case Studies, 7*, 287–300.

Sadler, O. W., & Merkert, F. (1977). Evaluating the Foxx and Azrin toilet training procedure for retarded children in a day training center. *Behavior Therapy, 8*, 499–500.

Sansosti, F. J., & Powell-Smith, K. A. (2008). Using computer-presented social stories and video models to increase the social communication skills of children with high-functioning autism spectrum disorders. *Journal of Positive Behavior Interventions, 10*, 162–178.

Sawyer, L. M., Luiselli, J. K., Ricciardi, J. N., & Gower, J. L. (2005). Teaching a child with autism to share among peers in an integrated preschool classroom: Acquisition, maintenance, and social validation. *Education and Treatment of Children, 28*, 1–10.

Scattone, D. (2007). Social skills interventions for children with autism. *Psychology in the Schools. Special Issue: Autism Spectrum Disorders, 44*, 717–726.

Self, T., Scudder, R. R., Weheba, G., & Crumrine, D. (2007). A virtual approach to teaching safety skills to children with autism spectrum disorder. *Topics in Language Disorders, 27*, 242–253.

Sewell, T. J., Collins, B. C., Hemmeter, M. L., & Schuster, J. W. (1998). Using simultaneous prompting within an activity-based format to teach dressing skills to preschoolers with developmental delays. *Journal of Early Intervention, 21*, 132–145.

Shipley-Benamou, R., Lutzker, J. R., & Taubman, M. (2002). Teaching daily living skills to children with autism through instructional video modeling. *Journal of Positive Behavior Interventions, 4*, 166–177.

Sigafoos, J., O'Reilly, M., Cannella, H., Edrisinha, C., de la Cruz, B., Upadhyaya, M., et al. (2007). Evaluation of a video prompting and fading procedure for teaching dish washing skills to adults with developmental disabilities. *Journal of Behavioral Education, 16*, 93–109.

Sisson, L. A., & Dixon, M. J. (1986). Improving mealtime behaviors through token reinforcement: A study with mentally retarded behaviourally disordered children. *Behavior Modification, 10*, 333–354.

Smith, P. (1979). A comparison of different methods of toilet training the mentally handicapped. *Behaviour, Research & Therapy, 17*, 33–43.

Solomon, M., Goodlin-Jones, B. L., & Anders, T. F. (2004). A social adjustment enhancement intervention for high functioning autism, Asperger's syndrome, and pervasive developmental disorder NOS. *Journal of Autism and Developmental Disorders, 34*, 649–668.

Stahmer, A. C., Ingersoll, B., & Carter, C. (2003). Behavioral approaches to promoting play. *Autism. Special Issue on Play, 7*, 401–413.

Stichter, J. P., Randolph, J., Gage, N., & Schmidt, C. (2007). A review of recommended social competency programs for students with autism spectrum disorders. *Exceptionality. Special Issue: Effective Practices for Children and Youth with Autism Spectrum Disorders, 15*, 219–232.

Stokes, J. V., Cameron, M. J., Dorsey, M. F., & Fleming, E. (2004). Task analysis, correspondence training, and general case instruction for teaching personal hygiene skills. *Behavioral Interventions, 19*, 121–135.

Strickland, D. C., McAllister, D., Coles, C. D., & Osborne, S. (2007). An evolution of virtual reality training designs for children with autism and Fetal Alcohol Spectrum Disorders. *Topics in Language Disorders, 27*, 226–241.

Taylor, B. A., Hughes, C. E., Richard, E., Hoch, H., & Rodriquez Coello, A. (2004). Teaching teenagers with autism to seek assistance when lost. *Journal of Applied Behavior Analysis, 37*, 79–82.

Thiemann, K. S., & Goldstein, H. (2004). Effects of peer training and written text cueing on social communication of school-age children with pervasive developmental disorder. *Journal of Speech, Language, and Hearing Research, 47*, 126–144.

van den Pol, R. A., Iwata, B. A., Ivancic, M. T., Page, T. J., Neef, N. A., & Whitley, F. P. (1981). Teaching the handicapped to eat in public places: Acquisition, generalization and maintenance of restaurant skills. *Journal of Applied Behavior Analysis, 14*, 61–69.

Wacker, D., & Berg, W. (1983). Effects of picture prompts on the acquisition of complex vocational tasks by mentally retarded adolescents. *Journal of Applied Behavior Analysis, 16*, 417–433.

Weiss, M. J., & Harris, S. L. (2001). Teaching social skills to people with autism. *Behavior Modification. Special Issue: Autism, Part 1, 25*, 785–802.

Williams White, S., Keonig, K., & Scahill, L. (2007). Social skills development in children with autism spectrum disorders: A review of the intervention research. *Journal of Autism and Developmental Disorders, 37*, 1858–1868.

Wolf, M. M. (1978). Social validity: The case for subjective measurement or how applied behavior analysis is finding its heart. *Journal of Applied Behavior Analysis, 11*(2), 203–214.

22

Nozomi Naoi

Autism spectrum disorders (ASD) are pervasive developmental disorders characterized by impairments in social interaction, communication, and restricted, repetitive, and stereotyped behaviors (DSM-IV, American Psychiatric Association, 1994). Symptoms exhibited by individuals diagnosed with ASD can manifest themselves over a wide variety of combinations of these three core behavioral deficits, with severities ranging from mild to severe. In addition, many individuals with ASD frequently evince at least one maladaptive behavior such as self-injury behavior (e.g., hand-biting, head-banging, face-slapping), property destruction, disruptions (e.g., tantrums), noncompliance, stereotypies (e.g., body rocking, hand flapping), and aggression toward others (Baghdadli, Pascal, Grisli, & Aussiloux, 2003; Horner, Carr, Strain, Todd, & Reed, 2002; Machalicek, O'Reilly, Beretvas, Sigafoos, & Lancioni, 2007; Matson & Nebel-Schwalm, 2007; Matson, Wilkins, & Macken, 2009; McClintock, Hall, & Oliver, 2003; Rojahn, Aman, Matson, & Mayville, 2003). These maladaptive behaviors can often cause physical injury to oneself and others, and, for that reason, many caregivers increase the use of restrictive procedures such as restraint, long-term residential care, and psychotropic medication to manage these problems (Harris, 1993; Singh, Matson, Cooper, Dixon, & Sturmey, 2005; Sturmey, Lott, Laud, & Matson, 2005). In addition, maladaptive behaviors often produce significant stress in others, including parents, siblings, peers, or teachers of individuals with ASD who display maladaptive behavior (Bägenholm & Gillberg, 1991; Block & Rizzo, 1995; Golden & Reese, 1996; Hastings & Brown, 2002; Hastings, 2002). Therefore, maladaptive behaviors interfere with an individual's social relationships, inclusion in his/her community, and prevent

the acquisition of new skills (Anderson, Lakin, Hill, & Chen, 1992; Chadwick, Piroth, Walker, Bernard, & Taylor, 2000). One approach for the treatment of maladaptive behavior is to identify the function of the behavior and teach the individual functional alternative behaviors or skills to replace the maladaptive behavior, known as "functional skill replacement training." The aim of this chapter is to provide a rationale methodology for replacing maladaptive behavior with more positive adaptive behaviors through functional skill replacement training.

Behavioral Approaches to the Treatment of Maladaptive Behavior

Researchers have developed a wide range of behavioral intervention strategies based on the principles of applied behavioral analysis (ABA) to decrease maladaptive behaviors in individuals with ASD and related developmental disorders (Matson & LoVullo, 2008). ABA is based on experimentally derived principles of behavior, such as operant conditioning (Skinner, 1938). In Skinner's (1938, 1953) analysis of behavior, human behaviors can be analyzed within the framework of a three-term contingency of operant conditioning, which includes the events that precede behavior (antecedents), the behavior itself, and the stimuli that follow the behavior (consequences). Recently, researchers have expanded the three-term contingency to also include establishing operations, such as reinforcer deprivation and satiation. To treat maladaptive behaviors, behavioral interventions based on ABA consistently focus on identifying establishing operations, antecedents, and consequences of the maladaptive behavior to determine the function of the behavior.

Several intervention methodologies are increasingly focused on manipulating antecedent events of maladaptive behaviors to prevent the occurrence of the behavior (Clarke, Dunlap, & Vaughn, 1999; Horner et al., 2002; Jolivette, Wehby, & Hirsch, 1999; Kern, Choutka, & Sokol, 2002; Mittenberger, 1998; Peck, Sasso, & Jolivette,

N. Naoi (✉)
Okanoya Emotional Information Project, Japan Science Technology Agency, ERATO, and Graduate School of Education, Kinki District Invention Center, 14 Yoshida-Kawara-cho, Sakyo-ku, Kyoto 606-8305, Japan
e-mail: nnaoi@educ.kyoto-u.ac.jp

J.L. Matson, P. Sturmey (eds.), *International Handbook of Autism and Pervasive Developmental Disorders*, Autism and Child Psychopathology Series, DOI 10.1007/978-1-4419-8065-6_22, © Springer Science+Business Media, LLC 2011

1997; Reeve & Carr, 2000). These antecedent-based intervention strategies, such as environmental modifications, task-related choice, and curricular modifications, are effective in reducing maladaptive behaviors (Brown, 1991; Conroy & Stichter, 2003; Duker & Rasing, 1989; Flannery & Horner, 1994; Golonka et al., 2000; Lohrmann-O'Rourke & Yurman, 2001; Lucyshyn, Albin, & Nixon, 1997; Luiselli, 1998; Mittenberger, 1998; Moes, 1998; Realon, Favell, & Cacace, 1995; Saunders, Saunders, Brewer, & Roach, 1996; Taylor, Ekdahl, Romanczyk, & Miller, 1994; Touchette, MacDonald, & Langer, 1985).

Other behavioral intervention methodologies focus on manipulating consequent events. When the presentation or removal of a stimulus following a behavior increases the likelihood that the behavior will be repeated in the future, that consequence is a reinforcer. On the other hand, when a consequence that follows a behavior decreases the probability that the behavior will be repeated in the future, the consequence is referred to as a punishment. In addition, when a behavior that in the past was reinforced by the presentation of a stimulus is no longer reinforced, the probability that the behavior will occur in the future also decreases (Ayllon & Haughton, 1964; Ducharme & Van Houten, 1994). This procedure is known as extinction.

Until the 1980s, maladaptive behaviors were more likely than current interventions to be treated with aversive punishment procedures (Axelrod & Apsche, 1983; Azrin, 1956; Carr & Lovaas, 1983; Guess, Helmstetter, Turnbull, & Knowlton, 1987; Iwata & Bailey, 1974; Lovaas & Simmons, 1969; Zeilberger, Sampen, & Sloane, 1968). The general efficacy of punishment procedures for individuals with ASD, as a way to decrease maladaptive behavior, has not been disputed; this approach does have significant limitations. The most frequently cited limitation is that the effects of punishment in decreasing maladaptive behaviors are generally short term and that the maladaptive behaviors often revert to a baseline or a higher level of responding when the contingency maintaining punishment is removed (Estes, 1944; Skinner, 1953). Another side effect of punishment procedures is that aversive techniques may generate an emotional response, such as aggression (LaVigna & Donnellan, 1986; Lohrman-O'Rourke & Zirkel, 1998). Furthermore, punishment is less accepted in community settings (Blampied & Kahan, 1992; Miltenberger, Suda, Lennox, & Lindeman, 1991). For these reasons, punishment procedures should be used only when positive procedures alone are not effective in reducing maladaptive behaviors, and even then, careful attention should be given to the severity of maladaptive behaviors, including potential harm to an individual with ASD or others, and to the benefits of procedures to reduce the maladaptive behavior (Davies, Howlin, Bernal, & Warren, 1998; Fisher et al., 1993; Hagopian, Fisher, Sullivan, Acquisto, & LeBlanc, 1998; Matson & LoVullo, 2008; Matson & Taras, 1989; Wacker et al., 1990).

Differential reinforcement procedures are often effective alternatives to punishment procedures for decreasing maladaptive behavior. A differential reinforcement procedure is defined as the reinforcement of one behavior but not the reinforcement of another behavior. When applied as a strategy to reduce behavioral problems, the response targeted for reinforcement includes adaptive responses, while the response targeted for extinction includes maladaptive responses. Differential reinforcement of other behavior (DRO) is a procedure in which a person receives reinforcement when he/she does not engage in the target maladaptive behavior for a specified period of time (Conyers, Miltenberger, Romaniuk, Kopp, & Himle, 2003; de Zubicaray & Clair, 1998; Friman, Barnard, Altman, & Wolf, 1986; Reynolds, 1961; Vollmer & Iwata, 1992). In a DRO procedure, any response in the person's existing behavioral repertoire other than the target maladaptive behaviors that occur during reinforcement intervals is reinforced. DRO procedures can reduce the frequency and the severity of the maladaptive behavior such as self-injurious behavior (Cowdery, Iwata, & Pace, 1990; Ragain & Anson, 1976; Taylor, Hoch, & Weissman, 2005; Tiger, Fisher, & Bouxsein, 2009) and aggression (Repp & Deitz, 1974; Vukelich & Hake, 1971).

There are, however, shortcomings in using DRO to decrease maladaptive behaviors. DRO results in the reinforcement of all behaviors other than the targeted maladaptive behaviors that occur during reinforcement intervals, including precursor behaviors and other maladaptive behaviors. Therefore, DRO procedures themselves are not necessarily optimal and do not necessarily result in the acquisition of alternative, more adaptive behavior (Bregman, Zager, & Gerdtz, 2005). In addition, it is practically difficult in terms of monitoring and counting behaviors to implement DRO procedures consistently in some clinical settings (Bregman et al., 2005). To address these shortcomings in using DRO, other differential reinforcement techniques have been developed.

Differential reinforcement of incompatible behavior (DRI) is a procedure in which behavior is reinforced contingent on the occurrence of a behavior that is topographically incompatible with the target behavior (Azrin, Besalel, Janner, & Caputo, 1988; Barmann, 1980; Denny, 1980; Favell, 1973; Friman et al., 1986; Mace, Kratochwill, & Fiello, 1983; McNally, Calamari, Hansen, & Keliher, 1988; Tarpley & Schroeder, 1979; Underwood, Figueroa, Thyer, & Nzeocha, 1989). For example, playing with a ball would be incompatible with head-banging because both activities require hand movements, and it is difficult to emit both behaviors simultaneously. Tarpley and Schroeder (1979) compared the effects of DRO and DRI to decrease self-injurious behavior (i.e., head-banging) in three individuals with severe intellectual disabilities. The authors found DRI to be more effective than DRO in rapidly decreasing head-banging behavior, even without them specifying the responses to be reinforced. The major disadvantage of DRI is that it may be difficult to select a behavior that is entirely incompatible with the target maladaptive behavior (Bregman et al., 2005).

Functional Skill Replacement Training

Recently, functional skill replacement training that focuses on identifying the function of maladaptive behaviors and teaches functional alternative behaviors to replace the maladaptive behaviors is increasingly used to treat individuals with ASD (Carr et al., 2002; Horner, 2000; Horner et al., 1990; Koegel, Koegel, & Dunlap, 1996). The rationale for this approach is that an increase in reinforcement of the alternative adaptive response with the same reinforcer that maintained the maladaptive response is likely to decrease the rate of that maladaptive response. (Catania, 1966; Parrish, Cataldo, Kolko, Neef, & Egel, 1986). The primary principle of functional skill replacement training is the functional equivalence of an alternative response and the maladaptive behavior to be replaced. Functional equivalence occurs when two or more topographically different behaviors have the same effect on the environment, and these behaviors comprise a response class (Carr, 1988; Catania, 1998; Johnston & Pennypacker, 1993). Any behavior, including maladaptive and adaptive behavior, can be viewed as choices among concurrently available response alternatives (Herrnstein, 1961, 1970; McDowell, 1982, 1988; Myerson & Hale, 1984). Similarly, interventions for maladaptive behavior can be viewed as a competition between either maladaptive behaviors or one or more concurrently available adaptive responses (Mace & Roberts, 1993).

The matching law (Baum, 1974; Herrnstein, 1961, 1970) provides a theoretical framework for response allocation or choice across concurrent schedules of reinforcement in which two or more different schedules operate simultaneously but independently, and consequences are delivered for different response alternatives (Baum & Rachlin, 1969; Mace & Roberts, 1993; McDowell, 1986, 1988; Myerson & Hale, 1984; Pierce & Epling, 1983). According to the matching law, response and time allocation across concurrently available response alternatives tends to be proportional to the number and magnitude of reinforcers provided for each response, reinforcer delay, and response effort for the maladaptive and replacement responses (Beardsley & McDowell, 1992; Herrnstein, 1970; Mace, McCurdy, & Quigley, 1990; McDowell, 1982, 1986; Myerson & Hale, 1984; Pierce & Epling, 1995; Redmon & Lockwood, 1986; Vollmer & Bourret, 2000).

Several applied researchers have evaluated the effects of concurrent schedules of reinforcement on the choice-making behavior of individuals who display maladaptive behavior. Although applied research indicated that direct applications of the matching law to applied settings is limited by differences between laboratory conditions and natural human environments (Baer, 1981; Fuqua, 1984), matching theory has been imported into applied work at a conceptual level. That is, individuals' choices are affected by various dimensions of reinforcement that are concurrently available for each response option (Fisher & Mazur, 1997; Mace & Roberts, 1993; McDowell, 1988). Dimensions of reinforcement are determined by variables such as rate of reinforcement (Davison & McCarthy, 1988; Herrnstein, 1970; Horner & Day, 1991; Neef, Mace, Shea, & Shade, 1992), quality of reinforcement (Neef et al., 1992; Peck et al., 1996), amount of reinforcement (Cooper et al., 1999; Martens & Houk, 1989; Martens, 1990; Martens, Halperin, Rummel, & Kilpatrick, 1990; Martens, Lochner, & Kelly, 1992), delay of reinforcement (Horner & Day, 1991; Neef, Mace, & Shade, 1993), and response effort (Horner & Day, 1991; Mace, Neef, Shade, & Mauro, 1996; Neef, Shade, & Miller, 1994; Richman, Wacker, & Winborn, 2001). In addition, these dimensions of reinforcement may also interact to influence the probability of particular responses (Lalli, Mace, Wohn, & Livezey, 1995; Neef & Lutz, 2001; Neef et al., 1992; 1994). Based on these findings, in functional skill replacement training, the parameters of reinforcement for each response option are manipulated to increase the likelihood of an alternative response (adaptive positive response) over the other responses (maladaptive behavior) (Dixon & Cummings, 2001; Fisher & Mazur, 1997; Harding et al., 1999; Lalli & Casey, 1996; Mace & Roberts, 1993; Mace et al., 1996; Neef & Lutz, 2001; Neef et al., 1993; 1992; Neef et al., 1994; Piazza et al., 1997).

One approach used in functional skill replacement training is differential reinforcement of alternative behavior (DRA) (Azrin, Kaplan, & Foxx, 1973; Dyer, 1987). DRA is a procedure in which reinforcement is contingent on the occurrence of a predetermined appropriate, alternative behavior (Vollmer & Iwata, 1992; Vollmer, Roane, Ringdahl, & Marcus, 1999). A DRA procedure is a similar protocol to DRI; however, in DRA, the behavior is reinforced and does not have to be completely topographically incompatible with the target behavior (Jones & Baker, 1989). The benefit of DRA is that the program can be used to teach the individual a variety of adaptive responses. Many of the alternative responses selected for an individual to be trained in using DRA involve communication skills (Petscher, Rey, & Bailey, 2009).

Functional communication training (FCT) is a variant of DRA in which appropriate communicative responses are shaped and maintained as an alternative to maladaptive behavior using the reinforcer that maintains maladaptive behavior (functional reinforcers), rather than an arbitrary reinforcer (Carr & Durand, 1985; Derby et al., 1997; Durand & Carr, 1992; Durand, 1990; Shirley, Iwata, Kahng, Mazaleski, & Lerman, 1997). FCT is based on a positive behavioral support intervention (Koegel et al., 1996) that states that the maladaptive behavior of a person with limited communication skills serves a communicative function (Carr & Durand, 1985; Durand, 1990). The goal of FCT is to teach a communicative behavior that is functionally equivalent to the maladaptive behavior for that individual.

An early example of FCT comes from Carr and Durand (1985) who taught four children with disabilities who displayed disruptive behavior that was motivated by escape from task demands and to get attention from others. During training, they received adult assistance by saying "I don't understand" during difficult tasks, and they gained verbal praise from adults by saying "Am I doing good work?" The result was a decline in the children's disruptive behavior. Durand and Crimmins (1987) taught a boy with ASD, who emitted inappropriate vocalizations, to say "Help me" as an appropriate escape response that was motivated by his desire to escape from task demands. The frequency of the inappropriate vocalizations decreased following the boy's acquisition of an alternative response, and he maintained a reduction in inappropriate vocalizations for 6 months following training and generalized this behavior to a different setting. In addition, stereotyped behaviors, such as body rocking and hand flapping, may respond to FCT (Durand & Carr, 1987). Durand and Carr (1987) taught four individuals with ASD who displayed escape-motivated stereotypy during difficult tasks, the phrase "Help me". This phrase was used to request assistance with difficult tasks and resulted in a significant decline in the frequency of stereotypy in these individuals.

Numerous studies have shown that function-based interventions are effective to reduce various forms of maladaptive behavior (Bird, Dores, Moniz, & Robinson, 1989; Carr & Durand, 1985; Day, Rea, Schussler, Larsen, & Johnson, 1988; Durand & Carr, 1991; Durand & Kishi, 1987; Durand, 1999; Fisher et al., 1993; Iwata, Pace, Cowdery, & Miltenberger, 1994; Lalli, Casey, & Kates, 1995; Richman et al., 2001; Shukla & Albin, 1996; Wacker et al., 1990; Worsdell, Iwata, Hanley, Thompson, & Kahng, 2000) in a variety of settings (Bowman, Fisher, Thompson, & Piazza, 1997; Braithwaite & Richdale, 2000; Brown et al., 2000; Carr & Durand, 1985; Durand & Carr, 1991; Durand, 1999; Frea, Arnold, & Vittimberga, 2001; Hirsch & Myles, 1996; Kennedy, Meyer, Knowles, & Shukla, 2000; Nuzzolo-Gomez, Leonard, Ortiz, Rivera, & Greer, 2002; Peterson et al., 2005; Schindler & Horner, 2005; Shirley et al., 1997; Taylor, Hoch, &Weissman, 2005; Wacker, Berg, Harding, & Cooper-Brown, 2009; Wacker et al., 2005). In addition, functional skill replacement training procedures such as DRA and FCT are often relatively less intrusive and are rated more positively than punishment-based approaches in community settings (Cowdery et al., 1990; Weigle & Scotti, 2000).

Methods of Functional Communication Training

Functional Behavioral Assessment

Most functional skill replacement training generally involves two major components. First, a functional assessment and/or functional analysis is conducted to identify the behavioral functions that maintain the maladaptive behaviors by identifying the antecedents and consequences of the behavior (Durand, 1990; Mace, 1994). The primary principle of functional skill replacement training is that the alternative communication response and maladaptive behavior should be controlled by the same variables; therefore, a functional behavioral assessment must be the basis for selecting the communicative response. The functional assessment is typically conducted by interviewing and making direct observations, and the functional analysis is conducted by systematically manipulating environmental events (Hanley, Iwata, & McCord, 2003; Hanley, Piazza, & Fisher, 1997; Homer, 1994; Iwata, Dorsey, Slifer, Bauman, & Richman, 1994; Kennedy et al., 2000; Potoczak, Carr, & Michael, 2007). Prior to a functional behavioral assessment, a maladaptive behavior must be clearly defined in objective, observable, and quantifiable terms such as "hair-pulling" and "hand-biting" rather than a behavior category such as "self-injurious behavior." Although there is a possibility that an individual may use multiple behaviors for the same function, there is also a possibility that the individual's various maladaptive behaviors are maintained by different functions. Furthermore, it is also possible that one form of maladaptive behavior may serve more than one function. For these reasons, grouping various maladaptive behaviors together may make it difficult to determine the function of each behavior (Edelson, Taubman, & Lovaas, 1983). In addition, objective and observable definitions of the target behaviors are necessary to measure behavior, implement intervention, and enhance accountability, which promote communication and collaboration among parents, teachers, and other professionals. During the functional assessment, the frequency, duration, severity of the target maladaptive behavior, immediate antecedent events (e.g., activities, settings, individuals, and objects), and the consequences that follow the behavior should be recorded. The functional assessment should also include information about the settings in which the behavior occurs most frequently, such as the physical setting, the social setting, and activities (O'Neill et al., 1997).

The functional analysis developed by Iwata et al. (1994) has involved the measurement of maladaptive behavior under several analogue conditions, each designed to examine the effects of particular consequences such as attention and automatic reinforcement (see Hanley et al., 2003, for a review). For example, to reduce maladaptive behaviors such as tantrums, a functional analysis of a child's environment is conducted to identify the variables that are likely to maintain the behavior. The behavioral functions that have been hypothesized to maintain the child's maladaptive behaviors include attention from others, access to tangible items and preferred activities, escape from an undesired situation or difficult instruction, and generation of sensory reinforcement (Carr & Durand, 1985; Carr, 1977; Derby et al., 1992; Durand & Carr, 1987; Hanley et al., 2003; Iwata et al., 1994; Mace & Belfiore, 1990). During the attention condition of the functional analysis, the child is permitted to interact with toys, and the adult delivers verbal reprimands contingent on target maladaptive behavior (e.g., the child's tantrums). During the demand condition, the child is presented with requests to complete academic tasks, but is allowed brief escape periods contingent on the occurrence of maladaptive behavior. During the tangible condition, the child is provided with food that he/she greatly enjoys contingent on an occurrence of target behavior. The rate of the child's tantrums is compared across conditions to ascertain the function of the behavior.

The length of a functional analysis can be an important consideration for therapists and caregivers who are dealing with an individual's maladaptive behavior. Participants will be exposed to an additional risk of self-injury and harm to others during lengthy assessment periods (Northup et al., 1991). One possible approach is that direct observations are made in natural settings, and that, based on these observations, brief functional analyses be conducted. In regard to this point, a functional analysis should be conducted by the relevant stakeholders in relevant settings. The functional analysis precludes the typical settings, and the relevant stakeholders may produce false negatives.

Selecting an Alternate Response

The selection of appropriate alternative communicative behaviors to replace maladaptive behavior is one of the most important aspects of successful intervention for decreasing maladaptive behavior. It is important to select a functionally equivalent, alternative communication response that serves to replace maladaptive behavior (Bosch & Fuqua, 2001; Rosales-Ruiz & Baer, 1997; Wacker et al., 1996). In addition, it is necessary that the alternative communicative response be more efficient than the maladaptive behavior that it is to replace (Carr & Durand, 1985; Horner & Day, 1991; Horner et al., 1990; Richman et al., 2001). Response efficiency is determined by the amount of physical effort to

emit, the time delay between a response and reinforcement, and the quality of reinforcement (Friman & Poling, 1995; Horner & Day, 1991; Horner et al., 1990; Mace & Roberts, 1993; O'Neill et al., 1997). Using existing responses in an individual's repertoire as alternative responses to teach may increase the efficiency in implementing treatment (Grow, Kelley, Roane, & Shillingsburg, 2008).

Some individuals with ASD have demonstrated limited comprehension and use of language. The augmentative and alternative communication (AAC) approach has been adapted for teaching nonverbal communication skills as alternative responses in functional skill replacement training for individuals with ASD who have limited or no verbal communication skills (Mirenda, 1997).

Studies using single-subject designs have demonstrated that individuals with ASD and related developmental disabilities show decreases in various maladaptive behaviors following the mastery of AAC, such as manual signs and a voice output communication aid (VOCA). For example, Day, Horner, and O'Neill (1994) reported that three individuals with severe intellectual disabilities, who displayed self-injury and aggression maintained by a desire to escape from difficult tasks and access to preferred items, were taught to use the manual sign for "want" and/or to give the trainer a card labeled with the word "break" or "help." After each participant was trained in functionally equivalent communication skills using AAC, his/her levels of maladaptive behavior decreased. Durand (1993) also evaluated the effects of FCT using VOCA to replace maladaptive behaviors in three individuals with severe disabilities who possessed little or no functional speech. The participants learned to request attention or escape using VOCA rather than to engage in self-injury or aggression. Durand (1999) extended these results with five other students with severe disabilities such as cerebral palsy and intellectual disabilities, to evaluate whether VOCA could be used successfully with untrained community members in novel community settings such as a local candy store, a local shopping mall, the movie theater, a book and magazine shop, and the library, following training in the classroom. Following a functional assessment, each of the students learned to use VOCA as the alternative behavior to express the functions that seemingly maintained their maladaptive behaviors. The students successfully used their VOCA to express the communicative functions that maintained their maladaptive behavior in novel community settings and their maladaptive behaviors were reduced. Similarly, Northup et al. (1994) trained four teachers to teach students with intellectual disabilities to use a VOCA and manual signs to request attention, tangibles, and escape. Results indicated that there was a decrease in maladaptive behavior and maintenance and generalization of acquired skills.

Teaching Procedures

Once the stimuli maintaining the maladaptive behavior are identified in a functional behavioral assessment, instruction in an alternative communicative response can produce the same consequences as maladaptive behaviors (Carr et al., 1994; Durand, 1990). Prior to a therapist implementing treatment, the current levels of the individual's maladaptive and alternative responses are measured as a baseline. During intervention, both the target maladaptive behavior and the alternative communicative behaviors are continuously measured in order to determine the effectiveness of the intervention, and, in general, the generalizations of acquired communication skills across settings are assessed following the individual's completion of training. In addition, follow-up data are frequently collected to evaluate the generalization and maintenance of the behavior.

To increase socially appropriate alternative behaviors rapidly, reinforcement for alternative behavior should be delivered continuously and immediately during the initial phase of intervention. Once maladaptive behavior begins to decrease and alternative behavior has become efficient, it will be necessary to thin the reinforcement schedule to make the treatment easier to implement and maintain in the natural environment (Hagopian, Contrucci, Kuhn, Long, & Rush, 2005).

Reinforcement Schedule Thinning

Schedule thinning refers to gradually increasing the number of responses required to obtain reinforcement. Several methods have been used to thin reinforcement schedules for alternative responses. One approach involves gradually increasing delays between the alternative response and the reinforcement (Fisher et al., 1993; Fisher, Thompson, Hagopian, Bowman, & Krug, 2000; Hagopian et al., 1998). Although increases in maladaptive behavior have been commonly observed as the delay is increased, providing an alternative activity during delay could facilitate schedule thinning (Fisher et al., 2000; Hagopian et al., 2005). A second approach involves progressively increasing the response requirement needed to obtain the reinforcer (Lalli et al., 1995). Furthermore, the use of discriminative stimuli signaling periods of reinforcement and extinction in a multiple schedule arrangement also facilitates reinforcement schedule thinning (Fisher, Kuhn, & Thompson, 1998; Hanley, Iwata, & Thompson, 2001).

In addition, the reinforcement schedule for maladaptive behavior can also be manipulated (DeLeon, Fisher, Herman, & Crosland, 2000; Vollmer et al., 1999; Worsdell et al., 2000). In the study by Worsdell et al. (2000), an alternative response was reinforced on continuous schedules, and the schedule of reinforcement for maladaptive behavior was thinned from a fixed ratio 1 (FR1) to FR 5 and so on until the participants acquired the alternative response and the rates of maladaptive behavior decreased. Another approach is the addition of noncontingent reinforcement, which was thinned over time (Goh, Iwata, & DeLeon, 2000; Marcus & Vollmer, 1996).

Functional skill replacement training has often been combined with other operant procedures, such as extinction (Carr & Durand, 1985; Durand & Carr, 1991; Lalli et al., 1995; Shirley et al., 1997) and/or punishment (Fisher et al., 1993; Hagopian et al., 1998; Hanley, Piazza, Fisher, & Maglieri, 2005; Wacker et al., 1990) to assist in the reduction of maladaptive behavior. For example, Shirley et al. (1997) studied three participants with developmental disabilities to compare the effectiveness of FCT with and without extinction in decreasing maladaptive behavior (self-injurious behavior) and in increasing an alternative response (a manual sign). Shirley et al. (1997) demonstrated that FCT with extinction resulted in more behavior reduction than FCT alone. Kelley, Lerman, and Van Camp (2002) and O'Neill and Sweetland-Baker (2001) also found similar results that supported the need for extinction for maladaptive behavior during FCT.

Wacker et al. (1990) examined the effects of extinction, punishment, and/or prompting in decreasing maladaptive behavior and in increasing an alternative response during FCT. Although participants demonstrated substantial decreases in maladaptive behaviors and increases in alternative communication behaviors following the completion of a treatment combined with extinction, punishment, and/or prompting, they demonstrated considerable increases in maladaptive behavior when extinction or punishment for maladaptive behavior was later removed. In addition, Wacker et al. (1990) found that treatment combined with a punishment procedure was superior to DRO with punishment to reduce maladaptive behavior and increase an alternative response.

Fisher et al. (1993) compared the effects of FCT alone, FCT with extinction, and FCT with punishment and found that FCT combined with a punishment procedure is superior to FCT with or without an extinction procedure in reducing maladaptive behavior and increasing an appropriate alternative response. Similarly, Hagopian et al. (1998) and Hanley et al. (2005) demonstrated that FCT with punishment was more effective than FCT with or without extinction.

While FCT with punishment and/or extinction procedures has proven useful in the treatment of maladaptive behaviors, it is often accompanied by certain undesirable side effects. As previously mentioned, there are limitations to using punishment to decrease maladaptive behaviors, such as the occurrence of an emotional response (LaVigna & Donnellan, 1986; Lohrman-O'Rourke & Zirkel, 1998). In terms of extinction, the most commonly cited undesirable effect of extinction is an extinction burst which is a temporary increase in the rate and magnitude of the target behavior that occurs at the beginning of extinction (Lerman & Iwata, 1995, 1996). Other characteristics related to undesirable side effects of extinction include increases in aggression and other emotional behavior such as crying (Azrin, Hutchinson, & Hake, 1966; Zeiler, 1971). Another possible side effect of extinction is related to extinction-induced resurgence, which is the recurrence of a previously reinforced behavior when another behavior is placed on extinction (Lieving, Hagopian, Long, & O'Connor, 2004). It is possible that previously reinforced maladaptive behavior may reemerge if reinforcement is not provided consistently for alternative responses.

Shirley et al. (1997) demonstrated with three participants that when both maladaptive behavior (self-injurious behavior) and an alternative response (manual sign) continued to produce reinforcement on an FR 1, all three participants continued to exhibit high baseline rates of self-injurious behavior and failed to acquire the alternative response; however, once the participants acquired the alternative response, obtaining reinforcement with appropriate behavior effectively competed with the ongoing reinforcement of maladaptive behavior for two of the three participants. Two other studies have examined the effects of providing intermittent reinforcement for maladaptive behavior during the acquisition of appropriate behavior (Kelley et al., 2002; Worsdell et al., 2000). In Worsdell et al. (2000), both maladaptive behavior and an alternative response were reinforced on continuous schedules during the acquisition phase of FCT. The reinforcement schedule for maladaptive behavior was then thinned until the participants acquired the alternative response and the rates of maladaptive behavior decreased.

Future Research Agenda

This chapter reviewed research findings on functional skill replacement training such as DRA and FCT for individuals with ASD and related disorders. Functional skill replacement training has been successful in reducing a variety of maladaptive behaviors for many participants, replacing maladaptive behaviors with appropriate behaviors that can enhance a participant's quality of life.

One disadvantage of functional skill replacement training is that for some individuals, a punishment and/or extinction procedure may be necessary to maintain their performance. Therefore, sometimes it is not simply sufficient to encourage an individual to adopt socially appropriate functional behaviors to replace maladaptive behavior; however, for those cases, schedule thinning has been shown to successfully reduce the maladaptive behavior (Fisher et al., 1993; O'Neill & Sweetland-Baker, 2001; Wacker et al., 1990).

Given that there is great heterogeneity among individuals with ASD, every such individual may benefit from different combinations of interventions. Thus, it is important to individualize interventions based on functional behavioral assessments.

In addition, interventions for individuals with ASD focus on interactions between the person and the environment. The environment should be structured so that the individual is more likely to engage in appropriate behaviors and to avoid maladaptive behaviors. It is also necessary to examine the applicability of functional skill replacement training in schools, communities, and home settings for individuals with ASD who live in countries outside the United States. Most functional skill replacement training generally involves a functional behavioral assessment and instruction in an alternative communicative response. It is possible that these intervention components are not conducted regularly due to a lack of well-trained professionals with the required knowledge, experience, and skills (Crawford, Brockel, Schauss, & Miltenberger, 1992; Durand & Crimmins, 1988). Instructional packages should be developed to train a variety of individuals such as teachers, teaching staffs, and caregivers to implement functional skill replacement training.

References

American Psychiatric Association. (1994). *Diagnostic and statistical manual of mental disorders* (4th ed.). Washington, DC: Author.

Anderson, D. J., Lakin, K. C., Hill, B. K., & Chen, T. H. (1992). Social integration of older persons with mental retardation in residential facilities. *American Journal on Mental Retardation, 96,* 488–501.

Axelrod, S., & Apsche, J. (1983). *The effects of punishment on human behavior.* New York: Academic Press.

Ayllon, T., & Haughton, E. (1964). Modification of symptomatic verbal behavior of mental patients. *Behaviour Research and Therapy, 2,* 87–97.

Azrin, N. H. (1956). Some effects of two intermittent schedules of immediate and non-immediate punishment. *Journal of Psychology, 42,* 3–21.

Azrin, N. H., Besalel, V. A., Janner, J. P., & Caputo, J. N. (1988). Comparative study of behavioral methods of treating severe self-injury. *Behavioral Residential Treatment, 3,* 119–152.

Azrin, N. H., Hutchinson, R. R., & Hake, D. F. (1966). Extinction induced aggression. *Journal of the Experimental Analysis of Behavior, 9,* 191–204.

Azrin, N. H., Kaplan, S. J., & Foxx, R. M. (1973). Autism reversal: Eliminating stereotyped self-stimulation of retarded individuals. *American Journal of Mental Deficiency, 78,* 241–248.

Baer, D. M. (1981). A flight of behavior analysis. *The Behavior Analyst, 4,* 85–91.

Baghdadli, A., Pascal, C., Grisli, S., & Aussiloux, C. (2003). Risk factors for self-injurious behaviours among 222 young children with autistic disorders. *Journal of Intellectual Disabilities Research, 47,* 622–627.

Barmann, B. C. (1980). Use of contingent vibration in the treatment of self-stimulatory handmouthing and ruminative vomiting behavior. *Journal of Behavior Therapy and Experimental Psychiatry, 11,* 307–311.

Baum, W. M. (1974). On two types of deviation from the matching law: Bias and undermatching. *Journal of the Experimental Analysis of Behavior, 22*, 231–242.

Baum, W. M., & Rachlin, H. (1969). Choice as time allocation. *Journal of the Experimental Analysis of Behavior, 12*, 861–874.

Beardsley, S. D., & McDowell, J. J. (1992). Application of Herrnstein's hyperbola to time allocation of naturalistic human behavior maintained by naturalistic social reinforcement. *Journal of the Experimental Analysis of Behavior, 57*, 177–185.

Bird, F., Dores, P. A., Moniz, D., & Robinson, J. (1989). Reducing severe aggressive and self-injurious behaviors with functional communication training. *American Journal of Mental Retardation, 94*, 37–48.

Blampied, N. M., & Kahan, E. (1992). Acceptability of alternative punishments. *Behavior Modification, 16*, 400–413.

Block, M. E., & Rizzo, T. (1995). Attitudes and attributes of physical educators associated with teaching individuals with sever and profound disabilities. *Journal of the Association for Persons with Severe Handicaps, 20*, 80–87.

Bosch, S., & Fuqua, R. W. (2001). Behavioral cusps: A model for selecting target behaviors. *Journal of Applied Behavior Analysis, 34*, 123–125.

Bowman, L. G., Fisher, W. W., Thompson, R. H., & Piazza, C. C. (1997). On the relation of mands and the function of destructive behavior. *Journal of Applied Behavior Analysis, 30*, 251–265.

Braithwaite, K. L., & Richdale, A. L. (2000). Functional communication training to replace challenging behaviors across two behavioral outcomes. *Behavioral Interventions, 15*, 21–36.

Bregman, J. D., Zager, D., & Gerdtz, J. (2005). Behavioral interventions. In F. R. Volkmar, R. Paul, A. Klin, & D. Cohen. (Eds.), *Handbook of autism and pervasive developmental disorders* (3rd ed., pp. 897–924). Hoboken, NJ: Wiley.

Brown, F. (1991). Creative daily scheduling: A nonintrusive approach to challenging behaviors in community residences. *Journal of the Association for Persons with Severe Handicaps, 16*, 75–84.

Brown, K. A., Wacker, D. P., Derby, K. M., Peck, S. M., Richman, D. M., Sasso, G. M., et al. (2000). Evaluating the effects of functional communication training in the presence and absence of establishing operations. *Journal of Applied Behavior Analysis, 33*, 53–71.

Bägenholm, A., & Gillberg, C. (1991). Psychosocial effects on siblings of children with autism and mental retardation: A population-based study. *Journal of Mental Deficiency Research, 35*, 291–307.

Carr, E. G. (1977). The motivation of self-injurious behavior: A review of some hypotheses. *Psychological Bulletin, 84*, 800–816.

Carr, E. G. (1988). Functional equivalence as a mechanism of response generalization. In R. Horner, G. Dunlap, & R. L. Koegel (Eds.), *Generalization and maintenance: Life-style changes in applied settings* (pp. 221–241). Baltimore: Paul H. Brookes.

Carr, E. G., Dunlap, G., Horner, R. H., Koegel, R. L., Turnbull, A. P., Sailor, W., et al. (2002). Positive behavior support: Evolution of an applied science. *Journal of Positive Behavior Interventions, 4*, 4–16.

Carr, E. G., & Durand, V. M. (1985). Reducing behavior problems through functional communication training. *Journal of Applied Behavior Analysis, 18*, 111–126.

Carr, E. G., Levin, L., McConnachie, G., Carlson, J. I., Kemp, D. C., & Smith, C. E. (1994). *Communication-based intervention for problem behavior: A user's guide for producing positive change*. Baltimore: Paul H. Brookes.

Carr, E. G., & Lovaas, O. I. (1983). Contingent electric shock as a treatment for severe behavior problems. In S. A. J. Apsche (Ed.), *Punishment: Its effects on human behavior* (pp. 221–245). New York: Academic Press.

Catania, A. C. (1966). Concurrent operants. In W. K. Honig (Ed.), *Operant behavior: Areas of research and application* (pp. 213–270). New York: Appleton-Century-Crofts.

Catania, A. C. (1998). *Learning* (4th ed.). Upper Saddle River, NJ: Prentice Hall.

Chadwick, O., Piroth, N., Walker, J., Bernard, S., & Taylor, E. (2000). Factors affecting the risk of behavior problems in children with severe intellectual disability. *Journal of Intellectual Disability Research, 44*, 108–123.

Clarke, S., Dunlap, G., & Vaughn, B. (1999). Family-centered, assessment-based intervention to improve behavior during an early morning routine. *Journal of Positive Behavior Interventions, 1*, 235–241.

Conroy, M. A., & Stichter, J. P. (2003). The application of antecedents in the functional assessment process: Existing research, issues, and recommendations. *The Journal of Special Education, 37*, 15–25.

Conyers, C., Miltenberger, R. G., Romaniuk, C., Kopp, B., & Himle, M. (2003). Evaluation of DRO schedules to reduce disruptive behavior in a preschool classroom. *Child and Family Behavior Therapy, 25*, 1–6.

Cooper, L. J., Wacker, D. P., Brown, K., McComas, J. J., Peck, S. M., Drew, J., et al. (1999). Useof a concurrent operants paradigm to evaluate positive reinforcers during treatment of food refusal. *Behavior Modification, 23*, 3–40.

Cowdery, G. E., Iwata, B. A., & Pace, G. M. (1990). Effects and side effects of DRO as treatment for self-injurious behavior. *Journal of Applied Behavior Analysis, 23*, 497–506.

Crawford, J., Brockel, B., Schauss, S., & Miltenberger, R. G. (1992). A comparison of methods for the functional assessment of stereotypic behavior. *Journal of the Association for Persons with Severe Handicaps, 17*, 77–86.

Davies, M., Howlin, P., Bernal, J., & Warren, S. (1998). Treating severe self-injury in a community setting: Constraints on assessment and intervention. *Child Psychology and Psychiatry Review, 3*, 26–32.

Davison, M., & McCarthy, D. (1988). *The matching law: A research review*. Hillsdale, NJ: Erlbaum.

Day, H. M., Horner, R. H., & O'Neill, R. E. (1994). Multiple functions of problem behaviors: Assessment and intervention. *Journal of Applied Behavior Analysis, 27*, 279–289.

Day, R. M., Rea, J. A., Schussler, N. G., Larsen, S. E., & Johnson, W. L. (1988). A functionally based approach to the treatment of self-injurious behavior. *Behavior Modification, 12*, 565–589.

DeLeon, I. G., Fisher, W. W., Herman, K. M., & Crosland, K. C. (2000). Assessment of a response bias for aggression over functionally equivalent appropriate behavior. *Journal of Applied Behavior Analysis, 33*, 73–77.

Denny, M. (1980). Reducing self-stimulatory behavior of mentally retarded persons by alternative positive practice. *American Journal of Mental Deficiency, 84*, 610–615.

Derby, K. M., Wacker, D. P., Berg, W., DeRaad, A., Ulrich, S., Asmus, J., et al. (1997). The long-term effects of functional communication training in home settings. *Journal of Applied Behavior Analysis, 30*, 507–531.

Derby, K., Wacker, D., Sasso, G., Steege, M., Northup, J., Cigrand, K., et al. (1992). Brief functional assessment techniques to evaluate aberrant behavior in an outpatient setting: A summary of 79 cases. *Journal of Applied Behavior Analysis, 25*, 713–721.

Dixon, M. R., & Cummings, A. (2001). Self-control in children with autism: Response allocation during delays to reinforcement. *Journal of Applied Behavior Analysis, 34*, 491–495.

Ducharme, J. M., & Van Houten, R. (1994). Operant extinction in the treatment of severe maladaptive behavior. *Behavior Modification, 18*, 139–170.

Duker, P. C., & Rasing, E. (1989). Effects of redesigning the physical environment on self-stimulation and on-task behavior in three autistic-type developmentally disabled individuals. *Journal of Autism and Developmental Disorders, 19*, 449–460.

Durand, V. M. (1990). *Severe behavior problems: A functional communication training approach*. New York: Guilford Press.

Durand, V. M. (1993). Functional communication training using assistive devices: Effects on challenging behavior and affect. *Augmentative and Alternative Communication, 9*, 168–176.

Durand, V. M. (1999). Functional communication training using assistive devices: Recruiting natural communities of reinforcement. *Journal of Applied Behavior Analysis, 32*, 247–267.

Durand, V. M., & Carr, E. G. (1987). Social influences on 'self-stimulatory' behavior: Analysis and treatment application. *Journal of Applied Behavior Analysis, 20*, 119–132.

Durand, V. M., & Carr, E. G. (1991). Functional communication training to reduce challenging behavior: Maintenance and application in new settings. *Journal of Applied Behavior Analysis, 24*, 251–264.

Durand, V. M., & Carr, E. G. (1992). An analysis of maintenance following functional communication training. *Journal of Applied Behavior Analysis, 25*, 777–794.

Durand, V. M., & Crimmins, D. B. (1987). Assessment and treatment of psychotic speech in an autistic child. *Journal of Autism and Developmental Disorders, 17*, 17–28.

Durand, V. M., & Crimmins, D. B. (1988). Identifying the variables maintaining self-injurious behavior. *Journal of Autism and Developmental Disorders, 18*, 99–117.

Durand, V. M., & Kishi, G. (1987). Reducing severe behavior problems among persons with dual sensory impairments: An evaluation of a technical assistance model. *Journal of the Association for Persons with Severe Handicaps, 12*, 2–10.

Dyer, K. (1987). The competition of autistic stereotyped behavior with usual and specially assessed reinforcers. *Research in Developmental Disabilities, 8*, 607–626.

Edelson, S. M., Taubman, M. T., & Lovaas, O. I. (1983). Some social contexts to self-destructive behavior. *Journal of Abnormal Child Psychology, 11*, 299–312.

Estes, W. K. (1944). An experimental study of punishment. *Psychological Monographs, 57*, (3, Whole No. 263).

Favell, J. E. (1973). Reduction of stereotypies by reinforcement of toy play. *Mental Retardation, 11*, 21–23.

Fisher, W. W., Kuhn, D. E., & Thompson, R. H. (1998). Establishing discriminative control of responding using functional and alternative reinforcers during functional communication training. *Journal of Applied Behavior Analysis, 31*, 543–560.

Fisher, W. W., & Mazur, J. E. (1997). Basic and applied research on choice responding. *Journal of Applied Behavior Analysis, 30*, 387–410.

Fisher, W. W., Piazza, C. C., Cataldo, M. F., Harrell, R., Jefferson, G., & Corner, R. (1993). Functional communication training with and without extinctions and punishment. *Journal of Applied Behavior Analysis, 26*, 23–26.

Fisher, W. W., Thompson, R. H., Hagopian, L. P., Bowman, L. G., & Krug, A. (2000). Facilitating tolerance of delayed reinforcement during functional communication training. *Behavior Modification, 24*, 3–29.

Flannery, K. B., & Horner, R. H. (1994). The relationship between predictability and problem behavior for students with severe disabilities. *Journal of Behavioral Education, 4*, 157–176.

Frea, W., Arnold, C., & Vittimberga, G. (2001). A demonstration of the effects of augmentative communication on the extreme aggressive behavior of a child with autism within an integrated preschool setting. *Journal of Positive Behavior Interventions, 3*, 194–198.

Friman, P. C., Barnard, J. D., Altman, K., & Wolf, M. M. (1986). Parent and teacher use of DRO and DRI to reduce aggressive behavior. *Analysis and Intervention in Developmental Disabilities, 6*, 319–330.

Friman, P. C., & Poling, A. (1995). Making life easier with effort: Basic and applied research on response effort. *Journal of Applied Behavior Analysis, 28*, 583–590.

Fuqua, R. W. (1984). Comments on the applied relevance of the matching law. *Journal of Applied Behavior Analysis, 17*, 381–386.

Goh, H., Iwata, B. A., & DeLeon, I. G. (2000). Competition between noncontingent and contingent reinforcement schedules during response acquisition. *Journal of Applied Behavior Analysis, 33*, 195–205.

Golden, J., & Reese, M. (1996). Focus on communication: Improving interaction between staff and residents who have sever or profound mental retardation. *Research in Developmental Disabilities, 17*, 363–382.

Golonka, Z., Wacker, D. P., Berg, W., Derby, K. M., Harding, J., & Peck, S. (2000). Effects of escape to alone versus escape to enriched environments on adaptive and aberrant behavior. *Journal of Applied Behavior Analysis, 33*, 243–246.

Grow, L. L., Kelley, M. E., Roane, H. S., & Shillingsburg, M. A. (2008). Utility of extinction induced response variability for the selection of mands. *Journal of Applied Behavior Analysis, 41*, 15–24.

Guess, D., Helmstetter, E., Turnbull, H. R., & Knowlton, S. (1987). Use of aversive procedures with persons who are disabled: A historical review and critical analysis. *Monograph of the Association for Persons with Severe Handicaps, 2*, 1–68.

Hagopian, L. P., Contrucci, Kuhn, S. A., Long, E. S., & Rush, K. S. (2005). Schedule thinning following communication training: Using competing stimuli to enhance tolerance to decrements in reinforcer density. *Journal of Applied Behavior Analysis, 34*, 17–38.

Hagopian, L. P., Fisher, W. W., Sullivan, M. T., Acquisto, J., & LeBlanc, L. A. (1998). Effectiveness of functional communication training with and without extinction and punishment: A summary of 21 inpatient cases. *Journal of Applied Behavior Analysis, 2*, 211–235.

Hanley, G. P., Iwata, B. A., & McCord, B. E. (2003). Functional analysis of problem behavior: A review. *Journal of Applied Behavior Analysis, 36*, 147–185.

Hanley, G. P., Iwata, B. A., & Thompson, R. A. (2001). Reinforcement schedule thinning following treatment with functional communication training. *Journal of Applied Behavior Analysis, 34*, 17–38.

Hanley, G. P., Piazza, C. C., & Fisher, W. (1997). Noncontingent presentation of attention and alternative stimuli in the treatment of attention-maintained destructive behavior. *Journal of Applied Behavior Analysis, 30*, 229–237.

Hanley, G. P., Piazza, C. C., Fisher, W. W., & Maglieri, K. A. (2005). On the effectiveness of and preference for punishment and extinction components of function-based interventions. *Journal of Applied Behavior Analysis, 38*, 51–65.

Harding, J. W., Wacker, D. P., Berg, W. K., Cooper, L. J., Asmus, J., Mlela, K., et al. (1999). An analysis of choice making in the assessment of young children with severe behavior problems. *Journal of Applied Behavior Analysis, 32*, 63–82.

Harris, P. (1993). The nature and extent of aggressive behavior amongst people with learning difficulties (mental handicap) in a single health district. *Journal of Intellectual Disability Research, 37*, 221–242.

Hastings, R. P. (2002). Parental stress and behaviour problems of children with developmental disability. *Journal of Intellectual & Developmental Disability, 27*, 149–160.

Hastings, R. P., & Brown, T. (2002). Coping strategies and the impact of challenging behaviors on special educators' burnout. *Mental Retardation, 40*, 148–156.

Herrnstein, R. J. (1961). Relative and absolute strength of response as a function of frequency of reinforcement. *Journal of the Experimental Analysis of Behavior, 4*, 267–272.

Herrnstein, R. J. (1970). On the law of effect. *Journal of the Experimental Analysis of Behavior, 13*, 243–266.

Hirsch, N., & Myles, B. S. (1996). The use of a pica box in reducing pica behavior in a student with autism. *Focus on Autism and Other Developmental Disabilities, 11*, 222–227.

Homer, R. H. (1994). Functional assessment: Contributions and future directions. *Journal of Applied Behavior Analysis, 28*, 401–404.

Horner, R. H. (2000). Positive Behavior Supports. *Focus on Autism and Other Developmental Disabilities, 15*, 97–105.

Horner, R. H., Carr, E. G., Strain, P. S., Todd, A. W., & Reed, H. K. (2002). Problem behavior interventions for young children with autism: A research synthesis. *Journal of Autism and. Developmental Disorders, 32*, 423–446.

Horner, R. H., & Day, H. M. (1991). The effects of response efficiency on functionally equivalent competing behaviors. *Journal of Applied Behavior Analysis, 24*, 719–732.

Horner, R. H., Dunlap, G., Koegel, R. L., Carr, E. G., Sailor, W., Anderson, J., et al. (1990). Toward a technology of "nonaversive" behavior support. *Journal of the Association for Persons with Severe Handicaps, 15*, 125–132.

Iwata, B. A., & Bailey, J. S. (1974). Reward versus cost token systems: An analysis of the effects on student and teacher. *Journal of Applied Behavior Analysis, 7*, 567–576.

Iwata, B. A., Dorsey, M., Slifer, K., Bauman, K., & Richman, G. (1994). Toward a functional analysis of self-injury. *Journal of Applied Behavior Analysis, 27*, 197–209.

Iwata, B. A., Pace, G. M., Cowdery, G. E., & Miltenberger, R. G. (1994). What makes extinction work: An analysis of procedural form and function. *Journal of Applied Behavior Analysis, 27*, 131–144.

Johnston, J. M., & Pennypacker, H. S. (1993). *Strategies and tactics of behavioral research* (2nd ed.). Hillsdale, NJ: Lawrence Erlbaum Associates.

Jolivette, K., Wehby, J. H., & Hirsch, L. (1999). Academic strategy identification for students exhibiting inappropriate classroom behaviors. *Behavioral Disorders, 24*, 210–221.

Jones, R. S., & Baker, L. J. (1989). Differential reinforcement and challenging behavior: A critical review of the DRI schedule. *Behavioural Psychotherapy, 18*, 35–47.

Kelley, M. E., Lerman, D. C., & Van Camp, C. M. (2002). The effects of competing reinforcement schedules on the acquisition of functional communication. *Journal of Applied Behavior Analysis, 35*, 59–63.

Kennedy, C. H., Meyer, K. A., Knowles, T., & Shukla, S. (2000). Analyzing the multiple functions of stereotypical behavior for students with autism: Implications for assessment and treatment. *Journal of Applied Behavior Analysis, 33*, 559–571.

Kern, L., Choutka, C. M., & Sokol, N. (2002). Assessment-based antecedent interventions used in natural settings to reduce challenging behavior: An analysis of the literature. *Education and Treatment of Children, 25*, 113–130.

Koegel, L. K., Koegel, R. L., & Dunlap, G. (1996). *Positive behavioral support: Including people with difficult behavior in the community*. Baltimore: Paul H. Brookes.

LaVigna, G. W., & Donnellan, A. M. (1986). *Alternatives to punishment: Solving behavior problems with non-aversive strategies*. New York: Irvington Publishers, Inc.

Lalli, J. S., & Casey, S. D. (1996). Treatment of multiply controlled problem behavior. *Journal of Applied Behavior Analysis, 29*, 391–395.

Lalli, J. S., Casey, S., & Kates, K. (1995). Reducing escape behavior and increasing task completion with functional communication training, extinction, and response chaining. *Journal of Applied Behavior Analysis, 28*, 261–268.

Lalli, J. S., Mace, F. C., Wohn, T., & Livezey, K. (1995). Identification and modification of a response-class hierarchy. *Journal of Applied Behavior Analysis, 28*, 551–559.

Lerman, D. C., & Iwata, B. A. (1995). Prevalence of the extinction burst and its attenuation during treatment. *Journal of Applied Behavior Analysis, 28*, 93–94.

Lerman, D. C., & Iwata, B. A. (1996). A methodology for distinguishing between extinction and punishment effects associated with response blocking. *Journal of Applied Behavior Analysis, 29*, 231–234.

Lieving, G. A., Hagopian, L. P., Long, E. S., & O'Connor, J. (2004). Response-class hierarchies and resurgence of severe problem behavior. *The Psychological Record, 54*, 621–634.

Lohrman-O'Rourke, S., & Zirkel, P. A. (1998). The case law on aversive interventions for students with disabilities. *Exceptional Children, 65*, 101–123.

Lohrmann-O'Rourke, S., & Yurman, B. (2001). Naturalistic assessment of and intervention for mouthing behaviors influenced by establishing operations. *Journal of Positive Behavior Interventions, 3*, 19–27.

Lovaas, O. I., & Simmons, J. Q. (1969). Manipulation of self-destruction in three retarded children. *Journal of Applied Behavior Analysis, 2*, 143–157.

Lucyshyn, J. M., Albin, R. W., & Nixon, C. D. (1997). Embedding comprehensive behavioral support in family ecology: An experimental, single case analysis. *Journal of Consulting and Clinical Psychology, 65*, 241–251.

Luiselli, J. K. (1998). Intervention conceptualization and formulation. In J. K. Luiselli & M. J. Cameron (Eds.) *Antecedent control: Innovative approaches to behavioral support* (pp. 29–44). Baltimore: Paul H. Brookes.

Mace, F. C. (1994). The significance and future of functional analysis methodologies. *Journal of Applied Behavior Analysis, 27*, 385–392.

Mace, F. C., & Belfiore, P. (1990). Behavioral momentum in the treatment of escape-motivated stereotypy. *Journal of Applied Behavior Analysis, 23*, 507–514.

Mace, F. C., Kratochwill, T. R., & Fiello, R. A. (1983). Positive treatment of aggressive behavior in a mentally retarded adult: A case study. *Behavior Therapy, 14*, 689–696.

Mace, F. C., McCurdy, B., & Quigley, E. A. (1990). A collateral effect of reward predicted by matching theory. *Journal of Applied Behavior Analysis, 23*, 197–206.

Mace, F. C., Neef, N. A., Shade, D., & Mauro, B. C. (1996). Effects of problem difficulty and reinforcer quality on time allocated to concurrent arithmetic problems. *Journal of Applied Behavior Analysis, 29*, 11–24.

Mace, F. C., & Roberts, M. L. (1993). Factors affecting selection of behavioral interventions. In J. Reichle & D. P. Wacker (Eds.), *Communicative alternatives to challenging behavior: Integrating functional assessment and intervention strategies* (pp. 113–133). Baltimore: Paul H. Brookes.

Machalicek, W., O'Reilly, M. F., Beretvas, N., Sigafoos, J., & Lancioni, G. (2007). A review of interventions to reduce challenging behavior in school settings for students with autism spectrum disorders. *Research in Autism Spectrum, 1*, 229–246.

Marcus, B. A., & Vollmer, T. R. (1996). Combining noncontingent reinforcement and differential reinforcement schedules as treatment for aberrant behavior. *Journal of Applied Behavior Analysis, 29*, 43–51.

Martens, B. K. (1990). A context analysis of contingent teacher attention. *Behavior Modification, 14*, 138–156.

Martens, B. K., Halperin, S., Rummel, J. E., & Kilpatrick, D. (1990). Matching theory applied to contingent teacher attention. *Behavioral Assessment, 12*, 139–156.

Martens, B. K., & Houk, J. L. (1989). The application of Herrnstein's laws of effect to disruptive and on-task behavior of a retarded adolescent girl. *Journal of the Experimental Analysis of Behavior, 51*, 17–27.

Martens, B. K., Lochner, D. G., & Kelly, S. Q. (1992). The effects of variable-interval reinforcement on academic engagement: A demonstration of matching theory. *Journal of Applied Behavior Analysis, 25*, 143–151.

Matson, J. L., & LoVullo, S. V. (2008). A review of behavioral treatments for self-injurious behaviors of persons with autism spectrum disorders. *Behavior Modification, 32*, 61–76.

Matson, J. L., & Nebel-Schwalm, M. S. (2007). Comorbid psychopathology with autism spectrum disorder in children: An overview. *Research in Developmental Disabilities, 28,* 341–352.

Matson, J. L., & Taras, M. E. (1989). A 20 year review of punishment and alternative methods to treat problem behaviors in developmentally delayed persons. *Research in Developmental Disabilities, 10,* 85–104.

Matson, J. L., Wilkins, J., & Macken, J. (2009). The relationship of challenging behaviors to severity and symptoms of autism spectrum disorders. *Journal of Mental Health Research in Intellectual Disabilities, 2,* 29–44.

McClintock, K., Hall, S., & Oliver, C. (2003). Risk markers associated with challenging behaviours in people with intellectual disabilities: A meta-analytic study. *Journal of Intellectual Disability Research, 47,* 405–416.

McDowell, J. J. (1982). The importance of Herrnstein's mathematical statement of the law of effect for behavior therapy. *American Psychologist, 37,* 771–779.

McDowell, J. J. (1986). On the falsifiability of matching theory. *Journal of the Experimental Analysis of Behavior, 45,* 63–74.

McDowell, J. J. (1988). Matching theory in natural human environments. *The Behavior Analyst, 11,* 95–109.

McNally, R. J., Calamari, J. E., Hansen, P. M., & Keliher, C. (1988). Behavioral treatment of psychogenic polydipsia. *Journal of Behavior Therapy and Experimental Psychiatry, 19,* 57–61.

Miltenberger, R. G., Suda, K. T., Lennox, D. B., & Lindeman, D. P. (1991). Assessing the acceptability of behavioral treatments to persons with mental retardation. *American Journal on Mental Retardation, 96,* 291–298.

Mirenda, P. (1997). Functional communication training and augmentative communication: A research review. *Augmentative and Alternative Communication, 13,* 207–225.

Mittenberger, R. G. (1998). Methods for assessing antecedent influences on challenging behaviors. In J. K. Luiselli & M. J. Cameron (Eds.), *Antecedent control procedures for the behavioral support of persons with developmental disabilities* (pp. 47–66). Baltimore: Paul H. Brookes.

Moes, D. R. (1998). Integrating choice-making opportunities within teacher-assigned academic tasks to facilitate the performance of children with autism. *Journal of the Association for Persons with Severe Handicaps, 23,* 319–328.

Myerson, J., & Hale, S. (1984). Practical implication of the matching law. *Journal of Applied Behavior Analysis, 26,* 367–380.

Neef, N. A., & Lutz, M. N. (2001). A brief computer-based assessment of reinforcer dimensions affecting choice. *Journal of Applied Behavior Analysis, 34,* 57–60.

Neef, N. A., Mace, F. C., & Shade, D. (1993). Impulsivity in students with serious emotional disturbance: The interactive effects of reinforcer rate, delay, and quality. *Journal of Applied Behavior Analysis, 26,* 37–52.

Neef, N. A., Mace, F. C., Shea, M. C., & Shade, D. (1992). Effects of reinforcer rate and reinforcer quality on time allocation: Extensions of matching theory to educational settings. *Journal of Applied Behavior Analysis, 2(5),* 691–699.

Neef, N. A., Shade, D., & Miller, M. S. (1994). Assessing influential dimensions of reinforcers on choice in students with serious emotional disturbance. *Journal of Applied Behavior Analysis, 27,* 575–583.

Northup, J., Wacker, D. P., Berg, W. K., Kelly, L., Sasso, G., & DeRaad, A. (1994). The treatment of severe behavior problems in school settings using a technical assistance model. *Journal of Applied Behavior Analysis, 27,* 33–47.

Northup, J., Wacker, D., Sasso, G., Steege, M., Cigrand, K., Cook, J., et al. (1991). A brief functional analysis of aggressive and alternative behavior in an outclinic setting. *Journal of Applied Behavior Analysis, 24,* 509–522.

Nuzzolo-Gomez, R., Leonard, M. A., Ortiz, E., Rivera, C. M., & Greer, R. D. (2002). Teaching children with autism to prefer books or toys over stereotypy or passivity. *Journal of Positive Behavioral Interventions, 4,* 80–87.

O'Neill, R. E., Horner, R. H., Albin, R. W., Sprague, J. R., Storey, K., & Newton, J. S. (1997). *Functional assessment and program development for problem behavior: A practical handbook* (2nd ed.). Pacific Grove, CA: Brooks/Cole Publishing.

O'Neill, R. E., & Sweetland-Baker, M. (2001). Brief report: An assessment of stimulus generalization and contingency effects in functional communication training in two students with autism. *Journal of Autism and Developmental Disorders, 31,* 235–240.

Parrish, J. M., Cataldo, M. F., Kolko, D. J., Neef, N. A., & Egel, A. L. (1986). Experimental analysis of response covariation among compliant and inappropriate behaviors. *Journal of Applied Behavior Analysis, 19,* 241–254.

Peck, J., Sasso, G., & Jolivette, K. (1997). Use of structural analysis hypothesis testing model to improve social interactions via peer-mediated interventions. *Focus on Autism and Other Developmental Disabilities, 12,* 219–230.

Peck, S. M., Wacker, D. P., Berg, W. K., Cooper, L. J., Brown, K. A., Richman, D., et al. (1996). Choice-making treatment of young children's severe behavior problems. *Journal of Applied Behavior Analysis, 29,* 263–290.

Peterson, S. M. P., Caniglia, C., Royster, A. J., Macfarlane, E., Plowman, K., Baird, S. J., et al. (2005). Blending functional communication training and choice making to improve task engagement and decrease problem behaviour. *Educational Psychology, 25,* 257–274.

Petscher, E. S., Rey, C., & Bailey, J. S. (2009). A review of empirical support for differential reinforcement of alternative behavior. *Research in Developmental Disabilities, 30,* 409–425.

Piazza, C. C., Fisher, W. W., Hanley, G. P., Remick, M. L., Contrucci, S. A., & Aitken, T. L. (1997). The use of positive and negative reinforcement in the treatment of escape-maintained destructive behavior. *Journal of Applied Behavior Analysis, 30,* 279–298.

Pierce, W. D., & Epling, W. F. (1983). Choice, matching, and human behavior: A review of the literature. *The Behavior Analyst, 6,* 57–76.

Pierce, W. D., & Epling, W. F. (1995). The applied importance of research on the matching law. *Journal of Applied Behavior Analysis, 28,* 237–241.

Potoczak, K., Carr, J. E., & Michael, J. (2007). The effects of consequence manipulation during functional analysis of problem behavior maintained by negative reinforcement. *Journal of Applied Behavior Analysis, 40,* 719–724.

Ragain, R. D., & Anson, J. E. (1976). The control of self-mutilating behavior with positive reinforcement. *Mental Retardation, 14,* 22–25.

Realon, R. E., Favell, J. E., & Cacace, S. (1995). An economical, humane, and effective method for short-term suppression of hand mouthing. *Behavioral Interventions, 10,* 141–147.

Redmon, W. K., & Lockwood, K. (1986). The matching law and organizational behavior. *Journal of Organizational Behavior Management, 8,* 57–72.

Reeve, C. E., & Carr, E. G. (2000). Prevention of severe behavior problems in children with developmental disorders. *Journal of Positive Behavior Interventions, 2,* 144–160.

Repp, A. C., & Deitz, S. M. (1974). Reducing aggressive and self-injurious behavior of institutionalized retarded children through reinforcement of other behaviors. *Journal of Applied Behavior Analysis, 7,* 313–325.

Reynolds, G. S. (1961). Behavioral contrast. *Journal of the Experimental Analysis of Behavior, 4,* 57–71.

Richman, D. M., Wacker, D. P., & Winborn, L. (2001). Response efficiency during functional communication training: Effects of effort on response allocation. *Journal of Applied Behavior Analysis, 34,* 73–76.

Rojahn, J., Aman, M. G., Matson, J. L., & Mayville, E. A. (2003). The Aberrant Behavior Checklist and the Behavior Problems Inventory: Convergent and divergent validity. *Research in Developmental Disabilities, 24*, 391–404.

Rosales-Ruiz, J., & Baer, D. M. (1997). Behavioral cusps: A developmental and pragmatic concept for behavior analysis. *Journal of Applied Behavior Analysis, 30*, 533–544.

Saunders, R. R., Saunders, M. D., Brewer, A., & Roach, T. (1996). The reduction of self injury in two adolescents with profound retardation by the establishment of a supported routine. *Behavioral Interventions, 11*, 59–86.

Schindler, H. R., & Horner, R. H. (2005). Generalized reduction of problem behavior of young children with autism: Building trans-situational interventions. *American Journal on Mental Retardation, 110*, 36–47.

Shirley, M. J., Iwata, B. A., Kahng, S. W., Mazaleski, J. L., & Lerman, D. C. (1997). Does functional communication training compete with ongoing contingencies of reinforcement? An analysis during response acquisition and maintenance. *Journal of Applied Behavior Analysis, 30*, 93–104.

Shukla, S., & Albin, R. W. (1996). Effects of extinction alone and extinction plus functional communication training on covariation of problem behaviors. *Journal of Applied Behavior Analysis, 29*, 565–568.

Singh, A. N., Matson, J. L., Cooper, C. L., Dixon, D., & Sturmey, P. (2005). The use of risperidone among individuals with mental retardation: Clinically supported or not? *Research in Developmental Disabilities, 26*, 203–218.

Skinner, B. F. (1938). *The behavior of organisms: An experimental analysis.* New York: Appleton-Century-Crofts.

Skinner, B. F. (1953). *Science and human behavior.* New York: Macmillan.

Sturmey, P., Lott, J. D., Laud, R., & Matson, J. L. (2005). Correlates of restraint use in an institutional population: A replication. *Journal of Intellectual Disability Research, 49*, 501–506.

Tarpley, H. D., & Schroeder, S. R. (1979). Comparison of DRO and DRI on rate of suppression of self-injurious behavior. *American Journal of Mental Deficiency, 84*, 188–194.

Taylor, B. A., Hoch, H., & Weissman, M. (2005). The analysis and treatment of vocal stereotypy in a child with autism. *Behavioral Interventions, 20*, 239–253.

Taylor, J. T., Ekdahl, M. M., Romanczyk, R. G., & Miller, M. L. (1994). Escape behavior in task situations: Task versus social antecedents. *Journal of Autism and Developmental Disorders, 24*, 331–344.

Tiger, J. H., Fisher, W. W., & Bouxsein, K. J. (2009). Therapist- and self-monitored DRO contingencies as a treatment for the self-injurious skin picking of a young man with Asperger syndrome. *Journal of Applied Behavior Analysis, 42*, 315–319.

Touchette, P. E., MacDonald, R. F., & Langer, S. N. (1985). A scatter plot for identifying stimulus control of problem behavior. *Journal of Applied Behavior Analysis, 18*, 343–351.

Underwood, L. A., Figueroa, R. G., Thyer, B. A., & Nzeocha, A. (1989). Interruption and DRI in the treatment of self-injurious behavior among mentally retarded and autistic self-restrainers. *Behavior Modification, 13*, 471–481.

Vollmer, T. R., & Bourret, J. (2000). An application of the matching law to evaluate the allocation of two- and three-point shots by college basketball players. *Journal of Applied Behavior Analysis, 33*, 137–150.

Vollmer, T. R., & Iwata, B. A. (1992). Differential reinforcement as treatment for behavior disorders: Procedural and functional variations. *Research in Developmental Disabilities, 13*, 393–417.

Vollmer, T. R., Roane, H. S., Ringdahl, J. E., & Marcus, B. A. (1999). Evaluating treatment challenges with differential reinforcement of alternative behavior. *Journal of Applied Behavior Analysis, 32*, 9–23.

Vukelich, R., & Hake, D. F. (1971). Reduction of dangerously aggressive behavior in a severely retarded resident through a combination of positive reinforcement procedures. *Journal of Applied Behavior Analysis, 4*, 215–225.

Wacker, D. P., Berg, W. K., Harding, J. W., Barretto, A., Rankin, B., & Ganzer, J. (2005). Treatment effectiveness, stimulus generalization, and acceptability to parents of functional communication training. *Educational Psychology, 25*, 233–256.

Wacker, D. P., Berg, W. K., Harding, J. W., & Cooper-Brown, L. J. (2009). Matching treatment to the function of destructive behavior. In P. Reed (Ed.), *Behavioral theories and interventions for autism* (pp. 3–21). New York: Nova Science.

Wacker, D. P., Harding, J., Cooper, L. J., Derby, K. M., Peck, S., Asmus, J., et al. (1996). The effects of meal schedule and quantity on problematic behavior. *Journal of Applied Behavior Analysis, 29*, 79–87.

Wacker, D. P., Steege, M. W., Northup, J., Sasso, G., Berg, W., Reimers, T., et al. (1990). A component analysis of functional communication training across three topographies of severe behavior problems. *Journal of Applied Behavior Analysis, 23*, 417–429.

Weigle, K. L., & Scotti, J. R. (2000). Effects of functional analysis information on ratings of intervention effectiveness and acceptability. *Journal of the Association for Persons with Severe Handicaps, 25*, 217–228.

Worsdell, A. S., Iwata, B. A., Hanley, G. P., Thompson, R. H., & Kahng, S. (2000). Effects of continuous and intermittent reinforcement for problem behavior during functional communication training. *Journal of Applied Behavior Analysis, 33*, 167–179.

Zeilberger, J., Sampen, S. E., & Sloane, H. N. (1968). Modification of a child's problem behaviors in the home with the mother as therapist. *Journal of Applied Behavior Analysis, 1*, 47–53.

Zeiler, M. D. (1971). Eliminating behavior with reinforcement. *Journal of the Experimental Analysis of Behavior, 16*, 401–405.

de Zubicaray, G., & Clair, A. (1998). An evaluation of differential reinforcement of other behavior, differential reinforcement of incompatible behavior, and restitution for time management of aggressive behaviors. *Behavioral Interventions, 13*, 157–168.

Verbal Behavior and Communication Training

23

Thomas S. Higbee and Tyra P. Sellers

Introduction

Communication deficits are a defining characteristic of autism spectrum disorders (ASD) (American Psychiatric Association, 2000). Thus, it is not surprising that improving communication skills is the primary focus of virtually all early intervention programs for children with ASD. Many of the most effective teaching strategies for building language come from the field of applied behavior analysis (ABA) (see Matson, Benavidez, Compton, Paclawskyj, & Baglio, 1996 for a review). ABA-based intervention programs typically use well-established behavior-analytic teaching/intervention techniques such as positive reinforcement, shaping, prompting/prompt fading, chaining, extinction, imitation, modeling, and other behavioral procedures to teach communicative behavior to children with ASD.

Historically, even in behavioral programs, instructional goals and teaching programs have been organized using traditional language categories such as receptive (understanding others' language) and expressive (using language to communicate) language. Traditional terms such as labels, requests, nouns, verbs, and prepositions have been used to describe the types of language being taught. While the choice of terms used to describe and organize instructional programs may seem relatively unimportant, there have been recent calls from within the behavior-analytic community to use a behavior-analytic conceptual/organizational framework (Sundberg & Michael, 2001).

Skinner's Analysis of Verbal Behavior

In his 1957 book, *Verbal Behavior*, B.F. Skinner outlined a behavioral model for understanding and studying language. In contrast to most theories of language which are primarily concerned with the structure, or topography, of language (e.g., syntax, grammar, etc.), Skinner's approach focused on the functional properties of language (i.e., why and under what circumstances it occurs). He proposed that language was learned behavior and, as such, was subject to the same principles of learning that account for other types of behavior, namely, reinforcement and punishment. He defined verbal behavior functionally, as behavior that is reinforced through the mediation of another person (Skinner, 1957). In other words, the consequences that control verbal behavior are provided by people within a person's environment, rather than by the environment directly. For example, a child asking a parent for a cookie and then receiving a cookie would be an instance of verbal behavior because the reinforcer (the cookie) was delivered by another person (the parent). In contrast, if the child picks up the cookie themselves, then this is not verbal behavior, since another person did not mediate the delivery of the reinforcer. This functional definition is not restricted by the form of the response and need not be vocal to be considered verbal. In the example above, a request made by exchanging a picture, making a manual sign, pressing a button on a voice output device, or even by making an unintelligible scream while pointing at the cookie jar would all be instances of verbal behavior because they all occur to produce a consequence that is delivered by another person – the parent gives the cookie. Verbal behavior simply consists of "social interactions between speakers and listeners, whereby speakers gain access to reinforcement and control their environment through the behavior of listeners" (Sundberg, 2007, p. 529).

Rather than categorizing language according to its form (e.g., verbs and nouns), Skinner proposed a classification system organized into functional categories based on

T.S. Higbee (✉)
Department of Special Education and Rehabilitation, Utah State University, Logan, UT 84322-2865, USA
e-mail: tom.higbee@usu.edu

the different environmental conditions that control different types of language. Skinner (1957) outlined several primary categories of language that he termed "elementary verbal operants." Four of these, echoics, mands, tacts, and intraverbals, warrant particular discussion here because of their utility in assessing and teaching language to children with ASD.

Echoics

Skinner (1957) defined echoic behavior as verbal behavior under the control of verbal stimuli where there is "point-to-point" correspondence between the verbal stimulus and verbal response (i.e., the verbal stimulus and response match precisely). For example, a toddler repeating "Mama" in response to her mother saying "Say, Mama" would be considered echoic behavior. Echoic behavior is maintained by what Skinner calls "generalized conditioned reinforcement" in the form of praise or attention from others or other conditioned reinforcers, such as tokens. A well-established echoic repertoire is essential for the development of more complex forms of verbal behavior. Being able to repeat the phonemes and words of others allows the speaker to come in contact with environmental consequences that can maintain the future production of verbal behavior in the absence of verbal models. Acquiring an effective echoic repertoire, sometimes called "generalized imitation," is critical for children with autism and other language delays, as most behavioral teaching procedures rely heavily on the use of echoic prompts (i.e., verbal models) to establish other forms of language.

Mands

Mands are verbal behavior under the control of specific motivational variables (called motivating operations or MOs) and specific behavioral consequences. That is, mands are specific requests made by a speaker that produce desired outcomes. For example, when thirsty, a child may request a glass of water from a parent by saying, "Can I have some water, please?" The reason this mand occurs is because the child is motivated (i.e., "thirsty") and because the parent has provided water when similar requests were made in the past (specific reinforcement). Because mands produce direct reinforcement for the speaker and allow individuals to control their environment by gaining access to desired items/activities and avoiding exposure to aversive items/activities, they are a particularly valuable form of verbal behavior for the speaker. If an individual has not acquired socially appropriate mand forms, then problem behavior may emerge to serve this purpose. That is, if a child has not

learned to verbally request a drink of water, he may throw a temper tantrum near the kitchen sink until a parent delivers water. Thus, it is important to begin mand training as early as possible.

Tacts

Tacts occur when an individual names stimuli (e.g., objects and actions) in his/her environment. They are instances of verbal behavior that are under the antecedent control of specific environmental stimuli. For example, saying "ball" in the presence of a ball or "book" in the presence of a book would be considered tacting. Anything that can be perceived through the senses can be tacted, including events that are not observable by others (e.g., pain). As with the echoic, tacts are maintained by generalized conditioned reinforcement (verbal praise would be one example of this type of reinforcement), which is not directly linked to the object being tacted. That is, a tact is not reinforced by gaining access to the item/event tacted; it is merely the verbal labeling of that event and is reinforced by nonspecific reinforcement (e.g., praise or a smile). Much of human language consists of labeling objects and events in our environment.

Intraverbals

Intraverbals are instances of verbal behavior that occur in response to other instances of verbal behavior. Skinner defined intraverbal behavior as verbal behavior evoked by verbal stimuli where there is no "point-to-point" correspondence between the verbal response and the verbal stimulus that evokes it (Skinner, 1957). In other words, the verbal stimulus and verbal response do not match each other directly. Answering a verbal question, such as "What is your favorite basketball team?" by saying "The Utah Jazz" is intraverbal behavior. Singing songs, describing activities, telling stories, explaining problems, and much academic behavior, such as answering factual questions, are common forms of intraverbal behavior that occur at high rates in typically developing children (Sundberg, 2007). Just like tacts, generalized conditioned reinforcement is what maintains intraverbal responding. In classroom situations, this reinforcement could take the form of teacher praise, points on a classwide reinforcement system, or simply the opportunity to move on to the next problem or activity (Sundberg, 2007). Conversations are largely composed of intraverbal behavior, making a well-developed intraverbal repertoire critically important for maintaining social interactions.

Rationale for Applying Skinner's Analysis of Verbal Behavior

A primary reason for adopting Skinner's model of verbal behavior, rather than traditional linguistic structures, as a programming guide for intervention programs for children with autism is because there is some evidence of functional independence between the different types of verbal operants. That is, if a child is taught to tact a particular object in his environment (e.g., say "water" while pointing to a glass of water), it does not mean that he will necessarily mand for that item (e.g., say "water" to request a drink of water when thirsty) without additional training. This idea was suggested by Skinner (1957) and subsequently demonstrated by multiple researchers across verbal operants including mands and tacts (Hall & Sundberg, 1987; LaMarre & Holland, 1985; Sigafoos, Doss, & Reichle, 1989) and tacts and intraverbals (Miguel, Petursdottir, & Carr, 2005). Recently, however, researchers have determined that this functional independence between operants is not absolute. For example, Petursdottir, Carr, and Michael (2005) demonstrated that following mand training, four out of four participants subsequently used the response forms taught with mand training as tacts. When the procedures were reversed and response forms established as tacts were evaluated to see if participants would use them as mands, the results were more inconclusive than in the first procedure.

Wallace, Iwata, and Hanley (2006) also showed that generalization from tacts to mands is at least partially determined by the reinforcing value of the items being tacted and manded. That is, when individuals were taught to tact high-preference items, they were more likely to subsequently mand for these items without additional training than low-preference items. Kelley, Shillingsburg, Castro, Addison, and LaRue (2007) conducted a study with three children with developmental disabilities as participants where they evaluated the extent to which responses taught as mands generalized to tacts, and vice versa, without additional training. They found that some responses generalized across verbal operants and others did not, both within and across participants, providing partial support for the notion of functional independence. In contrast, Shillingsburg, Kelley, Roane, Kisamore, and Brown (2009) recently demonstrated the functional independence of "yes" and "no" responses across verbal operants. While mastery of "yes" or "no" responses produced generalization to untaught items within verbal operant classes, generalization did not occur across verbal operants, demonstrating functional independence.

A second reason for using Skinner's (1957) model of verbal behavior is because of its potential implications for language assessment (Sundberg & Michael, 2001). Despite recent examples showing that functional independence between verbal operants might not always occur, given the existing evidence, it seems important to ensure that intensive intervention programs for children with autism include assessments and instructional programs that evaluate and teach all of the elementary verbal operants. Thus, communication assessments that survey a child's use of each of the basic verbal operants will likely provide more useful information for individuals working with children with autism than standardized language assessments. By assessing the strength of each of the verbal operants, the instructor would know in which areas to focus educational programming.

A final benefit of utilizing Skinner's (1957) verbal behavior framework is that it helps practitioners understand the importance of early mand training in intensive programs for young children with autism (Sundberg & Michael, 2001). As described previously, the mand is the only one of the basic verbal operants that produces direct, specific reinforcement for the speaker, rather than nonspecific generalized conditioned reinforcement, such as praise. Mands produce a direct benefit to the speaker by allowing him/her to gain access to desired items or activities or terminate exposure to aversive conditions. When children with autism learn to mand, they are then able to control their social environment, at least to a degree. Given the disconnect that is often present between children with autism and the social world, teaching manding may be a way of building an initial bridge across this social chasm and connecting the child with the social world. As will be seen in subsequent sections, mands can also be used to facilitate the acquisition of other forms of verbal behavior. Much of the research on Skinner's (1957) analysis of verbal behavior has focused on mand training. Because of its importance to early language training for children with autism, the research on mand training will be emphasized in this chapter.

In the sections that follow, we will briefly describe general teaching techniques for establishing echoics, mands, tacts, and intraverbals and present some of the recent research on each.

Echoic Training and Research

Verbally imitating words spoken by others is an important prerequisite skill that can facilitate the acquisition of other forms of verbal behavior. Many prompting procedures in intensive behavior intervention programs rely heavily on echoic prompting strategies. Thus, the primary reason to build an echoic repertoire in young children with autism is so that echoic prompts (i.e., verbal models) can be used to establish more complex verbal operants such as mands, tacts, and intraverbals (Sundberg, 2007).

Echoic behavior, called "verbal imitation" in many intensive behavioral programs, is usually taught using differential reinforcement and shaping procedures. The instructor models a specific sound or word (e.g., "Say 'ahhh'") and reinforcement is provided when the child correctly imitates or makes an approximation to the verbal model. Reinforcement is provided contingent upon verbal responses that become closer and closer to the verbal model. The instructor might also exaggerate oral motor movements or use physical prompting of the lips or tongue to produce the desired response. The instructor provides reinforcement for the imitation of more and more complex verbal stimuli until the child can imitate new words and word combinations (sometimes called "generalized verbal imitation"). For children who do not emit a variety of sounds, the instructor may need to begin by reinforcing all vocal behavior for some period of time before differentially reinforcing some response forms over others.

For some children with autism, this type of direct echoic training may be ineffective. Sundberg (2007) described an alternative procedure where a preferred item is used both as a non-verbal prompt and motivational tool to produce echoic behavior. In this procedure, the instructor conducts echoic teaching trials using a preferred item (e.g., a ball) while motivation for that item is high. The instructor shows the preferred item to the child while modeling the verbal response (e.g., "Say ball") and only provides access to it when the child makes a verbal approximation to the modeled response. As Sundberg (2007) points out, to transfer control from the item and motivating operations to the verbal model, the item will need to be faded out over time and replaced with general reinforcement. He suggests that this process may be facilitated by using a picture of the desired item rather than the item itself.

Drash, High, and Tudor (1999) provide an example of a procedure similar to that proposed by Sundberg (2007). In this study, the authors first established a manding repertoire in three children with autism who exhibited no functional language by creating establishing operations for preferred toys or edibles, by withholding the items for a period of time, and then placing them in view but out of reach of the children. The researchers then used verbal prompting and shaping procedures to teach the children to mand for preferred items by vocalizing. Once the children consistently vocalized to produce access to preferred items, echoic trials began in which the instructor provided verbal models of sounds that the children were already making and reinforced the production of these sounds using preferred items whose names shared sounds with those already being produced by the children (e.g., if a child said "bah" then a ball might be delivered as a reinforcer). As the children began imitating more sounds, additional items were introduced, including pictures of items, and reinforcement was

changed from delivery of the item whose name was produced in response to the verbal model to another preferred item or edible. In response to these procedures, all three children rapidly acquired an echoic repertoire.

While several studies have investigated how to establish basic echoic behavior, little research has been conducted to evaluate procedures to expand the complexity of echoics. Recently, Tarbox, Madrid, Aguilar, Jacobo, and Schiff (2009) conducted a study to evaluate such a procedure in children with autism. Their procedure involved breaking longer auditory stimuli (e.g., words) into smaller units (e.g., Monday was broken into two parts, "mun" + "day") and then teaching these units using a chaining procedure. During teaching trials, the instructor modeled the first unit (e.g., "Say 'mun'") and provided reinforcement if the child imitated the verbal model. The second unit (e.g., "Say 'day'") was immediately modeled by the instructor and reinforcement was again provided for correct imitation. Following reinforcement, the instructor immediately modeled the entire word (e.g., "Say 'Monday'") and again provided reinforcement for correct imitation of the target word. This three-component prompting procedure was repeated five times in each experimental session. All three participants acquired the complete echoic response via the chaining procedure and responding generally maintained after the three-component prompting procedure was withdrawn.

Kodak and Clements (2009) investigated the effectiveness of using echoics to facilitate acquisition of mands and tacts when the participant, a 4-year-old child with autism, had failed to acquire mands or tacts when they were taught separately. Initial training procedures consisted of the instructor providing a verbal prompt of "What do you want?" (mand) or "What is it?" (tact) in the presence of a preferred item, followed by an echoic model prompt of the correct word if the child did not respond correctly within 5 s. Correct responding produced reinforcement appropriate to the verbal operant being trained. When the participant failed to acquire mands or tacts following these traditional training procedures, the instructor inserted an echoic training session immediately before subsequent mand or tact training sessions. During the echoic training session, the instructor provided an echoic prompt in the absence of the target item (e.g., "Say 'music'") and provided brief general verbal praise and access to preferred items contingent on correct responding. When echoic training sessions preceded mand- or tact-training sessions, high levels of unprompted manding and tacting were observed.

Young, Krantz, McClahannan, and Poulson (1994) investigated the influence of response topography on generalized echoic responding in four children with autism. Researchers presented the children with models of three different response types: vocal only (no objects or actions), toy play (vocal model + toy and action), and pantomime (vocal model + action without toy). The authors found that while children acquired new echoics via reinforcement procedures, they were more likely to do so following models that were topographically similar to reinforced training models, indicating that echoic responding generalized only within each response type, rather than across response types. This study suggests the importance of training echoics in a variety of ways, with a variety of objects and activities, to produce generalized echoic responding.

Mand Training and Research

As previously mentioned, an effective, socially appropriate manding repertoire allows individuals to effect change on their environment and express their needs and desires. Individuals with ASD often experience deficits in their ability to effectively mand, often resulting in occurrences of problem behavior in an attempt to have their needs met. Mand training is generally addressed as early as possible in an individual's instructional program and is considered a critical repertoire to be developed.

Before mand training occurs, care providers and instructors decide on an appropriate form of manding for the individual based on skill level and learner characteristics (e.g., vocal, sign, an icon, or picture-based system). Mand training initially involves capitalizing on instances where an individual is motivated to access a particular highly preferred item (e.g., when he/she is hungry or thirsty and when he/she has not had access to a preferred item/activity for a period of time). Depending on the skill level of the individual learner, physical prompts, verbal/echoic prompts, visual cues, shaping, and fading may be used to establish independent manding (Sundberg & Partington, 1998).

Mand training often begins by making the desired item visually available to the individual and then providing some indirect verbal prompt (e.g., "What do you want?"). Eventually, the presence of the item is faded and the verbal instruction is removed, if possible, to ensure that motivation to access the item is controlling the mand. While mand training may begin in a structured setting, training and practice opportunities are quickly moved into the natural environment throughout the individual's day. Given the importance of this type of verbal behavior, it is not surprising that much of the research literature on teaching language to individuals with ASD consists of teaching manding.

Early researchers were concerned with increasing the language, particularly manding, of individuals with autism. Two studies in the early and mid-1980s demonstrated the utility of using various prompting, fading, and reinforcement strategies to increase the spontaneous language, in the form of requesting preferred items, of individuals with autism (Carr & Kologinsky, 1983; Charlop, Schreibman, and

Thibodeau, 1985). Carr and Kologinsky focused on teaching children with autism to request desired items using sign language. In that study, the researchers used model prompts, fading, and differential reinforcement (i.e., reinforcing one response class while placing another on extinction) to increase the participants' spontaneous mands for items in the presence of a communication partner. The researchers demonstrated that manding generalized across adults by introducing adults who had never participated in the training sessions. Following initial training procedures, all participants were able to mand using signs with the untrained adults.

In another study, researchers used echoic prompts and a time delay procedure to increase spontaneous vocal manding in young children with autism (Charlop et al., 1985). Time delay prompting involves initially presenting the echoic prompt immediately and then gradually increasing the delay between the instruction (e.g., "What do you want?") or presentation of the item to be manded for, and the echoic prompt. All of the participants in the study increased vocal manding in the presence of desired item and adult. In addition, vocal manding generalized across unfamiliar settings and untrained stimuli.

Given the empirical evidence suggesting that children with autism can learn to mand for desired items, researchers began to explore ways to make the process more efficient. Bourret, Vollmer and Rapp (2004) evaluated an assessment strategy geared toward identifying deficits related to vocal mands for desired items with individuals with autism and intellectual disabilities. The researchers then used the results from the assessment to develop and implement strategies to establish or increase vocal manding.

During the vocal mand assessment, a sequence of prompts was used to assist in determining a specific level of intervention that would likely result in the acquisition of unprompted manding. If the participant engaged in the targeted vocal mand at any point during the trial, he received access to the item for the remainder of the trial. If, however, he did not engage in a vocal mand, the prompt sequence was implemented. The prompt sequence moved from a non-specific, indirect verbal prompt to a full verbal model, to a partial verbal model (e.g., phonemic cue of the initial word sound). The results of the assessments indicated that varied interventions would be appropriate for teaching vocal manding across the three participants. The interventions that were subsequently tested included reinforcing prompted responses, shaping, and shaping plus prompt fading. The interventions resulted in acquisition of unprompted vocal mands for two of the three participants. One participant acquired a vocal mand, but continued to require prompting.

This study demonstrates that conducting a relatively brief assessment (6–11 sessions) could indicate effective strategies, tailored to an individual's particular strengths and deficits, for teaching vocal mands. All participants increased their vocal manding, to some degree, using strategies indicated by the initial assessment. Such an assessment could potentially streamline subsequent intervention procedures, making the teaching process more efficient and eliminating the need for a trial and error approach.

In a study by Pellecchia and Hineline (2007), researchers taught children with autism to mand to adults and then assessed if this skill would generalize to other individuals. Specifically, children were taught to vocally mand, using single words or the mand frame "I want _____," for desired items that were visually present using modeling and differential reinforcement of unprompted mands. Once the children could reliably mand independently with their teachers the researchers tested generalization with parents, siblings, and peers. All of the children demonstrated the ability to mand for preferred items with their parents without any training; however, none of the participants generalized manding to siblings or peers. After specific training with siblings and peers, all participants vocally manded with the targeted people. This research suggests that once individuals learn to successfully mand for items, this skill is likely to generalize to some people, but not to all individuals. To increase the ability to independently and functionally obtain desired items, it may be necessary to program generalization (Stokes & Baer, 1977), for example, by conducting mand training with a variety of individuals with whom a child is likely to interact.

Researchers have also expanded examinations of manding to include mands that are more complex than simply requesting a desired item. Children with autism, many of whom can reliably mand for access to preferred items, often experience deficits in ability to mand for information and social attention. In one such study, experimenters taught children with autism to ask "What's that?" in a variety of contexts (Taylor & Harris, 1995). Initially, children learned to mand for information related to a photograph of an unknown item. All participants acquired the skill and generalized to 3-D objects and to untrained adults in untrained settings. Next, the participants were taught to mand for information about items while on a walk around their school. All participants increased manding for information over baseline levels, manding about both target and untrained, novel items. The results indicate that children with autism can learn to mand for information about unknown items and can generalize this skill to natural settings.

Sundberg, Loeb, Hale and Eigenheer (2002) taught children with autism to mand for information using the words "where" and "who." The procedures involved allowing access to an item, subsequently distracting the child, and then asking the child to get the item. During the distraction time, the item was either placed in a container or given to a person. Children were taught to mand for the location of the item using verbal modeling, fading, and time delay. All of the participants learned to mand, using "where" and "who" across both preferred and non-preferred items. This study demonstrated that children with autism can learn to mand for items that are not visually available using more complex language in the form of questions. Recent replications of this procedure by Endicott and Higbee (2007) and Betz, Higbee, and Pollard (2010) have confirmed the utility of these procedures.

Researchers have also demonstrated that children with autism can learn to vocally mand for adult attention (Krantz & McClahannan, 1998; MacDuff, Ledo, McClahannan, & Krantz, 2007). Krantz and McClahannan used text scripts and fading to teach children with autism to mand for attention using the words "Look" or "Watch me" in the context of independent play. All participants learned to mand for attention and demonstrated this skill across novel activities. In a more recent study, children with autism learned to mand for joint attention from an adult (MacDuff, Ledo et al., 2007). In that investigation, MacDuff and colleagues used small, single button voice recorders, attached to interesting items placed in the hallway of the children's school. The researchers used physical prompting, script fading, and reinforcement to teach the children to vocally mand for joint attention (i.e., stating, "See" while pointing to the item in question and orienting to the adult). All participants demonstrated the ability to vocally mand for joint attention from their adult communication partner in the absence of audio scripts and generalized this skill across untrained settings and items.

While learning to mand for access to desired items, information, and adult attention is an important skill for individuals with autism, many individuals with autism engage in undesirable behaviors (e.g., crying, flopping to the ground, and aggression) in an attempt to have an undesirable item or activity removed. In a study by Yi, Christian, Vittimberga, and Lowenkron (2006), researchers taught children with autism to engage in socially acceptable mands for the removal of non-preferred items, instead of inappropriate behaviors. Two participants were taught to vocally mand, while the third was taught to mand using a sign. Strategies used to teach manding included verbal instruction, modeling the desired response, physical prompts, and time delays. All of the participants learned to appropriately mand for the removal of undesirable items and this skill generalized across untrained stimuli; however, the most aversive untrained items required some mand training. In addition to increasing the use of socially appropriate mands, occurrences of undesirable mands were reduced for all participants. This research suggests that children with autism can learn to affect changes in their environment, in the form of manding for the removal of aversive items, as a functional replacement for engaging in challenging behavior.

Researchers have also investigated teaching children with autism to mand to correct incorrect responses from a communication partner (Yamamoto & Mochizuki, 1988). In that study, participants were taught to mand for specific items. The researches then taught the participants to state "That's not it. Give me _____." when given an incorrect item (e.g., the participant asked for a pencil but the researcher handed over a piece of paper). Teaching procedures included verbal models of the correct response, prompt fading, and reinforcement for correct responding. All participants demonstrated the ability to state "That's not it" and mand again for the desired item when presented with an incorrect item. This skill generalized to an untrained, free play setting and maintained at a 2-month maintenance check. This study demonstrates that children with autism can learn to repair mands in a socially appropriate way when the incorrect item is produced.

Many individual with autism have deficits or a total lack of vocal language. Because of this, researchers have developed and investigated alternative means of communication for individuals with vocal communication deficits. A common strategy used to increase manding with such individuals involves having an individual hand a photo or illustration of the desired item to a communication partner. Charlop-Christy, Carpenter, Le, LeBlanc, and Kellet (2002) investigated the acquisition of the picture exchange communication system (PECS) and the effects on vocal speech, other communicative behavior, and challenging behavior with children with autism. All participants were taught to use the PECS through phases 5 and 6 (creating a sentence strip "I want ____" to mand and "I see ____" to tact). This involved the presentation of a vocal question (e.g., "What do you want?" or "What do you see?") and the use of physical prompting and fading to have the child first hand a picture card, eventually make a sentence strip, and hand it to the communication partner. The communication partner then delivered the item while verbally labeling it. All participants acquired these skills and were able to reliably mand and tact using the PECS sentence strips. In addition, the results indicate that, following PECS training, participants increased imitative and spontaneous speech and mean length of utterances, while occurrences of problem behavior decreased. Overall, this study provides empirical evidence that children with autism can be taught to mand using the PECS and that collateral effects are increased speech and decreased frequencies of challenging behavior.

In 2002, researchers again evaluated the use of PECS with children with autism (Ganz & Simpson, 2004). Children with autism were taught to mand, following the phases outlined in the PECS manual (Frost & Bondy, 2002). All of the participants learned to mand using sentence strips. In addition, the participants demonstrated an overall increase in number of intelligible words spoken, whereas prior to PECS training participants engaged in little to no intelligible vocal language.

In an interesting study by Markel, Neef, and Ferrari (2006), researchers evaluated the use of PECS to teach improvisational manding to children with autism. Researchers taught the participants to mand for items, following the question, "What do you want?" by using either a function, color, or shape related to the desired items. For example, instead of creating a sentence strip that read "I want cookie." the participant might mand by putting "eat" and "circle" together. Teaching procedures followed the PECS teaching format using physical prompts, fading, and access to the desired item. All participants demonstrated zero rates of manding using function, color, or shape in baseline. Following PECS training, all participants increased manding in this form and demonstrated generalization to untrained items.

Recently, Ben Chaabane, Alber-Morgan, and DeBar (2009) replicated and extended the study by Markel and colleagues by having parents train their children using PECS. Both participants learned to mand by requesting the function, color, or shape of the desired item and generalized this skill across untrained items. Taken together, the results of these two investigations indicate that children with autism can learn to problem solve, in the form of manding for items using PECS, when the noun card for the item is not available. Given these results, it is also possible that learning to mand in this more generalized manner could be beneficial when the child does not know the name of the desired item, but can effectively mand for the item by using descriptors.

In addition to teaching children with autism mand using vocal responses, or a PECS response, researchers have evaluated the use of voice output communication aids (VOCA) on manding. VOCA devices come in a variety of sizes and levels of complexity, but all produce some recorded or synthesized speech when the user presses a button. Schepis, Reid, Behrmann, and Sutton (1998) evaluated the use of VOCAs and naturalistic teaching to increase the communication skills of children with autism. The results of that study indicated that all participants increased their ability to mand using a VOCA device. The participants also demonstrated the ability to use the VOCA device to respond to questions and make social comments during a snack activity. In another study, researchers demonstrated that children with autism increased independent manding, using a VOCA, during a 5-min play period (Olive et al., 2007).

Given that both PECS and VOCA devices can be effective in increasing a child with autism's manding for desired items, Son and colleagues compared the two systems (Son, Sigafoos, O'Reilly, & Lancioni, 2006). Researchers taught children how to mand using both types of systems separately. There was a little difference in acquisition rates in learning to proficiently use the different systems. Once the children demonstrated mastery of the individual systems, researchers made both systems concurrently available. In other words, anytime the participants wanted to mand for a desired item, they could choose which communication system to use. Two of the participants chose the picture exchange system more frequently, demonstrating a preference for this mode of communication. The third participant engaged in more selections toward the VOCA device. The results of this investigation suggest that individual preferences might be important when selecting the mode of communication for individuals with autism.

Tact Training and Research

Much of human communication involves tacting objects, actions, concrete and abstract properties of objects and actions, relationships between objects (e.g., prepositions), and even private events (e.g., pain and emotions). Because of this, many intensive behavioral intervention programs focus on building an extensive tact repertoire (Sundberg, 2007). If an individual has a well-developed echoic repertoire, tact training is fairly straightforward. The instructor presents objects, or pictures of objects, along with a verbal instruction (e.g., "What is it?"). If the child responds correctly, praise and additional reinforcement are provided. If the child does not respond or makes an error, the learning trial can be repeated and an echoic prompt added following the verbal question (e.g., While holding a picture of an apple, the instructor says "What is it?" followed immediately by the echoic prompt "apple"). Over time, the echoic prompt can be faded to transfer control of the response to the presence of the visual stimulus and the verbal question rather than the echoic prompt. Differential reinforcement and shaping can also be effective tools in building simple tacts.

For children who fail to readily acquire tacts using basic teaching procedures such as those outlined above, pairing tact learning trials with manding trials may produce positive results. This combined procedure involves ensuring motivating operations are in place for gaining access to a particular item and then providing an echoic prompt to facilitate a mand for the item. Once the child verbally mands for the item and receives brief access to it, a tact trial begins using procedures similar to those outlined above. Mand and tact trials alternate in this fashion to facilitate tacting. Over time, echoic prompts are faded in both mand and tact components and reinforcement changes from direct item access to social praise. Carroll and Hesse (1987) investigated this procedure with typically developing children and documented its superiority to tact-only training conditions.

Arntzen and Almas (2002) conducted a replication of Carroll and Hesse (1987) using both typically developing children and children with developmental disabilities, including autism. In the study, the authors taught five children to tact objects or letters using tact-only training (verbal

instructions + echoic models) and the combined mand–tact procedure in which mand and tact trials alternated. On average, the mand–tact procedure was superior to the tact-only procedure, confirming the findings of Carroll and Hesse (1987).

Partington, Sundberg, Newhouse, and Spengler (1994) investigated a procedure for teaching tacts to a child with autism who had failed to acquire tacts using traditional teaching methods. A unique feature of this study was that the mode of communication was via manual signs, rather than vocal speech. The authors speculated that the verbal instruction used as part of the traditional tact training procedure "What is that?" interfered with the establishment of the tact relation because the participant attended exclusively to the vocal instruction rather than the object to be tacted. When the verbal instruction was replaced with a procedure where the instructor stated the participant's name, pointed to the item to be tacted, instead of providing a verbal instruction, and provided intraverbal (e.g., "Sign _____") or imitative (modeling the correct sign) prompts, the participant readily learned to tact the items using manual signs.

Barbera and Kubina (2005) demonstrated the effectiveness of using procedures to transfer stimulus control from verbal to non-verbal stimuli. Specifically, they used echoic prompts (verbal response under the control of a verbal stimulus) to teach a child with autism to tact (verbal response under the control of a non-verbal stimulus). The teaching procedure began with the presentation of a picture of the object to be tacted. The instructor then engaged in one of two prompting procedures. In the receptive-echoic-tact transfer procedure, the instructor asked the participant to select the item to be tacted from an array of three pictures (e.g., "Touch ball"). If the participant did not touch the correct item, he was prompted to do so. The participant typically echoed the name of the item while touching it in response to the verbal instruction from the instructor. The instructor then stated, "Right. What is it?" and provided an echoic prompt if the participant did not tact the item. When the participant reliably selected the correct item from the array, the instructors began using an echoic-tact transfer procedure where a picture of the object was held up and the instructor provided an echoic prompt (e.g., "Ball"). When the participant echoed the response, the instructor provided the verbal instruction, "Right. What is it?" Praise was provided contingent on correct responding and the instructor rapidly moved back and forth between the different prompting procedures. The participant rapidly acquired multiple tacts using this transfer of stimulus control procedure.

Another example of using one verbal operant repertoire to establish another is described in a study by Sundberg, Endicott, and Eigenheer (2000). In this study, the authors successfully used intraverbal prompts to teach tacting skills to children with autism who had previously failed to acquire the ability to tact. The researchers compared a common, general verbal prompt ("What is that?") with an intraverbal prompt ("Sign _____.") to teach the participants to tact common objects. Both prompts were faded so that simply holding up the item would elicit the tact response. The intraverbal procedure was more effective in establishing tact responses. In other words, participants engaged in fewer errors and reached mastery faster using the intraverbal prompting procedure.

Williams, Carnerero, and Perez-Gonzalez (2006) investigated the impact on generalization of including verbal instructions (e.g., "What is she doing?") while teaching children to tact actions. Each of the six participants in the study could echo phrases and sentences, mand for items, and tact most actions in pictures when given the verbal prompt, "What is he/she doing?"; however, none of the participants tacted actions or events in the absence of the verbal instruction. The authors used a combination of echoic prompts in both the absence and presence of the verbal instruction, in combination with prompt fading procedures, to teach the participants to tact behavior of actors performing actions. Once participants learned to tact the action in the absence of the verbal instruction in the presence of one action, the majority could subsequently tact the action without the verbal instruction in the presence of other modeled actions, demonstrating generalization. This study suggests that it may be important to teach tacting both with and without verbal instructions to promote spontaneous tacting in the absence of verbal instructions in the natural environment.

Intraverbal Training and Research

Intraverbal training is an essential part of increasing an individual with autism's verbal repertoire. Establishing verbal stimulus control over verbal responding can be more difficult than non-verbal stimulus control and some researchers have suggested that it should not be attempted until the learner has well-developed mand, tact, echoic, imitation, and matching-to-sample repertoires (Sundberg & Partington, 1998). Teaching intraverbals too early or that are too complex for a child's developmental level, e.g., "What is your name and phone number?" may be a mistake (Sundberg, 2007).

While advanced intraverbal training can be used to increase complex verbal repertoires and academic skills, early intraverbal training generally focuses on responses that are motivating, and may be very specific to the individual (Sundberg, 2007). For example, if an individual is highly reinforced by a particular song, jingle, rhyme, saying, movie, or book, the training may simply involve establishing responding by filling in a favorite word or line (e.g., the instructor states: "The wheels on the bus go" and the individual responds with "round and round"). Appropriate

approximations may be accepted and shaped in an attempt to begin to establish intraverbal skills. Teaching intraverbal skills can take place in a structured, trial-based format for many learners; however, many highly motivating opportunities are likely to arise in the individual's natural environment, and it may be necessary to take advantage of these during early intraverbal training. In addition, it is often helpful to sabotage naturally occurring activities to create the opportunity to work on intraverbal skills. For example, an adult might give a child a broken colored pencil when coloring a picture and later ask the child "What's the problem with your pencil" to elicit "It's broken."

When teaching intraverbal responses, it may be necessary to begin with an echoic prompt (e.g., a full verbal model of what the individual should say). Early on the echoic prompt should immediately follow the phrase to be filled in or the questions answered. Eventually, a time delay can be inserted to allow for more independent responding. In addition, the echoic prompt can be faded from a full prompt to partial verbal (e.g., a phonemic cue of the initial word sound). Other prompts that can be effective include gestures, such as providing an expectant look, exaggerated facial expressions, shrugged shoulders, or uplifted hand with palms turned up (as if to say "What's next?").

In initial intraverbal training, an item is often present to prompt correct responses. For example, when stating "A cow says" the instructor might also hold up a photo of a cow or a toy cow. Correct intraverbal responses are reinforced with general praise and other tangible items, if required. Eventually, the presence of the item is faded out, so that only the instructor's verbal behavior is controlling the response. For very early learners, access to the actual item is often provided, especially if using items that are highly reinforcing; however, reinforcement is quickly faded to nonspecific reinforcement (e.g., praise, tickles, or a non-related edible) in an attempt to ensure that the response is controlled by the instructor's verbal behavior.

The initial content of intraverbal training involves having the individual fill in the blank for motivating targets or common age-appropriate expressions (e.g., "Ready, set" and the individual fills in "Go!"). Other commonly targeted fill-in-the-blank intraverbals involve commonly heard phrases and animal and object sounds (e.g., "A dog says _____"). Once the ability to respond to the verbal behavior of another person is established and reliably demonstrated, the content levels can progress to classification, features, functions, associations, opposites, and questions ranging in complexity and required abstraction (Sundberg & Partington, 1998).

Children with autism often experience difficulties with the intraverbal behavior of providing contextually appropriate answers to questions. Given that these difficulties are shared by children with other types of communication disorders, and the relatively small number of studies completed on this topic, studies both with and without individuals with autism will be reviewed here.

Watkins, Pack-Teixeira, and Howard (1989) taught children with intellectual disabilities to engage in intraverbal responses when asked to name adjectives or nouns. Children were taught to produce a verbal response following a verbal instruction. The researchers used echoic prompting and positive reinforcement to establish responding. No visual stimuli were presented. In addition to teaching single responses (e.g., naming adjectives or nouns), the participants learned to emit multi-word responses (e.g., adjective + noun). Echoic prompting was effective in teaching all of the children to engage in intraverbal responding. Interestingly, multiple word responses did not occur without specific intraverbal training; however, once several two-word responses were trained, untrained multi-word responses did occur. This early study paved the way for teaching intraverbal skills, as it supported the need for direct intraverbal training and established that echoic prompting was effective at teaching this skill.

In another study by Secan, Egel, and Tilley (1989), researchers taught children with autism to answer why, what, and how questions. Children were taught to answer these questions using pictures and photographs via verbal modeling. Correct responses were reinforced, while incorrect responses resulted in a remedial trial. All participants acquired intraverbal responses for why, what, and how in relation to questions from storybooks and from naturally occurring opportunities (e.g., "How did you get to school today?"). More importantly, these skills generalized to untrained stimuli, with very few requiring brief supplemental training. In addition, these skills remained above baseline levels at maintenance probes ranging from 5- to 68-week post-intervention. The results of this investigation demonstrated that children with autism can learn to respond to direct "wh" questions about stories and pictures, as well as about naturally occurring events.

Partington and Bailey (1993) further demonstrated the need for specific intraverbal training. In this study, several typically developing preschoolers who learned to tact were assessed for intraverbal responding. Despite the fact that these children could tact items, none of them could provide intraverbal responses when presented with a verbal question. The children were taught using visual prompts (e.g., a photograph of the item was presented) and positive reinforcement. Following training, all children engaged in intraverbal responses for item names. Researchers then taught the children to tact items and classes of items (i.e., categories) and assessed if those skills transferred to intraverbal responding. Half of the children increased intraverbal responding following the tact training, but the other half required specific intraverbal training to engage in correct intraverbal responses. These results further indicate that

direct intraverbal training is effective and necessary for some individuals to increase intraverbal repertoires.

In a related study, researchers evaluated if receptive or tact training would transfer to intraverbal skills with typically developing preschool children (Miguel et al., 2005). Children did not engage in verbal responses following a verbal question related to categories (e.g., "What are some [tools/musical instruments]?"), even though they had learned to tact and receptively identify the items. Direct intraverbal training, in the form of visual cues (e.g., showing a photograph of the item) and echoic prompting plus reinforcement, was effective in establishing intraverbal responding for the children. This study further supports the need for specific intraverbal training to produce intraverbal responding.

An intraverbal repertoire is required to carry on a conversation, which is often an area of deficit for children with autism. Charlop and Milstein (1989) used video modeling to teach children with autism to have a conversation about a toy. The conversations consisted of asking and answering questions with an adult communication partner. Participants watched video clips of a conversation and then practiced until each participant was able to independently and accurately complete the modeled conversation. The researchers used corresponding scripted conversations to test generalization across topics (i.e., a conversation about a novel toy). Generalization across people and settings was assessed with untrained partners (peers and adults), including the participants' siblings, outside and in the participants' homes. Finally, the investigators tested generalization to "abstract" conversation topics where the item that was the topic of the conversation was not present.

In Charlop and Milstein (1989), researchers found that all participants mastered the conversations and generalized across topics, settings, and people. All participants also demonstrated some generalization to the abstract conversations. Another noteworthy result is that all participants maintained conversational skills above baseline levels at 15-month maintenance probes. Children with autism can increase their intraverbal repertoires, such that they can engage in conversational exchanges, via video modeling.

Krantz and McClahannan (1993) investigated the effects of printed scripts and script fading on the intraverbal skills of children with autism. While the primary behavior of concern was initiations to peers, the researchers also measured participant responses to their peers. Responses were contextually appropriate vocal responses controlled by the verbal behavior of the communication partner. All participants increased contextually appropriate intraverbal responses well above baseline levels. While not the primary measure in this study, the results indicate that children with autism can learn to increase their conversational intraverbal repertoires in response to their peers' vocal initiations using script-fading procedures.

In another investigation, researchers investigated the effects of text scripts to increase intraverbal conversational skills of children with autism with adult partners (Charlop-Christy & Kelso, 2003). Researchers used printed cue cards with reciprocal responses and questions. The topics did not relate to any items that were physically present. Instead, the scripts addressed abstract topics relating to recently completed activities and preferred leisure activities. The scripts were taught using verbal prompts (e.g., "read it."). The participants in this study all increased their intraverbal skills and generalized to untrained topics and an untrained communication partner in an untrained setting.

The above studies indicate that intraverbal skills can be taught using a variety of strategies (e.g., video modeling, text scripts, and verbal prompting). Investigators have compared instructional methods in an attempt to determine the best method of increasing intraverbal repertoires for children with autism. Finkel and Williams (2001) and Vedora, Meunier, and Mackay (2009) compared textual versus echoic prompts. Both studies taught participants to engage in intraverbal responding, in the form of answering questions. In both studies, the results indicated that participants acquired intraverbal responses faster when taught with text prompts. Additionally, during the text prompt teaching phase, participants engaged in fewer errors, resulting in faster acquisition and more frequent contact with positive reinforcement. These studies suggest that particular teaching methods (e.g., text prompts) may be more effective (i.e., faster acquisition and fewer errors) than other common strategies in teaching intraverbal skills with children with autism.

While intraverbal skills are useful in increasing an individual's verbal repertoire, responding verbally to other's verbal behavior can also be an effective means of teaching other verbal operants. This strategy is exemplified by the previously described study by Sundberg et al. (2000) in which intraverbal prompts were used to establish a tacting repertoire in children with autism who had failed to acquire tacts using other methods.

Summary and Future Directions

Skinner's (1957) analysis of verbal behavior has much to offer practitioners working with individuals with autism. His functional approach to understanding language provides a framework for the assessment and treatment of communication challenges in individuals with autism and related disorders. The evidence reviewed here suggests that it is important to evaluate the status of individual verbal operants in children with autism to ensure that all forms of verbal behavior are adequately addressed by intervention programs. As evidenced by the studies reviewed in this chapter, there is a growing body of research demonstrating the utility of interventions based on Skinner's framework.

While the logic of the approach is firmly based on behavioral theory and there exists a modest body of research providing support for its utility for treatment programs for individuals with autism, more research needs to be completed before definitive statements can be made about the superiority of this approach over others (Carr & Firth, 2005). Specifically, outcome studies on the long-term effectiveness of comprehensive behavioral intervention programs based on Skinner's (1957) analysis are needed. Assuming that these investigations provide additional evidence for the utility of this approach, researchers might then investigate strategies for training practitioners and parents to use this approach with their students and children. Recent studies by Lafasakis and Sturmey (2007) and Seiverling, Pantelides, Ruiz, and Sturmey (2010) on the behavioral skills training (BST) approach provide examples of one method that might be effective for providing this training. Given the positive outcomes demonstrated in the studies reviewed in this chapter, conducting this research appears to be a worthy pursuit.

References

American Psychiatric Association. (2000). *Diagnostic and statistical manual of mental disorders* (4th ed., Text Rev.). Washington, DC: Author.

Arntzen, E., & Almas, I. K. (2002). Effects of mand-tact training versus tact-only training on the acquisition of tacts. *Journal of Applied Behavior Analysis, 35*, 419–422.

Barbera, M.L., & Kubina, R. M. (2005). Using transfer procedures to teach tacts to a child with autism. *The Analysis of Verbal Behavior, 21*, 155–161.

Ben Chaabane, D. B., Alber-Morgan, S. R., & DeBar, R. M. (2009). The effects of parent-implemented PECS training on improvisation of mands by children with autism. *Journal of Applied Behavior Analysis, 42*, 671–677.

Betz, A.M., Higbee, T.S., & Pollard, J. S. (2010). Promoting generalization of mands for information used by young children with autism. *Research in Autism Spectrum Disorders, 4*, 501–508.

Bourret, J., Vollmer, T. R., & Rapp, J. T. (2004). Evaluation of vocal mand assessment and vocal mand training procedures. *Journal of Applied Behavior Analysis, 37*, 129–144.

Carr, E. G., & Kologinsky, E. (1983). Acquisition of sign language by autistic children II: Spontaneity and generalization effects. *Journal of Applied Behavior Analysis, 16*, 297–314.

Carr, J.E., & Firth, A.M. (2005). The verbal behavior approach to early and intensive behavioral intervention for autism: A call for additional empirical support. *Journal of Early and Intensive Behavioral Intervention, 2*, 18–27.

Carroll, R. J., & Hesse, B. E. (1987). The effect of alternating mand and tact training on the acquisition of tacts. *The Analysis of Verbal Behavior, 5*, 55–65.

Charlop-Christy, M. H., Carpenter, M., Le, L., LaBlanc, L. A., & Kellet, K. (2002). Using the picture communication exchange system (PECS) with children with autism: Assessment of PECS acquisition, social-communication behavior, and problem behavior. *Journal of Applied Behavior Analysis, 35*, 213–231.

Charlop-Christy, M. H., & Kelso, S. E. (2003). Teaching children with autism conversational speech using a cue card/written script program. *Education and Treatment of Children, 26*, 108–127.

Charlop, M. H., & Milstein, J. P. (1989). Teaching autistic children conversational speech using video modeling. *Journal of Applied Behavior Analysis, 22*, 275–285.

Charlop, M. H., Schreibman, L., & Thibodeau, M. G. (1985). Increasing spontaneous verbal responding in autistic children using a time delay procedure. *Journal of Applied Behavior Analysis, 18*, 155–166.

Drash, P. W., High, R.L., & Tudor, R. M. (1999). Using mand training to establish an echoic repertoire in young children with autism. *The Analysis of Verbal Behavior, 16*, 29–44.

Endicott, K., & Higbee, T. S. (2007). Contriving establishing operations to teach preschoolers with autism to mand for information. *Research in Autism Spectrum Disorders, 1*, 210–217.

Finkel, A. S., & Williams, R. L. (2001). A comparison of textual and echoic prompts on the acquisition of intraverbal behavior in a six-year-old boy with autism. *The Analysis of Verbal Behavior, 18*, 61–70.

Frost, L., & Bondy, A. (2002). *Picture Exchange Communication System training manual* (2nd ed). Newark, DE: Pyramid Educational Consultants.

Ganz, J. B., & Simpson, R. L. (2004). Effects on Communicative Requesting and Speech Development of the Picture Exchange Communication System in Children with Characteristics of Autism. *Journal of Autism and Developmental Disorders, 34*, 395–409.

Hall, G., & Sundberg, M. L. (1987). Teaching mands by manipulating conditioned establishing operations. *The Analysis of Verbal Behavior, 5*, 41–53.

Kelley, M. E., Shillingsburg, M. A., Castro, M. J., Addison, L. R., & LaRue, R. H. (2007). Further evaluation of emerging speech in children with developmental disabilities: Training verbal behavior. *Journal of Applied Behavior Analysis, 40*, 431–444.

Kodak, T., & Clements, A. (2009). Acquisition of mands and tacts with concurrent echoic training. *Journal of Applied Behavior Analysis, 42*, 839–843.

Krantz, P. J., & McClahannan, L. E. (1993). Teaching children with autism to initiate to peers: Effects of a script-fading procedure. *Journal of Applied Behavior Analysis, 26*, 121–132.

Krantz, P. J., & McClahannan, L. E. (1998). Social interaction skills for children with autism: A script-fading procedure for beginning readers. *Journal of Applied Behavior Analysis, 31*, 191–202.

LaMarre, J., & Holland, J.G. (1985). The functional independence of mands and tacts. *Journal of the Experimental Analysis of Behavior, 43*, 5–19.

Lafasakis, M. & Sturmey, P. (2007). Training parent implementation of discrete-trial teaching: Effects on generalization of parent teaching and child correct responding. *Journal of Applied Behavior Analysis, 40*, 685–689.

MacDuff, J. L., Ledo, R., McClahannan, L.E., & Krantz, P. J. (2007). Using scripts and script-fading procedures to promote bids for joint attention by young children with autism. *Research in Autism Spectrum Disorders, 1*, 281–290.

Markel, J. M., Neef, N. A., & Ferrari, S. J. (2006). A preliminary analysis of teaching improvisation with the picture exchange communication system to children with autism. *Journal of Applied Behavior Analysis, 39*, 109–115.

Matson, J. L., Benavidez, D. A., Compton, L. S., Paclawskyj, T., & Baglio, C. (1996). Behavioral treatment of autistic persons: A review of research from 1980 to the present. *Research in Developmental Disabilities, 17*, 433–465.

Miguel, C. F., Petursdottir, A. I., & Carr, J. E. (2005). The effects of multiple-tact and receptive-discrimination training on the acquisition of intraverbal behavior. *The Analysis of Verbal Behavior, 21*, 27–41.

Olive, M. L., de la Cruz, B., Davis, T. N., Chan, J. M., Lang, R. B., O'Reilly, M. F., & Dickson, S. M. (2007). The effects of enhanced milieu teaching and a voice output communication aid on the requesting of three children with autism. *Journal of Developmental Disorders, 37*, 1505–1513.

Partington, J. W., & Bailey, J. S. (1993). Teaching intraverbal behavior to preschool children. *The Analysis of Verbal Behavior, 11*, 9–18.

Partington, J. W., Sundberg, M. L., Newhouse, L., & Spengler, S. M. (1994). Overcoming an autistic child's failure to acquire a tact repertoire. *Journal of Applied Behavior Analysis, 27*, 733–744.

Pellecchia, M., & Hineline, P. N. (2007). Generalization of mands in children with autism from adults to peers. *The Behavior Analyst Today, 8*, 483–491.

Petursdottir, A. I., Carr, J.E., & Michael, J. (2005). Emergence of mands and tacts of novel objects among preschool children. *The Analysis of Verbal Behavior, 21*, 59–74.

Schepis, M. M., Reid, D. H., Behrmann, M. M., & Sutton, K. A. (1998). Increasing communicative interactions of young children with autism using a voice output communication aid and naturalistic teaching. *Journal of Applied Behavior Analysis, 31*, 561–578.

Secan, K. E., Egel, A. L., & Tilley, C. S. (1989). Acquisition, generalization, and maintenance of question-answering skills in autistic children. *Journal of Applied Behavior Analysis, 22*, 181–196.

Seiverling, L., Pantelides, M., Ruiz, H.H., & Sturmey, P. (2010). The effect of behavioral skills training with general-case training on staff chaining of child vocalizations within natural language paradigm. *Behavioral Interventions, 25*, 53–75.

Shillingsburg, M. A., Kelley, M. E., Roane, H. S., Kisamore, A, & Brown, M. R. (2009). Evaluating and training of yes-no responding across verbal operants. *Journal of Applied Behavior Analysis, 42*, 209–223.

Sigafoos J., Doss S., & Reichle J. (1989). Developing mand and tact repertoires in persons with severe developmental disabilities using graphic symbols. *Research in Developmental Disabilities, 10*, 183–200.

Skinner, B. F. (1957). *Verbal behavior.* Acton, MA: Copley.

Son, S-H., Sigafoos, J., O'Reilly, M., & Lancioni, G. E. (2006). Comparing two types of augmentative and alternative communication systems for children with autism. *Developmental Neurorehabilitation, 9*, 389–395.

Stokes, T. F., & Baer, D. M. (1977). An implicit technology of generalization. *Journal of Applied Behavior Analysis, 10*, 349–367.

Sundberg, M.L. (2007). Verbal behavior. In J.O. Cooper, T.E. Heron, & W.L. Heward, *Applied behavior analysis* (2nd ed, pp. 526–547). Upper Saddle River, NJ: Pearson/Merrill Prentice Hall.

Sundberg, M. L., Endicott, K., & Eigenheer, P. (2000). Using intraverbal prompts to establish tacts for children with autism. *The Analysis of Verbal Behavior, 17*, 89–104.

Sundberg, M. L., Loeb, M., Hale, L., & Eigenheer, P. (2002). Contriving establishing operations to teach mands for information. *The Analysis of Verbal Behavior, 18*, 15–29.

Sundberg, M. L. & Michael, J. (2001). The benefits of Skinner's analysis of verbal behavior for children with autism. *Behavior Modification, 25*, 698–724.

Sundberg, M. L., & Partington, J. W. (1998). *Teaching language to children with autism or other developmental disabilities (7.1).* Pleasant Hill, CA: Behavior Analysts, Inc.

Tarbox, J., Madrid, W., Aguilar, B., Jacobo, W., & Schiff, A. (2009). Use of chaining to increase complexity of echoics in children with autism. *Journal of Applied Behavior Analysis, 42*, 901–906.

Taylor, B. A., & Harris, S. L. (1995). Teaching children with autism to seek information: Acquisition of novel information and generalization of responding. *Journal of Applied Behavior Analysis, 28*, 3–14.

Vedora, J., Meunier, L., & Mackay, H. (2009). Teaching intraverbal behavior to children with autism: A comparison of textual and echoic prompts. *The Analysis of Verbal Behavior, 25*, 79–86.

Wallace, M.D., Iwata, B.A., & Hanley G. P. (2006). Emergence of mands following tact training as a function of reinforcer strength. *Journal of Applied Behavior Analysis, 39*, 17–24.

Watkins, C. L., Pack-Teixeira, L., & Howard, J. S. (1989). Teaching intraverbal behavior to severely retarded children. *The Analysis of Verbal Behavior, 7*, 69–81.

Williams, G., Carnerero, J. J., & Perez-Gonzalez, L. A. (2006). Generalization of tacting actions in children with autism. *Journal of Applied Behavior Analysis, 39*, 233–237.

Yamamoto, J., & Mochizuki, A. (1988). Acquisition and functional analysis of manding with autistic students. *Journal of Applied Behavior Analysis, 21*, 57–64.

Yi, J. I., Christian, L., Vittimberga, G., & Lowenkron, B. (2006). Generalized negatively reinforced manding in children with autism. *The Analysis of Verbal Behavior, 22*, 21–33.

Young, J. M., Krantz, P. J., McClahannan, L. E., & Poulson, C. L. (1994). Generalized imitation and response-class formation in children with autism. *Journal of Applied Behavior Analysis, 27*, 685–697.

Training Children with Autism and Pervasive Developmental Disorders to Comply with Healthcare Procedures: Theory and Research

24

Anthony J. Cuvo

Overview

All children should have scheduled visits to various healthcare providers. The American Academy of Pediatrics recommends 12 scheduled well-child care visits between 3–5 days of age and age 3, and yearly visits thereafter (Mozingo, 2009). General developmental surveillance should occur during these visits, as well as developmental screening, when indicated. The American Academy of Pediatrics (2010) also recommended an immunization schedule for children of age 0 through 6 years. The 2010 schedule includes 25 shots during the first 15 months of life that generally are given during the well care visits.

The American Academy of Pediatric Dentistry (2009) published periodicity dental recommendations for children and youth between 6 months and 12 years of age and older. The academy recommends that all infants receive an oral health risk assessment by 6 months of age and, either at the eruption of the first tooth or no later than 12 months, have a thorough oral exam. The academy also recommends during this age range clinical oral assessments every 6 months, assessment of oral growth and development, radiographic examinations, prophylaxis, and topical fluoride.

In addition to these medical and dental recommendations for routine services, there might be additional visits either for acute (e.g., otitis media) or chronic (e.g., asthma) healthcare conditions, or the need for healthcare services for other purposes. For example, children might be required to obtain a physical exam, as well as vision and hearing screening prior to entering school. Thus, there are numerous scheduled and unplanned encounters for all children with healthcare professionals, many of which involve aversive and sometimes inherently painful conditions.

Along with these routine and unscheduled healthcare visits, children either with developmental delay or suspected of having autism will be subjected to additional procedures. Screening specifically for autism should occur during well-child visits at 18 and 24 months and when parents raise concerns (Johnson & Myers, 2007). A formal audiologic hearing evaluation should occur for children with developmental delay or those being considered for an autism diagnosis (Filipek et al., 1999). Children with pica should also have a lead screen, which requires a blood draw. For the formal evaluation and diagnosis of autism, children should have a physical exam, including an unclothed search for dysmorphic features, neurologic abnormalities, and Wood's lamp examination of the skin (Johnson & Myers, 2007). Genetic, selective metabolic, and other laboratory testing might also be performed when indicated.

The National Survey of Children's Health compared the parent-reported prevalence of health conditions and healthcare use between children with and without autism (Gurney, McPheeters, & Davis, 2006). Findings indicated that children with autism had a greater prevalence of depression- or anxiety-related problems, behavioral or conduct problems, as well as respiratory, food, and skin allergies. Parents also reported a higher mean number of physician visits for preventative, nonemergency, and hospital emergency care over 1 year.

Support for some of these parent reports comes from file data of Medicaid-insured children with autism and pervasive developmental disorders, as well as typically developing peers (McDermott, Zhou, & Mann, 2008). The former had a higher relative rate of emergency or hospital treatment for injury, including that for the head, face, and neck. Children with autism were also more likely to have treatment for poisoning and self-inflicted injury.

Considering the number of scheduled routine medical and dental exams recommended for all children, the additional unplanned healthcare procedures that might arise, the greater prevalence of certain disorders, and the larger number of medical visits for children with autism, there are numerous

A.J. Cuvo (✉)
Center for Autism Spectrum Disorders, Southern Illinois University,
Carbondale, IL 62901, USA
e-mail: acuvo@siu.edu

J.L. Matson, P. Sturmey (eds.), *International Handbook of Autism and Pervasive Developmental Disorders*,
Autism and Child Psychopathology Series, DOI 10.1007/978-1-4419-8065-6_24, © Springer Science+Business Media, LLC 2011

opportunities for these children to experience aversive and possibly painful stimuli that can contribute to healthcare noncompliance.

The context in which health care is delivered can also be problematic for children with autism. Healthcare appointments alter children's typical daily routine, and that might function as a motivating operation (Michael, 2004) that increases the aversiveness of the healthcare context, as well as the likelihood of noncompliant behavior as a result of that heightened aversiveness. Often, children must stay an extended time in a waiting room with strangers in an unfamiliar environment before being called for their appointment. When called to the healthcare provider's office or operatory, the environment typically is unfamiliar or already is a conditioned aversive stimulus. It might have unusual and aversive sensory stimuli (e.g., sounds, odors) and a number of strangers in unfamiliar garb that seek to have close physical contact with the child who might be in some degree of undress. Furthermore, the healthcare providers might deliver painful primary aversive stimuli with unfamiliar equipment, make requests or demands for the child's compliance, and use physical means to achieve compliance if the child is noncompliant. Given the healthcare context cited and the frequency with which the children have healthcare experiences, it is understandable that they might be noncompliant under these conditions.

Compliance in the context of health care should be defined prior to a consideration of why it might not occur. Compliance has two forms. It can involve recipients merely tolerating a provider perform procedures without engaging in escape/avoidance (E/A) or other disruptive behavior that interferes with the implementation and completion of the healthcare activities. The recipient of care is not required to engage in active responding, but merely to allow the provider to emit healthcare behavior involving the recipient. For example, a physician might do auscultation of the body by applying a stethoscope to the child's chest or back or examine the individual's eyes or nose with an otoscope. In these situations, compliance would involve the recipient tolerating the provider performing these procedures without engaging in E/A or other forms of disruptive behavior that interferes with the healthcare procedures.

In addition to tolerance, the compliance response class might also involve active responding by the recipient emitting behavior that allows the provider to perform a healthcare routine. Patients initially might comply by opening their mouth when instructed by a dental hygienist and further comply by tolerating a mouth mirror being inserted in their mouth without engaging in behavior that would disrupt the oral examination. This example illustrates both members of the compliance response class.

Function of Healthcare Noncompliance

There are at least four major classes of functions for noncompliance to healthcare routines. Each of these classes has a number of specific additional functions that should be considered and assessed when possible. Given the typical community context of healthcare provision in which time and behavioral intervention resources are limited, attempts to ascertain the function of noncompliance to healthcare procedures most likely will be either descriptive (e.g., antecedent–behavior–consequence, continuous or narrative recording) or indirect (e.g., questionnaires) (Neef & Peterson, 2007). Nevertheless, given the necessary time, behavioral expertise, and other resources, more formal functional behavioral assessment could be performed.

Performance of each response of a healthcare routine, as well as the responses' antecedents and consequences, can be directly observed and scored. Based on an analysis of these observational data and the use of parent questionnaires, tentative hypotheses could be formed regarding why noncompliance might have occurred for specific steps of the routine. The following classes of factors that might account for healthcare noncompliance could occur either individually or in combination.

Characteristics of Disorder

The defining characteristics of autism could contribute to healthcare encounters being aversive and noncompliance occurring. Children with autism might not comply because of the core features of autism (i.e., impairments in communication and social behavior, restricted repetitive behavior), as well as associated characteristics and comorbid disorders (e.g., intellectual disability, attention deficit–hyperactivity disorder). For example, children with autism might not have the receptive and expressive language that would facilitate compliance. They might lack joint attention with the healthcare provider, be hyper- or hyposensitive to sensory stimuli, be impulsive, and escape or avoid physical contact with strangers, all of which might exacerbate the inherent aversiveness of the healthcare situation. The core characteristics of autism present on a continuum or spectrum of severity and can affect a child's compliance to varying degrees.

Motivation

Another function class that might account for noncompliance to health care is motivational. Motivating operations are environmental or contextual variables that temporarily change the reinforcing or punishing value of a stimulus or event and alter the behavior that has been influenced by that stimulus or event (Michael, 2004). Deprivation is a general form of motivating operation that can alter the context of health care and, as a result, change a child's behavior. Sleep deprivation because of an early morning appointment, for example, might decrease the reinforcing effectiveness of health care (or increase its punishing value) and increase the frequency of E/A behavior. A child's hunger or thirst because of time of day or the extended time required by healthcare procedures might operate in a similar fashion. A change in a child's routine the day of a healthcare procedure, likewise, might function as a motivating operation and increase the frequency of E/A behavior.

Behavioral Deficit

Another major function of noncompliance to healthcare procedures could be a limited behavioral repertoire. Noncompliance can be a function of lack of acquisition of the required behavior. For example, children with autism might not have acquired symbol or letter identity matching required for a vision screening or not be under instructional control when told to breathe deeply. Another learning-based hypothesis is that children might have acquired but no longer maintain a required response (e.g., letter matching at the time of vision screening). Lack of stimulus generalization is another possible learning deficit hypothesis to consider. Children might name letters correctly at home with flashcards, but do not do so at an optometrist's office when examined with visual acuity testing equipment. Lack of response fluency could be another type of learning deficit. A child might have acquired visual discriminations and naming responses, but cannot make the required responses rapidly enough to pass a screening test.

Escape/Avoidance

A child with autism might engage in noncompliant behavior during healthcare routines because the instrumental behavior has been reinforced by its consequences. For example, the noncompliant behavior might result in E/A from the healthcare procedure, which increases the likelihood that the behavior will reoccur under similar stimulus conditions. Noncompliance might also be reinforced by attention or tangible items provided by the parent or healthcare provider.

Learning Theory and Healthcare Compliance

Respondent Conditioning–Response Acquisition

E/A behavior in the healthcare context could be a product of respondent conditioning. For example, assume that pain caused by a vaccine injection is an unconditioned stimulus that elicits an unconditioned response class. The respondent might consist of covert behavior, such as increased heart rate and pulse, as well as adrenaline secretion. There might also be overt behavior of the respondent, such as arm withdrawal and crying. The class might be called "fear" or "anxiety." The healthcare provider who wears a white coat during the injection initially is a neutral stimulus. Because of the conditional or pairing relation between the person in the white coat and the pain caused by the injection, control of the respondent is transferred to the healthcare provider. The person in the white coat then becomes a conditioned stimulus that elicits a conditioned respondent that is similar to the unconditioned respondent. Thus, children might come to engage in respondent behavior when they enter the exam room and see the healthcare provider wearing a white coat. Because of the intensity of the pain caused by an injection, conditioning could occur in very few trials.

A respondent conditioning dental example might begin with a dental drill that produces pain (i.e., unconditioned stimulus) when used to drill a child's tooth. The pain elicits the unconditioned response class of crying, various autonomic responses, and an attempt to escape from the pain-inducing drill. After having a tooth drilled, the sight of the drill and its sounds become conditioned aversive stimuli that elicit conditioned responses similar to those of the unconditioned response class.

Respondent processes might also be used in the intervention for noncompliance with health care. Systematic desensitization traditionally includes a relaxation component to counter-condition the anxiety associated with the healthcare procedure. While relaxed, items from a fear hierarchy (e.g., steps to have an oral exam) are introduced step by step to the person. "If a response inhibitory of anxiety can be made to occur in the presence of anxiety-evoking stimuli it will weaken the bond between these stimuli and the anxiety" (Wolpe & Lazarus, 1966, p. 12). Giving the child access to preferred stimuli during the healthcare procedure might serve a counter-conditioning function similar to relaxation.

Higher-order respondent conditioning. Secondary conditioning, a form of higher-order conditioning, extends control of responding from a conditioned stimulus to other initially neutral stimuli associated with the conditioned stimulus, but not directly associated with the original unconditioned stimulus. In the previous example, stimuli physically associated with the person in the white coat (e.g., exam room, stethoscope, nurse) might become secondary conditioned stimuli and elicit the noncompliant respondent.

Operant conditioning–response acquisition. In the operant conditioning process, responses are reinforced or punished by their consequences. A likely example is the three-term contingency in which a discriminative stimulus signals that punishment will occur as a consequence if a response would be emitted in the presence of the discriminative stimulus. For example, the sight of the healthcare provider might signal that approach behavior by the child would result in aversive consequences. The child, therefore, might avoid entering the room with the healthcare provider and also engage in emotional behavior. The child behaves in a manner to avoid contacting punishment, and that behavior is negatively reinforced.

Under the same discriminative conditions, the child might not only engage in behavior to avoid contacting the aversive healthcare stimuli, but also run to his mother who hugs and comforts him. In this situation, the child's response class is negatively reinforced by avoiding contact with the aversive stimuli, and also may be positively reinforced by receiving attention from his parent. In this situation, the healthcare provider is discriminative for punishment and occasions the avoidance response class. Simultaneously, the mother is a discriminative stimulus for reinforcement and occasions approach because that response is likely to contact reinforcement.

Another operant process is the four-term contingency in which the three-term contingency operates in a particular context (i.e., the fourth term). Contextual variables or motivating operations, as previously described, either increase or decrease the reinforcing effectiveness of some stimuli, objects, or events and, as a result, alter the probability that behaviors reinforced by these stimuli, objects, or events will be emitted (Cooper, Heron, & Heward, 2007). In addition to the three- and four-term operant contingencies, most other operant processes are relevant to teaching healthcare compliance and reducing noncompliance (e.g., effective use of reinforcement, principles and procedures of stimulus control, including its transfer, prompting, shaping, differential reinforcement, extinction, self-management).

Stimulus generalization. After a three-term contingency has been established, the response class is under the stimulus control of the antecedent stimulus and response consequence. The discriminative stimulus, which predicts reinforcing or punishing response consequences, reliably evokes members of the response class. It might be the case that the response class is also evoked by stimuli that are physically similar to the initial discriminative stimulus, despite the lack of a history of reinforcement of the response under these novel antecedent conditions. Stimulus generalization could occur under either the respondent or operant paradigm. An operant example might be that of a child who has acquired E/A behavior in the presence of a specific medical provider who gave the child a physical examination while wearing a white coat. The child might come to emit similar E/A behavior in the presence of novel medical providers wearing white coats where there has been no history of punishing the child's compliant responses (e.g., approach provider). Healthcare providers who wear white coats have become a broad stimulus class that the child comes to avoid.

Respondent–operant interrelationships. Respondent and operant conditioning are distinct as defined by their operations; however, they might contribute to the same response class. Behavior that is acquired by respondent conditioning (e.g., crying, escape from pain-eliciting stimuli) might also be reinforced by its consequences, as previously cited in the medical and dental examples. Thus, the acquisition and maintenance of healthcare noncompliance might be a function of both types of conditioning.

Derived relational responding. Stimulus generalization can account for the spread of responding to stimuli that are physically similar to the discriminative stimulus in whose presence responses have had a history of either reinforcing or behavior-reducing consequences. A stimulus class can develop that includes members incorporated into the class as a result of individuals either directly experiencing the consequences or by stimulus generalization. That stimulus class, however, can be broadened even further by derived relations. Derived relations, as is the case with stimulus generalization, are not directly taught; however, unlike stimulus generalization, derived relations are not based on the physical similarity of stimuli in the class. Instead, they emerge as novel responses based on other types of relations among stimuli that have been learned. "Derived relations can be used to explain how nonspecific, temporal distal, and harmless events can set the occasion for the fearful responses that compose the particulars of fears/anxiety disorders" (Friman, 2007, p. 339).

Stimulus equivalence is a type of derived relation that might explain certain types of healthcare noncompliance. The logic of the stimulus equivalence model is that if A→B and B→C, then A→C. The former two relations are trained, if necessary, and after they are, the A→C relation is derived or emerges without training. All these relations are bidirectional. Most research studies use the match-to-sample procedure to study derived relations. In the match-to-sample procedure, there is a sample stimulus and, typically, several comparison stimuli. In the case of visual stimuli, such as words or pictures, the comparison stimuli might be placed in a horizontal array on a table top or computer screen and positioned a short distance from the sample stimulus. When auditory stimuli (e.g., words) are used, they are spoken. The task requires the learner to select one of the comparison stimuli that matches the sample stimulus in some predetermined fashion. For example, using the match-to-sample procedure, learners would be trained to select the comparison stimulus, picture of doctor (B), in the presence of the sample stimulus, spoken word "doctor" (A). Next, the picture of doctor would be the sample stimulus and the written word "doctor" (C) the comparison stimulus to be selected. After the A–B and B–C relations have been trained, the relationship between the spoken word "doctor" and the written word "doctor" (A–C) could emerge without direct training. The learner

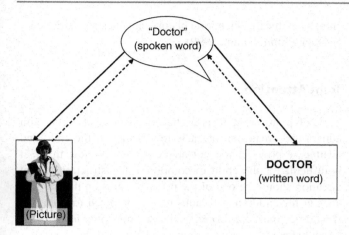

Fig. 24.1 Example of how a derived relation might occur during match-to-sample training. Derived relations are depicted by *dashed arrows* and trained relations by *solid arrows*

would select the written word "doctor" when presented the spoken word "doctor." In addition, the B–A and C–B relations that have not been directly trained should emerge. This example of derived relations is illustrated in Fig. 24.1. The figure shows both the trained and derived relations.

Derived relations can occur naturally in the environment and are not restricted to laboratory demonstrations. Derived relations can have clinical importance, such as accounting for fear of a class of stimuli, such as those in the previous stimulus equivalence illustration (Friman, 2007). Although research has not yet been conducted in this specific area, it is plausible that fearful responses could be emitted to networks of healthcare relations formed in natural environments. Those networks could include relations among actual healthcare providers, equipment in the healthcare context, the room and building where healthcare delivery occurs, thoughts about healthcare stimuli, as well as related pictures, written words, and spoken words. Fearful behavior that originates with an initial aversive encounter with a healthcare provider eventually could come to be emitted, not only in stimulus conditions that are physically similar to the original stimuli, but also under diverse and remote stimulus conditions that are products of derived relations. If a member of each of these classes comes into an equivalence relationship with each other, the result can be a large merged class of fearful stimuli (Friman, 2007). Furthermore, transfer of behavioral function among members of an equivalence class has been demonstrated (Dougher, Auguston, Markham, Greenway, & Wulfert, 1994). Transfer of behavioral function refers to members of an equivalence class taking on behavioral properties of other members of the class. For example, conditioned emotional responses elicited by a stimulus might also occur for other members of the equivalence class.

Although this conceptual analysis explains how fearful and E/A behavior might occur under multiple-stimulus conditions related to health care, there is no research directly

supporting this analysis. Studies, however, have demonstrated the acquisition of derived relations by participants with autism (Rehfeldt, Dillen, Ziomek, & Kowalchuck, 2007; Rehfeldt, Latimore, & Stromer, 2003). Since a verbal naming repertoire is considered important for deriving relations, these unlearned relations might account for the fear and E/A behavior of some individuals with autism who have verbal naming repertoires. Nevertheless, whether individuals with autism actually develop fear and E/A as presented in this conceptual analysis awaits empirical demonstration.

Application of Learning Theory to Train Healthcare Compliance: Pretraining Considerations

Prerequisite Behavior

Requiring participants to have certain prerequisite behaviors is a common inclusion criterion for skill training. This practice enables researchers and clinicians to focus on the target behaviors of interest more immediately because participants already have in their behavioral repertoires responses that are critical for training the target behaviors. In a study that investigated procedures to teach young children with autism to swallow pills, prerequisite skills included following one-step gross motor instructions and four specific basic oral-motor responses (Ghuman, Cataldo, Beck, & Slifer, 2004). Among the inclusion criteria for training children with autism to comply with medical (Cuvo, Reagan, Ackerlund, Huckfeldt, & Kelly, 2010) and dental (Cuvo, Godard, Huckfeldt, & DeMattei, 2010) exams were a demonstrated history of joint attention, as well as following a visual schedule and simple instructions. Joint attention refers to both the healthcare provider and person with autism attending to the same stimulus. In the context of vision screening, for example, the person with autism attends to the Snellen chart when instructed by the vision screener. Training prerequisite skills is not always possible in actual clinical situations, and clinicians must proceed without children having those skills. Unfortunately, that might necessitate the use of more restrictive procedures to ensure compliance.

Healthcare Behavioral History

It is helpful to have the history of a child's behavior in various healthcare contexts. The history should indicate under which stimulus conditions the child was and was not compliant, the challenging behaviors that occurred, and which procedures, if any, might have contributed to obtaining compliance. Was the child generally noncompliant in different healthcare contexts with different providers (e.g., medical office, dental operatory, hospital)? Was the child noncompliant with just certain providers and only under limited conditions? What members of the noncompliant response class were emitted? This behavioral history might help identify the degree of generality of noncompliance and efforts that might facilitate compliance.

Preference and Reinforcement Assessment Choice Making

The use of preferred objects, events, and activities plays a major role in the intervention of noncompliance with healthcare procedures for children with autism. Preferred objects and activities can be made freely available to divert the attention and, perhaps, provide an alternative motor activity for a child who is undergoing aversive healthcare procedures. Also, preferred objects and activities could be used as contingent response reinforcers, if they serve that function. Preference assessment can be conducted by parent interview (Fisher, Piazza, Bowman, & Amari, 1996), as well as by direct testing (DeLeon & Iwata, 1996). For example, multiple-stimulus-without-replacement preference assessment (DeLeon & Iwata, 1996) was used for (a) an 18-year-old boy diagnosed with autism, intellectual disabilities, and type 2 diabetes who was receiving treatment for needle phobia (Shabani & Fisher, 2006), (b) children with autism who were being trained to comply with medical (Cuvo, Reagan et al., 2010) and dental (Cuvo, Godard et al., 2010) exams; and (c) a 15-year-old girl with severe intellectual disabilities and uncontrolled epilepsy who was noncompliant with a ketogenic diet (Amari, Grace, & Fisher, 1995). Stimuli identified by preference assessment procedures subsequently could be tested for their effectiveness as reinforcers (Higbee, Carr, & Harrison, 2000).

In addition to preference assessment, another way that researchers have attempted to ensure that preferred stimuli would be used in training is to allow participants to make choices among alternatives. Allowing a participant with severe intellectual disabilities and uncontrolled epilepsy to make a choice with respect to the sequence with which she ate lower preferred foods, however, was not more effective than consumption of foods in a least to most preferred sequence (Amari et al., 1995).

Aversive Stimulus Assessment

Assessment of stimuli that might be aversive to a child in the healthcare environment could help identify items from which the child might attempt E/A and these items might be controlled. Aversive stimuli might be determined from the child's healthcare behavioral history and questionnaires, e.g., *Sensory Profile* (Dunn, 1999).

Joint Attention

Lack of joint attention is a characteristic of children with autism and creates an obstacle to learning. If the child and healthcare provider are not attending to the same thing, it is difficult for the child to comply with instructions. Joint attention should be one of the primary items on the training agenda for children with autism, and the need to train this should be considered when healthcare noncompliance is the target behavior.

Communication Assessment

All training requires communication with the child in some form, and the healthcare provider should determine how to communicate effectively with the child. The provider should have an understanding of the communication modality (e.g., speech, picture, sign) that is appropriate for the child and the level of the child's receptive and expressive language. A child might benefit from prompts (e.g., picture, gestures) that supplement some other form of communication.

Some Learning Deficit Interventions

Pre-teaching/Education/Priming

Various procedures have been used to provide information to healthcare participants prior to the implementation of intervention procedures. These procedures might involve brief exposure or preview of upcoming healthcare procedures or more substantive instruction of concepts and procedures. Education and training have been part of a number of studies on teaching children with autism and other disabilities to be compliant with healthcare procedures.

Parents, for example, have been educated about their children's disability and trained on how to implement healthcare procedures. A goal of such education and training is to extend responding to the home daily. An example of such intervention is from a study on the treatment of children with developmental disabilities and sleep apnea (Rains, 1995). Parents were educated regarding the symptoms of sleep apnea and its treatment. Additionally, they were trained on how to use and maintain nasal continuous positive airway pressure equipment, and implement behavior management procedures. In another research, typically developing children with asthma received education regarding asthma and its management (DaCosta, Rapoff, Lemanek, & Goldstein,

1997). Education, such as that cited for parents and typically developing children, might be considered for children with high-functioning autism and Asperger's disorder.

Priming refers to a response antecedent condition that is intended to affect responding to subsequent stimuli (Catania, 1998). For example, DVDs that demonstrated the compliant behavior of child undergoing a medical exam (Cuvo, Reagan et al., 2010) and a dental exam (Cuvo, Godard et al., 2010) were shown to children with autism who subsequently underwent those exams. Viewing the DVDs prior to the exams and during training was intended to prime the children's compliant behavior. Parents were asked to observe and rate their children's attention to the videos, as well as the frequency with which they watched the videos. A book with color prints of the behavioral sequence of visiting a dentist was similarly used for priming (Bäckman & Pilebro, 1999). A descriptive study explained a pre-teaching program to prepare children with developmental delay, including autism, for vision screening (Bachman, Bachman, Franzel, & Marcus, 1995). The materials and the sequence of procedures used with the children in advance of their screening were described to them.

Reinforced Practice

Acquisition training programs commonly have a series of discrete training trials in which a neutral stimulus programmed to become a discriminative stimulus is presented, the learner has the opportunity to respond, a response consequence follows, and a brief intertrial interval precedes a repetition of the preceding events. This process has been termed variously as reinforced practice, behavioral rehearsal, discrete trial training, practice trials, and training trials. For example, a series of "practice pills" trials was presented to children who had swallowing difficulties (Ghuman et al., 2004). During a trial, the children were prompted to swallow the pill, drink a preferred beverage, and then differential response consequences were provided. Similar reinforced practice procedures are used for behavior reduction, such as having repetitive trials on fading in aversive stimuli in a fear or desensitization hierarchy (Cuvo, Godard et al., 2010; Cuvo, Reagan et al., 2010).

Prompting and Transfer of Stimulus Control

Children with autism might not have the responses in their behavioral repertoires that are required to comply with a healthcare procedure. Natural discriminative stimuli do not evoke the desired responses, and some form of prompt is used as an artificial discriminative stimulus to occasion the responses. Research has demonstrated the role of various prompts to evoke healthcare compliance by children with autism and other developmental disabilities.

Verbal prompt. Verbal instruction is a basic component of teaching programs and generally has been incorporated in healthcare compliance research, such as studies on pill swallowing (Ghuman et al., 2004), medical exams (Cuvo, Reagan et al., 2010), dental procedures (Bäckman & Pilebro, 1999; Cuvo, Godard et al., 2010), and blood draws (Shabani & Fisher, 2006). Verbal instructions should be simple concrete requests, e.g., "open mouth," "sit" (Bäckman & Pilebro, 1999).

Positional prompt. The position of a stimulus can be manipulated to serve as a prompt for the correct response. For example, in a match-to-sample procedure to teach letter identity matching as part of a vision-screening training program, the neutral comparison stimulus (S+) correlating with reinforcement was positioned closer to the participant than the neutral comparison stimulus (S–) correlating with extinction (Simer & Cuvo, 2009).

Modeling. Modeling target responses has been used as a response prompt to occasion compliance with healthcare procedures. The function of modeling is to demonstrate the compliant responses to be learned. In vivo demonstration has been used to prompt pill swallowing (Ghuman et al., 2004) and compliance with nasal continuous positive airway pressure for children with developmental disabilities and sleep apnea (Rains, 1995). Video modeling has been employed to teach compliance with dental procedures to adults with intellectual disabilities (Conyers et al., 2004; Klepac, Lander, & Godding, 1984). The former study suggested that video modeling was less effective than in vivo desensitization. Video modeling by typically developing peers acting as patients was used to teach compliance to dental exams (Cuvo, Godard et al., 2010; Luscre & Center, 1996).

Visual prompt. Various types of visual prompts have been used as part of training programs for people with autism. These visual stimuli might be either representations of responses to be performed or they might make more salient natural discriminative stimuli. An example of the latter is a poster displaying pills of increasing sizes that were to be swallowed by children with autism who had swallowing difficulties (Ghuman et al., 2004). The poster also presented the objective of training, visual performance feedback, and a visual representation of the reinforcement playroom. In another research, photographic prompts have been used to show responses to be performed during medical (Cuvo, Reagan et al., 2010) and dental (Cuvo, Godard et al., 2010) exams, as well as for tooth brushing (Pilebro & Bäckman, 2005). The latter study also used color cues as prompts for which toothbrush to use for certain teeth (i.e., red for maxillary teeth and blue for mandibular teeth).

Physical prompting. Physical prompts, such as manual gestures, using the hand to shadow a participant's manual response, or full hand-over-hand manual guidance, have been used to occasion responding to healthcare procedures by children with autism and other developmental disabilities. Hand-over-hand manual guidance was used to prompt match-to-sample responding in a letter identity-matching task (Simer & Cuvo, 2009), and a child's hand and arm placement on a board as part of a needle phobia intervention (Shabani & Fisher, 2006).

Transfer of stimulus control. After a response comes under the stimulus control of a prompt, it is necessary to transfer that control from the prompt to the natural discriminative stimulus that eventually will evoke the response. There are several transfer of stimulus control procedures, and they will be illustrated from the literature on training healthcare compliance to children with autism and other developmental disabilities.

Stimulus fading, or gradual stimulus change, has been used to transfer control from training stimuli to the natural stimuli as part of a discrimination learning procedure. Stimulus fading was used in a simultaneous discrimination preparation to teach vision testing procedures to nonverbal children with autism and schizophrenia (Newsom & Simon, 1977). The stimulus-fading procedure involved gradually changing the brightness of the S− card until it was the same brightness as the S+ card. Ultimately, the vertical and horizontal stripes were changed to downward and left pointing Snellen "Es." The discrimination training phase was used to prepare participants to take the visual acuity test, during which cards with progressively smaller "Es" were presented until the size that participants could consistently discriminate was determined.

Stimulus fading was also used to train pill swallowing to children with autism and hyperactivity (Ghuman et al., 2004). Children were trained to swallow cake decorations and then practice capsules, both of progressively increasing sizes, until the children swallowed the criterion pill. Participants were required to make two consecutively successful swallows before the next increasing size practice decoration or pill was faded in.

Prompt fading has also been used in healthcare compliance research. Parents were trained to teach their children with developmental disabilities and sleep apnea to comply with nasal continuous positive airway pressure procedures (Rains, 1995). As the children became more compliant, the parents' assistance was faded and stimulus control was transferred to natural discriminative stimuli.

Discrimination Training

A simultaneous discrimination preparation was used to measure and teach vision screening to nonverbal children with autism and schizophrenia (Newsom & Simon, 1977). The implicit hypothesis was that the participants lacked the skill to meet the vision testing response requirements. A set of stimulus cards was constructed to train the discrimination between a Snellen chart "E" whose prongs pointed down (S+) and an "E" whose prongs pointed left (S−). The S+ training cards had three vertical black stripes that alternated with two white stripes; the height of the white stripes also differed across cards. The final training S+ card, which also served as the first test card, had a downward pointing Snellen "E."

A different set of cards was made to test participants' visual acuity threshold. Pairs of S+ and S− cards were constructed with black Snellen "Es" of the same size but different physical orientation. The S+ cards had "Es" that pointed down, and the "S−" cards had "Es" that pointed to the left.

A more recent study also used discrimination training procedures to teach children with autism to pass the state-required vision screening (Simer & Cuvo, 2009). The test initially required that children match-to-sample comparison flashcards, with the sample letters "H," "O," "T," and "V" presented on a chart. Next, the same four letters were presented on a Good-Lite HOTV Insta-Line instrument. Participants were instructed to point to the comparison letter that matched the blinking sample letter. The discrimination testing procedure was repeated with the participants wearing glasses with either the right or left lens occluded. Participants had a skill deficit with respect to making the required discriminations, and a package of training procedures was used to teach letter identity matching. The procedures for this study are described more fully below.

Reinforcement

Reinforcement of target responses is a standard component in healthcare compliance training programs. Reinforcement might take the form of descriptive praise, tangibles, activities, or other preferred consequences. For example, performance feedback, descriptive verbal praise, and tangible items were used as reinforcers in research on teaching children with autism to be compliant with vision screening (Simer & Cuvo, 2009).

Tokens have been used as reinforcers of target behaviors in a differential reinforcement procedure. Children with developmental disabilities, including autism, who were noncompliant with EEG procedures selected a sticker of their choice and exchanged it at the end of the session for a tangible reinforcer (Slifer, Avis, & Frutchey, 2008). Token reinforcers have also been used with typically developing children who were noncompliant with hemodialysis (Carton & Schweitzer, 1996; Magrab & Papadopoulou, 1977) and neuroimaging (Slifer, Cataldo, Cataldo, Llorente, & Gerson, 1993). In the latter study, edible items served as tokens that could be exchanged for toys as back-up reinforcers. Tokens have also been used as contingent reinforcers for typically developing children with asthma taking their medication (Da Costa et al., 1997). Tokens could also be used as reinforcers for children with autism for whom tokens have been conditioned to function as reinforcers.

The Premack (1962) principle has been applied to reinforce healthcare-related behavior of children with severe disabilities. This principle states that providing the opportunity for a person to engage in a high-probability response contingent on the occurrence of a low-probability response will function as a reinforcer for the latter. This principle was used in training an adolescent with severe intellectual disabilities and uncontrolled epilepsy to comply with a ketogenic diet (Amari et al., 1995). The procedure involved the presentation of more highly preferred foods contingent on the participant eating less preferred food. The former reinforced the consumption of the latter.

Shaping and Teaching Response Sequences

Healthcare routines have been task-analyzed into a sequence of components, and the individual components, in turn, into a series of discrete responses. The responses and components might be required to occur either in a fixed (i.e., chain) or flexible sequence. For example, a physical exam for children with autism was analyzed into a sequence of 10 components, including entering the exam room and complying with the examination of various body organs (Cuvo, Reagan et al., 2010). Task analysis of a dental exam for children with autism has been conducted in a similar manner (Cuvo, Godard et al., 2010; Kohlenberg, Greenberg, Reymore, & Hass, 1972). The task analysis procedure has also been used to teach tooth brushing. Color prints demonstrating the sequence for brushing all teeth and tooth surfaces were placed in the home bathrooms of children with autism (Pilebro & Bäckman, 2005). The 13 pictures in sequence could be used as visual prompts for whole or total task instruction to teach the complete sequence of behaviors to brush teeth.

Shaping responses, which involves reinforcement of successive approximations, has been used when noncompliance to healthcare procedures was attributed to a lack of skill. An example of shaping can be cited from a study training compliance to a medical exam (Cuvo, Reagan et al., 2010). The lung exam required the child to take six deep breaths, while tolerating the stethoscope on the back for 30 s. The breathing requirement was shaped from one, to three, to six deep breaths. For the mouth/throat exam, the participants' behavior was shaped to open the mouth and stick out the tongue for increasing durations (i.e., 1 s, 5 s, 10 s). Shaping has also been used to increase the duration of compliance with respiratory treatment by an 8-year-old boy with autism, intellectual disabilities, and cystic fibrosis (Hagopian & Thompson, 1999). Compliance involved the boy tolerating the respiratory mask being held to his face for a predetermined duration, which gradually increased in 5 s increments, from 5 to 20 s.

Maintaining Behavior

After healthcare compliance has been acquired, it is important for individuals to maintain that behavior. Healthcare appointments might be unpredictable and irregularly spaced over time; therefore, response maintenance can be problematic. A strategy to help maintain behavior is to thin reinforcement from a continuous (CRF) to an intermittent schedule (e.g., fixed ratio). Thinning schedules may also be more efficient for service personnel to administer. In a study to train youth with intellectual disabilities to be compliant with dental procedures, a CRF schedule was used initially, and then it was thinned to an FR2 and finally an FR3 schedule (Kohlenberg et al., 1972). Thinning schedules can be used effectively for persons with autism and for a variety of healthcare procedures. In another study involving children with autism, a delay of reinforcement was introduced during the final four steps of dental desensitization (Luscre & Center, 1996). Behavioral rehearsal or role playing in advance of future appointments could be useful tactics to promote response maintenance. Additionally, video modeling media could be viewed prior to an appointment.

Expanding Stimulus Classes

Training children with autism under natural healthcare stimulus conditions can be disruptive to that environment, as well as time consuming. To mitigate the disruption and time requirements, initial training might occur under noncriterion stimulus conditions, such as in analog or artificial settings, and with research personnel. Efforts should be made to broaden responding to appropriate members of the natural stimulus class, including the criterion physical environments and personnel in those environments. Training, therefore, should include procedures either to teach in criterion contexts after performance goals have been achieved under noncriterion conditions or to promote stimulus generalization to criterion contexts.

In a study to teach children with autism to comply with vision-screening requirements, training was conducted initially by an experimenter in an available school room (Simer & Cuvo, 2009). To expand responding to natural conditions, the experimenter then trained in the school's vision-screening room, and then the school's certified vision screener tested in the same room under the natural conditions. Similarly, compliance with respiratory treatment originally was conducted in a treatment room with research personnel, and then extended to a variety of settings and treatment personnel (Hagopian & Thompson, 1999).

Other studies have trained in contexts that physically simulated the criterion conditions (e.g., analog dental operatory using portable equipment in a university autism center) and tested for stimulus generalization in a member of the natural stimulus class (university dental clinic). If responding to the member of the natural stimulus class was not demonstrated by generalization, training was conducted in that environment (e.g., Cuvo, Godard et al., 2010).

Another approach has been to promote class expansion to natural conditions by parent training. Research personnel initially established stimulus control of pill swallowing by children with autism in a clinic setting, and then parents were taught to administer the procedures to their children at home (Ghuman et al., 2004). In another study, parents were trained at the outset to use nasal continuous positive airway pressure in the treatment of their children with various developmental disabilities who also had obstructive sleep apnea (Rains, 1995).

Escape/Avoidance Hypothesis Interventions

Distracting stimuli. Distracting stimuli have been incorporated in intervention packages when participants emit E/A or other noncompliant behavior. Distracting stimuli typically are discriminative stimuli correlated with reinforcement that compete for attention with the aversive healthcare stimuli. In addition, the goal of the distracting stimulus might be to evoke responses that are incompatible with E/A behavior or otherwise promote compliance. For example, children watched cartoons as a distracter in both a magnetic resonance simulator and actual scanner (Durston et al., 2009). A similar distracting video cartoon procedure was used as part of a behavioral package to control the motion of typically developing children who were undergoing neuroimaging (Slifer et al., 1993). In these examples, a two-choice situation was created. Children allocated their responding to cartoon watching, a reinforcing activity, more so than the aversive scanning procedures.

Children with autism who were being trained to comply with a dental exam had preferred objects available during the initial steps of all desensitization hierarchies when the aversive stimuli were being faded-in (Cuvo, Godard et al., 2010). These objects that participants could see and manipulate served as distracters to the aversive dental stimuli and as noncontingent reinforcers. The preferred objects might also have served to counter-condition the fear of the aversive dental stimuli. Kemp (2005) stated that distraction would be more effective if the person is actively engaged with the distracters (e.g., playing a video game), and the distractors are also used as differential reinforcers (i.e., available during compliance and removed contingent on noncompliance). The examples of watching cartoons as distractors show that active visual engagement can be effective, and incompatible motor responding is not essential. The type of distracter will have to be tailored to the healthcare procedure and the requirements for compliance.

Procedure simulation. Participating in magnetic resonance imaging (MRI) can create anxiety for individuals undergoing the procedure. Research has been conducted to test the efficacy of magnetic resonance simulation in reducing the anxiety of children diagnosed with, autism, attention-deficit/hyperactivity disorder, and typically developing children, who were subsequently tested with actual imagining equipment (Durston et al., 2009). Children were able to lie in the simulator and view cartoons while actual MRI equipment sounds played. Younger and more anxious children had access to a play tunnel that had the same diameter as the MRI scanner. A toy animal with a large head that could accommodate headphones was used in a play MRI simulation. Additionally, virtual simulation with a cartoon of the toy animal was available by Internet at home prior to going to the laboratory. The effectiveness of the procedure simulation in reducing anxiety not only for the simulation but also for the actual MRI was demonstrated. There was no difference among the three participant samples. Other researchers used a similar type of procedure simulation for children who were noncompliant with functional magnetic resonance imaging procedures (Slifer, Koontz, & Cataldo, 2002).

Maintenance task interspersal. Maintenance task interspersal involves intermixing test trials of already acquired responses with those of responses currently in training. Although task interspersal is often used to promote the maintenance of responses that have been learned, when used as an intervention for E/A responses it serves a different function. When E/A behavior occurs and maintenance tasks are interspersed during training trials, these tasks reduce response effort for those trials and increase the probability that participants will contact reinforcement. Maintenance trial interspersal might reduce the aversiveness of training and the motivation for E/A behavior. Maintenance tasks selected from previously mastered Individual Education Program goals were interspersed among training trials on average of every three trials to teach children with autism to comply with the response requirements for vision screening (Simer & Cuvo, 2009). Maintenance tasks were also presented if the final response in a trial block was incorrect.

Behavioral momentum. Behavioral momentum is a construct used to describe the increased compliance to a request that has had a history of noncompliance, when that request is preceded by a series of requests for which there has been a history of high compliance (Mace & Belfiore, 1990). A 22-month-old boy with developmental delay, short-bowel syndrome, and self-injurious behavior engaged in various forms of escape and disruptive behavior during the cleaning of his central-venous line (McComas, Wacker, & Cooper, 1998). Compliance with the request to "hold still" during the cleaning of his central-venous line was increased by preceding this request with a series of three to five high probability of compliance requests.

Reinforcement Variables

Differential reinforcement. Differential reinforcement is a common component in intervention packages described in the healthcare compliance literature. The purpose of differential reinforcement is to limit reinforcement to members of a designated response class and not provide reinforcement for responses that fall outside that class (e.g., E/O and noncompliant behavior). For example, praise and preferred items were provided when a boy with autism, intellectual disabilities, and cystic fibrosis was compliant with respiratory treatment during 1-min intertrial intervals (Hagopian & Thompson, 1999). The trial was terminated and reinforcement not provided contingent on aggression and avoidance behavior. In another study, an adolescent with autism and type 2 diabetes was provided access to preferred food contingent on 10 s of compliance with fading-in a lancet for a blood draw (Shabani & Fisher, 2006). If he did not meet the response requirement, the trial was terminated. In these studies, the consequence for noncompliance was escape from the training trial.

Differential reinforcement was part of a behavioral package to train compliance with a dental exam for children with autism (Cuvo, Godard et al., 2010). If the participants complied with the training requirements for 10 s, they were given descriptive praise. If they did not comply, praise was deferred until a 10-s interval occurred without noncompliance. Differential reinforcement was also used to train compliance with mock neuroimaging procedures for children with and without disabilities (Slifer et al., 1993; Slifer et al., 2002). Slifer et al. (2008) also used differential reinforcement for cooperation, instruction following, and tolerance of the application of EEG leads by children with developmental disabilities, including autism.

Differential Reinforcement of Other Behavior (DRO). DRO has been used as a component in healthcare compliance training programs. Children with autism were given access to preferred stimuli for 30 s after a specified interval terminated during which no problem behavior occurred during medical exam compliance training (Cuvo, Reagan et al., 2010). The generality of the DRO procedure in healthcare research extends to typically developing children who were given a token reinforcer contingent on 30-min without noncompliance with hemodialysis (Carton & Schweitzer, 1996).

Noncontingent reinforcement. Noncontingent reinforcement is a component of a number of behavioral packages for training compliance with healthcare procedures for children with developmental disabilities. This procedure has been implemented by making preferred tangible items and attention by therapists continuously available to participants. For example, noncontingent reinforcement was used to train compliance with wearing prescription glasses (DeLeon et al., 2008). Participants had continuous access to preferred items and attention by therapists. Providing noncontingent reinforcement might be considered when E/A behavior is a function of obtaining reinforcement.

Escape extinction. Escape extinction is a procedure that prevents an operant response that is maintained by negative reinforcement to contact that reinforcement; instead the aversive stimulus continues to occur (Cooper et al., 2007). As a consequence of extinction, the escape response is weakened. Escape extinction, such as blocking escape responses, has been used to prevent escape from healthcare aversive stimuli by children with autism. Examples include blocking (a) removal of glasses (DeLeon et al., 2008; Simer & Cuvo, 2009), (b) EEG equipment (Slifer et al., 2008), (c) medical instruments (Cuvo, Reagan et al., 2010), and (d) dental instruments (Cuvo, Godard et al., 2010).

Time Out

The temporary withdrawal of access to reinforcers has been used to reduce noncompliance with healthcare procedures. Slifer et al. (2008), for example, briefly withdrew reinforcing activities and provided response contingent feedback when children with developmental disabilities were noncompliant with EEG procedures. In another study, attention was withheld for 30 s from individuals with intellectual disabilities and comorbid disorders, including autism, when they attempted to remove eyeglasses (DeLeon et al., 2008.).

Response Cost

Response cost involves the contingent loss of reinforcers that results in behavior reduction (Cooper et al., 2007). Individuals with intellectual disabilities and comorbid disorders, including autism, lost preferred items when they attempted to remove eyeglasses (DeLeon et al., 2008.).

Graduated Exposure/Stimulus Fading/Systematic Desensitization

Gradual exposure to the aversive stimuli is a frequent component of intervention packages to train compliance with healthcare procedures when there is fear, E/A, or other problem behavior. A fear hierarchy is constructed and the stimuli are faded-in over the relevant aversive dimensions (e.g., proximity to participant, stimulus intensity) until compliance occurs. In addition, the participant might engage in relaxation exercises or have access to preferred tangible stimuli or an activity while the gradual stimulus exposure occurs. The function of relaxation and preferred stimuli is to counter-condition the effects of the aversive stimulus that might create fear or anxiety. Gradual exposure to aversive stimuli helps ensure compliant responses that could be reinforced, which could increase the reinforcement density. A dense reinforcement schedule could serve a counter-conditioning function. Also, engagement with preferred objects or activities could provide a source of reinforcement, and individuals might switch their response allocation from E/A behavior to engagement with preferred objects or activities. Desensitization could be conducted either in in vivo, analog, or artificial environments.

Research on training compliance with a medical exam by children with autism included contact desensitization (Cuvo, Reagan et al., 2010). Desensitization or fear hierarchies were created for each organ component of the exam (e.g., lung, heart, abdomen), and aversive stimuli (e.g., stethoscope, otoscope) were faded-in over the steps of the hierarchy. For example, there were 15 steps to train compliance to the lung exam. Over these 15 steps, the physical proximity between the stethoscope and the child was gradually reduced. Then, the stethoscope was applied to the child's back for increasing durations, first with toys present and then without them available. Finally, the number of deep breaths that the child was required to take was progressively increased with the stethoscope on the child's back. Participants also had preferred stimuli to hold, which was intended to serve a counter-conditioning function during the desensitization process. In another medical exam study, in vivo exposure using a graduated hierarchy of assessed fear stimuli was used with children with autism in their school nurse's office (Gillis, Natof, Lockshin, & Romanczyk, 2009). In still other medical studies, the proximity between a lancet and the finger of an adolescent with autism, intellectual disabilities, and type 2 diabetes was gradually faded-in over nine steps (Shabani & Fisher, 2006). Gradual exposure was also used to train compliance with an EEG exam (Slifer et al., 2008).

Children with autism were also trained to be compliant with a dental exam by a similar gradual exposure approach (Cuvo, Godard et al., 2010; Luscre & Center, 1996). In the latter study, desensitization with guided mastery and counter-conditioning with preferred stimuli were used. These "antianxiety stimuli" included music, a hand-held mirror, fruit, songs, and rhymes.

The generality of systematic desensitization procedures to train noncompliance with healthcare procedures by persons with other developmental disabilities has been demonstrated for several decades. This approach has been used to treat noncompliance with dental procedures by persons with intellectual disabilities (Altabet, 2002; Conyers et al., 2004; Klepac et al., 1984; Kohlenberg et al., 1972; Shabani & Fisher, 2006). In the Klepac et al. study, for example, the participant was a 20-year-old man with mild intellectual disabilities. Systematic desensitization was accomplished by videotape modeling of the steps to perform dental restoration and relaxation exercises. Systematic desensitization, including relaxation training, also was used to increase compliance to dental procedures by individuals with severe and profound intellectual disabilities (Altabet, 2002).

Intervention Packages

The procedures previously described have been incorporated in various combinations in intervention packages to train individuals with autism spectrum disorders to be compliant with healthcare procedures. Noncompliance might be attributable either to skill deficits, E/A, or both. An intervention package will be described to illustrate the integration of the behavioral components in a package to promote compliance with vision screening (Simer & Cuvo, 2009).

Teaching Compliance with Vision Screening. The American Academy of Pediatrics recommends vision screening for all children between 3 and 5 years of age, and states have mandated vision screening for all children. Children with autism and other developmental disabilities are often scored "could not test" on their vision screening. If these children cannot be tested successfully in school, they are referred to a vision-care professional. Research on children with autism or developmental delay has been conducted to demonstrate procedures that resulted in successful vision screening (Simer & Cuvo, 2009).

Participants initially were administered a preference assessment to identify items that could be used as response consequences. The natural vision screening administered in school by a certified technician served as the pretest; she also performed the same screening as a posttest. The screening procedures were subjected to a task analysis and the experimenter administered a pre-assessment based on the task analysis.

Discrimination training involved a series of shaping steps, including picture identity matching, picture identity matching with one eye occluded, and finally letter identity matching. Discrimination training included match-to-sample discrete trial training, prompting, transfer of stimulus control procedures, differential reinforcement, and choice making of preferred stimuli.

Participants also engaged in E/A behavior by attempting to prevent wearing or removing the glasses. Intervention procedures included gradually fading in the duration of wearing glasses, escape extinction, escape as a reinforcer, interspersing maintenance tasks with training trials, and reinforcement of alternative behavior. The research also included procedures to expand responding from experimental to natural testing conditions. Participants were successfully screened for vision, and their compliance generalized to the hearing screening for which they also had been scored "could not test."

Recommendations

Kemp (2005) reviewed the literature on nonpharmacologic approaches to increasing the cooperation of persons with special needs to aversive dental procedures, and he drew conclusions regarding characteristics of effective treatments. The current review supports his conclusions and extends them to aversive healthcare procedures more broadly for individuals with autism and pervasive developmental disorders.

First, an attempt should be made to determine the stimulus conditions under which healthcare noncompliance occurs. Is it limited to specific procedures that occur in certain settings, with only one or two healthcare providers, during restricted times of day, when specific alternative activities have to be foregone to attend healthcare, and so forth, or does noncompliance generally occur across all nonhealthcare conditions?

Next, each required healthcare response should be considered to determine whether noncompliance is a function of a skill deficit or environmental contingencies. Is the required response not emitted because there is a lack of response acquisition, maintenance, stimulus generalization, or fluency, and should a program to enhance the individuals' behavioral repertoire be initiated? Or, on the other hand, does the required behavior in the person's repertoire, but aversive stimuli elicit or evoke noncompliance? Is noncompliance reinforced by its consequences?

In the absence of demonstrations that single-component interventions alone are effective in achieving successful outcomes, evidence supports the use of multi-component treatment packages. Those treatment packages could include components to teach behavioral goals, as well as reduce noncompliant behavioral goals. Regardless of the specific goals, intervention packages should include components to ensure joint attention, effective communication, identification of reinforcers, use of them effectively, and repeated training trials.

When teaching behavior, the package components should be based on the general type of learning required (e.g., acquisition, maintenance). The package's components must be tailored further for the specific kind of learning (e.g., visual discrimination training, shaping a motor skill). All packages should include the use of appropriate prompting and transfer of stimulus control procedures. When behavior reduction is the goal of intervention, evidence supports the use of fading in aversive stimuli, availability of distracting reinforcing stimuli, differential reinforcement procedures, and additional behavior reduction procedures (e.g., escape extinction, time out from reinforcement, response cost).

Consideration should be given to programming for stimulus generalization, as necessary, and response maintenance. Training individuals with autism and pervasive developmental disabilities to be compliant under criterion conditions might not be feasible. The in vivo conditions might be highly aversive, training might require considerable time, and the natural healthcare facilities may not be available for an extended time to conduct training. Initial training in analog or artificial conditions that researchers or clinicians can control may be necessary. If this is the case, it is necessary to program to extend performance to the criterion conditions. This could involve programming for stimulus generalization as well as some training in the criterion environment. Response maintenance might be problematic because the healthcare visits are spaced over time and might be unpredictable with acute problems. Role play could be practiced at home with parents and video modeling media could be watched in an effort to maintain responding.

Given the frequency of healthcare opportunities, the inherent aversiveness of many of them, and the core characteristics of autism, it is not surprising that individuals with autism and pervasive developmental disabilities might be noncompliant with these procedures. There is relatively little research on this topic and efforts should be made to extend this line of study. Research should investigate compliance with the broader spectrum of health care and work on translating the existing research so that healthcare personnel could implement procedures in their environments with behavioral consultation. For example, intervention procedures could be manualized, and dental hygienists might be able to use the manual to implement desensitization and additional intervention procedures similar to those described. Likewise, with a manual and behavioral consultation school personnel might be able to implement vision and hearing screening procedures for children who have been scored "could not test." Given the increasing prevalence of autism in recent years and the importance of health care, there will be a greater need for evidence-based interventions for healthcare compliance by this population.

References

Altabet, S. (2002). Decreasing dental resistance among individuals with severe and profound mental retardation. *Journal of Developmental and Physical Disabilities, 14,* 297–305.

Amari, A., Grace, N. C., & Fisher, W. W. (1995). Achieving and maintaining compliance with the ketogenic diet. *Journal of Applied Behavior Analysis, 28,* 341–342.

American Academy of Pediatric Dentistry. (2009). *Guideline on periodicity of examination, preventative dental services, anticipatory guidance/counseling, and oral treatment for infants, children, and adolescents.* Retrieved from http://www.aapd.org/media/Policies_Guidelines/G_Periodicity.pdf

American Academy of Pediatrics. (2010). *Recommended immunization schedule for persons aged 0 through 6 years – United States 2010.* Retried from http://aapredbook.aappublications.org/resources/IZSchedule0-6yrs.pdf

Bachman, J. A., Bachman, W. G., Franzel, A. S., & Marcus, M. C. (1995). An easy-to-use preteaching program to assist vision screening for developmentally delayed preschoolers. *Journal of School Health, 65,* 71–72.

Bäckman, B., & Pilebro, O. C. (1999). Visual pedagogy in dentistry for children with autism. *Journal of Dentistry for Children, 14,* 325–331.

Carton, J. S., & Schweitzer, J. B. (1996). Use of token economy to increase compliance during hemodialysis. *Journal of Applied Behavior Analysis, 29,* 111–113.

Catania, A. C. (1998). *Learning* (4th ed.). Upper Saddle River, NJ: Prentice Hall.

Conyers, C., Miltenberger, R. G., Peterson, B., Gubin, A., Jurgens, M., Selders, A., et al. (2004). An evaluation of in vivo desensitization and video modeling to increase compliance with dental procedures in persons with mental retardation. *Journal of Applied Behavior Analysis, 37,* 233–238.

J. O. Cooper, T. E. Heron, W. A. Heward (Eds.). (2007). *Applied behavior analysis* (2nd ed.). Upper Saddle River, NJ: Pearson.

Cuvo, A. J., Godard, A., Huckfeldt, R., & DeMattei, R. (2010). Training children with autism spectrum disorders to be compliant with an oral assessment. *Research in Autism Spectrum Disorders, 4,* 681–696.

Cuvo, A. J., Reagan, A. L., Ackerlund, J., Huckfeldt, R., & Kelly, C. (2010). Training children with autism spectrum disorders to be compliant with a physical exam. *Research in Autism Spectrum Disorders, 4,* 168–185.

Da Costa, I. G., Rapoff, M. A., Lemanek, K., & Goldstein, G. L. (1997). Improving adherence to medication regimens for children with asthma and its effect on clinical outcome. *Journal of Applied Behavior Analysis, 30,* 687–691.

DeLeon, I. G., Hagopian, L. P., Rodriguez-Catter, V., Bowman, L. G., Long, E. S., & Boelter, E. W. (2008). Increasing wearing of prescription glasses in individuals with mental retardation. *Journal of Applied Behavior Analysis, 41,* 137–142.

DeLeon, I. G., & Iwata, B. A. (1996). Evaluation of a multiple-stimulus presentation format for assessing reinforcers preferences. *Journal of Applied Behavior Analysis, 29,* 519–533.

Dougher, M. J., Auguston, E., Markham, M. R., Greenway, D. E., & Wulfert, E. (1994). The transfer of respondent eliciting and extinction functions through stimulus equivalence classes. *Journal of Experimental Analysis of Behavior, 62,* 331–351.

Dunn, W. (1999). *The sensory profile.* San Antonio, TX: The Psychological Corporation.

Durston, S., Nederveen, H., van Dijk, S., van Dijk, B., de Zeeuw, P., Langen, M., et al. (2009). Magnetic resonance stimulation is effective in reducing anxiety related to magnetic resonance scanning in children. *Journal of the American Academy of Child and Adolescent Psychiatry, 48,* 206–207.

Filipek, P. A., Accardo, P. J., Baranek, G. T., Cook, E. H., Dawson, G., Gordon, B., et al. (1999). The screening and diagnosis of autistic spectrum disorders. *Journal of Autism and Developmental Disorders, 29,* 439–484.

Fisher, W., Piazza, C. C., Bowman, L. G., & Amari, A. (1996). Integrating caregiver report with a systematic stimulus preference assessment. *American Journal on Mental Retardation, 101,* 15–25.

Friman, P. C. (2007). The fear factor: A functional perspective on anxiety. In P. Sturmey (Ed.), *Functional analysis in clinical treatment* (pp. 335–355). Boston: Elsevier.

Ghuman, J. K., Cataldo, M. D., Beck, M. H., & Slifer, K. J. (2004). Behavioral training for pill-swallowing difficulties in young children with autistic disorder. *Journal of Child and Adolescent Psychopharmacology, 14,* 601–611.

Gillis, J. M., Natof, T. H., Lockshin, S. B., & Romanczyk, R. G. (2009). Fear of routine physical exams in children with autism spectrum disorders. *Focus on Autism and Other Developmental Disabilities, 24,* 156–168.

Gurney, J. G., McPheeters, M. L., & Davis, M. M. (2006). Parental report of health conditions and health care use among children with and without autism. *Archives of Pediatric and Adolescent Medicine, 160,* 826–830.

Hagopian, L. P., & Thompson, R. H. (1999). Reinforcement of compliance with respiratory treatment in a child with cystic fibrosis. *Journal of Applied Behavior Analysis, 32,* 233–236.

Higbee, T. S., Carr, J. E., & Harrison, C. D. (2000). Further evaluation of the multiple-stimulus preference assessment. *Research in Developmental Disabilities, 21,* 61–73.

Johnson, C. P., & Myers, S. M. (2007). Identification and evaluation of children with autism spectrum disorders. *Pediatrics, 120,* 1183–1215.

Kemp, F. (2005). Alternatives: A review of non-pharmacologic approaches to increasing the cooperation of patients with special needs to inherently unpleasant dental procedures. *The Behavior Analyst Today, 6,* 88–108.

Klepac, R. K., Lander, E. M., & Godding, P. R. (1984). Brief behavioral treatment for dental avoidance in a mentally handicapped adult. *Journal of the American Dental Association, 108,* 985–987.

Kohlenberg, R., Greenberg, D., Reymore, L., & Hass, G. (1972). Behavior modification and the management of mentally retarded dental patients. *Journal of Dentistry for Children, 39,* 61–67.

Luscre, D., & Center, D. (1996). Procedures for reducing dental fear in children with autism. *Journal of Autism and Developmental Disorders, 26,* 547–556.

Mace, F. C., & Belfiore, P. (1990). Behavioral momentum in the treatment of escape-motivated stereotypy. *Journal of Applied Behavior Analysis, 23,* 507–514.

Magrab, P. R., & Papadopoulou, Z. L. (1977). The effect of a token economy on dietary compliance for children on hemodialysis. *Journal of Applied Behavior Analysis, 10,* 573–578.

McComas, J. J., Wacker, D. P., & Cooper, L. J. (1998). Increasing compliance with medical procedures: Application of the high-probability request procedure to a toddler. *Journal of Applied Behavior Analysis, 31,* 287–290.

McDermott, S., Zhou, L., & Mann, J. (2008). Injury treatment among children with autism or pervasive developmental disorder. *Journal of Autism and Developmental Disorders, 38,* 626–633.

Michael, J. (2004). *Concepts and principles of behavior analysis* (rev. ed.). Kalamazoo, MI: Society for the Advancement of Behavior Analysis.

Mozingo, T. A. (2009). Well-child care-a check-up for success. *Healthy Children, Summer/Back to school,* 17–19.

Neef, N. A., & Peterson, S. M. (2007). Functional behavior assessment. In J. O. Cooper, T. E. Heron, & W. L. Heward (Eds.), *Applied behavior analysis* (2nd ed., pp. 500–524). Upper Saddle River, NJ: Pearson.

Newsom, C. D., & Simon, K. M. (1977). A simultaneous discrimination procedure for the measurement of vision in nonverbal children. *Journal of Applied Behavior Analysis, 10*, 633–644.

Pilebro, C., & Bäckman, B. (2005). Teaching oral hygiene to children with autism. *International Journal of Pediatric Dentistry, 15*, 1–9.

Premack, D. (1962). Reversibility of the reinforcement relation. *Science, 136*, 235–237.

Rains, J. C. (1995). Treatment of obstructive sleep apnea in pediatric patients: Behavioral intervention for compliance with nasal continuous positive airway pressure. *Clinical Pediatrics, 34*, 535–541.

Rehfeldt, R. A., Dillen, J. E., Ziomek, M. M., & Kowalchuck, R. (2007). Assessing relational learning deficits in perspective-taking in children with high-functioning autism spectrum disorder. *The Psychological Record, 57*, 23–47.

Rehfeldt, R. A., Latimore, D., & Stromer, R. (2003). Observational learning and the formation of classes of reading skills by individuals with autism and other developmental disabilities. *Research in Developmental Disabilities, 24*, 333–358.

Shabani, D. B., & Fisher, W. W. (2006). Stimulus fading and differential reinforcement for the treatment of needle phobia in a youth with autism. *Journal of Applied Behavior Analysis, 39*, 449–452.

Simer, N., & Cuvo, A. J. (2009). Training vision screening behavior to children with developmental disabilities. *Research in Autism Spectrum Disorders, 3*, 409–420.

Slifer, K. J., Avis, K. T., & Frutchey, R. A. (2008). Behavioral intervention to increase compliance with electroencephalographic procedures in children with developmental disabilities. *Epilepsy & Behavior, 13*, 189–195.

Slifer, K. J., Cataldo, M. F., Cataldo, M. D., Llorente, A. M., & Gerson, A. C. (1993). Behavior analysis of motion control for pediatric neuroimaging. *Journal of Applied Behavior Analysis, 26*, 469–470.

Slifer, K. J., Koontz, K. L., & Cataldo, M. F. (2002). Operant-contingency-based preparation of children for functional magnetic resonance imaging. *Journal of Applied Behavior Analysis, 35*, 191–194.

Wolpe., J. A., & Lazarus, A. A. (1966). *Behavior therapy techniques.* New York: Pergamum.

Kerri L. Staples, Greg Reid, Kyle Pushkarenko, and Susan Crawford

Intervention Strategies to Promote the Acquisition of Movement Skills

Participation in regular physical activity throughout childhood is essential for healthy growth and development of musculoskeletal tissues (i.e., bones, muscles, and joints), cardiovascular fitness, strength, and flexibility (Health Canada, 2009). In addition to the control and maintenance of body weight, regular physical activity also plays a preventative role in many chronic diseases, including cancer, heart disease and stroke, osteoporosis, and type 2 diabetes (Public Health Agency of Canada, 2010). Active living is a philosophy that places specific emphasis on empowering individuals to lead active and healthy lifestyles by gaining the requisite movement skills and knowledge needed to achieve health benefits from physical activity. The Canadian Society for Exercise Physiology (2003) supports this emphasis by highlighting the health benefits associated with maintaining an active lifestyle throughout the life span.

In order to achieve meaningful health benefits, the World Health Organization (2003) recommended that children and youth engage in a minimum target of 60 min of moderate to vigorous physical activity per day. Health Canada (2009) extended these recommendations by stating that children and youth should engage in at least 90 min of physical activity or 16,500 steps per day. A physically active lifestyle that meets and/or exceeds these recommendations is important for all children, including those with autism spectrum disorders (ASD). Yet, in 2007, an overwhelming 87% of Canadian children and adolescents aged 5–19 years did not achieve these recommendations. Based on the report card released by Active Healthy Kids Canada (2010), 88% of Canadian children and adolescents are still not meeting Canada's most recent guidelines (Canadian Fitness and Lifestyle Research Institute, 2008).

Active living, however, is more than just meeting recommended guidelines for frequency and intensity of exercise. Active living is about incorporating meaningful and enjoyable physical activity as an integral part of daily life (Seidl, 2003). Given that children and adolescents spend a significant portion of each day attending school, school is an obvious place for providing opportunities for acquisition of movement skills and promoting positive physical activity experiences. Patterns of physical activity that are acquired during childhood and adolescence are more likely to be maintained throughout the life span (World Health Organization, 2003), underscoring the importance of developing requisite movement skills and adopting an active lifestyle early. The foundations of fundamental movement skills are laid early in childhood; these skills are essential to successful participation in later physical activity pursuits contributing to an active lifestyle. However, many children with ASD have not mastered many of the requisite skills to successfully engage in physical activity (Pan, Tsai, & Chu, 2009; Staples & Reid, 2010), and parent reports suggest that physical activity participation among children and adolescents with ASD (aged 4–21 years) decreases with age (Rosser-Sandt & Frey, 2005). These findings demonstrate the importance of maximizing participation at school (World Health Organization, 2008) by providing positive experiences and learning opportunities for young children with ASD to develop the movement skills, knowledge, and confidence necessary for lifelong participation.

This chapter will begin with a brief overview of research examining movement behavior among children and adolescents with ASD, focusing on the movement skills that span play, recreation, and physical education. Current education-based interventions and instructional strategies that have been used to facilitate the acquisition and performance of these movement skills will be discussed.

K.L. Staples (✉)
Faculty of Kinesiology and Health Studies, University of Regina, Regina, SK, Canada S4S 0A2
e-mail: kerri.staples@uregina.ca

Movement Behavior

Motor delays and movement skill differences are recognized as deficit areas for many children and adolescents with ASD when compared to their typically developing peers, and these differences seemingly become more obvious with increasing age (for review, see Baranek, 2002; National Research Council, 2001). The availability of accurate information on the early development of movement skills among young children with ASD is limited, in part because until recently ASD was not diagnosed until pre-school age and few systematic investigations have examined the performance of movement skills among children with ASD. However, research suggests that many infants and children with ASD demonstrate delays in motor development and others show irregularity in terms of their developmental progressions (Provost, Lopez, & Heimerl, 2007; Teitelbaum, Teitelbaum, Nye, Fryman, & Maurer, 1998). Although our understanding of how movement skills develop is still very limited, it is this understanding that will advance instruction and facilitate the development of appropriate intervention programs that are directed toward improvement of these skills.

Early Motor Development

Early development has been examined by looking retrospectively at videotapes of babies who were later diagnosed with ASD (Baranek, 1999; Teitelbaum et al., 1998). Based on these videos and parental recollection, some infants with ASD were delayed in the attainment of motor milestones at 6 months of age and continued to show irregularity with respect to the order and timing of their developmental progressions (Ornitz, Guthrie, & Farley, 1977; Teitelbaum et al., 1998). For example, Ornitz et al. (1977) reported that sometimes there were short time periods (spurts) between the attainment of successive milestones and other times there were long delays. Consistent delays were also found when young children with ASD (aged 21–41 months) were assessed on the *Bayley Scales of Infant Development* (Bayley, 1993) and *Peabody Developmental Motor Scales* (Folio & Fewell, 2000), with all young children with ASD demonstrating delays in at least one area of motor development (Provost et al., 2007).

The recalled age of independent walking has been more equivocal, where one study reported that majority of children with ASD began walking within typical ranges (Mayes & Calhoun, 2003) and another reported that approximately 50% were slow to walk (Manjiviona & Prior, 1995). Lösche (1990) suggested that differences in movement become increasingly apparent following the ability to walk and increased opportunities to explore, when many young children with ASD become insistent on practicing and repeating well-known movements instead of learning to search and explore their environments with the purpose of developing new skills.

In addition to delays in the attainment of these milestones, abnormalities in postures and movement patterns have also been documented (Gepner & Mestre, 2002; Ornitz et al., 1977; Teitelbaum et al., 1998). Many of the early delays in sitting and walking likely reflect the inability of the infant to stabilize their head or maintain postural control for the particular movement. Similarly, postural adjustments during movement do not appear to be automatic. Teitelbaum et al. (1998) extended this idea of postural adjustment by suggesting that the early movements of infants and young children with ASD are asymmetrical, with movement differences typically being seen on the right side of the body. As a result of this asymmetry, some infants with ASD were not able to maintain a sitting position, becoming off balance and falling over when reaching for an object outside their base of support. Similarly, when crawling, the arm and leg on the right side of the body seem to be weaker than the left with the right leg often being carried passively. When one side of the body is more active than the other, the base of support progressively narrows and the infant eventually falls over to their right side. Overall, there appears to be general consensus that early motor development among young children with ASD may be delayed and show distinct qualitative differences when compared to typically developing children of the same age.

Motor Abilities

Motor abilities refer more generally to the underlying capacities (i.e., balance) that contribute to the performance of movement skills (Magill, 1998). Generally speaking, motor abilities can also refer to groupings of abilities (i.e., fine or gross motor) without consideration of the individual skills that make up each composite. The *Movement Assessment Battery for Children* (*mABC*; Henderson, Sugden, & Barnett, 2007) was designed to assess the motor abilities of children aged 4–12 years in three areas: manual dexterity, ball skills, and balance. For the most part, the majority of children with ASD demonstrate impairments on the *mABC*, with greater than 80% of children and adolescents with Asperger syndrome (AS) scoring below the 5th percentile and demonstrating significant motor impairment across all three areas (Green et al., 2002; Miyahara et al., 1997). Another study used an earlier version of the *mABC*, and although results demonstrated variability in performance, 50% of children and adolescents with AS and 67% with high-functioning autism showed clinically significant motor impairment (Manjiviona & Prior, 1995).

The *Bruininks–Oseretsky Test of Motor Proficiency* (*BOTMP*) also provides a measure of gross and fine motor skills for children and adolescents aged 4–14 years in the original (Bruininks, 1978) and 4–21 years in the second edition (Bruininks & Bruininks, 2005). In addition to an overall composite score, the later version provides composite scores in four motor areas: fine manual control, manual coordination, body coordination, and strength and agility (Bruininks & Bruininks, 2005). Children and adolescents with ASD demonstrated significant impairment on the *BOTMP* when scores were compared to normative data (Ghaziuddin & Butler, 1998; Ghaziuddin, Butler, Tsai, & Ghaziuddin, 1994) or to a comparison group comprised of typically developing children of similar age and IQ (Dewey, Cantell, & Crawford, 2007). Based on assessment using the short form of the *BOTMP*, 41% of the children and adolescents with ASD included in one study did not meet criteria for motor impairment (Dewey et al., 2007), although results may have been different had the complete assessment battery been used. Thus, while much of this research demonstrates that motor impairments are common among children and adolescents with ASD, these impairments do not appear to be universal.

Movement Skills

Despite the importance of movement skills to overall development and the importance of physical activity to overall health and well-being (World Health Organization, 2003), the majority of research examining the movement behavior of children and adolescents with ASD has been based on early motor development and motor abilities. Fundamental movement skills are the goal-directed, locomotor, and object control skills that emerge following walking (Burton & Miller, 1998) and are assumed to be the basis of more advanced or sport-specific skills. Movement skills can be evaluated in terms of the final outcome (i.e., how fast, how far, how accurate) or the movement pattern used (i.e., over- or under-hand, specific performance criteria). The *Test of Gross Motor Development* (*TGMD-2*) (Ulrich, 2000) provides a developmental framework for examining the performance of fundamental movement skills for children aged 3–10 years in terms of the movement patterns used. It includes movement skill sequences for 12 fundamental movement skills divided evenly into locomotor (run, gallop, hop, leap, jump, and slide) and object control (strike, dribble, catch, kick, throw, and roll) subtests.

Each skill is evaluated according to three to five performance criteria that represent the mature pattern for performance of that skill. Multiple criteria help children to receive credit for any aspect of the movement they are able to perform, which provides a more detailed understanding of how the movement skill is being performed. This detailed understanding informs the specific skill areas that need to be improved upon and should be targeted during intervention.

Although there is considerable variability and impaired performance of movement skills cannot be considered universal (Berkeley, Zittel, Pitney, & Nichols, 2001; Pan et al., 2009), immature throwing and catching patterns have been observed among many children and adolescents with ASD (DeMyer, 1976; Reid, Collier, & Morin, 1983). Based on *TGMD-2* performance and when compared to normative data, one study found that 70 and 30% of 6- to 8-year-old boys with ASD demonstrated delays on locomotor and object control skills, respectively (Berkeley et al., 2001). Staples and Reid (2010) extended these findings and suggested that performance of fundamental movement skills by majority of children with ASD is considerably delayed by late childhood. Performance on the *TGMD-2* of 9- to 12-year-old children with ASD was compared to three groups of typically developing children matched on chronological age, movement skill, or cognitive ability (Staples & Reid, 2010). Children with ASD performed similarly on locomotor and object control subtests, demonstrating significant delays relative to their chronological age, with the majority performing similar to children approximately half their age (4–6 years). These movement skill impairments were also greater than would be expected given their cognitive level. The findings of a study by Pan et al. (2009) also found significant group differences based on performance of both locomotor and object control skills between 6- to 10-year-old boys with ASD and their typically developing peers of similar age. This study also conducted separate analyses to examine the performance of individual skills in the *TGMD-2*; results demonstrated that children with ASD had particular difficulty with two locomotor (gallop and hop) and four object control (strike, dribble, catch, and roll) skills.

Based on observations across a variety of fundamental movement skills, many children with ASD experience difficulty performing multi-sequence movements (Bauman, 1992) and show difficulty with the overall timing and coordination of movements that may involve two or more limbs, or both sides of the body, at the same time (Ghaziuddin & Butler, 1998; Jones & Prior, 1985; Morin & Reid, 1985; Reid et al., 1983; Staples & Reid, 2010). Many children with ASD also had specific difficulty controlling the direction and force of the ball when throwing or kicking (Manjiviona & Prior, 1995). Generally speaking, many performance differences seem related to two concepts: momentum/force and timing/coordination (see Staples & Reid, 2010). Just as there is great heterogeneity in most behavior among children and adolescents with ASD, it is not unsurprising that they also demonstrate a wide range of movement behavior. Overall, the majority of children with ASD do not perform movement skills with the same level of proficiency as their typically developing peers, which underscores the importance of focusing efforts on provision of intervention that will facilitate the acquisition of these movement skills so that children with ASD can participate meaningfully in physical activity pursuits alongside their peers.

Intervention

Inclusion reflects a belief that all individuals, regardless of ability, should participate in an activity if they so choose to (Longmuir, 2003, p. 364). As such, intervention approaches that support successful inclusion in physical activity environments are far more than just physically placing a child with ASD in a gymnasium or extracurricular activity alongside their peers (Stainback & Stainback, 1990). While the importance of physical activity and motor development has frequently been overlooked when it comes to intervention for children with ASD (Machalicek et al., 2008), physical education, which can be successfully adapted for children with disabilities, is an essential component of the education curriculum. Similarly, it is important that individuals with ASD have similar opportunities to acquire movement skills as their typically developing peers. Inclusion is based on two key attitudes: (a) each student's educational objectives and learning needs are met through adaptations to the curriculum and (b) necessary supports are provided to meet the unique needs of each student (i.e., specialized equipment, individualized instruction, or additional educators), thereby increasing opportunities for each student to be successful in that environment (see Block, 2007, for review).

Furthermore, maintaining an active lifestyle depends on being motivated to continue participation, which is largely based on having had both enjoyable and successful experiences. Enjoyment primarily depends on the availability of activities that match the individual's interests, goals, and preferences. Success depends, in part, on matching the child's strengths and abilities with the demands of the activity. Children with ASD who experience repeated failure are likely to lose interest in the task and/or decrease responding to instruction (Dunlap, Koegel, & Egel, 1979). Thus, a challenge for instructors is to modify task goals, rules, and environment to maintain interest and ensure an adequate amount of successful experiences for each child with tasks that are meaningful to them. Individualized instruction based on prompting, feedback, and reinforcement specific to each child or adolescent's interests and current level of functioning is fundamental to their successful learning and generalization of movement skills (see Staples, Todd, & Reid, 2006 for a review of strategies).

Education-Based Intervention

In 2001, the National Research Council conducted a systematic review of research examining educational interventions for children with ASD from birth to 8 years of age. Based on this review, specific characteristics of effective interventions were identified: (a) early intervention; (b) intensive instructional programming, defined as 5 days per week, 25 h per week, and 12 months per year; (c) the use of systematic instruction; (d) one-to-one and small-group instruction; (e) instructional objectives addressing social, communication, adaptive living, recreation-leisure, cognitive, and academic skills; (f) ongoing monitoring of the effectiveness of interventions; (g) an emphasis on the generalization of skills; and (h) opportunities for supported interaction with typically developing students. While these characteristics are important for determining an effective intervention program, this report did not provide guidelines to differentiate among the varied intervention options and it only examined research that had been conducted with children up to 8 years of age.

The National Standards Report (National Autism Center, 2009) extended the National Research Council (2001) recommendations by reviewing research demonstrating the effectiveness of a multitude of educational and behavioral treatments targeting the core behaviors among individuals with ASD up to 22 years of age. In doing so, this report addressed the need for evidence-based guidelines to assist parents, educators, and service providers in making informed decisions regarding effective intervention practices for students with ASD. In an effort to review the research more objectively, they also developed more stringent methods of objectively evaluating the methods used in each study in order to provide specific information about the effectiveness of these treatments for teaching individuals with ASD (see National Autism Center, 2009, pp. 16–25).

Throughout this report, the term treatment referred to either specific intervention strategies, such as techniques that can be used alone, or intervention categories that were a combination of different intervention strategies that share similar characteristics. Whenever possible, intervention strategies were combined into categories as many treatment approaches consist of multiple intervention strategies. As such, sometimes the names of these treatment categories will seem unfamiliar because similar strategies have been grouped together based on common underlying characteristics. Based on this review, 11 intervention treatments were identified as being "established" according to several well-controlled studies demonstrating the use of these interventions to produce beneficial effects. These established treatments include (a) antecedent package, (b) behavioral package, (c) comprehensive behavioral treatment for young children, (d) joint attention intervention, (e) modeling, (f) naturalistic teaching strategies, (g) peer training package, (h) pivotal response treatment, (i) schedules, (j) self-management, and (k) story-based intervention package. Furthermore, both exercise and structured teaching were among the treatments identified as having "emerging" evidence – one or more studies to suggest their use may produce favorable outcomes among children with ASD.

The developmental trajectories of young children with ASD can be significantly influenced by the provision of individualized intervention programs that target specific learning areas. Given that many children with ASD are included in either full- or part-time public education systems and spend much of their waking hours at school, it is essential to examine research that demonstrates the effective implementation of interventions in the school system. This review will highlight three intervention approaches – applied behavior analysis, treatment and education of autistic and related communication – handicapped children (TEACCH), and pivotal response treatment – that support successful inclusion of children and adolescents with ASD in physical education and encourage active living – lifelong participation in physical activity. While not named explicitly, many of the principles underlying and the strategies used in each of these intervention approaches were included in the "established" treatments outlined in the National Standards Report (National Autism Center, 2009). The review of each of these intervention approaches should not be considered exhaustive; the strategies focus primarily on the acquisition of movement skills and behavior that are essential to participation.

Applied Behavior Analysis

Applied behavior analysis (ABA) is considered the scientific study of behavior, first documented by Skinner in 1938. The first indication of the effectiveness of ABA for children with autism was documented by Ferster (1961) who demonstrated that operant conditioning techniques, in this instance positive reinforcement, could promote learning. Conceptually, ABA is a group of methods, strategies, and principles rather than a specific program (Leaf & McEachin, 1999) that are consistently implemented in an effort to increase the probability that a specific behavior will occur again (Lovaas, 1981). ABA is also directed toward decreasing the frequency of aggressive behavior, attention deficits, and stereotyped behavior with the assumption that decreasing these behaviors will allow more opportunities for children to learn more desirable skills or behavior. Romanczyk and Matthews (1998) provided an overview of some of the techniques that can be used in various combinations across different age groups, levels of functioning, and environmental settings.

The general public interest in ABA grew after a study by Lovaas (1987) claimed that some preschool-aged children with ASD actually "recovered" following a 2-year intensive intervention. Results from that study showed significant gains for the children following the intensive 40-h per week program. Specifically, nine children (47%) of the group achieved educational and intellectual functioning similar to their typically developing classmates. A follow-up study examining the longevity or maintenance of these improvements 2 years later (McEachin, Smith, & Lovaas, 1993) reported that eight of the nine children who made the greatest progress in the original study (Lovaas, 1987) continued to showed progress and were indistinguishable from typically developing children on tests of intelligence and adaptive behavior. Several additional studies have replicated parts of the results of the original Lovaas study (Eikeseth, Smith, Jahr, & Eldevik, 2002; Sheinkopf & Siegel, 1998; Weiss, 1999). While these findings show the effective use of and positive outcomes associated with ABA when teaching academic skills, there is little empirical research documenting the efficacy of ABA in facilitating the acquisition of fundamental movement skills for children with ASD.

Interventions to Improve Physical Activity Skills

Although the original "ABA manual" dedicated less than one page to instruction related to "participating in recreational activities" (Lovaas, 1981, pp. 102–103), modeling was the primary strategy recommended for teaching movement skills to individuals with ASD, followed by physical prompting and reinforcement. For example, to teach a child to throw a ball the "teacher" should tell the child to "do this" and then model throwing the ball. If the child does not imitate the model, the instructor could begin instruction by first moving the child's arm through the desired movement pattern. Correct responses are reinforced and subsequently prompts are systematically faded.

Prompting is a technique that can be used prior to or at the same time as instruction, during the child's response, or following an incorrect response to help a child respond correctly. Prompts are verbalizations, gestures, demonstrations, or physical manipulations that assist the child during skill acquisition (MacDuff, Krantz, & McClannahan, 2001). They can be thought of in terms of a hierarchy where verbal cues or gestures would be considered as least intrusive and physical prompts as most, where the goal is to fade the use of prompts from most to least intrusive (Leaf & McEachin, 1999). Fading can also be achieved by placing less emphasis on, using a more subtle, or delaying the time before providing a prompt to allow the child more time to initiate their response independently. Fading is an important aspect of prompting because it is important that a child does not become dependent on the prompts being used or on an adult providing them. Just like other responses, it is important to reinforce correct responses to increase the probability of the correct answer for the next time.

Although the timing of the provision of prompts remains a matter of considerable debate within motor learning (see Hodges & Franks, 2002; Lee, Chamberlin, & Hodges, 2001; Williams & Hodges, 2005), prompting in physical activity programs has been recommended for many years (Watkinson & Wall, 1982). It would be a rare physical educator who would not speak, demonstrate, or even move a youngster's limb to prompt a correct response. Independence is achieved by systematic prompt fading.

The effective use of prompting was tested with six boys with ASD who performed 332 trials of a bowling task (Collier & Reid, 1987). Participants were randomly assigned to one of two instructional methods that included either (a) the provision of a hierarchy of physical, verbal, and visual prompts or (b) prompts that were embedded within the structure of the task such as barriers to guide the path of the ball and/or colored pathways leading to the bowling pins. Scoring was based on a 14-step task analysis relative to the distance to the pins (i.e., 5, 10, or 15 ft), the presence of barriers, and the presence and width of the path. In order to move to the next sequence, five pins had to be knocked down on five consecutive trials. The results, based on the sequences achieved in the task analysis, were clearly supportive of instruction being supported by the provision of a hierarchy of prompts. Reid, Collier, and Cauchon (1991) also ascertained whether the use of visual or physical prompts was more effective when two boys and two girls aged 11–15 years performed 240 trials (120 trials per instructional model) on a bowling task similar to the one used by Collier and Reid (1987). This study used a 19-step task analysis (steps 15–19 reflect the addition of 20 ft distance to the pins), including the same within-stimulus prompts outlined in the earlier study. Physical prompts were more effective than visual prompts in three of four students who showed greater improvements in the number of sequences achieved when verbal instructions were used in addition to physical guidance.

Crawford, MacDonncha, and Smyth (2007) conducted a preliminary evaluation of the effectiveness of an adapted physical activity intervention program, which included elements of ABA, for 17 children with autism and co-occurring intellectual disabilities to determine its effect on the performance of movement skills. The program lasted 10 weeks with three sessions per week. A non-active group of seven children with motor impairment and co-occurring learning disabilities was used as control. The program was set up as an obstacle course and included catching, throwing, striking, running, hopping, and balancing skills. Elements of applied behavior analysis included hand-over-hand prompting, modeling of skills, and use of primary and secondary reinforcement. Skills were broken into component parts as necessary. There were significant improvements in ball skills

and balance (static where children balanced on one foot and dynamic where participants walked on balance beams unaided) among the children who participated in the intervention but not among the children in the control group. Results of paired t tests indicated significant improvements occurred for the intervention group in ball skills, static and dynamic balance, social communication, social motivation, and autistic mannerisms. Overall results indicate the benefits of instruction, using components of applied behavior analysis in promoting movement ability and social responsiveness, for children with autism and co-occurring learning disabilities.

Antecedent Physical Activity

Physical activity has also been used as an antecedent intervention to reduce repetitive or stereotypical behaviors and promote positive responding. A considerable body of evidence suggests that these behaviors and interests may be socially stigmatizing, restrict social interactions, and interfere in many learning domains (Koegel & Covert, 1972).

The use of exercise to reduce such behaviors has a relatively long history in individuals with severe and profound developmental disabilities, including ASD (Elliott, Dobbin, Rose, & Soper, 1994; Lancioni & O'Reilly, 1998). For example, Watters and Watters (1980) investigated the impact of physical exercise on self-stimulation of five boys with autism. Language training sessions were preceded by exercise, TV watching, or typical academic activities. While the lowest level of self-stimulation followed the exercise condition with a reduction of 32.7%, none of the antecedent conditions had a differential impact on correct responding in the language training.

Kern, Koegel, Dyer, Blew, and Fenton (1982) examined the impact of a mildly strenuous jogging program lasting between 5 and 20 min on the behavior of children with ASD. Four children aged 4–7 years participated in a clinical environment, separate from their classmates and working individually with a therapist. Consistently, jogging decreased self-stimulatory behavior and increased ball play or academic responding for all participants during the 15 min following jogging compared to the 15 min prior to jogging. Academic responses were measured in the context of their typical classroom activities. To examine the practicality of implementing such a program in a classroom context, three additional children aged 9–14 years who were educated in a special education classroom participated. The jogging sessions were implemented at recess time and classroom behavior was scored as being either "on task" or "off task." Higher levels of "on-task" behavior were recorded for all three children after recess on the jogging days.

A subsequent study by Kern, Koegel, and Dunlap (1984) examined the type and intensity of exercise by comparing the effects of two antecedent exercise conditions, (a) 15 min of jogging and (b) 15 min of ball playing, on three children with ASD aged 7–11 years on behavior in the 90 min following exercise. Once again, jogging was followed by a reduction in stereotyped behaviors while playing ball had no influence. The results of this study replicate previous research (Celiberti, Bobo, Kelly, Harris, & Handleman, 1997) demonstrating the effectiveness of exercise intensity to reduce stereotypic behavior.

Another study compared the impact of three antecedent conditions, (a) sedentary behavior (i.e., no exercise), (b) general motor activities (i.e., riding an exercise bike and lifting weights on a universal gym), and (c) vigorous aerobic exercise (i.e., motorized treadmill moving at 4 miles/h), on the subsequent maladaptive and stereotypic behaviors of six adults with ASD and intellectual disability (Elliott et al., 1994). Twenty-minute experimental sessions were followed by 30 min of observation. The findings confirmed the benefits of vigorous exercise on subsequent behavior, although the authors acknowledged that two participants improved very little. Again this research supported the intensity of exercise as being a critical factor to consider in reducing maladaptive and stereotypic behaviors.

Levinson and Reid (1993) examined the intensity of exercise more specifically when three 11-year-old participants engaged in multiple baseline experiment in which treatment sessions consisted of either walking or jogging. Observations were recorded immediately following exercise and then for an additional 90 min. Heart rate results showed that walking and jogging were differentiated by intensity of exercise, but only jogging was followed by a reduction in stereotypic behavior. This was consistent with Kern and colleagues (1984) who also found that intensity of exercise was important; however, the impact of exercise on stereotypic behaviors was temporary as Levinson and Reid found this behavior returned to baseline levels within the 90 min following exercise.

Prupas and Reid (2001) acknowledged that the antecedent effects of exercise on stereotypic behaviors might be short-lived, but evaluated if these effects would continue to occur if exercise was repeated throughout the day. Four participants aged 5–9 years of age were exposed to two treatment conditions, either a single session of 10 min of exercise or three 10-min sessions of exercise interspersed throughout the school day. The single-frequency condition demonstrated a 51.6% reduction in stereotypic behavior, but this positive finding was temporary as in previous research (Levinson & Reid, 1993), whereas the multiple frequency condition produced only a slightly greater reduction in behavior at 58.9%, these benefits remaining throughout the day. These effects were further maximized when the exercise was followed by very structured learning environment. In summary, exercise of sufficient intensity is an effective means to reduce stereotypic behaviors, at least temporarily, and should be added to the list of treatments for these behaviors (see Luiselli, 1981).

Movement skills can be classified as being either open or closed (Shumway-Cook & Woollacott, 2007, p. 6) based on the context in which they are being performed. Basketball is an open movement task, requiring an individual to adapt their behavior to meet the demands of a constantly changing and perhaps unpredictable environment. Simply practicing shooting free throws would be a "closed" movement skill that is relatively stereotyped and has little variation because the environment changes very little, if at all. Of course it is easier to learn how to perform a skill under closed conditions; however, as learning continues, practice conditions should be varied and moved progressively closer to resembling a game context, by shooting from different locations on the court, dribbling the ball before taking a shot, or even driving to the basket and finishing with a lay-up. The skills practiced, and the manner in which they are practiced, ultimately influence how they are performed in a real-life context. Repeated practice in one particular context may not actually facilitate performance in other, less familiar contexts.

While ABA principles have been demonstrated as being effective in teaching "closed" or discrete movement skills (e.g., shooting a basketball or kicking a soccer ball), research to date has been limited with respect to the generalization of these skills within the context of organized games and activities alongside their peers. Similarly, the use of these natural learning opportunities would facilitate the generalization of skills and behaviors across contexts and afford multiple opportunities for children with ASD to learn to respond to multiple cues across a variety of situations (Stokes & Baer, 1977). Much of the ABA research done to date, however, has been criticized for overlooking the opportunities for learning that exist naturally within day-to-day activities – opportunities that could increase learning and practice of meaningful and functional skills that are primarily used during activities of daily living. Nonetheless, the evidence to support the effective use of behavioral techniques among children and adolescents with ASD has been reviewed extensively and ABA is regarded as an empirically evaluated intervention (National Autism Center, 2009; Simpson, 2005). Based on the extensive review conducted in the National Standards Report, it does seem that a competently designed ABA intervention program that specifically addresses generalization of movement skills could promote physical activity participation in the broader sense.

Treatment and Education of Autistic and Related Communication – Handicapped Children

The TEACCH program from North Carolina takes a developmental approach to understanding behavior and placing specific emphasis on each child's strengths and interests (Mesibov, Shea, & Schopler, 2006). Traditionally, TEACCH was used as an instructional method in segregated (i.e., special education) classrooms. These techniques and methods have also been successfully implemented in inclusive classrooms (see Lord & Schopler, 1994), home-based programs with parents serving as co-therapists (Ozonoff & Cathcart, 1998), and more recently to promote the acquisition of movement skills (Pan, 2010). The TEACCH program has continued to evolve beyond education curriculum and now includes services designed to meet the unique needs of adults with ASD by promoting life skills and supporting transitions into work environments (Mesibov et al., 2006).

TEACCH uses highly structured learning environment (Mesibov et al., 2006), which refers to providing additional structure to the existing learning environment to encourage learning of independent work skills and management of challenging behavior (Mesibov, Schopler, & Hearsey, 1994). Structure can be provided by actively organizing the physical environment, breaking down skills into bite-size pieces and sequences, implementing specific organizational strategies or schedules, choosing materials and tasks based on the child's strengths and interests, and then systematically arranging them so they are both meaningful and visually appealing to the child (Mesibov et al., 1994). While each of these components can be individualized for specific use with a child or adolescent with ASD, most of these strategies should also be effective at increasing independence of all students when implemented for the entire classroom. There are five distinct elements of structured teaching: (a) physical organization, (b) visual structure, (c) schedules, (d) individual work systems, and (e) routines (Mesibov et al., 1994; 2006). Each of these structural components and the research supporting their effective use for children and adolescents with ASD will be reviewed.

Physical organization refers to the physical layout of the environment, including the selection of work areas and the provision of boundaries (Mesibov et al., 1994). Schultheis, Boswell, and Decker (2000) provide a summary of strategies related to structure and physical organization that have been successfully implemented in a gymnasium. For example, visually clear divisions between locations for work and play will afford a child to understand what is expected of them within each particular area (Schopler, Mesibov, & Hearsey, 1995). The placement of mats on the floor of a gymnasium can designate specific areas for listening to instructions. The placement of equipment in specific areas of the gymnasium (i.e., each of the four corners) can be used to communicate what activity should take place and in which area. For example, targets and tennis balls could be placed in one corner and soccer balls and nets in another to work on aiming. A third corner could include scooters and a series of pylons to maneuver through, and an obstacle course requiring children to negotiate a series of horizontal barriers by moving over or under them could be set up in a fourth. Each area and the

activity to be performed is defined according to the equipment that is strategically placed there. These stations also facilitate transitions between activities because it is obvious what activity will happen next.

In addition to physical organization, removing mirrors, closing gymnasium doors, or simply returning equipment that is not currently being used to the storage room may facilitate focus for some children and adolescents with ASD when learning. Gymnasiums are distracting environments; some children and adolescents with ASD may fixate on school logos painted on the walls or in the middle of the gym floor or even on the championship banners that are proudly displayed hanging from the ceiling. Some of these distracters can simply be removed or covered, while others that are more permanent or too large cannot. In these instances, moving that child to work in an area of the gymnasium away from these distracters or structuring the activity so their back is turned to them may help to maintain their attention and (re)focus their learning back on the task at hand. Noise and interruptions from peers may also be distracting or even aversive. As such, some children or adolescents with ASD may prefer to work at a workstation or in their own corner on some occasions or when learning new skills that require increased attention to be paid. These modifications attempt to clarify the physical space and reduce environmental information that may disrupt student work (Howley, Preece, & Arnold, 2001).

Many children and adolescents with ASD learn more effectively using visual rather than verbal cues (Quill, 1997). Given these visual strengths, the provision of visual cues and structure are essential components of TEACCH. These include simple modifications, such as color coding to guide where items are to be returned to during cleanup or to help a child learn which foot goes where when learning to throw a ball. Provision of visual instruction and organization will help to make tasks more clear, meaningful, and easier to understand (Mesibov et al., 2006). The schedules implemented in the TEACCH program should be specific to each student's level of understanding and can be provided visually through a series of objects, pictures, or words that cue the child to a sequence of activities. A day or even an activity can be broken down into a series of events or steps to assist a child in understanding the progression of events (Mesibov et al., 1994). Because transitions from one activity to the next may be difficult, schedules can be individualized for each student or more general ones made for the entire class, affording students to look at the schedule, understand what is coming next, and then prepare for the next activity. Schedules can also be referred back to if the child happens to forget what comes next, thereby decreasing the amount of prompting required from the educator and in turn increasing the independence of the student.

While the physical organization of the environment and the schedule specify the activities, individual work systems inform students about each activity and what is expected of them (Mesibov et al., 1994). These systems aid in providing organizational strategies (Howley et al., 2001) and communicate four pieces of information: (a) what work they are supposed to do, (b) how much work there is, (c) how they will know when they are finished, and (d) what happens after the work is completed (Mesibov et al., 1994). Individual work systems are developed in the same manner as schedules and can serve as a checklist to monitor progress and guide each student in completing their work independently (Mesibov, Browder, & Kirkland, 2002).

Last, routines are systematic and consistent ways in which tasks are carried out (Mesibov et al., 1994). In addition to schedules, routines provide another strategy for facilitating transitions between activities and increasing the independence of children and adolescents with ASD (Howley et al., 2001). Although it is important to establish consistent routines, some degree of flexibility should be systematically introduced into them as the events of each day are not always predictable. For example, many physical educators include four essential components in every class: (a) begin with a warm-up, (b) followed by a period of specific instruction and skill development, (c) an organized activity or game to practice the skills just learned, and (d) finish the class up with free choice where the students select the activity and/or the equipment they would like to use. While the order and sequence of activities remain consistent, the actual skills being learned changes from class to class. Once the routine becomes familiar, a visual schedule can be used to outline which activities will be performed in that class.

There is evidence to support the effective use of an 18-month structured teaching program for children and adolescents with ASD and severe intellectual disability (aged 7–18 years) program that incorporated four key elements from the TEACCH program (i.e., physical organization, schedules, work systems, and task organization) for children and adolescents with ASD and severe intellectual disability (aged 7–18 years) (Panerai, Ferrante, Caputo, & Impellizzeri, 1998). Although this study did not include a control group to ascertain whether the improvements were related primarily to the structured teaching program, the effectiveness of this intervention was seen in terms of increased capacities for learning and the occurrence of spontaneous communication. There was also a reduction in behavioral problems that were measured at baseline, 12 months, and again following the intervention.

Research has also examined the impact of modifying the physical structure of the environment on learning; the use of physical boundaries to provide structure in a physical activity setting led to an increase in independence and reduced off-task behavior (Schultheis et al., 2000). While not examining the performance of movement skills per se, these studies (i.e., Panerai et al., 1998; Schultheis et al., 2000) found that

modifying the physical structure of the environment did lead to increased time spent on-task and therefore increased time with which the children and adolescents with ASD were able to learn movement skills.

Another element of structure that has proven successful in facilitating transitions between classroom activities is the use of schedules (e.g., Massey & Wheeler, 2000; Schmit, Apler, Raschke, & Ryndak, 2000). Using an ABAB design, the use of visual schedules and work systems was found to be an effective means of increasing the independence of two boys aged 5 and 7 years transitioning between activities and decreasing the amount of time it took for them to move between activities (Dettmer, Simpson, Smith Myles, & Ganz, 2000). Moreover, schedules have also been shown to be effective in self-managing behavior in the absence of supervision (Pierce & Schreibman, 1994), reducing teacher-delivered verbal and physical prompts (Dettmer et al., 2000) and maintaining high levels of on-task and on-schedule behavior (Bryan & Gast, 2000).

Physical education environments (i.e., gymnasiums or swimming pools) are inherently more open, noisy, and potentially more distracting than classrooms; research evidence supporting the effectiveness of structured teaching in such environments has also been conducted. Pushkarenko (2004) examined the effectiveness of using individual work systems and visual schedules with three boys with ASD (aged 11–17 years) during a school swimming program. Large schedules on the pool deck outlined the overall sequence of the swimming lesson (i.e., warm-up, instruction, relays, and free time) for all three boys. Individual works systems depicted specific activities within the scheduled instruction time for each boy (e.g., a series of three pictures depicting swimming using three different flotation devices). The effectiveness of these schedules and work systems was assessed using a single-subject design over the course of the 13-week swimming program. While two boys showed modest increases in time on-task throughout and maintained these increases following the program, all three spent significantly decreased time engaging in inappropriate behavior. Overall, the findings of this study support the effective use of visual schedules and work systems in physical activity programs to provide greater opportunities to both learn and practice aquatic skills.

Pan (2010) used similar methods to examine how a program using structured teaching strategies impacted the learning of swimming skills by 16 boys with ASD aged 6–9 years. The boys were divided into two groups, the first receiving the swimming program and the other serving as a control group, continuing their regular treatment and physical activity programs. Each condition was 10 weeks in length and the order was counterbalanced, with each group completing both 10-week regimens in order to examine the effects of the swimming program on skill acquisition. The swimming program consisted of two 90-min sessions per week. Each session was divided into four instructional categories: (a) out of pool warm-up, (b) small-group instruction (2 children:1 instructor), (c) group/cooperative games (8 children:4 instructors), and (d) cool-down activities. Structured teaching strategies (i.e., organization of physical environment, visual schedules, and individual work systems) were embedded in the instruction. Furthermore, the progression from instruction (2:1) to practicing the skills learned and engaging in cooperative games with their peers (8:4) facilitated generalization. Outcome was measured by a 32-item checklist that was developed according to an aquatics instructional approach called the Halliwick Method, a holistic approach which encompasses all aspects of a swimmer's development – physical, psychological, and social. This checklist grouped aquatic skills into five areas: introduction to water, rotations, balance, controlled movement, and independent movement. Overall, the swimming program resulted in improvements in four of five skill areas, demonstrating its effective use in facilitating the acquisition of swimming skills.

Overall, there is growing evidence to support the effective use of structured teaching (i.e., TEACCH) in physical activity contexts. Well-controlled evidence to support TEACCH is beginning to emerge at this time, although there are not currently a large number of well-controlled trials. TEACCH can be implemented effectively for both children with ASD and their typical classmates. While research examining structured teaching is in its infancy when it comes to the acquisition of movement skills, it has been promising in terms of promoting independence in physical activity engagement, another essential component of active living.

Pivotal Response Training

Pivotal response training (PRT) is also based on many of the principles of ABA. Instead of working on specific skills, PRT focuses on pivotal behaviors such as self-regulation and motivation that when targeted produce widespread improvements and often collateral changes in other untargeted areas of functioning and responding (Koegel, Koegel, Harrower, & Carter, 1999). The goal of this intervention program is to move children toward a typical developmental trajectory by providing opportunities for meaningful learning in their natural environments, including within the general education curriculum (Koegel & Koegel, 2006; Koegel, Koegel, & Carter, 1999). PRT emerged from the natural language paradigm (Koegel, O'Dell, & Koegel, 1987), and early empirical support was based on the acquisition of language skills in inclusive environments by following a typical developmental sequence of learning (Koegel & Koegel, 2006). Unlike most intervention models that rely heavily on the provision of intervention in highly structured environments by specific service providers, PRT encourages a coordinated

effort to provide consistent and ongoing intervention that is implemented across people, settings, and environments (Koegel & Koegel, 2006; R. L. Koegel et al., 1999). It gives everyone the child interacts with the skills necessary to play an integral role in their learning. PRT promotes both the acquisition and the maintenance of skills, as many of these techniques become a natural way of interacting with the child that can easily be integrated into daily routines and family life.

The most fundamental characteristics of individuals with ASD (i.e., social interaction, functional communication, and essential "people skills") are the most difficult to teach. It is these difficult to teach skills that are targeted in PRT (Koegel & Koegel, 2006). PRT uses discrete trials for teaching, in that clear instructions are given, the child responds, prompts may be used, and reinforcement is provided; however, instead of teaching one specific skill at a time, pivotal behaviors (i.e., self-regulation or motivation) are targeted and the reinforcements used are already found within the context of the task. This is achieved by targeting the fundamental skills that are needed in natural environments, such as going to the park with family for a picnic, having goals and objectives from the general education curriculum, or playing catch with a sibling. Instead of repeating the same stimulus–response trial (e.g., catch ball), a game of catch is organized among the family, and catching is practiced in the context of a natural interaction, along with turn-taking, throwing, and social communication. PRT does not provide the child with a specific stimulus to respond to, but creates multiple opportunities for them to initiate interaction and essentially makes them want to communicate and connect with others (R. L. Koegel et al., 1999).

The principles of PRT are based on skills or behavior that will generalize the most and contribute to overall functioning by targeting four specific pivotal areas: (a) motivation to engage, (b) responsivity to multiple cues, (c) social initiation, and (d) self-regulation (Koegel & Koegel, 2006). Each of these pivotal areas is not mutually exclusive and therefore each is difficult to operationalize. When children respond incorrectly or experience repeated failure, they become less likely to respond and lose motivation to engage further in the task (Koegel & Egel, 1979). Motivation is fundamental to learning and is at the heart of continuing to use these acquired skills. PRT motivates children with ASD to become increasingly responsive to everyday stimuli and tries to make these everyday activities intrinsically motivating.

One study targeted motivation through the symbolic play skills of seven boys with ASD aged 4–7 years using pivotal response methods (Stahmer, 1995). Symbolic play and language training were implemented, both of which took place for 1 h, three times per week, for 8 weeks. Measures were taken pre- and post-training as well as 3 months follow-up to examine maintenance of skills. The boys with ASD learned to perform complex and creative symbolic play at levels similar to typically developing, language-matched peers. Following training, they also began to respond more positively to initiations made by adults during play, suggesting possible generalization to other skills associated with the training; however, the children did not improve in responses to peer initiations and still did not initiate interaction very often following training.

The primary teaching techniques advocated for in PRT to target motivation are as follows: (a) the provision of choice, (b) providing direct and natural reinforcements, (c) reinforcing attempts, and (d) interspersing acquisition and maintenance tasks (Koegel & Koegel, 2006). While all of these techniques are fundamental characteristics of quality teaching, their consistent use across all learning opportunities and the structuring of the environment to create these learning opportunities are important elements of PRT.

The provision of choice is a technique to motivate a child to respond, or to select among multiple options, or to initiate an activity they prefer to engage in (Koegel et al., 1999). Some degree of choice can be integrated into almost any activity (Dunlap et al., 1994). By providing choice in terms of activities, task goals, or even the equipment they use, educators will learn what is meaningful to children and adolescents with ASD, allowing them to be involved in and take ownership of their learning (R. L. Koegel et al., 1999; Moes, 1998). Furthermore, the provision of choice is likely to increase interest in the activity (Dyer, Dunlap, & Winterling, 1990; Koegel, Dyer, & Bell, 1987) and ultimately motivation for continued participation. Three studies found that when three children with autism and intellectual disability were given choice of the reinforcers to be used and the tasks to be performed (Dyer et al., 1990) or the order in which the tasks were to be completed (Newman, Needelman, Reinecke, & Robek, 2002), significantly fewer disruptive behaviors were seen and participant engagement increased (Watanabe & Sturmey, 2003). Staples et al. (2006) provided an overview of several strategies that can be used to provide choice for children and adolescents with ASD during physical education.

Similarly, the provision of contingent reinforcement is used across majority of intervention models to teach all skills, but PRT is the use of reinforcements that are incorporated directly into the learning environment. For example, a child may be fixated on playing with a particular ball. So, when they complete their task of running around the gym three times, they get to play with the ball. This line of reinforcement could be compared to when they complete their task, they get to eat an M&M.

Task variation is an instructional strategy where the acquisition of new skills is interspersed with practice of well-learned skills. A study by Weber and Thorpe (1992) examined the acquisition of fundamental movement skills (i.e., dribble, kick, roll, throw, jump, slide) by 12 adolescents with ASD aged 11–15 years by comparing traditional teaching methods focused on learning one skill at a time (i.e., massed practice) versus task variation (i.e., distributed practice). They found that task variation provided opportunities to practice previously learned skills (i.e., run, hop, catch), which also provided a natural reinforcement in that successful performance was interspersed with learning. Interest was maintained by working on multiple skills divided into short time segments in which only 2–3 min were spent on any one skill and overall a greater frequency of success was experienced because they were also practicing skills they already knew. At baseline, there was no difference between the two groups on any of the six fundamental movement skills that were targeted. Following the 6 weeks of instruction, significant differences were found on all six skills, demonstrating task variation to be an effective instructional strategy.

When used together, these teaching techniques have been found to be effective. A recent study demonstrated that peers could effectively implement PRT strategies during recess to two boys with ASD aged 8 and 9 years, particularly initiations to gain the attention of or to play with peers and turn-taking (Blauvelt Harper, Symon, & Frea, 2008). In seven 20-min training sessions, classmates were taught PRT strategies to target the motivation and responding of their peers with ASD including gaining attention before giving directions, varying activities and providing choice, modeling appropriate play and providing appropriate commentary on their behavior, reinforcing attempts, and turn-taking (see Blauvelt et al., 2008 for review of peer training methods). Both boys with ASD increased in frequency of social interactions (measured by the number of attempts to initiate play, gain the attention of a peer, or engage in a turn-taking activity) with peers during recess. They also maintained these skills during a generalization phase and continued to improve after the intervention. Peer interactions may allow for better generalization of social skills and logically it would also be easier to generalize skills that were practiced and reinforced in varied environments, when participating in enjoyable activities alongside their peers. The results of this study demonstrated the important role that peers can play in facilitating social development among children with ASD and a reasonable extension of these findings would be to examine the role of peers in the acquisition of movement skills.

A recent work by Hutzler and Margalit (2009) investigated the acquisition of field hockey skills by seven students with ASD aged 15–16 years in an inclusive high school setting. There were four 45-min instructional sessions over a 2-week period. Pre- and post-testing occurred in periods one and four with instruction occurring in periods two and three. Instruction included the provision of verbal, visual, or physical prompts as necessary, verbal reinforcement, and peer tutors who served both as models and provided the prompting and reinforcement for the students with ASD. Despite the short instructional duration, the students with ASD demonstrated a significant improvement on one of the three skills being targeted, moving the field hockey ball around a cone as frequently as possible in 30 s. While improvements were not seen on the other two skills, a passing test for precision and negotiating the ball through a series of cones, the role of peers in guiding learning and motivating peers with ASD to participate does provide future direction with respect to implementation of peer-mediated intervention in the context of physical education.

Participation in physical activity can be limited for individuals with ASD due to difficulties in performance of movement skills (Pan et al., 2009; Staples & Reid, 2010) and low motivation (Koegel & Egel, 1979; Koegel, Koegel, & McNerney, 2001). The ability to self-monitor performance is also considered an important skill within the scope of PRT (Koegel et al., 1999). Furthermore, strategies that target motivation, by combining verbal cueing (i.e., prompts) and external reinforcement, in addition to self-monitoring, may be effective in encouraging physical activity participation (Todd & Reid, 2006). For example, Todd and Reid (2006) conducted an intervention using prompting, reinforcement, and systematic self-monitoring strategies of three males with ASD and severe intellectual disability (aged 15–20 years) to engage in sustained physical activity. The physical activity intervention built on their classroom activities which used structured teaching. The intervention sessions were twice per week for 6 months and included snowshoeing or walk/jogging around a diamond-shaped circuit that was created on a soccer field with colored flags to mark each of the four corners. A self-monitoring board enabled each participant to place a happy face after they completed each circuit. As the intervention progressed, the need for edible reinforcements and verbal cueing declined, while the number of circuits completed increased for each of the participants, highlighting the importance of self-monitoring to ongoing participation in physical activity pursuits. Furthermore, by the end of the program two of the participants jogged the majority of the 30 min, demonstrating that individuals with ASD can meet the recommended physical activity guidelines (World Health Organization, 2003) when provided with structured opportunities to do so.

Todd, Reid, and Butler-Kisber (2010) followed up their earlier study (Todd & Reid, 2006) by investigating self-monitoring, goal setting, and self-reinforcement in promoting cycling in three adolescents aged 15–17 years with ASD and severe intellectual disability who were non-verbal and used pictograms to communicate. The adolescents cycled around a 75 m circuit on an asphalt surface adjacent to the school, three times per week for approximately 4 months. A multiple baseline changing criterion design was used.

Participants selected their own bicycle, either a lowered bicycle with extra stabilizing wheels or an adult tricycle. A self-monitoring board similar to the one in Todd and Reid (2006) was used throughout, goal setting was introduced after baseline, and edible reinforcements were provided for the first 12 sessions to increase motivation. Two participants increased the number of circuits completed significantly over the program as judged by standard visual analyses guidelines, suggesting that they not only understood the concept of goal setting but also were able to monitor their progress and set increasingly challenging and realistic goals over the sessions; however, it is difficult to ascertain exactly which self-regulation strategy (i.e., monitoring or goal setting) might have been most effective or whether their interaction was the important mediator. As Bandura (1997) stated, the most effective results may occur when several self-regulation strategies are included simultaneously. Thus, overall the self-regulation strategies manipulated by Todd et al. (2010) and other factors in self-determination theory seem to have potential in promoting sustained physical activity in individuals with ASD and warrant additional research.

While research examining the effectiveness of PRT in the acquisition of movement skills and participation in physical activity is limited, findings are promising. PRT is a coordinated service delivery model that recognizes the opportunities for learning that exist within the day-to-day activities. Given the importance placed on family involvement in successful implementation of and positive outcomes associated with intervention models, it is especially promising to see that parents can learn to successfully implement PRT strategies throughout all interactions with their child, thereby increasing the number of opportunities for consistency, intensity, and sustainability of intervention (Bryson et al., 2007). Since learning occurs throughout the day, PRT aims to move the focus of intervention from being on specific skills predetermined by a service provider and targeted in a one-to-one context to recognizing opportunities for learning that naturally exist in everyday activities including school. Similarly, PRT targets both the development of individual skills and the use of those skills in the context of their natural environment, both of which are essential components of leading an active lifestyle.

Conclusions

The acquisition of, and meaningful experiences associated with, movement skills can be building blocks for subsequent development and learning. Physical activity can and should be built into a regular routine, being spread out throughout the day, becoming a lifestyle choice rather than another thing that needs to be done. While sustained physical activity is essential for healthy living, the effective use of exercise for individuals with ASD as a means to decrease stereotypical behavior has been documented (Elliott et al., 1994; Levinson & Reid, 1993). Similarly, the importance of young children with ASD developing movement skills early to be able to achieve these benefits is paramount, and in recent years researchers, educators, and parents have learned more about the use of effective interventions to facilitate this learning process. As a result, children and adolescents with ASD are being successfully included in educational and recreational programs more frequently. Despite this increasing knowledge, we still have a great deal to learn about the most effective means with which fundamental movement skills are acquired and physically active lifestyles are encouraged in the context of inclusive environments. There is no "one size fits all" approach to intervention, just as there is not one set of characteristics that describes all individuals with ASD. As such, it is a strength that multiple intervention models exist; research is beginning to demonstrate the effectiveness of each to provide empirical support for them. As professionals we must understand this research and advocate for use of intervention strategies that are both empirically sound and most effective for each child to achieve their fullest potential, while working within the constraints of what works best for them and their families. This chapter has provided an overview of three education-based intervention models that can be used to effectively promote movement skill acquisition and active living. The National Standards Report concluded that several ABA methods and PRT all meet criteria for "established" treatments and that TEACCH met criteria for an "emerging" treatment.

References

Active Healthy Kids Canada. (2010). 2010 report card on physical activity for children and youth. Retrieved April 27, 2010, from www.activehealthykids.ca

Bandura, A. (1997). *Self-efficacy: The exercise of personal control.* New York: Freeman.

Baranek, G. (1999). Autism during infancy: A retrospective video analysis of sensory-motor and social behaviors at 9–12 months of age. *Journal of Autism and Developmental Disorders, 29,* 213–224.

Baranek, G. T. (2002). Efficacy of sensory and motor interventions for children with autism. *Journal of Autism and Developmental Disorders, 32,* 397–422.

Bauman, M. L. (1992). Motor dysfunction in autism. In A. B. Joseph & R. R. Young (Eds.), *Movement disorders in neurology and neuropsychiatry* (pp. 660–663). Cambridge, MA: Blackwell Scientific Publications.

Bayley, N. (1993). *Bayley scales of infant development manual* (2nd ed.). San Antonio, TX: The Psychological Corporation.

Berkeley, S. L., Zittel, L. L., Pitney, L. V., & Nichols, S. E. (2001). Locomotor and object control skills of children diagnosed with autism. *Adapted Physical Activity Quarterly, 18,* 405–416.

Blauvelt Harper, C., Symon, J. B. G., & Frea, W. D. (2008). Recess is time-in: Using peers to improve social skills of children with autism. *Journal of Autism and Developmental Disorders, 38,* 815–826.

Block, M. (2007). *A teacher's guide to including children with disabilities in general physical education* (3rd ed.). Baltimore: Paul H. Brooks.

Bruininks, R. H. (1978). *Bruininks-Oseretsky test of motor proficiency.* Circle Pines, MN: American Guidance Service.

Bruininks, R. H., & Bruininks, B. D. (2005). *Bruininks-Oseretsky test of motor proficiency* (2nd ed.). Windsor: NFER-Nelson.

Bryan, L. C., & Gast, D. L. (2000). Teaching on-task and on-schedule behaviors to high-functioning children with autism via picture activity schedules. *Journal of Autism and Developmental Disorders, 30,* 553–567.

Bryson, S. E., Koegel, L. K., Koegel, R. L., Openden, D., Smith, I. M., & Nefdt, N. (2007). Large scale dissemination and community implementation of pivotal response treatment: Program description and preliminary data. *Research and Practice for Persons with Severe Disabilities, 32,* 142–153.

Burton, A. W., & Miller, D. E. (1998). *Movement skill assessment.* Champaign, IL: Human Kinetics.

Canadian Fitness and Lifestyle Research Institute. (2008). Canadian physical activity levels among youth (CANPLAY). Retrieved August 28, 2009, from http://www.cflri.ca/eng/statistics/surveys/documents/CANPLAY_2008

Canadian Society for Exercise Physiology. (2003). *The Canadian physical activity, fitness and lifestyle appraisal manual: CSEP's plan for healthy active living* (3rd ed.). Ottawa, ON: Author.

Celiberti, D. A., Bobo, H. E., Kelly, K. S., Harris, S. L., & Handleman, J. S. (1997). The differential and temporal effects of antecedent exercise on the self-stimulatory behavior of a child with autism. *Research in Developmental Disabilities, 18,* 139–150.

Collier, D., & Reid, G. (1987). A comparison of two models designed to teach autistic children a motor task. *Adapted Physical Activity Quarterly, 4,* 226–236.

Crawford, S., MacDonncha, C., & Smyth, P. J. (2007). *An examination of current provision and practice of adapted physical activity for children with disabilities and the subsequent application of an adapted physical activity intervention programme for children with autism and co-occurring learning disabilities.* Unpublished dissertation. Limerick: University of Limerick.

DeMyer, M. K. (1976). Motor, perceptual-motor, intellectual disabilities of autistic children. In L. Wing (Ed.), *Early childhood autism* (pp. 169–193). New York: Pergamon Press.

Dettmer, S., Simpson, R. L., Smith Myles, B., & Ganz, J. B. (2000). The use of visual supports to facilitate transitions of students with autism. *Focus on Autism and other Developmental Disabilities, 15,* 163–169.

Dewey, D., Cantell, M., & Crawford, S. G. (2007). Motor and gestural performance in children with autism spectrum disorders, developmental coordination disorder, and/or attention deficit hyperactivity disorder. *Journal of the International Neuropsychological Society, 13,* 246–256.

Dunlap, G., DePerczel, M., Clark, S., Wilson, D., Wright, S., White, R., et al. (1994). Choice-making to promote adaptive behavior for students with emotional and behavioral challenges. *Journal of Applied Behavior Analysis, 24,* 505–518.

Dunlap, G., Koegel, R. L., & Egel, A. L. (1979). Children with autism in school. *Exceptional Child, 45,* 522–528.

Dyer, K., Dunlap, G., & Winterling, V. (1990). Effects of choice making on the serious problem behaviors of students with severe handicaps. *Journal of Applied Behavior Analysis, 23,* 515–524.

Eikeseth, S., Smith, T., Jahr, E., & Eldevik, S. (2002). Intensive behavioral treatment at school for 4- to 7-year-old children with autism: A 1-year comparison controlled study. *Behavior Modification, 26,* 49–68.

Elliott, R. O., Jr., Dobbin, A. R., Rose, G. D., & Soper, H. V. (1994). Vigorous, aerobic exercise versus general motor training activities: Effects on maladaptive and stereotypic behaviors of adults with both autism and mental retardation. *Journal of Autism and Developmental Disorders, 24,* 565–576.

Ferster, C. B. (1961). Positive reinforcement and behavioral deficits of autistic children. *Child Development, 32,* 437–456.

Folio, M. R., & Fewell, R. R. (2000). *Peabody developmental motor scales examiner's manual* (2nd ed.). Austin, TX: PRO-ED.

Gepner, B., & Mestre, D. R. (2002). Brief report: Postural reactivity to fast visual motion differentiates autistic from children with Asperger syndrome. *Journal of Autism and Developmental Disorders, 32,* 231–238.

Ghaziuddin, M., & Butler, E. (1998). Clumsiness in autism and Asperger syndrome: A further report. *Journal of Intellectual Disability Research, 42,* 43–48.

Ghaziuddin, M., Butler, E., Tsai, L. Y., & Ghaziuddin, N. (1994). Is clumsiness a marker for Asperger syndrome. *Journal of Intellectual Disability Research, 38,* 519–527.

Green, D., Baird, G., Barnett, A. L., Henderson, L., Huber, J., & Henderson, S. E. (2002). The severity and nature of motor impairment in Asperger's syndrome: A comparison with specific developmental disorder of motor function. *Journal of Child Psychology and Psychiatry, 43*(5), 1–14.

Health Canada. (2009). Physical activity. Retrieved April 21, 2010, from www.hc-sc.gc.ca

Henderson, S. E., Sugden, D. A., & Barnett, A. L. (2007). *Movement assessment battery for children* (2nd ed.). London: Pearson Assessment.

Hodges, N., & Franks, I. M. (2002). Modelling coaching practice: The role of instruction and demonstration. *Journal of Sports Sciences, 20,* 793–811.

Howley, M., Preece, D., & Arnold, T. (2001). Multidisciplinary use of 'structured teaching' to promote consistency of approach for children with autistic spectrum disorder. *Educational and Child Psychology, 18,* 41–52.

Hutzler, Y., & Margalit, M. (2009). Skill acquisition in students with and without pervasive developmental disorder. *Research in Autism Spectrum Disorders, 3,* 685–694.

Jones, V., & Prior, M. P. (1985). Motor imitation abilities and neurological signs in autistic children. *Journal of Autism and Developmental Disorders, 15,* 37–46.

Kern, L., Koegel, R. L., & Dunlap, G. (1984). The influence of vigorous versus mild exercise on autistic stereotyped behaviors. *Journal of Autism and Developmental Disorders, 14,* 57–67.

Kern, L., Koegel, R. L., Dyer, K., Blew, P. A., & Fenton, L. R. (1982). The effects of physical exercise on self-stimulation and appropriate responding in autistic children. *Journal of Autism and Developmental Disorders, 12,* 399–419.

Koegel, L. K., Koegel, R. L., Harrower, J. K., & Carter, C. M. (1999). Pivotal response intervention I: Overview of approach. *Journal of the Association for Persons with Severe Handicaps, 24,* 174–185.

Koegel, R. L., & Covert, A. (1972). The relationship of self-stimulation to learning in autistic children. *Journal of Applied Behavior Analysis, 5,* 381–387.

Koegel, R. L., Dyer, K., & Bell, L. K. (1987). The influence of child-preferred activities on autistic children's social behavior. *Journal of Applied Behavior Analysis, 20,* 243–252.

Koegel, R. L., & Egel, A. L. (1979). Motivating autistic children. *Journal of Abnormal Psychology, 88,* 418–426.

Koegel, R. L., & Koegel, L. K. (2006). *Pivotal response treatments for autism: Communication, social, and academic development.* Paul H. Brookes: Baltimore.

Koegel, R. L., Koegel, L. K., & Carter, C. M. (1999). Pivotal teaching interactions for children with autism. *School Psychology Review, 28,* 576–594.

Koegel, R. L., Koegel, L. K., & McNerney, E. K. (2001). Pivotal areas in intervention for autism. *Journal of Clinical Child Psychology, 30,* 19–32.

Koegel, R. L., O'Dell, M. C., & Koegel, L. K. (1987). A natural language teaching paradigm for nonverbal autistic children. *Journal of Autism and Developmental Disorders, 17,* 187–200.

Lancioni, G. E., & O'Reilly, M. F. (1998). A review of research on physical exercise with people with severe and profound developmental disabilities. *Research in Developmental Disabilities, 19,* 477–492. doi: 10.1016/S0891-4222(98)00019-5.

Leaf, R., & McEachin, J. (1999). *A work in progress: Behavior management strategies and a curriculum for intensive behavioral treatment of autism.* New York: DRL Books.

Lee, T. D., Chamberlin, C. J., & Hodges, N. (2001). Practice. In R. N. Singer, H. A. Hausenblas, & C. M. Janelle (Eds.), *Handbook of sport psychology* (2nd ed, pp. 115–143). New York: Wiley.

Levinson, L. J., & Reid, G. (1993). The effects of exercise intensity on the stereotypic behaviors of individuals with autism. *Adapted Physical Activity Quarterly, 10,* 255–268.

Longmuir, P. E. (2003). Creating inclusive physical activity opportunities: An abilities-based approach. In R. D. Steadward, G. D. Wheeler, & E. J. Watkinson (Eds.), *Adapted physical activity* (pp. 363–381). Edmonton, AB: The University of Alberta Press.

Lord, C., & Schopler, E. (1994). TEACCH services for preschool children. In S. L. Harris & J. S. Handleman (Eds.), *Preschool education programs for children with autism* (pp. 87–106). Austin, TX: PRO-ED.

Lovaas, O. I. (1981). *Teaching developmentally disabled children: The ME book.* Baltimore: University Park Press.

Lovaas, O. I. (1987). Behavioral treatment and normal educational and intellectual functioning in young autistic children. *Journal of Consulting and Clinical Psychology, 55,* 3–9.

Luiselli, J. K. (1981). Behavior treatment of self-stimulation. *Education and Treatment of Children, 4,* 375–392.

Lösche, G. (1990). Sensorimotor and action development in autistic children from infancy to early childhood. *Journal of Child Psychology and Psychiatry, 31,* 749–761.

MacDuff, G. S., Krantz, P. J., & McClannahan, L. E. (2001). Prompts and prompt-fading strategies for people with autism. In C. Maurice, G. Green, & R. M. Foxx (Eds.), *Making a difference: Behavioral intervention for autism* (pp. 37–50). Austin, TX: PRO-ED.

Machalicek, W., O'Reilly, M. F., Beretvas, N., Sigafoos, J., Lancioni, G., Sorrells, A., et al. (2008). A review of school-based instructional interventions for students with autism spectrum disorders. *Research in Autism Spectrum Disorders, 2,* 396–416.

Magill, R. A. (1998). *Motor learning: Concepts and applications* (5th ed.). Boston: McGraw-Hill.

Manjiviona, J., & Prior, M. (1995). Comparison of Asperger syndrome and high-functioning autistic children on a test of motor impairment. *Journal of Autism and Developmental Disorders, 25,* 23–39.

Massey, N. G., & Wheeler, J. J. (2000). Acquisition and generalization of activity-schedules and their effects on task engagement in a young child with autism in an inclusive pre-school classroom. *Education and Training in Mental Retardation and Developmental Disabilities, 35,* 326–335.

Mayes, S. D., & Calhoun, S. L. (2003). Ability profiles in children with autism: Influence of age and IQ. *Autism, 7,* 65–80, doi: 10.1177/1362361303007001006

McEachin, J. J., Smith, T., & Lovaas, O. I. (1993). Long-term outcome for children with autism who received early intensive behavioral treatment. *American Journal on Mental Retardation, 97,* 359–372.

Mesibov, G. B., Browder, D. M., & Kirkland, C. (2002). Using individualized schedules as a component of positive behavioral support for students with developmental disabilities. *Journal of Positive Behavior Interventions, 4,* 73–79.

Mesibov, G. B., Schopler, E., & Hearsey, K. L. (1994). Structured teaching. In E. Schopler & G. B. Mesibov (Eds.), *Behavioral issues in autism* (pp. 195–207). New York: Plenum.

Mesibov, G. B., Shea, V., & Schopler, E. (2006). *The TEACCH approach to autism spectrum disorders*. New York: Springer.

Miyahara, M., Tsujii, M., Hori, M., Nakanishi, K., Kageyama, H., & Sugiyama, T. (1997). Brief report: Motor incoordination in children with Asperger syndrome and learning disabilities. *Journal of Autism and Developmental Disorders, 27*, 595–603.

Moes, D. R. (1998). Integrating choice-making opportunities within teacher-assigned academic tasks to facilitate the performance of children with autism. *Journal of the Association for Persons with Severe Handicaps, 23*, 319–328.

Morin, B., & Reid, G. (1985). A quantitative and qualitative assessment of autistic individuals on selected motor tasks. *Adapted Physical Activity Quarterly, 2*, 43–55.

National Autism Center. (2009). *National standards report*. Randolph, MA: Author.

National Research Council. (2001). *Educating children with autism: Report of the committee on educational interventions in children with autism*. Washington, DC: National Academy Press.

Newman, B., Needelman, M., Reinecke, D. R., & Robek, A. (2002). The effect of providing choices on skill acquisition and competing behavior of children with autism during discrete trial instruction. *Behavioral Interventions, 17*, 31–41.

Ornitz, E. M., Guthrie, D., & Farley, A. J. (1977). The early development of autistic children. *Journal of Autism and Childhood Schizophrenia, 7*, 207–229.

Ozonoff, S., & Cathcart, K. (1998). Effectiveness of a home program intervention for young children with autism. *Journal of Autism and Developmental Disorders, 28*, 25–32.

Pan, C. Y. (2010). Effects of water exercise swimming program on aquatic skills and social behaviors in children with autism spectrum disorders. *Autism, 14*, 9–28.

Pan, C. Y., Tsai, C. L., & Chu, C. H. (2009). Fundamental movement skills in children diagnosed with autism spectrum disorders and attention deficit hyperactivity disorder. *Journal of Autism and Developmental Disorders, 39*, 1694–1705. doi: 10.1007/s10803-009-0813-5

Panerai, S., Ferrante, L., Caputo, V., & Impellizzeri, C. (1998). Use of structured teaching for treatment of children with autism and severe and profound mental retardation. *Education and Training in Mental Retardation and Developmental Disabilities, 33*, 367–374.

Pierce, K. L., & Schreibman, L. (1994). Teaching daily living skills to children with autism in unsupervised settings through pictorial self-management. *Journal of Applied Behavior Analysis, 27*, 471–181.

Provost, B., Lopez, B. R., & Heimerl, S. (2007). A comparison of motor delays in young children: Autism spectrum disorder, developmental delay, and developmental concerns. *Journal of Autism and Developmental Disorders, 37*, 321–328.

Prupas, A., & Reid, G. (2001). Effects of exercise frequency on stereotypic behaviors of children with developmental disabilities. *Education and Training in Mental Retardation and Developmental Disabilities, 36*, 196–206.

Public Health Agency of Canada. (2010). Benefits of physical activity for children and youth. Retrieved May 3, 2010, from www.publichealth.gc.ca

Pushkarenko, K. (2004). *Enhancing the structure of a swimming program for three boys with autism through the use of activity schedules*. Montreal, QC: McGill University (Unpublished master's thesis).

Quill, K. A. (1997). Instructional considerations for young children with autism: The rationale for visually cued instruction. *Journal of Autism and Developmental Disorders, 27*, 697–714.

Reid, G., Collier, D., & Cauchon, M. (1991). Skill acquisition by children with autism: Influence of prompts. *Adapted Physical Activity Quarterly, 8*, 357–366.

Reid, G., Collier, D., & Morin, B. (1983). The motor performance of autistic individuals. In R. Eason, T. Smith, & F. Caron (Eds.), *Adapted physical activity* (pp. 201–218). Champaign, IL: Human Kinetics.

Romanczyk, R. G., & Matthews, A. L. (1998). Physiological state as antecedent: Utilization in functional analysis. In J. K. Lusiselli & M. J. Cameron (Eds.), *Antecedent control procedures for the behavioural support of persons with developmental disabilities*. New York: Paul H. Brookes.

Rosser-Sandt, D. D., & Frey, G. C. (2005). Comparison of physical activity levels between children with and without autistic spectrum disorders. *Adapted Physical Activity Quarterly, 22*, 146–159.

Schmit, J., Apler, S., Raschke, D., & Ryndak, D. (2000). Effects of using a photographic cueing package during routine school transitions with a child who has autism. *Mental Retardation, 38*, 131–137.

Schopler, E., Mesibov, G. B., & Hearsey, K. (1995). Structured teaching in the TEACCH system. In E. Schopler & G. B. Mesibov (Eds.), *Learning and cognition in autism* (pp. 243–268). New York: Plenum Publishing.

Schultheis, S. F., Boswell, B. B., & Decker, J. (2000). Successful physical activity programming for students with autism. *Focus on Autism and Other Developmental Disabilities, 15*, 159–162.

Seidl, C. M. (2003). Inclusive fitness appraisal developments. In R. D. Steadward, G. D. Wheeler, & E. J. Watkinson (Eds.), *Adapted physical activity* (pp. 383–406). Edmonton, AB: The University of Alberta Press.

Sheinkopf, S. J., & Siegel, B. (1998). Home-based behavioral treatment of young children with autism. *Journal of Autism and Developmental Disorders, 28*, 15–23.

Shumway-Cook, A., & Woollacott, M. H. (2007). *Motor control: Translating research into clinical practice*. Philadelphia: Lippincott, Williams, & Wilkins.

Simpson, R. L. (2005). Evidence-based practices and students with autism spectrum disorders. *Focus on Autism and Other Developmental Disabilities, 20*, 140–149.

Skinner, B. F. (1938). *The behavior of organisms*. New York: Appleton-Century.

Stahmer, A. C. (1995). Teaching symbolic play skills to children with autism using pivotal response training. *Journal of Autism and Developmental Disorders, 25*, 123–141.

Stainback, S., & Stainback, W. (1990). Inclusive schooling. In W. Stainback & S. Stainback (Eds.), *Support networks for inclusive schooling* (pp. 3–24). Baltimore: Paul H. Brookes.

Staples, K. L., & Reid, G. (2010). Fundamental movement skills and autism spectrum disorders. *Journal of Autism and Developmental Disorders, 40*, 209–217. doi: 10.1007/s10803-009-0854-9

Staples, K., Todd, T., & Reid, G. (2006). Physical activity instruction and autism spectrum disorders. *ACHPER Healthy Lifestyles Journal, 53*(3–4), 17–23.

Stokes, T. F., & Baer, D. M. (1977). An implicit technology of generalization. *Journal of Applied Behavior Analysis, 10*, 349–367.

Teitelbaum, P., Teitelbaum, O., Nye, J., Fryman, J., & Maurer, R. G. (1998). Movement analysis in infancy may be useful diagnosis of autism. *Proceedings of the National Academy of Sciences, 95*, 13982–13987.

Todd, T., & Reid, G. (2006). Increasing physical activity in individuals with autism. *Focus on Autism and Other Developmental Disabilities, 21*, 167–176.

Todd, T., Reid, G., & Butler-Kisber, L. (2010). Cycling for students with ASD: Self-regulation promotes sustained physical activity. *Adapted Physical Activity Quarterly, 27*, 226–241.

Ulrich, D. A. (2000). *Test of gross motor development* (2nd ed.). Austin, TX: PRO-ED.

Watanabe, M., & Sturmey, P. (2003). The effect of choice-making opportunities during activity schedules on task engagement of adults with autism. *Journal of Autism and Developmental Disorders, 33*, 535–538.

Watkinson, E. J., & Wall, A. E. (1982). *The PREP play program.* Ottawa, ON: CAHPER.

Watters, R. G., & Watters, W. E. (1980). Decreasing self-stimulatory behavior with physical exercise in a group of autistic boys. *Journal of Autism and Developmental Disorders, 10*, 379–387.

Weber, R. C., & Thorpe, J. (1992). Teaching children with autism through task variation in physical education. *Exceptional Children, 59*, 77–86.

Weiss, M. (1999). Differential rates of skill acquisition and outcomes of early intensive behavioural intervention for autism. *Behavioural Interventions, 14*, 3–22.

Williams, A. M., & Hodges, N. J. (2005). Practice, instruction and skill acquisition in soccer: Challenging tradition. *Journal of Sports Sciences, 23*, 637–650.

World Health Organization. (2003). *Health and development through physical activity and sport.* Geneva: Author.

World Health Organization. (2008). *School policy framework: Implementation of the WHO global strategy on diet, physical activity and health.* Geneva: Author.

Aggression, Tantrums, and Other Externally Driven Challenging Behaviors

26

Nirbhay N. Singh, Giulio E. Lancioni, Alan S.W. Winton, and Judy Singh

By definition, individuals with autism have severe difficulties in reciprocal relationships, verbal and nonverbal communication, unusual repetitive behavior, and restricted interests (American Psychiatric Association, 2000). Furthermore, in about 75–80% of cases, autism is comorbid with intellectual disabilities (National Research Council, 2001). Epidemiological studies indicate that 10–15% of individuals with intellectual disabilities engage in problem behaviors, or what is currently termed "challenging behaviors" (Holden & Gitlesen, 2006; Lowe et al., 2007; Murphy et al., 2005). Challenging behaviors have been defined as "culturally abnormal behavior(s) of such intensity, frequency or duration that the physical safety of the person or others is likely to be placed in serious jeopardy, or behavior which is likely to seriously limit use of, or result in the person being denied access to, ordinary community facilities" (Emerson, 2001, p. 3). Aggression, tantrums, property destruction, disruptive behavior, and self-injury are examples of challenging behavior often displayed by individuals with autism and pervasive developmental disorders (PDD).

Challenging behaviors have received considerable attention in the research literature, as well as in clinical practice, because of negative educational, vocational, and social consequences for the individual. Furthermore, depending on severity, challenging behaviors can significantly impair the quality of life of not only the individual but also parents, siblings, and care staff (Hastings, 2002). Individuals exhibiting challenging behaviors are more likely to be refused community placements of their choice and be more frequently readmitted to institutions or other restrictive settings (Borthwick-Duffy, Eyman, & White, 1987). If they do remain in the community, they may not receive appropriate services because their severe challenging behaviors cannot be well managed by staff, reduce their social network,

and lessen opportunities for community-integrated activities (Anderson, Larkin, Hill, & Chen, 1992). A critical reason for effectively treating challenging behaviors, however, is that they serve as a major impediment to learning in integrated school settings, as well as in the family home (Chadwick, Piroth, Walker, Bernard, & Taylor, 2000), and ineffective or no treatment places these individuals on a very restrictive life trajectory. Additionally, although stereotyped behaviors are not as problematic as other challenging behaviors, they may be precursors to self-injury (Morrison & Rozales-Ruiz, 1997) and produce similar negative consequences such as aggression and self-injury, but they receive minimal attention and are often left untreated (Matson, Benavidez, Compton, Paclawskyj, & Baglio, 1996).

Research indicates that individuals who engage in challenging behaviors often exhibit more than one of these behaviors. For example, Emerson et al. (2001) reported that up to two-thirds of individuals who engage in challenging behavior exhibit two or more such behaviors, with the three most common forms being aggression, self-injury, and property destruction. In addition, each of these behaviors may have multiple topographies. For example, aggression may be present as hitting, kicking, scratching, slapping, and biting, among others. In terms of risk factors, males are more likely to exhibit aggression (Tyrer et al., 2006), but it is unclear if gender per se is a risk factor for challenging behavior. Although, in general, the challenging behaviors of individuals with intellectual disabilities appear to peak between ages 15 and 34 (Oliver, Murphy, & Corbett, 1987), and are much less prevalent in individuals over 40 years of age (Holden & Gitlesen, 2006), they may occur independent of age in individuals with autism (Murphy, Healy, & Leader, 2009). Furthermore, the prevalence of challenging behaviors increases with the degree of intellectual disability, with the highest rates being evident in those with profound intellectual disabilities (Borthwick-Duffy, 1994).

N.N. Singh (✉)
American Health and Wellness Institute, Verona, VA 24484, USA
e-mail: nirbsingh52@aol.com

J.L. Matson, P. Sturmey (eds.), *International Handbook of Autism and Pervasive Developmental Disorders*,
Autism and Child Psychopathology Series, DOI 10.1007/978-1-4419-8065-6_26, © Springer Science+Business Media, LLC 2011

Treatment Approaches

In the first comprehensive survey of treatments used by parents of children with autism, Green et al. (2006) reported data from 552 parents who responded to each of 111 treatments as being one they (a) currently used, (b) used previously but not presently, and (c) never used. The 111 treatments were grouped into seven categories: (a) medications, (b) vitamin supplements, (c) special diets, (d) medical procedures, (e) educational/therapy approaches (e.g., applied behavior analysis, speech therapy, and music therapy), (f) alternative therapy/medicine (e.g., acupuncture and aromatherapy), and (g) combined programs (e.g., TEACCH and Giant Steps). Of the 111 listed treatments, 108 were being used, or had been used in the past, by one or more parents. The mean number of current and past treatments was 7 and 8, respectively. The five most frequently used treatments included standard therapies (e.g., speech and music; 70%), followed by other skill-based therapies (e.g., Fast ForWard and social stories; 61%), skill-based training based on principles of applied behavior analysis (56%), medication (53%), and physiological therapies (e.g., auditory integration training and sensory integration) (47%). As this study did not parse out what the therapies targeted, it is not possible to separate treatments for skill deficits from those for behavioral excesses.

In a similar but much more detailed survey, Goin-Kochel, Myers, and Mackintosh (2007) reported findings from 479 parents of children with autism spectrum disorders (ASD). About 43% of the parents reported that their children had tried pharmacological treatments and about 32% had been on special diets. Behavioral and other interventions included applied behavior analysis [including picture exchange communication system (PECS)], early intervention services, floor time, music therapy, occupational therapy, physical therapy, sensory integration, and speech therapy. Overall, the children were receiving between four and six treatments and had tried a mean of eight treatments in the past, replicating the findings of Green et al. (2006). As in the Green et al. study, data were not presented in terms of what the therapies targeted (i.e., skill deficits or behavioral excesses); however, most parents rated the treatments and therapies they used as being effective for their children (Goin-Kochel, Mackintosh, & Myers, 2009). For example, almost 77 and 73% of the parents rated applied behavior analysis and positive behavior support as being effective, respectively. Different classes of medication were rated as effective for 50–80% of children.

Our knowledge of treatments for individuals with ASD has grown exponentially in the last few decades; however, not all of our knowledge is derived from well-designed scientific research. For example, we have an abundance of subjective evidence from parents and other caregivers, as mentioned above, but on closer scrutiny, these have often been found to be unreliable (Green, 1996). Furthermore, even when controlled studies have shown treatments or therapies to be ineffective, parents and other caregivers continue to use them in the hope that their child will be an exception and will benefit from using them. The use of facilitated communication (Jacobson, Mulick, & Schwartz, 1995; Mostert, 2001) and secretin (Sturmey, 2005; Williams, Wray, & Wheeler, 2005) is probably the most glaring example of discredited treatment that continues to be used. Fortunately, there are now guidelines for determining empirically validated treatments (Beutler, Moleiro, & Talebi, 2002; Chambless & Hollon, 1998). Data for well-established treatments are typically derived from randomized controlled trials, as is evidenced by some of the psychopharmacological studies discussed in this chapter, and from small N experimental studies (Chambless & Hollon, 1998).

Aggression and Other Challenging Behaviors

In this chapter, we focus on the treatment of aggression, tantrums, and other externally driven challenging behaviors of individuals with ASD. Our focus is on current evidence-based behavioral, cognitive–behavioral, and pharmacological therapies, and on the current status of treatment research.

Behavioral Interventions

Most interventions for aggressive and other externally driven challenging behaviors of individuals with ASD are based on principles and procedures derived from applied behavior analysis and positive behavior support (Carr, 2007; Carr et al., 2002). Although some research predates it, most effective behavioral interventions are based on a functional assessment technology that enables researchers and clinicians to derive testable hypotheses about the functions of the behavior in specific settings (Matson & Nebel-Schwalm, 2007; Matson, 2009). At least one intervention is clearly aligned with the key function of a challenging behavior. The interventions vary in scope, ranging from a single focus (e.g., to eliminate aggressive behavior) to multiple foci (e.g., to eliminate aggressive behavior, teach social interaction skills, and improve quality of life).

Behavioral interventions for aggression, tantrums, and other externally driven challenging behaviors in individuals with autism can be broadly divided into three groups: (a) antecedent strategies; (b) instructional strategies; and (c) contingency management strategies. Antecedent strategies are used when a functional assessment suggests that the challenging behavior is maintained by environmental, biological, or other setting events (Luiselli, 1998). The behavioral intervention involves manipulating the antecedents in order to preempt the occurrence of the challenging behavior. The essence of this approach is that the assessment provides information on what is the causal risk factor for the occurrence of a behavior and enables the clinician to develop and implement procedures that would reduce the probability of the individual needing to engage in the behavior to achieve an outcome that reinforces the behavior; outcomes such as changing staff behavior, the environment, or other contextual conditions which may be behavioral or biological. Ideally, proactive antecedent manipulations provide individuals with an environment that encourages and reinforces healthy, socially acceptable behaviors, without them having to engage in challenging behaviors (Luiselli, 2006).

Instructional strategies can be used to teach the individual alternative ways of achieving similar outcomes to those obtained through engaging in challenging behaviors, thus making the problem behavior inefficient. This approach, based on the concept of *functional equivalence* (Carr, 1988), teaches an individual more efficient and socially acceptable behavior that functions in an equivalent way to the challenging behavior. Functional communication training (FCT) is the most commonly used method for teaching an individual an acceptable form of communication (e.g., speech, sign language, gesture, and picture exchange) as a functionally equivalent alternative to challenging behavior (Carr et al., 1994; Durand, 1990).

Another way of doing this is by teaching self-management skills to the individual. Skinner (1953) conceptualized self-management in terms of controlling and controlled where "One response, the *controlling response*, affects variables in such a way as to change the probability of the other, the *controlled response*. The controlling response may manipulate any of the variables of which the controlled response is a function; hence there are a good many different forms of self-control" (p. 231). In this context, the controlled response would include aggression, tantrums, and other externally driven behaviors, and the controlling response would include counting to 10, relaxing, enduring increasing delay of gratification, enhancing social skills, and using mindfulness-based techniques (Halle, Bambara, & Reichle, 2005; Singh et al., in press). Teaching the individual that engaging in the challenging behavior is not going to produce the intended effects (e.g., a tangible reinforcer) is another method of decreasing or eliminating the behavior by making it ineffective (Crone & Horner, 2003).

Contingency management strategies use consequences to produce behavior change. For example, positive reinforcers are used to increase socially acceptable or desirable behaviors and punishers are used to decrease undesirable behaviors. In some cases, when a behavior threatens imminent harm to self or others, a graduated series of consequences may be programmed, such as verbal redirection, blocking, and physical redirection, in an effort to terminate the response chain that may lead to aggressive behavior. If these actions are not effective, then more restrictive consequences may have to be applied.

Antecedent Strategies

Antecedent strategies include those that manipulate environmental conditions to preempt the occurrence of a behavior. These changes may involve rearranging the actual conditions that lead to the occurrence of a behavior (e.g., overcrowding and placement of furniture) or artificially manipulating the conditions to show performance of a behavior that is not firmly established in the individual's repertoire. For example, video self-modeling (VSM) enables an individual to view himself behaving in situations in more advanced ways than his current functioning. That is, a person who stutters can view himself as not having a stutter, a person who responds with anger in a given situation can view himself as responding with calmness, and so on. VSM has been used to treat a number of clinical conditions (e.g., depression, elective mutism, and stuttering) and to enhance educational performance (e.g., in math, life skills, social behaviors, and language). In one of three studies, Buggey (2005) assessed the effects of VSM on the behavior of two boys aged almost 7 and 8 years. The first boy had a diagnosis of Asperger's disorder and the other boy had autism, and both engaged in tantrums (e.g., flailing arms and legs, weeping, and disruptive muttering). When the boys viewed their VSM tapes immediately prior to each class, their tantrums decreased significantly in the classroom. The reductions in tantrums were maintained at follow-up. This study suggests that VSM might provide a technological solution to behavior change in children with ASD.

Much like picture prompts, social stories provide cues to the individual regarding his anticipated response to particular environmental conditions. They provide social information that informs the individual about an expected response. For example, the story may involve a sequence of activities expected of the individual in a classroom, and the sentence "When class begins, I need to be seated quietly at my desk" informs the student that he should sit quietly. In some ways it is like PECS, where the teacher may provide the child with a picture cue for anticipated behavior. Kuttler, Myles, and Carlson (1998) reported a study that tested the effects of social stories on the precursors to tantrum behavior of a 12-year-old boy with autism. Two social stories were constructed, one for each of two settings, and the relevant story was read to the boy, prior to his engaging in activities in that setting. Using a reversal design, the effects of the social stories were tested on two precursors to tantrums – inappropriate vocalizations, and dropping to the floor. During the social stories condition, the boy's behaviors were at a zero level in one setting and at very low rates in the other. This study suggests that providing advance cues to children with autism may assist them in responding appropriately to specific environmental conditions.

Noncontingent reinforcement (NCR) is another antecedent intervention used to reduce maladaptive behavior by presenting a stimulus with known reinforcing properties on a fixed- or variable-time schedule, independent of the target behaviors. For example, Ingvarsson, Kahng, and Hausman (2008) assessed the effects of NCR on the maladaptive behavior of an 8-year-old girl with autism, whose behavior was maintained by escape from demands and access to edible items. The girl engaged in aggression (e.g., hitting, scratching, pinching, biting, kicking, and pushing), disruptions (e.g., banging on objects, swiping objects off surfaces, and throwing, breaking, or otherwise damaging or destroying objects), and self-injury. They tested the comparative effects of high-density NCR (i.e., an edible delivered before every demand) and low-density NCR (i.e., an edible delivered prior to every fourth demand), and high-density NCR with differential reinforcement of alternative behavior (DRA). Results showed that NCR was effective in reducing the rate of maladaptive behaviors and in increasing task completions following verbal instructions and model prompts. Furthermore, both high- and low-density NCR schedules were found to be equally effective, and the high-density NCR and DRA differed minimally in effectiveness.

In another study, Mueller, Wilczynski, Moore, Fusilier, and Trahant (2001) assessed the effects of relative preference of restricted and noncontingently available stimuli on the aggressive behavior (e.g., hitting, kicking, slapping, biting, pinching, and head butting) of an 8-year-old boy with autism. A functional assessment indicated that his aggression was maintained by access to tangible items. His aggressive behavior was recorded when high, medium, or low preference materials were restricted or were noncontingently available with alternate high, medium, or low preference materials. Results showed that his aggressive behavior was highest when highly preferred materials were restricted, regardless of the preference level of the noncontingently available alternative items. Furthermore, moderate levels of aggression occurred when less preferred stimuli were restricted even when the alternative items were more preferred.

Instructional Strategies

During FCT, individuals are taught a socially acceptable form of communication as a functional alternative to the challenging behavior. Sigafoos and Meikle (1996) reported

using FCT to treat the challenging behaviors of two boys with autism. The boys were 8 years old and their challenging behaviors included aggression (e.g., hitting, pushing, biting, and pinching), self-injury, and property destruction (e.g., breaking, ripping, and throwing objects). A functional analysis showed that these behaviors had multiple functions, most prominent being obtaining attention and tangible reinforcers. Sigafoos and Meikle taught the children two communication responses as functional alternatives to engaging in these behaviors and tested the effects of the FCT within a multiple baseline design. When the children used alternative functional communication strategies, their maladaptive behaviors decreased to zero or near-zero levels.

Thompson, Fisher, Piazza, and Kuhn (1998) used direct and indirect methods of functional assessment with a 7-year-old boy who had PDD, severe intellectual disabilities, and severe hemophilia, and who showed several topographies of aggression (e.g., hitting, kicking, pinching, scratching, and grinding his chin against others). Functional assessments indicated that his aggression was maintained by attention, but his chin grinding was independent of social contingencies. Using an FCT methodology, the boy was taught to hand a picture communication card to the therapist to gain 30 s of verbal and physical attention, as an alternative to aggression. When he engaged in aggression, it was ignored (i.e., put on an extinction schedule). When the FCT plus extinction treatment was implemented, all topographies of aggression were greatly reduced except for chin grinding, which was subsequently treated using response blocking and an alternative form of chin stimulation.

Durand (1999) reported a study on five students that needed an assistive device for communication, who engaged in challenging behaviors. One of these students was a 9.5-year-old boy with autism and severe intellectual disabilities. He was very aggressive toward his teachers, peers, and family members. A functional assessment showed that low adult attention was correlated with aggressive behavior. When he was taught to use an assistive device to recruit adult attention, his aggressive behavior was reduced from a mean of 42 to 0.5% of intervals. Furthermore, he was able to use, without prompting, his assisted communication device to access adult attention in the community, without engaging in aggressive behavior. Similar results were obtained with another boy with autism and severe intellectual disabilities. This study demonstrated the utility of FCT not only in controlling aggressive behavior but also in its generalized application to novel community settings.

Braithwaite and Richdale (2000) assessed the effects of combining FCT with extinction on the aggressive and self-injurious behavior of a 7-year-old boy with autism and mild to moderate intellectual disability. He was at a special school in an integrated setting and engaged in aggression (e.g., hitting and head butting) and self-injury. A functional analysis suggested that aggression and self-injury provided escape from difficult tasks and access to preferred tangibles. As alternative responses to aggression and self-injury, prior to intervention for access to preferred items, he was taught to say "I want ____, please," and prior to intervention for escape, he was taught to say "I need help, please." All occurrences of maladaptive behavior were subjected to extinction. During the access condition, his maladaptive behaviors decreased from a mean rate of 94% of trials to 1.3%, and his correct use of the alternative response increased from 0% to a mean of 96%. During the escape condition, his maladaptive behaviors decreased from a mean rate of 92% of trials to 9.6%, and his correct use of the alternative response increased from 0% to a mean of 79%. The most significant findings were that the maladaptive behaviors decreased very rapidly and were maintained at zero levels when the delay of reinforcement was increased.

Hagopian, Wilson, and Wilder (2001) conducted two consecutive functional analyses on a 6-year-old boy with autism and mild intellectual disabilities, to determine the nature of the negative reinforcement that maintained his aggression (e.g., hitting, kicking, scratching, and head butting), disruption (e.g., screaming, throwing objects, swiping objects off tables, and tearing objects), and other maladaptive behaviors. These behaviors were maintained by escape from attention and access to preferred tangible items. As a first step, he was taught to say "play by myself" to terminate attention and "toys please" to access toys. Once this functional communication was established, a treatment plan consisting of FCT, extinction following the occurrence of the maladaptive behaviors, delay to reinforcement (i.e., waiting to receive toys following a request), and NCR was implemented. Results showed substantial (96%) decreases in aggressive and disruptive behaviors in both escape from attention and access to tangible items. Furthermore, communication increased during both conditions.

Schindler and Horner (2005) assessed the impact of FCT in a school setting with three children enrolled in an early intervention program for children with ASD. Two of the children were 4 years old and the other was 5 years old. They engaged in aggression (e.g., pinching, biting, and hair pulling), tantrums, and other maladaptive behaviors (e.g., screaming and noncompliance). Functional assessments suggested that aggression and/or tantrums were maintained by access to preferred activities for one child, escape from aversive features of an activity in another, and avoidance of transitions to unpredictable activities in the third child. The children were taught specific functional communication skills that they could use as alternatives to engaging in maladaptive behavior. Results showed substantial decreases in maladaptive behavior for all three children.

Vollmer, Borrero, Lalli, and Daniel (1999) described a study that looked at the relationship between impulsiveness and self-control. The study involved two children, one of whom was a 9-year-old boy with autism who engaged in severe aggression (i.e., hitting, slapping, and pushing others). A functional analysis suggested that his aggression was maintained by access to material items. Based on the functional assessment findings, a treatment plan was developed that included FCT and FCT with delay. (Further assessments were undertaken to better understand the mechanisms involved in his impulsive behavior and self-control in terms of reinforcer magnitude, but that discussion is beyond the scope of the present chapter.) Reinforcing appropriate alternative communication decreased the boy's aggressive behavior.

Schmit, Alper, Raschke, and Ryndak (2000) assessed the effects of using a modified PECS to control the tantrums of a 6-year-old boy with autism. The boy would engage in tantrums (e.g., screaming, hitting an adult, falling to the ground, and refusing to walk) when making a transition from one activity to another. He had a single word in his verbal repertoire (i.e., "no"), which he used appropriately and in context. He was taught to use the PECS prior to the study. Immediately preceding the anticipated transition to a new activity, he was given verbal and photographic cues of the next activity. The effects of the PECS were assessed across three school contexts, within a multiple baseline design. Results showed substantial decreases in tantrums across all three contexts, and the positive changes in the boy's behavior were evident during a maintenance condition.

In a related study, Dooley, Wilczenski, and Torem (2001) used PECS to decrease aggressive behavior, and increase cooperative behavior, in a 3-year-old boy with PDDs. He engaged in both aggression (e.g., hitting, kicking, and biting) and tantrums (loud, distressed vocalizations). A functional analysis suggested that this was because he found transitions from one activity to the next confusing and distressing, and engaging in aggression and tantrums allowed him to exert maladaptive control over his environment. In the first intervention, his use of PECS was paired with reinforcement for task completion, and in the second intervention, PECS was used by itself. His aggression and tantrums decreased from a mean of 13 incidents per day during baseline to only 10 incidents during the first 3 days on intervention, and was at zero levels thereafter for the next 3 days. When PECS was used by itself, there were only two instances of maladaptive behavior over 9 days on intervention. Concomitantly, compliance with his teacher's directions increased dramatically.

Frea, Arnold, and Vittimberga (2001) assessed the effects of using PECS and choice-making opportunities on the aggressive behavior of a 4-year-old nonverbal child with autism and moderate mental retardation. His uncontrolled aggression (e.g., biting, kicking, and hitting), toward peers and adults, put him at risk for losing his integrated school placement. Prior to formal intervention, he was taught to use PECS, phases 1–3, to make requests of his choosing. Once he mastered this, Frea et al. assessed its effects on the boy's aggressive behavior, using a multiple baseline across settings design. Aggression decreased rapidly to a zero level by the 6th day in the first setting and by the 3rd day in the second setting. Concomitantly, the use of picture communication during the 10-min sessions increased from a zero level during baseline to an average of 5.5 in the first setting, and to an average of 6.2 in the second setting. These results ensured continued placement at the integrated school.

Heckaman, Alber, Hooper, and Heward (1998) investigated the effects of two instructional strategies on the disruptive behavior of four boys, aged 6–9 years, all diagnosed with autism and moderate to severe disabilities. During classroom instruction, the boys engaged in disruptive behaviors that included aggression, screaming, whining, banging hands or objects on desktops, and throwing objects. Hechaman et al. compared the effects of a least-to-most prompting procedure (LTM) to those of a progressive time delay (PTD) procedure, on errors and disruptive behaviors when difficult tasks were presented. The PTD procedure more effectively reduced both error rate and disruptive behavior, for all four boys. This study indicated that aggression, and other externally driven behaviors that students exhibit during instruction, might be amenable to change via instructional technology. Unfortunately, very little work has been done with this method of behavior change.

Contingency Contracting

Contingency contracting is an agreement, or clinical contract, made between an individual (the person whose behavior is to be changed) and a parent, a teacher, or a therapist. The contract specifies the behaviors that will be consequated. Although contingency contracts have been widely used in the clinical literature, there is a dearth of research on individuals with ASD. Mruzek, Cohen, and Smith (2007) assessed the effects of contingency contracting with a 9-year-old boy with autism and a 10-year-old boy with Asperger's disorder who exhibited tantrums, physical aggression, and antisocial vocalizations. Mruzek et al. developed written contingency contracts with the two boys that promoted adherence to rules of conduct, as opposed to a direct focus on engagement in maladaptive behaviors. The assumption was that, by focusing on socially acceptable alternatives, the boys' maladaptive behaviors would decrease and eventually be eliminated. They assessed the effects of the contingency contracts using a changing criterion design. Results showed that the contingency contracts were successful in reducing the target behaviors in both children.

Multiple Component Strategies

In addition to these three broad groups of interventions, some researchers used multi-component treatment procedures to control challenging behaviors. For example, Paisey, Fox, Curran, Hooper, and Whitney (1991) used a package of treatments with a 11-year-old girl with autism who engaged in screaming, foot stamping, property destruction, and physical aggression. The treatment package, which targeted all of her maladaptive behaviors, included differential reinforcement of other behavior (DRO), publically posted good behavior rules, physical management training, and redirection to relaxation. The treatment was delivered by both trained professionals and the girl's mother. Results showed that both the professional staff and the mother were able to successfully implement the treatment, but the mother was unable to achieve or maintain the clinical outcomes in the absence of the professional staff.

Foxx and Garito (2007) used a comprehensive behavioral intervention protocol to treat severe behavior problems of a 12-year-old preadolescent boy with autism. He exhibited a number of challenging behaviors, including aggression, disruption, and self-injury. A large number of behavioral techniques had been used prior to the current interventions, including discrimination training, extinction, DRA, DRO, facial screening, and physical restraint, all without much success. In this clinical case study, Foxx and Garito developed a four-phase intervention: phase 1 (Baseline) consisted of two interventions that had been developed by an inpatient facility. The child's school day was divided into 15-min segments in which he could spend 5 min in self-directed behaviors and 10 min in teacher- or parent-directed activities. Phase 2 (home and community-based program) included differential reinforcement of appropriate behaviors, token economy for compliance with classroom rules, response cost for aggression and self-injury, redirection, and physical restraint. Phase 3 (community-based program) included refining phase 2 procedures and adding contingent physical exercise for aggressive behavior, overcorrection for dangerous and disruptive behaviors, and contingent movement for off-task classroom behaviors. Phase 4 (transition to public school classroom) included phase 3 procedures, but with contingent movement replaced by a modified response cost procedure. Aggressive and disruptive behaviors were highest during baseline and gradually decreased across the remaining three phases to near-zero level in phase 4. This successful treatment was maintained for 2 years.

In a similar clinical case study, Foxx and Meindl (2007) used a multi-component behavioral intervention to treat the aggressive behavior of a 13-year-old preadolescent with autism. His aggressive behavior included hitting, kicking, pinching, and especially biting and head butting. He also engaged in property destruction. Previous unsuccessful interventions for aggression included extinction, time-out, restraint, token economy, and DRO. An informal functional assessment suggested that aggression functioned primarily to escape academic or social demands, and to obtain desired items. The new interventions included a token economy system, DRO, response cost, overcorrection, and physical restraint. Aggressive behavior decreased from a mean of 102 incidents per day during baseline to a mean of about 5 incidents per day during the first month of intervention, to a mean of 0.29 incidents per day by the end of the sixth month of intervention. Aggressive behavior remained at or near-zero levels for another 6 months.

These three case studies illustrate how multi-component packages can be used to produce good clinical outcomes; however, they were not controlled investigations, and it is impossible to determine the contribution of each of the multiple components of treatment, or to determine if all components were necessary. While the authors make a case for using restrictive procedures, such procedures are generally eschewed in current practice.

Other research using multi-component strategies, but under controlled conditions, shows how less restrictive procedures can be very effective in reducing target behaviors, including aggression. For example, Kern, Carberry, and Haidara (1997) assessed the effects of an intervention package that included gradually increasing the delay to reinforcement, mand training (i.e., developing an appropriate alternative communicative behavior to replace the maladaptive behavior), and extinction on the self-injury and aggressive behavior (e.g., grabbing clothing of another individual, typically around the neck) of a 15-year-old girl with autism and severe intellectual disabilities. Functional assessment suggested that self-injury allowed her access to food at mealtimes, and aggression allowed her to escape from tasks. Based on these findings, a treatment package was developed and tested using a reversal design. The treatment package was effective in decreasing self-injury but was more effective with aggression when the gradual delay procedure was removed from the package.

Hagopian, Bruzek, Bowman, and Jennett (2007) assessed and treated the maladaptive behavior of three children with autism. The participants were a 12-year-old boy who engaged in aggression (e.g., pinching, scratching, hitting, kicking, and hitting others with objects), disruption (e.g., throwing objects, banging on hard objects, and kicking and hitting walls), and self-injury; a 6-year-old boy who engaged in aggression (e.g., hitting, kicking, pinching, scratching, grabbing), disruption (e.g., hitting or kicking surfaces, throwing objects), self-injury, and screaming; and a 12-year-old girl who engaged in aggression (e.g., hair pulling, pinching, hitting, and kicking). When a formal functional analysis proved inconclusive, further observations and analyses

suggested response interruption occasioned the maladaptive behaviors. Based on this finding, the treatment package included differential and noncontingent reinforcement without interruption, extinction, and a demand fading procedure. This package successfully reduced the maladaptive behaviors to low levels and generalized the treatment across settings, people, and time.

Cognitive–Behavioral Strategies

Many symptoms of psychological distress may arise from an individual's irrational thinking that leads to problems in cognition, behavior, and affect. An individual can use one of a number of cognitive behavior therapy approaches, such as self-monitoring, reality testing, and other cognitive restructuring approaches, to modify his or her irrational or negative thinking. The particular technique chosen will depend on the nature of the psychological distress (e.g., psychiatric disorder and maladaptive behavior), and mediating and moderating variables (e.g., status of medical and psychological distress, cognitive level of the individual, motivation for therapeutic change, and ability to shift the focus of one's attention).

Mindfulness-based techniques, a recent addition to cognitive behavior therapy, generally aim to change the individual's relationship to thoughts and feelings instead of changing the individual's response to irrational thoughts (Shapiro & Carlson, 2009). Like cognitive behavior therapy itself, mindfulness-based approaches encompass a wide range of techniques that are customized to the needs of the individual. Mindfulness has been described not only as a Buddhist practice but also as a state, a trait, a process, and an outcome (Singh, Lancioni, Wahler, Winton, & Singh, 2008). It ranges from Gunaratana's (2009, p. 197) almost too brief definition, "the quality of mind that notices and recognizes," to Nyanaponika Thera's (1996, p. 30) description of mindfulness as "the clear and single-minded awareness of what actually happens to us and in us, at successive moments of perception. It is called "bare" because it attends just to the bare facts of a perception as presented either through the five physical senses or through the mind . . . without reacting to them by deed, speech or by mental comment which may be one of self-reference (like, dislike, etc.), judgment, or reflection." We have defined mindfulness as "the awareness and nonjudgmental acceptance by a clear, calm mind of one's moment-to-moment experience, without either pursuing the experience or pushing it away" (Singh et al., in press).

In the context of individuals with challenging behaviors, there is an emerging body of research that attests to the effectiveness of mindfulness-based procedures in assisting individuals with intellectual disabilities to self-manage their challenging behaviors (Singh et al., in press; Singh et al., 2006). A mindfulness-based procedure, *Meditation on the*

Soles of the Feet, has been shown to be reasonably effective for self-management of aggression, disruption, and property destruction by individuals with intellectual disabilities (Singh et al., in press). In a translational study, Adkins, Singh, Winton, McKeegan, and Singh (2010) extended this work by having a community-based therapist teach this procedure to three individuals with intellectual disabilities to control their maladaptive behaviors that included verbal aggression, disruptive behavior, and physical aggression. They were taught to shift the focus of their attention from the negative emotions that triggered their maladaptive behavior to a neutral stimulus, the soles of their feet. All three individuals were able to reduce their maladaptive behaviors to near-zero levels and maintain their community placement, which had been in jeopardy due to their maladaptive behavior.

In a recent study, Adkins (2010) taught three adolescents with Asperger's syndrome to use *Meditation on the Soles of the Feet* to control their physical aggression in the family home and during outings in the community. The adolescents had moderate rates of aggression (i.e., between 2 and 6 incidents per week) prior to training in the mindfulness-based procedure. During mindfulness practice, which lasted between 17 and 24 weeks, their mean rates of aggression decreased to 0.9, 1.09, and 0.88 incidents per week, respectively, for the three boys, with no incidents during the last 3 weeks of practice. During a 4-year follow-up, no episodes of physical aggression occurred. This study suggests that adolescents with Asperger's syndrome can successfully use a mindfulness-based procedure to control their aggressive behavior.

In a novel use of mindfulness training, Singh et al. (2006) taught three mothers of children diagnosed with autism the philosophy and practice of mindfulness in a 12-week course and assessed the outcome of the training on their children's behavior. In addition to monitoring changes in the children's behavior, the mothers rated satisfaction with their parenting skills and the interactions with their children. Mothers' mindful parenting decreased their children's aggression, noncompliance, and self-injury and also increased the mothers' satisfaction with their parenting skills and interactions with their children. Positive changes occurred in the children's behavior, without their parents actively focusing on specific contingencies that might govern their adaptive or maladaptive behavior. This study suggests that training mothers in mindfulness might produce measurable beneficial behavior change in their children because of the positive mother and child transactions that result from such training.

In sum, there is growing evidence from single-subject experimental studies that behavioral and cognitive–behavioral interventions can be used to reduce aggression, tantrums, and property destruction in children with ASD. Although the data are not from randomized controlled trials,

based on the current evidence, we can state confidently that these are well-established treatments for aggression and other externalizing behaviors in this population.

Pharmacological Interventions

There are no well-established pharmacological treatments for the core symptoms of ASD, but there is a growing literature on psychopharmacological interventions for specific behavioral symptoms associated with these disorders. Although a few drug studies have targeted the core symptoms of autism, most target symptoms that are associated with ASD, such as aggression, self-injury, tantrums, irritability, and hyperactivity. These behaviors interfere with learning and daily functioning, and compete with habilitation efforts. By reducing these behaviors, pharmacotherapy makes the individuals more amenable to educational and psychosocial interventions (Filipek, Steinberg-Epstein, & Book, 2006; Stigler, Posey, & McDougle, 2002). Studies show that typical antipsychotics, such as the dopamine receptor antagonist haloperidol, have statistically significant effects in controlling externally driven behaviors such as aggression, disruption, and property destruction by children and adolescents, but the clinical effects are very modest. Moreover, there has been considerable concern over these drugs because of frequently observed dyskinesias and other extrapyramidal symptoms. Therefore, these drugs have been gradually replaced by the new generation antipsychotics (e.g., risperidone, olanzapine, quetiapine, clozapine, ziprasidone, aripiprazole), dopamine, and serotonin receptor antagonists that purportedly present a lower risk of acute extrapyramidal symptoms and tardive dyskinesia but pose a much greater risk for metabolic syndrome (De Leon, Greenlee, Barber, Sabaawi, & Singh, 2009).

Although a wide range of drugs have been tested, the most promising drugs for treating aggression, tantrums, disruptive behavior, and property destruction in individuals with ASD appear to be the new generation antipsychotics and some antidepressants (Chavez, Chavez-Brown, & Rey, 2006; Malone & Waheed, 2009; Stachnik & Nunn-Thompson, 2007). Our review will focus only on these two drug classes and only on those studies in which aggression, tantrums, and other externally driven challenging behaviors were the primary targets of the drug trials. Even within these two drug classes, we do not cover the entire gamut of drugs because of the very limited evidence for some of them in treating the maladaptive behavior of individuals with ASD. In effect, we cover one typical antipsychotic (i.e., haloperidol), six atypical or new general antipsychotics (i.e., risperidone, olanzapine, quetiapine, clozapine, ziprasidone, and aripiprazole), and three antidepressants (i.e., fluvoxamine, fluoxetine, and sertraline).

Antipsychotic Medications

Haloperidol

In a series of early studies in children with autism, Campbell et al. (1978, 1982) showed that haloperidol reduced behavioral symptoms and facilitated learning in an enriched psychosocial environment. In a double-blind, placebo-controlled study, Anderson et al. (1984) administered 0.5–4.0 mg/day of haloperidol to 40 children with autism, aged 2–7 years. When compared to placebo, this resulted in general clinical improvement, facilitation and retention of discrimination learning, and decreased behavioral symptoms, including angry affect on the Children's Psychiatric Rating Scale (CPRS; Guy, 1976). These findings were replicated in a 4-week double-blind, placebo-controlled trial of haloperidol by Anderson et al. (1989) in a sample of 45 children with autism, aged 2–8 years, at dosages ranging from 0.25 to 4.0 mg/day (mean, 0.84 mg/day). The use of haloperidol has waned in recent years, however, because of its potential for significant adverse effects, including excessive sedation, acute dystonic reactions, and tardive dyskinesia.

Risperidone

The Food and Drug Administration (FDA) has approved risperidone for the treatment of symptoms associated with autistic disorder, including irritability, aggression, self-injury, and tantrums in children and adolescents with autistic disorder, aged 5–16 years. Until recently, most of the investigations involving the new generation antipsychotics in individuals with intellectual disabilities involved risperidone. The early case studies found the drug to be effective in treating aggression and other externally driven challenging behaviors across a wide age range and suggested that controlled trials may be warranted.

McDougle et al. (1995) used risperidone to treat two adults with autistic disorder (aged 20 and 31 years) and one adult with pervasive developmental disorder not otherwise specified (PDD NOS) (aged 44 years) for impulsive aggression, social relatedness, and repetitive thoughts and behavior. The dosage started at 1 mg/day and was titrated up until therapeutic effects were observed, with the final dosages ranging from 2 to 8 mg/day. Significant reductions in impulsive aggression were observed in all three adults, and these improvements were maintained for a minimum of 1 year.

Demb (1996) treated three children with PDDs and intellectual disabilities (aged 5, 7, and 10 years) with risperidone for aggression, tantrums, self-injury, and other maladaptive behaviors. They were treated with 3, 1, and 1 mg/day of risperidone, respectively, together with other psychotropic drugs. The authors reported significant reductions in maladaptive behaviors, especially aggression, self-injury, and agitation.

Fisman and Steele (1996) treated 14 children and adolescents with PDD, aged 9–17 years (mean age, 12.7 years), with risperidone. The dosage was started at 0.5 mg/day and was increased, in 0.25 mg/day increments, every 5–7 days, with the final dosages ranging from 0.75 to 1.5 mg/day, as clinically indicated. While the data presentation was sparse, a significant decrease in the disruptive behavior of the children and adolescents was noted.

In a 12-week, open-label study, McDougle et al. (1997) investigated the short-term effectiveness and safety of risperidone in 18 children and adolescents with PDD, aged 5–18 years (mean age, 10.2 years), for aggression and impulsivity. Risperidone was initiated at 0.5 mg/day and increased by 0.5 mg every week, as clinically indicated, with the dosage ranging from 1 to 4 mg/day (mean dosage, 1.8 ± 1.0 mg/day). All children and adolescents completed the trial, and 12 of the 18 were considered clinical responders on the Clinical Global Impression (CGI) scale [National Institute of Mental Health (NIMH), 1985]. Among other findings, there was a statistically significant reduction in aggression and impulsivity among the responders. The most frequent side effects included weight gain by 12 children and adolescents, ranging from 10 to 35 lb (mean weight, 17.8 ± 7.5 lb), and sedation.

In an open-label study, Horrigan and Barnhill (1997) treated 11 male outpatients with autistic disorder and moderate to severe intellectual disabilities, aged 6–34 years (mean age, 18.3 years), with risperidone for severe explosive aggression. The drug was initiated at 0.5 mg/day and titrated up in 0.25–0.5 mg increments every 5–7 days until therapeutic or adverse effects were observed. The dosages ranged from 0.5 to 1.5 mg/day, with a modal dosage of 0.5 mg/day at 4 weeks and 4 months. Risperidone was given as monotherapy for five participants and as adjunctive medication for the remaining six. The final dose of risperidone was achieved within 4 weeks of beginning the trial. Two participants dropped out of the trial, one at week 2 for medication nonadherence and one at week 10 for a possible chemical hepatitis. All remaining participants showed statistically significant decreases in aggression, as well as in self-injury and overactivity. An average weight gain of 0.47 kg/week was a serious side effect with eight participants, but no other extrapyramidal symptoms were reported.

In an open-label study, Perry, Pataki, Munoz-Silva, Armenteros, and Silva (1997) evaluated the effectiveness of risperidone in six children and adolescents with PDD, aged 7–14 years (mean age, 10.7 years). For five participants, the targets were aggression and, for four of these, also tantrums. All but one had multiple trials of medications (e.g., haloperidol and clomipramine) but their behavior had proven refractory to these medications. Risperidone was initiated at 0.5 or 1.0 mg/day and was increased by 0.5 mg/day every few days until therapeutic or adverse effects were observed. The dosages ranged from 1 to 6 mg/day (mean dosage, 2.7 mg/day). Aggression and tantrums were reduced in all five participants, and three of them continued to show a good response to the drug for 2 years. The most serious side effect was that five of the six participants showed a mean weight gain of 12 lb, over 7 weeks.

In an 8-week, open-label study, Findling, Maxwell, and Wiznitzer (1997) evaluated the effectiveness and tolerability of risperidone monotherapy in six children with autistic disorder, aged 5–9.5 years (mean age, 7.4 years). The children's target behaviors included aggression, tantrums, restlessness, irritability, and fearfulness. The starting dosage was 0.25 mg/day and titrated up in 0.25 mg increments at weekly intervals until therapeutic or adverse effects were observed. By the end of the 4th week, the mean daily dosage was 1.1 mg (range, 0.75–1.5 mg/day). All participants completed the trial and were clinically responsive to the drug. In each case, aggression and tantrums were ameliorated with individualized dosages of risperidone. The most common side effect was weight gain. One participant developed extrapyramidal symptoms (i.e., parkinsonism) that were alleviated with a reduction in dosage from 1.0 to 0.075 mg/day.

In a 12-week, open-label trial, Nicolson, Awad, and Sloman (1998) evaluated the effectiveness and side effects of risperidone in 10 children with autistic disorder, aged 4.5–10.8 years (mean age, 7.2 years). Risperidone was initiated at 0.5 mg/day and increased weekly by this amount until therapeutic or adverse effects were observed. The mean dosage was 1.3 ± 0.5 mg/day, with a maximum dosage of 6 mg/day or 0.1 mg/kg/day, whichever was less. Eight of the 10 children were rated as clinical responders on the CGI scale (NIMH, 1985). Behavioral ratings showed clinically significant reductions in aggression and/or tantrums in four of the five children who exhibited these behaviors.

Posey, Walsh, Wilson, and McDougle (1999) treated two very young children with autistic disorder, aged 23 and 29 months, with risperidone for their severe and persistent aggression and irritability that had not responded to previous treatments. The dosage for the 23-month-old boy was 0.25 mg twice daily, and his aggression and self-injury decreased at this dose; however, he also had persistent tachycardia and QTc interval prolongation that was found to be dose related and which could result in fatal ventricular arrhythmias (Moss, 1993). [QTc is an electrocardiographic metric of the time for ventricular depolarization and repolarization.]. With the 29-month old, his aggression and self-injurious behavior improved following 1 month on 0.25 mg bedtime dosage of risperidone, and his self-injury was eliminated at a 0.5-mg/day dose. Dosage was further increased

to 1.25 mg/day over the following year to control his continuing tantrums. Follow-up of the toddlers at 5 and 13 months, respectively, showed that the behavior of both children remained significantly improved, with no new side effects.

In a 6-month, open-label study with a 12-month follow-up, Zuddas, Di Martino, Muglia, and Cianchetti (2000) evaluated the safety and effectiveness of risperidone in 11 children and adolescents with PDDs, aged 7–17 years (mean age, 12.3 years), who exhibited aggression, tantrums, hyperactivity, stereotypy, and sleep abnormalities. Risperidone was initiated at 0.5 mg/day and titrated up in increments of 0.5 mg/day every 5 days until therapeutic or adverse effects were observed. The maximum dosage was 6 mg/day or 0.1 mg/kg/day, whichever was less. Risperidone therapy was terminated for those whose target behaviors persisted or worsened with 2 months of therapy. Ten of the 11 participants were rated as clinical responders on the CGI scale (NIMH, 1985) and were treated for 6 months, with 7 of the 10 followed up at 12 months. All participants showed clinically significant decreases in their target behaviors, including aggression and tantrums, at both 6 and 12 months. Weight gain over time was the most notable side effect (a 15% mean increase in 6 months). Following 6 months of therapy, two participants developed mild to moderate facial dystonia that was treated by decreasing the dose for one and discontinuing the drug for the other.

In a 6-month, open-label study, Diler, Firat, and Avci (2002) evaluated the effectiveness and tolerability of risperidone in 20 children with autistic disorder, aged 3–7.5 years (mean age, 4.95 years), who had previously not been treated with medication. The mean dosage of risperidone was 1.53 mg/day (range, 0.04–0.11 mg/kg/day). Although not a target behavior for these children, aggression was exhibited by two children as a side effect of risperidone and was resolved with its discontinuation.

In a two-phase, open-label study, Malone, Maislin, Choudhury, Gifford, and Delaney (2002) investigated the effectiveness and safety of risperidone in the short term and neuroleptic-related dyskinesias in the long term, with 22 outpatient children and adolescents with autistic disorder, aged 2.9–16.3 years (mean age, 7.1 years). Risperidone was started at 0.5 mg/day and titrated up until optimal effectiveness or minimal side effects emerged. The overall upper dosage limit was 6 mg/day. By the end of the 1-month short-term phase, the dosage ranged from 0.5 to 2.5 mg/day (mean dosage, 1.2 ± 0.6 mg/day), and by the end of the 6-month long-term phase, the dosage ranged from 0.5 to 4.0 mg/day (mean dosage, 1.8 ± 1.1 mg/day). Following short-term treatment, 17 of the 22 participants were deemed clinical responders on the CGI scale (NIMH, 1985). There was significant improvement in the anger factor of the 14 selected items of the CPRS (NIMH, 1985). Eleven of the

13 participants who completed the long-term phase maintained this improvement. None of the participants developed dyskinesias during the short term, but two did so during the long-term treatment. The dyskinesias ceased within 2 and 3 weeks, respectively, in these two individuals.

In a three-phase, open-label study, Troost et al. (2005) evaluated the effects of risperidone on 36 children and adolescents with ASD, aged 5–17 years. The study design included an 8-week open-label treatment phase ($N = 36$), a 16-week phase for treatment responders ($N = 24$), and a double-blind discontinuation phase ($N = 24$), which consisted of either 3 weeks of taper plus 5 weeks of placebo, or continued treatment with risperidone. Risperidone was started at 0.5 mg/day and titrated up in 0.5 mg/day increments to a maximum of 2.5 mg/day for those below 45 kg in weight and 3.5 mg/day for those above it. Two children dropped out of the study during the open-label phase because of large weight gains, and after 24 weeks of the open-label phase, 18 participants were rated as clinical responders on the CGI scale (NIMH, 1985). In the discontinuation phase, 67% of those randomized to placebo relapsed compared to 25% of those who continued treatment with risperidone. In terms of target behaviors, those on risperidone showed continued reductions in tantrums, aggression, and self-injurious behavior. Weight gain was the most notable side effect.

In a 12-week, double-blind, placebo-controlled study, McDougle and colleagues (1998) evaluated the short-term efficacy and safety of risperidone in 31 adults with autistic disorder, aged 18–43 years (mean age, 28.1 years). Risperidone or placebo was started at 1 mg/day and titrated up in increments of 1 mg/day every 3–4 days to a maximum of 10 mg/day, as clinically indicated. The optimum dosage of risperidone was achieved in 5 weeks and participants were maintained on this dose for 7 weeks. The participants could be prescribed chloral hydrate for agitation (2 g/day), but no other medication during the trial. Fifteen adults were randomly assigned to risperidone and 16 to placebo, 14 of whom were subsequently given open-label risperidone for 12 weeks following their participation in the double-blind placebo phase of the trial. Thirty adults completed at least 4 weeks of the trial and 24 completed the entire 12 weeks. Risperidone was statistically superior to placebo in reducing physical aggression, property destruction, and self-injurious behavior. Significant differences between the two groups emerged at week 4 of the trial, and again at weeks 8 and 12, with the largest differences being evident at week 12. Similar findings were reported for those who were included in the open-label risperidone treatment that followed the double-blind trial.

In an 8-week, double-blind, placebo-controlled trial, Shea et al. (2004) investigated the efficacy and safety of risperidone in 79 children with autistic and other PDDs, aged 5–12 years (mean age, 7.5 years). The children's target behaviors included aggression, self-injury, and stereotypy. Oral solution of risperidone or placebo was started at 0.01 mg/kg/day for the first 2 days and increased to 0.02 mg/kg/day on day 3. Depending on clinical indications, the dosage could be adjusted incrementally by 0.02 mg/kg/day, with a maximum allowable dosage of 0.06 mg/kg/day. The mean daily dosage during the trial was 0.04 mg/kg/day, with the study endpoint dosage of 0.05 mg/kg/day. Forty children were randomized to the drug condition and 39 to placebo. Of these 79, seven dropped out of the study – two from the drug condition and five from placebo. Of the two that withdrew from the drug condition, one was because of adverse effects and the other was because of insufficient response. Target behaviors, measured using the Irritability subscale of the Aberrant Behavior Checklist (ABC; Aman, Singh, Stewart, & Field, 1985), showed an improvement of 64% in the risperidone group, compared to 30.7% in the placebo group. Only 5 of the 40 children in the risperidone-treated group had severe adverse effects, 1 each of hyperkinesias, somnolence, weight gain, aggression, and extrapyramidal symptoms as a result of accidental overdose.

In a two-phase, 8-week, double-blind, placebo-controlled study, the Research Units on Pediatric Psychopharmacology Autism Network (RUPPAN, 2002) evaluated the short-term efficacy and safety of risperidone in 101 children with autistic disorder, aged 5–17 years (mean age, 8.8 years). The children exhibited aggression, tantrums, and self-injurious behaviors. Depending on pre-trial weight, risperidone was started at either 0.25 mg/day (weight under 20 kg) or 0.5 mg/day (weight between 20 and 45 kg) and titrated up in increments of 0.5 mg/day to a maximum of 2.5 mg/day or 3.5 mg/day by day 29, respectively. Dosage reductions could occur as clinically indicated, but no dosage increases were allowed beyond day 29. In the first phase, 49 children were randomized to the risperidone condition and 52 to the placebo condition. In the risperidone group, 34 of the 49 children were deemed clinical responders, and they were maintained on risperidone for 6 months during the second phase of the trial. Improvement, which was measured as reduction on the ABC Irritability subscale, was 56.9% for the risperidone group compared to 14.1% for the placebo group. In terms of positive response, it was 69% for the risperidone group compared to 12% for placebo. Of the 34 clinical responders in the first phase, 23 continued to show improvement at 6 months during the second phase. Side effects included weight gain, increased appetite, fatigue, drowsiness, dizziness, drooling, tremor, and constipation.

There were two follow-up reports from this rather extensive multisite study, as well as a two-part follow-up study using a subsample of the children from the original study. The first follow-up report showed that risperidone was effective in controlling the most common behavioral symptoms in the children (i.e., tantrums, aggression, and hyperactivity) as identified by parents (Arnold et al., 2003). The other report indicated that while risperidone has significant effects on externally driven behaviors, such as aggression, severe tantrums, and self-injury, it may also improve restricted, repetitive, and stereotyped patterns of behavior but have little effect on social interaction and communication deficits (McDougle et al., 2005). The two-part, follow-up study (RUPPAN, 2005) included 63 of the 101 children from the original 8-week protocol (RUPPAN, 2002), aged 5–17 years (mean age, 8.6 years), who had shown a positive response to risperidone. They were enrolled in a new 4-month, open-label trial, thus giving a total drug exposure time of 6 months, followed by a placebo-controlled, double-blind, 8-week placebo substitution discontinuation protocol. One of the aims of this study was to ascertain if the short-term effects of risperidone on aggression, tantrums, and self-injurious behavior would persist over an extended treatment period. In part one, the dosage was 1.96 mg/day for 16 weeks. Fifty-one of the 63 participants completed the 16-week study. Although there were minor changes in the target variables, there was essentially no decrease in the effectiveness of risperidone in controlling the children's target behaviors. A total of 38 children was enrolled in part two of the study – the discontinuation phase. Data comparing clinical outcomes on the children's target behaviors showed the relapse rate was significantly higher in the placebo-treated children as compared to risperidone-treated children. This multisite study suggests risperidone is well tolerated and has short- and long-term efficacy in treating aggression, tantrums, and self-injury in children with autistic disorder.

Overall, from the numerous case studies, open-label, observational, and retrospective reports, and the double-blind, placebo-controlled trials, there is a strong suggestion that risperidone is effective in treating aggression, tantrums, irritability, hyperactivity, and stereotypy. This effectiveness is maintained for up to 6 months, and probably as long as 12 months, while the individuals continue to adhere to the medication regimen at an individually titrated dosage. Risperidone is not effective, however, in enhancing social interaction or communication skills, or widening the markedly restricted repertoire of activities and interests that are cardinal features of individuals with ASD. The most common adverse effects of risperidone are weight gain, ranging from 1 to 10 kg, and transient sedation at the initiation of therapy and with dosage increase.

Olanzapine

Olanzapine has not been used much in individuals with ASD. Horrigan, Barnhill, and Courvoisie (1997) reported

successfully using olanzapine in two children with developmental disabilities. One was a 10-year-old boy diagnosed with autistic disorder, severe intellectual disabilities, and bipolar disorder not otherwise specified, who experienced cyclical increases in motor activity and diminished need for sleep. He showed physical aggression toward others, and explosive rage outbursts, hand flapping, and vocalizations. Trials with the following medications were not effective in controlling his behaviors: carbamazepine, valproic acid, fluoxetine, clomipramine, clonidine, molindone, haloperidol, risperidone, naltrexone, and buspirone. A clinically estimated 40% reduction in the frequency and severity of his behaviors was achieved on a regimen that included 150 mg/day thioridazine, 1,500 mg/day lithium carbonate, and 40 mg/day fenfluramine. The positive effects lasted less than 6 months, so the thioridazine and fenfluramine were replaced with 10 mg/day olanzapine. There was a 75% reduction in his target behaviors by the third day, and with increased dosage (i.e., 20 mg/day) by the third week, his behavior had stabilized, without sedation, or extrapyramidal signs or symptoms.

In another case study, Malek-Ahmadi and Simonds (1998) reported the treatment of an 8-year-old boy diagnosed with autistic disorder who exhibited hyperactivity and aggressive behavior. His hyperactivity had been treated unsuccessfully with methylphenidate, clomipramine, carbamazepine, haloperidol, and thioridazine, with methylphenidate actually worsening his behavior. Immediately prior to the drug trial, he was on buspirone 5 mg twice a day, but when the dosage was increased to 15 mg/day, his hyperactivity increased and the drug was discontinued. Olanzapine was prescribed at 5.0 mg/day, and increased to 7.5 mg/day 2 days later. His hyperactivity decreased and aggressive behavior was eliminated, with no reported side effects from the medication. No mention was made of weight gain due to medication, even though this has been a ubiquitous finding in virtually all studies of olanzapine with children, regardless of diagnosis (Krishnamoorthy & King, 1998).

In a 12-week, open-label study, Potenza, Holmes, Kanes, and McDougle (1999) evaluated the effectiveness and tolerability of olanzapine in eight children, adolescents, and adults with autistic disorder ($N = 5$) and PDD NOS ($N = 3$). By the 12th week of the trial, they were on a mean daily dosage of 7.8 ± 4.7 mg/day (dosage range, 5–20 mg/day). Seven of the eight individuals completed the trial, and six of the seven were clinical responders (i.e., they were rated as much improved, or very much improved, on the global item of the CGI). The six clinical responders showed significant improvements not only in aggression and irritability or anger but also in self-injurious behavior. In terms of adverse effects, six individuals gained weight and there was evidence of sedation in three. The issue of weight gain with this drug (a mean of 18.44 lb in this study) may limit its usefulness in this population (Stigler, Potenza, Posey, & McDougle, 2004).

In a 6-week, open-label study, Malone, Cater, Sheikh, Choudhury, and Delaney (2001) evaluated the comparative effectiveness and safety of olanzapine and haloperidol in 12 children with autistic disorder (mean age, 7.8 years). Using a parallel group design, they randomized the children to receive a final mean dosage of 7.9 ± 2.5 mg/day of olanzapine and 1.4 ± 0.7 mg/day of haloperidol. On the CGI scale (National Institute of Mental Health, 1985), all six children in the olanzapine group, and three of the six children in the haloperidol group, were clinical responders. Of interest here is that there was a significant decrease in the Anger/Uncooperativeness factor on the CRPS scale for children on olanzapine but not for those on haloperidol. Weight gain was noted in 11 of the 12 children, with weight loss for one child who was on haloperidol.

In a 3-month, open-label study, Kemner, Willemsen-Swinkels, De Jonge, Tuynman-Qua, and Van Engeland (2002) investigated the effectiveness and safety of olanzapine in 25 children and adolescents with autistic disorder, or PDD NOS, aged 6.4–16.6 years (mean age, 11.2 years). Olanzapine was initiated at 2.5 mg every other day and then increased to 2.5 mg/day. The dosage was increased by 2.5 or 5.0 mg/day every other week, until a maximum dosage of 15 or 20 mg/day was achieved for children who were under or over 55 kg, respectively. Dosage could be titrated down, as clinically indicated. At the end of the trial, the mean dosage was 10.7 mg/day (range, 2.5–20 mg/day). Only 3 of the 22 children and adolescents who completed the trial were deemed clinical responders on the CGI scale (NIMH, 1985). As measured on the ABC (Aman et al., 1985), the Irritability subscale score was significantly lower with olanzapine compared to baseline. Significant side effects included weight gain, asthenia, and increased appetite.

In an 8-week, double-blind, placebo-controlled trial, Hollander et al. (2006) evaluated the efficacy of olanzapine in 11 children and adolescents with PDDs, aged 6–14 years (mean age, 9 years). Depending on the weight of each participant, dosage was started at 2.5 mg every day, or every other day, and increased in 5 mg increments weekly to a maximum of 20 mg/day, as clinically indicated. The final mean dosage ranged from 7.5 to 12.5 mg/day (mean dosage, 10 ± 2.04 mg/day). Eight of the 11 participants completed the trial. On the CGI scale (NIMH, 1985), 50% of the participants on olanzapine, and 20% of the participants on placebo, were clinical responders; however, there was no significant difference between the active drug and placebo conditions in terms of aggression. Side effects due to olanzapine included sedation and increased appetite, as well as weight gain (mean weight, 7.5 lb), but no extrapyramidal symptoms or dyskinesias were reported.

Overall, the two cases studies, three open-label, and one double-blind study suggest that some children and adolescent may benefit from olanzapine in reducing aggression and other externally driven challenging behaviors, but the weight gain (up to a mean of 18 lb in a 12-week study) should be a major clinical consideration in its use in this population.

Quetiapine

In a 16-week, open-label study, Martin, Koenig, Scahill, and Bregman (1999) evaluated the effectiveness and safety of quetiapine in six children and adolescents with autistic disorder (mean age, 10.9 years). Quetiapine dosages ranged from 100 to 350 mg/day (mean dosage, 225 mg/day). Two of the six children completed the 16-week trial and were considered clinical responders on the CGI scale (NIMH, 1985); three others dropped out of the trial because of lack of response and sedation, and the remaining participant dropped out during the fourth week of treatment because of a possible seizure. Although no direct behavioral measures were taken, no change was observed on the Irritability subscale of the ABC (Aman et al., 1985) which is highly correlated with aggressive and other maladaptive behaviors, such as self-injury.

In a 12-week, open-label study, Findling et al. (2004) evaluated the effectiveness of quetiapine in nine adolescents with autistic disorder (mean age, 14.6 years). These adolescents had multiple maladaptive behaviors, including irritability, tantrums, and aggression. Quetiapine was started at a dosage of 50 mg/day for the first 3 days of treatment, and then the dosages were increased to 100 mg/day for the first 2 weeks of the study. Thereafter, dosage was increased by 100 mg/day every other week until a target dosage of 300 mg/day was reached. Dosages could be increased, as clinically indicated, up to a maximum of 750 mg/day or decreased to minimize treatment-emergent side effects. Three adolescents dropped out of the study; one was lost to follow-up after the first week and two due to side effects (i.e., increased aggression/agitation and drowsiness). Of the remaining six adolescents, two were deemed clinical responders on the CGI scale (NIMH, 1985) and showed decreased aggression and tantrums on quetiapine. The other four showed minimal or no improvement.

In a retrospective analysis of 857 medical records, Corson, Barkenbus, Posey, Stigler, and McDougle (2004) found 20 individuals with PDD, aged 5–28 years (mean age, 12.1 years), who had received treatment with quetiapine for at least 4 weeks. These individuals received dosages of quetiapine ranging from 25 to 600 mg/day (mean dosage, 248.7 ± 198.4 mg/day) for 4–180 weeks (mean duration, 59.8 ± 55.1 weeks). Their target symptoms included aggression, self-injury, irritability, and hyperactivity. Eight of the

20 individuals were deemed clinical responders on the CGI scale (National Institute of Mental Health, 1985) and showed decreases in the target behaviors. Ten of the 20 individuals reported adverse effects of the drug, with three so severe that their drug was discontinued. Two had their drug discontinued because of intolerable weight gain.

Overall, in the two open-label studies and one retrospective study, 12 of the 35 children and adolescents showed some clinical response to quetiapine. Current research suggests that quetiapine is not indicated for children, adolescents, and adults with autism because it is not very effective, is poorly tolerated, and has serious side effects.

Clozapine

This drug has not been used much at all in individuals with ASD. Zuddas, Ledda, Fratta, Muglia, and Cianchetti (1996) reported using clozapine with two boys (aged 8 years) and a girl (aged 12 years) diagnosed with autistic disorder. They had high rates of hyperactivity and fidgetiness or aggressiveness, and had made minimal progress on typical antipsychotics. Clozapine was administered at progressively increasing dosages and modified according to clinical response. After 3 months of treatment, there was 40% improvement in their target behaviors. The two boys were on 200-mg/day maintenance dose following 8 months of treatment, with their target behaviors still under control. After 5 months on treatment at a maximum dosage of 450 mg/day, the girl's behavior regressed to baseline levels.

Chen, Bedair, McKay, Bowers, and Mazure (2001) reported the short-term use of clozapine in treating the aggressive behavior of a 17-year-old adolescent with autistic disorder and severe intellectual disabilities. His aggression had been poorly controlled with quetiapine, olanzapine, and risperidone in the past. Prior to his treatment with clozapine, he was maintained in four-point restraints due to his aggressive behavior. Clozapine was initiated at 12.5 mg/day and titrated up to a dosage of 275 mg/day by the 10th day. His aggression decreased substantially, and on the 10th day, he was removed from restraints for 3 days. The only reported side effects were mild constipation and drooling. The results of this case report should be interpreted conservatively because it was a very short trial, with no controls.

Currently, there is no good scientific evidence for using clozapine with this population. Furthermore, clozapine's propensity to lower seizure threshold, and the risk of agranulocytosis, should be seriously considered before using this drug in individuals with ASD.

Ziprasidone

In an open-label study, McDougle, Kem, and Posey (2002) evaluated the effectiveness and safety of ziprasidone in 12 youths with autistic disorder, aged 8–20 years (mean age, 11.62 years). The trial ranged from 6 to 30 weeks (mean duration, 14.5 ± 8.29 weeks), with dosages ranging from 20 to 120 mg/day (mean dosage, 59.23 ± 34.76 mg/day). Only 6 of the 12 youths were deemed clinical responders on the CGI scale (NIMH, 1985), with significant decreases in their aggression, property destruction, self-injury, and irritability. Adverse effects included transient sedation but no weight gain or cardiovascular side effects.

In a 6-week, open-label study, Malone, Delaney, Hyman, and Cater (2007) evaluated the effectiveness and safety of ziprasidone in 15 adolescents with autistic disorder, aged 12.1–18.5 years (mean, 14.5 years). Three adolescents dropped out of the trial before they received the study medication, thus reducing the sample to 12 adolescents. Dosage was clinically titrated, with the final dosage ranging from 40 to 160 mg/day (mean, 98.3 ± 40.4 mg/day). On the CGI scale (NIMH, 1985), 9 of the 12 adolescents were rated as responders, and on the Irritability subscale of the ABC (Aman et al., 1985), the effect of ziprasidone was statistically superior to baseline and indicated that the drug produced decreases in disruptive behaviors, such as irritability, aggression, and hyperactivity. Weight was not a side effect and the increase in QTc remained within accepted safety parameters.

Ziprasidone has a major advantage over some of the other new generation antipsychotics (such as risperidone and olanzapine) in that it does not pose a risk for weight gain, but it is associated with prolongation of the QTc interval.

Aripiprazole

In an open-label study, Stigler, Posey and McDougle (2004) evaluated the effectiveness and tolerability of aripiprazole in five youths with pervasive developmental disorders, aged 5–18 years (mean, 12.2 years). The trial ranged from 8 to 16 weeks (mean duration, 12 weeks), with dosages ranging from 10 to 15 mg/day (mean dosage, 12.0 mg/day). All five youths were deemed to be clinical responders on the CGI scale (NIMH, 1985). Aggression and other externalizing behaviors of all five youths were well controlled with individualized dosages of aripiprazole. The drug was well tolerated, with minimal side effects.

In a retrospective chart review, Valicenti-McDermott and Demb (2006) reported on the effectiveness and side effects of aripiprazole in 32 children, aged 5–19 years (mean, 10.9 years). This sample consisted of 24 children with a diagnosis of autistic disorder or PDD, and 8 with mental retardation. Their target symptoms included aggression ($N = 28$), hyperactivity, impulsivity, and self-injury, among others. The initial dosage of aripiprazole ranged from 1.25 to 10 mg/day (mean dosage, 7.1 ± 0.32 mg/day) and was titrated to an acceptable clinical response. The maintenance dosage ranged from 1.25 to 30 mg/day (mean dosage, 10.55 ± 6.9 mg/day). Eighteen of the 32 children were clinical responders, with 9 of these 18 having autistic disorder. Improvements in aggression were reported in 15 of the 28 who were aggressive at baseline; 7 with autistic disorder showed clinically significant decreases in aggression. Half of the 32 children reported side effects, with the most frequent being sleepiness and weight gain.

In a 14-week, open-label study, Stigler et al. (2009) investigated the effectiveness and tolerability of aripiprazole in 25 children and adolescents with PDD NOS ($N = 21$) and Asperger's disorder ($N = 4$), aged 5–17 years (mean, 8.6 years). The participants' target behaviors included aggression, self-injury, and tantrums. Initial dosing started at 1.25 mg/day for 3 days, increased to 2.5 mg/day for 2 weeks, and further increased to a maximum dosage of 15 mg/day over the next 4 weeks, depending on clinical response or emergence of side effects. The optimal dosage (range, 2.5–15 mg/day) was maintained for 8 weeks. Only three participants did not complete the study; of these, two completed 8 weeks and one completed 6 weeks, prior to exiting the study protocol. The remaining 22 were deemed clinical responders on the CGI scale (NIMH, 1985). When compared to baseline, aripiprazole produced a statistically significant improvement in the target symptoms. The drug was well tolerated, with ECGs showing no clinically significant changes (including the QTc interval). While parents reported extrapyramidal symptoms in nine children, the treating physicians reported none. There was no clinically significant weight gain.

In a retrospective chart review, Masi et al. (2009) evaluated the clinical outcomes and adverse effects of aripiprazole in 34 children and adolescents with PDDs ($N = 24$) and autistic disorder ($N = 10$), aged 4.5–15 years (mean, 10.2 years). Their target behaviors were aggression, self-injury, hyperactivity, and severe impulsiveness. For preschool children, aripiprazole dosage was started at 2.5 mg/kg and titrated up in 1.25 mg/day increments every 5 days, until optimal clinical response or adverse effects emerged. A higher starting dose (i.e., 2.5 or 5.0 mg/day) was used with the older children and adolescents. Of the 34 participants, 11 were clinical responders on the CGI scale (NIMH, 1985). In terms of side effects, five reported severe agitation, associated with self-injury, and another five reported insomnia. Weight gain was not reported except in one adolescent who gained 9 kg during the study period.

In an 8-week, double-blind, placebo-controlled, parallel-group study, Owen et al. (2009) evaluated the short-term

efficacy and safety of aripiprazole in the treatment of irritability in 98 children and adolescents with autistic disorder, aged 6–17 years (mean, 9.3). Their target behaviors included aggression, tantrums, and self-injurious behavior. Of the 98 participants, 47 received aripiprazole treatment and 51 placebo, with 36 and 39, respectively, completing the study. Aripiprazole was initiated at 2 mg/day and titrated up to a maximum of 15 mg/day, with no dosage increases following week 6 of the trial; however, decreases were allowed, depending on clinical indication. During the last week of treatment, active medication dosages ranged from 2 to 15 mg/day. At week 8, there was a statistically significant improvement in irritability with aripiprazole, compared to placebo, with about 53% responders in the active drug condition compared to 14% in the placebo condition. Although some mild to moderate side effects were reported for both groups, none was considered serious; however, three and five participants from the placebo- and aripiprazole-treated groups, respectively, discontinued the trial.

In an 8-week, fixed-dose, placebo-controlled, double-blind study, Marcus et al. (2009) evaluated the efficacy and safety of aripiprazole in treating irritability in 218 children and adolescents with autistic disorder, aged 6–17 years. The participants' target behaviors included irritability, agitation, self-injurious behavior, or a combination of these symptoms. Aripiprazole, at fixed dosages of 5, 10, and 15 mg/day, produced significantly better outcomes in the participants' irritability when compared to placebo; however, irritability was not defined in this study as including aggression or tantrums, and thus no conclusions can be drawn regarding the effects on these target behaviors of aripiprazole, at the fixed dosages.

Antidepressant Medications

Fluvoxamine

In a 12-week, double-blind, placebo-controlled trial, McDougle et al. (1996) investigated the efficacy of fluvoxamine in 30 adults diagnosed with autistic disorder, aged 18–53 years (mean, 30.1 years). Fluvoxamine was initiated at 50 mg/day and increased every 3 or 4 days to a maximum dosage of 300 mg/day, as clinically indicated. Maximum dosage was reached within 3 weeks and maintained for 9 weeks. All 30 individuals completed the trial, with 15 receiving fluvoxamine and 15 placebo. Eight of the 15 in the fluvoxamine group, and none of the 15 in the placebo group, were deemed clinical responders on the CGI scale (NIMH, 1985). Their clinical response was not correlated with age, level of autistic behavior, or IQ. On the Brown Aggression Scale (Brown, Goodwin, Ballenger, Goyer, & Major, 1979), fluvoxamine was significantly better than placebo in reducing aggression by the 8th week of the trial, although a clear trend toward decreased aggression was evident from the 4th week. There was no significant reduction in aggression in the placebo group at any time. An unpublished study by the same group (see Potenza et al., 1999), as well as a 10-week, open-label study of low-dose fluvoxamine by Martin, Koenig, Anderson, and Scahill (2003), indicated that fluvoxamine is neither effective nor well tolerated by children and adolescents with PDD. However, in a small open-label study, Yokoyama, Hirose, Haginoya, Munakata, and Iinuma (2002) reported that fluvoxamine was effective in reducing aggression and self-injury in three of five children with autistic disorder.

Fluoxetine

In an open trial, Cook, Rowlett, Jaselskis, and Leventhal (1992) treated 39 children and adults with autistic disorder and intellectual disability (autistic disorder, 23; intellectual disability, 16) with fluoxetine ranging from 20 mg every other day to 80 mg/day. Fifteen of the 23 with autistic disorder showed improvement in fluoxetine on the CGI scale (NIMH, 1985) including decreased rates of aggression, destructive behavior, decreased severity and intensity of tantrums, and decreased irritability. Ten of the 16 with intellectual disability showed similar improvements. Six of the 23 with autistic disorder and 3 of the 16 with intellectual disability exhibited adverse effects that significantly interfered with their functioning or outweighed the drug's therapeutic effects. It should be noted that the raters were the treating clinicians, to were not blind to study conditions.

Sertraline

Buck (1995) described the use of sertraline in two adults who were very violent. One was a 33-year-old man with PDD NOS who had engaged in self-injury and aggression toward others since the age of 2 years. His self-injury and aggression were severe enough to require use of restraints for imminent danger to himself and others. He was on a medication regimen of perphenazine and lorazepam, which inadequately controlled his target behaviors. Sertraline was added to this regimen, titrated up to 200 mg/day, and then reduced to 100 mg/day for the best clinical response. His self-injury and aggression were reported to be less frequent and severe after 8 months of treatment.

In a small open trial, Hellings, Kelley, Gabrielli, Kilgore, and Shah (1996) evaluated the effectiveness of sertraline in nine adults with intellectual disability, five of whom also had autistic disorder. Sertraline was given in dosages ranging

from 25 to 150 mg/day, based on each individual's clinical response to the drug and to target self-injury and aggression. Eight of the nine adults, deemed clinical responders based on the CGI scale (NIMH, 1985), showed significant decreases in self-injury and aggression. Sertraline was discontinued after 18 weeks of treatment in one person, due to agitation and worsening of self-injury.

Steingard, Zimnitzky, DeMaso, Bauman, and Bucci (1997) reported a series of nine cases of children with autistic disorder, aged 6–12 years, who were treated with sertraline for transition-related anxiety and agitation. Eight of the nine also exhibited aggressive behavior. A low dose of sertraline (range, 25–50 mg/day) was prescribed as clinically indicated for each individual. Initially, eight of the nine individuals showed improvements in their target behaviors, which included aggression and explosive outbursts. For three of these eight, the effects diminished after 3–7 months, despite increased dosage; however, five were able to be maintained on sertraline for between 4 and 12 months after the introduction of the drug.

In a 12-week, open-label trial, McDougle et al. (1998) investigated the short-term effectiveness and tolerability of sertraline in 42 adults with PDD (autistic disorder, 22; Asperger's disorder, 6; PDD NOS, 14). The participants' mean age was 26.1 years (range, 18–39 years). Sertraline was started at 50 mg/day and increased to 200 mg/day, as clinically indicated. They reached their maximum dosage within 3 weeks and then received this dosage for 9 weeks. Thirty seven of the 42 completed the trial and 5 dropped out; 3 because of increased anxiety/agitation, 1 because of a syncopal episode of undetermined cause, and 1 because of medication nonadherence. Twenty-four of the 42 were clinical responders: 15 with autistic disorder and 9 with PPD NOS. Sertraline was effective in decreasing the adults' aggressive symptoms, as measured on the CGI scale (NIMH, 1985). No adverse cardiovascular effects, extrapyramidal signs or symptoms, or seizures were reported, suggesting sertraline was well tolerated in this adult population.

Overall, drug treatment with new generation antipsychotics and selected antidepressants appears to result in statistically significant improvement in some behaviors associated with ASD, including aggression, tantrums, and other externally driven challenging behaviors. The best controlled studies are from trials of risperidone, aripiprazole, and olanzapine, with limited trials on the other drugs.

Current Status

Current research indicates that behavioral technology is demonstrably effective in treating aggression, tantrums, and other externally driven behaviors of individuals with ASD (Machalicek, O'Reilly, Beretvas, Sigafoos, & Lancioni,

2007; Matson, 2009). When applied consistently and systematically, behavioral treatments are capable of decreasing or eliminating even the most severe maladaptive behavior in this population. While this achievement is impressive, it must be balanced against the reality of the current research. Most extant behavioral studies are demonstrations and refinements of behavioral technology, and could have used any population with the same maladaptive behaviors. The majority of studies used very short sessions (usually less than 1 h), with a few specifically selected participants, in tightly controlled contexts, and with treatments delivered by highly trained specialists. In fact, the central aim of many studies reviewed was not to treat the individuals but was to gain a better understanding of the mechanisms that underlie a specific treatment, the parameters of chosen treatments, and the methods for deriving assessment-based treatments, or was to assess the comparative effectiveness of alternative behavioral treatments. Indeed, the extant literature dealing with behavioral treatment of aggression in individuals with ASD provides very modest evidence in regard to the process of functional assessment, the development of testable hypotheses, the alignment of the treatments with the stated functions of the behavior, and the development and implementation of behavioral treatments for use by parents and care staff under community living conditions. Most studies are clinic, school, or institution based, where the findings might not translate to home or other community contexts. This is not to imply that parents and care staff cannot use these technologies; it is just that there is little empirical demonstration of this process in the current literature.

The behavioral field needs to research methodologies that enable parents and care staff to design and implement behavioral interventions that encompass most of the child's waking hours. Such research should focus on how behavioral technology can enhance the quality of life of an individual in real time and move beyond simply demonstrating that it can be achieved in short, well-controlled, treatment sessions. What is needed is research showing how the findings from tightly controlled studies can be translated into interventions that can be implemented effectively in the real world, outside of clinics and institutions. Adkins et al. (2010) provided a good example of this kind of research by showing that a community therapist could successfully use a research-based cognitive behavioral technique in her daily work. In addition, it cannot be emphasized enough that, at some point, behavioral researchers must move on from simply examining the same procedures with minor variations (e.g., new settings, populations, or parameters) and investigate the clinical utility of these procedures in the day-to-day lives of children, adolescents, and adults with ASD. We need to demonstrate that when parents and care staff are treating individuals with

ASD on a 24-h/day basis, these procedures work as effectively as they do in tightly controlled short sessions in the clinic, school, or institution.

A great model for this kind of research is provided by the early intensive behavioral interventions for infants, toddlers, and children with autistic disorder (Lovaas, 1987; Matson & Smith, 2008; McEachin, Smith, & Lovaas, 1993; Sallows & Graupner, 2005; Schreibman, 2000). Perry et al. (2008) has recently provided an excellent example of the effectiveness of an intensive behavioral intervention in a large community-based program with 332 children aged 2–7 years. Their data show both statistically and clinically significant improvements in a number of domains, including a reduction in autism severity, gains in cognitive and adaptive skills, and the doubling of the children's rate of development. At least 75% of the children showed overall gains, and 11% actually achieved average functioning. When this kind of approach is used early, intensively, and consistently, it puts the lives of the participating children and their families on a much more positive trajectory for life. By employing behavioral interventions at the front end, when the children are developmentally young and have greater plasticity in their brain development, we can teach them appropriate behaviors and communication systems so that later they will not have to use maladaptive behavior to communicate with their parents, families, care staff, and teachers. This approach may preempt the later emergence of maladaptive behavior and the need for labor-intensive behavior support plans.

The emerging field of mindfulness-based interventions (Shapiro & Carlson, 2009) is a new addition to the ASD literature and shows some promise. The current studies on mindfulness with intellectual disabilities suggest that procedures like *Meditation on the Soles of the Feet* could be used more broadly with children, adolescents, and adults with ASD (Singh et al., in press). Just how useful mindfulness-based procedures will prove to be in this population remains to be investigated, but early studies with parents of children with autism, and adolescents with autism, provide some reason for optimism; however, extant studies are from only one research group and await verification by other researchers.

There is just enough research data to suggest new generation antipsychotic drugs are useful in reducing maladaptive behaviors, especially irritability, aggression, disruption, self-injury, and hyperactivity, as well as improving overall functioning, in individuals with ASD. However, it must be remembered that the proportion of children and adolescents who responded to the target drug in each of the drug studies was small, and there was more of an emphasis on statistical vs clinical outcomes. There is much less robust data supporting the use of a few antidepressant drugs to achieve similar outcomes. While pharmacotherapy with ASD is promising, there are several issues that need highlighting.

First is the issue of the specificity of the participant sample used in the drug studies. In many studies, the diagnosis of the participants was made by the treating psychiatrists and not confirmed with standardized diagnostic instruments, such as the Autism Diagnostic Interview-Revised (Lord, Rutter, & Le Coteur, 1994), which is often seen as the gold standard for PDD diagnosis. The study sample in many studies was treated as homogenous and not divided into subtypes of ASD, thereby reducing the precision of the findings for various diagnostic groups. The number of subjects in many studies was relatively small, thus precluding generalization to the ASD population as a whole. This is further complicated by having unbalanced numbers in the samples – both in terms of subgroups with different diagnoses (i.e., autistic disorder, PDD, and PDD NOS) and age groups (i.e., children, adolescents, and adults). Future studies should consider using larger sample sizes that would enable stratification by subject profiles (e.g., by subgroups based on diagnosis, age, target behaviors, gender, and IQ).

An additional issue concerns participants being on multiple medications during a drug trial. While some studies used monotherapy, many allowed the study participants to stay on their current medications, during the testing of a new medication. Our knowledge of drug–drug interactions is so incomplete that having participants on different multiple medications poses immense problems for data interpretation. Furthermore, many participants have comorbid disorders—hence the need for multiple medications—which also pose data interpretation problems. We do not know, for example, if a child with only autistic disorder reacts to a specific drug in the same way as a child with additional psychiatric disorders. In a typical drug trial, the participants may have many different comorbid disorders, thus compounding the problem. Both of these issues impact the reliability and validity of the findings.

Second is the nature of the experimental design used in the drug studies. There is a preponderance of uncontrolled case reports, retrospective chart reviews, and open-label studies. Case studies are useful as a first step in establishing the utility of a drug in specific cases. Chart reviews provide actuarial data on the number of individuals who are clinical responders on a specific drug for a specific disease, disorder, or target behavior. Open-label studies provide the basis for randomized control trials, the gold standard for evidence-based treatment. The problem with case studies, retrospective chart reviews, and open-label studies is that bias and placebo effects cannot be controlled, and these could be significant factors in accounting for the positive findings. An additional problem, specific to retrospective studies, is that they usually do not have fixed endpoints for evaluating treatment outcomes. Also, these studies have an inherent problem of selection bias that can result from discontinuation of the drug treatment in the first few weeks, due to adverse effects. This bias can preclude comparison of findings across similar retrospective studies. In open-label studies, the absence of control groups limits firm conclusions regarding safety and tolerability of the drug in the study population. Thus, data from case reports, retrospective chart reviews, and open-label studies should be interpreted with great caution.

Third is the issue of measurement of target variables. Most often improvements are measured through global measures (e.g., the CGI scale) rather than by direct observations (e.g., as in Kemner et al., 2002), behavior-specific rating scales, or parental reports. While the data from global measures provide an overall picture of improvement (i.e., very much improved, much improved, minimally improved, or unchanged), they are not specific to target behaviors in terms of number, duration, intensity, or severity.

Fourth is that the metric used for weight gain in most studies has been the number of pound or kilograms of weight gained during the study period. Given that many of these studies used children and adolescents as participants, body mass index may be a better metric, because it adjusts weight for height (e.g., Malone et al., 2007). Weight gain in children and adolescents may be an indication of developmental growth, and this needs to be factored in when analyzing weight gain data in this population. While it may not be an issue for short-term studies (e.g., a few weeks), it would certainly affect interpretation of the data for longer term studies (e.g., a few months). Weight gain is a risk factor for many health conditions, including diabetes and cardiovascular and pulmonary disorders. Significant weight gain may adversely affect self-esteem and treatment compliance in children and adolescents, particularly if they are on long-term maintenance regimen. Thus, it is imperative to analyze the causative factors of weight gain in drug studies.

Fifth, there has always been a call that psychotropic drugs be used as an adjunctive treatment to behavioral, psychosocial, and educational interventions (e.g., Malone & Waheed, 2009). The reality of the situation is that drug trials do not typically consider other treatments when evaluating the effectiveness or efficacy of a new drug. Thus, we have no data about the utility of drugs when used as adjunctive therapy.

Finally, we need to consider the interactive effects of two or more concomitant therapies. Typically, behavioral interventions and pharmacotherapy are concurrently prescribed to control, manage, or treat severe challenging behaviors, but we have little understanding of their interactive effects. Over 25 years ago, Schroeder, Lewis, and Lipton (1983) presented a conceptual methodology to evaluate interactive effects, by adopting the minimum standards of drug research suggested by Sprague and Werry (1971) and incorporating the neuropsychopharmacology research model for studying the interactions between pharmacotherapy and psychotherapy advanced by Uhlenhuth, Lipman, and Covi (1969). With the exception of a handful of studies (e.g. Crosland et al.,

2003; Valdovinos, Ellringer, & Alexander, 2007; Valdovinos et al., 2002; Zarcone et al., 2004), this call for investigating the interaction between behavioral interventions and pharmacotherapy has gone unheeded, even though it is clear how such studies will assist clinicians to choose the best available treatments for people with challenging behaviors. Hopefully, such studies will become commonplace in the literature in the near future.

References

Adkins, A. D. (2010, April). *Adolescents with Asperger's syndrome use mindfulness-based strategy to control their anger*. Paper presented at the NADD 2010 International Congress, Toronto, Canada.

Adkins, A. D., Singh, A. N., Winton, A. S. W., McKeegan, G. F., & Singh, J. (2010). Using a mindfulness-based procedure in the community: Translating research to practice. *Journal of Child and Family Studies, 19*, 175–183.

Aman, M. G., Singh, N. N., Stewart, A. W., & Field, C. J. (1985). The Aberrant Behavior Checklist: A behavior rating scale for the assessment of treatment effects. *American Journal on Mental Deficiency, 89*, 485–491.

American Psychiatric Association. (2000). *Diagnostic and statistical manual of mental disorders,* (4th ed., Text Revision). Washington, DC: Author.

Anderson, D. J., Larkin, K. C., Hill, B. K., & Chen, T. H. (1992). Social integration of older persons with mental retardation in residential facilities. *American Journal on Mental Retardation, 96*, 488–501.

Anderson, L. T., Campbell, M., Adams, P., Small, A. M., Perry, R., & Shell, J. (1989). The effects of haloperidol on discrimination learning and behavioral symptoms in autistic children. *Journal of Autism and Developmental Disorders, 19*, 227–239.

Anderson, L. T., Campbell, M., Grega, D. M., Perry, R., Small, A. M., & Green, W. H. (1984). Haloperidol in the treatment of infantile autism: Effects on learning and behavioral symptoms. *American Journal of Psychiatry, 141*, 1195–1202.

Arnold, L. E., Vitiello, B., McDougle, C. J., Scahill, L., Shah, B., Gonzalez, N. M., et al. (2003). Parent-defined target symptoms respond to risperidone in RUPP Autism study: Customer approach to clinical trials. *Journal of the American Academy of Child and Adolescent Psychiatry, 42*, 1443–1450.

Beutler, L. E., Moleiro, C., & Talebi, H. (2002). How practitioners can systematically use empirical evidence in treatment selection. *Journal of Clinical Psychology, 58*, 1199–1212.

Borthwick-Duffy, S. A. (1994). Prevalence of destructive behaviors: A study of aggression, self-injury, and property destruction. In T. Thompson & D. B. Gray (Eds.), *Destructive behavior in developmental disabilities: Diagnosis and treatment* (pp. 3–23). Thousand Oaks, CA: Sage.

Borthwick-Duffy, S. A., Eyman, R. K., & White, J. F. (1987). Client characteristics and residential placement patterns. *American Journal on Mental Deficiency, 92*, 24–30.

Braithwaite, K. L., & Richdale, A. L. (2000). Functional communication training to replace challenging behaviors across two behavioral outcomes. *Behavioral Interventions, 15*, 21–36.

Brown, G. L., Goodwin, F. K., Ballenger, J. C., Goyer, P. F., & Major, L. F. (1979). Aggression in humans correlated with cerebrospinal fluid amine metabolites. *Psychiatric Research, 1*, 131–139.

Buck, O. D. (1995). Sertraline for reduction of violent behavior. *American Journal of Psychiatry, 152*, 953.

Buggey, T. (2005). Video self-modeling applications with students with autism spectrum disorder in a small private school setting. *Focus on Autism and Other Developmental Disabilities, 20*, 52–63.

Campbell, M., Anderson, L. T., Small, A. M., Perry, R., Green, W. H., & Caplan, R. (1982). The effects of haloperidol on learning and behavior in autistic children. *Journal of Autism and Developmental Disorders, 12*, 167–175.

Carr, E. G. (1988). Functional equivalence as a mechanism of response generalization. In R. H. Horner, G. Dunlap, & R. L. Koegel (Eds.), *Generalization and maintenance: Lifestyle changes in applied settings* (pp. 221–241). Baltimore: Paul H. Brookes.

Carr, E. G. (2007). The expanding vision of positive behavior support: Research perspectives on happiness, helpfulness, hopefulness. *Journal of Positive Behavior Interventions, 9*, 3–14.

Carr, E. G., Dunlap, G., Horner, R. H., Koegel, R. L., Turnbull, A. P., Sailor, W., et al. (2002). Positive behavior support: Evolution of an applied science. *Journal of Positive Behavior Interventions, 4*, 4–16, 20.

Carr, E. G., Levin, L., McConnachie, G., Carlson, J. I., Kemp, D. C., & Smith, C. E. (1994). *Communication-based interventions for problem behavior: A user's guide for producing positive change*. Baltimore: Paul H. Brookes.

Chadwick, O., Piroth, N., Walker, J., Bernard, S., & Taylor, E. (2000). Factors affecting the risk of behavior problems in children with severe intellectual disability. *Journal of Intellectual Disability Research, 44*, 108–123.

Chambless, D. L., & Hollon, S. D. (1998). Defining empirically supported therapies. *Journal of Consulting and Clinical Psychology, 66*, 7–18.

Chavez, B., Chavez-Brown, M., & Rey, J. A. (2006). Role of risperidone in children with autism spectrum disorder. *The Annals of Pharmacotherapy, 40*, 909–916.

Chen, N. C., Bedair, H. S., McKay, B., Bowers, M. B., & Mazure, C. (2001). Clozapine in the treatment of aggression in an adolescent with autistic disorder. *Journal of Clinical Psychiatry, 62*, 479–480.

Cook, E. H., Rowlett, R., Jaselskis, C., & Leventhal, B. L. (1992). Fluoxetine treatment of children and adults with autistic disorder and mental retardation. *Journal of the American Academy of Child and Adolescent Psychiatry, 31*, 739–745.

Corson, A. H., Barkenbus, J. E., Posey, D. J., Stigler, K. A., & McDougle, C. J. (2004). A retrospective analysis of quetiapine in the treatment of pervasive developmental disorders. *Journal of Clinical Psychiatry, 65*, 1531–1536.

Crone, D. A., & Horner, R. H. (2003). *Building positive behavior support systems in schools: Functional behavioral assessment*. New York: Guilford.

Crosland, K. A., Zarcone, J. R., Lindauer, S. E., Valdovinos, M. G., Zarcone, T. J., Hellings, J. A., et al. (2003). Use of functional analysis methodology in the evaluation of medication effects. *Journal of Autism and Developmental Disabilities, 33*, 271–279.

De Leon, J., Greenlee, B., Barber, J., Sabaawi, M., & Singh, N. N. (2009). Practical guidelines for the use of new generation antipsychotic drugs (except Clozapine) in individuals with intellectual disabilities. *Research in Developmental Disabilities, 30*, 613–669.

Demb, H. B. (1996). Risperidone in young children with pervasive developmental disorders and other developmental disabilities. *Journal of Child and Adolescent Psychopharmacology, 6*, 79–80.

Diler, R. S., Firat, S., & Avci, A. (2002). An open-label trial of risperidone in children with autism. *Current Therapeutic Research, 63*, 91–102.

Dooley, P., Wilczenski, F. L., & Torem, C. (2001). Using an activity schedule to smooth school transitions. *Journal of Positive Behavior Interventions, 3*, 57–61.

Durand, V. M. (1990). *Severe behavior problems: A functional communication training approach*. New York: Guilford.

Durand, V. M. (1999). Functional communication training using assistive devices: Recruiting natural communities of reinforcement. *Journal of Applied Behavior Analysis, 32,* 247–267.

Emerson, E. (2001) *Challenging behavior: Analysis and intervention in people with severe intellectual disabilities* (2nd ed.). Cambridge: Cambridge University Press.

Emerson, E., Kiernan, C., Alborz, A., Reeves, D., Mason, H., Swarbrick, R., et al. (2001). The prevalence of challenging behaviors: A total population study. *Research in Developmental Disabilities, 22,* 77–93.

Filipek, P. A., Steinberg-Epstein, R., & Book, T. (2006). Intervention for autism spectrum disorders. *NeuroRX, 3,* 207–216.

Findling, R. L., Maxwell, K., & Wiznitzer., M. (1997). An open clinical trial risperidone monotherapy in young children with autistic disorder. *Psychopharmacology Bulletin, 33,* 155–159.

Findling, R. L., McNamara, N. K., Gracious, B. L., O'Riordan, M. A., Reed, M. D., Demeter, C., et al. (2004). Quetiapine in nine youths with autistic disorder. *Journal of Child and Adolescent Psychopharmacology, 14,* 287–294.

Fisman, S., & Steele, M. (1996). Use of risperidone in pervasive developmental disorders: A case series. *Journal of Child and Adolescent Psychopharmacology, 6,* 177–190.

Foxx, R. M., & Garito, J. (2007). The long term successful treatment of the very severe behaviors of a preadolescent with autism. *Behavioral Interventions, 22,* 69–82.

Foxx, R. M., & Meindl, J. (2007). The long term successful treatment of the aggressive/destructive behaviors of a preadolescent with autism. *Behavioral Interventions, 22,* 83–97.

Frea, W. D., Arnold, C. L., & Vittimberga, G. L. (2001). A demonstration of the effects of augmentative communication on the extreme aggressive behavior of a child with autism within an integrated preschool setting. *Journal of Positive Behavior Interventions, 3,* 194–198.

Goin-Kochel, R. P., Mackintosh, V. H., & Myers, B. J. (2009). Parental reports on the efficacy of treatments and therapies for their children with autism spectrum disorders. *Research in Autism Spectrum Disorders, 3,* 528–537.

Goin-Kochel, R. P., Myers, B. J., & Mackintosh, V. H. (2007). Parental reports on the use of treatments and therapies for children with autism spectrum disorders. *Research in Autism Spectrum Disorders, 1,* 195–209.

Green, G. (1996). Early behavioral intervention for autism: What does research tell us? In C. Maurice, G. Green, & S. C. Luce (Eds.), *Behavioral intervention for young children with autism: A Manual for parents and professionals* (pp. 29–44). Austin, TX: PRO-ED.

Green, V. A., Pituch, K. A., Itchon, J., Choi, A., O'Reilly, M., & Sigafoos, J. (2006). Internet survey of treatments used by parents of children with autism. *Research in Developmental Disabilities, 27,* 70–84.

Gunaratana, B. H. (2009). *Beyond mindfulness in plain English.* Boston: Wisdom Publications.

Guy, W. (1976). *ECDEU assessment manual for psychopharmacology.* Rockville, MD: US National Institute of Health, Psychopharmacology Research Branch.

Hagopian, L. P., Bruzek, J. L., Bowman, L. G., & Jennett, H. K. (2007). Assessment and treatment of problem behavior occasioned by interruption of free-operant behavior. *Journal of Applied Behavior Analysis, 40,* 89–103.

Halle, J., Bambara, L. M., & Reichle, J. (2005). Teaching alternative skills. In L. M. Bambara & L. Kern (Eds.), *Individualized supports for students with problem behaviors: Designing positive behavior support plans* (pp. 237–274). New York: Guilford.

Hastings, R. P. (2002). Parental stress and behaviour problems in children with developmental disability. *Journal of Intellectual and Developmental Disability, 27,* 149–160.

Heckaman, K. A., Alber, S., Hooper, S., & Heward, W. L. (1998). A comparison of least-to-most prompts and progressive time delay on the disruptive behavior of students with autism. *Journal of Behavioral Education, 8,* 171–201.

Hellings, J. A., Kelley, L. A., Gabrielli, W. F., Kilgore, E., & Shah, P. (1996). Sertraline response in adults with mental retardation and autistic disorder. *Journal of Clinical Psychiatry, 57,* 333–336.

Holden, B., & Gitlesen, J. P. (2006). A total population study of challenging behavior in the county of Hedmark, Norway: Prevalence and risk markers. *Research in Developmental Disabilities, 27,* 456–465.

Hollander, E., Wasserman, S., Swanson, E. N., Chaplin, W., Schapiro, M. L., Zagursky, K., et al. (2006). A double-blind placebo-controlled pilot study of olanzapine in childhood/adolescent pervasive developmental disorder. *Journal of Child and Adolescent Psychopharmacology, 16,* 541–548.

Horrigan, J. P., & Barnhill, L. J. (1997). Risperidone and explosive aggressive autism. *Journal of Autism and Developmental Disorders, 27,* 313–323.

Horrigan, J. P., Barnhill, L. J., & Courvoisie, H. E. (1997). Olanzapine in PDD. *Journal of the American Academy of Child and Adolescent Psychiatry, 36,* 1166–1167.

Ingvarsson, E. T., Kahng, S., & Hausman, N. L. (2008). Some effects of noncontingent positive reinforcement on multiply controlled problem behavior and compliance in a demand context. *Journal of Applied Behavior Analysis, 41,* 435–440.

Jacobson, J. W., Mulick, J. A., & Schwartz, A. A. (1995). A history of facilitated communication: Science, pseudoscience, and anti-science working group on facilitated communication. *American Psychologist, 50,* 750–765.

Kemner, C., Willemsen-Swinkels, S. H. N., De Jonge, M., Tuynman-Qua, H., & Van Engeland, H. (2002). Open-label study of olanzapine in children with pervasive developmental disorder. *Journal of Clinical Psychopharmacology, 22,* 455–460.

Kern, L., Carberry, N., & Haidara, C. (1997). Analysis and intervention with two topographies of challenging behavior exhibited by a young woman with autism. *Research in Developmental Disabilities, 18,* 275–287.

Krishnamoorthy, J., & King, B. H. (1998). Open-label olanzapine treatment in five preadolescent children. *Journal of Child and Adolescent Psychopharmacology, 8,* 107–113.

Kuttler, S., Myles, B. S., & Carlson, J. K. (1998). The use of social stories to reduce precursors to tantrum behavior in a student with autism. *Focus on Autism and Other Developmental Disabilities, 13,* 176–182.

Lord, C., Rutter, M., & Le Coteur, A. M. (1994). Autism diagnostic interview revised: A revised version of a diagnostic interview for caregivers of individuals with possible pervasive developmental disorders. *Journal of Autism and Developmental Disorders, 24,* 659–685.

Lovaas, O. I. (1987). Behavioral treatment and normal educational and intellectual functioning in young autistic children. *Journal of Consulting and Clinical Psychology, 55,* 3–9.

Lowe, K., Allen, D., Jones, E., Brophy, S., Moore, K., & James, W. (2007). Challenging behaviors: Prevalence and topographies. *Journal of Intellectual Disability Research, 51,* 625–636.

Luiselli, J. K. (1998). Intervention conceptualization and formulation. In J. K. Luiselli & M. J. Cameron (Eds.), *Antecedent control: Innovative approaches to behavioral support* (pp. 29–44). Baltimore: Paul H. Brookes.

Luiselli, J. K. (2006). *Antecedent assessment and intervention: Supporting children and adults with developmental disabilities in the community.* Baltimore: Paul H. Brookes

Machalicek, W., O'Reilly, M. F., Beretvas, N., Sigafoos, J., & Lancioni, G. E. (2007). A review of interventions to reduce challenging behavior in school settings for students with autism spectrum disorders. *Research in Autism Spectrum Disorders, 1,* 229–246.

Malek-Ahmadi, P., & Simonds, J. F. (1998). Olanzapine for autistic disorder with hyperactivity. *Journal of the American Academy of Child and Adolescent Psychiatry, 37*, 902–903.

Malone, R. P., Cater, J., Sheikh, R. M., Choudhury, M. S., & Delaney, M. A. (2001). Olanzapine versus haloperidol in children with autistic disorder: An open pilot study. *Journal of the American Academy of Child and Adolescent Psychiatry, 40*, 887–893.

Malone, R. P., Delaney, M. A., Hyman, S. B., & Cater, J. R. (2007). Ziprasidone in adolescents with autism: An open-label pilot study. *Journal of Child and Adolescent Psychopharmacology, 17*, 779–790.

Malone, R. P., Maislin, G., Choudhury, M. S., Gifford, C., & Delaney, M. A. (2002). Risperidone treatment in children and adolescents with autism: Short- and long-term safety and effectiveness. *Journal of the American Academy of Child and Adolescent Psychiatry, 41*, 140–147.

Malone, R. P., & Waheed, A. (2009). The role of antipsychotics in the management of behavioral symptoms in children and adolescents with autism. *Drugs, 69*, 535–548.

Marcus, R. N., Owen, R., Kamen, L., Manos, G., McQuade, R. D., Carson, W. H., et al. (2009). A placebo-controlled, fixed-dose study of aripiprazole in children and adolescents with irritability associated with autistic disorder. *Journal of the American Academy of Child and Adolescent Psychiatry, 48*, 1110–1119.

Martin, A., Koenig, K., Anderson, G. M., & Scahill, L. (2003). Low-dose fluvoxamine treatment of children and adolescents with pervasive developmental disorders: A prospective, open-label study. *Journal of Autism and Developmental Disorders, 33*, 77–85.

Martin, A., Koenig, K., Scahill, L., & Bregman, J. (1999). Open-label quetiapine in the treatment of children and adolescents with autistic disorder. *Journal of Child and Adolescent Psychopharmacology, 9*, 99–107.

Masi, G., Cosenza, A., Millediedi, S., Muratori, F., Pari, C., & Salvadori, F. (2009). Aripiprazole monotherapy in children and young adolescents with pervasive developmental disorders: A retrospective study. *CNS Drugs, 23*, 511–521.

Matson, J. L. (2009). Aggression and tantrums in children with autism: A review of behavioral treatments and maintaining variables. *Journal of Mental Health Research in Intellectual Disabilities, 2*, 169–187.

Matson, J. L., Benavidez, D. A., Compton, L. S., Paclawskyj, T., & Baglio, C. (1996). Behavioral treatment of autistic persons: A review of research from 1980 to the present. *Research in Developmental Disabilities, 17*, 433–465.

Matson, J. L., & Nebel-Schwalm, M. (2007). Assessing challenging behaviors in children with autism spectrum disorders: A review. *Research in Developmental Disabilities, 28*, 567–579.

Matson, J. L., & Smith, K. R. M. (2008). Current status of intensive behavioral interventions of young children with autism and PDD-NOS. *Research in Autism Spectrum Disorders, 2*, 60–74.

McDougle, C. J., Brodkin, E. S., Naylor, S. T., Carlson, D. C., Cohen, D. J., & Price, L. H. (1998). Sertraline in adults with pervasive developmental disorders: A prospective open-label investigation. *Journal of Clinical Psychopharmacology, 18*, 62–66.

McDougle, C. J., Brodkin, E. S., Yeung, P. P., Naylor, S. T., Cohen, D. J., & Price, L. H. (1995). Risperidone in adults with autism or pervasive developmental disorder. *Journal of Child and Adolescent Psychopharmacology, 5*, 273–283.

McDougle, C. J., Holmes, J. P., Bronson, M. R., Anderson, G. M., Volkmar, F. R., Price, L. H., et al. (1997). Risperidone treatment of children and adolescents with pervasive developmental disorders: A prospective, open-label study. *Journal of the American Academy of Child and Adolescent Psychiatry, 36*, 685–693.

McDougle, C. J., Holmes, J. P., Carlson, D. C., Pelton, G. H., Cohen, D. J., & Price, L. H. (1998). A double-blind, placebo-controlled study of risperidone in adults with autistic disorder and other pervasive developmental disorders. *Archives of General Psychiatry, 55*, 633–641.

McDougle, C. J., Kem, D. L., & Posey, D. J. (2002). Case Series: Use of ziprasidone for maladaptive symptoms in youths with autism. *Journal of the American Academy of Child and Adolescent Psychiatry, 41*, 921–927.

McDougle, C. J., Naylor, S. T., Cohen, D. J., Volkmar, F. R., Heninger, G. R., & Price, L. H. (1996). A double-blind, placebo-controlled study of fluvoxamine in adults with autistic disorder. *Archives of General Psychiatry, 53*, 1001–1008.

McDougle, C. J., Scahill, L., Aman, M. G., McCracken, J. T., Tierney, E., Davis, M., et al. (2005). Risperidone for the core symptom domains of autism: Results from the study by the Autism Network of the Research Units on Pediatric Psychopharmacology. *American Journal of Psychiatry, 162*, 1142–1148.

McEachin, J. J., Smith, T., & Lovaas, O. I. (1993). Long-term outcome for children with autism who received early intensive behavioral treatment. *American Journal on Mental Retardation, 97*, 359–372.

Morrison, K., & Rosales-Ruiz, J. (1997). The effect of object preferences on task performance and stereotypy in a child with autism. *Research in Developmental Disabilities, 18*, 127–137.

Moss, A. J. (1993). Measurement of the QT interval and the risk associated with QTc interval prolongation: A review. *American Journal of Cardiology, 72*, 23B–25B.

Mostert, M. P. (2001). Facilitated communication since 1995: A review of published studies. *Journal of Autism and Developmental Disorders, 31*, 287–313.

Mruzek, D. W., Cohen, C., & Smith, T. (2007). Contingency contracting with students with autism spectrum disorders in a public school setting. *Journal of Developmental and Physical Disabilities, 19*, 103–114.

Mueller, M. M., Wilczynski, S. M., Moore, J. W., Fusilier, I., & Trahant, D. (2001). Antecedent manipulations in a tangible condition: Effects of stimulus preference on aggression. *Journal of Applied Behavior Analysis, 34*, 237–240.

Murphy, G. H., Beadle-Brown, J., Wing, L., Gould, J., Shah, A., & Holmes, N. (2005). Chronicity of challenging behaviors in people with severe intellectual disabilities and/or autism: A total population sample. *Journal of Autism and Developmental Disorders, 35*, 405–418.

Murphy, O., Healy, O., & Leader, G. (2009). Risk factors for challenging behaviors among 157 children with autism spectrum disorder in Ireland. *Research in Autism Spectrum Disorders, 3*, 474–482.

National Institute of Mental Health. (1985). Rating scales and assessment instruments for use in pediatric psychopharmacology research. *Psychopharmacology Bulletin, 21*, 839–843.

National Research Council. (2001). *Educating children with autism. Committee on Education and Interventions for Children with Autism. Division of Behavioral and Social Sciences and education.* Washington, DC: National Academy Press.

Nicolson, R., Awad, G., & Sloman, L. (1998). An open trial of risperidone in young autistic children. *Journal of the American Academy of Child and Adolescent Psychiatry, 37*, 372–376.

Oliver, C., Murphy, G. H., & Corbett, J. A. (1987). Self-injurious behavior in people with mental handicap: A total population survey. *Journal of Mental Deficiency Research, 31*, 147–162.

Owen, R., Sikich, L., Marcus, R. N., Corey-Lisle, P., Manos, G., McQuade, R. D., et al. (2009). Aripiprazole in the treatment of irritability in children and adolescents with autistic disorder. *Pediatrics, 124*, 1533–1540.

Paisey, T. J., Fox, S., Curran, C., Hooper, K., & Whitney, R. (1991). Case study: Reinforcement control of severe aggression exhibited by a child with autism in a family home. *Behavioral Residential Treatment, 6*, 289–302.

Perry, A., Cummings, A., Geier, J. D., Freeman, N. L., Hughes, S., LaRose, L., et al. (2008). Effectiveness of intensive behavioral intervention in a large, community-based program. *Research in Autism Spectrum Disorders, 2*, 621–642.

Perry, R., Pataki, C., Munoz-Silva, D. M., Armenteros, J., & Silva, R. R. (1997). Risperidone in children and adolescents with pervasive developmental disorder: Pilot trial and follow-up. *Journal of Child and Adolescent Psychopharmacology, 7*, 167–179.

Posey, D. J., Walsh, K. H., Wilson, G. A., & McDougle, C. J. (1999). Risperidone in the treatment of two very young children with autism. *Journal of Child and Adolescent Psychopharmacology, 4*, 273–276.

Potenza, M. N., Holmes, J. P., Kanes, S. J., & McDougle, C. J. (1999). Olanzapine treatment of children, adolescents, and adults with pervasive developmental disorders: An open-label pilot study. *Journal of Clinical Psychopharmacology, 19*, 37–44.

Research Units on Pediatric Psychopharmacology Autism Network. (2002). Risperidone in children with autism and serious behavior problems. *New England Journal of Medicine, 347*, 314–321.

Research Units on Pediatric Psychopharmacology Autism Network. (2005). Risperidone treatment of autistic disorder: Longer-term benefits and blinded discontinuation after 6 months. *American Journal of Psychiatry, 162*, 1361–1369.

Sallows, G. O., & Graupner, T. D. (2005). Intensive behavioral treatment for children with autism: Four-year outcome and predictors. *American Journal on Mental Retardation, 110*, 417–438.

Schindler, H. R., & Horner, R. H. (2005). Generalized reduction of problem behavior of young children with autism: Building transsituational interventions. *American Journal on Mental Retardation, 110*, 36–47.

Schmit, J., Alper, S., Raschke, D., & Ryndak, D. (2000). Effects of using a photographic cueing package during routine school transitions with a child who has autism. *Mental Retardation, 38*, 131–137.

Schreibman, L. (2000). Intensive behavioral/psychoeducational treatments for autism: Research needs and future directions. *Journal of Autism and developmental Disorders, 30*, 373–378.

Schroeder, S. R., Lewis, M. H., & Lipton, M. A. (1983). Interactions of pharmacotherapy and behavior therapy among children with learning and behavioral disorders. *Advances in Learning and Behavioral Disabilities, 2*, 179–225.

Shapiro, S. L., & Carlson, L. E. (2009). *The art and science of mindfulness: Integrating mindfulness into psychology and the helping professions.* Washington, DC: American Psychological Association.

Shea, S., Turgay, A., Carroll, A., Schulz, M., Orlik, H., Smith, I., et al. (2004). Risperidone in the treatment of disruptive behavioral symptoms in children with autistic and other pervasive developmental disorders. *Pediatrics, 114*, e634–e641.

Sigafoos, J., & Meikle, B. (1996). Functional communication training for the treatment of multiply determined challenging behavior in two boys with autism. *Behavior Modification, 20*, 60–84.

Singh, N. N., Lancioni, G. E., Wahler, R. G., Winton, A. S. W., & Singh, J. (2008). Mindfulness approaches in cognitive behavior therapy. *Behavioural and Cognitive Psychotherapy, 36*, 659–666.

Singh, N. N., Lancioni, G. E., Winton, A. S. W., Adkins, A. D., Singh, A. N., & Singh, J. (in press). Mindfulness-based approaches. In J. L. Taylor, W. R. Lindsay, R. Hastings, & C. Hatton (Eds.), *Psychological therapies for adults with intellectual disabilities.* Chichester, West Sussex: Wiley.

Singh, N. N., Lancioni, G. E., Winton, A. S. W., Fisher, B. C., Wahler, R. G., McAleavey, K., et al. (2006). Mindful parenting decreases aggression, noncompliance and self-injury in children with autism. *Journal of Emotional and Behavioral Disorders, 14*, 169–177.

Singh, N. N., Winton, A. S. W., Singh, J., McAleavey, K., Wahler, R. G., & Sabaawi, M. (2006). Mindfulness-based caregiving and support. In J. K. Luiselli (Ed.), *Antecedent assessment and intervention:*

Supporting children and adults with developmental disabilities in community settings (pp. 269–290). Baltimore: Paul H. Brookes.

Skinner, B. F. (1953). *Science and human behavior.* New York: MacMillan

Sprague, R. L., & Werry, J. S. (1971). Methodology of psychopharmacological studies with the retarded. In N. R. Ellis (Ed.), *International review of research in mental retardation* (vol. 5, pp. 147–219). New York: Academic Press.

Stachnik, J. M., & Nunn-Thompson, C. (2007). Use of atypical antipsychotics in the treatment of autistic disorder. *The Annals of Pharmacotherapy, 41*, 626–634.

Steingard, R. J., Zimnitzky, B., DeMaso, D. R., Bauman, M. L., & Bucci, J. P. (1997). Sertraline treatment of transition-associated anxiety and agitation in children with autistic disorder. *Journal of Child and Adolescent Psychopharmacology, 7*, 9–15.

Stigler, K. A., Diener, J. T., Kohn, A. E., Li, L., Erickson, C. A., Posey, D. J., et al. (2009). Aripiprazole in pervasive developmental disorder not otherwise specified and Asperger's disorder: A 14-week, prospective, open-label study. *Journal of Child and Adolescent Psychopharmacology, 19*, 265–274.

Stigler, K. A., Posey, D. J., & McDougle, C. J. (2002). Recent advances in the pharmacotherapy of autism. *Expert Review of Neurotherapeutics, 2*, 499–510.

Stigler, K. A., Posey, D. J., & McDougle, C. J. (2004). Aripiprazole for maladaptive behavior in pervasive developmental disorders. *Journal of Child and Adolescent Psychopharmacology, 14*, 455–463.

Stigler, K. A., Potenza, M. N., Posey, D. J., & McDougle, C. J. (2004). Weight gain associated with atypical antipsychotic use in children and adolescents: Prevalence, clinical relevance, and management. *Paediatric Drugs, 6*, 33–44.

Sturmey, P. (2005). Secretin is an ineffective treatment for pervasive developmental disabilities: A review of 15 double-blind randomized controlled trials. *Research in Developmental Disabilities, 26*, 87–97.

Thera, N. (1996). *The heart of Buddhist meditation.* Kandy, Sri Lanka: Buddhist Publication Society.

Thompson, R. H., Fisher, W. W., Piazza, C. C., & Kuhn, D. E. (1998). The evaluation and treatment of aggression maintained by attention and automatic reinforcement. *Journal of Applied Behavior Analysis, 31*, 103–116.

Troost, P. W., Lahuis, B. E., Steenhuis, M. -P., Ketelaars, C. E. J., Buitelaar, J. K., Van Engeland, H., et al. (2005). Long-term effects of risperidone in children with autism spectrum disorders: A placebo discontinuation study. *Journal of the American Academy of Child and Adolescent Psychiatry, 44*, 1137–1144.

Tyrer, F., McGrother, C. W., Thorp, C. F., Donaldson, M., Bhaumik, S., Watson, J. M., et al. (2006). Physical aggression towards others in adults with learning disabilities: Prevalence and associated factors. *Journal of Intellectual Disability Research, 50*, 295–304.

Uhlenhuth, E. H., Lipman, R. S., & Covi, L. (1969). Combined pharmacotherapy and psychotherapy. *Journal of Nervous and Mental Disease, 148*, 52–64.

Valdovinos, M. G., Ellringer, N. P., & Alexander, M. L. (2007). Changes in the rate of problem behavior associated with the discontinuation of the antipsychotic quetiapine. *Mental Health Aspects of Developmental Disabilities, 10*, 64–67.

Valdovinos, M. G., Napolitano, D. A., Zarcone, J. R., Hellings, J. A., Williams, D. C., & Schroeder, S. R. (2002). Multimodal evaluation of risperidone for destructive behavior: Functional analysis, direct observation, rating scales, and psychiatric impressions. *Experimental and Clinical Psychopharmacology, 10*, 268–275.

Valicenti-McDermott, M. R., & Demb, H. (2006). Clinical effects and adverse reactions of off-label use of aripiprazole in children and adolescents with developmental disabilities. *Journal of Child and Adolescent Psychopharmacology, 16*, 549–560.

Vollmer, T. R., Borrero, J. C., Lalli, J. S., & Daniel, D. (1999). Evaluating self-control and impulsivity in children with severe behavior disorders. *Journal of Applied Behavior Analysis, 32,* 451–466.

Williams, K. J., Wray, J. J., & Wheeler, D. M. (2005). Intravenous secretin for autism spectrum disorder. *Cochrane Database of Systematic Reviews,* (3), Art. No.: CD003495. doi: 10.1002/14651858.CD003495.pub2

Yokoyama, H., Hirose, M., Haginoya, K., Munakata, M., & Iinuma, K. (2002). Treatment with fluvoxamine against self-injury and aggressive behavior in autistic children. *No to Hattatsu [Brain and Development], 34,* 249–253.

Zarcone, J. R., Lindauer, S. E., Morse, P. S., Crosland, K. A., Valdovinos, M. G., McKerchar, T. L., et al. (2004). Effects of risperidone on destructive behavior of persons with developmental disabilities: III. Functional analysis. *American Journal on Mental Retardation, 109,* 310–321.

Zuddas, A., Di Martino, A., Muglia, P., & Cianchetti, C. (2000). Long-term risperidone for pervasive developmental disorder: Efficacy, tolerability, and discontinuation. *Journal of Child and Adolescent Psychopharmacology, 10,* 79–90.

Zuddas, A., Ledda, M. G., Fratta, A., Muglia, P., & Cianchetti, C. (1996). Clinical effects of clozapine on autistic disorder. *American Journal of Psychiatry, 153,* 738.

Campbell, M., Anderson, L. T., Meier, M., Cohen, I. L., Small, A. M., Samit, C., et al. (1978). A comparison of haloperidol and behavior therapy and their interaction in autistic children. *Journal of the American Academy of Child Psychiatry, 17,* 640–655.

Hagopian, L. P., Wilson, D. M., & Wilder, D. A. (2001). Assessment and treatment of problem behavior maintained by escape from attention and access to tangible items. *Journal of Applied Behavior Analysis, 34,* 229–232.

Frederick Furniss, Asit B. Biswas, Bradley Bezilla, and Aaron A. Jones

Self-injurious behavior (SIB) is a serious problem for some people with pervasive developmental disorders (PDDs) which is a common focus of clinical treatment and has received extensive attention in the research literature. This is the first of two related chapters. The first provides an overview of SIB and behavioral approaches to its treatment. The second reviews pharmacological approaches to treatment of SIB and then work which attempts to integrate behavioral and pharmacological treatments. Although other approaches to treatment of SIB, such as psychotherapy, counseling, and sensory approaches, may be used in practice, there is little research evidence to review on their efficacy in people with ASDs. Additionally, single-case experiments suggest that reported effects of interventions such as sensory integration with particular individuals may be more parsimoniously explained by the social interaction or reduction in task demands associated with the therapy and that function-based behavioral interventions are equally or more effective in reducing SIB (Devlin, Leader, & Healey, 2009; Mason & Iwata, 1990). Hence, these two chapters focus on behavioral and pharmacological interventions.

Overview

PDDs include autistic disorder, Asperger's disorder, childhood disintegrative disorder (CDD), Rett's disorder, and PDD-not otherwise specified (NOS) (American Psychiatric Association, 1994); however, Rett's and childhood disintegrative disorders are rare, and participants with these diagnoses are often not included in clinical research with people with autism spectrum disorders (ASDs) (Posey, Stigler, Erickson, & McDougle, 2008). In this chapter, the term ASDs will, in general, only refer to autistic disorder,

Asperger's disorder, and PDD-NOS. Where research studies describe participants as persons with autism or PDDs or ASDs without clarifying which specific diagnoses are included and excluded, we generally refer to those participants as persons with ASDs or use the description employed by the authors. Where, however, participants in group studies are limited to those with a single diagnosis or those with a diagnosis of autistic disorder are specifically excluded, we use more specific terms. SIB, which is generally defined as comprising non-accidental, self-inflicted acts causing damage to or destruction of body tissue and carried out without suicidal ideation or intent (Yates, 2004), is relatively common both in people with severe intellectual disabilities (IDs) and in those with ASDs (Lecavalier, 2006; Lowe et al., 2007; Oliver, Murphy, & Corbett, 1987). In both groups SIB may present as repetitive head banging or face slapping, biting hands or other body parts, removing scabs from old wounds, self-pinching or scratching, hair-pulling, and eye-poking. Often one person presents multiple forms of SIB.

Although a prevalence of 53% has been reported in a clinical sample of children diagnosed with "infantile autism" using ICD-10 criteria (Baghdadli, Pascal, Grisi, & Aussilloux, 2003), the overall prevalence of SIB in persons with ASDs does not appear to differ markedly from that in persons with IDs, with rates of 10–12% typically reported in large-scale population-based studies when all forms of SIB are included (Lecavalier, 2006; Lowe et al., 2007). Presence of ASD has been identified as a risk factor for SIB in people with IDs (Collacott, Cooper, Branford, & McGrother, 1998; McClintock, Hall, & Oliver, 2003), but this may be accounted for by the association between presence of ASD and severity of ID (Bhaumik, Branford, McGrother, & Thorp, 1997). Studies controlling experimentally or statistically for ability find that although lower ability predicts presentation of SIB, presence of ASD does not (Chadwick, Piroth, Walker, Bernard, & Taylor, 2000; Cooper et al., 2009). With ability controlled for, young children with ASDs show higher rates of various restrictive and repetitive behaviors (RRBs) than those with other developmental disabilities,

F. Furniss (✉)
School of Psychology, University of Leicester, Leicester LE1 7LT, UK
e-mail: fred.furniss@hesleygroup.co.uk

J.L. Matson, P. Sturmey (eds.), *International Handbook of Autism and Pervasive Developmental Disorders*, Autism and Child Psychopathology Series, DOI 10.1007/978-1-4419-8065-6_27, © Springer Science+Business Media, LLC 2011

but comparable prevalence and severity of SIB (Richler, Bishop, Kleinke, & Lord, 2007).

Cohen et al. (2010) presented evidence from a large-scale study suggesting that persons with ASDs score higher than persons with IDs but no diagnosis of ASD on a measure of self-injury. This was particularly marked in females. Since ASDs are highly variable and their causation multifactorial, although a clinical diagnosis of an ASD per se may not increase risk for SIB, the presence or the severity of specific features of ASD may do so. Matson and Rivet (2008) measured the severity of features of autism and ASD-NOS in 298 adults with severe IDs using the Autism Spectrum Disorders-Diagnosis for Adults (ASD-DA) (Matson, Boisjoli, González, Smith, & Wilkins, 2007). Multivariate analysis of covariance with measures of communication, daily living, and social skills as covariates showed that participants with higher ASD-DA scores had higher scores on the SIB subscale of the Autism Spectrum Disorders-Behavior Problems for adults (Matson & Rivet, 2007), and subsequent analyses showed that with measures of communication, daily living, and social skills controlled for, severity of RRBs showed a significant, albeit moderate, relationship with severity of SIB.

Given that the knowledge base on causes of and intervention for SIB in persons with IDs (Schroeder et al., 2001) currently exceeds that for persons with ASDs (Matson & LoVullo, 2008), the question arises as to the extent to which approaches to assessment and intervention developed with people with IDs can be directly extended to those with ASDs. Adaptations to interventions helpful for people with IDs to SIB in persons with ASDs might be required if (a) SIBs in the latter population represent one form of the RRBs which are a defining feature of the disorder (Gal, Dyck, & Passmore, 2009), (b) SIBs in people with ASDs are underpinned by other emotional and behavioral disorders for which persons with ASDs are at specifically enhanced risk, or (c) the cognitive and social dimensions of ASD require specific modifications of intervention methods developed for persons with IDs.

Factor analyses of data from descriptive assessments of maladaptive behaviors in persons with IDs and ASDs do not in general support the hypothesis that SIBs are members of a broader class of stereotyped movements, since SIB and other stereotyped movements usually emerge as separate factors (Brinkley et al., 2007; Lam & Aman, 2007; Rojahn, Matson, Naglieri, & Mayville, 2004). Brinkley et al. (2007), however, factor analyzing the Aberrant Behavior Checklist (ABC) scores (Aman & Singh, 1994) of 275 individuals with ASDs, found that in a subsample of 59 individuals with more severe SIB the three items comprising a self-injury factor in the total sample loaded onto a factor otherwise reflecting stereotypy. The findings of Brinkley et al. (2007) suggest that there may be a relationship between RRBs and severity

and/or chronicity of SIB in persons with ASDs. Studies considering whether presence of an ASD predicts chronicity of SIB and other behavioral difficulties have yielded mixed results. Emerson et al. (2001) in a 7-year follow-up of 95 people with ID presenting severe SIB found that a diagnosis of autism at the time of the original study did not predict SIB at follow-up in a logistic regression analysis. Cooper et al. (2009) followed up 34 adults with ID out of a group of 50 who presented SIB in a total population study 2 years previously and found that 21 (62%) continued to present SIB. Melville et al. (2008), drawing on the same data set as Cooper et al. (2009), did not study individual topographies of problem behavior, but found that over the 2-year period only one (5.9%) of the 17 people with autism presenting various topographies of problem behavior ceased to do, whereas 12 (37.5%) of 32 control participants without autism, and matched to participants with autism for gender, ability level, age, and presence or absence of Down's syndrome, ceased to present such behaviors. Baghdadli et al. (2008) followed up 185 children with "infantile autism" diagnosed according to ICD-10 criteria and a mean age of 8 years out of a sample of 222 first assessed at a mean age of 5 years. Seventy-nine (42.7%) of the children did not show SIB at either time point, 44 (23.8%) initially showing SIB did not do so at follow-up, 48 (25.9%) showed SIB at both initial assessment and follow-up, and 14 (7.6%) did not present SIB initially but did so at follow-up. Logistic regression identified severity of features of autism at initial assessment as measured by the Childhood Autism Rating Scale (Schopler, Reichler, DeVellis, & Daly, 1980) and lower speech level as risk factors for presentation of SIB at follow-up.

Both young people and adults with ASDs experience high rates of emotional and behavioral disturbances including conduct problems, anxiety, hyperactivity, RRBs, and SIB (Bhaumik et al., 1997; Lecavalier, 2006). Less clear is whether the prevalence of such difficulties in people with ASDs who have IDs is higher than those in people with IDs not diagnosed with ASDs. Tsakanikos et al. (2006), comparing 147 adults with ID and ASD with 605 adults with ID alone, found that rates of clinical diagnosis of schizophrenia spectrum disorder, anxiety, depressive disorder, and adjustment reaction did not differ between the groups. Several studies using screening questionnaires for psychiatric difficulties suggest, however, that persons with ASD are at particularly enhanced risk of experiencing mania, stereotyped behaviors, which are of course a defining feature of the disorder, and anxiety, while impulse control problems may be associated with ID, rather than specifically with ASD (Bradley, Summers, Wood, & Bryson, 2004; Hill & Furniss, 2006; Matson et al., 1996). Although the reliance on screening questionnaires in these studies leaves open the issue of whether the difficulties observed would meet formal diagnostic criteria, the context of comorbid emotional and behavioral difficulties experienced by a person with ASD presenting SIB may have implications for intervention. For example, Aman et al. (2005) have suggested that risperidone may be useful primarily in treatment of "impulsive" rather than "compulsive" forms of SIB. Assessment of emotional/behavioral comorbidity, with particular reference to impulsivity, mood disturbance, anxiety, and severity and phenomenology of RRBs, may therefore be useful both in selecting interventions targeted at SIB and for identification of possible related difficulties which may be amenable to psychosocial or pharmacological interventions.

Given the evidence base for function-based behavioral interventions for problem behavior in persons with IDs and ASDs (Campbell, 2003; Didden, Duker, & Korzilius, 1997; Didden, Korzilius, Van Oorsouw, & Sturmey, 2006; Herzinger & Campbell, 2007), research on the implications of the cognitive and social difficulties of persons with ASDs for such interventions has primarily concerned the possibility that problem behavior in this population may frequently serve different functions from those typical for other persons with developmental disabilities. Reese, Richman, Belmont, and Morse (2005) categorized the functions of problem behavior in 46 children with and without ASDs into six categories, three of which were described as "standard" functions (gain attention, escape demand, or gain tangible item) and three hypothesized by Reese et al. (2005) to be "more directly related to particular characteristics of children with autism" (p. 422) (i.e., gain item for repetitive behavior, escape demand while engaged in repetitive behavior, and escape sensory stimulation). The problem behaviors of boys and girls without ASDs, and of girls with ASDs, were assessed as serving almost exclusively "standard" functions. The problem behaviors of boys with ASDs were assessed as serving both "standard" functions and functions hypothesized to be related to characteristics of autism, with the latter identified more frequently than the former. Love, Carr, and LeBlanc (2009) reviewed data from 32 functional assessments of problem behavior in children with ASDs aged 2–12 years. Consistent with results from studies involving participants with varied developmental disabilities (Asmus et al., 2004; Derby et al., 1992; Iwata et al., 1994; Kurtz et al., 2003), in most cases (88%) problem behavior had a social function, although a greater proportion of cases (45%) than typically reported in previous studies were identified as showing behavior controlled by more than one type of reinforcement. In contrast, O'Reilly et al. (2010) conducted experimental functional analyses (EFAs) with 10 children with ASDs aged from 4 to 8 years and found results consistent with functions of gaining access to tangibles and demand avoidance in two cases and largely undifferentiated patterns of responding across conditions in 8 others. Undifferentiated

responding is consistent not only with behavior being automatically reinforced (i.e., the reinforcing consequence being produced mechanically by the behavior without social mediation) but also with control by multiple sources of reinforcement and/or control by processes not modeled in standard EFA conditions (for a description of EFA methodology see Section "Behavioral Interventions").

Irrespective of the eventual resolution of these discrepant findings, two preliminary conclusions seem warranted. First, in some persons with ASDs, problem behaviors, including SIB, may be maintained by sources of reinforcement not evaluated by standardized rating scales such as the Questions About Behavioral Function (QABF) scale (Vollmer & Matson, 1995) or by EFAs using only the conditions originally designed by Iwata, Dorsey, Slifer, Bauman, and Richman (1982) to assess functions of SIB commonly identified in children with diverse developmental disabilities. Functional assessment of SIB in persons with ASDs should therefore begin with a broad descriptive assessment of possible antecedents and maintaining consequences before proceeding to assessments designed to test specific hypotheses. Second, SIB in persons with ASDs may be multiply controlled and/or automatically reinforced in a substantial number of cases. Both possibilities are likely to pose additional challenges to the design and implementation of effective behavioral interventions (O'Reilly et al., 2010).

Implications for Assessment and Intervention

Despite the relatively limited body of relevant research, four conclusions are warranted when considering assessment and intervention in SIB presented by persons with ASDs. First, in general, current evidence suggests that SIBs represent a comorbid behavior disorder which should be a target for intervention rather than one set of topographies of the RRBs which are a diagnostic feature of ASD. Second, methods developed to assess and intervene with SIBs in persons with IDs will have substantial applicability with persons with ASDs, but function-based interventions may need to address issues of identifying and matching sources of automatic reinforcement, identifying idiosyncratic maintaining variables, and training caregivers to respond appropriately to multiply controlled behavior. Third, effective intervention for SIB may require direct intervention targeted at the SIB plus adjunctive intervention targeted at other comorbid emotional or behavioral difficulties, especially anxiety, impulsivity, mania, and RRBs. Finally, successful treatment of SIBs may be more difficult than is the case with people with other developmental disabilities, perhaps because in complex cases the SIB may be related to RRBs which may be relatively difficult to replace in

440   F. Furniss et al.

persons with ASDs or perhaps due to the additional complexities involved in function-based interventions with this population.

Behavioral Interventions

In the remainder of this chapter we review behavioral interventions for SIB in persons with ASDs. Any attempt to treat SIB, whether by behavioral or pharmacological methods, should be preceded by a comprehensive assessment covering social and medical contextual factors, history, phenomenology, including comorbidity with other emotional and behavioral difficulties, and detailed assessment of functional relationships between SIB and antecedent and consequent environmental events. An early overview of possible underlying mechanisms or causes of SIB in a particular individual may, however, enable short-term management to be initiated quickly to prevent or limit further injury while assessment proceeds.

Initial Assessment and Screening of Contributing Medical Conditions

Medical conditions which may impact on SIB include otitis media (Luiselli, Cochran, & Huber, 2005; O'Reilly, 1997) and pain related to a variety of other conditions (Symons, 2002). Examination for and treatment of possible related physical complaints are therefore indicated in initial assessment of SIB. Sleep deprivation and disturbance are associated with SIB (O'Reilly & Lancioni, 2000; Symons, Davis, & Thompson, 2000), and in some cases behavioral intervention to stabilize sleep patterns may have a beneficial effect on SIB (DeLeon, Fisher, & Marhefka, 2004). Attention to conditions such as menstrual discomfort may be useful in designing multi-component interventions (Carr, Smith, Giacin, Whelan, & Pancari, 2003).

Rationale for Behavioral Interventions

Behavioral interventions approach SIB as a learned behavior (Baumeister & Rollings, 1976). Specifically, it has been suggested that in people with IDs, SIB may develop from early repetitive behaviors through a process in which those behaviors first develop homeostatic functions in regulating overall degree of stimulation and are then shaped into SIB through socially mediated operant reinforcement (Guess & Carr, 1991; Kennedy, 2002). SIB may then increase in severity through a process of shaping in which carers progressively reinforce increasingly severe forms of the behavior by ceasing to respond to milder forms but reinstating their response

to the more severe and/or frequent behavior which occurs in the ensuing extinction burst (Oliver & Head, 1990).

In the behavioral conceptualization, the fundamental, long-term cause of SIB is thus a process of positive or negative reinforcement which maintains the behavior. Two other processes are, however, conceptualized as affecting the probability of a person engaging in SIB on a minute-to-minute or hour-by-hour basis. Motivating operations (MOs) (Laraway, Snycerski, Michael, & Poling, 2003) alter the extent to which stimuli occurring or ceasing consequent on SIB are effective in reinforcing the behavior (value-altering effect) and simultaneously tend to directly increase or decrease the probability of the behavior occurring (behavior-altering effect). O'Reilly et al. (2008) for example observed the SIB of a 16-year old with severe IDs and marked features of autism as he engaged in leisure sessions. Prior assessment of the function of the young man's SIB and aggression to others suggested that these problem behaviors were reinforced by contingent access to savory snacks. Levels of problem behavior were higher by a factor of 10 during leisure sessions preceded by 15 min without access to savories by comparison with sessions preceded by a 15-min period of continuous access to savories. Since problem behaviors were never reinforced by snacks during leisure sessions, although snacks were present, the impact on SIB was due to the behavior-altering effect of the MO of access to/deprivation of savories. Had SIB been reinforced by allowing contingent access to savories during the leisure session, such access may additionally have strengthened SIB more following pre-session deprivation of access to savories than following pre-session access, an effect which, if observed, would reflect the value-altering effect of the MO.

The second antecedent process which may be involved in control of SIB is stimulus control. Stimulus control is defined when, with motivating operations and reinforcement contingencies held constant, a response which has been reinforced in the presence of a stimulus thereafter occurs more frequently when that stimulus, thereby defined as a positive discriminative stimulus or S^D, is present than when it is absent. By contrast, inhibitory stimulus control is defined when a response which has not been reinforced in the presence of a stimulus thereafter occurs less frequently when that stimulus, thereby defined as a negative discriminative stimulus or S^Δ, is present than when it is absent. Stimulus control differs from the behavior-altering effect of an MO in that the S^D or S^Δ exerts its control by virtue of a history of association with a particular response being reinforced or not reinforced. Changing the reinforcement contingencies associated with a discriminative stimulus will therefore change the control exerted by that stimulus. Appropriate changes to discriminative stimuli may, however, accelerate or support behavior change produced by changes in reinforcement contingencies.

Early Interventions

Early attempts to intervene with SIB presented by persons with developmental disabilities focused on differential reinforcement approaches, using reinforcers chosen without reference to the consequences presumed to be maintaining the challenging behavior (Cowdery, Iwata, & Pace, 1990). Methods included differential reinforcement of other behavior (DRO) in which reinforcement is provided contingent on the absence or omission of the target behavior, differential reinforcement of alternative behavior (DRA) in which reinforcement is delivered contingent on the occurrence of a specified alternative behavior, or differential reinforcement of incompatible behavior (DRI) in which reinforcement is delivered contingent on the occurrence of a behavior which is physically incompatible with the SIB (e.g., performing a manual task using both hands for SIB comprising head-hitting). In the early stages of implementation of differential reinforcement procedures, the individual may be assisted to engage in the alternative responses by prompting or physical guidance. Differential reinforcement procedures have, for example, been used to replace self-injurious, disruptive, and aggressive behaviors with self-care skills (Vollmer, Iwata, Smith, & Rodgers, 1992).

Interventions Based on Functional Assessment and Analysis

Substantial impetus was given to the development of behavioral interventions for SIB by Carr (1977), who reviewed evidence suggesting that SIB was maintained by a variety of consequences in different individuals and argued that treatment should therefore be individualized with respect to behavioral function. Carr and his colleagues demonstrated, for example, that the SIB and aggression to others of some children with IDs and autistic features were reinforced by escape from task demands and could be reduced by signaling the withdrawal of such demands, allowing escape from demands contingent on a nonaggressive response or not allowing such escape contingent on aggression (Carr, Newsom, & Binkoff, 1976, 1980). The foundation for the widespread application of the principle of basing intervention on behavioral function was, however, provided when Iwata et al. (1982) described a method for assessing behavioral function prior to treatment planning. Iwata et al.'s (1982) method, variously described as EFA or "analogue assessment" involves briefly exposing clients to highly structured combinations of MOs, S^Ds, and reinforcement contingencies, each of which is designed to evoke high rates of problem behavior maintained by specific contingencies (see Vollmer, Sloman, & Borrero, 2009, for a detailed discussion). Iwata et al. (1982) described four conditions, one (unstructured play) being a control condition involving positive social interaction and non-demanding encouragement to engage with leisure materials and the others designed to test hypotheses regarding functions of self-injury based on Carr's (1977) review of previous studies of this question. In the "social disapproval" condition, a carer is present (S^D) but carer attention is withheld (MO), being delivered to the client only contingent on occurrence of SIB (reinforcement). In "task demand," the client is required to participate in challenging educational activities, with escape from task demands allowed contingent on occurrence of SIB. Finally, the "alone" condition involves absence of social or material stimulation. A consistently higher level of SIB in the "social disapproval" condition is interpreted as supporting a hypothesis that the target behavior is maintained by positive social reinforcement in the person's natural environment. A consistently higher level of the behavior in the "task demand" condition is taken to indicate a function of escape from task demands for the behavior in the natural environment, while a higher level of the behavior in the "alone" condition is generally interpreted as suggesting that the behavior is maintained by automatic reinforcement. An undifferentiated pattern of responding, consisting of similar levels of the target behavior in all conditions, may indicate that the behavior is multifunctional, that it is maintained by automatic reinforcement, or that it is maintained by some other process not modeled by the analogue conditions. In a review of application of EFA in 152 cases of SIB in persons with developmental disabilities, Iwata et al. (1994) reported that social-negative reinforcement maintained SIB in 38.1% of the sample, social-positive reinforcement maintained SIB for 26.3%, automatic reinforcement accounted for 25.7%, and 5.3% had SIB maintained by multiple controlling variables.

Key elements in behavioral interventions frequently include modification of MOs in order to reduce the probability of SIB and reduce the reinforcing value of the events which have previously reinforced SIB, use of stimulus control procedures to reduce the probability of SIB, teaching and/or increasing the density of reinforcement for prosocial behaviors which compete with SIB for the reinforcer(s) which have maintained the SIB, and increasing the effort involved in SIB and reducing or eliminating reinforcement of the behavior (Iwata, Roscoe, Zarcone, & Richman, 2002). Starting from the assumption that similar processes are involved in the establishment and maintenance of SIB and other problem and prosocial behaviors and that common processes control the behavior of persons with and without ASDs, behavioral approaches to treatment of SIB in persons with ASDs therefore apply the same principles used in interventions with persons with other or no developmental disabilities and for other topographies of problem behavior.

Examples given here accordingly draw on intervention studies on SIB and other problem behavior both in persons with ASDs and those with other disabilities.

Assessing the Function of SIB

Identification of the reinforcement processes maintaining SIB is an essential first step in behavioral intervention. The methods employed in this process of functional assessment include interviews or questionnaires used to request information including generic descriptions of events which typically precede and follow occurrences of SIB from third parties who spend considerable time with the client, descriptive observational methods which involve gathering information by observing sequences of events including SIB in the person's natural environment, and EFAs. Vollmer et al. (2009) have recently provided an excellent overview of each of these approaches including specific methodologies and the advantages and current limitations of each approach in assessing SIB. The focus here therefore will be on issues specific to applying these methods in working with persons with ASDs.

There are two common complications to be expected in functional assessment of the SIB of persons with ASDs. First, in persons with ASDs problem behavior may be maintained by relatively idiosyncratic sources of reinforcement, such as access to items used in specific repetitive behaviors or escape from idiosyncratically aversive sensory stimulation (Reese et al., 2005). Second, automatic and/or multiple reinforcement processes may frequently be important in maintenance of problem behavior (Love et al., 2009; O'Reilly et al., 2010). The first difficulty may be addressed by using descriptive analyses to identify relevant potential reinforcers which may then be evaluated in experimental analyses (Carr, Yarbrough, & Langdon, 1997; Vollmer & Smith, 1996) and/or by further investigation of unexpected results from initial experimental assessments. For example, Hagopian, Wilson, and Wilder (2001) and Tiger, Fisher, Toussaint, and Kodak (2009) both reported cases in which boys diagnosed with autism showed high levels of problem behavior in the EFA "unstructured play" condition. In both cases the researchers hypothesized that high rates of problem behavior unexpectedly seen in this condition might indicate that problem behavior was maintained by escape from social interaction. They confirmed this hypothesis by demonstrating high rates of problem behavior in a subsequent EFA condition in which social interaction was briefly terminated following occurrence of problem behavior.

The second difficulty relates to interpretation of EFA results when responding is high in all conditions. Such a pattern of results is often interpreted as suggestive of automatic, i.e., nonsocially mediated, reinforcement, but is also consistent with SIB having multiple functions. Healey, Ahearn,

Graff, and Libby (2001), having observed undifferentiated responding across conditions in an initial EFA with a man diagnosed with autism, conducted a further EFA with the addition of a "sensory" condition in which the client was alone in a room with a variety of preferred sensory toys. SIB was lower in this condition than others, consistent with the hypothesis of automatic reinforcement. McKerchar, Kahng, Casioppo, and Wilson (2001), also observing undifferentiated levels of SIB across EFA conditions in a boy diagnosed with autism, followed an alternative strategy. The assessment was repeated, but the boy wore a soft-padded helmet and all attempts to engage in SIB were blocked, a procedure which the researchers hypothesized would eliminate automatic consequences of the behavior. Under these conditions, SIB occurred at a higher rate in the contingent attention condition of the EFA than in others, consistent with the hypothesis that the behavior was maintained both by automatic and by social-positive reinforcement. Such extended assessments may be necessary to differentiate situations in which SIB is maintained solely by nonsocial reinforcement from those in which the behavior is maintained by multiple reinforcement processes.

Treating SIB Maintained by Socially Mediated Reinforcement

Two types of socially mediated positive reinforcement have frequently been reported to be involved in maintenance of SIB in people with ASDs: interaction with carers (Love et al., 2009) and caregiver delivery of tangible items (e.g., toys) (O'Reilly et al., 2010). The negative reinforcement process which has received most attention is escape from or avoidance of task demands, although escape from or avoidance of a variety of other aversive events and from people or situations which have been associated with such events is also frequently implicated in maintenance of SIB (Reese et al., 2005).

Modification of MOs

Fixed-time (FT) schedules, sometimes referred to as noncontingent reinforcement (NCR), deliver the consequence maintaining SIB on a predetermined schedule irrespective of the occurrence of the target behavior. Vollmer, Iwata, Zarcone, Smith, and Mazaleski (1993) treated the long-established SIB (head banging and hitting, body hitting, or hand-mouthing) of three women with severe/profound IDs, which had been shown by EFA to be reinforced by contingent attention, by providing attention on an FT schedule, initially continuously, then gradually reducing to 10 s of attention each 5 min, with reduction contingent upon on low rates of SIB in the previous session. Van Camp, Lerman, Kelley, Contrucci, and Vorndran (2000) demonstrated that variable-time schedules, with inter-reinforcement intervals varied randomly around a mean value, were as effective as corresponding FT schedules, increasing the feasibility of this approach for applied settings in which FT schedules might be difficult to sustain. Kahng, Iwata, DeLeon, and Wallace (2000) further demonstrated that schedule thinning could be achieved more rapidly than using the fixed-step approach of Vollmer et al. (1993), and without compromising intervention effectiveness, by a procedure in which the interval between reinforcer delivery for each session was set to equal the mean interval between SIBs for the previous three sessions, subject to a maximum increase of 100% in the inter-reinforcer interval from one session to the next. Time-based schedules have also been used to reduce SIB maintained by socially mediated tangible reinforcement, such as access to food (Ingvarsson, Kahng, & Hausman, 2008) and by socially mediated negative reinforcement (escape from instructional activities) (Vollmer, Marcus, & Ringdahl, 1995).

FT schedules may not only reduce motivation to engage in SIB by providing the reinforcer freely but also reduce SIB by extinction (removing the contingency between SIB and the reinforcer) and by increasing tolerance of delay to reinforcement during schedule thinning (Vollmer et al., 1998), thereby producing reductions in the level of problem behavior extending beyond the period in which the motivating operation is modified. The risk of maintaining SIB through adventitious reinforcement when SIB occurs immediately before a scheduled reinforcer delivery can be avoided by briefly postponing reinforcement when this situation occurs (Carr & LeBlanc, 2006).

Where MOs cannot be directly modified, it may be possible to increase tolerance of them or neutralize their effects. McCord, Iwata, Galensky, Ellingson, and Thomson (2001) reduced problem behavior, including SIB, maintained by escape from noise by progressive exposure to increasing noise levels, extinction, by engineering that problem behavior did not lead to noise termination, and, in one case, DRO in the presence of noise. Horner, Day, and Day (1997) reduced the escape-maintained aggression and SIB of two of three children with severe IDs, which occurred in response to error correction only following earlier delay or postponement of planned, preferred activities, by providing individually developed calming routines following such events.

Modifications of Instructional Conditions

SIB maintained by escape from or avoidance of scheduled tasks or activities may be reduced by modifying those activities. Many demonstrations of such effects have used multi-element interventions and in some cases the processes

underlying their effectiveness remain to be fully elucidated. Pace, Iwata, Cowdery, Andree, and McIntyre (1993) produced rapid and substantial reductions in levels of SIB for three young people with IDs by initially completely withdrawing demands and then gradually increasing these over sessions to baseline levels while preventing escape from activities contingent on SIB (escape extinction). Extinction appears to be necessary if reduction of SIB is to be maintained as demand levels increase (Zarcone, Iwata, Smith, Mazaleski, & Lerman, 1994). Other instructional procedures which may be helpful in reducing levels of demand-escape maintained SIB include identifying specific tasks which elicit SIB and interspersing requests to complete these among tasks less likely to elicit SIB (Horner, Day, Sprague, O'Brien, & Heathfield, 1991), increasing levels of reinforcement for task engagement (Hoch, McComas, Thompson, & Paone, 2002; Lalli et al., 1999), or preceding demands which elicit SIB by a sequence of demands with which the person typically cooperates while preventing escape from the demand contingent on SIB (Zarcone, Iwata, Mazaleski, & Smith, 1994).

Assessing and Manipulating Stimulus Control

Lalli, Mace, Livezey, and Kates (1998), working with a 10-year old with severe intellectual disabilities, identified physical contact with a carer as the reinforcer maintaining her SIB. Hypothesizing that the physical proximity of an adult might be an S^D controlling her SIB, Lalli et al. (1998) demonstrated that the level of SIB observed varied inversely with the distance between child and carer. A treatment package comprising a time-based schedule of physical contact, withholding physical contact contingent on SIB (i.e., extinction), and the child's mother managing the controlling stimulus by maintaining a distance of 9 m from the child during periods when she was unable to implement the time-based schedule, resulted in a substantial reduction in SIB.

Teaching and Reinforcing Competing Prosocial Responses

Functional Communication Training (FCT) is a version of DRA in which problem behavior is replaced with verbal phrases or non-vocal communicative responses which serve the same social function as the problem behavior (Carr & Durand, 1985). Carr and Durand (1985) reduced the behavior problems, including aggression, tantrums, and SIB, of four children with developmental disabilities who presented problem behavior maintained by socially mediated positive or negative reinforcement (escape from difficult tasks) by teaching them to verbally solicit attention and/or assistance from adults. Carr and Durand (1985) showed that the efficacy of FCT depended on teaching the child to verbally request the reinforcer maintaining the problem behavior and that the positive effects of training on the children's behavior problems also occurred with carers unaware of the purpose of the study, arguing that this latter effect of FCT offered an important potential advantage by comparison with approaches which required systematic changes in carer behavior. Especially with individuals with limited behavioral repertoires, a single topography of problem behavior may be maintained by several distinct reinforcers. Day, Horner and O'Neill (1994) demonstrated that the SIB and aggression of three individuals with autism or severe IDs was in each case maintained both by escape from tasks and by access to preferred items and showed that establishing a communicative response appropriate to each function was necessary to reduce problem behavior across both contexts in which problem behavior was displayed. Since the limited evidence to date suggests that control of problem behavior by multiple sources of reinforcement may be common in people with ASDs (Love et al., 2009; O'Reilly et al., 2010), FCT may be a particularly valuable component in interventions for this client group. In cases of multiply controlled SIB, modification of MOs requires carers to assess the current importance of different sources of reinforcement to the maintenance of the behavior, whereas FCT enables the client to indicate which reinforcer is currently critical.

There is, however, no reason to expect that acquisition of a prosocial functional equivalent to SIB, even if that response is consistently reinforced, will necessarily reduce the level of SIB. If both behaviors elicit qualitatively similar responses from carers, the proportion of responses which are prosocial and SIB will be determined by the effort associated with each response (Richman, Wacker, & Winborn, 2001) and other factors including reinforcer magnitude, reinforcer latency, and schedule value (Symons, Hoch, Dahl, & McComas, 2003). A number of studies have found that FCT reduced problem behavior only when extinction or time-out contingencies were in effect for problem behavior in addition to positive reinforcement of the communicative response (Shirley, Iwata, Kahng, Mazaleski, & Lerman, 1997; Wacker et al., 1990). Even if the alternative response is well established simultaneously with SIB being placed on extinction, levels of SIB may increase to pre-treatment levels if it is again reinforced (Shirley et al., 1997). Worsdell, Iwata, Hanley, Thompson, and Kahng (2000), treating the SIB of five adults with profound IDs, showed that for four participants substantial reductions in SIB were achieved only when the appropriate communication was continuously reinforced and the rate of reinforcement of SIB was reduced, in two cases to one reinforcement per 20 SIBs. These are important considerations in planning behavioral treatment programs in many settings, where even given a high level of training and

support for families and other carers, SIB may be at least intermittently reinforced. Additionally, both appropriate and problem behavior may belong to the same functional class, and if a member of that class is selected as the prosocial behavior to be reinforced in FCT, the entire functional class including SIB may be strengthened (Derby, Fisher, Piazza, Wilke, & Johnson, 1998). For optimal effect, FCT should therefore preferably teach a novel communicative response which has no history of membership of the same functional class as SIB (Winborn, Wacker, Richman, Asmus, & Geier, 2002). To avoid or minimize the possibility of the communicative response joining the same functional class as SIB, reinforcement of SIB should be eliminated or minimized and clinicians should consider the possibility that SIB may be maintained by reinforcement of other, apparently unproblematic, members of the preexisting functional class (Derby et al., 1998).

Implementation of FCT may result in the client using the alternative communicative response so frequently that to reinforce every occurrence is impracticable. Hanley, Iwata, and Thompson (2001) employed a stimulus control intervention to address this problem following FCT treatment of the SIB and aggression of three adults with profound IDs. Having established the communicative response using continuous reinforcement they then introduced and progressively lengthened periods of signaled extinction in which presence of a colored card indicated that the communicative response would not be reinforced.

Reducing or Eliminating Reinforcement of SIB

Although eliminating or reducing the reinforcement maintaining SIB is likely to be essential to successful treatment using FCT, any attempt to treat SIB using extinction alone faces major ethical and practical problems. The transition from reinforcement to extinction of operant behavior without other treatment procedures may be accompanied by an extinction burst, a temporary increase in the rate and intensity of the behavior, and by aggression and negative emotional behavior such as crying (Lerman, Iwata, & Wallace, 1999). Lerman et al. (1999) found evidence for extinction bursts in 62% of 41 data sets for children and adults with moderate to profound IDs whose SIB was treated by extinction alone versus only 15% of cases in which antecedent change and/or reinforcement procedures were combined with extinction.

Treatment of SIB Maintained by Automatic Reinforcement

Experimental epidemiological studies implicate nonsocially mediated reinforcement maintaining SIB and other problem behavior in approximately one-quarter to one-third of cases (Derby et al., 1992; Iwata et al., 1994). As noted above, automatic sources of reinforcement may frequently be implicated in maintaining problem behaviors in persons with ASDs (O'Reilly et al., 2010). Assessment and treatment of automatically reinforced behavior is challenging because it is difficult to identify precisely the nature of the reinforcement maintaining the behavior (Vollmer, 1994) and to manipulate that putative reinforcer. Some success has, however, been reported with behavioral interventions, examples of which we next review, analogous to those used with socially reinforced behavior.

Modification of MOs

In EFAs, automatic reinforcement of SIB may be inferred if rates of SIB are highest when the client is left alone without activities or if SIB occurs at a high rate in all conditions; however, such an analysis provides no information regarding the nature of the reinforcer. In the absence of this information, the most frequently investigated behavioral intervention has been provision of non-contingent access to sensory and other stimuli. The items used are typically selected using structured preference assessments in which the client's preferences from a range of sources of stimulation are assessed by systematically observing either choices when items are presented simultaneously in pairs (Fisher et al., 1992) or the length of time for which the client interacts with items presented individually (DeLeon, Iwata, Conners, & Wallace, 1999) or simultaneously (Roane, Vollmer, Ringdahl, & Marcus, 1998). Vollmer, Marcus, and LeBlanc (1994) showed that non-contingent access to preferred items reduced levels of SIB in three young children with developmental disabilities, although additional procedures, including 5 s restraint of one child's hands, were also necessary to achieve acceptable reductions in SIB for two of the children. Vollmer et al. (1994) noted that treatment effectiveness might reduce owing to satiation if such treatments were used over extended time periods; however, subsequent studies have reported that providing access to a variety of sources of stimulation and/or rotating the objects provided can produce long-term reductions of SIB (DeLeon, Anders, Rodriguez-Catter, & Neidert, 2000; Lindberg, Iwata, Roscoe, Worsdell, & Hanley, 2003). Van Camp, Vollmer, and Daniel (2001), working with a boy diagnosed with autism whose SIB involved placing harmful substances into his eyes, showed that increasing the effort involved in SIB relative to that involved in accessing a preferred keyboard, by ensuring that items required to engage in SIB were further away from him than the keyboard, produced greater reduction in SIB than providing the keyboard alone.

Teaching and Reinforcing Competing Prosocial Responses

Early studies suggested that even where stimuli to potentially compete with stimulation provided by SIB could be identified, attempts to use them in differential reinforcement programs were ineffective, presumably due to the effort required to make the alternative response (Shore, Iwata, DeLeon, Kahng, & Smith, 1997). Steege, Wacker, Berg, Cigrand, and Cooper (1989) reduced the damaging hand-mouthing of a child with severe multiple disabilities by reducing the response effort required to produce alternative stimulation by teaching him to use a microswitch to activate a radio or a fan.

Reducing or Eliminating Reinforcement of SIB

A number of studies in which apparently automatically reinforced SIB was reduced by blocking SIB, or application of protective clothing, have interpreted consequent reductions in SIB in terms of reduction of automatic reinforcement produced by the behavior (Mazaleski, Iwata, Rodgers, Vollmer, & Zarcone, 1994; Moore, Fisher, & Pennington, 2004; Van Houten, 1993). The mechanisms involved in such effects are, however, often obscure and may include punishment.

Pica

Pica has been variously defined as eating of non-food items or as compulsive eating of specific food items (Albin, 1977; Matson & Bamburg, 1999). Items ingested may include stones, nails, dirt, buttons, feces, coins, plant matter such as grass or twigs, string, and paper. Pica is considered to be a serious and potentially life-threatening behavior (Danford & Huber, 1982). It may result in a variety of medical risks including blockage or puncture of the digestive tract, infestation by gastrointestinal parasites, and poisoning (Fisher et al., 1994; Foxx & Martin, 1975; Serour, Witzling, Frenkel-Laufer, & Gorenstein, 2008; Winton & Singh, 1983). Pica may also result in serious negative social consequences such as avoidance by others (Foxx & Martin, 1975) and recommendations for use of mechanical restraints.

Although pica is a relatively common problem for persons with IDs, overall prevalence is uncertain. Matson and Bamburg (1999) identified 45 cases (6%) among 790 persons with IDs in institutional care, whereas Swift, Paquette, Davison, and Saeed (1999) identified 152 cases (22%) among 689 residents of another institution serving persons with IDs. Hardan and Sahl (1997) reported 10 cases (4%) of pica among 233 children and adolescents with IDs referred to a clinical program. Although there is common agreement that pica is more prevalent among persons with severe or profound intellectual disabilities, little is known regarding its prevalence in persons with ASDs. Kinnell (1985) reviewed the case records of 70 children and adults with ASDs and 70 adults with Down syndrome and reported that 42 (60%) of the ASD group had engaged in pica at some time as compared to only 3 (4%) of the group with Down syndrome, 2 of whom were themselves described as "autistic." Matson and Bamburg (1999) reported that stereotypic movement disorder was present in 15, and autistic disorder in 9, of the 45 cases of pica identified. Lecavalier (2006) in the large-scale community study described above found that 12.2% of parents of young people with ASDs rated "gouges self, puts things in ears, nose, etc., or eats inedible things" as a moderate or severe problem. As with other forms of SIB, therefore, it is currently unclear as to whether presence of ASDs is a risk factor for pica independent of severity of ID.

Treatment of Pica

Individuals engaging in pica have been shown to have plasma levels of zinc and iron reduced by comparison with levels in persons not displaying pica; however, whether trace metal deficiencies motivate pica or pica results in malabsorption of zinc and iron remains unresolved (Danford, Smith, & Huber, 1982; Swift et al., 1999). Convincing demonstrations of successful treatment of pica by dietary supplementation remain few in number (Bugle & Rubin, 1993; Lofts, Schroeder, & Maier, 1990; Pace & Toyer, 2000). Nevertheless, thorough medical investigation including, where appropriate, tests to identify potential mineral deficiencies (Ellis, Singh, & Ruane, 1999) should be considered in preparation for development of a treatment package.

Reports of successful psychopharmacological treatment (Lerner, 2008) are limited to uncontrolled case reports. The evidence base for successful interventions relates primarily to behavioral interventions, and as with other forms of SIB, it relates mainly to pica in individuals with ID. Again, however, treatment protocols developed for persons with IDs might assist in the treatment of pica in individuals with ASD.

McAdam, Sherman, Sheldon, and Napolitano (2004), reviewing behavioral intervention studies published to that date, identified interventions including punishment, such as overcorrection and contingent visual blocking, negative practice, DRO, DRI, and FT schedules (Ausman, Ball, & Alexander, 1974; Duker & Nielen, 1993; Foxx & Martin, 1975; Mace & Knight, 1986; Mulick, Barbour, Schroeder, & Rojahn, 1980; Singh & Bakker, 1984; Singh & Winton, 1984; Smith, 1987). A functional analysis of variables maintaining pica was conducted in only 4 of the 26 studies reviewed, possibly due to ethical concerns in respect of

conducting EFAs with a behavior that can be so dangerous. Such concerns can, however, be at least partially addressed by methods such as "baiting" the assessment environment with items which resemble the client's typically preferred pica items but which can safely be ingested, or by measuring latency to engage in pica rather than frequency, thus allowing the behavior to be blocked during assessment (McAdam et al., 2004). Despite the difficulties involved, EFA should be used where appropriate in order to determine the most appropriate function-based intervention (McAdam et al., 2004).

Pica has in some cases been shown to be at least partly maintained by socially mediated reinforcers (Mace & Knight, 1986; Piazza et al., 1998). In many cases, however, the behavior appears to be maintained by automatic reinforcement (Applegate, Matson, & Cherry, 1999; Matson et al., 2005; Piazza et al., 1998; Piazza, Hanley, & Fisher, 1996; Wasano, Borrero, & Kohn, 2009), and intervention must contend with the difficulties noted above in precisely identifying and then effectively competing with the specific source of reinforcement maintaining the behavior (Kennedy & Souza, 1995; Kern, Starosta, & Adelman, 2006). Progress made in assessing automatically reinforced behavior (LeBlanc, Patel, & Carr, 2000) has, however, been applied to treatment of pica.

A functional analysis of the pica of three persons conducted by Piazza et al. (1998) led the researchers to hypothesize that pica was primarily or partially maintained by automatic reinforcement. Systematic stimulus preference assessments and consideration of the properties of items favored for pica by each person enabled the researchers to identify specific items which could be provided non-contingently to compete with the automatic reinforcement of pica. For example, for one participant the oral stimulation provided by hard items was hypothesized to reinforce pica, which was reduced in frequency by allowing non-contingent access to rice cakes, but not by access to soft food items.

In some cases, however, provision of alternative stimulation, even if matched closely to that hypothesized to be maintaining pica, will not reduce the behavior to clinically acceptable levels (Piazza et al., 1998). In such cases it may be combined with physically blocking completion of the response, which should prevent it from producing reinforcing consequences. Although response blocking has been shown to be effective in reducing SIB maintained by automatic reinforcement (Lerman & Iwata, 1996), it has produced mixed results when addressing pica. Rapp, Dozier, and Carr (2001) indicated that response blocking alone failed to reduce pica to an acceptable level and McCord, Grosser, Iwata, and Powers (2005) reported that response blocking may only be effective when other interventions are included and the blocking is implemented as early as possible in the response chain. The aggression which response blocking may elicit can be reduced by combining blocking with redirection to a preferred edible (Hagopian & Adelinis, 2001).

The effectiveness of interventions may depend critically on the relative effort required to obtain pica items or the treatment alternative. Piazza, Roane, Keeney, Boney, and Abt (2002) manipulated the response effort required for automatically reinforced pica and to obtain appropriate highly preferred food items and toys, for three young people with severe IDs. Pica levels reduced when alternative items were present irrespective of the response effort required for pica, or when response effort for pica was increased, even when alternative items were not present. Increasing the effort required to obtain alternative items, or decreasing the effort to engage in pica, resulted in increased levels of pica. Clinicians should therefore consider environmental variables which may affect the response effort required to engage in pica and alternatives to pica and may be manipulated to reduce the behavior.

Although most intervention studies have used non-contingent and often continuous access to alternative sources of stimulation in attempting to compete with pica, Kern et al. (2006) demonstrated that systematic stimulus preference assessments could also identify effective reinforcers for use in a differential reinforcement intervention. Two young people with severe IDs and one also with an ASD learned to hand pica items to carers in exchange for highly preferred edible snacks. The frequency of exchanges was then reduced by thinning the schedule of reinforcement and increasing the delay between the student handing over the pica item and obtaining the edible, although only limited progress in schedule thinning was achieved.

Many interventions for pica require substantial caregiver effort, and stimulus control procedures have been applied to extend treatment effects to periods where the client is not directly supervised. Piazza et al. (1996) paired non-contingent food availability and a response interruption procedure with presence of a purple card and demonstrated that thereafter, giving a 17-year old with a severe ID and ASD a purple card to carry maintained low rates of cigarette pica even when the interruption contingency was not in operation. Falcomata, Roane, and Pabico (2007), however, reported on the case of a 12-year old with an ASD in which reduced levels of pica inadvertently came under the control of presence of the therapist rather than with the wearing of wristbands which had been intended to be associated with implementation of a visual screening intervention.

Although some progress has been made toward developing effective, non-aversive, function-based interventions for pica in persons with ASDs, there are still few studies which demonstrate successful intervention in everyday settings for extended periods of time. Currently, effective long-term control of pica will in some cases require not only individual intervention but also systematic efforts to

minimize the availability of preferred pica items (Williams, Kirkpatrick-Sanchez, Enzinna, Dunn, & Borden-Karasack, 2009). Meanwhile, behavioral approaches may be useful in making decisions regarding default interventions, for example by demonstrating whether hypothesized punishment procedures such as reprimands or brief physical restraint are actually effective (McAdam et al., 2004) or whether use of potentially socially stigmatizing protective equipment such as helmets or face guards, which may reduce social interactions (Rojahn, Schroeder, & Mulick, 1980) actually decrease or increase rate of pica (Mace & Knight, 1986). Decisions regarding short-term management of pica will need to consider impact on the behavior and on the client's quality of life together with feasibility of implementation by the client's carers. LeBlanc, Piazza, and Krug (1997) present a clinical decision-making model addressing these factors.

Behavioral Treatment: Conclusions

Reviewing studies on behavioral treatment of SIB published between 1964 and 2000, Kahng, Iwata, and Lewin (2002) noted that most reported that SIB was reduced by at least 80% from baseline to the end of treatment; however, a number of issues arise in considering these impressive results. First, although complex interventions can be successfully implemented by service staff such as teachers (Sigafoos & Meikle, 1996), some of the evidence for treatment effectiveness comes from interventions implemented by highly skilled staff during defined time periods, and only a minority of studies report data on generalization and maintenance of treatment effects (DeLeon, Rodriguez-Catter, & Cataldo, 2002; Kahng et al., 2002). The extent to which such generalization requires careful planning (Stokes & Baer, 1977) at the beginning of treatment design and implementation and/or systematic re-implementation of treatment across carers, settings, and tasks varies substantially across individuals (Shore, Iwata, Lerman, & Shirley, 1994). Second, although behavioral interventions are less associated with adverse events than most psychopharmacological treatments, problems, including inadvertent reinforcement of functional classes including SIB, extinction bursts, emergence of new topographies of SIB, and difficult-to-manage levels of alternative responses taught to replace SIB, may occur. Behavioral interventions therefore require supervision by professional staff with the expertise to predict, recognize, and appropriately manage such events. Finally, only in a minority of cases do behavioral interventions completely eliminate SIB (DeLeon et al., 2002). Potentially seriously dangerous forms of SIB including pica remain, therefore, in many cases, difficult-to-treat problems for which improved methods for assessment and intervention are urgently needed.

Behavioral interventions remain the most widely researched approaches to treating SIB in people with ASD. Contemporary approaches to behavioral treatment emphasize treatments based on functional assessment and analysis that focus on teaching other appropriate behavior, especially behavior that serves the same function as SIB. Challenges that face behavioral interventions include training and maintaining staff and family member behavior over extended periods of time and integrating behavioral and pharmacological treatments. The next chapter addresses pharmacological and integrated treatments.

References

Albin, J. B. (1977). The treatment of pica (scavenging) behavior in the retarded: A critical analysis and implications for research. *Mental Retardation, 15*, 14–17.

Aman, M. G., Arnold, L. E., McDougle, C. J., Vitiello, B., Scahill, L., Davies, M., et al. (2005). Acute and long-term safety and tolerability of risperidone in children with autism. *Journal of Child and Adolescent Psychopharmacology, 15*, 869–884.

Aman, M. G., & Singh, N. N. (1994). *Aberrant behavior checklist – community: Supplementary manual.* East Aurora, NY: Slosson Educational Publications.

American Psychiatric Association. (1994). *Diagnostic and statistical manual of mental disorders* (4th ed.). Arlington, VA: American Psychiatric Publishing Inc.

Applegate, H., Matson, J. L., & Cherry, K. E. (1999). An evaluation of functional variables affecting severe problem behaviors in adults with mental retardation by using the questions about behavioral function scale (QABF). *Research in Developmental Disabilities, 20*, 229–237.

Asmus, J. M., Ringdahl, J. E., Sellers, J. A., Call, N. A., Andelman, M. S., & Wacker, D. P. (2004). Use of a short-term inpatient model to evaluate aberrant behavior: Outcome data summaries from 1996 to 2001. *Journal of Applied Behavior Analysis, 37*, 283–304.

Ausman, J., Ball, T. S., & Alexander, D. (1974). Behavior therapy of pica with a profoundly retarded adolescent. *Mental Retardation, 12*, 16–18.

Baghdadli, A., Pascal, C., Grisi, S., & Aussilloux, C. (2003). Risk factors for self-injurious behaviours among 222 young children with autistic disorders. *Journal of Intellectual Disability Research, 47*, 622–627.

Baghdadli, A., Picot, M. C., Pry, R., Michelon, C., Burzstejn, C., Lazartigues, A., et al. (2008). What factors are related to a negative outcome of self-injurious behaviour during childhood in pervasive developmental disorders? *Journal of Applied Research in Intellectual Disabilities, 21*, 142–149.

Baumeister, A. A., & Rollings, J. P. (1976). Self-injurious behavior. In N. R. Ellis (Ed.), *International review of research in mental retardation* (Vol. 8, pp. 1–34). New York: Academic Press.

Bhaumik, S., Branford, D., McGrother, C., & Thorp, C. (1997). Autistic traits in adults with learning disabilities. *British Journal of Psychiatry, 170*, 502–506.

Bradley, E. A., Summers, J. A., Wood, H. L., & Bryson, S. E. (2004). Comparing rates of psychiatric and behavior disorders in adolescents and young adults with severe intellectual disability with and without autism. *Journal of Autism and Developmental Disorders, 34*, 151–161.

Brinkley, J., Nations, L., Abramson, R. K., Hall, A., Wright, H. H., Gabriels, R., et al. (2007). Factor analysis of the aberrant behavior checklist in individuals with autism spectrum disorders. *Journal of Autism and Developmental Disorders, 37*, 1949–1959.

Bugle, C., & Rubin, H. B. (1993). Effects of a nutritional supplement on coprophagia: A study of three cases. *Research in Developmental Disabilities, 14*, 445–456.

Campbell, J. M. (2003). Efficacy of behavioral interventions for reducing problem behavior in persons with autism: A quantitative synthesis of single-subject research. *Research in Developmental Disabilities, 24*, 120–138.

Carr, E. G. (1977). The motivation of self-injurious behavior: A review of some hypotheses. *Psychological Bulletin, 84*, 800–816.

Carr, E. G., & Durand, V. M. (1985). Reducing behavior problems through functional communication training. *Journal of Applied Behavior Analysis, 18*, 111–126.

Carr, E. G., Newsom, C. D., & Binkoff, J. A. (1976). Stimulus control of self destructive behaviour in a psychotic child. *Journal of Abnormal Child Psychology, 4*, 139–153.

Carr, E. G., Newsom, C. D., & Binkoff, J. A. (1980). Escape as a factor in the aggressive behaviour of two retarded children. *Journal of Applied Behavior Analysis, 13*, 101–117.

Carr, E. G., Smith, C. E., Giacin, T. A., Whelan, B. M., & Pancari, J. (2003). Menstrual discomfort as a biological setting event for severe problem behavior: Assessment and intervention. *American Journal on Mental Retardation, 108*, 117–133.

Carr, E. G., Yarbrough, S. C., & Langdon, N. A. (1997). Effects of idiosyncratic stimulus variables on functional analysis outcomes. *Journal of Applied Behavior Analysis, 30*, 673–686.

Carr, J. E., & LeBlanc, L. A. (2006). Noncontingent reinforcement as antecedent behavior support. In J. K. Luiselli (Ed.), *Antecedent assessment and intervention* (pp. 147–164). Baltimore: Paul H. Brookes.

Chadwick, O., Piroth, N., Walker, J., Bernard, S., & Taylor, E. (2000). Factors affecting the risk of behaviour problems in children with severe intellectual disability. *Journal of Intellectual Disability Research, 44*, 108–123.

Cohen, I. L., Tsiouris, J. A., Flory, M. J., Kim, S. -Y., Freedland, R., Heaney, G., et al. (2010). A large scale study of the psychometric characteristics of the IBR modified overt aggression scale: Findings and evidence for increased self-destructive behaviors in adult females with autism spectrum disorder. *Journal of Autism and Developmental Disorders, 40*, 599–609.

Collacott, R. A., Cooper, S. -A., Branford, D., & McGrother, C. (1998). Epidemiology of self-injurious behaviour in adults with learning disabilities. *British Journal of Psychiatry, 173*, 428–432.

Cooper, S. -A., Smiley, E., Allan, L. M., Jackson, A., Finlayson, J., Mantry, D., et al. (2009). Adults with intellectual disabilities: Prevalence, incidence and remission of self-injurious behaviour, and related factors. *Journal of Intellectual Disability Research, 53*, 200–216.

Cowdery, G. E., Iwata, B. A., & Pace, G. M. (1990). Effects and side effects of DRO as treatment for self-injurious behaviour. *Journal of Applied Behavior Analysis, 23*, 497–506.

Danford, D. E., & Huber, A. M. (1982). Pica among mentally retarded adults. *American Journal of Mental Deficiency, 87*, 141–146.

Danford, D. E., Smith, J. C., Jr., & Huber, A. M. (1982). Pica and mineral status in the mentally retarded. *American Journal of Clinical Nutrition, 35*, 958–967.

Day, H. M., Horner, R. H., & O'Neill, R. E. (1994). Multiple functions of problem behaviors: Assessment and intervention. *Journal of Applied Behavior Analysis, 27*, 279–289.

DeLeon, I. G., Anders, B. M., Rodriguez-Catter, V., & Neidert, P. L. (2000). The effects of noncontingent access to single-versus multiple-stimulus sets on self-injurious behavior. *Journal of Applied Behavior Analysis, 33*, 623–626.

DeLeon, I. G., Fisher, W. W., & Marhefka, J. (2004). Decreasing self-injurious behaviour associated with awakening in a child with autism and developmental delays. *Behavioral Interventions, 19*, 111–119.

DeLeon, I. G., Iwata, B. A., Conners, J., & Wallace, M. D. (1999). Examination of ambiguous stimulus preferences with duration-based measures. *Journal of Applied Behavior Analysis, 32*, 111–114.

DeLeon, I. G., Rodriguez-Catter, V., & Cataldo, M. F. (2002). Treatment: Current standards of care and their research implications. In S. R. Schroeder, M. L. Oster-Granite, & T. Thompson (Eds.), *Self-injurious behavior: Gene-brain-behavior relationships* (pp. 81–91). Washington, DC: American Psychological Association.

Derby, K. M., Fisher, W. W., Piazza, C. C., Wilke, A. E., & Johnson, W. (1998). The effects of noncontingent and contingent attention for self-injury, manding, and collateral responses. *Behavior Modification, 22*, 474–484.

Derby, K. M., Wacker, D. P., Sasso, G., Steege, M., Northup, J., Cigrand, K., et al. (1992). Brief functional assessment techniques to evaluate aberrant behavior in an outpatient setting: A summary of 79 cases. *Journal of Applied Behavior Analysis, 25*, 713–721.

Devlin, S., Leader, G., & Healey, O. (2009). Comparison of behavioral intervention and sensory-integration therapy in the treatment of self-injurious behavior. *Research in Autism Spectrum Disorders, 3*, 223–231.

Didden, R., Duker, P. C., & Korzilius, H. (1997). Meta-analytic study on treatment effectiveness for problem behaviors with individuals who have mental retardation. *American Journal on Mental Retardation, 101*, 387–399.

Didden, R., Korzilius, H., Van Oorsouw, W., & Sturmey, P. (2006). Behavioral treatment of challenging behaviors in individuals with mild mental retardation: Meta-analysis of single-subject research. *American Journal on Mental Retardation, 111*, 290–298.

Duker, P. C., & Nielen, M. (1993). The use of negative practice for the control of pica behavior. *Journal of Behavior Therapy and Experimental Psychiatry, 24*, 249–253.

Ellis, C. R., Singh, N. N., & Ruane, A. L. (1999). Nutritional, dietary, and hormonal treatments for individuals with mental retardation and developmental disabilities. *Mental Retardation and Developmental Disabilities Research Reviews, 5*, 335–341.

Emerson, E., Kiernan, C., Alborz, A., Reeves, D., Mason, H., Swarbrick, R., et al. (2001). Predicting the persistence of severe self-injurious behavior. *Research in Developmental Disabilities, 22*, 67–75.

Falcomata, T. S., Roane, H. S., & Pabico, R. R. (2007). Unintentional stimulus control during the treatment of pica displayed by a young man with autism. *Research in Autism Spectrum Disorders, 1*, 350–359.

Fisher, W., Piazza, C. C., Bowman, L. G., Hagopian, L. P., Owens, J. C., & Slevin, I. (1992). A comparison of two approaches for identifying reinforcers for persons with severe and profound disabilities. *Journal of Applied Behavior Analysis, 25*, 491–498.

Fisher, W. W., Piazza, C. C., Bowman, L. G., Kurtz, P. F., Sherer, M. R., & Lachman, S. R. (1994). A preliminary evaluation of empirically derived consequences for the treatment of pica. *Journal of Applied Behavior Analysis, 27*, 447–457.

Foxx, R. M., & Martin, E. D. (1975). Treatment of scavenging behavior (coprophagy and pica) by overcorrection. *Behaviour Research and Therapy, 13*, 153–162.

Gal, E., Dyck, M. J., & Passmore, A. (2009). The relationship between stereotyped movements and self-injurious behavior in children with developmental or sensory disabilities. *Research in Developmental Disabilities, 30*, 342–352.

Guess, D., & Carr, E. (1991). Emergence and maintenance of stereotypy and self-injury. *American Journal on Mental Retardation, 96*, 299–319.

Hagopian, L. P., & Adelinis, J. D. (2001). Response blocking with and without redirection for the treatment of pica. *Journal of Applied Behavior Analysis, 34*, 527–530.

Hagopian, L. P., Wilson, D. M., & Wilder, D. A. (2001). Assessment and treatment of problem behavior maintained by escape from attention and access to tangible items. *Journal of Applied Behavior Analysis, 34*, 229–232.

Hanley, G. P., Iwata, B. A., & Thompson, R. H. (2001). Reinforcement schedule thinning following treatment with functional communication training. *Journal of Applied Behavior Analysis, 34*, 17–38.

Hardan, A., & Sahl, R. (1997). Psychopathology in children and adolescents with developmental disorders. *Research in Developmental Disabilities, 18*, 369–382.

Healey, J. J., Ahearn, W. H., Graff, R. B., & Libby, M. E. (2001). Extended analysis and treatment of self-injurious behavior. *Behavioral Interventions, 16*, 181–195.

Herzinger, C. V., & Campbell, J. M. (2007). Comparing functional assessment methodologies: A quantitative synthesis. *Journal of Autism and Developmental Disorders, 37*, 1430–1445.

Hill, J., & Furniss, F. (2006). Patterns of emotional and behavioural disturbance associated with autistic traits in young people with severe intellectual disabilities and challenging behaviours. *Research in Developmental Disabilities, 27*, 517–528.

Hoch, H., McComas, J. J., Thompson, A. L., & Paone, D. (2002). Concurrent reinforcement schedules: Behavior change and maintenance without extinction. *Journal of Applied Behavior Analysis, 35*, 155–169.

Horner, R. H., Day, H. M., & Day, J. R. (1997). Using neutralizing routines to reduce problem behaviors. *Journal of Applied Behavior Analysis, 30*, 601–614.

Horner, R. H., Day, H. M., Sprague, J. R., O'Brien, M., & Heathfield, L. T. (1991). Interspersed requests: A nonaversive procedure for reducing aggression and self-injury during instruction. *Journal of Applied Behavior Analysis, 24*, 265–278.

Ingvarsson, E. T., Kahng, S. W., & Hausman, N. L. (2008). Some effects of noncontingent positive reinforcement on multiply controlled problem behavior and compliance in a demand context. *Journal of Applied Behavior Analysis, 41*, 435–440.

Iwata, B. A., Dorsey, M. F., Slifer, K. J., Bauman, K. E., & Richman, G. S. (1982). Toward a functional analysis of self-injury. *Analysis and Intervention in Developmental Disabilities, 2*, 3–20.

Iwata, B. A., Pace, G. M., Dorsey, M. F., Zarcone, J. R., Vollmer, T. R., Smith, R. G., et al. (1994). The functions of self-injurious behavior: An experimental-epidemiological analysis. *Journal of Applied Behavior Analysis, 27*, 215–240.

Iwata, B. A., Roscoe, E. M., Zarcone, J. R., & Richman, D. M. (2002). Environmental determinants of self-injurious behavior. In S. R. Schroeder, M. L. Oster-Granite, & T. Thompson (Eds.), *Self-injurious behavior: Gene-brain-behavior relationships* (pp. 93–103). Washington, DC: American Psychological Association.

Kahng, S., Iwata, B. A., DeLeon, I. G., & Wallace, M. D. (2000). A comparison of procedures for programming noncontingent reinforcement schedules. *Journal of Applied Behavior Analysis, 33*, 223–231.

Kahng, S., Iwata, B. A., & Lewin, A. B. (2002). Behavioral treatment of self-injury, 1964 to 2000. *American Journal on Mental Retardation, 107*, 212–221.

Kennedy, C. H. (2002). Evolution of stereotypy into self-injury. In S. R. Schroeder, M. L. Oster-Granite, & T. Thompson (Eds.), *Self-injurious behavior: Gene-brain-behavior relationships* (pp. 133–143). Washington, DC: American Psychological Association.

Kennedy, C. H., & Souza, G. (1995). Functional analysis and treatment of eye poking. *Journal of Applied Behavior Analysis, 28*, 27–37.

Kern, L., Starosta, K., & Adelman, B. E. (2006). Reducing pica by teaching children to exchange inedible items for edibles. *Behavior Modification, 30*, 135–158.

Kinnell, H. G. (1985). Pica as a feature of autism. *British Journal of Psychiatry, 147*, 80–82.

Kurtz, P. F., Chin, M. D., Huete, J. M., Tarbox, R. S. F., O'Connor, J. T., Paclawskyj, T. R., et al. (2003). Functional analysis and treatment of self-injurious behavior in young children: A summary of 30 cases. *Journal of Applied Behavior Analysis, 36*, 205–219.

Lalli, J. S., Mace, F. C., Livezey, K., & Kates, K. (1998). Assessment of stimulus generalization gradients in the treatment of self-injurious behavior. *Journal of Applied Behavior Analysis, 31*, 479–483.

Lalli, J. S., Vollmer, T. R., Progar, P. R., Wright, C., Borrero, J., Daniel, D., et al. (1999). Competition between positive and negative reinforcement in the treatment of escape behavior. *Journal of Applied Behavior Analysis, 32*, 285–296.

Lam, K. S. L., & Aman, M. G. (2007). The repetitive behavior scale-revised: Independent validation in individuals with autism spectrum disorders. *Journal of Autism and Developmental Disorders, 37*, 855–866.

Laraway, S., Snycerski, S., Michael, J., & Poling, A. (2003). Motivating operations and terms to describe them: Some further refinements. *Journal of Applied Behavior Analysis, 36*, 407–414.

LeBlanc, L. A., Patel, M. R., & Carr, J. E. (2000). Recent advances in the assessment of aberrant behavior maintained by automatic reinforcement in individuals with developmental disabilities. *Journal of Behavior Therapy and Experimental Psychiatry, 31*, 137–154.

LeBlanc, L. A., Piazza, C. C., & Krug, M. A. (1997). Comparing methods for maintaining the safety of a child with pica. *Research in Developmental Disabilities, 18*, 215–220.

Lecavalier, L. (2006). Behavioral and emotional problems in young people with pervasive developmental disorders: Relative prevalence, effects of subject characteristics, and empirical classification. *Journal of Autism and Developmental Disorders, 36*, 1101–1114.

Lerman, D. C., & Iwata, B. A. (1996). A methodology for distinguishing between extinction and punishment effects associated with response blocking. *Journal of Applied Behavior Analysis, 29*, 231–234.

Lerman, D. C., Iwata, B. A., & Wallace, M. D. (1999). Side effects of extinction: Prevalence of bursting and aggression during the treatment of self-injurious behavior. *Journal of Applied Behavior Analysis, 32*, 1–8.

Lerner, A. J. (2008). Treatment of pica behavior with olanzapine. *CNS Spectrums, 13*, 19.

Lindberg, J. S., Iwata, B. A., Roscoe, E. M., Worsdell, A. S., & Hanley, G. P. (2003). Treatment efficacy of noncontingent reinforcement during brief and extended application. *Journal of Applied Behavior Analysis, 36*, 1–19.

Lofts, R. H., Schroeder, S. R., & Maier, R. H. (1990). Effects of serum zinc supplementation on pica behavior of persons with mental retardation. *American Journal on Mental Retardation, 95*, 103–109.

Love, J. R., Carr, J. E., & LeBlanc, L. A. (2009). Functional assessment of problem behavior in children with autism spectrum disorders: A summary of 32 outpatient cases. *Journal of Autism and Developmental Disorders, 39*, 363–372.

Lowe, K., Allen, D., Jones, E., Brophy, S., Moore, K., & James, W. (2007). Challenging behaviours: Prevalence and topographies. *Journal of Intellectual Disability Research, 51*, 625–636.

Luiselli, J. K., Cochran, M. L., & Huber, S. A. (2005). Effects of otitis media on a child with autism receiving behavioral intervention for self-injury. *Child and Family Behavior Therapy, 27*, 51–56.

Mace, F. C., & Knight, D. (1986). Functional analysis and treatment of severe pica. *Journal of Applied Behavior Analysis, 19*, 411–416.

Mason, A. A., & Iwata, B. A. (1990). Artifactual effects of sensory-integrative therapy on self-injurious behavior. *Journal of Applied Behavior Analysis, 23*, 361–370.

Matson, J. L., Baglio, C. S., Smiroldo, B. B., Hamilton, M., Paclawskyj, T., Williams, D., et al. (1996). Characteristics of autism as assessed by the Diagnostic Assessment for the Severely Handicapped-II (DASH-II). *Research in Developmental Disabilities, 17*, 135–143.

Matson, J. L., & Bamburg, J. W. (1999). A descriptive study of pica behavior in persons with mental retardation. *Journal of Developmental and Physical Disabilities, 11*, 353–361.

Matson, J. L., Boisjoli, J. A., González, M. L., Smith, K. R., & Wilkins, J. (2007). Norms and cut off scores for the autism spectrum disorders diagnosis for adults (ASD-DA) with intellectual disability. *Research in Autism Spectrum Disorders, 1*, 330–338.

Matson, J. L., & LoVullo, S. V. (2008). A review of behavioral treatments for self-injurious behaviors of persons with autism spectrum disorders. *Behavior Modification, 32*, 61–76.

Matson, J. L., Mayville, S. B., Kuhn, D. E., Sturmey, P., Laud, R., & Cooper, C. (2005). The behavioral function of feeding problems as assessed by the questions about behavioral function (QABF). *Research in Developmental Disabilities, 26*, 399–408.

Matson, J. L., & Rivet, T. T. (2007). A validity study of the autism spectrum disorders-behavior problems for adults (ASD-BPA) scale. *Journal of Developmental and Physical Disabilities, 19*, 557–564.

Matson, J. L., & Rivet, T. T. (2008). The effects of severity of autism and PDD-NOS symptoms on challenging behaviors in adults with intellectual disabilities. *Journal of Developmental and Physical Disabilities, 20*, 41–51.

Mazaleski, J. L., Iwata, B. A., Rodgers, T. A., Vollmer, T. R., & Zarcone, J. R. (1994). Protective equipment as treatment for stereotypic hand mouthing: Sensory extinction or punishment effects? *Journal of Applied Behavior Analysis, 27*, 345–355.

McAdam, D. B., Sherman, J. A., Sheldon, J. B., & Napolitano, D. A. (2004). Behavioral interventions to reduce the pica of persons with developmental disabilities. *Behavior Modification, 28*, 45–72.

McClintock, K., Hall, S., & Oliver, C. (2003). Risk markers associated with challenging behaviours in people with intellectual disabilities: A meta-analytic study. *Journal of Intellectual Disability Research, 47*, 405–416.

McCord, B. E., Grosser, J. W., Iwata, B. A., & Powers, L. A. (2005). An analysis of response-blocking parameters in the prevention of pica. *Journal of Applied Behavior Analysis, 38*, 391–394.

McCord, B. E., Iwata, B. A., Galensky, T. L., Ellingson, S. A., & Thomson, R. J. (2001). Functional analysis and treatment of problem behavior evoked by noise. *Journal of Applied Behavior Analysis, 34*, 447–462.

McKerchar, T. L., Kahng, S., Casioppo, E., & Wilson, D. (2001). Functional analysis of self-injury maintained by automatic reinforcement: Exposing masked social functions. *Behavioral Interventions, 16*, 59–63.

Melville, C. A., Cooper, S. -A., Morrison, J., Smiley, E., Allan, L., Jackson, A., et al. (2008). The prevalence and incidence of mental ill-health in adults with autism and intellectual disabilities. *Journal of Autism and Developmental Disorders, 38*, 1676–1688.

Moore, J. W., Fisher, W. W., & Pennington, A. (2004). Systematic application and removal of protective equipment in the assessment of multiple topographies of self-injury. *Journal of Applied Behavior Analysis, 37*, 73–77.

Mulick, J. A., Barbour, R., Schroeder, S. R., & Rojahn, J. (1980). Overcorrection of pica in two profoundly retarded adults: Analysis of setting effects, stimulus, and response generalization. *Applied Research in Mental Retardation, 1*, 241–252.

Oliver, C., & Head, D. (1990). Self-injurious behaviour in people with learning disabilities; determinants and interventions. *International Review of Psychiatry, 2*, 99–114.

Oliver, C., Murphy, G. H., & Corbett, J. A. (1987). Self-injurious behaviour in people with mental handicap: A total population study. *Journal of Mental Deficiency Research, 31*, 147–162.

O'Reilly, M. F. (1997). Functional analysis of episodic self-injury correlated with recurrent otitis media. *Journal of Applied Behavior Analysis, 30*, 165–167.

O'Reilly, M. F., & Lancioni, G. (2000). Response covariation of escape-maintained aberrant behavior correlated with sleep deprivation. *Research in Developmental Disabilities, 21*, 125–136.

O'Reilly, M., Rispoli, M., Davis, T., Machalicek, W., Lang, R., Sigafoos, J., et al. (2010). Functional analysis of challenging behavior in children with autism spectrum disorders: A summary of 10 cases. *Research in Autism Spectrum Disorders, 4*, 1–10.

O'Reilly, M. F., Sigafoos, J., Lancioni, G., Rispoli, M., Lang, R., Chan, J., et al. (2008). Manipulating the behavior-altering effect of the motivating operation: Examination of the influence on challenging behavior during leisure activities. *Research in Developmental Disabilities, 29*, 333–340.

Pace, G. M., Iwata, B. A., Cowdery, G. E., Andree, P. J., & McIntyre, T. (1993). Stimulus (instructional) fading during extinction of self-injurious escape behavior. *Journal of Applied Behavior Analysis, 26*, 205–212.

Pace, G. M., & Toyer, E. A. (2000). The effects of a vitamin supplement on the pica of a child with severe mental retardation. *Journal of Applied Behavior Analysis, 33*, 619–622.

Piazza, C. C., Fisher, W. W., Hanley, G. P., LeBlanc, L. A., Worsdell, A. S., Lindauer, S. E., et al. (1998). Treatment of pica through multiple analyses of its reinforcing functions. *Journal of Applied Behavior Analysis, 31*, 165–189.

Piazza, C. C., Hanley, G. P., & Fisher, W. W. (1996). Functional analysis and treatment of cigarette pica. *Journal of Applied Behavior Analysis, 29*, 437–450.

Piazza, C. C., Roane, H. S., Keeney, K. M., Boney, B. R., & Abt, K. A. (2002). Varying response effort in the treatment of pica maintained by automatic reinforcement. *Journal of Applied Behavior Analysis, 35*, 233–246.

Posey, D. J., Stigler, K. A., Erickson, C. A., & McDougle, C. J. (2008). Antipsychotics in the treatment of autism. *Journal of Clinical Investigation, 118*, 6–14.

Rapp, J. T., Dozier, C. L., & Carr, J. E. (2001). Functional assessment and treatment of pica: A single-case experiment. *Behavioral Interventions, 16*, 111–125.

Reese, R. M., Richman, D. M., Belmont, J. M., & Morse, P. (2005). Functional characteristics of disruptive behavior in developmentally disabled children with and without autism. *Journal of Autism and Developmental Disorders, 35*, 419–428.

Richler, J., Bishop, S. L., Kleinke, J. R., & Lord, C. (2007). Restricted and repetitive behaviors in young children with autism spectrum disorders. *Journal of Autism and Developmental Disorders, 37*, 73–85.

Richman, D. M., Wacker, D. P., & Winborn, L. (2001). Response efficiency during functional communication training: Effects of effort on response allocation. *Journal of Applied Behavior Analysis, 34*, 73–76.

Roane, H. S., Vollmer, T. R., Ringdahl, J. E., & Marcus, B. A. (1998). Evaluation of a brief stimulus preference assessment. *Journal of Applied Behavior Analysis, 31*, 605–620.

Rojahn, J., Matson, J. L., Naglieri, J. A., & Mayville, E. (2004). Relationships between psychiatric conditions and behavior problems among adults with mental retardation. *American Journal on Mental Retardation, 109*, 21–33.

Rojahn, J., Schroeder, S. R., & Mulick, J. A. (1980). Ecological assessment of self protective devices in three profoundly retarded adults. *Journal of Autism and Developmental Disorders, 10*, 59–66.

Schopler, E., Reichler, R. J., DeVellis, R. F., & Daly, K. (1980). Toward objective classification of childhood autism: Childhood autism rating scale (CARS). *Journal of Autism and Developmental Disorders, 10*, 91–103.

Schroeder, S. R., Oster-Granite, M. L., Berkson, G., Bodfish, J. W., Breese, G. R., Cataldo, M. F., et al. (2001). Self-injurious behavior: Gene-brain-behavior relationships. *Mental Retardation and Developmental Disabilities Research Reviews, 7*, 3–12.

Serour, F., Witzling, M., Frenkel-Laufer, D., & Gorenstein, A. (2008). Intestinal obstruction in an autistic adolescent. *Pediatric Emergency Care, 24*, 688–690.

Shirley, M. J., Iwata, B. A., Kahng, S., Mazaleski, J. L., & Lerman, D. C. (1997). Does functional communication training compete with ongoing contingencies of reinforcement? An analysis during response acquisition and maintenance. *Journal of Applied Behavior Analysis, 30*, 93–104.

Shore, B. A., Iwata, B. A., DeLeon, I. G., Kahng, S. W., & Smith, R. G. (1997). An analysis of reinforcer substitutability using object manipulation and self-injury as competing responses. *Journal of Applied Behavior Analysis, 30*, 21–41.

Shore, B. A., Iwata, B. A., Lerman, D. C., & Shirley, M. J. (1994). Assessing and programming generalized behavioral reduction across multiple stimulus parameters. *Journal of Applied Behavior Analysis, 27*, 371–384.

Sigafoos, J., & Meikle, B. (1996). Functional communication training for the treatment of multiply determined challenging behavior in two boys with autism. *Behavior Modification, 20*, 60–84.

Singh, N. N., & Bakker, L. W. (1984). Suppression of pica by overcorrection and physical restraint: A comparative analysis. *Journal of Autism and Developmental Disorders, 14*, 331–341.

Singh, N. N., & Winton, A. S. W. (1984). Effects of a screening procedure on pica and collateral behaviors. *Journal of Behavior Therapy and Experimental Psychiatry, 15*, 59–65.

Smith, M. D. (1987). Treatment of pica in an adult disabled by autism by differential reinforcement of incompatible behavior. *Journal of Behavior Therapy and Experimental Psychiatry, 18*, 285–288.

Steege, M. W., Wacker, D. P., Berg, W. K., Cigrand, K. K., & Cooper, L. J. (1989). The use of behavioral assessment to prescribe and evaluate treatments for severely handicapped children. *Journal of Applied Behavior Analysis, 22*, 23–33.

Stokes, T. F., & Baer, D. M. (1977). An implicit technology of generalization. *Journal of Applied Behavior Analysis, 10*, 349–367.

Swift, I., Paquette, D., Davison, K., & Saeed, H. (1999). Pica and trace metal deficiencies in adults with developmental disabilities. *British Journal of Developmental Disabilities, 45*, 111–117.

Symons, F. J. (2002). Self-injury and pain: Models and mechanisms. In S. R. Schroeder, M. L. Oster-Granite, & T. Thompson (Eds.), *Self-injurious behavior: Gene-brain-behavior relationships* (pp. 223–234). Washington, DC: American Psychological Association.

Symons, F. J., Davis, M. L., & Thompson, T. (2000). Self-injurious behavior and sleep disturbance in adults with developmental disabilities. *Research in Developmental Disabilities, 21*, 115–123.

Symons, F. J., Hoch, J., Dahl, N. A., & McComas, J. J. (2003). Sequential and matching analyses of self-injurious behavior: A case of overmatching in the natural environment. *Journal of Applied Behavior Analysis, 36*, 267–270.

Tiger, J. H., Fisher, W. W., Toussaint, K. A., & Kodak, T. (2009). Progressing from initially ambiguous functional analyses: Three case examples. *Research in Developmental Disabilities, 30*, 910–926.

Tsakanikos, E., Costello, H., Holt, G., Bouras, N., Sturmey, P., & Newton, T. (2006). Psychopathology in adults with autism and intellectual disability. *Journal of Autism and Developmental Disorders, 36*, 1123–1129.

Van Camp, C. M., Lerman, D. C., Kelley, M. E., Contrucci, S. A., & Vorndran, C. M. (2000). Variable-time reinforcement schedules in the treatment of socially maintained problem behavior. *Journal of Applied Behavior Analysis, 33*, 545–557.

Van Camp, C. M., Vollmer, T. R., & Daniel, D. (2001). A systematic evaluation of stimulus preference, response effort, and stimulus control in the treatment of automatically reinforced self-injury. *Behavior Therapy, 32*, 603–613.

Van Houten, R. (1993). The use of wrist weights to reduce self-injury maintained by sensory reinforcement. *Journal of Applied Behavior Analysis, 26*, 197–203.

Vollmer, T. R. (1994). The concept of automatic reinforcement: Implications for behavioural research in developmental disabilities. *Research in Developmental Disabilities, 15*, 187–207.

Vollmer, T. R., Iwata, B. A., Smith, R. G., & Rodgers, T. A. (1992). Reduction of multiple aberrant behaviors and concurrent development of self-care skills with differential reinforcement. *Research in Developmental Disabilities, 13*, 287–299.

Vollmer, T. R., Iwata, B. A., Zarcone, J. R., Smith, R. G., & Mazaleski, J. L. (1993). The role of attention in the treatment of attention-maintained self-injurious behavior: Noncontingent reinforcement and differential reinforcement of other behavior. *Journal of Applied Behavior Analysis, 26*, 9–21.

Vollmer, T. R., Marcus, B. A., & LeBlanc, L. (1994). Treatment of self-injury and hand mouthing following inconclusive functional analyses. *Journal of Applied Behavior Analysis, 27*, 331–344.

Vollmer, T. R., Marcus, B. A., & Ringdahl, J. E. (1995). Noncontingent escape as treatment for self-injurious behavior maintained by negative reinforcement. *Journal of Applied Behavior Analysis, 28*, 15–26.

Vollmer, T. R., & Matson, J. L. (1995). *User's guide: Questions about behavioral function (QABF)*. Baton Rouge, LA: Scientific Publishers, Inc.

Vollmer, T. R., Progar, P. R., Lalli, J. S., Van Camp, C. M., Sierp, B. J., Wright, C. S., et al. (1998). Fixed-time schedules attenuate extinction-induced phenomena in the treatment of severe aberrant behavior. *Journal of Applied Behavior Analysis, 31*, 529–542.

Vollmer, T. R., Sloman, K. N., & Borrero, C. S. W. (2009). Behavioral assessment of self-injury. In J. L. Matson, F. Andrasik, & M. L. Matson (Eds.), *Assessing childhood psychopathology and developmental disabilities* (pp. 341–369). New York: Springer.

Vollmer, T. R., & Smith, R. G. (1996). Some current themes in functional analysis research. *Research in Developmental Disabilities, 17*, 229–249.

Wacker, D. P., Steege, M. W., Northup, J., Sasso, G., Berg, W., Reimers, T., et al. (1990). A component analysis of functional communication training across three topographies of severe behavior problems. *Journal of Applied Behavior Analysis, 23*, 417–429.

Wasano, L. C., Borrero, J. C., & Kohn, C. S. (2009). Brief report: A comparison of indirect versus experimental strategies for the assessment of pica. *Journal of Autism and Developmental Disorders, 39*, 1582–1586.

Williams, D. E., Kirkpatrick-Sanchez, S., Enzinna, C., Dunn, J., & Borden-Karasack, D. (2009). The clinical management and prevention of pica: A retrospective follow-up of 41 individuals with intellectual disabilities and pica. *Journal of Applied Research in Intellectual Disabilities, 22*, 210–215.

Winborn, L., Wacker, D. P., Richman, D. M., Asmus, J., & Geier, D. (2002). Assessment of mand selection for functional communication training packages. *Journal of Applied Behavior Analysis, 35*, 295–298.

Winton, A. S. W., & Singh, N. N. (1983). Suppression of pica using brief-duration physical restraint. *Journal of Mental Deficiency Research, 27*, 93–103.

Worsdell, A. S., Iwata, B. A., Hanley, G. P., Thompson, R. H., & Kahng, S. W. (2000). Effects of continuous and intermittent reinforcement for problem behavior during functional communication training. *Journal of Applied Behavior Analysis, 33*, 167–179.

Yates, T. M. (2004). The developmental psychopathology of self-injurious behavior: Compensatory regulation in posttraumatic adaptation. *Clinical Psychology Review, 24*, 35–74.

Zarcone, J. R., Iwata, B. A., Mazaleski, J. L., & Smith, R. G. (1994). Momentum and extinction effects on self-injurious escape behavior and noncompliance. *Journal of Applied Behavior Analysis, 27*, 649–658.

Zarcone, J. R., Iwata, B. A., Smith, R. G., Mazaleski, J. L., & Lerman, D. C. (1994). Reemergence and extinction of self-injurious escape behavior during stimulus (instructional) fading. *Journal of Applied Behavior Analysis, 27*, 307–316.

Self-Injurious Behavior: II. Pharmacological and Integrated Treatments

28

Frederick Furniss, Asit B. Biswas, Bradley Bezilla, and Aaron A. Jones

This is the second of two chapters reviewing treatment of self-injurious behavior (SIB) in people with pervasive developmental disabilities (PDDs). The preceding chapter reviewed the general characteristics of SIB in people with PDDs and behavioral treatment of SIB. The present chapter goes on to review pharmacological and combined pharmacological and behavioral treatments. The final section of this chapter points out directions for future research in the treatment of SIB. As in the previous chapter, the term autistic spectrum disorders (ASDs) will, in general, be used to refer to autistic disorder, Asperger's disorder, and pervasive developmental disorder-not otherwise specified (PDD-NOS); where participants in group studies are limited to those with a single diagnosis, or those with a diagnosis of autistic disorder are specifically excluded, we use more specific terms.

Pharmacological Treatment

Rationales for Pharmacological Treatment

Neurotransmitter systems including the serotonin, dopamine, opioid, and noradrenaline systems, acting alone or in combination, have been implicated in SIB. Although a variety of psychotropic medications have been used in attempts to treat SIB in persons with ASDs and intellectual disabilities (IDs), the empirical evidence regarding the effectiveness of anti-epileptics, mood stabilizers, and anti-anxiety medications is both limited in quantity and comprised primarily of studies with significant methodological limitations (Deb & Unwin, 2007). The most specific rationales for psychopharmacological treatments of SIB relate to the dopamine, serotonin, and opioid systems, and this chapter reviews available evidence for effectiveness of drugs targeting these systems. The rationales for treatments primarily targeting each system are presented for each major class of pharmacological agents discussed below.

Atypical Antipsychotics

Interest in the role of dysregulation of the dopamine system and the possible utility of atypical antipsychotics in treating SIB was stimulated by findings of reduced levels of striatal dopamine in individuals with Lesch-Nyhan disease, an X-linked genetic disorder involving reduced levels of hypoxanthine-guanine phosphoribosyl transferase and with characteristic presentation including ID and behavioral disturbance including SIB (Schretlen et al., 2005). Further, in a series of studies reviewed by Breese et al. (2005), it was demonstrated that rats in whom dopaminergic neurons were destroyed in the neonatal period using 6-hydroxydopamine show severe self-biting when given L-DOPA in maturity. The SIB produced by L-DOPA is mainly produced by activation of the D_1 dopamine receptor subtype, although activation of the D_2 subtype, while not leading to SIB in isolation, may facilitate expression of SIB produced by D_1 activation. In addition to depletion of dopamine levels, neonatal lesioning of dopaminergic neurons results in increases in striatal serotonin, and a variety of evidence suggests that both serotonin modulation of D_1 receptor activity and changes in $GABA_A$ receptor function in the substantia nigra reticulata may be involved in the increased susceptibility to SIB in neonatally 6-hydroxydopamine-lesioned rats (Breese et al., 2005).

Clozapine, olanzapine, and quetiapine all block both D_1 and D_2 dopamine receptor subtypes, together with several types of 5-HT receptor and a variety of other receptors including adrenergic receptors, while risperidone blocks D_2, 5-HT, and adrenergic receptors (Aman & Madrid, 1999). In a systematic review of studies using atypical antipsychotics to treat persons with IDs and/or ASDs published

F. Furniss (✉)
School of Psychology, University of Leicester, Leicester LE1 7LT, UK
e-mail: fred.furniss@hesleygroup.co.uk

J.L. Matson, P. Sturmey (eds.), *International Handbook of Autism and Pervasive Developmental Disorders*, Autism and Child Psychopathology Series, DOI 10.1007/978-1-4419-8065-6_28, © Springer Science+Business Media, LLC 2011

up to and including 1999, Aman and Madrid (1999) identified 14 studies including at least some participants with ASDs, one also including 1 participant with childhood disintegrative disorder (CDD), 12 on risperidone and 1 each on olanzapine and clozapine. Several reported improvement in SIB in some participants; however, the majority had multiple methodological problems. Sedation and weight gain were frequently observed and dyspepsia and hyperprolactemia were also reported. Since Aman and Madrid's review a number of better-controlled studies of the use of atypical antipsychotics with people with ASDs, especially of risperidone, have appeared.

Risperidone

In an 8-week, double-blind, placebo-controlled study, Scahill et al. (2002) examined the effect of risperidone in doses between 0.5 and 3.5 mg/day at the end of the study on the behavior of 49 children with autistic disorder, 76% of whom had mild-severe IDs, compared with 52 children receiving placebo. Participants were aged between 5 and 17 years and engaged in tantrums, aggression, SIB, or multiple behavior problems. Repeated assessment on the Aberrant Behavior Checklist (ABC) (Aman & Singh, 1994) irritability subscale showed a significant group by time interaction, with a mean 57% decrease in irritability score in the risperidone-treated group compared with a 14% decrease in the placebo group. The ABC stereotypy and hyperactivity subscales also showed significantly greater reductions for the risperidone than the placebo group. Reports of increased appetite, fatigue, and drowsiness were significantly associated with risperidone treatment, and weight gain was significantly greater in the risperidone group. Clinical assessment using structured scales showed no extrapyramidal symptoms in either group. Parental reports of tremor and tachycardia were significantly associated ($p = 0.06$) with risperidone usage. A 16-week open-label follow-up (Research Units on Pediatric Psychopharmacology Autism Network, 2005) of 63 children previously treated with risperidone in the double-blind trial, or given 8 weeks of open-label treatment following placebo, showed small but significant increases in ABC irritability subscale score, although the mean score remained well below the baseline level of the double-blind phase. Participants showed a mean 6-month weight increase of 5.1 (SD = 3.6) kg. A subsequent 8-week double-blind placebo-substitution phase showed relapse rates of 13% with ongoing risperidone and 63% with placebo substitution. Anderson et al. (2007) confirmed that although initially increasing prolactin levels decreased over the course of treatment, approximately one-third of participants had values above the normal range at 22 months of treatment. Shea et al. (2004) reported results from an 8-week, double-blind, placebo-controlled trial involving 79 children, aged between 5 and 12, all with PDD, including 1 with CDD, with 69% having diagnosis of autistic disorder. Forty participants, 30 of whom had mild-severe IDs,

received risperidone and 39 participants, including 29 with ID, received placebo. At study endpoint all ABC subscales showed significantly greater decreases for the risperidone than for the placebo group, as did the conduct problem, hyperactive, insecure/anxious, and overly sensitive subscales of the Nisonger Child Behavior Rating Form (NCBRF) (Tassé, Aman, Hammer, & Rojahn, 1996). There were no significant differences between groups in change on the self-isolated/ritualistic or self-injurious/stereotypic subscales of the NCBRF. Somnolence was reported for over 70% of the risperidone group, but was reported to resolve in most cases, usually following dose rescheduling or reduction. Increases in weight, pulse rate, and systolic blood pressure were all significantly greater at study endpoint for the risperidone versus the placebo group.

While the above studies have produced evidence suggestive of a beneficial effect of risperidone on the behavior of children with ASDs and behavior problems, they provide little evidence specifically relevant to the impact of risperidone on SIB. Arnold et al. (2003), however, asked parents of 87 children participating in the Scahill et al. (2002) study to describe and quantify at baseline their two greatest concerns regarding their child's behavior. SIB was selected as a primary concern by parents of 11 children receiving placebo and 8 receiving risperidone. After 4 and 8 weeks, descriptions of the child's current status with respect to these problems were rated for degree of change by a panel of clinical judges blind to treatment group. The mean improvement rating for SIB was significantly higher for the children receiving risperidone, showing the greatest effect size of all target symptoms.

Subsequent studies including younger children as participants (Luby et al., 2006; Nagaraj, Singhi, & Malhi, 2006) have produced mixed evidence concerning possible benefits of risperidone for core features of ASDs, but again contribute little to the evidence base for its efficacy in reducing SIB. Evidence regarding the effectiveness of risperidone for treating adults with ASDs is substantially less than that available for children. McDougle et al. (1998) reported data from 30 adults with ASDs and a mean age of 28 years randomized to treatment with either risperidone (mean dose 2.0 mg/day) or placebo over a period of 12 weeks. Risperidone treatment was associated with greater improvement than placebo on Clinical Global Impression, repetitive behavior as assessed by a modified form of the Yale-Brown Obsessive-Compulsive Scale (Y-BOCS) (Goodman et al., 1989), and structured clinician ratings of problem behaviors.

Other Atypical Antipsychotics

There is considerably less evidence regarding the effectiveness of the other atypical antipsychotics for behavioral difficulties in people with ASDs. Use of clozapine is associated with risks of agranulocytosis and seizures (McDougle, Stigler, Erickson, & Posey, 2006) and the need for frequent blood samples for white cell counts is particularly undesirable in people with ASDs.

Olanzapine has a high affinity for dopamine D_1, D_2, and D_4 receptors as well as various 5-HT, alpha-1 adrenergic, H_1 histaminic, and multiple muscarinic receptor subtypes (McDougle et al., 2006). A short-term open-label study of 8 children and adults with ASDs, most with IDs (Potenza, Holmes, Kanes, & McDougle, 1999) reported improvements on the ABC irritability and hyperactivity subscales. Malone, Cater, Sheikh, Choudhury, and Delaney (2001) randomized 12 children with ASDs, 11 of whom had IDs, to 6 weeks of open treatment with olanzapine or haloperidol. The Children's Psychiatric Rating Scale (National Institute of Mental Health, 1985) showed improvement for the olanzapine, but not the haloperidol group, on anger/uncooperativeness and hyperactivity factors. A 12-week open-label study reporting efficacy data from 22 children with ASDs (mean age 11.2 years; mean I.Q. 98) treated with olanzapine (mean dose 10.7 mg/day) for 12 weeks reported significant improvement on ABC irritability, hyperactivity, and inappropriate speech subscales (Kemner, Willemsen-Swinkels, De Jonge, Tuynman-Qua, & Van Engeland, 2002); however, only three participants were rated as much improved, although this may be related to the relatively low severity of disruptive behavior pre-treatment (Posey, Stigler, Erickson, & McDougle, 2008). A small double-blind placebo-controlled trial with six children with ASDs, four of whom had IDs, receiving olanzapine, found no evidence for an effect of olanzapine on standardized measures of irritability or aggression (Hollander et al., 2006). All the above studies noted problems with weight gain and sedation. There have to date been no published controlled studies of the atypical antipsychotics quetiapine and ziprasidone with people with ASDs; McDougle et al. (2006), Stachnik and Nunn-Thompson (2007), and Posey et al. (2008) have reviewed relevant retrospective and open-label studies. An outline of the relevant studies is provided in Table 28.1.

A number of recent studies have evaluated the efficacy of aripiprazole for treatment of behavior problems in persons with ASDs. Aripiprazole is a partial D_2 and 5-HT$_{1A}$ agonist as well as a 5-HT$_{2A}$ antagonist (Posey et al., 2008). Following promising results, including a significant mean ABC irritability subscale score reduction from 29 at baseline to 8.1 at week 14, from an open-label study of aripiprazole in young people diagnosed with PDD-NOS or Asperger's disorder (Stigler et al., 2009), two randomized, placebo-controlled, double-blind, parallel-group studies have evaluated the impact of aripiprazole on problem behaviors presented by young people with ASDs. Marcus et al. (2009) randomized 218 young people (ages 6–17 years) with autistic disorder, a minimum ABC irritability subscale score of 18, and problem behaviors including SIB to 8 weeks of treatment with placebo or one of three fixed dose levels of aripiprazole

(5, 10, or 15 mg/day). A total of 178 participants (82%) completed the study, with completion rates similar across groups. All three doses of aripiprazole produced significantly greater baseline–week 8 reductions in ABC irritability, stereotypy, and hyperactivity subscale scores than did placebo. The rate of positive response, defined by a 25% or greater reduction in ABC irritability score and a Clinical Global Impression of Severity rating of "much improved" or "very much improved," at week 8 was significantly greater than for placebo only for the 5 mg/day aripiprazole group. A variety of adverse events were associated with aripiprazole treatment, the most commonly reported being sedation, fatigue, vomiting, increased appetite, tremor, and nasopharyngitis. Over 20% of each group taking aripiprazole showed adverse events related to treatment-emergent extrapyramidal symptoms, tremor and extrapyramidal disorder being most commonly reported. All aripiprazole groups gained significantly more weight over the course of the study than the placebo group (mean change from baseline, observed cases: placebo 0.4 kg, aripiprazole 5 mg/day 1.5 kg, aripiprazole 10 mg/day 1.4 kg, aripiprazole 15 mg/day 1.6 kg). Aripiprazole 5 and 15 mg/day were associated with higher rates of clinically significant weight gain than placebo. All doses of aripiprazole were associated with significant reductions in serum prolactin over the course of the study, and aripiprazole treatment was not associated with clinically significant changes in vital sign measurements or ECG abnormalities. In another 8-week study, Owen et al. (2009) randomized 98 young people aged 6–17 years with autistic disorder and problem behaviors such as tantrums, aggression, and SIB to treatment with either placebo or flexibly dosed aripiprazole (starting dose 2 mg/day, maximum dose 15 mg/day). Results in terms of mean improvement on ABC irritability, hyperactivity, and stereotypy subscales, emergent extrapyramidal symptoms, other adverse events, weight gain, and reduction in serum prolactin were similar to those of Marcus et al. (2009).

Atypical Antipsychotics: Conclusions

Despite a considerable amount of well-controlled research indicating a beneficial effect of risperidone on behavioral difficulties of children and adolescents with ASDs, and some evidence from adults, it remains difficult to evaluate the specific effectiveness of risperidone for treatment of SIB. The one study which has used reported clinician ratings of change in specifically described behavior problems (Arnold et al., 2003) reported a larger effect size for risperidone treatment related to SIB than for any other behavior problem considered, but this figure relates to only 8 children treated with risperidone and 11 given placebo, and Shea et al. (2004) found no advantage for risperidone over placebo on the self-injury/stereotypic subscale of the NCBRF. Further research on this question is clearly warranted, given the mixed results to date and because the 6-hydroxydopamine-lesioned rat

Table 28.1 Open-label prospective and retrospective studies of quetiapine and ziprasidone for persons with ASDs

Drug	Studies	Clinical Global Impression response rate	Main side effects reported
Quetiapine	No RCTs, four open-label studies: Martin, Koenig, Scahill & Bregman, 1999; Findling et al., 2004; Corson, Barkenbus, Posey, Stigler & McDougle, 2004; Hardan, Jou & Handen 2005. Participant numbers: 6, 9, 20, 10	Martin et al.: 33% Findling et al.: 22%	Agitation, sedation, weight gain
		Corson et al.: 40%	
		Hardan et al.: 60%	
		Positive impact reported on challenging behavior, inattention, and hyperactivity in responders	
Ziprasidone	No RCTs, two open-label studies: McDougle, Kem & Posey, 2002; Cohen, Fitzgerald, Khan & Khan, 2004.	McDougle et al.: 50%	Transient sedation, weight gain (but most patients lost weight on switch to ziprasidone from other atypical antipsychotics)
	Participant numbers: 12, 10	Cohen et al.: 70% improvement or no change on switch from other atypical antipsychotics	
		Positive impact reported on aggression, agitation, and irritability in responders	

model of SIB would suggest that owing to its lack of affinity for the D_1 type receptor risperidone may be a less effective treatment for this specific behavior than other atypical antipsychotics. In one-third of cases it appears that risperidone treatment can be successfully withdrawn after periods of up to 6 months from children with ASDs who have been judged to respond positively to initial treatment (Research Units on Pediatric Psychopharmacology Autism Network, 2005; Troost et al., 2005). The current evidence base therefore suggests that if risperidone is used in treatment of SIB its effects should be carefully monitored, there should be frequent review to determine whether medication can be withdrawn without negative effects on behavior, and prescription of risperidone should be accompanied by behavioral interventions.

Despite the specific rationale for use of dopamine D_1 receptor blockers in treatment of SIB, there is no stronger evidence for the effectiveness of olanzapine than for risperidone in the treatment of SIB, and side effects of weight gain, sedation, and increases in prolactin levels are of equal concern. Evidence for the potential utility of the other atypical antipsychotics in behavior disorders in people with ASDs is currently very limited. There is preliminary evidence to suggest that ziprasidone use is less likely to be associated with weight gain problems than is the case for the other atypical antipsychotics, but the potential for QTc interval prolongation has led to the warning that ziprasidone should not be used with persons with cardiac arrhythmias or long QT syndrome or who use other medications which may prolong

the QTc interval (Posey et al., 2008). (The QTc interval, the interval from the beginning of the Q wave to the end of the T wave in the heart's electrical cycle corrected for heart rate, measures the time taken for the heart to re-polarize following a heartbeat, and its prolongation represents a risk factor for ventricular arrhythmias and possible sudden death.) The effectiveness and safety of aripiprazole for persons with ASDs has to date only been evaluated in short-term studies. The reduction in serum prolactin apparently associated with its use may result from its action as a partial dopamine agonist, and longer term evaluation of this effect is needed.

A retrospective review of the introduction of atypical antipsychotics for 31 adults with IDs, 17 of whom were diagnosed with ASDs, concluded that aggression to others, but not SIB, improved when atypical antipsychotics replaced or supplemented previously prescribed medications (Ruedrich et al., 2008). Low-dose antipsychotics, nonetheless, have a role to play for some persons with ASD and significant SIB. As adverse reactions can be significant, starting with a low dose and careful and incremental change in dose of the atypical antipsychotic drug is recommended as a general rule.

Specific Serotonin Reuptake Inhibitors

Interest in the possible utility of serotonin reuptake inhibitors (SRIs) in treatment of SIB in people with ASD has been strengthened by the evidence for abnormalities of serotonin function in persons with ASDs and IDs (Aman, Arnold, & Armstrong, 1999; Masi, 2004; Posey, Erickson, Stigler, & McDougle, 2006), and the possibility that in some cases SIB may have similarities to obsessional behavior (King, 1993).

Aman et al. (1999) reviewed studies to that date on use of clomipramine and the SSRIs (specific serotonin reuptake inhibitors) with people with developmental disabilities, noting the preponderance of case reports or uncontrolled trials and suggesting the need among others for further study of possible age differences in responsivity. The potential serious side effects of clomipramine (Aman et al., 1999) have led to more recent interest being focused on the SSRIs, with most evidence available regarding fluvoxamine and fluoxetine. Reviews by McDougle et al. (2006) and Posey et al. (2006) suggested that although there may be some evidence for the effectiveness of SSRIs in treating repetitive behavior in adults with developmental disabilities there are still few well-controlled studies, while for children the results of both open-label and double-blind placebo-controlled studies of fluvoxamine suggest limited effectiveness and frequent adverse reactions including insomnia, behavioral activation, and aggression. Henry et al. (2009), in a retrospective chart review of 22 young people with ASDs who were treated with an SSRI following a clinically unsuccessful trial of a previous SSRI, reported that over two-thirds showed activation side effects, which may include agitation, impulsivity, hyperactivity, and insomnia, with the second SSRI. For children with ASDs the lack of evidence of effectiveness, frequent occurrence of adverse reactions, and uncertainties about appropriate dosage (Posey et al., 2006) do not support the utility of currently available SSRIs in treatment of SIB. For some adults with ASDs, however, SSRIs may have a role in treatment of SIB presenting with features of compulsivity. The clinician should, however, be aware of possible side effects including elevated mood, reduced sleep, hyperactivity, and aggression in adults with IDs (Biswas, Bhaumik, & Branford, 2001).

Naltrexone hydrochloride

A variety of evidence has suggested dysregulation of the hypothalamic–pituitary–adrenal stress system in persons with ASDs and others with developmental disabilities who engage in SIB (Sandman & Touchette, 2002), with recent interest focused on the pro-opiomelanocortin (POMC) system. Enzyme cleavage converts the POMC molecule into a number of biologically active products including the opioid β-endorphin and adrenocorticotrophin (ACTH), and in adults plasma levels of these products of the POMC molecule are normally highly correlated. Recent studies have suggested however that this normal coupling of β-endorphin and ACTH

is reduced following episodes of SIB in adults with developmental disabilities (Sandman, Touchette, Lenjavi, Marion, & Chicz-DeMet, 2003), with levels of β-endorphin elevated with respect to levels of ACTH. It has been argued that this phenomenon may indicate that persons showing SIB experience enhanced opioid-mediated analgesia and/or that SIB produces an opioid-induced state of euphoria.

Administration of the opiate antagonist naltrexone hydrochloride would be expected to reduce both of the above effects. Naltrexone may cause a number of side effects including liver toxicity (Matson et al., 2000); however, signs of possible toxicity have been observed in people without disabilities treated for addictions and using substantially larger doses than those used to treat SIB in people with IDs (Symons, Thompson, & Rodriguez, 2004).

Reports on the effectiveness of naltrexone in treatment of SIB have been mixed. Symons et al. (2004) reviewed 27 studies from which information on individual participants could be extracted, noting that 30 (35%) of the total of 86 children and adults treated with naltrexone were reported to be diagnosed with an ASD. Comparison of quantitative measures of SIB during baseline and during naltrexone administration showed that 47% of participants showed improvement of 50% or greater, and a further 33% showed smaller SIB decreases, during naltrexone treatment. Presence of an ASD was not associated with outcome of naltrexone treatment. Further, there is some evidence that for some people limited-term administration of naltrexone can produce reductions in SIB which persist after the medication is withdrawn (Crews, Bonaventura, Rowe, & Bonsie, 1993; Sandman et al., 2000).

Despite this promising overall picture, however, in addition to many reports of cases in which naltrexone has not improved SIB (e.g., Bodfish et al., 1997), there are also reports of paradoxical worsening of frequency and/or severity of SIB during naltrexone treatment (Benjamin, Seek, Tresise, Price, & Gagnon, 1995). The specific mechanism of action of naltrexone is not well understood. Dose–response relationships appear to be complex (Symons et al., 2004), and people showing long-term improvement in SIB following time-limited naltrexone treatment may show worsening of SIB if treated again with naltrexone (Sandman et al., 2000). Topography of SIB does not appear to predict response to naltrexone (Symons et al., 2004). Sandman and his colleagues (Sandman et al., 2000, 2003; Sandman, Touchette, Marion, Lenjavi, & Chicz-Demet, 2002) have suggested that baseline levels of β-endorphin relative to ACTH may be associated with patterns of SIB suggesting relative insensitivity to social/environmental events and may predict response to naltrexone; however, the relationship between the direct opiate blocking effect, possible adjustments in receptor sensitivity, and operant learning mechanisms in the effect of naltrexone remains to be elucidated. Benjamin et al. (1995), reporting a case in which naltrexone appeared to markedly worsen severity of SIB in a young adult with autism, suggested that his deterioration in behavior might be an operant extinction-induced process caused by the failure of SIB to produce β-endorphin-related effects. Although there is good evidence that naltrexone can be helpful in some cases of SIB, response to treatment and most effective dosage are difficult to predict, little is known regarding optimal duration of treatment, and paradoxical effects are possible. Particular attention to objective evaluation of treatment effect and dose parameters, as well as consideration of sensitivity to liver toxicity, is therefore needed with any trial of naltrexone in treatment of SIB.

Conclusions

The most direct rationales for psychopharmacological treatments of SIB relate to the dopaminergic and opioidergic systems, and to date the strongest available evidence of treatment effectiveness relates to drugs targeting these systems. Despite a substantial number of well-controlled studies, the evidence regarding the utility of atypical antipsychotics specifically for treatment of SIB in both children and adults with ASDs remains inconclusive, mainly owing to the reliance of most studies on global ratings of improvement and generalized behavior rating scales. Increases in weight, with the possible exception of ziprasidone, raised prolactin levels, with the possible exception of aripiprazole, and somnolence/sedation are frequently reported adverse events associated with treatment with atypical antipsychotics. Other side effects including effects on heart rate have also been reported. The possible long-term health consequences of these effects require further study and warrant serious consideration when use of an atypical antipsychotic is considered. Extrapyramidal symptoms have been reported in up to 26% of participants in 1-year follow-ups of children without PDDs using risperidone (Turgay, Binder, Snyder, & Fisman, 2002), and longer term research will be needed on the question of whether long-term use of risperidone and other atypical antipsychotics may be associated with development of tardive dyskinesia. Monitoring for other less frequent adverse events such as neuroleptic malignant syndrome remains important.

In cases where SIB is chronic and assessment does not identify functional relationships with social/environmental events, consideration of naltrexone treatment may be warranted. The effects of naltrexone, however, vary dramatically across individuals, are clinically difficult to predict for the individual case, and include the potential for adverse as well as beneficial effects on SIB. Again, therefore, careful monitoring of effectiveness and frequent review are appropriate where naltrexone is used in treatment of SIB. The evidence regarding adverse events with naltrexone is largely drawn

from its use with nondisabled adults and close monitoring for possible such events is appropriate where the drug is considered for use with persons with ASDs. Naltrexone use may increase SIB-related pain and/or decrease SIB-related euphoria, and its use has been reported to increase signs of negative affect during SIB (Benjamin et al., 1995). Given that some level of SIB will usually continue to occur in most cases even of successful treatment with naltrexone, and that social/environmental factors may be implicated in the maintenance of the behavior (Symons et al., 2001), it is therefore both practically and ethically important that consideration of naltrexone use in cases of SIB is accompanied by behavioral intervention.

Integrating Behavioral and Psychopharmacological Interventions

Assessment and treatment with SIB should generally first involve screening for possible contributing physical illness and a thorough functional assessment to indicate directions for behavioral treatment. Where initial treatment fails, this should be regarded as indicating the need for more detailed and individualized functional assessment to identify possible idiosyncratic functional relationships (Harding, Wacker, Berg, Barretto, & Ringdahl, 2005). In general, current best practice is to consider psychopharmacological approaches only where detailed functional assessment suggests insensitivity of the SIB to environmental contingencies or where individualized behavioral interventions repeatedly fail to reduce levels of SIB.

Behavioral interventions have a substantial evidence base for efficacy, but their wide-scale effectiveness in routine clinical practice is much less studied. Psychopharmacological treatments are of demonstrated benefit to some individuals, but with little evidence regarding impact on specific behaviors. Exploration of how these approaches might most effectively be combined would seem to offer the greatest possibilities for increasing treatment efficacy and effectiveness (Napolitano et al., 1999). In fact, however, studies on this issue are few in number (Weeden, Ehrhardt, & Poling, 2009). In the remainder of this chapter we will review some of the examples of, and possibilities for, systematic integration of behavioral and psychopharmacological approaches.

One way in which behavioral and psychopharmacological approaches might usefully be combined is by use of standardized behavior rating scales in choosing psychopharmacological intervention. Currently, initial choice of intervention is often determined on the basis of clinical impression. As noted in the previous chapter, impulsivity, stereotypy, compulsivity, mania, and anxiety have all been identified as disorders either possibly characteristic of ASDs and/or associated with ASDs, and the latter four of these conditions

Table 28.2 Subtypes of possibly "biologic" SIB together with indications for potential psychopharmacological treatment, based on subtypes proposed by Mace and Mauk (1995)

Clinical subtype	Presentation	Mechanism	Choice of drug (under specialist supervision)
SIB with extreme self-mutilation	Severe SIB with severe tissue damage, extensive and multiple wounds, and scarring	Insensitivity to pain mediated by β-endorphins	*Opiate antagonists*, e.g., naltrexone
Stereotypic SIB	Repetitive, rhythmic pattern of SIB	Dopaminergic pathways–mesolimbic and mesocortical	*Low-dose atypical or typical antipsychotics*, e.g., risperidone, olanzapine, haloperidol, aripiprazole, chlorpromazine
Compulsive SIB	Compulsive pattern of SIB which escalates on attempts to block/intervene or if interrupted	Serotonergic pathways	*SSRIs*, e.g., paroxetine, fluoxetine, fluvoxamine, sertraline
SIB with agitation and high anxiety	SIB presenting with psychomotor agitation and high psychological and physiological arousal	Noradrenergic pathways	*Beta blockers*, e.g., propranolol; *mood stabilizers*, e.g., carbamazepine, lithium carbonate, sodium valproate, lamotrigine, gabapentin; *others*, e.g., trazodone
SIB with mixed processes	Clinical features in different combinations, as above	Several of the above	One or more of the drugs as above depending on presentation

clearly map on to Mace and Mauk's (1995) proposed subtyping of "biologic" SIB and suggested initial interventions (see Table 28.2). Given that all of these difficulties are likely to be salient for many persons with ASDs, assessment of relative severity and initial choice of psychopharmacological treatment might well be aided by use of structured and norm-referenced assessments such as the Diagnostic Assessment for the Severely Handicapped-Revised (DASH-II) (Matson, 1995). This approach may in fact already have been selectively applied in much of the research suggesting possible utility of risperidone in the treatment of SIB, in which a high score on the ABC irritability subscale is a criterion for inclusion in the study. Risperidone may be useful primarily in treatment of "impulsive" rather than "compulsive" forms of SIB (Aman et al., 2005), and selecting participants on the basis of high ABC irritability subscale score may effectively be selecting participants whose SIB is likely to be "impulsive" in nature. More systematic assessment of behavioral and emotional comorbidity with SIB might improve choice of clinical intervention and enable subtyping of participants in larger-scale intervention studies with a view to evaluating clinical predictors of response to alternative interventions.

A further refinement of such an approach would be to select psychopharmacological interventions, and then to analyze their effectiveness, using functional analysis methodologies. Zarcone et al. (2004) for example conducted repeated experimental functional analyses (EFAs) (see preceding chapter) with 13 individuals with ASDs and IDs participating in a research evaluation of the impact of risperidone on

behaviors such as aggression, SIB, and disruption (tearing, breaking, or throwing materials). For most participants use of risperidone was associated with a generalized reduction in rates of these behaviors across EFA conditions. For one participant presenting SIB, however, a "high" dose of risperidone (0.25 mg/kg bodyweight/day), although not a "low" dose, was associated with a reduction in rate of SIB in the attention condition of the EFA by comparison with an initial placebo phase. Rates of SIB in the escape, tangible, ignore (a modified form of Iwata, Dorsey, Slifer, Bauman, and Richman's (1982) "alone" condition), and play conditions however did not change, consistent with the medication selectively affecting SIB dependent on its function. Such analyses may assist clinicians in titrating medication dosage and considering supplementary interventions. In a hypothetical case similar to that reported by Zarcone et al. (2004), for example, a clinician might conclude that risperidone had no effect on the client's behavior or might conclude that risperidone had a slight effect and be inclined to increase dosage. If, however, medication has selectively reduced SIB under one set of social conditions but not others, then continuing with the medication while introducing additional behavioral or other interventions might be more helpful to the client.

The most substantial effort to date to evaluate the effect of combined behavioral and psychopharmacological treatment has applied a model in which psychopharmacological intervention is conceptualized as directly reducing "irritability" as shown by behaviors such as tantrums, aggression, and SIB, whereas behaviorally oriented parent training impacts on these problems indirectly by improving compliance with carer requests and thereby improving adaptive functioning (Scahill et al., 2009). Aman et al. (2009) evaluated this model in a study in which 124 children with ASDs, aged between 4 and 13 years of age and with an ABC irritability subscale score of 18 or over, were randomized unequally to treatment with medication alone or medication plus parent training. Treatment with medication initially consisted of risperidone, which might be switched to aripiprazole if risperidone did not produce a positive response. Final group sizes were 49 for treatment with medication alone, 40 of whom completed the entire study, and 75 for combined treatment, 55 of whom completed. Parent training involved 11 core, 3 optional, and up to 3 "booster" sessions of 60–90 min, delivered individually to families by doctorally prepared or masters-level clinicians using a manualized program. Topics included use of positive reinforcement, teaching compliance, functional communication training, and teaching specific adaptive skills (Research Units on Pediatric Psychopharmacology Autism Network, 2007). Methods included direct instruction, use of video vignettes, practice activities, role-play, and behavior rehearsal with feedback. Optional sessions were chosen based on the child's specific needs and level of functioning. After 24 weeks of intervention, mean scores on a modified version of the Home Situations Questionnaire (Barkley, Edwards, & Robin, 1999) declined by 71% in the combined treatment group and 60% in the medication only group, showing a significantly greater rate of change in favor of combined treatment.

Future Directions

SIB remains a serious and relatively common problem for children and adults with ASDs. Relatively little is understood concerning its etiology and natural history. Although integrated bio-behavioral intervention has been advocated for many years (Mace & Mauk, 1995), further research on how to most effectively combine behavioral and psychopharmacological approaches is required. Improvement of methods for designing intervention based on the detailed phenomenology of the SIB presented, and salient comorbidity, appears likely to be a fruitful path for further clinical research.

References

Aman, M. G., Arnold, L. E., & Armstrong, S. C. (1999). Review of serotonergic agents and perseverative behavior in patients with developmental disabilities. *Mental Retardation and Developmental Disabilities Research Reviews, 5,* 279–289.

Aman, M. G., Arnold, L. E., McDougle, C. J., Vitiello, B., Scahill, L., Davies, M., et al. (2005). Acute and long-term safety and tolerability of risperidone in children with autism. *Journal of Child and Adolescent Psychopharmacology, 15,* 869–884.

Aman, M. G., & Madrid, A. (1999). Atypical antipsychotics in persons with developmental disabilities. *Mental Retardation and Developmental Disabilities Research Reviews, 5,* 253–263.

Aman, M. G., McDougle, C. J., Scahill, L., Handen, B., Arnold, L. E., Johnson, C., et al. (2009). Medication and parent training in children with pervasive developmental disorders and serious behavior problems: Results from a randomized clinical trial. *Journal of the American Academy of Child and Adolescent Psychiatry, 48,* 1143–1154.

Aman, M. G., & Singh, N. N. (1994). *Aberrant behavior checklist – Community: Supplementary manual.* East Aurora, NY: Slosson Educational Publications.

Anderson, G. M., Scahill, L., McCracken, J. T., McDougle, C. J., Aman, M. G., Tierney, E., et al. (2007). Effects of short- and long-term risperidone treatment on prolactin levels in children with autism. *Biological Psychiatry, 61,* 545–550.

Arnold, L. E., Vitiello, B., McDougle, C., Scahill, L., Shah, B., Gonzalez, N. M., et al. (2003). Parent-defined target symptoms respond to risperidone in RUPP autism study: Customer approach to clinical trials. *Journal of the American Academy of Child and Adolescent Psychiatry, 42,* 1443–1450.

Barkley, R. A., Edwards, G. H., & Robin, A. L. (1999). *Defiant teens: A clinician's manual for assessment and intervention.* New York: Guilford Press.

Benjamin, S., Seek, A., Tresise, L., Price, E., & Gagnon, M. (1995). Case study: Paradoxical response to naltrexone treatment of self-injurious behavior. *Journal of the American Academy of Child and Adolescent Psychiatry, 34,* 238–242.

Biswas, A. B., Bhaumik, S., & Branford, D. (2001). Treatment-emergent behavioural side effects with selective serotonin re-uptake inhibitors in adults with learning disabilities. *Human Psychopharmacology: Clinical and Experimental, 16,* 133–137.

Bodfish, J. W., McCuller, W. R., Madison, J. M., Register, M., Mailman, R. B., & Lewis, M. H. (1997). Placebo, double-blind evaluation of long-term naltrexone treatment effects for adults with mental retardation and self-injury. *Journal of Developmental and Physical Disabilities, 9,* 135–152.

Breese, G. R., Knapp, D. J., Criswell, H. E., Moy, S. S., Papadeas, S. T., & Blake, B. L. (2005). The neonate-6-hydroxydopamine-lesioned rat: A model for clinical neuroscience and neurobiological principles. *Brain Research Reviews, 48,* 57–73.

Cohen, S. A., Fitzgerald, B. J., Khan, S. R. F., & Khan, A. (2004). The effect of a switch to ziprasidone in an adult population with autistic disorder: Chart review of naturalistic, open-label treatment. *Journal of Clinical Psychiatry, 65,* 110–113.

Corson, A. H., Barkenbus, J. E., Posey, D. J., Stigler, K. A., & McDougle, C. J. (2004). A retrospective analysis of quetiapine in the treatment of pervasive developmental disorders. *Journal of Clinical Psychiatry, 65,* 1531–1536.

Crews, W. D., Jr., Bonaventura, S., Rowe, F. B., & Bonsie, D. (1993). Cessation of long-term naltrexone therapy and self-injury: A case study. *Research in Developmental Disabilities, 14,* 331–340.

Deb, S., & Unwin, G. L. (2007). Psychotropic medication for behaviour problems in people with intellectual disability: A review of the current literature. *Current Opinion in Psychiatry, 20,* 461–466.

Findling, R. L., McNamara, N. K., Gracious, B. L., O'Riordan, M. A., Reed, M. D., Demeter, C., et al. (2004). Quetiapine in nine youths with autistic disorder. *Journal of Child and Adolescent Psychopharmacology, 14,* 287–294.

Goodman, W. K., Price, L. H., Rasmussen, S. A., Mazure, C., Fleischmann, R. L., Hill, C. L., et al. (1989). The Yale-Brown obsessive compulsive scale. I. Development, use and reliability. *Archives of General Psychiatry, 46*, 1006–1011.

Hardan, A. Y., Jou, R. J., & Handen, B. L. (2005). Retrospective study of quetiapine in children and adolescents with pervasive developmental disorders. *Journal of Autism and Developmental Disorders, 35*, 387–391.

Harding, J., Wacker, D. P., Berg, W. K., Barretto, A., & Ringdahl, J. (2005). Evaluation of relations between specific antecedent stimuli and self-injury during functional analysis conditions. *American Journal on Mental Retardation, 110*, 205–215.

Henry, C. A., Shervin, D., Neumeyer, A., Steingard, R., Spybrook, J., Choueiri, R., et al. (2009). Retrial of selective serotonin reuptake inhibitors in children with pervasive developmental disorders: A retrospective chart review. *Journal of Child and Adolescent Psychopharmacology, 19*, 111–117.

Hollander, E., Wasserman, S., Swanson, E. N., Chaplin, W., Schapiro, M. L., Zagursky, K., et al. (2006). A double-blind placebo-controlled pilot study of olanzapine in childhood/adolescent pervasive developmental disorder. *Journal of Child and Adolescent Psychopharmacology, 16*, 541–548.

Iwata, B. A., Dorsey, M. F., Slifer, K. J., Bauman, K. E., & Richman, G. S. (1982). Toward a functional analysis of self-injury. *Analysis and Intervention in Developmental Disabilities, 2*, 3–20.

Kemner, C., Willemsen-Swinkels, S. H. N., De Jonge, M., Tuynman-Qua, H., & Van Engeland, H. (2002). Open-label study of olanzapine in children with pervasive developmental disorder. *Journal of Clinical Psychopharmacology, 22*, 455–460.

King, B. H. (1993). Self-injury by people with mental retardation: A compulsive behavior hypothesis. *American Journal on Mental Retardation, 98*, 93–112.

Luby, J., Mrakotsky, C., Stalets, M. M., Belden, A., Heffelfinger, A., Williams, M., et al. (2006). Risperidone in preschool children with autistic spectrum disorders: An investigation of safety and efficacy. *Journal of Child and Adolescent Psychopharmacology, 16*, 575–587.

Mace, F. C., & Mauk, J. E. (1995). Bio-behavioral diagnosis and treatment of self-injury. *Mental Retardation and Developmental Disabilities Research Reviews, 1*, 104–110.

Malone, R. P., Cater, J., Sheikh, R. M., Choudhury, M. S., & Delaney, M. A. (2001). Olanzapine versus haloperidol in children with autistic disorder: An open pilot study. *Journal of the American Academy of Child and Adolescent Psychiatry, 40*, 887–894.

Marcus, R. N., Owen, R., Kamen, L., Manos, G., McQuade, R. D., Carson, W. H., et al. (2009). A placebo-controlled, fixed-dose study of aripiprazole in children and adolescents with irritability associated with autistic disorder. *Journal of the American Academy of Child and Adolescent Psychiatry, 48*, 1110–1119.

Martin, A., Koenig, K., Scahill, L., & Bregman, J. (1999). Open-label quetiapine in the treatment of children and adolescents with autistic disorder. *Journal of Child and Adolescent Psychopharmacology, 9*, 99–107.

Masi, G. (2004). Pharmacotherapy of pervasive developmental disorders in children and adolescents. *CNS Drugs, 18*, 1031–1052.

Matson, J. L. (1995). *The diagnostic assessment for the severely handicapped-revised (DASH-II)*. Baton Rouge, LA: Scientific Publishers.

Matson, J. L., Bamburg, J. W., Mayville, E. A., Pinkston, J., Bielecki, J., Kuhn, D., et al. (2000). Psychopharmacology and mental retardation: A 10 year review (1990–1999). *Research in Developmental Disabilities, 21*, 263–296.

McDougle, C. J., Holmes, J. P., Carlson, D. C., Pelton, G. H., Cohen, D. J., & Price, L. H. (1998). A double-blind, placebo-controlled study of risperidone in adults with autistic disorder and other pervasive developmental disorders. *Archives of General Psychiatry, 55*, 633–641.

McDougle, C. J., Kem, D. L., & Posey, D. J. (2002). Case series: Use of ziprasidone for maladaptive symptoms in youths with autism. *Journal of the American Academy of Child and Adolescent Psychiatry, 41*, 921–927.

McDougle, C. J., Stigler, K. A., Erickson, C. A., & Posey, D. J. (2006). Pharmacology of autism. *Clinical Neuroscience Research, 6*, 179–188.

Nagaraj, R., Singhi, P., & Malhi, P. (2006). Risperidone in children with autism: Randomized, placebo-controlled, double-blind study. *Journal of Child Neurology, 21*, 450–455.

Napolitano, D. A., Jack, S. L., Sheldon, J. B., Williams, D. C., McAdam, D. B., & Schroeder, S. R. (1999). Drug-behavior interactions in persons with mental retardation and developmental disabilities. *Mental Retardation and Developmental Disabilities Research Reviews, 5*, 322–334.

National Institute of Mental Health. (1985). Special feature: Rating scales and assessment instruments for use in pediatric psychopharmacology research. *Psychopharmacological Bulletin, 21*, 839–843.

Owen, R., Sikich, L., Marcus, R. N., Corey-Lisle, P., Manos, G., McQuade, R. D., et al. (2009). Aripiprazole in the treatment of irritability in children and adolescents with autistic disorder. *Pediatrics, 124*, 1533–1540.

Posey, D. J., Erickson, C. A., Stigler, K. A., & McDougle, C. J. (2006). The use of selective serotonin reuptake inhibitors in autism and related disorders. *Journal of Child and Adolescent Psychopharmacology, 16*, 181–186.

Posey, D. J., Stigler, K. A., Erickson, C. A., & McDougle, C. J. (2008). Antipsychotics in the treatment of autism. *Journal of Clinical Investigation, 118*, 6–14.

Potenza, M. N., Holmes, J. P., Kanes, S. J., & McDougle, C. J. (1999). Olanzapine treatment of children, adolescents, and adults with pervasive developmental disorders: An open-label pilot study. *Journal of Clinical Psychopharmacology, 19*, 37–44.

Research Units on Pediatric Psychopharmacology Autism Network. (2005). Risperidone treatment of autistic disorder: Longer-term benefits and blinded discontinuation after 6 months. *American Journal of Psychiatry, 162*, 1361–1369.

Research Units on Pediatric Psychopharmacology Autism Network. (2007). Parent training for children with pervasive developmental disorders: A multi-site feasibility trial. *Behavioral Interventions, 22*, 179–199.

Ruedrich, S. L., Swales, T. P., Rossvanes, C., Diana, L., Arkadiev, V., & Lim, K. (2008). Atypical antipsychotic medication improves aggression, but not self-injurious behaviour, in adults with intellectual disabilities. *Journal of Intellectual Disability Research, 52*, 132–140.

Sandman, C. A., Hetrick, W., Taylor, D. V., Marion, S. D., Touchette, P., Barron, J. L., et al. (2000). Long-term effects of naltrexone on self-injurious behavior. *American Journal on Mental Retardation, 105*, 103–117.

Sandman, C. A., & Touchette, P. (2002). Opioids and the maintenance of self-injurious behavior. In S. R. Schroeder, M. L. Oster-Granite, & T. Thompson (Eds.), *Self-injurious behavior: Gene-brain-behavior relationships* (pp. 191–204). Washington, DC: American Psychological Association.

Sandman, C. A., Touchette, P., Lenjavi, M., Marion, S., & Chicz-DeMet, A. (2003). β-Endorphin and ACTH are dissociated after self-injury in adults with developmental disabilities. *American Journal on Mental Retardation, 108*, 414–424.

Sandman, C. A., Touchette, P., Marion, S., Lenjavi, M., & Chicz-Demet, A. (2002). Disregulation of proopiomelanocortin and contagious maladaptive behavior. *Regulatory Peptides, 108*, 179–185.

Scahill, L., Aman, M. G., McDougle, C. J., Arnold, L. E., McCracken, J. T., Handen, B., et al. (2009). Trial design challenges when combining medication and parent training in children with pervasive developmental disorders. *Journal of Autism and Developmental Disorders, 39*, 720–729.

Scahill, L., McCracken, J. T., McGough, J., Shah, B., Cronin, P., Hong, D., et al. (2002). Risperidone in children with autism and serious behavioral problems. *New England Journal of Medicine, 347*, 314–321.

Schretlen, D. J., Ward, J., Meyer, S. M., Yun, J., Puig, J. G., Nyhan, W. L., et al. (2005). Behavioral aspects of Lesch-Nyhan disease and its variants. *Developmental Medicine and Child Neurology, 47*, 673–677.

Shea, S., Turgay, A., Carroll, A., Schulz, M., Orlik, H., Smith, I., et al. (2004). Risperidone in the treatment of disruptive behavioral symptoms in children with autistic and other pervasive developmental disorders. *Pediatrics, 114*, e634–e641.

Stachnik, J. M., & Nunn-Thompson, C. (2007). Use of atypical antipsychotics in the treatment of autistic disorder. *Annals of Pharmacotherapy, 41*, 626–634.

Stigler, K. A., Diener, J. T., Kohn, A. E., Li, L., Erickson, C. A., Posey, D. J., et al. (2009). Aripiprazole in pervasive developmental disorder not otherwise specified and Asperger's disorder: A 14-week, prospective, open-label study. *Journal of Child and Adolescent Psychopharmacology, 19*, 265–274.

Symons, F. J., Tapp, J., Wulfsberg, A., Sutton, K. A., Heeth, W. L., & Bodfish, J. W. (2001). Sequential analysis of the effects of naltrexone on the environmental mediation of self-injurious behavior. *Experimental and Clinical Psychopharmacology, 9*, 269–276.

Symons, F. J., Thompson, A., & Rodriguez, M. C. (2004). Self-injurious behavior and the efficacy of naltrexone treatment: A quantitative synthesis. *Mental Retardation and Developmental Disabilities Research Reviews, 10*, 193–200.

Tassé, M. J., Aman, M. G., Hammer, D., & Rojahn, J. (1996). The Nisonger child behavior rating form: Age and gender effects and norms. *Research in Developmental Disabilities, 17*, 59–75.

Troost, P. W., Lahuis, B. E., Steenhuis, M., Ketelaars, C. E. J., Buitelaar, J. K., Van Engeland, H., et al. (2005). Long-term effects of risperidone in children with autism spectrum disorders: A placebo discontinuation study. *Journal of the American Academy of Child and Adolescent Psychiatry, 44*, 1137–1144.

Turgay, A., Binder, C., Snyder, R., & Fisman, S. (2002). Long-term safety and efficacy of risperidone for the treatment of disruptive behavior disorders in children with subaverage IQs. *Pediatrics, 110*, e34.

Weeden, M., Ehrhardt, K., & Poling, A. (2009). Conspicuous by their absence: Studies comparing and combining risperidone and applied behavior analysis to reduce challenging behavior in children with autism. *Research in Autism Spectrum Disorders, 3*, 905–912.

Zarcone, J. R., Lindauer, S. E., Morse, P. S., Crosland, K. A., Valdovinos, M. G., McKerchar, T. L., et al. (2004). Effects of risperidone on destructive behavior of persons with developmental disabilities: III. Functional analysis. *American Journal on Mental Retardation, 109*, 310–321.

Autism Spectrum Disorders: Comorbid Psychopathology and Treatment

29

Sarah Mohiuddin, Sara Bobak, Daniel Gih,
and Mohammad Ghaziuddin

Autism spectrum disorders (ASD), labeled as pervasive developmental disorders (PDD) in the DSM-IV-TR (APA, 2000), are characterized by a distinct pattern of social and communication deficits with rigid ritualistic interests. While autism (Kanner, 1943) is the main category, other conditions include Asperger syndrome (Asperger, 1944) and pervasive developmental disorder not otherwise specified (PDDNOS). Rett disorder and childhood disintegrative disorder, although classified in the same category, are often not referred to as ASDs. As discussed elsewhere in this volume, the DSM-V is likely to collapse autism, Asperger syndrome, and PDDNOS into a single category called ASD. Although autism is almost always a lifelong disorder, its core symptoms change in severity over time. Thus, a child's language may continue to evolve as he grows older and his idiosyncratic interests may change their focus. Simultaneously, additional medical and psychiatric disorders may emerge. For example, about 30% of individuals with autism suffer from seizures, which usually emerge during the pre-school years or at the time of puberty. Although several studies have explored its medical comorbidity, relatively little has been published on its mental health aspects. This topic is important because symptoms such as hyperactivity, anxiety, and depression not only affect its presentation but also modify its treatment and its long-term outcome. In this chapter, we provide a selective review of the presentation and treatment of common psychiatric disorders that occur in persons with ASD across their life span.

What Are Psychiatric Disorders?

First, it is important to clarify the meaning of the term psychiatric disorder. In general, any sustained disturbance of behavior that results in significant degree of functional impairment of the individual and causes distress to his family or to the community at large is called a psychiatric disorder. Thus, the concept of impairment is central to any definition of a psychiatric disorder. A related issue is the definition of normality, which depends as much on the cultural context as on the quality of behavior. Another issue is whether psychiatric conditions are best conceptualized as categories or dimensions. For example, does depression constitute a distinct disorder or does it form part of a continuum? Although there are strong reasons to support a dimensional approach to mental disorders, for practical aspects, such as deciding whom to treat and whom not to treat, and for the purpose of third-party payment of treatment, the categorical system is more appropriate than the dimensional system.

There are two main categorical systems of psychiatric classification: The American Diagnostic and Statistical Manual system (DSM) and the International Classification of Diseases (ICD) system. While a detailed discussion of the merits of each is beyond the scope of this chapter, two points are worth emphasizing. First, both the ICD and the DSM follow a multi-axial approach to classification. For example in the DSM system, the first axis relates to the description of the clinical diagnosis; the second discusses the underlying personality disorder or intellectual disability ([ID] mental retardation) (if any); the third lists the presence of any relevant medical disorder; the fourth deals with the coding of psychosocial stressors and life events; and the fifth assigns a score to the child's level of functioning in the previous year. For example, a depressed adolescent with autism who has ID and seizure disorder will be classified as follows: axis I: autistic disorder and depression; axis II: mental retardation (mild, moderate, severe, or profound); axis III: seizure disorder. The fourth axis would record the presence

S. Mohiuddin (✉)
Department of Psychiatry, The University of Michigan, Ann Arbor, MI 48109, USA
e-mail: smohiudd@umich.edu

J.L. Matson, P. Sturmey (eds.), *International Handbook of Autism and Pervasive Developmental Disorders*, Autism and Child Psychopathology Series, DOI 10.1007/978-1-4419-8065-6_29, © Springer Science+Business Media, LLC 2011

of any psychosocial stressors (such as bereavement, parental divorce, and change of schools) and the fifth would document the patient's level of functioning in the previous year as defined by the Clinical Global Impressions (CGI) scale from 0 to 100. (Note that in DSM-V intellectual disability will replace the term "mental retardation.")

Second, both the ICD and the DSM take a phenomenological approach to diagnosis based on a detailed description of the clinical signs and symptoms and not on the putative cause. This is because the cause of autism is not known or unclear in the majority of cases and because the clinical features of a psychiatric disorder are often independent of the underlying cause. For example, an episode of depression can be precipitated by the loss of a loved object or by moving to a different city; yet, the clinical features are almost identical. Another point in favor of a phenomenological approach is that there is no psychiatric disorder that can be diagnosed solely on the basis of a biological test. A rigorous, detailed, and systematic psychiatric examination, therefore, remains the gold standard in arriving at a psychiatric diagnosis.

What Is Comorbidity?

Although there are several ways of defining the concept of comorbidity, comorbidity is here defined as the simultaneous occurrence of two or more disorders. Several factors might be responsible for this phenomenon. First, the disorders might be related to the same underlying cause. Thus, condition A causes condition B. Second, the disorders may arise from the same underlying factors. For example, a patient with diabetes may develop eye symptoms and kidney complications. Third, the conditions might occur by coincidence. Fourth, referral bias may contribute to comorbidity. For example, the more severely ill a patient is, the more likely he is to have co-occurring conditions and complications. Finally, a combination of factors might be at work.

Psychiatric Comorbidity of ASD

Medical and psychiatric comorbidity is the rule in persons with ASD. As discussed elsewhere in this book, at least 10% of individuals with ASD have known medical conditions such as fragile X syndrome and tuberous sclerosis. Clinic-based studies suggest that at least 70% of individuals with ASD also have additional psychiatric disorders. A recent community-based study of ASD in the UK found that 71% of the sample could be diagnosed with a psychiatric disorder (Simonoff et al., 2008).

Several reasons account for the high rates of psychiatric comorbidity in persons with ASD. First is the presence of ID. Since a substantial number of patients with ASD have ID, they are more likely to have co-occurring mental disorders. In addition, there is preliminary data suggesting that higher functioning individuals with ASD may be more vulnerable to certain types of psychiatric disorders, such as depression, than those who are lower functioning, because insight and intellectual awareness may increase the risk of psychopathology. Second is the presence of medical disorders. Chronic medical conditions, such as epilepsy, which is found in about 30% of persons with ASD, increase the risk of psychiatric disorders. Third, persons with ASD may be vulnerable to unique life stressors and unpleasant events that place them at an increased risk of psychopathology including history of abandonment in childhood and exposure to abuse and neglect. Fourth, genetic factors may also play a role in increasing the risk of psychiatric disorders in this population. For example, patients with ASD who also have fragile X syndrome are more prone to anxiety disorders. Finally, a combination of factors may be responsible.

General Principles of Treatment of Psychiatric Comorbidity in ASD

The goal of the treatment of psychiatric comorbidity in the setting of ASD is not to cure the symptoms of autism, but to improve the quality of life of the individual and decrease the burden of care of the family and caregivers (Ghaziuddin, 2005). When problem behaviors are recognized as manifestations of a comorbid psychiatric disorder, rather than as part of ASD, perception of the individual and his problems is altered which itself is often therapeutic to the family and other caregivers. In addition, standard autism treatments work more efficiently and result in improved functioning, when comorbid disorders are treated in a timely and systematic manner (Simonoff et al., 2008).

The complexity of psychiatric disorders in individuals with ASD calls for a multidisciplinary and coordinated approach to treatment from different perspectives. There is no single medication or psychotherapeutic intervention that works in all cases. As a rule, multiple approaches are used which combine both medical and psychosocial strategies. This position is in line with the standard of practice in general psychiatry, as well as with the standard of care of individuals with ID (Benson & Havercamp, 2007; Dosen, 2007; Pratt, Gill, Barrett, & Roberts, 2007). According to this approach, the aim is to treat the whole person, i.e., the treatment is not only directed at the symptoms of the disorder but also at restoring the person's mental well-being and improving their global quality of life. Thus, psychiatric service is only one component of the wider range of provisions required. Clinical experience suggests that individualized treatments of persons with autism are associated with greater improvement in functioning than general interventions (Leyfer et al., 2006). It is important to make environmental adjustments, such as incorporating structure and predictability, and psychosocial and educational interventions on a case-by-case basis.

Adapting Treatment Methods from General Psychiatry

There is emerging evidence that individuals with psychiatric disorders benefit from specific treatments related to their specific disorder (Lehman & Steinwachs, 1998; Pratt et al., 2007); the same applies to individuals with ASD. Although systematic treatment studies for persons with ASD are only now beginning to be published, promising steps have already been taken to adapt treatment methods from general psychiatry to persons with ASD, with or without ID.

Thus, for individuals with ASD, therapy used is often direct and supportive in nature. Insight-oriented and psychodynamic psychotherapy aimed at uncovering inner conflicts is generally not useful, especially in the presence of disturbed behavior resulting from abnormal ideas or beliefs (Ghaziuddin, 2005). Behavior analytic and cognitive behavioral treatment approaches, adapted to the individuals' level of functioning, are most frequently used combined with traditional social work, consisting of helping the individual with problems of everyday living.

Among adults with ASD, approximately three out of four are treated with psychotropic medications (Myers, 2007), although there is no evidence that psychotropic medications can treat the core features of autism (Stachnik & Nunn-Thompson, 2007). The probability of being placed on psychotropic medications increases with poorer social skills, increased level of challenging behavior, living independently of parents, and advancing age; however, specific medications for specific psychiatric disorders should be used. Thus, medications should be ideally used not for management of non-specific behaviors, such as aggression or self-injury, but for the treatment of clearly identified symptom clusters, as in anxiety disorders, obsessive–compulsive disorder (OCD), psychotic disorders, and depression (Ghaziuddin, 2005; Tsai, 2006).

Specialized Mental Health Services

Despite increasing awareness of the psychiatric needs of persons with ASD, only a few specialized centers exist for treating their mental health problems (Royal College of Psychiatrists, 2006). Although individuals with ASD represent a small subgroup within the psychiatric hospital populations, their clinical needs may not be met (Lunsky, Gracey, & Bradley, 2009) because treatment facilities and therapy methods are often not adapted to their special needs. Persons with ASD may find the usual psychiatric clinical environment distressing and unhelpful lack of structure and specialized nursing help (Royal College of Psychiatrists, 2006) underscoring the need for improved professional training, better liaison between specialists, and systematic development of specialist services (Royal College of Psychiatrists, 2006). Professionals involved in the diagnosis and treatment of psychiatric disorders in people with ASD should have expertise both in ASD and in general psychiatry. When ASD appears in combination with ID, more specialized services are required. The current trend of providing community care to individuals with disabilities with mental health problems highlights the need to develop novel treatment approaches (Martin et al., 2005) and sophisticated models for training carestaff in the sectors of supportive living and adult residential care (Costello, Bouras, & Davies, 2007; McDonnell et al., 2008).

Common Psychiatric Disorders

Attention Deficit Hyperactivity Disorder

Attention deficit hyperactivity disorder (ADHD) is the most common psychiatric disorder of childhood, occurring in about 5–7% of children in the United States. Problems of hyperactivity, impulsivity, and distractibility are often present in children with ASD; however, few studies have focused on the occurrence of ADHD in ASD because DSM IV does not allow for the simultaneous diagnosis of ADHD and ASD because of the mistaken belief that ADHD-like symptoms are an integral part of ASD; and most studies of ADHD often exclude patients with ASD and ID.

Prevalence

Despite the above limitations, some studies have examined the association between ADHD and ASD. Clinical samples of children with ADHD have suggested that at least 10% of children referred to specialty clinics have from comorbid ASD. Conversely, in children with ASD, ADHD constitutes the most common psychiatric disorder. Preliminary reports have suggested that at least 60–70% of people with ASD referred to clinics may be diagnosed with ADHD. This figure is probably higher in low-functioning individuals, although exact figures are not available.

Clinical Features

The symptoms of ADHD in the setting of ASD depend on the general level of functioning, level of verbal skills, and presence of other medical and psychiatric conditions. Before the age of 5, severe hyperactivity and distractibility can co-exist with symptoms of social and communication impairment. In some children, ADHD-like symptoms may be the presenting features of ASD. Extreme hyperactivity is more likely to occur in those who are also cognitively impaired and in those who have seizures and language deficits. Between 7 and 13 years of age, ADHD-like symptoms are particularly disabling and are often the cause of academic and social failures. Children with Asperger syndrome and PDDNOS often show these symptoms at this age. As the child grows older and steps into puberty, ADHD symptoms may be complicated by depression, anxiety disorders, and increasing academic difficulties. Most patients with ASD and ADHD, however, do not show marked hyperactivity as they reach late adolescence and early adulthood. In fact, some patients in this category may become markedly slowed down in their movements.

Long-term studies of the comorbidity of ADHD with ASD have not been performed. Although ADHD is a childhood onset disorder, like ASD, its symptoms often persist into adulthood; however, these symptoms often change in form and severity. Persons with ASD who are hyperactive as children may grow into adults with normal or reduced levels of activity. Impulsivity and inattention may persist, however. The outcome also depends on the level of functioning and the presence of additional medical or psychological conditions.

Neurobiology

Because of methodological difficulties, studies have not examined the nature of the neurobiological deficit in those patients who have both ASD and ADHD. Studies conducted in the non-ASD population have implicated such areas of the brain as the corpus striatum and the prefrontal cortex. For example, children with ADHD show reduced activation of the corpus striatum during a "go-no-go" task compared with typical control children. A reduction in the size of the corpus callosum has also been reported in children and adolescents with pure ADHD. Some studies have found a reduction in the size of the right and the left caudate nucleus. Also, both children and adults with ADHD may show reduced prefrontal volumes.

Diagnosis

Although, according to the DSM-IV-TR, a diagnosis of ADHD should not be given to individuals with ASD (APA, 2000), in clinical practice the two diagnoses are often given together, especially in those individuals with ASD who have average intelligence. Recognizing the comorbidity of ASD and ADHD has clinical and research implications. Children with ASD who suffer from comorbid ADHD may fare worse than those who do not have these symptoms and require a different set of interventions, such as medications. Thus, when symptoms of ADHD result in a substantial degree of impairment to the child and problems for the family and community at large, an additional diagnosis of ADHD must be given. A screening instrument, such as the *Social and Communication Questionnaire* (SCQ; Rutter, Bailey, Berument, Lord, & Pickles, 2003), can help differentiate between the broad categories of autism and ADHD; however, a reliable diagnosis can only be made by a combination of rating scales, structured interviews, and clinical observation.

Psychopharmacologic Treatment of ADHD Symptoms

The treatment of ADHD in autism spectrum disorders consists of the combination of medications with behavioral and other forms of psychosocial interventions. The following section deals with the psychopharmacologic treatment of ADHD in the setting of ASD; psychosocial interventions are covered elsewhere in this volume.

As discussed above, a significant number of children and adolescents with ASD show inattention, distractibility, and hyperactivity, consistent with a diagnosis of ADHD. However, in some cases, because of accompanying severe intellectual disability, a diagnosis of ADHD is difficult to make. In such cases, categories such as impulse control disorder not otherwise are used. Medications for this purpose fall into one or more of the following categories: stimulants; alpha 2 agonists; atypical antipsychotic agents; and a miscellaneous group consisting of desyrel, strattera, etc. Thus far, placebo-controlled trials for methylphenidate, atomoxetine, and alpha 2 agonists have shown improvement in ASD symptoms (see below). All placebo-controlled trials reported to date have involved immediate release of methylphenidate; there are no data on sustained release of methylphenidate preparations. No placebo-controlled studies have been reported with dexamphetamine. Data from case series of patients treated with dexamphetamine have generally been equivocal, some even reporting a worsening of symptoms, though this should be systematically studied to further assess its utility in this population.

Methylphenidate

Handen, Johnson, and Lubetsky (2000) conducted a three-group placebo-controlled crossover trial of 13 pre-pubertal patients involving placebo and two different doses (0.3 and 0.6 mg/kg) of methylphenidate for 7 days. Sixty-two percent of patients were deemed responders based on a 50% reduction in the Hyperactivity Index scores on the Connors Teachers scale. Adverse event data were not systematically collected though both treatment groups reported poor appetite and irritability.

In 2005, the Research Units on Pediatric Psychopharmacology Autistic Disorder Network conducted the largest trial thus far with methylphenidate, including 72 patients from multiple sites. The trial included three different phases over a period of 13 weeks. Children were initially given a 1-week test dose to assess tolerability and were then randomized to a 4-week crossover trial with methylphenidate doses of 0.125 mg, 0.250 mg, or 0.500 mg/kg per dose, administered three times a day. Thirty-five (49%) of the 72 children enrolled in the study responded best to one of the three active doses of methylphenidate using the Clinical Global Impressions (CGI) (Guy, 1976) and the Aberrant Behavior Checklist (ABC) hyperactive subscale (Aman, Singh, Stewart, & Field, 1985) to measure response. Parent ratings indicated the greatest benefit of methylphenidate compared with placebo at 0.250 mg/kg per dose while teacher ratings indicated the greatest benefit at 0.500 mg/kg per dose.

Atomoxetine

There has been one randomized placebo-controlled crossover trial of atomoxetine in children with ASD (Arnold et al., 2006). This 6-week trial included 16 children with ASD, though the majority completed 3 weeks of each test condition. Atomoxetine was superior to placebo on the hyperactivity subscale of the ABC, which was used as the primary outcome measure; however, it had no statistically significant effect on nine DSM-IV ADHD inattentive symptoms.

Alpha-2 Adrenergic Agonists

There have been two placebo-controlled trials conducted on clonidine, though only one showed improvement in hyperactivity in people with ASD. Jaselskis, Cook, Fletcher, and Leventhal (1992) studied eight children with significant hyperactivity. They randomized them to 7 weeks of either placebo or oral clonidine. They found that both the parent ratings on the Conners Abbreviated Parent–Teacher Questionnaire and teacher ratings on the ABC hyperactivity scale favored clonidine over placebo; however, clonidine was associated with a significant increase in drowsiness compared to placebo. This contrasts with a negative finding of placebo crossover study of transdermal clonidine by Fankhauser et al. (1992); however, this study was also based on a small sample ($N = 9$), including a broad age range (5–33 years), and did not differentiate participation based on the degree of hyperactivity.

Impulse Control Disorders Including Aggression

Based on the DSM-IV-TR, an impulse control disorder (ICD) is a condition that occurs when an individual does not or cannot resist an impulse. If left untreated, it may result in a significant degree of distress to either the individual or others. Implicit in the definition is the premise that the individual has little or no control over his behavior, which is often not premeditated. While anyone can indulge in an impulsive act, such as stealing, the diagnostic label is often reserved for those who have other psychiatric disorders or medical disabilities, which can range from schizophrenia and autism to traumatic brain injury and ID. Thus, an important purpose of the assessment is to determine if there is a mitigating factor to explain the impulsive behavior.

Persons with ASD are diagnosed with impulse control disorders when the behavioral episodes cause a significant amount of distress to themselves to others. Examples include repeated aggressive acts against others (hitting, kicking, spitting, pushing, etc.), sexually inappropriate behaviors (exhibitionism, public masturbation, groping, etc.), and repeated use of profanities, indulging in arson. When severe physical aggression is the cardinal problem, the term intermittent explosive disorder is used. Assessment should include a careful search for psychiatric causes, such as depression or psychosis, or for any medical factors, such as brain injury and ID. The treatment is based on a comprehensive behavioral analysis; psychotropic medications are often used. If the behavior is dangerous to others and is not better accounted for by any mental or physical factors, referral to forensic services may be necessary. Treatment and outcome are often not satisfactory. The following section deals with the pharmacologic treatment of aggression in the setting of an impulse control disorder. It should also be underscored that medications must always be combined with appropriate behavioral and psychological interventions.

Pharmacologic Treatment of Aggression in ASD

Aggression and self-injury often occur in persons with ASD and can result from a variety of causes. The treatment of aggression is multimodal consisting of behavioral and pharmacological interventions. At least 21 trials with 12 medications have been studied. Out of these, six medications (tianeptine, methylphenidate, risperidone, clonidine, aripiprazole, and naltrexone) produced significant improvement as compared to placebo. Only three (risperidone, aripiprazole, and methylphenidate) have shown results that have been replicated in at least two studies. These medications are discussed in detail below.

Risperidone

Three RCTs utilized a standardized outcome measure of aggression to examine the efficacy of risperidone, a combined dopamine and serotonin antagonist, in children with autism. In 2002, the Research Units on Pediatric Psychopharmacology Autism Network first published results from a double-blind, placebo-controlled, parallel-group trial in 101, 5- to 17-year-old children with autism over 8 weeks

(McCracken et al., 2002). Risperidone was administered at a mean dose of 1.8 mg/day for 8 weeks. ABC-I, which measures irritability symptoms associated with autistic disorder, such as aggression toward others, deliberate self-injuriousness, temper tantrums, and quickly changing moods, was the dependent variable. Risperidone demonstrated significantly greater reductions in the mean irritability subscore of the ABC-I compared to placebo (56.9% vs. 14.1%).

Troost et al. (2005) conducted the second RCT that used a standardized measure of aggression to examine the efficacy of risperidone in children and adolescents with ASD. After an initial 24-week open-label phase, 24 responders were identified for entry into an 8-week double-blind, placebo-controlled, parallel-group discontinuation phase. For subjects who remained on risperidone, the mean dose was 1.81 mg/day. At study end point, significantly more subjects relapsed in the placebo group (67%) compared to those who continued to receive risperidone (25%). Over the duration of the discontinuation phase, 60% of subjects who received placebo also showed an increase in ABC-I subscore (60%) compared to 14% of those receiving risperidone.

The third RCT of risperidone was conducted in 80 children and adolescents with pervasive developmental disorders by Shea et al. (2004) using a double-blind, placebo-controlled, parallel-group design over 8 weeks. Subjects ranged in age from 5 to 12 years (mean 7.5 years). Risperidone was administered at a mean dose of 1.17 mg/day. Over the duration of the study period, subjects receiving risperidone had approximately twice the mean decrease in ABC-I subscore as compared to placebo.

Aripiprazole
The approval for the use of this drug in aggression was based on data from two, 8-week, randomized, placebo-controlled multicenter studies that evaluated the efficacy of oral aripiprazole for improving mean scores on the caregiver-rated ABC-I subscale. For the first study, aripiprazole was initiated at a dose of 2 mg/day and titrated weekly for the first 6 weeks to a mean of 8.6 mg/day, with most patients receiving either 5 or 10 mg/day. Aripiprazole was significantly more effective than placebo for improving mean scores on the ABC-I subscale ($p < 0.001$). Adjusted mean scores on the Clinical Global Impression Improvement scale, a secondary outcome measure, were likewise significantly improved ($p < 0.001$). The second study was a fixed dose trial in which patients were randomly assigned to receive 5, 10, or 15 mg/day of aripiprazole or placebo; active treatment was initiated at a dose of 2 mg/day and titrated by 5 mg weekly until the assigned dose was achieved. All aripiprazole doses were more effective than placebo for improving mean ABC-I subscale scores (5 mg, $p < 0.05$; 10 mg, $p < 0.01$; 15 mg, $p = 0.001$). Differences between dose groups were not evaluated.

Methylphenidate
Two RCTs have utilized a primary outcome measure of aggression to examine the efficacy and tolerability of methylphenidate, a dopaminergic agonist, in children and adolescents with autism. Quintana et al. (1995) conducted the first study in ten subjects 7–11 years of age with autism over 4 weeks using a double-blind, placebo-controlled, crossover design. Methylphenidate was administered in divided doses equaling 20 and 40 mg/day. The two primary outcomes were the ABC-I subscale and self-injurious behavior (SIB) and were completed independently by two psychiatrists during 3-h observation sessions that included a simulated structured classroom situation with classroom tasks and free play. From a mean baseline subscore, methylphenidate produced significant improvements in ABC-I mean endpoint subscore compared to placebo mean endpoint score. Tolerability was assessed using a side-effects checklist and no significant differences were found in the rates of side effects between methylphenidate and placebo.

Handen et al. (2000) conducted the second RCT of methylphenidate in 13 children from 5 to 11 years of age diagnosed with autism or PDDNOS over 7 days using a double-blind, placebo-controlled, crossover design. Methylphenidate was administered in low (0.3 mg/kg per dose) and high (0.6 mg/kg per dose) doses two to three times daily. Primary outcome measures of aggression were the ABC-I subscale and the aggression subscale of the IOWA Conners' Teacher Rating Scale. Subjects who received methylphenidate showed significant improvement on both outcome measures compared to those receiving placebo. A side-effects checklist was used to assess tolerability. A relatively high number of subjects (9 of 12) experienced some side effects while on placebo. Five children experienced severe side effects while receiving methylphenidate, including social withdrawal, dullness, sadness, irritability, and skin picking. These side effects caused three subjects to be discontinued from the study.

Ineffective Medications
Negative placebo-controlled studies have been reported for haloperidol, clomipramine, valproate, lamotragine, levecitram, secretin, and omega 3-fatty acids in the treatment of aggression in persons with ASD. Of the five published placebo-controlled trials of secretin, an endogenous gastrointestinal polypeptide, none improved aggression, with one study reporting significant negative side effects of secretin. Clomipramine also failed to demonstrate significant improvement in aggression and SIB, but this trial represents the only attempt to systematically study a serotonin reuptake inhibitor for aggression in autism. This is despite evidence from several open-label and placebo-controlled studies of selective serotonin reuptake inhibitors (SSRIs) in treating associated symptoms of autism, such as repetitive

behavior (Couturier & Nicolson, 2002; Fatemi, Realmuto, Khan, & Thuras, 1998; Namerow, Thomas, Bostic, Prince, & Monuteaux, 2003; Owley et al., 2005).

Depression

Depression occurs in about 15% of the general population. It is the most common psychiatric disorder whose prevalence increases after puberty. As opposed to transient states of depressed mood, depression is a distinct medical condition characterized by a combination of psychological and physical symptoms. These consist of persistent depressed mood, loss of interest in pleasurable activities, a tendency to focus on negative aspects of life, excessive preoccupation with sad themes, thoughts of recurrent self-harm, and death and suicidal behavior. Other features include problems with attention and concentration, distractibility, impairment of short-term memory, self-blame, and ruminations of guilt. Depressed patients tend to isolate themselves and have difficulties with relationships and employment.

Prevalence

Persons with ASD are prone to depressive episodes, especially after puberty. Clinic-based studies suggest that depression is the most common psychiatric disorder in persons with ASD during their life span. A recent study gave a lifetime rate of 53% for mood disorders in consecutively recruited adults with average IQ ASD referred to two centers specializing in the assessment of childhood-onset neuropsychiatric disorders (Hofvander et al., 2009). Compared to community-matched children, those with IQ's greater than 70, autism or Asperger's syndrome (AS) may have higher rates of anxiety and mood conditions, which often occur together (Kim, Szatmari, Bryson, Streiner, & Wilson, 2000). Previous estimates of comorbid depression in ASD ranged from 4 to 38% (Lainhart, 1999). When DSM-IV criteria for major depressive disorder were utilized, Leyfer and colleagues found a rate of approximately 10% in autistic children using a modified *Kiddie Schedule for Affective Disorders and Schizophrenia* (Leyfer et al., 2006). The rate of depression was approximately 20% in a cross-sectional study of adolescents and young adults with Asperger's syndrome (Shtayermman, 2007). Thus, most reports are derived from small, clinical samples that are often seen in tertiary care centers. Large-scale epidemiologic studies on representative samples have not been done.

Etiology of Depression in ASD

Several factors may contribute to the occurrence of depression in ASD. Excessive negative life events may precede depression similar to that seen in the general population (Ghaziuddin, Alessi, & Greden, 1995). Two types of stressors seem to contribute to the emergence of depressive symptoms: Exposure to general life events, that is, events that are common to all and that are known to be associated with depression such as bereavement and parental divorce, and exposure to specific life events, that is, life events which are unique to people with ASD such as change of schools, problems with dating, and socializing. Associated medical conditions, such as seizure disorder, increase the risk of all forms of psychopathology in persons with ASD, including depression. Genetic factors may also account for the occurrence of depression in persons with ASD. For example, depressed children with ASD are more likely to have parents with depression.

Phenomenology of Depression in ASD

The presentation of depression in persons with ASD depends mainly on the level of functioning. In those who are lower functioning, the main features consist of a change in behavior, such as regression of skills, weight loss, and mutism. In those who are higher functioning, that is, in those who have relatively good language, the clinical features are the same as those in depressed persons in the general population. Anhedonia is often present. For example, Stewart, Barnard, Pearson, Hasan, and O'Brien (2006) reviewed the presentation of depression in ASD and found that loss of interest was mentioned as a prominent feature in 7 of the 13 reports. In addition, affected ASD persons may show certain special features. These often consist of an increase in social withdrawal beyond what is typical for that particular individual, a change in the tone and flavor of autistic preoccupations, and a decrease in physical movements sometimes leading to catatonia (see below).

Bipolar Disorder

Bipolar disorder is characterized by cycles of disturbance of mood and behavior. Typically, the patient shows episodes of elation or excessively happy mood alternating with periods of persistent sadness or depression. The duration of the episodes varies; they often range from 1–2 weeks to a few days or less. Elation may be replaced by irritability or aggression. A host of biological features are often present depending on the mood state. Thus, during periods of elation, the patient often has a decreased need for sleep; may appear more focused on goal-oriented activities, etc. Depressed patients, on the other hand, may suffer from insomnia, have impaired appetite, and lose weight. If untreated, patients going through the elated phase may lapse into hypomania or mania. Judgment may be impaired leading to deviant or reckless behavior of various kinds. Suicidal behavior may also occur.

While depression is the most common mood disorder occurring in persons with ASD, those with high-functioning autism and Asperger syndrome may be at a higher risk for bipolar disorder. In a two-site community study designed to evaluate the validity of the *Autism Comorbidity Interview-Present and Lifetime Version*, 2% of children with autism, diagnosed by *Autism Diagnostic Interview-Revised* (ADI-R), *Autism Diagnostic Observation Schedule* (ADOS), and DSM-IV-TR (APA, 2000), met criteria for bipolar I disorder (Leyfer et al., 2006). Similarly in another study, 8% of adults with average intelligence and ASD also had bipolar disorder (Hofvander et al., 2009). A recent report (Munesue et al., 2008) suggested that bipolar disorder was more common than depression in high-functioning ASD. Whether average intelligence is a risk factor for bipolar disorder or allows for better detection is unknown.

As with depression, the diagnosis of bipolar disorder can be difficult and pediatric bipolar disorder is a controversial category (Leibenluft & Rich, 2008). A patient with rigid interests may be excitable and appear grandiose which may be interpreted as a manic state. Cyclical patterns or distinct changes in activity, behavior, and interests should trigger the consideration of a bipolar diagnosis (Frazier, Doyle, Chiu, & Coyle, 2002). When evaluating for the presence of bipolar disorder, new behavioral problems must be evaluated in the context of sensory disturbances and environmental changes that can also generate "mood swings." The presence of a family history of bipolar disorder may influence the mood profile in a child with ASD. In one family study, children with bipolar disorder were found to have extremes of affect, cyclicity, intense or obsessive interests, neuro-vegetative disturbances, and regression after a period of apparently average or precocious development compared to children without bipolar disorder (DeLong, 1994). Antidepressant-induced hypomania, considered a soft sign of bipolarity, has been described in persons with ASD with subsequent positive response to divalproex sodium (Damore, Stine, & Brody, 1998).

Assessment of Mood Disorders

While it is important to be aware of the risk of depression in persons with ASD, it is also critical to note that symptoms such as increased social withdrawal, oppositional behavior, and aggression may be mistaken for clinical depression. The sine qua non of major depression in DSM-IV-TR, depressed mood or anhedonia, may not be readily evident in a person with ASD. Such patients can be quiet, withdrawn, and minimally responsive in affect without having an underlying mood disorder. Communication difficulties in many individuals with ASD limit the ability to ascertain an internal mood state by self-report (Skokauskas & Gallagher, 2010). While verbally intact individuals may be reliably diagnosed

with a comorbid mood condition, clinicians should be reluctant to diagnose mood disorders in individuals with greater communication impairment. Due to the inherent challenges in diagnosing comorbid affective conditions, treatment may be delayed for years despite frequent medical evaluations. Depression can impair family activities and relationships (Kim et al., 2000). As such, a high index of suspicion for depression is critical for timely diagnosis and treatment.

There are no universally accepted scales to assess for depression in persons with ASD. Typically, in younger persons, the *Children's Depression Inventory* (Kovacs, 1985) and *Reynold's Adolescent Scale for Depression* (Reynolds, 1986) are used as screening measures, especially in those who are higher functioning. In those who are less verbal, the diagnosis is much more difficult and may need to be based on behavioral observations alone. The reader is referred to relevant sections in this volume dealing with the assessment of behavioral symptoms in persons with intellectual disabilities.

Pharmacologic Treatment of Mood Disorders in ASD

Despite ongoing data of high rates of comorbid mood disorders in persons with ASD, there has been little empirical research on the psychopharmacologic treatment of specific mood disorders in people with ASD. Overall, the data regarding pharmacologic treatment of comorbid mood disorders in people with ASD are sparse and are mostly extracted from other pharmacologic studies in people with ASD. Of note, not a single trial has been conducted on DSM-IV-specific mood disorders, including depression, bipolar disorder, or other mood disorders in people with ASD; however, a number of blinded psychopharmacologic trials have looked at irritability in these populations, which is sometimes regarded as an index of depression. The primary outcome measure in the studies looking at risperidone, aripiprazole, and methylphenidate in treatment of irritability was caregiver-rated ABC-I. Though irritability may not indicate a true comorbid mood disorder, these trials do provide some evidence for the use of risperidone, aripiprazole, and methylphenidate treatment of irritability as a mood symptom.

Few case reports have described the treatment of depression in patients with ASD with medications such as fluoxetine and amitriptiline (Ghaziuddin, Tsai, & Ghaziuddin, 1991; Pollard & Prendergast, 2004). One report described the use of mirtazapine and contraceptives in a patient with autism and depression related to the menstrual cycle (Skinner, Ng, McDonald, & Walters, 2005). A large open-label trial of fluoxetine in people with ASD by DeLong, Ritch, and Burch (2002) found that 89 of 129 subjects had good or excellent response, which was partially characterized by improved emotional stability and increased happiness, thereby possibly treating an underlying mood disorder. The finding that fluoxetine response correlated with the family history of a major affective disorder substantiates this theory.

Though pharmacological treatment is still considered the main treatment for depression reported for persons with ASD (Lainhart & Folstein, 1994), the combination of medication and milieu therapy, including communication facilitation and positive staff support (Long, Wood, & Holmes, 2000), proved to be effective in one case report, where the staff was guided by psychiatric experts. CBT reported a good treatment outcome in a young man with Asperger syndrome and depression (Hare, 1997). Effective light therapy of seasonal depression has also been reported for two patients (Cooke & Thompson, 1998), and electroconvulsive therapy (ECT) has been successfully used to treat catatonia in one case study (Zaw, Bates, Vijaya, & Bentham, 1999). ECT has been documented to be effective for severe depression, especially when psychotic features are involved (Bertagnoli & Borchardt, 1990) and also for individuals with ID (Aziz, Maixner, Dequardo, Aldridge, & Tandon, 2001).

Supportive Psychotherapy for Depression

Supportive psychotherapy is often used for persons with ASD, though it has been subjected to limited systematic investigation. Only higher functioning and verbal persons with ASD recognize unpleasant emotions and report them when depressed. In a review, only 1 out of 17 persons with ASD diagnosed with depression reported changes as mood related (Lainhart & Folstein, 1994). The aim of supportive psychotherapy is to help the patient recognize his/her own emotions and learn skills to deal with them effectively. The therapy should be highly structured (Ghaziuddin, Ghaziuddin, & Greden, 2002; Kestenbaum, 2008). In one case management project, 4 of 18 clients with psychiatric diagnoses received supportive psychotherapy (Bakken, Foss, Helverschou, Kalvenes, & Martinsen, 2008). The psychotherapy was closely linked to milieu therapy given by care staff. The authors described the case of a man in his thirties with ASD, mild ID, anxiety symptoms, and a severe depressive episode. Following his admission to a psychiatric ward, supportive psychotherapy was provided twice a week. Due to the patient's unrest, the first six sessions were conducted while walking around the hospital area. Initially the session lasted 5 min as the patient would hardly speak; however, gradually he began to be more forthcoming, and the sessions were accordingly increased to 30–60 min. The sessions were often used to solve misunderstandings caused by the patient's idiosyncratic and repetitive speech. For example, he frequently asked his caregivers "Are you strong?" and got upset if they answered in the affirmative. When it was revealed that he was afraid of being held tightly on the floor by staff, caregivers were counseled to answer the patient "Yes I'm strong, but I will not hold you on the floor." After 3 weeks, he stopped asking this question and became more cooperative on the unit. It is important to note in this context that the close co-operation between the therapist and the care

staff that is often necessary when the patient has cognitive impairment raises questions of confidentiality that should be addressed appropriately.

Anxiety Disorders

Anxiety symptoms must be distinguished from anxiety disorders. While the former can occur in most of us, the latter are persistent, severe, and disabling in nature. The most common types are general anxiety disorder (GAD), separation anxiety disorder (SAD), and OCD. Others include selective mutism and specific phobias. A variety of anxiety disorders occur in persons with ASD across the life span. Detecting comorbid anxiety disorders in the ASD population is complicated by the considerable overlap between the symptoms of ASD and those of the comorbid conditions – obsessions/compulsions versus repetitive behaviors, tics versus stereotypies, etc. (Ghaziuddin, Ghaziuddin, & Greden, 2002; Hutton, Goode, Murphy, Le Couteur, & Rutter, 2008). In addition, anxiety symptoms may be difficult to identify because of the communication deficits and associated problems with emotional recognition (Leyfer et al., 2006; Wood et al., 2009). It is important to diagnose and treat these symptoms of their impact on assessment, case conceptualization, and treatment planning. In addition, anxiety disorders often co-occur with other conditions, such as ADHD and mood disorders, leading to complex presentations (De Bruin, Ferdinand, Meesters, de Nijs, & Verheij, 2007; Muris, Steerneman, Merckelbach, Holdrinet, & Meesters, 1998; Wood & McLeod, 2008).

Treatment of Anxiety Disorders

There is some overlap between the principles of treatment of ASD and anxiety disorder. For example, the standard treatment of individuals with ASD without psychiatric comorbidity emphasizes structure, predictability, and gradual adjustments, to new tasks and environments. These correspond to the basic principles of anxiety management and are particularly important when co-occurring anxiety problems are identified in persons with ASD. Strategies to increase social understanding and problem solving are also general strategies in ASD treatment, which become especially important when the individual has anxiety problems.

Important components in specific anxiety treatment include strategies to achieve arousal regulation in anxiety-provoking situations, such as relaxation, and self-monitoring strategies to control behavior and decrease dependency on external contingencies (Groden, Baron, & Groden, 2006; Helverschou, 2006). Anxiety reactions usually increase if the individual is pressured to confront the aversive situation or object. Several practical strategies for managing anxiety reactions and panic attack in individuals with ASD and for preventing them have been suggested (Myles, 2003) including identifying each individual's unique stressors.

Behavior and Cognitive Behavior Therapies

Behavioral and cognitive–behavioral therapy (CBT) are those most frequently described and generally recognized as successful methods for treating anxiety disorders including OCD in general psychiatry (James, Soler, & Weatherall, 2005; March, Frances, Kahn, & Carpenter, 1997; Scott, Mughelli, & Deas, 2005). CBT includes some of the strategies described above. With the aid of psychoeducation, cognitive restructuring, relaxation strategies, exposure, and response prevention, the individual becomes more conscious of the relationship between thoughts, emotions, and behavior, and the treatment aims at changing the way of thinking and teaching new strategies for self-monitoring and coping. The primary treatment components include teaching the patient about their reactions and sorting them in a hierarchical manner, and then teaching them to confront the anxiety or OCD symptoms by means of exposure and response prevention (Tsai, 2006). In OCD treatment, exposure and response prevention are especially effective.

Several studies of small groups of individuals have reported successful treatment of anxiety disorders or OCD with the aid of CBT in higher functioning individuals with ASD (Cardaciotto & Herbert, 2004; Chalfant, Rapee, & Carroll, 2007; Reaven et al., 2009; Sofronoff, Attwood, & Hinton, 2005; Sze & Wood, 2007; White, Ollendick, Scahill, Oswald, & Albano, 2009; Wood et al., 2009). Overall, results are encouraging, showing a marked decrease in symptoms at post-treatment and follow-up; however, more research is needed because of the methodological limitations of these studies, such as small sample sizes, lack of adequate controls, poor validity of the diagnosis of anxiety disorders, and the use of non-standardized assessment tools to evaluate the efficacy of treatment. Furthermore, CBT should be adjusted to the special needs of individuals with ASD (Howlin, Goode, Hutton, & Rutter, 2004). Treatment manuals for CBT (e.g., March & Mulle, 1998) have also been adapted for use in persons with ASD (Attwood, 2004; Sofronoff & Attwood, 2003; Sofronoff et al., 2005; White et al., 2009; Wood & McLeod, 2008). Because CBT includes both behavioral and cognitive components, it is difficult to determine which components are the most effective in this population (Sturmey, 2004).

One study recently utilized a modified CBT for treatment of anxiety disorders in children with ASD (Wood et al., 2009). Children with ASD aged 7–11 years receiving a modified 16-session CBT trial were compared to children with ASD on a 3-month waitlist. The modified CBT group also received social skills training. The results showed that 78.5% of the CBT group met Clinical Global Impressions-Improvement scale criteria for positive treatment response at post-treatment, as compared to only 8.7% of the waitlist group. This study is important as it shows the possibility of using other treatment modalities to specifically target both the symptoms of ASD and anxiety.

Adjustments reported in the use of CBT in individuals or groups with ASD include adapting the cognitive components to the person's developmental level; increasing the time spent on emotional education and stress management; using the individuals' special interests as a starting point; using a structured treatment plan and describing it more thoroughly to the patient; employing visual aids to improve attention span and focus such as the use of drawings or cartoons to concretize; providing access to specific social training; and increasing the involvement of parents and teachers to secure generalization and completing exercises at home (Cardaciotto & Herbert, 2004; Lehmkuhl, Storch, Bodfish, & Geffken, 2008; Lord, 1996). The involvement of parents, in particular, seems to improve the outcome (Sofronoff & Attwood, 2003; Sofronoff et al., 2005).

Specific Adaptations for Individuals with ASD and Intellectual Disability

Adaptations are particularly indicated for individuals with ASD who additionally have ID. Many of these individuals do not talk, use only a few words and short sentences, or communicate with alternative communication techniques, such as visual or manual signs. It is a challenge to adjust methods to this group of people, and collaboration with care staff and family who know the person well is required. Nevertheless, successful interventions employing techniques similar to those used with the general population and in higher functioning individuals with ASD have been reported. Examples include the use of a gradual exposure procedure with modeling, treatment of dog phobia, and the use of an individualized fear hierarchy followed by graded exposure and relaxation training in individuals with ID (Benson & Havercamp, 2007). Procedures for reducing dental fear have also been reported as successful in children with ASD and ID (Luscre & Center, 1996). This is in line with our clinical experience. A report from 19 case management projects indicates that similar adaptations seem to work in individuals with ASD and ID (Bakken et al., 2008). For example, the development of an individualized fear hierarchy in a collaboration between carestaff and experienced clinicians and in vivo exposure training in treating dog phobia in an adult man with AD and severe ID. In a previously reported case story of a girl with autism and severe ID (Helverschou, 2006), a manual sign, "finished," was used to give her control and the possibility to escape from anxiety-provoking situations and activities. Once the use of the sign was established, she gradually learned to take part in activities previously assumed impossible for her, such as going to the dentist, hairdresser, cafés, and gymnastics and swimming group in her spare time.

Pharmacologic Treatment of Anxiety Disorders

Similar to the available data in mood disorders, there has been little systematic research on pharmacological intervention in the treatment of anxiety disorders in ASD populations, despite ongoing evidence of high rates of anxiety disorder comorbidity. Although SSRIs are now considered the mainstay of pharmacologic treatment of anxiety disorders in both children and adults, it is surprising that few studies on the use of SSRIs in people with ASD have used an anxiety rating scale as part of their outcome measures; however, one open-label study of fluvoxamine (Martin, Koenig, Anderson, & Scahill, 2003) did not find any significant differences in anxiety rating scales, global functioning, or repetitive behaviors between the treatment and placebo groups.

Schizophrenia

There is more than a causal historical relationship between schizophrenia and autism. When autism was first described, it was regarded as a psychological condition caused mainly by mothers. Many authorities regarded it as a form of schizophrenia; in fact, the labels infantile psychosis and childhood schizophrenia were used to describe children who would today be diagnosed with autism. Studies done later in the UK by Kolvin and colleagues were instrumental in clarifying the differences between autism and schizophrenia. As summarized by Rutter (1972), these two conditions can be differentiated on the basis of the age of onset, signs and symptoms, family history, association with seizure disorder and ID, course and treatment response. Thus, people with schizophrenia typically have the onset of their illness in late adolescence or early adulthood, have symptoms of hallucinations and/or delusions, a family history of schizophrenia or schizophrenia spectrum disorders, and no clear association with epilepsy or ID. Although the course is often chronic, it may sometimes be punctuated by periods of almost complete recovery. On the other hand, autism is characterized by an onset almost always before 3 years of age; a high family history of autism spectrum disorders; a close relationship with epilepsy and ID; and a chronic course where medication treatments are generally not successful.

Pharmacological Treatment of Psychosis in ASD

The mainstay of treatment of schizophrenia in autism is the use of antipsychotic medications as in the rest of the population. As discussed elsewhere, these consist of typical and atypical antipsychotic drugs. The trend currently is to use atypical antipsychotic agents, such as riperidone; however, data are limited on their long-term effects necessitating a close monitoring of their effects on the cardiovascular system and metabolism.

Psychosocial Treatment of Psychosis in ASD

Interventions for psychosis and mood disorder share core elements. In both disorders, the prominent shifts between normal functioning and prominent psychiatric symptoms in the affected persons appear as episodes. Thus, acute and long-term interventions are somewhat different because the intervention approaches change slightly when the client has passed the most acute phase.

In general psychiatry, psychosocial approaches, such as multidisciplinary assessment, supportive psychotherapy, milieu therapy, multi-family groups, and CBT, have been found to be effective in individuals with psychosis and mood disorders, especially in combination with medical treatment (McFarlane, Dixon, Lukens, & Lucksted, 2003; Sin & Lyubomirsky, 2009; Toth & King, 2008; van Os & Kapur, 2009). Newer antipsychotic medications seem to improve the outcome of psychosocial interventions and followed by fewer relapses when the two interventions are used in combination (van Os & Kapur, 2009) and psychosocial treatments may permit lower doses of antipsychotics (Mojtabai, Nicholson, & Carpenter, 1998).

Studies investigating treatment of psychosis in persons with ASD still consist of case studies or case series only (Bakken, Friis, Lovoll, Smeby, & Martinsen, 2007; Bølte & Bosch, 2005; Clarke, Baxter, Perry, & Prasher, 1999; Clarke, Littlejohns, Corbett, & Joseph, 1989; Petty, Ornitz, Michelman, & Zimmerman, 1984; Shastri, Lakshmiramana, & Sabaratnam, 2006; Skinner et al., 2005; Sverd, Montero, & Gurevich, 1993; Toth & King, 2008; Yapa & Clarke, 1989); however, these papers suggest that using interventions found to be effective for adolescents and adults without ASD works for people with ASD. A combination of medication and psychosocial treatment for clients with ASD and new-onset psychosis is generally recommended.

Efficient milieu therapy variables for people with ASD and additional severe psychiatric illness will for the most part include the same core elements as are used for non-autistic individuals (Bakken, Eilertsen, Smeby, & Martinsen, 2008a, b; Røssberg, 2005). In a report of 19 case management projects, 9 clients with psychosis or depression were given systematic conventional psychiatric milieu therapy, though all interventions were adapted to the individual client's idiosyncratic communication style and cognitive level (Bakken et al., 2008).

Social Interplay

Core therapeutic variables include creating a highly structured environment, creating a plan for early warning signs, such as increasing social withdrawal, odd behavior, and sleep disturbance, eliminating demands and tasks that the patient is not capable of performing, reinforcing autonomy, and improving feedback. Effective staff communication is critical, especially if the patient is psychotic (Bakken et al., 2008a, b). Staff members need to be familiar with the phenomenology of different psychiatric illnesses in order to be able to adapt their communication to the patient's shifting symptoms (Bakken et al., 2007). An empirical study of staff communication in social interplay with adults with ASD, ID, and psychosis revealed that some staff communication acts are effective with disorganized client behavior and decreased social client activity (Bakken et al., 2007). Four dimensions of staff communication termed *effective communication* were investigated. When a member of staff *responds meaningfully*, it seems to encourage initiatives in patients, but has the least impact on disorganized behavior. When a member of staff encourages the client to achieve *joint attention*, this seems to have a positive, diminishing effect on disorganized patient behavior. This result provides support for the importance of getting into contact with the patient in order to help him/her focus on objects or tasks. *Task sustentation* seems to have the most pronounced effect on disorganized behavior in this sample, but makes the patient passive. When task sustentation is used to help a strongly confused patient, he/she may become less frustrated and will experience the caregiver as both emotionally and practically supportive. *Emotional support* elicited initiative from the clients, but had no substantial effect on disorganized behavior.

Treatment Phases

In the acute phase, individuals with ASD and psychosis are often in a chaotic state characterized by stress symptoms, anxiety, disorganization, and aggravated social withdrawal. They may not be able to maintain basic self-care tasks such as eating, going to the bathroom or dressing, or social relationships (Bakken et al., 2007). A wholly compensatory care system is required, where the caregivers provide help and support in performing tasks around the clock (Meleis, 1997). When caregivers provide such compensatory and comprehensive care during the acute phase of mental illness, they might worry about the patient losing skills, such as dressing or washing himself; however, according to clinical experience, individuals with ASD, including people with ID, will again master previously learned skills when the most acute phase has passed (Bakken et al., 2008). Such concerns and misunderstandings might urge caregivers to make unrealistic demands, which may increase the patient's frustration and anxiety, and possibly cause an aggressive reaction. Being closely followed through the day might in turn increase the patient's frustration, as persons with ASD do not master complex social settings well. This applies particularly when they are in an acute phase of psychosis.

Wholly compensatory care will aim first and foremost at anxiety relief. The patient may need to be sheltered from strong stimulation such as crowds of people, loud music, or horror movies. Sick leave from work or daily activities

is needed. Caregivers should stay close to the client and be available. Limiting the setting or seclusion may be indicated when the patient is severely confused or shows strong deviant behavior. Referral to a psychiatric hospital may be necessary (Bakken et al., 2007; Bølte & Bosch, 2005).

Long-term interventions may be provided when the patient has passed the most acute phase. Standard treatment of ASD such as structure and predictability is an important component in the treatment plan, as well as effective communication regarding social interaction, autonomy, and meaningful activities. The goals for performing tasks should be small, making it easy for patients to succeed and experience mastering.

Relapse occurs frequently in schizophrenia. A description of early warning signs may prevent a new episode or at least keep the symptoms at the lowest level possible (Birchwood, Spencer, & McGovern, 2000; Herz & Melville, 1980). For example, Bakken, Foss, and colleagues (2008) found that crisis intervention plans were useful for 18 of 19 clients included in a project on case management. A plan for crisis intervention should cover warning signs in different stages of a progressing episode, as most people with ASD are not capable of recognizing these signs by themselves, as is common in neurotypical persons with psychosis (Birchwood et al., 2000). The intervention plan must correspond to the stage the client is in, indicated by the warning signs as described above.

Catatonia

Catatonia is a serious disorder characterized by a marked slowing of body movements and a decline in general level of functioning. If left untreated, death may occur due to starvation. Most cases of catatonia are precipitated by psychiatric causes such as depression and psychosis; however, in a small number of cases, catatonia may be associated with medical factors, such as chronic infections. In some cases, the cause of catatonia may not be apparent. Occasionally, catatonia may occur repeatedly in the same patient, a condition known as periodic catatonia. About 15% of persons with autism are said to develop catatonia during late adolescence and early adulthood (Wing & Shah, 2000).

Etiology

Why catatonia occurs in persons with autism is not clear. It may be related to undiagnosed medical factors. Co-existing psychiatric disorders, such as depression, may also be responsible. In addition, there is growing evidence that the use of antipsychotic medications may increase the risk of catatonia and of neuroleptic malignant syndrome, a related condition. It is important for clinicians to be aware that one of the long-term effects of the use of antipsychotic medications is the occurrence of catatonia.

Treatment

If not treated, catatonia can become a life-threatening condition; thus, it is important that all adolescents with ASD who display increasing behavioral problems are screened for this condition. Rating scales, such as the *Bush-Francis Rating Scale* (Bush, Fink, Petrides, Dowling, & Francis, 1996), may be tried although this is not specific to persons with ASD. A comprehensive medical and psychiatric examination should be performed along with relevant laboratory tests, such as creatinine phosphokinase levels in the blood. All antipsychotic medications should be stopped. Benzodiazepines should be given in acute phases. When the condition does not respond to these interventions, ECT may be necessary (Ghaziuddin, Gih, Barbosa, Maixner, & Ghaziuddin, 2010; Zaw et al., 1999).

Suicidal Behavior

Patients with ASD sometimes engage in suicidal behavior. This should be differentiated from repetitive self-injurious behavior that is described elsewhere in this volume. The latter is more common in low-functioning persons with ASD, especially those with severe ID. Correct estimates of true suicidal behavior in ASD are not available. No systematic studies have been done on this topic; however, a few case reports have been described in the media. In a report on the life experiences of adults with autism, the National Autistic Society of the UK found that 8% had felt suicidal or attempted suicide (Barnard, 2001).

A Medline search with the keywords of suicide, autism, and Asperger syndrome revealed only 20 relevant publications. Most of the reported cases of suicidal behavior have focused on high-functioning adults with autism or those with Asperger syndrome. While the reasons are not clear, this is probably linked to their greater verbal skills and level of intelligence. For example, in her description of 34 patients with Asperger syndrome, Wing (1981) reported that 11% had attempted suicide. Depression is often the underlying reason. Note that in Wing's series 23% showed signs of an affective illness while 11% attempted suicide. A few reports of suicidal behavior and completed suicide have been described in persons with ID, some of whom may have had comorbid autism. Clinicians and caregivers should be aware of the risk of suicidal behavior in this population. Instead of calling the behavior "manipulative" or "hystrionic," efforts should be made to identify the behavior and treat any underlying mood disorder.

Forensic Aspects

Persons with ASD sometimes get into trouble with the law for a variety of offences and sometimes indulge in violent acts; however, their violence usually lacks malicious intent, as a result of which, they are often not prosecuted. On the other hand, higher functioning individuals are known to commit crime acts, including serious acts, such as sexual assaults and killing people. Because most of the data on this topic are derived from captive populations in special hospitals, it is difficult to conclude that there is a real association between criminal violence and high-functioning autistic disorders; however, there is enough preliminary evidence to suggest that a subgroup of high-functioning individuals with ASD do commit acts of criminal violence, sometimes repeatedly so. Thus, the question is not whether some patients with ASD commit criminal acts but why? A recent review found that when individuals with ASD commit violent crime, they usually tend to do so when they are suffering from comorbid psychiatric disorders suggesting that it is the presence of psychiatric disorders and not of ASD per se that increases the risk of indulging in crime (Newman & Ghaziuddin, 2008) thus underscoring the need for early diagnosis and treatment of comorbid psychiatric disorders in these patients.

Conclusions

Persons with ASD are vulnerable to a range of psychiatric disorders. Because autism is a lifelong diagnosis, its symptoms change over time, and so does its psychiatric comorbidity. Although limited information exists about the prevalence of autism in the community, the most common co-existing disorder in children with autism is ADHD while the disorder that is most commonly seen in adolescents is depression, mirroring the rates of psychiatric disorders in the general population. Factors that influence the emergence of psychiatric disorders in persons with autism include genetic factors, environmental stressors, and medical causes. While these factors are the same as those that affect the occurrence of psychiatric disorders in the general population, some factors may be more specific to those with ASD, such as parental stress; however, there do not appear to be any major differences between affected autistic persons and affected non-ASD persons, at least in those who are of average intelligence and reasonably good verbal skills, underlying the role of these two factors in the phenomenology of psychiatric illness in this population.

Although several recent studies have focused on the psychopathology of persons with autism, several limitations exist that need to be addressed. First, there is a tendency to avoid using the term "psychiatric" in favor of non-specific terms, such as "behavioral," which has often proved to be a barrier to access to services. Caregivers and professionals should be educated about the comorbidity of autism and the risks associated for not recognizing it. Second, systematic studies should be done to estimate the prevalence of psychiatric disorders in the community.

Third, assessment tools should be developed specifically for this purpose, especially in those who have comorbid ID. Finally, more research should be undertaken to clarify the phenomenology of psychiatric disorders in this population; study their precipitating and maintaining factors; and devise appropriate assessment tools and treatment strategies.

References

Aman, M. G., Singh, N. N., Stewart, A. W., & Field, C. J. (1985). The aberrant behavior checklist: A behavior rating scale for the assessment of treatment effects. *American Journal of Mental Deficiency, 89*, 485–491.

American Psychiatric Association. (2000). *Diagnostic and statistical manual of mental disorders* (4th ed., text revision). Washington, DC: Author.

Arnold, L., Aman, M., Cook, A., Witwer, A., Hall, K., Thompson, S., et al. (2006). Atomoxetine for hyperactivity in autism spectrum disorders: Placebo-controlled crossover pilot trial. *Journal of the American Academy of Child and Adolescent Psychiatry, 45*, 1196–1205.

Asperger, H. (1944). Die autistischen Psychopathen im Kindersalter. *Archiv fur Psychiatrie und Nervenkrankheiten, 117*, 76–136.

Attwood, T. (2004). Cognitive behavior therapy for children and adults with Asperger's syndrome. *Behavior Change, 21*, 147–161.

Aziz, M., Maixner, D. F., Dequardo, J., Aldridge, A., & Tandon, R. (2001). ECT and mental retardation: A review and case reports. *Journal of ECT, 17*, 149–152.

Bakken, T. L., Eilertsen, D. E., Smeby, N. A., & Martinsen, H. (2008a). Observing communication skills in staffs interacting with adults suffering from intellectual disability, autism and schizophrenia. *Nordic Journal of Nursing Research and Clinical Studies, 28*, 30–35.

Bakken, T. L., Eilertsen, D. E., Smeby, N. A., & Martinsen, H. (2008b). Effective communication related to psychotic disorganized behavior in adults with intellectual disability and autism. *Nordic Journal of Nursing Research and Clinical Studies, 88*, 9–13.

Bakken, T. L., Foss, N. E., Helverschou, S. B., Kalvenes, G., & Martinsen, H. (2008). *Psychiatric disorders in adults with autism and intellectual disability – Experiences from 19 case management projects.* Oslo: The National Autism Unit, Rikshospitalet, Oslo University Hospital. [Published in Norwegian]

Bakken, T. L., Friis, S., Lovoll, S., Smeby, N. A., & Martinsen, H. (2007). Behavioral disorganization as an indicator of psychosis in adults with intellectual disability and autism. *Mental Health Aspects of Developmental Disabilities, 10*, 37–46.

Barnard, J. (2001). *Ignored or ineligible? The reality for adults with autism spectrum disorders.* London: National Autism Society.

Benson, B. A., & Havercamp, S. M. (2007). Behavioral approaches to treatment: Principles and practices. In N. Bouras & G. Holt (Eds.), *Psychiatric and behavioral disorders in intellectual and developmental disabilities* (pp. 283–309). Cambridge: Cambridge University Press.

Bertagnoli, M. D., & Borchardt, C. M. (1990). A review of ECT for children and adolescents. *Journal of American Academy of Child and Adolescent Psychiatry, 29*, 129–136.

Birchwood, M., Spencer, E., & McGovern, D. (2000). Schizophrenia: Early warning signs. *Advances in Psychiatric Treatment, 6*, 93–101.

Bølte, S., & Bosch, G. (2005). The long-term outcome in two females with autism spectrum disorder. *Psychopathology, 38*, 151–154.

Bush, G., Fink, M., Petrides, G., Dowling, F., & Francis, A. (1996). Catatonia. I. Rating scale and standardized examination. *Acta Psychiatrica Scandinavica, 93*, 129–136.

Cardaciotto, L., & Herbert, J. D. (2004). Cognitive behavior therapy for social anxiety disorder in the context of Asperger's syndrome: A single-subject report. *Cognitive and Behavioral Practice, 75*, 75–81.

Chalfant, A., Rapee, R., & Carroll, L. (2007). Treating anxiety disorders in children with high-functioning autism spectrum disorders: A controlled trial. *Journal of Autism and Developmental Disorders, 33*, 283–298.

Clarke, D., Baxter, M., Perry, D., & Prasher, V. (1999). The diagnosis of affective and psychotic disorders in adults with autism: Seven case reports. *Autism, 3*, 149–164.

Clarke, D. J., Littlejohns, C. S., Corbett, J. A., & Joseph, S. (1989). Pervasive developmental disorders and psychoses in adult life. *British Journal of Psychiatry, 155*, 692–699.

Cooke, L. B., & Thompson, C. (1998). Seasonal affective disorder and response to light in two patients with learning disability. *Journal of Affective Disorders, 48*, 145–148.

Costello, H., Bouras, N., & Davies, H. (2007). Evaluation of mental health training for care staff supporting people with intellectual disabilities. *Journal of Applied Research in Intellectual Disabilities, 20*, 118–135.

Couturier, J. L., & Nicolson, R. (2002). A retrospective assessment of citalopram in children and adolescents with pervasive developmental disorders. *Journal of Child and Adolescent Psychopharmacology, 12*, 243–248.

Damore, J., Stine, J., & Brody, L. (1998). Medication-induced hypomania in Asperger's disorder. *Journal of the American Academy of Child and Adolescent Psychiatry, 37*, 248–249.

De Bruin, E., Ferdinand, R., Meesters, S., de Nijs, P., & Verheij, F. (2007). High rates of psychiatric co-morbidity in PDD-NOS. *Journal for Autism and Developmental Disorders, 37*, 877–886.

DeLong, G. R., Ritch, C. R., & Burch, S. (2002). Fluoxetine response in children with autistic spectrum disorders: Correlation with familial major affective disorder and intellectual achievement. *Developmental Medicine and Child Neurology, 44*, 652–659.

DeLong, R. (1994). Children with autistic spectrum disorder and a family history of affective disorder. *Developmental Medicine and Child Neurology, 36*, 674–687.

Dosen, A. (2007). Integrative treatment in persons with intellectual disability and mental health problems. *Journal of Intellectual Disability Research, 51*, 66–74.

Fankhauser, M. P., Veeraiah, M. S., Karumanchi, V. C., German, M. L., Yates, A., & Devi Karumanchi, S. (1992). A double-blind, placebo controlled study of the efficacy of transdermal clonidine in autism. *Journal of Clinical Psychiatry, 53*, 77–82.

Fatemi, S. H., Realmuto, G. M., Khan, L., & Thuras, P. (1998). Fluoxetine in treatment of adolescent patients with autism: A longitudinal open trial. *Journal of Autism and Developmental Disorders, 28*, 303–307.

Frazier, J. A., Doyle, R., Chiu, S., & Coyle, J. T. (2002). Treating a child with Asperger's disorder and comorbid bipolar disorder. *The American Journal of Psychiatry, 159*, 13–21.

Ghaziuddin, M. (2005). *Mental health aspects of autism and Asperger syndrome.* London: Jessica Kingsley Press.

Ghaziuddin, M., Alessi, N., & Greden, J. F. (1995). Life events and depression in children with pervasive developmental disorders. *Journal of Autism and Developmental Disorders, 25*, 495–502.

Ghaziuddin, M., Ghaziuddin, N., & Greden, J. (2002). Depression in persons with autism: Implications for research and clinical care. *Journal of Autism and Developmental Disorders, 32*, 299–306.

Ghaziuddin, M., Tsai, L., & Ghaziuddin, N. (1991). Fluoxetine in autism with depression. *Journal of the American Academy of Child and Adolescent Psychiatry, 30*, 508–509.

Ghaziuddin, N., Gih, D., Barbosa, V., Maixner, D. F., & Ghaziuddin, M. (2010). Onset of catatonia at puberty: Electroconvulsive therapy response in two autistic adolescents. *Journal of ECT, 26*(4), 274–277. [Epub ahead of publication; accessed online August 18, 2010]

Groden, J., Baron, M. G., & Groden, G. (2006). Assessment and coping strategies. In M. G. Baron, J. Groden, G. Groden, & L. P. Lipsitt (Eds.), *Stress and coping in autism* (pp. 15–41). Oxford: Oxford University Press.

Guy, W. (1976). *ECDEU Assessment manual for psychopharmacology—Revised* (DHEW Publ No ADM 76-338). Rockville, MD: U.S. Department of Health, Education, and Welfare, Public Health Service, Alcohol, Drug Abuse, and Mental Health Administration, NIMH Psychopharmacology Research Branch, Division of Extramural Research Programs.

Handen, B., Johnson, C., & Lubetsky, M. (2000). Efficacy of methylphenidate among children with autism and symptoms of attention-deficit hyperactivity disorder. *Journal of Autism and Developmental Disorders, 30*, 245–255.

Hare, D. J. (1997). The use of cognitive-behavioural therapy with people with Asperger syndrome: A case study. *Autism, 1*, 215–225.

Helverschou, S. B. (2006). Structure, predictability and manual sign teaching as strategies in regulation of emotions and anxiety. In S. von Tetzchner, E. Grindheim, J. Johannessen, D. Smørvik, & V. Ytterland (Eds.), *Biologiske forutsetninger for kulturalisering (Biological presuppositions to culturalization)*. Oslo: Autismeforeningen og Universitetet i Oslo. (The Autism Society and University of Oslo) [Published in Norwegian]

Herz, M., & Melville, C. (1980). Relapse in schizophrenia. *American Journal of Psychiatry, 137*, 801–812.

Hofvander, B., Delorme, R., Chaste, P., Nydén, A., Wentz, E., Ståhlberg, O., et al. (2009). Psychiatric and psychosocial problems in adults with normal-intelligence autism spectrum disorders. *BMC Psychiatry, 9*, 35.

Howlin, P., Goode, S., Hutton, J., & Rutter, M. (2004). Adult outcome for children with autism. *Journal of Child Psychology and Psychiatry, 45*, 212–229.

Hutton, J., Goode, S., Murphy, M., Le Couteur, A., & Rutter, M. (2008). New-onset psychiatric disorders in individuals with autism. *Autism: The International Journal of Research and Practice, 12*, 373–390.

James, A., Soler, A., & Weatherall, R. (2005). Cognitive behavioral therapy for anxiety disorders in children and adolescents. *Cochrane Database Systematic Reviews, 19*(4) (Art. No.: CD004690. 004610)

Jaselskis, C., Cook, E., Fletcher, K., & Leventhal, B. (1992). Clonidine treatment of hyperactive and impulsive children with autistic disorder. *Journal of Clinical Psychopharmacology, 12*, 322–327.

Kanner, L. (1943). Autistic disturbances of affective contact. *Nervous Child, 2*, 217–250.

Kestenbaum, C. J. (2008). Autism, Asperger's and other oddities...Thoughts about treatment approaches. *Journal of American Academy of Psychoanalysis and Dynamic Psychiatry, 36*, 279–294.

Kim, J. A., Szatmari, P., Bryson, S. E., Streiner, D. L., & Wilson, F. J. (2000). The prevalence of anxiety and mood problems among children with autism and Asperger syndrome. *Autism, 4*, 117–132.

Kovacs, M. (1985). The children's depression, inventory (CDI). *Psychopharmacology Bulletin, 21*(4), 995–998.

Lainhart, J. (1999). Psychiatric problems in individuals with autism, their parents and siblings. *International Review of Psychiatry, 11*, 278–298.

Lainhart, J. E., & Folstein, S. (1994). Affective disorders in people with autism: A review of published cases. *Journal of Autism and Developmental Disorders, 24*, 592–601.

Lehman, A. F., & Steinwachs, D. M. (1998). Translating research into practice: The schizophrenia patient outcome research team (PORT) treatment recommendations. *Schizophrenia Bulletin, 24*, 1–10.

Lehmkuhl, H. D., Storch, E. A., Bodfish, J. W., & Geffken, G. R. (2008). Brief report: Exposure and response prevention for obsessive-compulsive disorder in a 12-year-old with autism. *Journal of Autism and Developmental Disorders, 38*, 977–981.

Leibenluft, E., & Rich, B. A. (2008). Pediatric bipolar disorder. *Annual Review of Clinical Psychology, 4*, 163–187.

Leyfer, O. T., Folstein, S. E., Bacalman, S., Davis, N. O., Dinh, E., Morgan, J., et al. (2006). Comorbid psychiatric disorders in children with autism: Interview development and rates of disorders. *Journal of Autism and Developmental Disorders, 36*, 849–861.

Long, K., Wood, H., & Holmes, N. (2000). Presentation, assessment and treatment of depression in a young woman with learning disability and autism. *British Journal of Learning Disabilities, 28*, 102–108.

Lord, C. (1996). Treatment of a high-functioning adolescent with autism. A cognitive-behavioral approach. In M. A. Reineke, F. M. Dattilio, & A. Freeman (Eds.), *Cognitive therapy with children and adolescents* (pp. 394–404). New York: The Guilford Press.

Lunsky, Y., Gracey, C., & Bradley, E. (2009). Adults with autism spectrum disorders using psychiatric hospitals in Ontario: Clinical profile and service needs. *Research in Autism Spectrum Disorders, 3*, 1006–1013.

Luscre, D., & Center, D. B. (1996). Procedures for reducing dental fear in children with autism. *Journal of Autism and Developmental Disorders, 26*, 547–556.

March, J. S., Frances, A., Kahn, D. A., & Carpenter, D. (1997). The expert consensus guidelines: Treatment of obsessive-compulsive disorder. *Journal of Clinical Psychiatry, 58*, 1–72.

March, J. S., & Mulle, K. (1998). *OCD in children and adolescents. A cognitive-behavioral treatment manual.* New York: The Guilford Press.

Martin, A., Koenig, K., Anderson, G., & Scahill, L. (2003). Low-dose fluvoxamine treatment of children and adolescents with pervasive developmental disorders: A prospective, open-label study. *Journal of Autism and Developmental Disorders, 33*, 77–85.

Martin, G., Costello, H., Leese, M., Slade, M., Bouras, N., Higgins, S., et al. (2005). An exploratory study of assertive community treatment for people with intellectual disability and psychiatric disorders: Conceptual, clinical, and service issues. *Journal of Intellectual Disability Research, 49*, 516–524.

McCracken, J. T., McGough, J., Shah, B., Cronin, P., Hong, D., Aman, M. G., et al. (2002). Risperidone in children with autism and serious behavioral problems. *The New England Journal of Medicine, 347*, 314–321.

McDonnell, A., Sturmey, P., Oliver, C., Cunningham, J., Hayes, S., Galvin, M., et al. (2008). The effects of staff training on staff confidence and challenging behavior in services for people with autism spectrum disorders. *Research in Autism Spectrum Disorders, 2*, 311–319.

McFarlane, W. R., Dixon, L., Lukens, E., & Lucksted, A. (2003). Family psychoeducation and schizophrenia: A review of the literature. *Journal of Marital and Family Therapy, 29*, 223–245.

Meleis, A. I. (1997). *Theoretical nursing: Development and progress.* Philadelphia: Lippincott.

Mojtabai, R., Nicholson, R. A., & Carpenter, B. N. (1998). Role of psychosocial treatments in management of schizophrenia: A meta-analytic review of controlled outcome studies. *Schizophrenia Bulletin, 24*, 569–587.

Munesue, T., Ono, Y., Mutoh, K., Shimoda, K., Nakatani, H., Kikuchi, M., et al. (2008). High prevalence of bipolar disorder comorbidity in adolescents and young adults with high-functioning autism spectrum disorder: A preliminary study of 44 outpatients. *Journal of Affective Disorders, 111*, 170–175.

Muris, P., Steerneman, P., Merckelbach, H., Holdrinet, I., & Meesters, C. (1998). Comorbid anxiety symptoms in children with pervasive developmental disorders. *Journal of Anxiety Disorders, 12*, 387–393.

Myers, S. M. (2007). The status of pharmacotherapy for autism spectrum disorders. *Expert Opinion on Pharmacotherapy, 8*, 1579–1603.

Myles, B. S. (2003). Behavioural forms of stress management for individuals with Asperger syndrome. *Child and Adolescent psychiatric Clinics, 12*, 123–141.

Namerow, L. B., Thomas, P., Bostic, J. Q., Prince, J., & Monuteaux, M. C. (2003). Use of citalopram in pervasive developmental disorders. *Journal of Developmental and Behavioral Pediatrics, 24*, 104–108.

Newman, S. S., & Ghaziuddin, M. (2008). Violent crime in Asperger syndrome: The role of psychiatric comorbidity. *Journal of Autism and Developmental Disorders, 38*, 1848–1852.

Owley, T., Walton, L., Salt, J., Guter, S. J., Jr., Winnega, M., Leventhal, B. L., et al. (2005). An open label trial of escitalopram in pervasive developmental disorders. *Journal of the American Academy of Child and Adolescent Psychiatry, 44*, 343–348.

Petty, L. K., Ornitz, E. M., Michelman, J. D., & Zimmerman, E. G. (1984). Autistic children who become schizophrenic. *Archives of General Psychiatry, 41*, 129–135.

Pollard, A. J., & Prendergast, M. (2004). Depressive pseudodementia in a child with autism. *Developmental Medicine and Child Neurology, 46*, 485–489.

Pratt, C. W., Gill, K. J., Barrett, N. M., & Roberts, M. M. (2007). *Psychiatric rehabilitation* (2nd ed.). Amsterdam: Elsevier Academic Press.

Quintana, H., Birmaher, B., Stedge, D., Lennon, S., Freed, J., Bridge, J., et al. (1995). Use of methylphenidate in the treatment of children with autistic disorder. *Journal of Autism and Developmental Disorders, 25*, 283–294.

Reaven, J. A., Blakeley-Smith, A., Nichols, S., Dasari, M., Flanigan, E., & Hepburn, S. (2009). Cognitive-behavioral group treatment for anxiety symptoms in children with high-functioning autism spectrum disorders. A pilot study. *Focus on Autism and Other Developmental Disabilities, 24*, 27–37.

Reynolds, W. (1986). *Reynolds adolescent depression scale*. Florida: Psychological Assessment Resources, Inc.

Royal College of Psychiatrists. (2006). *Psychiatric services for adolescents and adults with Asperger syndrome and other autistic-spectrum disorders*. Council report CR 136, London.

Røssberg, J. I. (2005). *Evaluations of inpatient units with emphasis on the ward atmosphere scale* Doctoral dissertation, Ullevaal University Hospital, Oslo.

Rutter, M. (1972). Childhood schizophrenia reconsidered. *Journal of Autism and Childhood Schizophrenia, 2*, 315–337.

Rutter, M., Bailey, A., Berument, S. K., Lord, C., & Pickles, A. (2003). *Social communication questionnaire (SCQ). Lifetime version*. Los Angeles, CA: Western Psychological Services.

Scott, R. W., Mughelli, K., & Deas, D. (2005). An overview of controlled studies of anxiety disorders treatment in children and adolescents. *Journal of the National Medical Association, 97*, 13–24.

Shastri, M., Lakshmiramana, A., & Sabaratnam, M. (2006). Aripiprazole use in individuals with intellectual disability and psychotic disorders: A case series. *Psychopharmalogica, 20*, 863–867.

Shea, S., Turgay, A., Carroll, A., Schulz, M., Orlik, H., Smith, I., et al. (2004). Risperidone in the treatment of disruptive behavioral symptoms in children with autistic and other pervasive developmental disorders. *Pediatrics, 114*, 634–641.

Shtayermman, O. (2007). Peer victimization in adolescents and young adults diagnosed with Asperger's syndrome: A link to depressive symptomatology, anxiety symptomatology and suicidal ideation. *Issues in Ccomprehensive Pediatric Nursing, 30*, 87–107.

Simonoff, E., Pickles, A., Charman, T., Chandler, S., Loucas, T., & Baird, G. (2008). Psychiatric disorders in children with autism spectrum disorders: Prevalence, comorbidity, and associated factors in a population-derived sample. *Journal of the American Academy of Child and Adolescent Psychiatry, 47*, 921–929.

Sin, N. L., & Lyubomirsky, S. (2009). Enhancing well-being and alleviating depressive symptoms with positive psychology interventions: A practice-friendly meta-analysis. *Journal of Clinical Psychology: In Session, 65*, 467–487.

Skinner, S. R., Ng, C., McDonald, A., & Walters, T. (2005). A patient with autism and severe depression: Medical and ethical challenges for an adolescent medicine unit. *The Medical Journal of Australia, 183*, 422–424.

Skokauskas, N., & Gallagher, L. (2010). Psychosis, affective disorders and anxiety in autistic spectrum disorder: Prevalence and nosological considerations. *Psychopathology, 43*, 8–16.

Sofronoff, K., & Attwood, T. (2003). A cognitive behavior therapy intervention for anxiety in children with Asperger's syndrome. *GAP (National Autistic Society), 4*, 2–8.

Sofronoff, K., Attwood, T., & Hinton, S. (2005). A randomized controlled trial of a CBT intervention for anxiety in children with Asperger syndrome. *Journal of Child Psychology and Psychiatry, 46*, 1152–1160.

Stachnik, J. M., & Nunn-Thompson, C. (2007). Use of atypical antipsychotics in the treatment of autistic disorder. *The Annals of Pharmacotherapy, 41*, 626–634.

Stewart, M. E., Barnard, L., Pearson, J., Hasan, R., & O'Brien, G. (2006). Presentation of depression in autism and Asperger syndrome: A review. *Autism, 10*, 103–116.

Sturmey, P. (2004). Cognitive therapy with people with intellectual disabilities: A selective review and critique. *Clinical Psychology and Psychotherapy, 11*, 223–232.

Sverd, J., Montero, G., & Gurevich, N. (1993). Brief report: Cases for an association between Tourette syndrome, autistic disorder, and schizophrenia-like disorder. *Journal of Autism and Developmental Disorders, 23*, 407–413.

Sze, K. M., & Wood, J. J. (2007). Cognitive behavioral treatment of comorbid anxiety disorders and social difficulties in children with high-functioning autism: A case report. *Journal of Contemporary Psychotherapy, 37*, 133–143.

Toth, K., & King, B. H. (2008). Asperger's syndrome: Diagnosis and treatment. *Treatment in Psychiatry, 165*, 958–963.

Troost, P. W., Lahuis, B. E., Steenhuis, M. P., Ketelaars, C. E., Buitelaar, J. K., van Engeland, H., et al. (2005). Long-term effects of risperidone in children with autism spectrum disorders: A placebo discontinuation study. *Journal of the American Academy of Child and Adolescent Psychiatry, 44*, 1137–1144.

Tsai, L. (2006). Diagnosis and treatment of anxiety disorders in individuals with autism spectrum disorders. In M. G. Baron, J. Groden, G. Groden, & L. P. Lipsitt (Eds.), *Stress and coping in autism* (pp. 388–440). Oxford: Oxford University Press.

van Os, J., & Kapur, S. (2009). Schizophrenia. *Lancet, 374*, 635–645.

White, S. W., Ollendick, T., Scahill, L., Oswald, D., & Albano, A. M. (2009). Preliminary efficacy of a cognitive-behavioral treatment program for anxious youth with autism spectrum disorders. *Journal of Autism and Developmental Disorder, 39*, 1652–1662.

Wing, L. (1981). Asperger's syndrome: A clinical account. *Psychological Medicine, 11*, 115–129.

Wing, L., & Shah, A. (2000). Catatonia in autistic spectrum disorders. *British Journal of Psychiatry, 176*, 357–362.

Wood, J. J., Drahota, A., Sze, K., Har, K., Chiu, A., & Langer, D. A. (2009). Cognitive behavioral therapy for anxiety in children with autism spectrum disorders: A randomized, controlled trial. *Journal of Child Psychology and Psychiatry, and Allied Disciplines, 50*, 224–234.

Wood, J. J., & McLeod, B. (2008). *Child anxiety disorders: A treatment manual for practitioners*. New York: Norton.

Yapa, P., & Clarke, D. J. (1989). Schizophreniform psychosis associated with delayed grief in a man with moderate mental handicap. *Mental Handicap Research, 2*, 211–212.

Zaw, F. K. M., Bates, G. D. L., Vijaya, M., & Bentham, P. (1999). Catatonia, autism and ECT. *Developmental and Medical Child Neurology, 41*, 843–845.

Joel E. Ringdahl

Introduction

Rituals, stereotypies, and obsessive-compulsive behavior are all terms used to describe one of the core symptoms of autistic disorder and autism spectrum disorders (ASDs; Militerni, Bravaccio, Falco, Fico, & Palermo, 2002). Their inclusion in the symptomatology related to ASDs can be traced back to Kanner's (1943) description of the disorder, which included various forms of repetition such as rituals, motor stereotypy, compulsions, and obsessions (Bodfish, Symons, Parker, & Lewis, 2000). Bodfish et al. and Bodfish (2007) point out that there is a lack of consensus regarding the terminology used to refer to such behavior. For example, Bodfish et al. report that the same topography (e.g., hand flapping) of behavior may be variously termed "stereotypic," "ritualistic," or "perseverative." In any event, these types of behavior (rituals, stereotypies, and obsessive-compulsive responses) can uniformly be described as "repetitive behavior disorders" (Ringdahl, Wacker, Berg, & Harding, 2001). While each may have some distinction with respect to physiological bases (Militerni et al., 2002), they do share the common feature of seemingly occurring in the absence of social sources of reinforcement in most cases.

The purpose of this chapter is to provide an overview of treatments that are effective to reduce such repetitive behavior exhibited by individuals diagnosed with ASDs. The chapter will begin with a description of repetitive behavior problems and their expression in the population of individuals with ASDs. Next, a brief discussion will be provided regarding the behavioral assessment of repetitive behavior disorders. Finally, the remainder of the chapter will focus on a discussion and description of the behavioral treatment strategies that have been effective in reducing the occurrence of repetitive behavior disorders. Examples in application of each treatment strategy will be provided. To the extent possible, these examples will be those implemented with individuals diagnosed with ASD.

Description and Expression

Rituals, stereotypy, and obsessive-compulsive behavior can be more inclusively described as repetitive behavior disorders (Bodfish, 2007; Ringdahl et al., 2001; Turner, 1999). Such behavior problems can vary in topography and include body rocking (Pyles, Riordan, & Bailey, 1997), hand flapping (Ringdahl et al., 2002), mouthing (Vollmer, Marcus, & LeBlanc, 1994), pica (Goh, Iwata, & Kahng, 1999), echoic speech (Charlop, 1983), lining up objects (Sigafoos, Green, Payne, O'Reilly, & Lancioni, 2009), and vocal stereotypy (Ahearn, Clark, MacDonald, & Chung, 2007). Several theories have been posited to explain why such behavior is exhibited. For example, psychoanalytic researchers such as Spitz and Wolfe (1949) described repetitive behavior disorders as manifestations of sexual impulses. Baumeister (1978) and Baumeister and Forehand (1973) provided organic explanations of repetitive behavior, including (a) chemical or structural brain pathology and (b) the maintenance of optimal stimulation levels to such behavior. Another organic explanation for repetitive behavior disorders is that they result in altered states of consciousness (Stone, 1964) or other pleasurable experiences, such as opiate-induced euphoria or pain attenuation (Thompson, Hackenberg, Cerutti, Baker, & Axtell, 1994). Finally, repetitive behavior has been described from an operant standpoint by Lovaas, Newsom, and Hickman (1987), among others. Lovaas et al. specifically hypothesized that repetitive behavior may be maintained by the reinforcing sensory consequences it produce. More generally, an operant explanation suggests that repetitive behavior may occur to access and be maintained by reinforcers directly produced by the behavior, sensory or otherwise. The

J.E. Ringdahl (✉)
Psychology Division, Department of Pediatrics, University of Iowa
Children's Hosptial, Iowa City, IA 52242, USA
e-mail: joel-ringdahl@uiowa.edu

J.L. Matson, P. Sturmey (eds.), *International Handbook of Autism and Pervasive Developmental Disorders*,
Autism and Child Psychopathology Series, DOI 10.1007/978-1-4419-8065-6_30, © Springer Science+Business Media, LLC 2011

putative reinforcers could be the sensory stimulation produced by the behavior (e.g., auditory stimulation produced by repetitive speech) or the decrease in anxiety produced by performance of obsessive-compulsive routines. For example, a child with ASD may engage in a behavior such as hand flapping because it directly produces visual stimulation that is reinforcing (Rapp & Vollmer, 2006). This type of operant relationship is known as "automatic reinforcement" (Vaughn & Michael, 1982).

To a degree, every individual diagnosed with autistic disorder will engage in some form of repetitive behavior. The Diagnostic and Statistical Manual IV-TR (DSM IV-TR; American Psychiatric Association [APA], 2000) indicates that individuals receiving the diagnosis of autistic disorder (299.00) must display restricted repetitive and stereotyped patterns of behavior, interests, and activities, as manifested by at least one of the following: (a) encompassing preoccupation with one or more stereotyped patterns of interest that is abnormal either in intensity or focus; (b) apparently inflexible adherence to specific, nonfunctional routines or rituals; (c) stereotyped and repetitive motor mannerisms (e.g., hand of finger flapping or twisting, or complex whole-body movements); and (d) persistent preoccupation with parts of objects. The diagnostic criteria for other disorders that fall under the umbrella of pervasive developmental disorders include similar language with respect to the required presence of these or similar repetitive behavior disorders as a necessity to achieve the diagnosis.

While repetitive behaviors may constitute a core feature of ASD, they are not uniformly exhibited across the population of individuals with ASD. Militerni et al. (2002) found that repetitive behavior varied as a function of age and IQ scores. Specifically, younger children were more likely to exhibit repetitive motor behavior, such as trunk and limb movement, while older children more frequently engaged in complex motor movements such as filling and emptying. Sensory behavior was more prevalent with individuals with low IQ (< 35), while complex motor sequences were more frequent in the sample population with high IQ (> 70). In addition, the types of repetitive behavior exhibited by individuals with ASD may differ from repetitive behavior problems with non-ASD diagnoses. For example, McDougle et al. (1995) reported that adults with ASD were more likely to exhibit the repetitive behavior including repeating, ordering, hoarding, and touching than adults diagnosed with OCD.

Behavioral Assessment of Repetitive Behavior Disorders: Functional Analysis

Since the application of functional analysis methodology (Iwata, Dorsey, Slifer, Bauman, & Richman, 1994) to the identification of the functional relationships between self-injurious behavior (SIB) and various consequences, this assessment methodology has become the standard for identifying the conditions under which problem behavior occurs, as well as its maintaining variables. Functional analysis allows for a more tailored approach to designing behavioral treatment than simply basing the treatment on the topography of the challenging behavior. A comprehensive discussion of functional analysis is not the purview of this chapter, as that topic was handled in Chapter 18 and elsewhere in this text. However, there are some particular considerations that will likely need to be kept in mind when assessing repetitive behavior problems via a functional analysis.

A functional analysis of problem behavior often consists of individually comparing the effects on behavior of several socially mediated consequences (e.g., attention and escape from instruction) and no programmed social consequences (e.g., when the individual is alone) to the effects of a control condition (e.g., ongoing access to alternative stimuli and attention in the absence of instruction, often termed "free play"). Results typically point to one of three broad classes of reinforcement related to the maintenance of problem behavior, based on the response pattern obtained: social positive reinforcement, social negative reinforcement, and automatic reinforcement. Often, repetitive behavior, such as those covered in this chapter, will have no apparent social function. That is, the behavior is not exhibited to obtain social positive reinforcers, such as attention or access to preferred items, and is not exhibited to obtain social negative reinforcement, such as avoidance or escape nonpreferred activities (e.g., academic instruction). Instead, the behavior may occur across conditions or be differentially more frequent when social consequences are not programmed. In such instances, the behavior can be said to be maintained by automatic reinforcement.

There are instances when repetitive behavior described as stereotypic or ritualistic does indeed serve a social function. Mace and Belfiore (1990) reported on the stereotypic touching exhibited by a woman diagnosed as functioning in the severe range of intellectual disability. Stereotypic touching was defined as the repetitive (response occurring less than 15 s apart), nonadaptive contact between the individual's hand or foot and another individual or object. A descriptive analysis, based on the identification of antecedents and consequence correlated with stereotypic touching, suggested that this individual's stereotypic behavior was motivated by escape from activities. In a similar vein, the presence of an automatic reinforcement function for the behavior does not rule out the potential for the behavior to be sensitive to other, social sources of reinforcement. Smith, Iwata, Vollmer, and Zarcone (1993) demonstrated that, for two of three participants whose problem behavior (in this case, SIB) was maintained by automatic reinforcement, a social function could also be identified.

Thus, while it may be a safe bet to progress toward treatment of repetitive behavior based on an assumption that the behavior is maintained by automatic reinforcement, it is still best practices to conduct the functional analysis prior to beginning treatment. This assessment process may be beneficial for a number of reasons. First, the assessment can identify whether or not the behavior is exclusively maintained by automatic reinforcement. This information is important for developing comprehensive treatment strategies. Second, the assessment may be helpful in identifying the influence of idiosyncratic stimuli on repetitive behavior. Third, the assessment may be helpful in identifying conditions under which the behavior does not occur (i.e., the free play condition when the presence of alternative stimuli competes with the expression of problem behavior). This information may be useful for identifying a starting point for treatment (e.g., ongoing access to competing items). Finally, this assessment provides a baseline against which the effects of treatment strategies can be compared.

When conducting a functional analysis, settling on an automatic reinforcement function can be difficult. In fact, many researchers and clinicians are uncomfortable with the determination that a behavior is maintained by automatic reinforcement because it represents a "default" decision. That is, the conclusion that behavior is maintained by automatic reinforcement is arrived at less because of what is observed (i.e., a distinct response–reinforcer or antecedent–response relationship), and more because of what is not observed (i.e., a lack of differentiation with respect to environmental antecedents or consequences). With that said, several researchers have provided guidelines for reaching the conclusion that a behavior is maintained by automatic reinforcement. More specifically, Iwata et al. (1994) indicated that an automatic reinforcement function is most likely demonstrated when target responding continues in the absence of social contingencies. Asmus et al. (2004) applied this logic and identified automatic reinforcement functions when behavior (a) occurred differentially or exclusively during the alone/ignore (i.e., no alternative stimuli and no programmed consequence) condition of a functional analysis or (b) occurred across all conditions of the functional analysis, including those associated with no programmed consequences (i.e., alone/ignore and free play conditions).

When assessing repetitive behavior, it may be necessary to make idiosyncratic modifications to the functional analysis test conditions. Often, these modifications will include the presence of specific stimuli that are reported to be included in the target response, consumed while engaging in the target response, or otherwise evocative of the target response. For example, Van Camp et al. (2000) reported on the influences of idiosyncratic stimuli on the functional analysis outcomes related to the problem behavior (SIB or hand flapping) exhibited by two young children with developmental disabilities. Results of this investigation indicated that idiosyncratic antecedent stimuli set the occasion for problem behavior that was demonstrated to then persist in the absence of social sources of reinforcement (i.e., maintained by automatic reinforcement). For one participant, repetitive behavior was occasioned by the presence of a specific toy (a Bumble Ball). For the second participant, repetitive behavior was occasioned by the ongoing presentation of toys and attention. In the absence of these stimuli, repetitive behavior was unlikely to occur.

Given results such as those reported by Van Camp et al. (2000), it may be important to identify specific stimuli to include in the functional analysis or other behavioral assessment. Van Camp et al. identified the idiosyncratic stimulus for one of the participants by noting the stimulus with which engagement and problem behavior were most highly correlated during the play condition of the functional analysis. In a similar study conducted by Carr, Yarbrough, and Langdon (1997), idiosyncratic stimuli demonstrated to be correlated with socially motivated problem behavior were identified via a more formal process of descriptive analyses. Specifically, naturalistic observations were conducted during which stimuli associated with the occurrence or omission of problem behavior were conducted. Functional analyses were conducted with and without these stimuli present for three individuals. Results of the functional analyses suggested that the socially motivated problem behavior exhibited by the participants was differentially affected by the presence of these particular stimuli.

Once the function of the behavior has been identified, whether it is automatic reinforcement, social reinforcement, or some combination thereof, treatment strategies can be developed to reduce and/or replace the problem behavior.

Behavioral Treatment of Repetitive Behavior Problems

There are a number of behavioral treatments that have been developed and successfully used to decrease repetitive behavior disorders such as rituals, stereotypies, and obsessive-compulsive behavior displayed by individuals with ASDs. This portion of the chapter will provide an overview of those treatment strategies. Four general approaches to behavioral treatment will be discussed and include (1) antecedent-based treatments, (2) consequence-based treatment, (3) extinction-based treatments, and (4) combinations of treatment strategies. As mentioned previously, an effort was made to provide examples of application with individuals diagnosed with ASDs; however, in some instances, examples are provided in which the individual(s) for whom the treatment was applied did not have an ASD diagnosis, or the diagnosis was unknown. Such cases do not necessarily impeach the utility of the treatment described for the population of individuals with ASDs. As many researchers have noted (Matson & Dempsey, 2009), repetitive behavior disorders are observed across diagnostic categories. Effective behavior-based treatment is more likely tied to the effective arrangement of environment, consequences, and/or extinction than it is to specific diagnosis.

Antecedent-Based Treatments

Antecedent-based treatments are those treatments that have an effect without intervening at the response–reinforcer level. These treatments are put in place prior to or regardless of the occurrence of the repetitive behavior. Their therapeutic effects may come about due to changes in the value of the automatic reinforcers maintaining problem behavior (Vollmer, 1994) or the increased opportunity to engage in alternative activities. Several antecedent-based treatments that have been demonstrated to reduce the occurrence of repetitive behavior disorders range from the noncontingent delivery of known reinforcers (sometimes called enriched environment [EE] and noncontingent reinforcement [NCR]; Horner, 1980), to the use of environmental supports such as warnings (Tustin, 1995) and structured activities (Sigafoos et al., 2009).

Noncontingent Reinforcement/Environmental Enrichment

Noncontingent reinforcement (NCR) or enriched environment (EE) is among the most common treatment strategies employed to reduce repetitive behavior. This approach to treatment is based on the notion that the reinforcers responsible for maintaining repetitive behavior may be able to be either diminished in value or effectively competed with through the availability of alternative sources of reinforcement. NCR/EE has been successfully used to decrease a wide range of repetitive behavior and has some practical utility. Specifically, when this treatment is an effective one for any given individual's repetitive behavior, its implementation is straightforward. Implementation requires only that alternative stimuli be identified and then placed in the individual's environment.

One of the first implementations of NCR/EE as treatment for repetitive behavior was demonstrated by Horner (1980). In this seminal study, the effects of enriched environments (i.e., environments that were structured to include a large number of toys and objects) were compared on the object-, self-, and other-directed inappropriate behavior

exhibited by five children with profound developmental disabilities. Behavior problems exhibited by the participants were wide-ranging and included such repetitive behavior as body rocking and tearing objects. Lower levels of inappropriate object- and self-directed behavior were displayed across the participants during enriched conditions as compared to baseline. Reductions in other-directed inappropriate behavior required the addition of contingency-based treatment components; however, the results suggested that repetitive behavior that may be stereotypic or otherwise maintained by automatic reinforcement may be reduced by a relatively simple procedure: increasing the availability of toys and other objects in the environment.

Since the Horner (1980) study, the use of NCR/EE as a treatment strategy for reducing repetitive behavior has gone on to widespread use. For example, Sidener, Carr, and Firth (2005) implemented an NCR-based environmental enrichment program to reduce the stereotypic behavior exhibited by two young girls diagnosed with autism. In this particular study, a treatment approach referred to as *reinforcer displacement* (described later in this chapter) was implemented with no change in the level of stereotypic responding relative to baseline. Environmental enrichment was then implemented across participants. The NCR-based treatment decreased levels of repetitive behavior exhibited by both participants.

NCR/EE is not effective in all cases. For example, Ringdahl, Vollmer, Marcus, and Roane (1997) demonstrated that NCR/EE was ineffective in the treatment of stereotypic SIB displayed by two of the three children included in that study. Several researchers have since developed strategies that predict when NCR will be an effective treatment or have developed assessments that help identify under what stimulus conditions NCR can be an effective treatment. The Ringdahl et al. study demonstrated that response allocation during free operant situations could be predictive of later success with NCR-based treatments. Specifically, for each of the participants, responding during a pre-treatment free operant assessment was indicative of NCR/EE treatment effectiveness. When responding during the free operant assessment was exclusively allocated to engagement with alternative items relative to engagement in stereotypic SIB, NCR/EE was shown to be effective. When responding during the free operant assessment was allocated across those two options (stereotypic SIB and toy or object manipulation), NCR was demonstrated to be ineffective.

Vollmer et al. (1994) demonstrated that the relative preference of the stimuli incorporated into NCR/EE treatments impacted effectiveness. In this study, three individuals diagnosed with developmental disabilities who engaged in repetitive behavior demonstrated to be maintained by automatic reinforcement were referred for assessment and treatment. The effects of NCR/EE with highly preferred alternative stimuli were directly compared to the effects of NCR/EE with low preferred stimuli for one of the three participants using a reversal design. This participant's treatment evaluation indicated that NCR/EE was an effective treatment only when the alternative stimuli available in the environment were those identified as highly preferred via a pre-treatment stimulus preference assessment.

This notion of preference and its impact on treatment success is one that has been explored further in the literature. Understanding the relevance to the development of NCR-based treatments has helped to make them as successful as possible. Piazza et al. (1998) and Piazza, Adelinis, Hanley, Goh, and Delia (2000) evaluated the utility of including stimuli matched to the purported sensory consequences of repetitive behavior. Piazza et al. (1998) demonstrated that NCR treatments incorporating matched stimuli hypothesized to correspond with the oral reinforcement provided by pica maintained by automatic reinforcement were more effective than NCR treatments that included stimuli that were not matched to these hypothesized sources of reinforcement. Piazza et al. (2000) applied the same logic to the treatment of other repetitive behavior problems, including saliva play and hand mouthing, exhibited by individuals with a wide range of developmental disabilities. Specifically, alternative stimuli were identified that were either matched or unmatched to the hypothesized automatic reinforcers maintaining problem behavior. These stimuli were then made available within two different NCR-based treatments: (a) matched alternatives and (b) unmatched alternatives (a third condition was included for one participant such that there were two separate matched-alternatives treatments). As with their 1998 study, Piazza et al. (2000) found that problem behavior occurred at lower levels during the NCR-based treatments that included matched alternatives.

Rapp (2007) provided another demonstration of the utility of matched stimuli to decrease repetitive behavior. Rapp used NCR-based treatments to reduce the vocal stereotypy exhibited by two young boys diagnosed with autism and intellectual disabilities. In this study, results for one individual suggested that toys producing auditory stimulation were effective in reducing vocal stereotypy while identical toys that did not produce auditory stimulation were ineffective. The second individual's results suggested that auditory and non-auditory toys were both ineffective in reducing vocal stereotypy; however, ongoing access to auditory stimulation provided by a CD player was effective in reducing this behavior. These results suggested that simply identifying and providing a matched stimulus may not effectively reduce repetitive behavior. Further evaluation may be needed to identify the specific matched stimulus that is most effective in making treatment gains. In particular, matched stimuli may also need to compete with repetitive behavior for effective treatment to take place.

Ahearn, Clark, DeBar, and Florentino (2005) extended the research regarding the inclusion of matched and unmatched stimuli in NCR/EE-based treatments designed to reduce repetitive behavior. In their study, a young man diagnosed with autism was referred for assessment and treatment of problem behavior including motor and vocal stereotypy. Preferred stimuli were identified that were both matched and unmatched to the hypothesized automatic reinforcers maintaining problem behavior; however, both classes of stimuli were demonstrated to effectively compete with the problem behavior during assessment. That is, the alternative items were relatively more reinforcing, and thus, resulted in more interaction, than the problem behavior. Ahearn et al. then compared the results of NCR-based treatments that included either matched, high-preference or unmatched, high-preference stimuli to baseline (i.e., no alternative stimuli available and no programmed consequences provided for problem behavior). Both treatments resulted in decreases in problem behavior relative to the baseline condition, with the unmatched, high-preference condition resulting in relatively greater decreases. This finding makes intuitive sense: if under free operant conditions (i.e., during a preference assessment) the individual will allocate responding to the alternative stimuli, then those stimuli are likely to be effective when presented in a NCR-based treatment, regardless of their hypothesized match. Thus, for some individuals, reinforcer competition may be a more important variable for effective treatment than reinforcer match.

While NCR-based treatments often require little effort on the part of care providers to implement, they may sometimes require additional supports to be effective. Britton, Carr, Landaburu, and Romick (2002) described the implementation of NCR/EE to reduce the repetitive behavior exhibited by three individuals with various developmental disabilities including autism. In this study, head rocking, face rubbing, and repetitive body movements were demonstrated to be maintained by automatic reinforcement. Sensory products were identified that appeared to match the sensory-based reinforcement produced by the repetitive behavior. NCR/EE was then implemented under two conditions: with and without therapist-delivered prompts for the participants to interact with the alternative sensory products that were freely available. NCR/EE resulted in larger reductions of repetitive behavior when the participants received prompts to interact with the alternative stimuli.

One drawback to NCR-based treatments is that the treatment can be difficult to fade. That is, ongoing and easy access to the competing stimuli is often required to maintain the treatment effects achieved through NCR/EE. Shore, Iwata, DeLeoin, Kahng, and Smith (1997) implemented NCR/EE to reduce the repetitive behavior exhibited by three individuals with developmental disabilities. The treatment was initially effective in reducing target behavior when alternative stimuli were made readily available (e.g., placed in the participants' hands); however, as the response requirement to gain access to the stimuli was increased by moving the stimuli incrementally further away from the participants, repetitive behavior reemerged. One potential reason for the inability to fade such treatments is that the response–reinforcer contingency maintaining the repetitive behavior is never eliminated. Because the reinforcers maintaining repetitive behavior are readily available, as stimuli are removed (either for short time periods or placed farther away), response allocation may change to favor repetitive behavior.

Other Antecedent-Based Treatments

Other antecedent-based treatments that do not rely on the delivery or provision of competing or otherwise reinforcing stimuli have also been demonstrated to reduce repetitive behavior exhibited by individuals with ASD. Dib and Sturmey (2007) demonstrated that enhancing teachers' implementation of a certain type of instructional method resulted in the decrease of repetitive behavior exhibited by three students diagnosed with ASD. In this study, staff training was conducted to teach educators how to implement discrete-trial training as part of their classroom activities. Staff training included, in order, (1) providing the educators with a behavior checklist of the responses they would be expected to exhibit as part of discrete-trial training; (2) providing immediately, directive, and spoken feedback during implementation of discrete-trial training followed by review of performance data; (3) describing and modeling the exact way to present tasks, prompt, and provide reinforcement; and (4) continuing feedback and modeling until the educator could successfully implement the teaching strategy with 100% integrity for two consecutive observations. Following the training of the educators on this teaching strategy, each of the targeted students demonstrated a decrease in repetitive behavior exhibited during instructional situations.

Tustin (1995) demonstrated that reductions in repetitive behavior were achieved when activity transitions were delivered in advance as opposed to immediately upon transition. Specifically, this study evaluated the influence of providing immediate versus advance prompts to change activities on the stereotypic body rocking and hand flapping exhibited by a man with ASD. Results of the study demonstrated decreased levels of repetitive behavior during the "advance" condition relative to the "immediate" condition.

The use of structured leisure opportunities has been demonstrated to be an effective approach to reducing repetitive behavior. Sigafoos et al. (2009) implemented structured leisure opportunities as a treatment approach to reduce the obsessive-repetitive behavior (constant rearrangement of objects) exhibited by a 15-year-old boy with ASD.

Pre-treatment assessments were conducted to identify alternative activities that were reinforcing or preferred for the participant. In addition, a pre-treatment assessment was conducted that indicated opportunities to engage in leisure activities were minimal prior to intervention. The structured opportunities to engage in leisure activities and social interaction resulted in decreased levels of the obsessive-repetitive behavior of object rearrangement. Similar results were observed during follow-up visits 6 weeks and 3 months following treatment evaluation.

Collectively, Dib and Sturmey (2007), Tustin (1995), and Sigafoos et al. (2009) are of interest in that they demonstrate that antecedent-based treatments can be effective simply by rearranging the environment or components of the environment, without the need to conduct additional assessments to identify preferred items or items that effectively compete with target problem behavior under free operant conditions; however, similar to NCR/EE-based treatments, these other antecedent-based treatments do not programmatically establish and increase alternative, appropriate behavior repertoires. While such changes may emerge during treatment, they are not programmed. In some therapeutic environments, one requirement of treatment may be the establishment of alternative, appropriate behavior. This goal can be achieved through the use of consequence-based treatments.

Consequence-Based Treatments

Differential Reinforcement

In typical application, differential reinforcement entails the identification of the reinforcer(s) that maintain problem behavior. This consequence is then arranged to be withheld or withdrawn when the target behavior occurs (i.e., extinction is in place) and presented following the omission of target behavior for a pre-specified time (differential reinforcement of omission; DRO), or following an alternative response (differential reinforcement of alternative responding; DRA). DRA strategies can be further divided to include a strategy that specifies the reinforcement of incompatible responses (differential reinforcement of incompatible behavior, or DRI). Finally, differential procedures may specify the delivery of reinforcement following low rates of the target behavior (differential reinforcement of low rates, or DRL). Such treatments may be effective because they disrupt the response–reinforcer relationship relative to problem behavior and establish or strengthen a response–reinforcer relationship relative to an alternative, appropriate response or set of responses.

Differential Reinforcement of Alternate Behavior. In typical application, differential reinforcement of alternative behavior entails (a) identifying the reinforcer maintaining challenging behavior, (b) identifying an alternative appropriate response to increase, and (c) differentially providing the reinforcer relevant to challenging behavior contingent on the alternative appropriate response (i.e., reinforcement for alternative, extinction for challenging). When this strategy is applied to the treatment of repetitive behavior, the often automatic reinforcement nature of its maintenance requires its implementation is amended to some extent. Specifically, (a) the reinforcer responsible for maintenance of the repetitive behavior is typically not the consequence provided for alternative responding, and (b) extinction for the repetitive behavior may not be possible (more on extinction-based procedures will be presented later in this chapter). Thus, when DRA is used to treat a behavior maintained by social positive reinforcement (e.g., attention), the DRA schedule refers to the manner in which the functional reinforcer (i.e., attention) is delivered and/or withheld. When DRA is used to treat a behavior maintained by automatic reinforcement, the DRA schedule refers to the manner in which some other known reinforcer unrelated to the function of problem behavior (i.e., an arbitrary reinforcer) is delivered or and/or withheld.

Berg et al. (in revision) applied a differential reinforcement-based treatments, including DRA, to reduce the repetitive behavior exhibited by individuals with autism and other developmental disabilities. The differential reinforcement procedure included the contingent provision of a preferred alternative stimulus following an appropriate response (e.g., communicative request or task completion). Access to the preferred stimulus was allowed until problem behavior occurred. Following any occurrence of problem behavior, the preferred stimulus was removed for a specified time period. The stimulus was represented following the next appropriate response. This type of DRA procedure was effective in reducing repetitive behavior exhibited by some, but not all, participants in the study.

Differential Reinforcement of Incompatible Behavior. As mentioned, DRI can be considered as a subset of DRA. One difference is that DRI specifies that the alternative response to be reinforced must be incompatible with the challenging behavior. For example, the behavior of clasping hands would be incompatible with the repetitive behavior of hand flapping. Thus, in a DRI-based treatment designed to reduce hand flapping maintained by automatic reinforcement, some known (i.e., arbitrary) reinforcer would be provided contingent on hand clasping, and withheld or withdrawn when hand clasping was not occurring. This strategy has been used to reduce the repetitive or other behavior maintained by automatic reinforcement exhibited by individuals with ASD including pica and stereotypy. Smith (1987) reported the effectiveness of using a DRI schedule to reduce occurrences of pica exhibited by a young adult diagnosed with autism. Instances of pica were reduced when food, drinks, or brief access to favorite activities were provided after each

approximately 15-min period during which the participant engaged in keeping his hands on his work and staying in the work area (responses incompatible with pica) while keeping his mouth clear.

Jones (1999) reported on a long-term follow-up of the effects of DRI used to reduce repetitive behavior exhibited by individuals with a wide range of developmental disabilities. The initial application of the treatment, as reported in previous studies by Jones and colleagues, indicated DRI was an effective treatment; however, at 10-year follow-up, results suggested that stereotypic behavior was an, "intractable, chronic, and long-standing behavior" (p. 49), with several of the participants continuing to engage in the behavior at high levels. Though levels or repetitive behavior were reduced for other participants, some repetitive behavior was reported to continue for each. While this study may indicate the intractable nature of stereotypic behavior, it may also indicate that the reductions in stereotypic and other repetitive behavior observed when DRI is implemented as treatment cannot be expected to be maintained if treatment is withdrawn.

Differential Reinforcement of Low Rates of Behavior. This approach to behavior change is somewhat different than the previously described differential reinforcement programs. Specifically, DRL does not require the omission of the target behavior for reinforcement to be achieved or earned. Instead, DRL treatments allow for the delivery of reinforcers following behavior that is preceded by increasingly longer intervals of time without a response. The goal, then, with a DRL program is to reduce the rate of a response that occurs too frequently, as opposed to eliminating a response altogether, as may be the goal with a DRO treatment (Cooper, Heron, & Heward, 2007). For example, Handen, Apolito, and Seltzer (1984) provided a demonstration of this type of approach to the reduction of repetitive speech exhibited by an adolescent diagnosed with ASD. In this example, tokens were provided to the participant contingent on increasingly lower rates of verbal repetition (starting at 4.4 repetitions per min and ending with 0.3 repetitions per min). The DRL schedule was successful in reducing repetitive verbal statements well below baseline levels.

DRO. This strategy differs somewhat from DRA-based approaches in that it does not specify what alternative response must be exhibited prior to the delivery of reinforcement. Instead, DRO-based treatments specify what response may not happen prior to delivery of reinforcement, as well as the specific window of time for which the individual must refrain from that behavior. Thus, in its application to the treatment of repetitive behaviors maintained by automatic reinforcement, DRO-based treatments specify the delivery of some identified reinforcing consequences after a pre-specified interval without target behavior. The time interval is usually "resetting" meaning that any instance of the target behavior resets the DRO timer to 0.

Several studies have demonstrated the utility of DRO-based treatment to reduce repetitive behavior (Patel, Carr, Kim, Robles, & Eastridge, 2000; Ringdahl et al., 1997; Taylor, Hoch, & Weissman, 2005). Ringdahl et al. (1997) implemented DRO as the sole or as one component of treatment to reduce the stereotypic SIB exhibited by two individuals diagnosed with developmental disabilities. DRO was effective by itself (Barry) or in combination with another DR schedule (David) in reducing these individuals' stereotypic SIB. Similar findings were obtained by Taylor et al. (2005) who compared the effectiveness of contingent reinforcement (i.e., a DRO) and NCR on the vocal stereotypy exhibited by a young girl diagnosed with autism. Both treatments' reinforcement intervals were set at 1 min. Thus, during DRO, the reinforcer was delivered following 1 min without vocal stereotypy. During the NCR treatment, the reinforcer was delivered on a fixed-time (FT) 1-min schedule, regardless of the occurrence or nonoccurrence of vocal stereotypy. The DRO arrangement reduced vocal stereotypy while the NCR arrangement did not. Another note of interest is that matched stimuli were identified and used as reinforcers in the Taylor et al. study. Thus, this study provides an example of the effectiveness of the contingent (as opposed to noncontingent or continuously available as discussed in the *Antecedent-Based Treatment* section of this chapter) delivery of matched stimuli as a method for reducing repetitive behavior.

Punishment

Consequence-based strategies do not only include those focused on the contingent delivery of reinforcement. Several examples of punishment-based strategies can be found in the literature related to the treatment of repetitive behavior. Punishment-based strategies are those that include the contingent presentation or removal of stimuli that result in a decreased likelihood of the response. When used in the treatment of repetitive behavior, the aversive event is delivered (i.e., positive punishment) or the reinforcing event is discontinued (i.e., negative punishment) contingent on the occurrence of the repetitive behavior. Examples of such strategies in the literature include contingent application of an aversive such as electric shock (Lovaas, Schaeffer, & Simmons, 1965) and overcorrection (Foxx & Axrin, 1973). The use of contingent aversives such as slaps and electric shock has by and large been abandoned as treatment strategies to address repetitive and other behavior problems, and will not be further addressed here.

Overcorrection can include (a) the restitution of the environment to its state prior to the exhibition of a disruptive response, termed *restitutional overcorrection*, contingent on that response (i.e., washing table tops following the occurrence of saliva play on the table) or (b) the practice of a

correct form of the behavior, termed *positive practice overcorrection*, contingent on the response (i.e., brushing teeth following an occurrence of hand or object mouthing). Foxx and Azrin (1973) implemented overcorrection to reduce the repetitive behavior (hand mouthing, head turning, and hand clapping) exhibited by four children with developmental disabilities, including ASD. Results of the study demonstrated the utility of this approach and included a demonstration that treatment gains could be maintained by providing a verbal warning upon first occurrence of the target behavior, in lieu of immediate implementation of the various overcorrection procedures. These findings related to the effectiveness of overcorrection have been replicated in numerous subsequent studies (Doke & Epstein, 1975; Harris & Wolchik, 1979; Maag, Rutherford, Wolchik, & Parks, 1986).

Punishment procedures can also be arranged in such a way that the consequence for repetitive behavior is the removal of a reinforcer or other preferred stimulus (i.e., negative punishment). Falcomata, Roane, Hovanetz, Kettering, and Keeney (2004) implemented a negative punishment procedure to reduce the repetitive inappropriate vocalizations exhibited by a young man diagnosed with ASD. The specific procedure entailed the response-contingent removal of a preferred stimulus (radio) for 5 s following occurrences of inappropriate vocalizations. This procedure was compared to an NCR/EE-based treatment that also incorporated the radio. The negative punishment procedure was more effective in reducing inappropriate vocalizations exhibited by this individual.

For a variety of reasons, the use of punishment procedures is not typically the first line of treatment to address repetitive behavior problems. Tiger, Toussaint, and Kliebert (2009) provided a brief but thorough discussion of the variables to consider prior to implementing a punishment procedure. These variables include aversiveness and immediacy of the consequence and socially acceptable nature of the procedure. More specifically, the consequence should be of sufficient aversiveness to impact behavior. As well, during the initial application of punishment, the consequence should be delivered immediately and following each occurrence of the target response. Finally, other, reinforcement-based components should continue to be in place and the treatment should be acceptable to the caregivers to ensure integrity with the procedure.

Inhibitory Stimulus Control

One interesting extension of punishment-based treatments is the possibility of continuing treatment effects in the absence of the punishment contingency. Rapp, Patel, Ghezzi, O'Flaherty, and Titterington (2009) attempted to achieve this outcome by pairing unique stimuli with punishers delivered contingent on the repetitive behavior (vocal stereotypy) exhibited by three children diagnosed with ASD.

Specifically, following an assessment demonstrating the automatic reinforcement function of the behavior, positive punishment (verbal reprimand) or negative punishment were paired with the presence of a red card. These punishment procedures effectively reduced repetitive behavior. The punishment contingencies were then discontinued, while the red card remained in place. The goal here was to determine if the mere presence of the card, as opposed to the contingent presentation of the punisher, could maintain treatment gains. Treatment gains maintained for one of the three participants when the red card was present, but in the absence of the punishment contingency. While not uniform across participants, these results suggested that, under some circumstances, stimuli associated with punishment contingencies (i.e., the red card) could come to exert inhibitory stimulus control over responding when the punishment contingency was discontinued. Such an approach to treatment may be more acceptable to care providers unwilling, reluctant, or unable to implement punishment procedures over a long time period.

Extinction

Sensory Extinction. Repetitive behavior maintained by automatic reinforcement can be reduced and eliminated through extinction. In the context of these types of problem behavior, the process is referred to as sensory extinction, as extinction targets the sensory consequences maintaining the behavior. Several strategies can be used to achieve sensory extinction. They include environmental modifications to eliminate the response–reinforcement relationship, the use of protective equipment to eliminate the response–reinforcement relationship, or strategies to otherwise dampen the response–reinforcement relationship.

Rincover, Newsom, and Carr (1979) described the application of sensory extinction to reduce the compulsive-like repetitive behavior (light switching) exhibited by two children with developmental disabilities. The treatment strategies consisted of visual sensory extinction (participant MS and RR) and auditory sensory extinction (participant RR). During visual sensory extinction, the light switch was disabled such that moving it up or down did not have any effect. Thus, behavior no longer produced the visual consequence. This procedure resulted in a decrease in the light switching exhibited by MS, but not RR, who had a significant visual impairment. During auditory sensory extinction, layers of carpet were fixed around the faceplate of the light switch and immediate wall surface so that the auditory feedback provided by the light switching behavior was eliminated. This treatment resulted in decreased light switching behavior exhibited by RR. Numerous additional examples of this strategy exist in the literature (Rincover, 1978; Rincover, Cook, Peoples, & Packard, 1979).

The use of protective equipment is sometimes used as a method to bring about sensory extinction. Kennedy and

Souza (1995) demonstrated the effectiveness of goggles as a strategy to mask the sensory consequences of and reduce the repetitive eye poking exhibited by a young man with developmental disabilities. When wearing the goggles, attempts at eye poking decreased relative to when goggles were not in place. It was hypothesized that the eye goggles effectively eliminated the reinforcers available for finger-to-eye contact. Similarly, Deaver, Miltenberger, and Stricker (2001) used the noncontingent application of mittens to reduce the hair twirling exhibited by a young girl. Attempts at hair twirling were reduced to near-zero levels when mittens were worn. In the absence of mittens, hair twirling continued. Similar response patterns (i.e., low response levels when mittens were worn and elevated when mittens were not) were observed across two settings, bedroom and day care.

Sensory extinction may also be achieved by dampening the effects of the repetitive response. Van Houten (1993) evaluated a somewhat different procedure to bring about extinction effects for repetitive behavior. In this study, the stereotypic SIB (face slapping) exhibited by a boy with developmental disabilities and "autistic features" was reduced through the use of noncontingent application of wrist weights. Data on the frequency of face slaps were collected for 5 min prior to each application of wrist weights, during wrist weight application, and for 5 min after wrist weights were removed. Wrist weight applications started at 10 min and were systematically increased to 60 min across observations. Wearing the wrist weights resulted in reductions in face slapping to 0 or near-zero levels. In addition, the wrist weights did not appear to interfere with the participant's ability to engage in toy play that required fine muscle movement. Similarly, the wrist weights did not appear to decrease gross motor activity (e.g., playing on a play ground). The study did not allow for a precise determination of the operant mechanisms responsible for response reduction; however, the wrist weights were correlated with lower levels of responding, suggesting that the automatic reinforcers responsible for maintaining face slapping were unavailable when wrist weights were worn. In essence, the response–reinforcer relationship was disrupted. This disruption can be considered a form of extinction.

Finally, sensory extinction may be achieved through procedures that interrupt and/or redirect the repetitive behavior. This strategy includes the physical or other interruption of repetitive behavior and often includes redirection to other, more appropriate stimuli and/or responses (Ahearn et al., 2007). Liu-Gitz and Banda (2010) used response interruption and redirection (RIRD) to decrease vocal stereotypy exhibited by a boy diagnosed with ASD. A functional analysis demonstrated that the vocal stereotypy was maintained by automatic reinforcement. The RIRD procedure was implemented by having the participant's teacher immediately interrupt vocal stereotypy as soon as it happened (interruption component) followed by the teacher asking a series of questions (redirection component). Specifically, contingent on the target response, the teacher would first say the student's name to interrupt and gain his attention, then ask a series of questions. This intervention effectively reduced vocal stereotypy to zero or near-zero levels.

Despite the apparent effectiveness of strategies designed to reduce or eliminate the sensory consequences of repetitive behavior, such treatment approaches may not always be effective. Maag et al. (1986) demonstrated that sensory extinction was an effective intervention in the reduction of repetitive behavior exhibited by two young children with autism; however, the effects of the treatment did not generalize well to a novel setting. The addition of another treatment component (e.g., overcorrection) was needed to bring about reductions in this novel setting. Another drawback to sensory extinction as a treatment approach is that the individual receiving the treatment is a passive participant. That is, they are not required to exhibit any appropriate behavior during treatment (such as would be required during DR-based treatments), and opportunities for other sources of reinforcement are not necessarily available (such as would be available during NCR/EE-based treatments). Thus, the use of sensory extinction as a treatment approach may best be pursued when (a) other reinforcement-based treatment strategies have been demonstrated to be ineffective and/or (b) some sort of protection from the immediate physical consequences of the behavior, such as in the case of severe stereotypic SIB, are needed.

Reinforcer Displacement. One unique extinction-based program to reduce repetitive behavior is reinforcer displacement. This strategy is based on the notion that responding maintained on continuous schedule of reinforcement (CRF), i.e., each response is followed by the delivery of a reinforcer, will decrease quickly when extinction is implemented. The difference with reinforcer displacement relative to other extinction-based procedures related to repetitive behavior is that an arbitrary reinforcer is initially delivered contingent on the repetitive response. The response–arbitrary reinforcer relationship is then discontinued during extinction. The relationship between the repetitive response and the automatic reinforcers that maintain it are not manipulated. The hypothesis is that the repetitive response will come under the control of the arbitrary, as opposed to automatic, reinforcers. When this relationship is discontinued during extinction, the repetitive behavior will decrease.

Neisworth, Hunt, Gallop, and Madle (1985) provided the initial demonstration of reinforcer displacement to decrease repetitive behavior. In this study, the repetitive behavior (hand flapping and finger flicking) exhibited by two individuals diagnosed with developmental disabilities was evaluated. Reinforcing stimuli (edibles for each participant) were identified and delivered following each repetitive response

during the CRF phase. When extinction was implemented, both participants exhibited decreases in repetitive behavior. This reduction was maintained for one of the participants; however, the second participant exhibited what the authors called "recovery." The term "recovery" refers to responding that returns to a previously observed level of responding after it has been reduced by an operation such as extinction (Catania, 1999); however, an alternative explanation is that the repetitive behavior re-contacted the automatic reinforcement contingencies that had previously maintained it, resulting in the observed reemergence of repetitive behavior during the extinction condition.

Combined Approaches to Treatment

Often, behavioral treatment strategies to address repetitive behavior will incorporate more than one of the above summarized treatment strategies. Athens, Vollmer, Sloman, and St. Peter Pipkin (2008) used a combined treatment approach to decrease the vocal stereotypy exhibited by a child with ASD and Down syndrome. The treatment package consisted of noncontingent attention, delivery of instructions contingent on target behavior (positive punishment), and removal of preferred toys for 10 s (negative punishment) contingent on target behavior. The treatment package was effective in reducing the repetitive behavior.

Paisey, Whitney, and Wainczak (1993) provided another example of a combined treatment approach to reduce the repetitive behavior exhibited by a young girl with Rett syndrome. The treatment package consisted of DRI plus response interruption. The combined treatment was effective in both reducing repetitive behavior (hand mouthing) and increasing appropriate toy play; however, the DRI component was ineffective in reducing hand mouthing when implemented in the absence of the interruption component. Thus, the interruption component was needed to affect behavior change related to hand mouthing.

Summary

Individuals with ASDs are likely to exhibit some form of repetitive behavior problems, whether described as rituals, stereotypies, or obsessive-compulsive behavior, as this behavioral symptom is a core feature of this set of disorders. These behavior problems pose particular challenges for treatment because they are typically maintained by automatic reinforcement, which increases the difficulty of controlling the reinforcers that maintain repetitive behavior during behavior-based treatment; however, there is a long history of behavioral treatments that have proven to be effective in addressing these behavior problems. In addition, the menu of treatment strategies at the disposal of clinicians is quite varied. Not every treatment will be effective in every situation, though. Thus, care must be taken to attempt to choose the best treatment option based on the conditions under which the repetitive behavior is most likely to occur and the information that can be gleaned from other assessments (see Ringdahl et al., 1997; Berg et al., in revision for examples of this process). As research continues to be conducted in this area, further clarifications will likely be provided regarding the assessments that should be conducted and how their results influence what treatments should be selected.

References

Ahearn, W. H., Clark, K. M., DeBar, R., & Florentino, C. (2005). On the role of preference in response competition. *Journal of Applied Behavior Analysis, 38*, 247–250.

Ahearn, W. H., Clark, K. M., MacDonald, R. P. F., & Chung, B. (2007). Assessing and treating vocal stereotypy in children with autism. *Journal of Applied Behavior Analysis, 40*, 263–275.

American Psychiatric Association. (2000). *Diagnostic and Statistical Manual of Mental Disorders-Text Revision* (4th ed.). Washington, DC: Author.

Asmus, J. M., Ringdahl, J. E., Sellers, J. A., Call, N. A., Andelman, M. S., & Wacker, D. P. (2004). Use of a short-term inpatient model to evaluate aberrant behavior: Outcome data summaries from 1996 to 2001. *Journal of Applied Behavior Analysis, 37*, 283–304.

Athens, E. S., Vollmer, T. R., Sloman, K. N., & Peter Pipkin, C., St. (2008). An analysis of vocal stereotypy and therapist fading. *Journal of Applied Behavior Analysis, 41*, 291–297.

Baumeister, A. A. (1978). Origins and control of stereotyped movements. In C. E. Meyers (Ed.), *Quality of life in severely and profoundly mentally retarded people: Research foundations for improvement* (pp. 353–384). Washington, DC: American Association on Mental Deficiency.

Baumeister, A. A., & Forehand, R. (1973). Stereotyped acts. In N. R. Ellis (Ed.), *International review of research in mental retardation*. New York: Academic Press.

Berg, W. K., Wacker, D. W., Ringdahl, J. E., Stricker, J., Vinquist, K., Dutt, A., et al. (in revision). An analysis of conditions that promote allocation of responding toward alternative stimuli over problem behavior maintained by automatic reinforcement. *Journal of Applied Behavior Analysis*.

Bodfish, J. W. (2007). Stereotypy, self-injury, and related abnormal repetitive behaviors. In J. Jacobson, J. Mulikc, & J. Rojahn (Eds.), *Handbook of intellectual and developmental disabilities. Issues in clinical child psychology* (pp. 481–505). US: Springer.

Bodfish, J. W., Symons, F. J., Parker, D. E., & Lewis, M. H. (2000). Varieties of repetitive behavior in autism: Comparisons to mental retardation. *Journal of Autism and Developmental Disorders, 30*, 237–243.

Britton, L. N., Carr, J. E., Landaburu, H. J., & Romick, K. S. (2002). The efficacy of non-contingent reinforcement as treatment for automatically reinforced stereotypy. *Behavioral Interventions, 17*, 93–103.

Carr, E. G., Yarbrough, S. C., & Langdon, N. A. (1997). Effects of idiosyncratic stimulus variables on functional analysis outcomes. *Journal of Applied Behavior Analysis, 30*, 673–686.

Catania, A. C. (1999). *Learning* (4th ed.). Upper Saddle River, NJ: Prentice Hall.

Charlop, M. H. (1983). The effects of echolalia on acquisition and generalization of receptive labeling in autistic children. *Journal of Applied Behavior Analysis, 16*, 111–126.

Cooper, J. O., Heron, T. E., & Heward, W. L. (2007). *Applied behavior analysis* (2nd ed.). Upper Saddle River, NJ: Prentice Hall.

Deaver, C. M., Miltenberger, R. G., & Stricker, J. M. (2001). Functional analysis and treatment of hair twirling in a young child. *Journal of Applied Behavior Analysis, 34*, 535–538.

Dib, N., & Sturmey, P. (2007). Reducing student stereotypy by improving teachers' implementation of discrete-trial teaching. *Journal of Applied Behavior Analysis, 40*, 339–343.

Doke, L. A., & Epstein, L. H. (1975). Oral overcorrection: Side effects and extended applications. *Journal of Experimental Child Psychology, 20*, 496–511.

Falcomata, T. S., Roane, H. S., Hovanetz, A. N., Kettering, T. L., & Keeney, K. M. (2004). An evaluation of response cost in the treatment of inappropriate vocalizations maintained by automatic reinforcement. *Journal of Applied Behavior Analysis, 37*, 83–87.

Foxx, R. M., & Axrin, N. H. (1973). The elimination of autistic self-stimulatory behaviour by overcorrection. *Journal of Applied Behavior Analysis, 6*, 1–14.

Goh, H. L., Iwata, B. A., & Kahng, S. W. (1999). Multicomponent assessment and treatment of cigarette pica. *Journal of Applied Behavior Analysis, 32*, 297–316.

Handen, B. L., Apolito, P. M., & Seltzer, G. B. (1984). Use of differential reinforcement of low rates of behavior to decrease repetitive speech in an autistic adolescent. *Journal of Behavior Therapy and Experimental Psychiatry, 15*, 359–364.

Harris, S. L., & Wolchik, S. A. (1979). Suppression of self-stimulation: Three alternative strategies. *Journal of Applied Behavior Analysis, 12*, 185–198.

Horner, D. (1980). The effects of an environmental "enrichment" program on the behavior of institutionalized profoundly retarded children. *Journal of Applied Behavior Analysis, 13*, 473–491.

Iwata, B. A., Dorsey, M. F., Slifer, K. J., Bauman, K. E., & Richman, G. S. (1994). Toward a functional analysis of self-injury. *Journal of Applied Behavior Analysis, 27*, 197–209. (Reprinted from *Analysis and Intervention in Developmental Disabilities, 2*, 3–20, 1982).

Jones, R. S. P. (1999). A 10 year follow-up of stereotypic behavior with eight participants. *Behavioral Interventions, 14*, 45–54.

Kanner, L. (1943). Autistic disturbances of affective contact. *Nervous Child, 2*, 217–250.

Kennedy, C. H., & Souza, G. (1995). Functional analysis and treatment of eye poking. *Journal of Applied Behavior Analysis, 28*, 27–37.

Liu-Gitz, L., & Banda, D. R. (2010). A replication of the RIRD strategy to decrease vocal stereotypy in a student with autism. *Behavioral Interventions, 25*, 77–87.

Lovaas, O. I., Newsom, C. D., & Hickman, C. (1987). Self-stimulatory behavior and perceptual reinforcement. *Journal of Applied Behavior Analysis, 20*, 45–68.

Lovaas, O. I., Schaeffer, B., & Simmons, J. Q. (1965). Building social behavior in autistic children by use of electric shock. *Journal of Experimental Research in Personality, 1*, 99–109.

Maag, J. W., Rutherford, R. B., Wolchik, S. A., & Parks, B. T. (1986). Sensory extinction and overcorrection in suppressing self-stimulation: A preliminary comparison of efficacy and generalization. *Education & Treatment of Children, 9*, 189–201.

Mace, F. C., & Belfiore, P. (1990). Behavioral momentum in the treatment of escape-motivated stereotypy. *Journal of Applied Behavior Analysis, 23*, 507–514.

Matson, J. L., & Dempsey, T. (2009). The nature and treatment of compulsions, obsessions, and rituals in people with developmental disabilities. *Research in Developmental Disabilities, 30*, 603–611.

McDougle, C. J., Kresch, L. E., Goodman, W. K., Naylor, S. T., Volkmar, D. J., Cohen, D. J., et al. (1995). A case-controlled study of repetitive thoughts and behavior in adults with autistic disorder and obsessive-compulsive disorder. *The American Journal of Psychiatry, 152*, 772–777.

Militerni, R., Bravaccio, C., Falco, C., Fico, C., & Palermo, M. T. (2002). Repetitive behaviors in autistic disorder. *European Child & Adolescent Psychiatry, 11*, 210–218.

Neisworth, J. T., Hunt, F. M., Gallop, H. R., & Madle, R. A. (1985). Reinforcer displacement: A preliminary study of the clinical application of the CRF/EXT effect. *Behavior Modification, 9*, 103–115.

Paisey, T. J., Whitney, R. B., & Wainczak, S. M. (1993). Noninvasive behavioral treatment of self-injurious hand stereotypy in a child with Rett syndrome. *Behavioral Residential Treatment, 8*, 133–145.

Patel, M. R., Carr, J. E., Kim, C., Robles, A., & Eastridge, D. (2000). Functional analysis of aberrant behavior maintained by automatic reinforcement: Assessments of specific sensory reinforcers. *Research in Developmental Disabilities, 21*, 393–407.

Piazza, C. C., Adelinis, J. D., Hanley, G. P., Goh, H. L., & Delia, M. D. (2000). An evaluation of the effects of matched stimuli on behavior maintained by automatic reinforcement. *Journal of Applied Behavior Analysis, 33*, 13–27.

Piazza, C. C., Fisher, W. W., Hanley, G. P., LeBlanc, L. A., Worsdell, A. S., Lindauer, S. E., et al. (1998). Treatment of pica through multiple analyses of its reinforcing functions. *Journal of Applied Behavior Analysis, 31*, 165–189.

Pyles, D. A. M., Riordan, M. M., & Bailey, J. S. (1997). The stereotypy analysis: An instrument for examining environmental variables associated with differential rates of stereotypic behavior. *Research in Developmental Disabilities, 18*, 11–38.

Rapp, J. T. (2007). Further evaluation of methods to identify matched stimulation. *Journal of Applied Behavior Analysis, 40*, 73–88.

Rapp, J. T., Patel, M. R., Ghezzi, P. M., O'Flaherty, C. H., & Titterington, C. J. (2009). Establishing stimulus control of vocal stereotypy displayed by young children with autism. *Behavioral Interventions, 24*, 85–105.

Rapp, J. T., & Vollmer, T. R. (2006). Stereotypy I: A review of behavioral assessment and treatment. *Research in Developmental Disabilities, 26*, 527–547.

Rincover, A. (1978). Sensory extinction: A procedure for eliminating self-stimulatory behavior in developmentally disabled children. *Journal of Abnormal Child Psychology, 6*, 299–310.

Rincover, A., Cook, R., Peoples, A., & Packard, D. (1979). Sensory extinction and sensory reinforcement principles for programming multiple adaptive behaviour change. *Journal of Applied Behavior Analysis, 12*, 221–233.

Rincover, A., Newsom, C. D., & Carr, E. G. (1979). Using sensory extinction procedures in the treatment of compulsivelike behavior of developmentally disabled children. *Journal of Consulting and Clinical Psychology, 47*, 695–701.

Ringdahl, J. E., Andelman, M. S., Kisukawa, K., Winborn, L. C., Barretto, A., & Wacker, D. P. (2002). Evaluation and treatment of covert stereotypy. *Behavioral Interventions, 17*, 43–49.

Ringdahl, J. E., Vollmer, T. R., Marcus, B. A., & Roane, H. S. (1997). An analogue evaluation of environmental enrichment: The role of stimulus preference. *Journal of Applied Behavior Analysis, 30*, 203–216.

Ringdahl, J. E., Wacker, D. P., Berg, W. K., & Harding, J. W. (2001). Repetitive behaviour disorders in persons with developmental disabilities. In D. Woods & R. Miltenberger (Eds.), *Tic disorders, trichotillomania, and other repetitive behavior disorders:*

Behavioral approaches to analysis and treatment (pp. 297–314). Boston: Kluwer.

Shore, B. A., Iwata, B. A., DeLeoin, I. G., Kahng, S. W., & Smith, R. G. (1997). An analysis of reinforcer substitutability using object manipulation and self-injury as competing responses. *Journal of Applied Behavior Analysis, 30*, 21–41.

Sidener, T. M., Carr, J. E., & Firth, A. M. (2005). Superimposition and withholding of edible consequences as treatment for automatically reinforced stereotypy. *Journal of Applied Behavior Analysis, 38*, 121–124.

Sigafoos, J., Green, V. A., Payne, D., O'Reilly, M. E., & Lancioni, G. E. (2009). A classroom-based antecedent intervention reduces obsessive-repetitive behavior in an adolescent with autism. *Clinical Case Studies, 8*, 3–13.

Smith, M. D. (1987). Treatment of pica in an adult disabled by autism by differential reinforcement of incompatible behavior. *Journal of Behavior Therapy and Experimental Psychiatry, 18*, 285–288.

Smith, R. G., Iwata, B. A., Vollmer, T. R., & Zarcone, J. R. (1993). Experimental analysis and treatment of multiply controlled self-injury. *Journal of Applied Behavior Analysis, 26*, 183–196.

Spitz, R. A., & Wolfe, K. M. (1949). Autoeroticism. *Psychoanalytic Studies of the Child, 3*, 85–120.

Stone, A. A. (1964). Consciousness: Altered levels in blind retarded children. *Psychomatic Medicine, 26*, 14–19.

Taylor, B. A., Hoch, H., & Weissman, M. (2005). The analysis and treatment of vocal stereotypy in a child with autism. *Behavioral Interventions, 20*, 239–253.

Thompson, T., Hackenberg, T., Cerutti, D., Baker, D., & Axtell, S. (1994). Opioid antagonist effects on self-injury in adults with mental retardation: Response form and location as determinants of medication effects. *American Journal on Mental Retardation, 99*, 85–102.

Tiger, J. H., Toussaint, K. A., & Kliebert, M. L. (2009). Rituals and stereotypies. In J. Matson (Ed.), *Applied behavior analysis for children with autism spectrum disorders*. New York: Springer.

Turner, M. (1999). Annotation: Repetitive behavior in autism: A review of psychological research. *Journal of Child Psychology and Psychiatry, 40*, 839–849.

Tustin, R. D. (1995). The effects of advance notice of activity transitions on stereotypic behavior. *Journal of Applied Behavior Analysis, 28*, 91–92.

Van Camp, C. M., Lerman, D. C., Kelley, M. E., Roane, H. S., Contrucci, S. A., & Vorndran, C. M. (2000). Further analysis of idiosyncratic antecedent influences during the assessment and treatment of problem behavior. *Journal of Applied Behavior Analysis, 33*, 207–221.

Van Houten, R. (1993). The use of wrist weights to reduce self-injury maintained by sensory reinforcement. *Journal of Applied Behavior Analysis, 26*, 197–203.

Vaughn, M. E., & Michael, J. E. (1982). Automatic reinforcement: An important but ignored concept. *Behaviorism, 10*, 217–227.

Vollmer, T. R. (1994). The concept of automatic reinforcement: Implications for behavioural research in developmental disabilities. *Research in Developmental Disabilities, 15*, 187–207.

Vollmer, T. R., Marcus, B. A., & LeBlanc, L. (1994). Treatment of self-injury and hand mouthing following inconclusive functional analyses. *Journal of Applied Behavior Analysis, 27*, 331–344.

Interventions to Treat Feeding Problems in Children with Autism Spectrum Disorders: A Comprehensive Review

31

Laura J. Seiverling, Keith E. Williams, John Ward-Horner, and Peter Sturmey

Feeding problems in children with autism spectrum disorder (ASD) are common and can be distressing for parents and other caregivers who are concerned that their children's diets are nutritionally inadequate and who often face mealtime behavior problems. This chapter will (a) review the definition and epidemiology of common feeding problems found in children with ASD as well as the interventions to treat them; (b) examine feeding problems in terms of functional analyses, treatment components, and component analyses of treatment packages; (c) discuss the measurement of long-term treatment gains, parent training, generalization, inclusion of social validity measures, initial assessments, and measurement of corollary responses in the current intervention literature; and (d) suggest areas for future researchers.

Definitions and Etiology of Common Feeding Problems

The most commonly researched feeding problem in children with ASD is food selectivity, which is the refusal to eat certain types of foods (e.g., meats, vegetables) or textures (e.g., crunchy) and has been associated with mealtime behavior problems (e.g., aggression, tantrums, throwing food) (McCartney, Anderson, & English, 2005). Williams and Foxx (2007) proposed that food selectivity may be an example of stereotypical responding, a characteristic of ASD. Environmental variables such as family diet, parent–child interactions, mealtime habits, mealtime structure, as well as biological factors such as gastroesophageal reflux and physical impairment, are associated with the development, maintenance, and exacerbation of food selectivity (Ahearn, Kerwin, Eicher, & Lukens, 2001). Children classified with

total food refusal eat nothing or almost nothing. One could also conceptualize food refusal as an extreme variant of food selectivity in that a child may refuse to eat a majority of foods that fall outside a narrow range of food items. The latter definition seems to be the case for many children with ASD. Therefore, in this review, we classified interventions for food selectivity and food refusal together.

Another feeding problem is liquid avoidance, the failure to consume sufficient fluids (Patel, Piazza, Kelly, Ochsner, & Santana, 2001). Like food selectivity and refusal, children who avoid liquids may also exhibit maladaptive behavior when presented with non-preferred or new liquids. In addition to constipation, potential effects of failure to consume adequate fluids are vomiting, and restricted caloric intake (Luiselli, Ricciardi, & Gilligan, 2005).

Packing involves the retention of food in the mouth for protracted durations (Buckley & Newchok, 2005). Patel, Piazza, Layer, Coleman, and Swartzwelder (2005) conducted a study examining the effects of texture on packing and suggested that while packing may occasionally be an avoidance behavior, similar to crying, head-turning, or pushing away the spoon, packing may also occur because the child does not have the requisite oral motor skills needed to eat higher texture foods. Thus, packing may be a function of response effort required to consume higher textures.

The least researched feeding problem in those with ASD is rapid eating, which occurs when one eats a meal in a very short period of time. Side effects include vomiting, aspiration, and social stigmatization. McGimsey (1977) reported that rapid eating is common in those with developmental disabilities. Several studies have evaluated treatments for rapid eating in those without ASD (Lennox, Miltenberger, & Donnelly, 1987; Wright & Vollmer, 2002), and Anglesea, Hoch, and Taylor (2008) conducted the first study on this problem in adolescents with ASD.

L.J. Seiverling (✉)
Department of Psychology, Queens College and The Graduate Center, City University of New York, Flushing, NY 11367, USA
e-mail: ljs1284@gmail.com

J.L. Matson, P. Sturmey (eds.), *International Handbook of Autism and Pervasive Developmental Disorders*, Autism and Child Psychopathology Series, DOI 10.1007/978-1-4419-8065-6_31, © Springer Science+Business Media, LLC 2011

Prevalence

Ledford and Gast (2006) found seven descriptive studies examining the prevalence of feeding problems in children with ASD (Ahearn, Castine, Nault, & Green, 2001; Bowers, 2002; Collins et al., 2003; Cornish, 1998, 2002; Field, Garland, & Williams, 2003; Shreck, Williams, & Smith, 2004). The incidence of feeding problems in these studies ranged from 46 to 89% of children with ASD. No studies have reported the prevalence of feeding problems in adults with ASD. Ledford and Gast defined feeding problems as the selective acceptance of food or refusal to eat many or most foods with no known medical explanation. This definition is limited in a number of ways. First, while it defined food selectivity and food refusal, it did not address other feeding problems, such as liquid avoidance, packing, and rapid eating. Second, the definition did not account for the medical or biological etiologies that have been shown to precipitate or maintain many feeding problems (Ahearn, Kerwin, et al., 2001). Feeding problems may be better defined if researchers use the presence of the behavior and not the etiology to classify feeding problems because medical issues may or may not precipitate a feeding problem.

Often, prevalence studies of feeding problems among children with ASD used questionnaires and anecdotal evidence. Ahearn, Castine, et al. (2001) criticized this approach by claiming that subject selection procedures were often not well specified and third-party reports could be inaccurate. Thus, Ahearn and his colleagues addressed these criticisms through direct assessment of food acceptance in 30 children, aged 3–14 years, with autism or pervasive developmental disorder-not otherwise specified (PDD-NOS) using Munk and Repp's (1994) procedure. Ahearn and colleagues presented 12 food items (i.e. three fruits, vegetables, starches, and proteins) with one item in each session presented in puree texture across six sessions. They presented children with 120 bites during the assessment, with 30 of the bites presented in pureed texture. They classified low acceptance as eating less than 30 bites and moderate acceptance as acceptance of 31–60 bites. To assess food selectivity, Ahearn and colleagues analyzed acceptance within food groups. Of the children assessed, 87% exhibited low or moderate food acceptance and 57% exhibited particular forms of food selectivity by type (e.g., eating primarily starches) or texture (e.g., only crunchy foods).

Both Ledford and Gast's review and Ahearn, Castine, et al.'s studies indicated that feeding problems are common in children with ASD. While previous research examined prevalence of food selectivity, future research should also examine prevalence of other less researched feeding problems such as liquid avoidance, packing, and rapid eating. The prevalence of these additional feeding problems is unknown.

Functional Analyses

The following section discusses the development, maintenance, and treatment of feeding problems in terms of functional analyses. A functional analysis involves the manipulation of antecedent and consequent variables to determine their influence on a problem behavior (Miltenberger, 2004). Often, researchers conduct functional analyses in order to evaluate possible functions of problem behavior.

Najdowski, Wallace, Doney, and Ghezzi (2003) and Levin and Carr (2001) conducted functional analyses to examine the function of mealtime problem behavior prior to intervention. The functional analysis conducted by Najdowski et al. (2003) involved four conditions: no interaction, attention, play, and escape conditions. In the no interaction condition, the participant's mother presented five bites of foods not chosen during a preference assessment (i.e., non-preferred foods), gave no demands to take bites, and provided no consequences for refusal. In the attention condition, again, the mother presented bites and gave no demands; however, when the participant engaged in refusal responses, the mother delivered attention (e.g., "I know the food is so gross."). During the play condition, the mother presented both preferred items and non-preferred items; there were no consequences for refusal and the mother provided non-contingent positive attention every 30 s. In the escape condition, the mother provided several prompts to initiate self-feeding. She delivered praise when food was accepted and removed the plate of non-preferred foods temporarily contingent on food refusal. In Levin and Carr's (2001) functional analysis, they presented bite-sized portions of foods determined as either preferred (e.g., items selected during an initial preference assessment) or non-preferred (i.e., items not selected during the preference assessment) to the child. If the child consumed a bite, the experimenter praised the child and offered more bites. If the child did not eat the bite, the experimenter presented the bite again every 10 s; however, if the child engaged in problem behavior, the experimenter temporarily removed the food and turned away from the child. In both studies, researchers identified escape from the demand of eating non-preferred foods as the function of maladaptive mealtime behavior.

Despite the small number of intervention studies which included functional analyses, escape from non-preferred or new foods appears to be a common function of the problem behavior. Although data to date support this conclusion, it may be possible that for some children escape from pain or escape from foods with a history of being paired with pain (e.g., gastroesophageal reflux) may also be an important function. Ahearn (2003) suggested that if a feeding problem is not maintained by escape or if a feeding problem is mild, escape extinction (EE), the typical treatment for escape-maintained behavior, may not be a necessary component for intervention. When planning future interventions, researchers may find functional analyses useful in identifying the most appropriate treatment components.

Motivating Operations

Several studies have speculated the role of motivating operations in feeding problems. According to Michael (2007), a motivating operation is an environmental variable that alters the reinforcing effects of a stimulus and alters the current frequency of all behavior reinforced by that stimulus. Often in intervention studies, researchers do not report the use of behavior change tactics such as appetite manipulation prior to intervention meals. Two exceptions are Ahearn, Kerwin, et al. (2001) and Piazza et al. (2002). When describing behavioral treatments for pediatric feeding disorders, Linscheid (2006) stated "Whereas natural consequence and specific behavioral procedures are important in treatment... inducing hunger in the child is almost always as or more important for success than the specific behavioral contingencies utilized," (p. 13). Satiation may occur as a result of a child drinking or eating between meals or scheduled snacks. Unfortunately, this practice is common and may undermine interventions for food selectivity if children consume foods prior to treatment meals because any extra caloric intake may decrease motivation to eat during the meal. Levin and Carr (2001) specifically manipulated access to preferred foods prior to an intervention involving positive reinforcement to increase acceptance of non-preferred foods to evaluate the role of appetite manipulation in combination with a treatment package. Participants increased consumption of non-preferred foods only when researchers limited prior access to preferred foods, indicating that appetite manipulation influences treatment efficacy. Thus, future researchers should continue to examine the role of motivating operations perhaps by varying periods of deprivation prior to treatment meals as well as examine the effects of deprivation prior to various treatments, particularly those with and without the use of EE.

Piazza et al. (2002) and Ahearn (2003) also discussed the role of potential motivating operations within simultaneous presentation treatment packages. Piazza and her colleagues argued that a non-preferred food may act as an aversive stimulus and thus, by combining the non-preferred food with the preferred food, the aversiveness may reduce through flavor–flavor conditioning in which preference for novel foods occurs as a result of being paired with preferred foods. This notion of flavor–flavor conditioning indicates a potential respondent mechanism involved in the treatment of food selectivity and refusal. In general, studies on conditioned food preferences involve conditioning phases in which researchers present preferred foods either simultaneously or sequentially with a flavor. Next, they present the flavor alone in a test phase to determine if preference has developed for the flavor. Studies in both humans and non-human animals have shown that increased preferences for new foods may develop after pairing the novel foods with preferred foods (Holman, 1975; Zellner, Rozin, Aron, & Kulish, 1983). For instance, Zellner et al. (1983) presented college students with a variety of teas, some with sweetener and some without. Next, they presented the students with all of the teas without sweetener and found students preferred the teas that had previously been mixed with sweetener.

In order to examine flavor–flavor conditioning, the experimenter must test the non-preferred food in the absence of the preferred food to determine if the participant has developed a preference for the initial non-preferred food. Whereas Piazza et al.'s (2002) study did not do so, Ahearn (2003) did this when conducting a study in which he presented preferred condiments with non-preferred items. When Ahearn removed the condiments, consumption reduced back to baseline levels. Thus, Ahearn rejected the notion of flavor–flavor conditioning as a mechanism involved in simultaneous presentation because had flavor–flavor conditioning occurred, the participant would have consumed the non-preferred item when Ahearn removed the preferred condiment. Ahearn's (2003) study was the first to directly examine flavor–flavor conditioning in children with food selectivity and although his findings do not support the notion of conditioned preferences developing through flavor–flavor conditioning, future researchers should further examine the potential role of flavor–flavor conditioning in treatment of food selectivity. Specifically, it may be interesting to see if the use of different preferred foods (e.g., candy instead of condiments) paired with non-preferred foods renders similar results.

Stimulus Control

While not specifically discussed in the feeding intervention literature, feeding problems may also be viewed in terms of stimulus control. Stimulus control occurs when the frequency, latency, duration, or amplitude of a behavior is altered by the presence or absence of an antecedent stimulus (Cooper, Heron, & Heward, 2007). Thus, particularly in the case of food selectivity and food refusal as well as liquid avoidance, a small number of items (e.g., crunchy foods or a limited number of highly preferred foods) may exert strong stimulus control over feeding behavior. Researchers often use fading as a component of treatment packages for feeding problems. Fading may assist in transfer of stimulus control to a larger number of foods or portions. It involves gradually increasing the bite size of non-preferred foods or by reducing the preferred foods presented as done in some studies on simultaneous presentation. Those delivering the meal may also exert stimulus control. For instance, when Patel et al. (2001) introduced the participant's mother into the session, the participant's mouth cleans (no visible food or liquid in the participant's mouth 30 s after acceptance) decreased from 100 to 0%. Following the parent-implemented session, experimenters reintroduced the therapist to the session. They then slowly faded the mother's presence into the treatment sessions in the following fading steps: (a) the mother was in the room with the therapist, (b) the mother conducted sessions with the therapist present, and (c) the mother conducted sessions alone. While other factors may have been related to the reduction in percentage of the child's mouth cleans (e.g., parent not implementing the procedure properly), it may also be the case that the therapist had acquired stimulus control over the mouth clean response and the mother had not. Using this assumption, the experimenters faded in the presence of the mother in order to transfer stimulus control from the therapist to the parent.

Summary

Examining feeding problems in terms of functional analyses, motivating operations, and transfer of stimulus control may enhance the understanding of why certain treatment packages are more effective than other packages at treating feeding problems. Examining interventions in terms of functional analyses and motivating operations may help identify potential treatment components necessary for successful intervention. Emphasizing transfer of stimulus control to novel foods, to portion sizes, and to novel people implementing meals will enhance generalization of treatment gains. Thus, future researchers should consider the behavior analytic mechanisms that may play a role in the amelioration of feeding problems in those with ASD.

Literature Search

The first author conducted a systematic literature review using PsychInfo ©. The search used combinations of the following terms: autism, pervasive developmental disorder, eating, feeding, pediatric feeding disorder, food selectivity, food acceptance, food consumption, and fluid consumption. This search identified 20 peer-reviewed intervention studies. There were 14 food selectivity studies, three liquid avoidance studies, two packing studies, and one rapid eating study (See Table 31.1). Some included additional participants without an ASD diagnosis (Ahearn, Kerwin, et al.,

2001; McCartney et al., 2005; Patel et al., 2005) and many had participants with dual diagnoses of ASD and other disabilities or medical problems (Ahearn, 2003; Anderson & McMillan, 2001; Anglesea et al., 2008; Freeman & Piazza, 1998; Hagopian, Farrell, & Amari, 1996; Levin & Carr, 2001; McCartney et al., 2005; Patel et al., 2005; Piazza et al., 2002). Interventions for feeding problems included antecedent- and consequence-based treatment components. Most interventions were multi-component packages and involved both antecedent- and consequence-based components. The following section first defines various intervention methods. Subsequent sections identify various components and packages to treat specific feeding problems.

Consequence-Based Interventions

Common consequence manipulations included use of differential reinforcement, escape extinction (EE), response cost (RC), and reinforcement fading/schedule thinning (e.g., increasing number of bites before reinforcement is delivered). Differential reinforcement entailed (a) the delivery of verbal praise, tangibles, preferred foods, or meal termination following the display of a desired behavior, such as eating a bite, and/or (b) removal of reinforcement for undesired behavior (Ledford & Gast, 2006). The papers generally described differential reinforcement procedures as differential reinforcement of alternative responses (DRA); these papers generally did not specify other procedures, such as differential reinforcement of other responses (DRO) and differential reinforcement of incompatible responses (DRI); however, the procedures may often be conceptualized as DRI, for example, an acceptance response could be considered an incompatible response to food refusal. Sometimes, researchers use the term sequential food presentation to describe using preferred food items to reinforce eating non-preferred items (Kern & Marder, 1996; Piazza et al., 2002). Completion of a non-preferred or low-probability response such as eating a non-preferred bite before allowing access to a preferred activity such as eating a preferred food is also an example of the Premack principle (Premack, 1962).

Escape from eating by crying, yelling, hitting, or simply waiting and failing to consume food may maintain feeding problems. Escape extinction (EE) also known as escape prevention (Ahearn, 2002; Paul, Williams, Riegel, & Gibbons, 2007) involves not allowing a child to leave the meal until the child has consumed a specific quantity of food – sometimes only one bite. EE typically involves non-removal of spoon until the child consumes the food and sometimes involves physical guidance, which consists of manually guiding acceptance of presented food often by placing pressure in the front of the mandibular junction of the jaw (Ahearn, Kerwin, et al., 2001). EE is often combined with other

Table 31.1 Feeding intervention studies in children with autism

Study	Research design	Procedures	Parent training	Participant/s	Results	Feeding problem
Gentry and Luiselli (2008)	Changing criterion	Goal setting, high-probability demands, PR, fading	Yes	4-year-old boy w/PDD	Increase in acceptance	Food selectivity
Patel et al. (2007)	ABAB design	High-probability demands, PR, fading	Yes	4-year-old boy w/PDD	Increase in acceptance	Food selectivity
Paul et al. (2007)	Changing criterion	Repeated taste exposure, EE, fading	Yes	3½-year-old boy w/autism 5-year-old girl w/autism	Increase in acceptance	Food selectivity
Buckley et al. (2005)	Multielement	Response cost with NCP or DR, fading	No	5-year-old boy w/autism	Increase in acceptance	Food selectivity
McCartney et al. (2005)	Changing criterion	EE, DR, fading	Yes	7-year-old boy w/autism and mild ID w/significant visual impairment 5-year-old boy w/autism 5-year-old boy w/autism and mild ID 1 other participant (not ASD)	Increase in acceptance	Food selectivity
Ahearn (2003)	Multiple baseline across stimuli, ABAB	Simultaneous presentation	No	14-year-old boy w/autism and profound ID	Increase vegetable acceptance	Food selectivity
Najdowski et al. (2003)	Changing criterion across settings	DR, EE, fading	Yes	5-year-old boy/autism	Increase in acceptance	Food selectivity
Ahearn (2002)	Changing criterion	DR, EE	No	4 boys, 2 girls; 4–11 years old 4 autism; 2 PDD-NOS	Increase in acceptance	Food selectivity
Piazza et al. (2002)	Alternating treatments	Simultaneous and sequential presentation, EE, PR	No	10-year-old boy/autism 11-year-old girl w/PDD-NOS, severe to profound ID, and seizure disorder 8-year-old boy w/PDD-NOS, ADHD, severe ID	Increase in acceptance	Food selectivity
Ahearn et al. (2001)	ABAC	Two forms of EE, PR	Yes	4-year-old boy w/PDD-NOS 1 other participant (not ASD)	Increase in acceptance	Food selectivity
Anderson and McMillan (2001)	ABAB	DR, EE, fading	Yes	5-year-old boy w/PDD-NOS and severe ID	Increase in fruit acceptance	Food selectivity
Levin and Carr (2001)	Multiple baseline across participants changing criterion	DR, establishing operations, fading, Premack principle	No	6-year-old boy w/autism 5-year-old boy/w autism 6-year-old girl w/PDD-NOS *All participants had moderate to severe ID	Increase in acceptance	Food selectivity
Freeman and Piazza (1998)	Alternating treatments	DR, EE, fading	No	6-year-old girl w/autism moderate ID, cerebellar atrophy and mild right hemiplegia	Increase in acceptance	Food selectivity
Kern and Marder (1996)	Adapted alternating treatments	Simultaneous and sequential presentation, EE	Yes	7-year-old boy w/PDD	Increase in acceptance	Food selectivity
Luiselli et al. (2005)	Changing criterion	Liquid fading, paced instructional prompting, EE, PR	No	4-year-old girl w/autism	Increase in consumption	Liquid avoidance
Patel et al. (2001)	Reversal and CC	DR, EE, fading, PR, modeling	Yes	6-year-old boy w/PDD	Increase in consumption	Liquid avoidance

Table 31.1 (continued)

Study	Research design	Procedures	Parent training	Participant/s	Results	Feeding problem
Hagopian et al. (1996)	Reversal and CC	Backward chaining, fading, PR	No	12-year-old boy w/autism, moderate MR, life-threatening GI conditions	Increase in consumption	Liquid avoidance
Buckley and Newchok (2005)	Reversal design	Simultaneous presentation DR, response cost	No	9-year-old girl w/autism	Reduced packing	Packing
Patel et al. (2005)	Reversal design	Texture manipulation	Yes	4-year-old boy with GER and autism 2 other participants (not ASD)	Reduced packing	Packing
Anglesea et al. (2008)	ABAB design	Pager prompt	No	15-year-old boy w/autism with rumination and GER 19-year-old boy w/autism with rumination and GER 15-year-old boy w/autism	Reduction in rapidity	Rapid eating

CC – Changing criterion
DR – Differential reinforcement
EE – Escape extinction
ID – Intellectual disability
NCP – Non-contingent presentation
PR – Positive reinforcement

intervention components such as DRA and stimulus fading. It has also become increasingly popular to attempt to treat feeding problems using alternatives to EE if possible (Ahearn, 2002, 2003; Gentry & Luiselli, 2008; Levin & Carr, 2001; Najdowski et al., 2003); however, when some of these treatments have failed, researches have implemented EE to the treatment components already in place.

The functions of treatment components are not always obvious. While authors often used the term "EE," reduction of escape responses by physical guidance or non-removal of spoon following escape responses may also be conceptualized as positive punishment. Further, interventionists may find physical guidance challenging to implement due to initial high-frequency interfering responses. Further, physical guidance is sometimes associated with pain or even injury (Gentry & Luiselli, 2008). Non-removal of spoon may also be difficult to implement as meals must be extended until the child consumes the required bite(s) prior to meal termination, which could potentially take hours. Due to these challenges when implementing EE, parents may be unsuccessful when trying to implement EE in the home and they may consider EE unacceptable (Gentry & Luiselli, 2008; McCartney et al., 2005).

RC is another consequence-based intervention which involves allowing the participant to engage in a preferred activity (e.g., watching a video) before presentation of a low-probability request (e.g., eating a bite) and removal of the preferred activity contingent upon non-compliance. In an intervention to reduce packing, RC involved removing a preferred item to which the child had access (e.g., video) when packing occurred (Buckley, Strunck, & Newchok, 2005).

Antecedent-Based Interventions

Researchers implement antecedent-based interventions prior to responses occurring. Antecedent interventions in the feeding literature included simultaneous food presentation (Ahearn, 2003), stimulus fading (Luiselli et al., 2005), repeated taste exposure (Paul et al., 2007), and techniques based on high-probability instructional sequences (Gentry & Luiselli, 2008; Patel et al., 2007). Simultaneous presentation involves embedding a non-preferred food within a preferred food (Piazza et al., 2002) or placing the undisguised, non-preferred food with the preferred item on the same spoon (Kern & Marder, 1996).

Antecedent stimulus fading procedures involve transfer of stimulus control from preferred to non-preferred stimuli. These procedures may involve gradually increasing bite sizes, gradually manipulating food texture, and gradually decreasing the amount of preferred food presented with the non-preferred food item (Kern & Marder, 1996). Repeated taste exposure is a recently used antecedent manipulation. Wardle, Herrera, Cooke, and Gibson (2003) exposed typically developing children to one of the three conditions; (a) they gave some children a sticker when tasting a red pepper repeatedly, (b) they repeatedly presented slices of red pepper without reinforcement to another group, and (c) they gave children in the control group two exposures to the pepper in pre- and post-test sessions. Children in the first and second groups reported liking the red pepper more than control group children. Thus, mere exposure to novel foods may lead to liking novel foods, regardless of reinforcement contingencies. Paul et al. (2007) successfully extended this procedure when they used repeated taste exposure, fading, and EE procedure to treat food selectivity in children with ASD.

Using a high-probability request sequence, also known as behavioral momentum, involves the presentation of preferred activities, or high-probability responses, before presentation of non-preferred activities or low-probability responses (Ledford & Gast, 2006). A few studies used this procedure to treat feeding problems in children with ASD (Gentry & Luiselli, 2008; Patel et al., 2007).

Food Selectivity and Refusal

Differential Reinforcement, Escape Extinction, and Fading Packages

Most food selectivity/food refusal treatment studies used treatment packages. For example, Freeman and Piazza (1998) combined stimulus fading, reinforcement, and EE to treat food refusal in a 6-year-old girl with ASD and moderate intellectual disability (ID) who did not reliably eat. Differential reinforcement involved termination of the meal following acceptance and fading involved gradually increasing the amount of food presented by 5 or 10% increments. EE involved manual guidance if the child did not comply. In this study, researchers terminated treatment meals if the child ate the food presented or after 45 min, even if the food was not eaten. Therapists first presented fruits because parents reported that the participant accepted fruits more than other items. When the child consumed 50% or more of an age-appropriate portion of fruit, therapists subsequently added proteins, starches, and vegetables in a multi-element design alternating between baseline and treatment sessions. Following intervention, the child ate more food and complied with prompting procedures.

Anderson and McMillan (2001) demonstrated that parental implementation of a similar treatment package, which involved EE, differential reinforcement, and fading increased acceptance of pureed fruits and reduced meal-related problem behavior in a 5-year-old boy with ASD and severe ID. Parents presented both preferred and non-preferred foods during mealtimes. Differential reinforcement involved statements of praise (e.g., "good job taking your bite!") and access to a preferred item (i.e., milk) when the child accepted a bite. EE included non-removal of spoon and placement of the bite into the child's mouth when he opened it, even if it was to cry or yawn. Fading involved gradually increasing number of bites of fruit required before

meal termination and was based on a 60% reduction in disruptive responses for two consecutive sessions; however, parents often increased the required bites prior to this criterion being met. Following intervention, the participant consumed age-appropriate amounts of fruit (approximately 4 oz per meal).

Najdowski et al. (2003) trained parents to conduct both a functional analysis and a treatment package to reduce food selectivity in a 5-year-old boy with ASD. As mentioned earlier, after an initial functional analysis, researchers concluded that removal of non-preferred foods maintained the food refusal. Treatment included (a) DRA using meal termination following acceptance; (b) reinforcement schedule thinning, involving increasing the number of bites required to consume prior to meal termination; (c) EE in both home and restaurant settings. In addition, Najdowski et al. systematically introduced multiple non-preferred foods to simulate a dinner meal composed of multiple foods. Treatment led to an increase in consumption of five target non-preferred foods in both home and restaurant environments.

McCartney et al. (2005) also trained caregivers to conduct a differential reinforcement (i.e., verbal praise, access to preferred foods, and meal termination when reinforcement criterion was met), EE, and fading treatment package to increase food acceptance in three children with ASD and one typically developing child, all of whom had food selectivity. They taught caregivers to ignore all interruptions and expulsions and to present the instruction "take a bite" approximately once per minute contingent on refusal. Originally, meals were one bite of one target food. When latency until acceptance was less than 20 s and there were no expulsions, they increased the reinforcement criterion by one bite. Initially, trained therapists presented meals. Parents/caregivers then presented meals when their child accepted eight bites of two target foods with latency until acceptance of each bite less than 20 s during therapist-fed meals. When caregivers began sessions, the reinforcement criterion started again at one bite of the first target food before gradually increasing reinforcement criterion. All children increased acceptance of target foods, expelled fewer bites, and exhibited a decrease in latency to accept bites. When the participant accepted eight bites of each target food in caregiver-fed meals the intervention was complete. Experimenters instructed caregivers to continue using the procedure with various foods at home.

Differential Reinforcement and Escape Extinction Packages

Ahearn, Kerwin, et al. (2001) compared the effectiveness of two forms of EE, non-removal of spoon and physical guidance, on food refusal in one 4-year-old boy with ASD and another participant without ASD. In all conditions, they reinforced eating bites without expulsion with contingent social interaction and access to preferred items. They presented 20 bites of four pureed foods, one from each of the four food categories during each meal. They also used non-removal of spoon before physical guidance with one participant and physical guidance followed by non-removal of spoon with another participant. Thus, the experimenter used ABAC and ACAB designs with the first child and the second child, respectively. In the A phase, they presented the spoon simultaneously with the verbal prompt to open; they presented social interaction and access to preferred items following acceptance, and refusal led to removal of the spoon from the lip and no access to preferred stimuli. In the B phase, they implemented EE using non-removal of the spoon. In the C phase, physical guidance was used. Both forms of EE led to an increase in percentage of bites accepted; however, physical guidance facilitated acquisition of acceptance. All responding was slightly more variable during EE with non-removal of spoon. When given a choice as to which treatment parents would like to be trained to implement, both parents chose the second treatment implemented with their child. Ahearn, Kerwin, et al. mentioned that the sequence of treatment implementation could have influenced parental choice since acquisition of acceptance and reduction in disruptive responses were faster during the second treatment phase.

Ahearn (2002) further examined differential reinforcement and EE in the treatment of food selectivity in six children with ASD. They assigned children to either single food item (e.g., banana) or multi-food items (e.g., banana, grape, orange) from the same food group and randomized the order of food presentation. When first presented with differential reinforcement without EE, the children's food acceptance did not meet criterion of at least 80% acceptance and less than 20% of bites with disruption and expulsion. Therefore, the authors assigned participants to either EE with non-removal of spoon or physical guidance. When the children met reinforcement criterion, they presented a new food or food group during generalization probes; the authors then targeted the probed foods. When participants consumed three foods in each of four food groups, intervention was complete. Although acquisition of acceptance was faster for the single food item group, participants in the second group exhibited better generalization of acceptance to previously rejected items.

Response Cost

Buckley et al. (2005) compared two forms of RC to treat food selectivity in a 5-year-old boy with ASD: RC with non-contingent presentation (NCP) of preferred items and RC plus DRA. The RC component involved removal of

a preferred video to which the child had access for 30 s prior to bites; however, researchers could only implement RC if they returned the video to the participant prior to bite presentation so that the video could be removed. Buckley et al. explained that they wanted to examine the use of NCP because of the potential limitation of DRA in which the participant may not meet the criterion for returning the preferred item. In DRA plus RC, they only re-presented the video when the child exhibited a clean mouth following the subsequent bite. In NCP plus RC condition, they presented materials non-contingently. While both procedures increased swallowing and reduced problem behavior, NCP plus RC was superior, perhaps because returning preferred materials non-contingently provided more opportunities to implement RC. Buckley et al. mentioned that they also used fading to increase bite sizes following the completion of the study.

Simultaneous Presentation

In a study involving only an antecedent-based intervention, Ahearn (2003) examined simultaneous presentation in the treatment of mild food selectivity in a 14-year-old boy with ASD. Ahearn conducted a multiple baseline design across non-preferred foods to examine the effectiveness of simultaneous presentation of preferred condiments (e.g., ketchup). During baseline, no condiments were presented. During intervention, Ahearn put condiments on the non-preferred foods and implemented reversals to baseline, in which condiments were not present. Ahearn did not use positive reinforcement (Piazza et al., 2002) or EE (Kern & Marder, 1996) in conjunction with the simultaneous food presentation. The participant's percentage of bites accepted ranged from 0 to 40% during baseline sessions and increased to 100% of bites accepted during simultaneous presentation of preferred condiments with vegetables. Thus, simultaneous presentation alone may be effective in increasing acceptance; however, Ahearn only demonstrated these findings in one participant with mild refusal, and thus, future research with those with more severe selectivity is warranted.

Differential Reinforcement, Fading, and Establishing Operations

Levin and Carr (2001) examined the role of deprivation of preferred food items, prior to intervention meal sessions to treat food selectivity in three children with ASD, all of whom had moderate to severe ID. The intervention involved a multi-component treatment of differential reinforcement and fading. During a preliminary functional analysis, all participants exhibited many problem behaviors in the presence of non-preferred and novel items. Levin and Carr exposed participants to a series of four conditions in the same ABCD sequence in a multiple baseline design. In condition A, researchers gave participants access to preferred foods during the 2 h prior to meals. They also gave access to the foods that would be used as reinforcers during meals for 5 min before the meal began. Thus, they allowed each child to eat one-third to one-half of his or her preferred lunchtime foods freely throughout the morning and during a midmorning snack. Additionally, there was no positive reinforcement for consumption of non-preferred items. They presented a small portion of a non-preferred food and terminated meals either after consumption of the food or after 5 min. In condition B, they permitted no access to preferred foods before meals and no positive reinforcement for consumption of bites. In condition C, they gave access to preferred foods before meals and provided positive reinforcement in which they gave the child a small bite of a preferred food item following consumption of a non-preferred item. In condition D, they gave no access to preferred items before meals and implemented the positive reinforcement contingency. In all conditions, if the child ate the portion of a target food for three consecutive days, the experimenters increased the portion of the target food. Each participant consumed little or none of the target food during conditions A, B, and C. In condition D, all participants consumed the target food and subsequently consumed more grams of the target food as reinforcement criterion increased.

Levin and Carr (2001) conducted a second intervention to control for possible order effects in the first intervention, in which they targeted a second non-preferred food for each participant and removed conditions B and C. They used condition A as a baseline before implementing condition D. They also collected data on problem behavior. Results resembled those in the first intervention and all participants exhibited a higher mean frequency of problem behavior during baseline than during intervention. Thus, this second study eliminated possible order effects as an explanation of the results of experiment 1 and replicated those results with a second non-preferred food. Levin and Carr concluded that the Premack principle-based intervention was only effective when (a) a positive reinforcement contingency was in place and (b) when therapists did not present preferred foods during the interval preceding the training meal. They also suggested this procedure as an alternative to procedures involving EE.

Simultaneous and Sequential Presentation and Escape Extinction

Kern and Marder (1996) compared simultaneous presentation and delayed (sequential) reinforcement in the treatment of food selectivity in a 7-year-old boy with ASD. During the simultaneous presentation condition, the authors presented a

preferred chip simultaneously with non-preferred fruits. In the sequential reinforcement condition, they presented the chip after bites of non-preferred vegetables were eaten. They implemented EE in both conditions and used reinforcement fading (i.e., reducing chip size) in both conditions based on non-occurrence of self-injurious behavior. While both procedures produced an increase in acceptance of non-preferred foods, simultaneous presentation led to a more rapid increase and greater overall increase in acceptance. Although simultaneous presentation appeared to be the superior treatment, the rapid increase may have been a function of food type as participants may have preferred the sweeter taste of fruits compared to vegetables.

Simultaneous and Sequential Presentation and Positive Reinforcement

Piazza et al. (2002) also compared simultaneous and sequential presentation of non-preferred and preferred foods to reduce food selectivity in three children with ASD. They included positive reinforcement in both procedures. For two children, they presented two foods from four food groups with simultaneous presentation and two foods from each of the food groups in sequential presentation. They evaluated only one non-preferred item for an additional participant. Thus, they targeted eight foods in each procedure. For two of the participants, simultaneous presentation led to a rapid increase in acceptance. For the other participant, there was an increase in acceptance for simultaneous presentation after implementing EE with physical guidance. There was an increase in acceptance in the sequential presentation condition for the child exposed to only one non-preferred food, but only after acceptance increased during the simultaneous presentation condition. After exposure to both the simultaneous and the sequential presentation procedure in a multi-element design, they presented the participants with the foods initially presented in the sequential condition in a simultaneous procedure alone. Acceptance immediately increased, indicating that the simultaneous procedure and not just the foods presented within that condition led to an increase in acceptance.

High-Probability Instructional Sequence, Positive Reinforcement, and Fading

Patel et al. (2007) examined the use of a high-probability instructional sequence to increase compliance to treat food selectivity in a 4-year-old boy with ASD. They targeted acceptance of one fruit, vegetable, and protein in puree form. They implemented an ABAB design which compared a low-probability instruction (A) and a high-probability instruction condition (B). In the A phase, they presented a participant with one spoonful of food placed on a spoon in the bowl and presented a verbal prompt, "take a bite," two times before they removed the bite. In the B phase, they delivered the verbal prompt with three presentations of an empty spoon preceding the presentation of a spoon containing food. Prior to treatment, Patel et al. found that the participant regularly accepted an empty spoon and classified acceptance of the empty spoon as a high-probability response. Thus, in the B phase, they presented an instruction to perform a high-probability response before the low-probability response, whereas in the A phase, they presented only instructions to perform a low-probability response. In each condition, they presented verbal praise and light physical touch following compliance. All sessions terminated after presentation of five low-probability bites. Compliance was zero during the low-probability request condition and 100% during the high-probability condition. Following evaluation of the high-probability sequence, Patel et al. anecdotally noted that additional new foods were gradually presented and mealtime length and volume requirements were increased; however, they did not present data on these fading components. Patel et al. proposed the use of a high-probability instructional sequence as a potential alternative to EE.

In another study involving the use of a high-probability instructional sequence, Gentry and Luiselli (2008) trained a mother to conduct two multi-component procedures to treat food selectivity in her 4-year-old son with ASD. In the first intervention, the mother placed two preferred foods and one non-preferred food in three sections on a paper plate. Next, the mother presented her child with a "Mystery Motivator" game in which the child had to spin a game arrow to determine how many bites of each food he was required to eat. To incorporate the high-probability instructional sequence, the mother suggested that her son eat the required bites from the preferred foods before eating the non-preferred foods. When the child ate the required bites of non-preferred foods, she praised his behavior and gave him access to a preferred activity. She also allowed him to eat the remainder of the food or ask for additional foods. If the "Mystery Motivator" game arrow landed on a question mark, the child was immediately given access to a preferred toy from a gift box and his mother allowed him to play with the toy. She also only gave him access to preferred foods during the meal. If her child did not eat the required number of non-preferred bites, the mother withheld praise, had him stay in his chair for 5 min, and then allowed him to leave the table. Thus, EE was not part of this intervention. The experimenter systematically increased the number of required bites on the "Mystery Motivator" game. The child did not consume any of the non-preferred foods during baseline. During intervention, he gradually consumed more bites of non-preferred foods when the number of bites specified by the "Mystery Motivator"

spinner systematically increased. The experimenter terminated the intervention when the child was consuming six bites of non-preferred foods during sessions.

Gentry and Luiselli trained the mother to conduct a second intervention because the mother wanted the child to clear his plate of all non-preferred food items. In this procedure, the child's mother provided a specific number of bites of a non-preferred foods and she instructed her son to eat. If her child ate all of the required bites and did not engage in interfering responses, she gave him access to a preferred activity. The experimenter terminated the second intervention when the child was eating five bites of non-preferred foods during sessions.

Repeated Exposure and Escape Extinction

In the first study to examine repeated exposure to treat food selectivity in children with ASD, Paul et al. (2007) used a combined procedure involving repeated taste exposure and EE in a 3-year-old boy and a 5-year-old girl, both with ASD. To minimize response effort and increase compliance, they initially presented a single pea-sized bite of food. They presented fruits, vegetables, meats, dairy products, and starches that parents reported as non-preferred in a rotating fashion. Researchers provided small drinks of various liquids during sessions, but based reinforcement criterion on eating the target bite. Expulsions led to re-presentation of the same food. After bite acceptance, the participant exited the treatment room for a minimum of 5 min and went to areas in which books, toys, and the child's parents sat. The experimenters increased bite size for a particular food to half spoonfuls and finally full spoonfuls when the participant accepted three out of four bites within 30 s of presentation with no disruptive behavior. When the child met mastery criterion for full spoonfuls of several foods, the experimenters presented probe meals, in which three to four spoonfuls of mastered foods and new foods were presented on a plate for 10 min. They told the child to take bites but the child was not required to eat bites during the meal. They presented uneaten foods in probe meals during subsequent taste sessions. Trained therapists conducted treatment for the first week and then parents implemented the procedure. After 15 days of intensive treatment, one participant who accepted two foods prior to treatment met mastery criterion with 65 foods and the other participant met criterion for 49 foods after being totally dependent on a gastrostomy tube for feedings before treatment.

While all of these studies demonstrate an increase in consumption of non-preferred foods or previously rejected items, the number of foods eaten following treatment by the participants in the study by Paul et al. (2007) far exceeds the number of foods consumed by participants exposed to other interventions. Thus, repeated taste exposure combined with EE is a promising new technique for treating food selectivity.

Liquid Avoidance

There is only a small literature on liquid avoidance interventions in children with ASD; however, various treatment packages have been successful at treating this problem. All interventions to increase liquid consumption have used antecedent fading procedures within multi-component treatment packages. For example, Hagopian et al. (1996) used backward chaining, reinforcement, and stimulus fading to treat total liquid refusal in a 12-year-old boy with ASD who was currently receiving nutrients through a central line. Hagopian et al. task analyzed the target response of drinking from a cup into the following response chain: (a) bringing cup of water to mouth, (b) accepting water into mouth, and (c) swallowing. First, researchers reinforced the participant's swallowing when prompted without water being present. Next, they reinforced the participant's swallowing after placing an empty syringe in his mouth and then after the syringe delivered water into his mouth. During the last step in the chain, the researchers reinforced swallowing only after the participant drank 3 cc of water from a cup. Hagopian et al. terminated the procedure when the participant drank from a cup containing 30 cc of water on 100% of trials. Finally, the researchers used stimulus fading to gradually add juice to the water. Follow-up data indicated that the participant was reliably drinking from a cup containing 90 cc.

Patel et al. (2001) used stimulus fading, differential reinforcement, and EE to increase intake of a calorie-dense fluid, Carnation Instant Breakfast™ (CIB), in a 6-year-old boy with ASD. Prior to treatment, the participant accepted water from a cup, but refused other liquids. Prior to introducing a fading component, Patel et al. implemented DRA and EE with physical guidance using milk and CIB followed by sessions alternating milk with chocolate and vanilla Pediasure™. DRA and EE alone without fading involved a verbal prompt (e.g., "take a drink") and a model of a drinking response prior to providing physical guidance. When needed, the therapist provided physical guidance and re-presented expelled drinks. Sessions were 5 min or until the participant finished the last drink presented within the session. This procedure without stimulus fading lead to 0% mouth cleans (no visible liquid in the participant's mouth 30 s after acceptance). Thus, to increase the percentage of mouth cleans, the researchers substituted milk with water. Stimulus fading included the following steps: (a) consistent consumption of water, (b) gradually increasing the concentration of CIB in water, and (c) gradually increasing the concentration of milk in the water with the CIB. At the end of the intervention, the

participant exhibited mouth cleans for 100% of trials when the fluid was 100% milk and CIB.

Luiselli et al. (2005) also used stimulus fading, reinforcement, and paced instructional prompting to establish milk consumption in a 4-year-old girl with ASD. Prior to treatment, the participant accepted Pediasure™ alone or as a blend with 50% milk, but would not accept the blend if the quantity of milk was increased or if milk was presented alone. The researchers used fading to gradually increase the milk to Pediasure™ ratio by adding one tablespoon (approximately 6.25%) of milk. Paced instructional prompting involved the delivery of the prompt "drink" any time 60 s elapsed without the participant drinking. Probe assessments involved periodically presenting 100% of milk. Gradual fading increased milk consumption and the consumption of 100% of milk occurred by the third probe.

Packing

This review identified two studies that have examined packing. In an antecedent-based intervention, Patel et al. (2005) evaluated the use of texture manipulation to decrease packing in a 4-year-old boy with ASD and two other participants without ASD. An occupational therapist affiliated with the study reported that higher textures were inappropriate relative to the oral motor skills of the participants. In a reversal design, Patel et al. presented four foods (one from each food group) to each participant. They presented one participant with foods in either puree form (i.e., regular table foods placed in a blender and blended until smooth) in the A condition or as wet ground (i.e., pureed foods with small chunks) in the B condition. Patel et al. exposed another participant to puree form (A condition), wet ground (B condition), or baby food (C condition). They presented the third participant with foods in puree form (A condition) or table foods chopped into small pieces (B condition). The authors provided brief praise for bite acceptance and re-presented bites if expulsions occurred. For two participants, Patel et al. required them to finish their last bite before session termination. Overall, the percentage of trials with packing decreased and the total grams consumed increased when Patel et al. presented participants with food in puree form. Although the researchers did not present formal data collection on fading, they gradually increased texture during follow-up visits for two participants.

Buckley and Newchok (2005) evaluated the use of simultaneous presentation and differential reinforcement with RC to reduce packing in 9-year-old girl with ASD who packed bites of new or non-preferred foods regardless of texture. They presented four target foods in various conditions. In the first phase, Buckley and Newchok provided positive reinforcement for mouth clean and implemented RC by (a) presenting a preferred video for 30 s prior to the first presented bite; (b) removing the video if packing occurred; and (c) returning the video following a mouth clean. The second phase was the same as the first, except that they used a simultaneous presentation procedure wherein they placed a bite of cookie behind the target food. A third phase evaluated simultaneous presentation only. All treatment phases led to a reduction in packed intervals per session with simultaneous presentation leading to superior reductions in packing compared to other treatment conditions. However, order effects may have played a large role in this reduction as simultaneous presentation followed the other two conditions.

As with studies on liquid avoidance, there is a dearth of studies examining packing. It appears that the function of packing varies from avoidance to oral motor difficulties and therefore it may be beneficial for future researchers studying packing to conduct functional analyses as well as oral motor assessments prior to implementation of intervention.

Rapid Eating

Anglesea, Hoch, and Taylor (2008) conducted the only study found in this review that addresses rapid eating in those with ASD. The participants were three teenagers with ASD who all exhibited self-feeding skills and had a history of rapid food consumption. The target food for each participant was one eaten regularly during lunch. First, researchers timed a typically developing adult man eating each target food to determine an average time between bites. Participants learned to take a bite of snack foods when a pager vibrated on a variable interval schedule by having the teacher deliver praise for waiting until the pager vibrated and blocking attempts to take bites before the pager vibrated. The researchers then activated the pager prompt during meals with target foods and all participants increased the duration of their total eating time to that of a typical adult. A limitation of the study was that the researchers did not fade out the vibrating pagers following intervention. Additional research should examine fading procedures to eventually remove the vibrating pagers as well as examine other interventions that may be successful at treating this feeding problem.

As discussed earlier, a variety of treatments, typically multi-component treatment packages, have been used to treat feeding problems such as food selectivity, liquid avoidance, packing, and rapid eating. A potential criticism of a majority of the studies examining feeding problems in those with ASD is the use of a treatment package, which makes it difficult to determine the active treatment components responsible for behavior change. Often, researchers mention that component analyses should be conducted to evaluate individual components of treatment packages. Two published component analyses have examined multi-component treatments

for feeding problems (Cooper et al., 1995; Hoch et al., 2001), but neither used participants with ASD.

Caregiver Training

Parents and caregivers are often responsible for preparing and presenting meals for their children, yet few of the above interventions involved parent/caregiver training. This review found only 10 studies that have done so (Ahearn, Kerwin, et al., 2001; Anderson & McMillan, 2001; Gentry & Luiselli, 2008; Kern & Marder, 1996; McCartney et al., 2005; Najdowski et al., 2003; Patel et al., 2007, 2001, 2005; Paul et al., 2007). Of these 10 studies, researchers often omitted or provided vague descriptions of specific parent-training techniques. Further, researchers often did not report procedural integrity of parent performance; thus, it is unclear if parents performed the procedure correctly. This issue of procedural integrity is particularly problematic regarding feeding interventions because changes in child performance following the introduction of the parent into the session may be related to how well parents implemented the procedure and not the procedure itself.

Two of the 10 studies (Anderson & McMillan, 2001; McCartney et al., 2005) reported data on parent/caregiver performance and provided details regarding parent training. Anderson and McMillan (2001) used verbal and written instructions, modeling, videotape review, and feedback during weekly home visits to train parents to implement EE, DRA, and fading. Parents role-played the procedure with one another acting as the participant, watched a video of the experimenter implement the procedure with the participant, and received verbal feedback during the first three meals. After the first three meals, researchers gave parents feedback during one meal per week, reviewed segments of videotaped meals, and discussed key points. Anderson and McMillan mentioned that feedback was not immediate because tapes were reviewed only once per week, and thus parents may have implemented parts of the procedure incorrectly for several meals before receiving feedback. When parents faced mealtime problem behavior by their children during the first meal, the experimenters instructed them to implement the procedure with only preferred foods for the next five meals. Overall, parents delivered a reinforcer (i.e., praise or access to a favorite drink) following a mean of 95% of accepted bites of preferred foods and 93% of accepted bites of fruit (non-preferred) while only allowing escape following 1% of bites of preferred foods and 3% of bites of fruit. Although providing data on parent performance is a strength of this study, Anderson and McMillan did not report the duration of time to train parents and specific training criterion. They did mention that parents often increased reinforcement criteria before specified criterion was met; a problem with procedural integrity that would not be identified in the parental data presented. Further, the researchers gave parents feedback throughout treatment. Therefore, it is unclear if initial training techniques were effective as parents may have relied on experimenter feedback throughout the intervention to perform the procedure correctly.

McCartney et al. (2005) trained parents/caregivers to implement a differential reinforcement, EE, and demand fading procedure. They faded parents/caregivers into clinical trials. The experimenters first presented the parent/caregivers with a video of therapist-conducted clinic meals. Then, the therapist reviewed the video with the parent/caregiver and explained the EE procedure. Next, the parent/caregiver observed several meals through an observation mirror and then observed one meal in the session room before implementing the procedure. Prior to each meal fed by the parent/caregiver, an experimenter reviewed the intervention. In addition, an experimenter provided feedback following each meal. McCartney et al. required each participant to eat only one bite of the first target food during the initial caregiver-/parent-fed meal. They calculated treatment integrity on proportion of bites (a) accepted; (b) not accepted; (c) expelled; and (d) with interruptions followed by attention. Both therapists and parents/caregivers performed the procedure accurately with therapists performing the procedure slightly better than parents. It is important to note, however, that as with Anderson and McMillan (2001), McCartney et al. provided feedback to parents/caregivers throughout the entire intervention.

While caregivers have learned to implement feeding interventions through various behavioral skills training packages that typically involve various combinations of instructions, modeling, rehearsal, and feedback, it is still unclear whether parents can receive training in the home or clinic and perform the procedure correctly without ongoing feedback following training. Further, accurate parental implementation of procedures often seems implied by the absence of procedural integrity information. Collecting procedural integrity will help determine (a) whether parents/caregivers correctly perform procedures, (b) which procedures parents/caregivers have most difficulty in implementing, and (c) whether parents can perform the procedures without ongoing supervision.

Maintenance

Six food selectivity/refusal studies, (Anderson & McMillan, 2001; Buckley et al., 2005; Freeman & Piazza, 1998; Kern & Marder, 1996; Patel et al., 2005; Piazza et al., 2002), one liquid avoidance study, (Patel et al., 2001), and the one study on rapid eating (Anglesea et al., 2008) failed to report any follow-up data on long-term treatment gains following

intervention. Patel et al. (2005) presented follow-up data for two out of three participants, but not for the participant who had ASD. Thus, 40% of these feeding intervention studies with those with ASD do not include any follow-up. Four food selectivity (Ahearn, 2002, 2003; Levin & Carr, 2001; Paul et al., 2007), one liquid avoidance (Luiselli et al., 2005), and one packing study (Buckley & Newchok, 2005) included anecdotal follow-up. Of these, Paul et al. included perhaps the most thorough anecdotal follow-up. At a 3-month follow-up appointment following the repeated taste exposure and EE procedure, parents indicated which foods their children ate from a list of 139 foods and added any foods not on the list. Parents of the participant eating 49 foods immediately following intervention reported that the participant was eating 47 foods. Parents of the participant eating 65 foods following treatment indicated that he was eating 53 foods at the 3-month follow-up; however, the experimenters explained that this was due to the parents' decision to become vegetarians. Further, the experimenters reported that both children ate foods not eaten prior to treatment in a meal during a follow-up appointment.

Five food selectivity (Ahearn, Kerwin, et al., 2001; Gentry & Luiselli, 2008; McCartney et al., 2005; Najdowski et al., 2003; Patel et al., 2007) and one liquid refusal study (Hagopian et al., 1996) presented empirical data on maintenance. Ahearn, Kerwin, et al. (2001) collected 3-month follow-up data for one participant after the initial exposure to EE. At the 3-month follow-up, the participant ate 100% of presented bites of 10 oz of pureed food and snacks of chopped table foods. At 9-month follow-up, the participant self-fed 10–11 oz of chopped table foods. The other participant accepted 100% of bites of 3–3.5 oz of pureed food at 2 months and consumed 9.5 oz of chopped foods and would occasionally self-feed at 9-month follow-up. Thus, the participants maintained treatment gains 9 months following intervention.

Gentry and Luiselli (2008) presented follow-up data for four sessions approximately 30 days following the termination of the second intervention. The participant continued to eat the same number of bites required at the end of the second intervention (i.e., 5 bites) during follow-up sessions. Patel et al. (2007) collected data during a 3-month follow-up appointment. At that time, the mother had discontinued the use of the high-instructional sequence and provided a prompt to take a bite if the participant did not take the bite independently. Patel et al. reported acceptance of bites to be 100% during follow-up, despite the discontinuation of the procedure. Najdowski et al. (2003) reported that the participant's mother fed the participant normal-sized portions of new foods and continued to use the treatment procedure. Further, Najdowski et al. collected follow-up data at 2, 4, 6, and 12 weeks following intervention; however, data from these sessions did not appear in the research report.

McCartney et al. (2005) presented follow-up data for two participants and anecdotal follow-up for an additional participant after caregiver/parent implementation of EE, fading, and differential reinforcement. Four weeks following the intervention, one participant ate all bites offered of two target foods during the follow-up meal, even though a new person was feeding him. Researchers collected follow-up data approximately 1 year following the intervention for the other participant who accepted eight bites each of two target foods in each of three follow-up meals. For the participant unavailable for follow-up data collection, the mother reported that the participant was willingly consuming both target foods and novel foods following the intervention.

Hagopian et al. (1996) provided follow-up data following the backward chaining and fading procedure to treat total liquid refusal, but did not mention when they conducted follow-up sessions. They conducted follow-up generalization sessions in a different environment (living unit). During these sessions, the participant consumed up to 90 cc of water and juice; however, it is unclear if these data should be considered maintenance data as the sessions may have occurred immediately following the termination of the procedure.

To consider an intervention to be successful, it is important to collect follow-up data to determine long-term effects of treatment. After all, investigators compromise the applied value of the research if participants do not maintain treatment gains over time. Future researchers should collect and report maintenance data.

Generalization

Generalization of treatment gains to new foods is another consideration when examining the efficacy of a feeding intervention. Six of 20 studies formally assessed generalization to novel foods or full portions of target foods throughout treatment: three for liquid avoidance/refusal (Hagopian et al., 1996; Luiselli et al., 2005; Patel et al., 2001), two for food selectivity (Ahearn, 2002; Paul et al., 2007), and one for rapid eating (Anglesea et al., 2008).

Two studies on liquid avoidance (Luiselli et al., 2005; Patel et al., 2001) conducted full-portion probes throughout intervention to determine if researchers could discontinue fading and to demonstrate experimental control. The target goal was consumption of 100% milk in Luiselli et al.'s study and 100% milk with CIB in the Patel et al.'s study. Thus, periodically throughout treatment involving the fading of Pediasure™ out of a Pediasure™/milk mix or increasing milk into a water/CIB mix until water was replaced with milk, researchers presented probes of 100% milk or 100% milk/CIB. A decrement in consumption during initial probes demonstrated experimental control of the fading procedure; however, eventually participants consumed the full portions, which indicated that additional fading was unnecessary. The

full-portion probes involved different combinations of the same liquids. Thus, it is unclear how participants would have responded to probes of new fluids (e.g., various juices, sports drinks, soda).

Similarly, Hagopian et al. (1996) presented 10 cc of water as probes throughout treatment. When the participant successfully consumed 10 cc of water, Hagopian et al. increased the reinforcement criterion to 30 cc of water. Following the intervention, the experimenters presented the participant with a cup containing 90 cc of water in a novel setting. Hagopian et al. reported that they gradually added juice to the water; however, they did not report data on consumption during this additional fading procedure. Thus, again, this study appears to have generalization to novel portions but lacks empirical data assessing different fluids.

Ahearn (2002) and Paul et al.'s (2007) treatment studies for food selectivity used probes to formally assess generalization to new foods. For example, Ahearn (2002) included generalization probes to novel foods when examining the effects of presenting either single food items or multiple food items. When criteria were met (> 80% acceptance, < 20% disruption, < 20% expulsion) for either the single target food item or food group, Ahearn introduced probes by presenting a new item for the last 5 trials of a 20-trial session. During probes, baseline contingencies, which entailed differential reinforcement for acceptance, were in place. During generalization probes, Ahearn presented foods that had not been accepted during initial assessments. He considered consumption of two or more bites during the five trial probe as generalization of acceptance to the new food. Findings from the probes suggested that presentation of multiple foods from the same food group facilitated generalization of acceptance to new foods compared to single food item presentation.

Paul et al. (2007) conducted probe meals throughout the repeated exposure and EE procedure when the participant met criterion (three out of four sessions in which the participant ate a full teaspoon of the food within 30 s) for at least three foods. During probe meals, the researchers presented the participant with three tablespoons each of three to four foods on a plate. They presented either new foods, foods presented in previous probe meals, or foods presented in previous taste sessions; however, none of the probe foods had been in the participant's pre-treatment diet. The therapist instructed the child to take a bite, but the child was not required to eat the food. Probe meals lasted 10 min and the therapist delivered praise if the participant took bites. If the participant ate an entire portion of a food during a probe meal, Paul et al. no longer presented that food during taste sessions. Parents conducted generalization probe meals following treatment to determine novel food acceptance outside of the clinic setting.

Anglesea et al. (2008) trained the participants to use the pager prompt with various snack foods, and following training the participants used the pager prompt with a target food that had not been present during training. Thus, all sessions following training were generalization sessions; however, only one target food was selected for each participant following training, and thus Anglesea et al. only assessed generalization for one target food per participant.

Studies have examined stimulus generalization to novel stimuli, such as novel foods, portion sizes, people, and settings. Many studies appear to tacitly assume these are examples of stimulus generalization: The literature on feeding problems is silent on the issue of response generalization. Yet, it seems likely that response generalization is intimately bound up in procedures that present novel foods and utensils. For example, the way a child chews yogurt with no fruit in it is not the same response as chewing yogurt with lumps of fruit in it and the way a child places his or her lips around a sippy cup is not quite the same response as placing his or her lips around a regular cup. Interventions for feeding problems have not explicitly addressed response generalization. Although this may present some challenges to measure behavior, future studies should do so.

Social Validity

Wolf (1978) explained that the purpose of the *Journal of Applied Behavior Analysis* (*JABA*) was to publish applications of the analysis of behavior to problems of social importance. Measures of social validity in feeding studies are often missing or researchers report them in a vague manner. This is particularly surprising considering that some view EE as controversial and have suggested alternative procedures whenever possible; however, it appears, at least in the feeding literature in those with ASD, researchers have rarely assessed the social validity of such procedures and the perceived unacceptability of procedures remains speculative.

Two of the 20 studies reported the administration of social validity questionnaires to parents/caregivers of the participants (McCartney et al., 2005; Paul et al., 2007). Paul et al. (2007) mentioned that parents of both children in the study rated the intervention of repeated taste exposure and EE as acceptable and effective through use of a satisfaction questionnaire. McCartney et al. also provided satisfaction questionnaires based on a Likert scale to each of the caregiver/parent and reported the questions and results of the questionnaire. Caregivers rated the intervention as effective in decreasing mealtime problem behaviors and increasing consumption of a variety of foods. Parents also reported that they would recommend the intervention to others who had children with mealtime difficulties; however, three of four caregivers/parents reported that mealtimes were still stressful and difficult. Thus, the results of this type of questionnaire can provide additional information regarding the procedures; for instance, even if a particular feeding problem improves, child behavior may still disrupt family mealtime.

Several studies provide statements regarding social validity but do not include direct measures. For instance, Gentry and Luiselli (2008) mentioned that although they did not formally assess social validity, the parent's desire to maintain the intervention suggested that she was satisfied with the procedures and the results. In the study that involved parent choice of training in one of the two forms of EE, Ahearn, Kerwin, et al. (2001) mentioned that caregivers continued to implement the procedure during outpatient and follow-up appointments. Further, Ahearn, Kerwin, et al. suggested that giving caregivers a choice may have long-term benefits for the child with feeding problems because the caregiver has an active role in treatment selection. Ahearn (2002) suggested that the results of the study with regard to presenting single food or multiple food presentations indicate that if rapid acquisition and weight gain are more pressing than response generalization, then clinicians and researchers should target one food item; however, if response generalization is more desirable than rapid acquisition, then they should target multiple food items. Thus, although Ahearn does not directly assess social validity, he makes statements regarding social implications of the findings. Future research will be more informative if researchers provide and discuss social validity measures administered to parents/caregivers.

Assessments

Ahearn, Castine, et al. (2001) argued that assessments based on direct observation are often more informative and accurate than those based on third-party reports. For example, Ahearn, Castine, et al. (2001) conducted an assessment based on direct observation to determine acceptance and rejection of foods and to examine various forms of food selectivity (e.g., food category or food texture); however, feeding intervention studies rarely report the use of such assessments. Direct observation may (a) help confirm parental statements regarding the problem behavior, (b) provide guidance for setting initial reinforcement criterion, and (c) help determine which foods to target. Preference assessments could be especially helpful if preferred foods are to be used as reinforcers in order to determine which foods to use as reinforcers during an intervention. Occasionally, such assessments may not be necessary, perhaps in the case of total food/liquid refusal. Also, parents often have strong opinions regarding which foods they would like to have targeted for intervention in their children.

Two intervention studies (Ahearn, 2002, 2003) used Ahearn, Castine, and colleague's (2001) direct observation assessment to examine feeding problems prior to intervention. In addition to performing the assessment, Ahearn (2002) also conducted a 2-week diet history in the child's natural eating environment. As a result of this diet history, Ahearn presented foods during the assessment and treatment that parents would expect the child to eat during meals following treatment. Ahearn, Kerwin, et al. (2001) mentioned that one participant presented with type and texture food selectivity according to Munk and Repp's (1994) assessment. McCartney et al. (2005) conducted a different type of assessment prior to intervention in which parents were asked to conduct several baseline probes. During these probes, the experimenters told parents to prompt their children to eat bites of a non-preferred and a preferred food using strategies typically used during meals. These sessions took place prior to therapist-fed baseline. This type of initial assessment allowed experimenters to examine parent–child dynamics during mealtimes. The same non-preferred foods used in probes were targeted during intervention.

Levin and Carr (2001) and Najdowski et al. (2003) conducted preference assessments to determine preferred and non-preferred foods while Buckley et al. (2005) and Ahearn, Kerwin, et al. (2001) conducted preference assessments to identify preferred items (not foods) to use as reinforcers during the intervention. Two studies used parental food history questionnaires (Gentry & Luiselli, 2008; Paul et al., 2007). The remaining studies involved either parental verbal report or unspecified methods for gathering information prior to intervention.

Depending on the type of problem behavior and intervention implemented, different types of initial assessments may be helpful. In the study evaluating food textures on packing, an occupational therapist assessed oral motor skills with each participant prior to intervention. In the study involving a high-probability instructional sequence to increase compliance, Patel et al. (2007) conducted a pre-treatment compliance assessment to determine that acceptance of an empty spoon was a high-probability response. As mentioned earlier, Najdowski et al. (2003) and Levin and Carr (2001) included functional analyses to examine the function of the problem behavior prior to intervention. These different types of formal assessments may help (a) determine reinforcers; (b) identify target foods to present in intervention; (c) determine variables maintaining problem behaviors; and (d) provide additional information that may lead to more effective treatment. Thus, we suggest future researchers to include these types of assessments as opposed to relying primarily on parental report.

Collateral Behavior

Often, failure to accept foods is accompanied by corollary behaviors such as negative vocalizations (e.g., "no!"), self-injurious behavior (e.g., hitting or biting oneself), expulsions (e.g., spitting out food), and disruptive responses (e.g., pushing the spoon away, turning away). Six studies on food selectivity (Ahearn, Kerwin, et al., 2001; Anderson & McMillan,

2001; Buckley et al., 2005; Freeman & Piazza, 1998; Levin & Carr, 2001; Paul et al., 2007), one study on packing (Patel et al., 2005), one study on liquid refusal (Hagopian et al., 1996), and the study on rapid eating (Anglesea et al., 2008) measured various corollary behaviors. Levin and Carr (2001) did not formally measure corollary behaviors during the first intervention, but after anecdotally observing problem behavior, they collected data on problem behavior in the second intervention. In one study that omitted corollary behaviors as dependent measures, Ahearn (2002) explicitly stated that corollary problem behaviors did not interfere with appropriate eating behavior of the participants and therefore were not included as measures. Nevertheless, it appears that studies would benefit from having these additional dependent measures, particularly if corollary behaviors do not reduce as acceptance increases, which could indicate potential limitations of a procedure. Two additional studies (Anglesea et al., 2008; Patel et al., 2005) reported multiple dependent measures, but not on disruptive corollary responses. Anglesea et al. (2008) measured number of bites eaten per session and time taken to eat bites while Patel et al. (2005) measured percentage of trials with packing and total grams consumed per session.

Collecting data on corollary disruptive behaviors may enhance the social validity of feeding studies. For instance, caregivers may rate a treatment as more effective and acceptable if disruptive corollary responses decrease as food consumption increases. Without measuring these responses, the effects of treatment on the disruptive responses that often make mealtimes difficult for parents are unknown. Including these supplementary dependent measures allows researchers to make additional conclusions regarding the efficacy and social validity of treatment.

Conclusions

Functional analyses (Levin & Carr, 2001; Najdowski et al., 2003) have identified that feeding problems are often maintained by escape as opposed to attention or tangibles. While motivational operations such as satiation and deprivation certainly play a role in the development and exacerbation of feeding problems, the effects of hunger and deprivation have been seldom assessed. Future research should further explore the role of appetite manipulation as the integration of this type of motivating operation into interventions could probably enhance their effectiveness. Feeding problems may also be a function of narrow stimulus control and in the case of food selectivity, a limited number of foods may exert strong stimulus control over acceptance. Thus, treatment components such as fading may enhance the transfer of stimulus control to a larger array of stimuli (e.g., gradually presenting more foods, different textures, larger portion sizes). The literature has clearly shown that treatment packages involving both antecedent-based components (i.e., simultaneous presentation, stimulus fading, repeated taste exposure, and high-probability instructional sequences) and consequence-based components (i.e., differential reinforcement, EE, reinforcement fading, and RC) have successfully treated a variety of feeding problems. Future research should explore which of the components are necessary or which components can enhance the effectiveness of other components.

A limitation of the feeding intervention literature in children with ASD is the lack of caregiver/parent involvement in the treatment. Further, in the studies that report parent involvement, researchers often fail to describe the techniques used to teach parents/caregivers and fail to report data on parent/caregiver performance. Thus, future research should examine various techniques for training caregivers and collect data on caregivers' performance in addition to the children's behavior to determine if caregivers can accurately implement the intervention. Suggestions for future researchers also include assessing long-term treatment gains and generalization to new foods. Further, administering social validity questionnaires to caregivers following treatment will provide additional information regarding the acceptability and outcomes of treatment. The use of formal preference assessments prior to intervention may help confirm parent reports regarding a child's feeding behavior and identify potential reinforcers to be used in the intervention. Lastly, the measurement of corollary responses could help determine the effects of treatment on behaviors associated with the primary dependent variable.

References

Ahearn, W. H. (2002). Effect of two methods of introducing foods during feeding treatment on acceptance of previously rejected items. *Behavioral Interventions, 17*, 111–127.

Ahearn, W. H. (2003). Using simultaneous presentation to increase vegetable consumption in a mildly selective child with autism. *Journal of Applied Behavior Analysis, 36*, 361–365.

Ahearn, W. H., Castine, T., Nault, K., & Green, G. (2001). An assessment of food acceptance in children with autism or pervasive developmental disorder-not otherwise specified. *Journal of Autism and Developmental Disorders, 31*, 505–511.

Ahearn, W. H., Kerwin, M., Eicher, P. S., & Lukens, C. T. (2001). An ABAC comparison of two intensive interventions for food refusal. *Behavior Modification, 25*, 385–405.

Anderson, C. M., & McMillan, K. (2001). Parental use of escape extinction and differential reinforcement to treat food selectivity. *Journal of Applied Behavior Analysis, 34*, 511–515.

Anglesea, M. M., Hoch, H., & Taylor, B. A. (2008). Reducing rapid eating in teenagers with Autism: Use of a pager prompt. *Journal of Applied Behavior Analysis, 41*, 107–111.

Bowers, L. (2002). An audit of referrals of children with autistic spectrum disorder to the dietetic service. *Journal of Human Nutrition and Dietetics, 14*, 141–144.

Buckley, S. D., & Newchok, D. K. (2005). An evaluation of simultaneous presentation and differential reinforcement with response cost to reduce packing. *Journal of Applied Behavior Analysis, 38*, 405–409.

Buckley, S. D., Strunck, P. G., & Newchok, D. K. (2005). A comparison of two multicomponent procedures to increase food consumption. *Behavioral Interventions, 20*, 139–146.

Collins, M. S., Kyle, R., Smith, S., Laverty, A., Roberts, S., & Eaton-Evans, J. (2003). Coping with the unusual family diet: Eating behavior and food choices of children with Down's syndrome, autistic spectrum disorders or Cri du Chat syndrome and comparison groups of siblings. *Journal of Learning Disabilities, 7*, 137–155.

Cooper, J. O., Heron, T. E., & Heward, W. L. (2007). *Applied behavior analysis* (2nd ed.). Saddle River, NJ: Pearson Education, Inc.

Cooper, L. J., Wacker, D. P., McComas, J. J., Brown, K., Peck, S. M., Richman, D., et al. (1995). Use of component analyses to identify active variables in treatment packages for children with feeding disorders. *Journal of Applied Behavior Analysis, 28*, 139–153.

Cornish, E. (1998). A balanced approach towards healthy eating in autism. *Journal of Human Nutrition and Dietetics, 11*, 501–509.

Cornish, E. (2002). Gluten and casein free diets in autism: A study of the effects on food choice and nutrition. *Journal of Human Nutrition and Dietetics, 15*, 261–269.

Field, D., Garland, M., & Williams, K. (2003). Correlates of specific childhood feeding problems. *Journal of Pediatrics and Child Health, 39*, 299–304.

Freeman, K. A., & Piazza, C. C. (1998). Combining stimulus fading, reinforcement, and extinction to treat food refusal. *Journal of Applied Behavior Analysis, 31*, 691–694.

Gentry, J. A., & Luiselli, J. K. (2008). Treating a child's selective eating through parent implemented feeding intervention in the home setting. *Journal of Developmental and Physical Disabilities, 20*, 63–70.

Hagopian, L. P., Farrell, D. A., & Amari, A. (1996). Treating total liquid refusal with backward chaining and fading. *Journal of Applied Behavior Analysis, 29*, 573–575.

Hoch, T. A., Babbitt, R. L., Farrar-Schneider, D., Berkowitz, M. J., Owens, C. J., Knight, T. L., et al. (2001). Empirical examination of a multicomponent treatment for pediatric food refusal. *Education and Treatment of Children, 24*, 176–198.

Holman, E. W. (1975). Immediate and delayed reinforcers for flavor preferences in rats. *Animal Learning and Behavior, 6*, 91–100.

Kern, L., & Marder, T. J. (1996). A comparison of simultaneous and delayed reinforcement as treatments for food selectivity. *Journal of Applied Behavior Analysis, 29*, 243–246.

Ledford, J. R., & Gast, D. L. (2006). Feeding problems in children with autism spectrum disorders: A review. *Focus on Autism and Other Developmental Disabilities, 21*, 153–166.

Lennox, D. B., Miltenberger, R. G., & Donnelly, D. R. (1987). Response interruption and DRL for the reduction of rapid eating. *Journal of Applied Behavior Analysis, 20*, 279–284.

Levin, L., & Carr, E. G. (2001). Food selectivity and problem behavior in children with developmental disabilities: Analysis and intervention. *Behavior Modification, 25*, 443–470.

Linscheid, T. R. (2006). Behavioral treatments for pediatric feeding disorders. *Behavior Modification, 30*, 6–23.

Luiselli, J. K., Ricciardi, J. N., & Gilligan, K. (2005). Liquid fading to establish milk consumption by a child with autism. *Behavioral Interventions, 20*, 155–163.

McCartney, E. J., Anderson, C. M., & English, C. L. (2005). Effect of brief clinic-based training on the ability of caregivers to implement escape extinction. *Journal of Positive Behavior Interventions, 7*, 18–32.

McGimsey, J. F. (1977). A brief survey of eating behaviors of 60 severe/profoundly retarded individuals. Unpublished manuscript, Western Carolina Center. Cited in J. E. Favell, J. F. McGimsey, &

M. L. Jones. (1980). Rapid eating in the retarded: Reduction by nonaversive procedures. *Behavior Modification, 4*, 481–492.

Michael, J. (2007). Motivating operations. In J. O. Cooper, T. E. Heron, & W. L. Heward (Eds.), *Applied behavior analysis* (2nd ed., pp. 374–391). Saddle River, NJ: Pearson Education, Inc.

Miltenberger, R. G. (2004). *Behavior modification: Principles and procedures* (3rd ed.). Belmont, CA: Wadsworth.

Munk, D. D., & Repp, A. C. (1994). Behavioral assessment of feeding problems of individuals with severe disabilities. *Journal of Applied Behavior Analysis, 27*, 241–250.

Najdowski, A. C., Wallace, M. D., Doney, J. K., & Ghezzi, P. M. (2003). Parental assessment and treatment of food selectivity in natural settings. *Journal of Applied Behavior Analysis, 36*, 383–386.

Patel, M. R., Piazza, C. C., Kelly, M. L., Ochsner, C. A., & Santana, C. M. (2001). Using a fading procedure to increase fluid consumption in a child with feeding problems. *Journal of Applied Behavior Analysis, 34*, 357–360.

Patel, M. R., Piazza, C. C., Layer, S. A., Coleman, R., & Swartzwelder, D. M. (2005). A systematic evaluation of food textures to decrease packing and increase oral intake of children with pediatric feeding disorders. *Journal of Applied Behavior Analysis, 38*, 89–100.

Patel, M., Reed, G. K., Piazza, C. C., Mueller, M., Bachmeyer, M. H., & Layer, S. A. (2007). Use of a high-probability instructional sequence to increase compliance to feeding demands in the absence of escape extinction. *Behavioral Interventions, 22*, 305–310.

Paul, C., Williams, K. E., Riegel, K., & Gibbons, B. (2007). Combining repeated taste exposure and escape extinction. *Appetite, 49*, 708–711.

Piazza, C. C., Patel, M. R., Santana, C. M., Goh, H. L., Delia, M. D., & Lancaster, B. (2002). An evaluation of simultaneous and sequential presentation of preferred and nonpreferred food to treat food selectivity. *Journal of Applied Behavior Analysis, 35*, 259–270.

Premack, D. (1962). Reversibility of the reinforcement relation. *Science, 136*, 255–257.

Shreck, K. A., Williams, K., & Smith, A. F. (2004). A comparison of eating behaviors between children with and without autism. *Journal of Autism and Developmental Disorders, 34*, 433–438.

Wardle, J., Herrera, M. L., Cooke, L., & Gibson, E. L. (2003). Modifying children's food preferences: The effects of exposure and reward on acceptance of an unfamiliar vegetable. *European Journal of Clinical Nutrition, 57*, 341–348.

Williams, K. E., & Foxx, R. M. (2007). *Treating eating problems of children with autism spectrum disorders and developmental disabilities.* Austin, TX: Pro-Ed.

Wolf, M. M. (1978). Social validity: The case for subjective measurement or how applied behavior analysis is finding its heart. *Journal of Applied Behavior Analysis, 11*, 203–214.

Wright, C. S., & Vollmer, T. R. (2002). Evaluation of a treatment package to reduce rapid eating. *Journal of Applied Behavior Analysis, 35*, 89–93.

Zellner, D. A., Rozin, P., Aron, M., & Kulish, D. (1983). Conditioned enhancement of humans' liking for flavors paired with sweetness. *Learning and Motivation, 14*, 338–350.

Training Staff and Parents: Evidence-Based Approaches

Dennis H. Reid and Wendy H. Fitch

The benefits of relying on evidence-based treatment for people with autism spectrum disorders (ASD) have become increasingly apparent. Most notably, reliance on treatment approaches with an established evidence base significantly enhances the likelihood that treatment will be effective and desired outcomes will result for people with ASD. Although controversy continues over what represents a sufficient evidence base in some cases (Detrich, Keyworth, & States, 2008; Shriver & Allen, 2008, Chapter 2), it is clear that many treatment strategies currently exist for people with ASD that are well supported by scientific evidence (see Cuvo & Vallelunga, 2007; Rosenwasser & Axelrod, 2001; Steege, Mace, Perry, & Longenecker, 2007, for summaries).

The existence of treatment approaches with sound evidence to support their utility is the basic foundation for providing evidence-based treatment for people with ASD; however, the availability of these treatment strategies alone is not sufficient to ensure the success of treatment. The strategies must also be appropriately implemented on a day-to-day basis with individuals who have ASD. Specifically, there must be adequate *treatment integrity* (Fisk, 2008; Vollmer, Sloman, & Peter Pipkin, 2008). Treatment integrity refers to the degree to which a respective treatment strategy is carried out in the manner in which it is designed to be implemented.

The integrity with which caregivers implement treatment procedures with individuals who have ASD is a significant concern in both the research literature and routine practice. Concern over treatment integrity in this regard stems from two related sources. First, a number of investigations have demonstrated that the effectiveness of a given treatment strategy tends to be associated with the degree to which the strategy is carried out in the manner in which it is designed (see Fisk, 2008, for a summary). Second, investigations also

have indicated that a significant number of treatment strategies are not carried out very accurately or consistently in common practice (Codding, Livanis, Pace, & Vaca, 2008; DiGennaro, Martens, & Kleinmann, 2007; Wilder, Atwell, & Wine, 2006). The end result in the latter case is that people with ASD are not truly receiving evidence-based treatment, and the likelihood that various treatment strategies will be successful is diminished.

Although there are several reasons why treatment strategies are not implemented appropriately, one of the most fundamental is inadequate caregiver training. In short, many people who are expected to carry out treatment strategies have not been adequately trained in how to implement the procedures (Reid, 2004; Steege et al., 2007). The lack of effective caregiver training takes on heightened significance when considering who actually provides the bulk of treatment services for people with ASD on a day-to-day basis. Treatment services are often provided by people who have no formal education specifically related to working with individuals with ASD (e.g., graduate and undergraduate courses or supervised practica or internships). For example, many intensive early intervention services, such as discrete-trial teaching within an applied behavior analysis (ABA) framework, are carried out by parents or paraprofessional "therapists." In school settings, many teaching and other program services are implemented by teacher assistants in classrooms or other paraeducators employed to provide one-to-one support as personal instructors or "shadows" (Lerman, Tetreault, Hovanetz, Strobel, & Garro, 2008). For adults with ASD, in many cases implementation of treatment strategies is the responsibility of paraprofessional, direct support personnel in residential or day habilitation settings such as adult activity centers, sheltered workshops, and adult education programs (Reid, Parsons, Lattimore, Towery, & Reade, 2005).

Parents and paraprofessionals who routinely carry out treatment programs for people with ASD must have opportunities to acquire relevant knowledge and skills to be able to implement the programs proficiently. Because these caregivers rarely have had formal training in treatment

D.H. Reid (✉)
Carolina Behavior Analysis and Support Center, Morganton, NC 28680, USA
e-mail: drhmc@vistatech.net

approaches as just indicated, they must be provided with opportunities for in vivo or on-the-job training. More importantly, they must have opportunities to receive *effective* training.

Caregiver training is most likely to be effective if there is an established evidence base to support the effectiveness of the procedures constituting training, just as treatment for people with ASD is most likely to be effective if that treatment is evidence-based. It is counterproductive to emphasize provision of evidence-based treatment for people with ASD if caregivers cannot provide such treatment proficiently due to lack of effective training – training that is not evidence-based. Although much less investigatory attention has been directed to evidence-based training procedures for caregivers relative to the development of evidence-based treatment strategies for people with ASD, information resulting from research that has been reported on caregiver training is significant.

The purpose of this chapter is to describe what constitutes an evidence-based approach to training staff and parents. The intent is to summarize what research has demonstrated to represent effective means of training caregivers. Common obstacles to providing effective caregiver training will also be reviewed. Recommended ways to overcome such obstacles likewise will be presented, along with suggested directions for future research. The premise for the latter discussion is that although an evidence-based approach to training staff and parents currently exists, common practice in many settings is not evidence-based and caregivers are not well prepared to provide desired supports and services for people with ASD (Reid, O'Kane, & Macurik, in press; Schell, 1998; Steege et al., 2007; Sturmey, 1998). Consequently, continued investigation in this area is warranted.

Chapter Organization

Initially, an overview of what research has indicated to represent effective caregiver training will be provided, along with a summary of the overall role of training within services intended to affect desired caregiver performance. A primary focus of the overview will be issues specifically related to effectively training *staff* in human service agencies providing supports for people with ASD, though reference to training *parents* will also be made where relevant. Subsequently, issues relating more directly to training parents and other family members who implement treatment programs for people with ASD in home-based programs will be discussed. The rationale for the latter section is that although the basic training procedures are the same for staff and parent caregivers, there are also special circumstances affecting training needs among parents in homes with their sons and daughters versus paid staff in human service agencies.

Evidence-Based Caregiver Training Procedures

Preparing caregivers to carry out treatment and related interventions with people who have ASD involves providing them with knowledge about the interventions and skills to implement the interventions proficiently. Although the methods involved in effectively providing caregivers with relevant knowledge and implementation skills overlap, there are also important differences. Providing caregivers with a knowledge base is often considered as *verbal training* whereas equipping caregivers with the skills to actually carry out treatment procedures is considered *performance training* (Reid & Parsons, 2000). One of the earliest and most noted research findings on caregiver training is that *both these types of training approaches are usually needed to effectively train caregivers* (Gardner, 1972). Verbal training approaches are typically necessary for informing caregivers about various treatment procedures and the conditions in which the procedures are warranted, and performance training approaches are necessary for preparing them to implement the treatment procedures. This finding has been discussed extensively and is a critical consideration in designing evidence-based training programs for caregivers (Reid & Parsons; Shriver & Allen, 2008; Weiss, 2005).

Verbal training procedures involve rather traditional instructional approaches with caregivers such as lecture- and discussion-based methods as well as presentation of written information (Reid & Parsons, 2000). Performance training procedures involve actually performing skills targeted by the training. The latter strategies include modeling or demonstrations by a trainer, supervised practice by caregiver trainees in implementing targeted interventions or treatment, and some form of feedback (Reid & Parsons). Our focus here is with procedures that effectively train caregivers to actually implement respective interventions. The rationale for such a focus is several-fold. First, it is what caregivers do with people who have ASD that represents evidence-based treatment or not (i.e., it is of little benefit if caregivers are knowledgeable about a treatment intervention but cannot implement it accurately). Second, typical training provided for caregivers is frequently much more verbal- than performance-based; caregivers are informed about a respective treatment intervention but not adequately prepared to actually carry it out (Reid et al., in press; Sturmey, 1998). For example, a relatively common approach for training direct support staff in residential centers to carry out a treatment plan to reduce an individual's challenging behavior is for a psychologist or other clinician who developed the plan to meet with staff, review the plan, and answer any questions of staff. Essentially, this type of training is exclusively verbal in nature as referred to earlier and frequently is not consistently effective for ensuring each staff trainee can adequately implement the plan (Reid & Parsons, 2002, Chapter 7; Weiss, 2005).

In accordance with the focus of this chapter on performance training with caregivers, the primary concern is training caregivers how to carry out evidence-based treatment interventions with individuals who have ASD, and particularly for implementing treatment strategies for teaching functional skills and preventing or reducing challenging behavior. As well indicated in other chapters in this text and elsewhere (Koegel & Koegel, 2006; Powers, 2000; Symon, 2005), there are many other types of knowledge and skills needed by caregivers to provide optimal supports and services for people with ASD. These include, for example, how to secure appropriate medical and related services, advocate with schools and other organizations for necessary services, and cope with the stress that often occurs when living or working with individuals with ASD. Although providing information in these areas is of critical importance for caregivers, it is nonetheless beyond the scope of this chapter.

Before summarizing the essential components of performance-based caregiver training, attention is warranted on the overall role of such training when attempting to affect caregiver performance. In essence, training is often necessary to prepare caregivers to effectively carry out treatment interventions for individuals with ASD but it is rarely sufficient (Greene, Willis, Levy, & Bailey, 1978; Harchik & Campbell, 1998; Reid & Parsons, 2006, Chapter 4; Smith, Parker, Taubman, & Lovaas, 1992). Effective training equips caregivers with necessary skills for providing quality treatment services but does not ensure the treatment strategies subsequently are actually applied or applied appropriately. Research has repeatedly demonstrated that on-the-job supervision is almost always needed following caregiver training programs to ensure newly acquired skills are applied effectively and maintained over time (Alavosius & Sulzer-Azaroff, 1990; Brackett, Reid, & Green, 2007; DiGennaro et al., 2007; Montegar, Reid, Madsen, & Ewell, 1977; Parsons & Reid, 1995; Petscher & Bailey, 2006).

Supervision of caregiver performance following training is necessary for a variety of reasons, and particularly to assist caregivers in modifying treatment interventions based on the responses of the recipients of the treatment (i.e., individuals with ASD). Supervision is likewise usually necessary to provide support to maintain proficient caregiver treatment intervention over time (Reid & Parsons, 2000, 2002; Sturmey, 1998). How to provide effective supervision in this regard, relying on a developing technology of evidence-based supervision, is described in a number of sources (e.g., Reid & Parsons, 2000; Reid, 2004; Sturmey, 1998). The point of concern here is that the focus on training caregivers should not be interpreted to mean that training should be provided in isolation. Training represents just one component of helping caregivers provide quality treatment services for people

with ASD. Nevertheless, it is a critical and necessary component for reasons described earlier and, as such, warrants significant attention in its own right.

In light of the importance of caregiver training, a considerable amount of research has been reported on developing effective training programs for providing caregivers with the skills necessary to carry out various treatment procedures (see Adkins, 1996; Demchak, 1987; Jahr, 1998; Reid & Parsons, 2000; Reid, 2004, for reviews). Although each caregiver training program investigated varies to some degree, there is a rather remarkable similarity among the core training methods used within programs that have successfully trained performance skills to caregivers. When used in combination with each other, these methods represent what is generally referred to as performance-based training (Reid & Parsons, 2000) or, more recently, behavioral skills training (Miles & Wilder, 2009; Sarokoff & Sturmey, 2004; Weiss, 2005). A prototypical, performance-based training program is represented in Table 32.1. This type of training approach has repeatedly been demonstrated through applied research to effectively train important performance skills to caregivers working with people with ASD including, for example, how to conduct discrete-trial teaching (Sarokoff & Sturmey, 2004), embed teaching within natural community routines (Parsons, Reid, & Lattimore, 2009; Schepis, Reid, Ownbey, & Parsons, 2001), and promote follow-through on job assignments in supported work (Reid et al., 2005).

The performance-based training process summarized in Table 32.1 begins with presentation of a rationale regarding the importance and relevance of the skills that will be trained to caregiver trainees. For example, when training caregivers to conduct discrete-trial teaching with young children with ASD, the importance of specifically teaching basic skills is stressed along with the necessity of teaching in a precise manner. Next, the skills to be trained to the caregivers are verbally described by the trainer. The third step entails presenting each trainee with a succinct, written summary of the target skills. The fourth step involves the trainer demonstrating for the trainees how to perform each aspect

Table 32.1 Procedural steps of performance- and competency-based caregiver training

Step	Trainer action
1.	Describe rationale and relevance regarding skills to be trained
2.	Describe performance steps constituting the skills
3.	Provide written summary of performance steps constituting the skills
4.	Demonstrate how to perform the skills
5.	Have trainee(s) practice performing the skills and provide feedback
6.	Repeat steps 2, 4, and 5 until trainee(s) demonstrate proficiency in performing the skills

of the target skills. The demonstration can be conducted in a scripted, role-play fashion and/or in vivo in the actual situation in which a trainee is expected to apply the skills being trained (Parsons, Reid, & Green, 1996). Following the demonstration, the fifth step consists of trainee practice in demonstrating the skills themselves while the trainer observes the practice and provides supportive and/or corrective feedback (Parsons & Reid, 1995) as necessary. Finally, the second, fourth, and fifth steps are repeated until each trainee performs the skills competently.

The final steps of the training process just described represent the *competency-based* aspect of evidence-based caregiver training (Reid et al., 2003). Specifically, the process continues until each trainee demonstrates competence in performing the target skills. If trainee practice of the skills occurs in a role-play situation, then that part of the training process continues in an in vivo manner in which each trainee carries out the treatment procedures addressed in the training with an individual with ASD. This latter step is critical to successful caregiver training; the training should never be considered complete until each respective trainee is observed to perform the skills competently with the individual with ASD.

Depending on the specific situation in which caregiver training is provided, variations in conducting each of the steps of performance- and competency-based training may be warranted. To illustrate, if the skills to be trained are complex or involve many performance steps, such as with many intervention procedures to reduce challenging behavior of a person with ASD, the skills may be broken down into component steps and each one introduced using the entire training process (e.g., the rationale for one component is presented followed by description, demonstration, and practice with feedback and then the entire process is repeated for each of the remaining components). Descriptions of variations with the steps of the overall training process are provided in a number of sources (Jahr, 1998; Reid & Parsons, 2000; Weiss, 2005).

Overcoming Common Obstacles to Evidence-Based Caregiver Training

As indicated previously, despite the repeatedly demonstrated effectiveness of the approach to caregiver training just summarized, it is not used in many human service agencies for training staff in relevant skills for providing treatment services for agency clients with ASD. The approach is also not used routinely for training many parents of children with ASD. There are two main reasons for the lack of evidence-based training of caregivers in this regard. First, people responsible for training staff and/or parents are not knowledgeable about evidence-based caregiver training procedures

(Reid et al., 2005). Second, the training process can be relatively time consuming and laborious in some situations (Phillips, 1998). The following two sections address each of these reasons, respectively, and how they may be addressed to potentially enhance more widespread application of evidence-based caregiver training procedures.

Informing caregiver trainers about evidence-based training. Human service personnel who are responsible for training caregivers of individuals with ASD have diverse backgrounds. Frequently, clinicians such as psychologists, occupational therapists, or speech and language pathologists are expected to train caregivers in designated treatment interventions. A common example is with clinicians who direct home-based intervention programs for children with ASD. These clinicians usually are the ones who train parents or paraprofessional "therapists" to implement the treatment programs they design. Clinicians also frequently train staff in service agencies to carry out various training programs to reduce challenging behavior among agency clients with ASD or to conduct teaching programs for developing adaptive skills. Supervisors and administrators in human service agencies likewise often assume staff training responsibilities. These personnel may have received training or education in any number of human service disciplines (e.g., social work, education administration, psychology). The formal training or education they have received, however, rarely focuses on use of evidence-based training procedures with caregivers (Reid et al., 2005; Schell, 1998). That is, they are trained to design and implement treatment programs with individuals with ASD, but not in how to train others to carry out such programs.

The lack of formal preparation of human service personnel in evidence-based caregiver training procedures represents a significant obstacle in many agencies for effectively training caregivers in treatment procedures for people with ASD. There is a rather pervasive, though infrequently recognized, misconception about professional skills necessary for training caregivers. It is assumed that if a clinician, for example, is skilled in a respective treatment procedure for application with a person with ASD, the clinician can pass on those skills to caregivers. Indeed, being skilled in conducting a treatment procedure is usually a prerequisite for training others to implement the procedure; however, it is not sufficient. Carrying out a treatment procedure and training others to carry out the procedure involve skills that overlap in part but are also different. Consequently, being skilled in implementing a treatment procedure does not ensure that an individual can effectively train someone else to carry out the procedure proficiently (McGimsey, Greene, & Lutzker, 1995; Parsons & Reid, 1995).

To promote more widespread application of evidence-based training procedures with caregivers, personnel expected to train caregivers must have opportunities to be trained themselves in how to effectively train others. Hence, more programs for training clinicians and other human service personnel in evidence-based caregiver training methods are warranted (Sturmey & Stiles, 1996). Such programs are needed in university and college courses in the human services as well as in on-the-job training opportunities in human service agencies. The latter training opportunities are especially needed for supervisory personnel in human service settings. Many human service supervisors are promoted from the ranks of direct support personnel and, as such, have no formal educational background in a human service discipline or in training the caregivers whom they supervise.

In considering the need for training of caregiver trainers, it should also be noted that such a need has recently begun to be addressed more frequently relative to what has occurred historically. Most notably, the rapid expansion of ABA services for individuals with ASD (Rosenwasser & Axelrod, 2001) has been accompanied by increases in university and college courses for training behavior analysts to provide those services. Formal training in behavior analysis, or at least training that leads to certification in behavior analysis, frequently addresses evidence-based caregiver training due in large part to the inclusion of this topic in the certification exam for aspiring behavior analysts (Moore & Shook, 2001). Additionally, the American Association on Intellectual and Developmental Disabilities has recently sponsored the development of a supervisor training curriculum that includes evidence-based caregiver training procedures (Reid, Parsons, & Green, 2011).

In addressing the need to expand adoption of evidence-based caregiver training procedures among human service personnel who provide such training, special consideration is warranted on the nature of what it means to be *evidence-based*. One component of maintaining an evidence base involves obtaining evidence to document that what is done results in the desired outcome (Reid et al., in press). In this case, observable evidence must be obtained to indicate that once trainees have received the training they can then perform the skills addressed in the training while on the job. Caregiver trainers must be held accountable for obtaining evidence that their trainees do indeed perform the targeted skills competently as they work with people with ASD. Such accountability is equally as important, though not as readily recognized, as the accountability imposed on clinicians and teachers who carry out treatment interventions themselves with clients and students with ASD. Just as a clinician's or teacher's effectiveness should be judged by improvement in the functioning of his/her clients or students, the effectiveness of caregiver trainers should be judged by the degree of improvement in the skills of the caregivers they train. Systematic observation of trainee on-the-job performance must be conducted to obtain evidence that following training, caregivers can demonstrate proficient application of the skills targeted by the training.

Reducing time and effort involved in evidence-based caregiver training. Evidence-based caregiver training usually requires increased time and effort of trainers and trainees relative to more commonly used verbal-based training procedures. As indicated previously, verbal-based training procedures focus on presentation of spoken and written information. Evidence-based training includes these components, yet requires the addition of the performance-based components. The latter training procedures often require much more time to complete than the former procedures.

The increased time and effort often inherent in evidence-based training procedures is well illustrated in situations in which clinicians who develop behavior support plans for challenging behavior must train residential staff who provide supports for clients with ASD and are expected to implement the plans. Most residential settings employ direct support staff who work on different shifts. Because staff on each shift are usually expected to implement the plans, all of these staff must be trained by the clinician. Hence, the clinician typically must be present to train staff on the day and evening work shifts as well as the night shift in many cases, which requires multiple training sessions by the clinician at different times of the day. Because various staff work different days to cover a 7-day week, training must also occur on different days to include all staff. The process becomes even more time consuming when there are staff from other parts of the agency who require training because they periodically work with a given client (e.g., they are temporarily re-assigned to cover staff absences). Training time is further expanded if a client's plan must be implemented by staff in different locations, such as by staff in the client's residence and day treatment or education site. To adequately train all of these staff, a clinician must spend time with each staff person across the various times and locations.

The amount of time required to provide evidence-based caregiver training in situations such as those just described can make it difficult for a trainer to find the necessary time to conduct the training adequately. In other situations, trainers simply are reluctant to exert the increased time and effort required for adequate caregiver training and resort to relying on less effortful – and less effective – training strategies. Financial considerations also can impede a trainer's likelihood of carrying out training in an evidence-based manner. Some human service agencies are reluctant to support large amounts of clinician time, for example, to train staff relative to time spent working directly with clients themselves. In a related vein, private practitioners may not be able to bill or receive financial remuneration for time spent training caregivers relative to time spent working more directly with individuals who have ASD.

In light of growing recognition of the need for evidence-based training of caregivers (Reid, 2004; Reid et al., in press; Weiss, 2005) and the amount of time and effort such training can entail, ways to reduce trainer time and effort have been explored. One of the earliest approaches used to reduce the workload of a respective trainer is a pyramidal training strategy (Demchak & Browder, 1990; Green & Reid, 1994; Jones, Fremouw, & Carples, 1977; Page, Iwata, & Reid, 1982; Shore, Iwata, Vollmer, Lerman, & Zarcone, 1995). A pyramidal approach to caregiver training generally involves a trainer training supervisors or related personnel to assist in caregiver training through a train-the-trainers method. To illustrate, a clinician may train supervisors in a group home and day support setting to assist in training staff to implement a respective client's behavior support plan. The time required of the supervisors to train staff is reduced relative to that of the clinician because the supervisors are usually present with the staff in their routine work setting and can provide the training without having to travel to different locations.

Several investigations have supported the effectiveness of pyramidal training approaches with caregivers (Green & Reid, 1994; Page et al., 1982; Shore et al., 1995). An additional benefit of this type of training is that the process can enhance relevant skills of those personnel (e.g., staff supervisors) who function as caregiver trainers after having been trained by someone else (e.g., a clinician) in a given treatment procedure for an individual with ASD. That is, the process can help the supervisors maintain their own skills in applying the treatment procedure (van den Pol, Reid, & Fuqua, 1983). In contrast, one potential obstacle with the pyramidal approach is that it requires time and effort of those personnel who are expected to assist with caregiver training beyond their typically expected work duties, and not all personnel welcome such increased responsibilities (van den Pol et al., 1983).

A variation on the pyramidal model of caregiver training involving staff supervisors is a peer training approach (Neef, 1995) in which staff (or parents) assume the responsibility of training their caregiver peers. This approach entails essentially the same advantages and disadvantages of involving supervisors as trainers of their staff; however, the issue of support staff desiring to function in a training capacity with their staff peers, and particularly when they are not relieved of other duties to allow time for peer training, can become more problematic relative to supervisors functioning as staff trainers (van den Pol et al., 1983). Supervisors generally have more control over how they spend their work time than do direct support staff and, consequently, usually can more easily arrange work time for staff training purposes.

More recent attempts to expedite evidence-based caregiver training have focused on use of visual technology, such as training videos and DVDs (Catania, Almeida, Liu-Constant, & Reed, 2009; Moore & Fisher, 2007). To illustrate, Macurik, O'Kane, Malanga, and Reid (2008) prepared computer videos that described the components of behavior support plans for clients. Residential staff who were to be trained to implement the plans were scheduled to view the videos on agency computers during their routine work days. The presence of the clinicians who developed the plans and were responsible for training the staff was not required for this portion of the training. The videos in the Macurik et al. investigation in essence provided the *verbal-based* components of the training steps represented in Table 32.1 (i.e., the rationale for the plans and summary of the plans' constituent procedures). Clinicians then conducted the *performance-based* components with individual staff while on the job (the demonstrations, trainee practice, and feedback). Macurik et al. found that use of the videos for a portion of the staff training was just as effective as more traditional live training by the clinicians, yet required less time for both trainers and trainees.

Use of visual technology appears to offer considerable promise for facilitating caregiver training. The technology is becoming more commonplace in many human service settings and is increasingly more affordable and exportable (Buzhardt & Heitzman-Powell, 2005; Neef, Trachtenberg, Loeb, & Sterner, 1991). Caution is also warranted though with this approach to training pending additional research. There is currently a plethora of training videos, web-based training programs, and DVDs available for caregivers of people with ASD; however, the vast majority of the training programs have not been thoroughly evaluated to determine the extent to which caregivers actually learn how to perform skills addressed in the programs (Macurik et al., 2008).

Concern over the effectiveness of visual technology becomes heightened when considering existing research as summarized earlier that supports the need for *performance-based* training components. Video-based training materials tend to focus on verbal (spoken and/or written) material, although relevant performance demonstrations can also be included. To date, these approaches to training generally do not include the performance practice and feedback components that are usually critical for effective caregiver training. Some research has indicated that without the latter performance-based components, video training is not sufficiently effective (Neef et al., 1991; Nielsen, Sigurdsson, & Austin, 2009), although contradictory results have also been reported that support the effectiveness of exclusive reliance on video training (Catania et al., 2009). Continued research is needed on various types of visual-based technology for caregiver training, both to evaluate general effectiveness and to delineate the conditions under which such approaches to training are and are not sufficiently effective in helping caregivers acquire new performance skills.

In considering research on the utility of visual-based technology for training caregivers, an area that warrants attention in addition to effectiveness is the *acceptability* of the training. Acceptability refers to the degree to which caregiver trainees like or enjoy the training process (Parsons, 1998). Caregiver acceptance of a training program, as well as trainer acceptance associated with conducting the training, can impact the likelihood of the program's long-term survival in an agency (Parsons). Relatedly, enhancing the degree of acceptance of a particular approach to caregiver training may make it more likely that the approach will be used by more caregiver trainers (Balcazar, Shupert, Daniels, Mawhinney, & Hopkins, 1989).

To date, acceptability research on the types of performance-based training programs summarized earlier has generally indicated that the programs are well received by caregivers (see Reid & Parsons, 2000, for a summary). Research has also indicated that different components of the training process, or variations in how the components are conducted, have differential effects on trainee acceptance of the training. For example, how quickly feedback is provided by a trainer following trainee practice of target skills as part of the training process seems to impact trainee acceptance, with somewhat more acceptance of immediate versus delayed feedback (Reid & Parsons, 1996). There is also some indication that live demonstrations by trainers are more preferred by trainees than video-taped demonstrations (Macurik et al., 2008); however, there is concern over the methodology used to evaluate trainee acceptance of training programs in which they participate (Parsons, 1998; Reid & Parsons, 1995), such that conclusions about the acceptability of respective training programs and their constituent procedures should be considered cautiously at this point. Continued research seems needed to better evaluate the acceptability of caregiver training programs, as well as to develop programs that are maximally effective and acceptable.

Issues Related to Parent Training

Parents of course play a vital role in the development of children with ASD. Other family members such as grandparents and siblings also frequently impact a child's development. For family members to be maximally successful in assisting children with ASD in overcoming the numerous obstacles ASD typically presents, family members often must be well versed in evidence-based treatment strategies. For example, family members need knowledge and skills for helping children develop and functionally use language, social, and self-help skills. Family members also usually need to help children overcome various types of challenging behavior. When children enter school, family members likewise must possess various knowledge and skills to help in the extension, generalization, and maintenance of skills taught in school settings.

The importance of the skills of family members of children with ASD in applying evidence-based treatment strategies is well illustrated in early intervention services within an ABA format. These types of services generally are considered to represent the most scientifically established, effective means of promoting the development of children with ASD and helping them overcome obstacles presented by this disability (Cuvo & Vallelunga, 2007; Rosenwasser & Axelrod, 2001). In turn, ABA services are more likely to be maximally effective for children living at home when family members are integrally involved in, and skillfully provide, ABA interventions (Matson, Mahan, & Matson, 2009; Symon, Koegel, & Singer, 2006). The latter outcome is due to the need to provide rather intensive amounts of ABA teaching services beyond what can be provided within schools and other day programs (Cuvo & Vallelunga, 2007) and to provide consistency in preventing and decreasing challenging behavior throughout a child's waking hours (Symon et al., 2006).

When parents are not well equipped in evidence-based treatment strategies, not only is the development of their children likely to be diminished but the overall quality of life of the family at large is likely to be negatively impacted (Symon, 2001). This is particularly the case with challenging behavior that can seriously limit family opportunities to participate in typical social and community experiences. The day-to-day functioning of the family within the home can likewise become difficult and stressful (Symon, 2001).

In light of the important role parents as well as other family members play in the development and socialization process of children with ASD, there has been a very considerable amount of research on how to train parents for assisting their children in this regard (see Matson et al., 2009; Shriver & Allen, 2008; Symon, 2001, 2005, for reviews and summaries). As indicated earlier, the basic components of effectively training parents and other family members in important knowledge and skills for helping children with ASD are the same as those for training other caregivers (see also Shriver & Allen, Chapter 5); however, there are also special issues and circumstances to consider in training parents relative to training paid staff who work in agencies providing supports and services for individuals with ASD. Particular issues to consider include ensuring parents are knowledgeable about what constitutes evidence-based practices for individuals with ASD, accessing resources to receive training in these evidence-based treatment strategies, and assisting parents in providing effective training for other parents and family members.

Determining What Constitutes Evidence-Based Practices

As presented in other chapters in this text as well as elsewhere (Cuvo & Vallelunga, 2007; Dyer, Martino, & Parvenski, 2006; Matson et al., 2009), both the number of children diagnosed with ASD and public awareness of ASD have increased dramatically in recent years. Commensurate with such increases has been increased availability of, and access to, information about this disability. The number of available books, manuals, compact disks, and videotapes relating to ASD has grown rapidly. Internet and related media have likewise become a significant source of information for parents and other family members. Ready access to information about ASD and methods to help people with ASD can be very beneficial for family members; however, there are also some accompanying disadvantages about the relative ease with which parents can access such information.

The most notable disadvantage of the rapidly increasing amount of available information about ASD is difficulties parents and other family members can encounter in determining if the information will be truly helpful in assisting children who have ASD. Some of the information has a strong evidence base as referred to in the introductory comments to this chapter: the information is based on valid scientific research to support its efficacy and specifies the conditions in which the information is likely to be helpful for respective people with ASD. There is also a large amount of information though that has no such evidence base and its true usefulness is unknown at best and at worst, harmful. Much information continues to be disseminated about ASD that includes a variety of fads, quick "cures," and totally unvalidated treatment recommendations (Cuvo & Vallelunga, 2007; Pelios & Lund, 2001).

It is only natural that parents, as well as other concerned family members, would strongly desire information to help their children with ASD. When the information has no acceptable evidence to support its utility though, parents can spend tremendous amounts of time and financial resources on treatment approaches and other supports that are not likely to be of any significant benefit. Additionally, when time is spent providing interventions that are not effective, individuals with ASD are deprived of other, evidence-based treatment services that are likely to be helpful. Spending time on noneffective treatments is especially problematic during the early years of children with ASD. In essence, the longer effective early intervention is delayed, the amount of expected progress in the children's functioning correspondingly tends to decrease (Koegel, Nefdt, Koegel, Bruinsma, & Fredeen, 2006).

Due to the importance of effective treatments, and particularly as part of early intervention for children with ASD, it is critical that parents have opportunities to receive information and training on what constitutes evidence-based treatment. The importance of providing information to parents on how to evaluate the evidence basis for recommended treatment approaches is becoming increasingly recognized, and some useful information sources are available (see Koegel & Koegel, 2006; Shriver & Allen, 2008, for representative samples); however, much work is needed in this area to provide parents with more ready access to valid means of determining the evidence base of the numerous treatment approaches currently advertised for individuals with ASD (Crockett, Fleming, Doepke, & Stevens, 2007).

Increasing Evidence-Based Training Opportunities

A rather pervasive obstacle many parents and other family members of children with ASD face is where to find services that will give them the knowledge and skills to provide evidence-based treatment strategies for their children. Although many good services exist across the United States (Crockett et al., 2007; Matson et al., 2009; Shriver & Allen, 2008; Chapter 2), numerous gaps exist in service availability in most states and particularly in more rural areas (Symon, 2001; Symon et al., 2006).

It is likewise important that services be made available that provide not only applicable information on evidence-based treatment strategies for individuals with ASD, but also evidence-based training of parents themselves in how to use effective treatment strategies (Matson et al., 2009). Parents warrant training about evidence-based interventions that is effective, and that training generally must be both performance- and competency-based as summarized earlier. As also noted earlier regarding effective training of staff working with individuals with ASD, such training almost always must be accompanied by follow-up services to support parent application of skills acquired in parent training programs. Until more of these types of services become available, many parents will likely encounter serious difficulty in providing maximally effective home-based support for their children with ASD.

As the number of children diagnosed with ASD has increased and public recognition of ASD has grown, the number of public school programs offering evidence-based treatment services such as ABA-based interventions has increased (Steege et al., 2007). Public schools represent one potentially very helpful source of training for parents and other family members. In many cases though, school programs providing evidence-based services for students with ASD offer little in the way of formal parent training. Often the training that is provided is the responsibility of classroom teachers who may or may not have had formal training in evidence-based services for students with ASD, much less training in how to effectively train parents (Ingersoll & Dvortcsak, 2009). The parent training that is provided is often informal, consisting of brief discussions at the end of the school day or quickly prepared notes or e-mail messages concerning classroom activities and student responses to the activities. A significant need exists for school systems to offer more formal training programs for parents and to use evidence-based strategies for training the parents in how to help their children with ASD (Ingersoll & Dvortcsak, 2009). A number of models for providing these types of parent training services currently exist (e.g., Crockett et al., 2007; Cuvo & Vallelunga, 2007; Dyer et al., 2006; Neef, 1995), though a much more comprehensive adoption of the approaches is needed across school systems in most parts of the United States.

Improved Preparation of Parents as Trainers of Other Parents

One of the most useful and frequently relied upon sources of information for parents is other parents of children with ASD (Neef, 1995; Symon, 2005). Numerous support groups exist specifically for parents to provide information on treatment interventions as well as to provide needed advocacy support. As with other issues specifically related to parents though, often the information that is provided is not evidence-based. In the worst case scenario, parents are provided with information that may be locally popular but has no established evidence base and, as such, is not likely to be of significant benefit to the parent recipients and their children.

Several issues seem paramount to address if parents are to function effectively as trainers of other parents. First, parents must have opportunities to become knowledgeable about what constitutes evidence-based treatment for individuals with ASD as summarized earlier. Second, parents must also have opportunities to become skilled in effective strategies for training others. Addressing these two needs on a much broader scale than what currently exists represents an area in which many human service agencies and schools could provide a very useful service.

Summary

Effective training of caregivers is a critical component in the overall provision of evidence-based treatment for individuals who have ASD. In turn, training of caregivers is most likely to be effective if the training itself is evidence-based. We have summarized what currently constitutes an evidence-based approach to caregiver training, focusing on performance- and competency-based training procedures.

The approach to training discussed in this chapter is well supported by applied research, having been successfully implemented and carefully evaluated in numerous investigations with both staff and parent caregivers; however, more work needs to be done to extend what research and application have demonstrated into more common practice. Specific obstacles to providing more evidence-based training of caregivers that warrant resolution include training more people who train caregivers in how to provide evidence-based training, making the existing training technology more practical and efficient by reducing the time and effort required of both trainers and trainees, and providing more caregivers with ready access to both evidence-based treatment strategies for individuals with ASD and evidence-based training in how to apply those strategies. Addressing these issues through research and systematic action could help prepare more caregivers to provide effective treatment services and lead to better outcomes and overall life quality for people who have ASD.

References

Adkins, V. K. (1996). Discussion: Behavioral procedures for training direct care staff in facilities serving dependent populations. *Behavioral Interventions, 11*, 95–100.

Alavosius, M. P., & Sulzer-Azaroff, B. (1990). Acquisition and maintenance of health-care routines as a function of feedback density. *Journal of Applied Behavior Analysis, 23*, 151–162.

Balcazar, F. E., Shupert, M. K., Daniels, A. C., Mawhinney, T. C., & Hopkins, B. L. (1989). An objective review and analysis of ten years of publication in the Journal of Organizational Behavior Management. *Journal of Organizational Behavior Management, 10*, 7–37.

Brackett, L., Reid, D. H., & Green, C. W. (2007). Effects of reactivity to observations on staff performance. *Journal of Applied Behavior Analysis, 40*, 191–195.

Buzhardt, J., & Heitzman-Powell, L. (2005). Training behavioral aides with a combination of online and face-to-face procedures. *Teaching Exceptional Children, 37*, 20–26.

Catania, C. N., Almeida, D., Liu-Constant, B., & Reed, F. D. D. (2009). Video modeling to train staff to implement discrete-trial instruction. *Journal of Applied Behavior Analysis, 42*, 387–392.

Codding, R. S., Livanis, A., Pace, G. M., & Vaca, L. (2008). Using performance feedback to improve treatment integrity of classwide behavior plans: An investigation of observer reactivity. *Journal of Applied Behavior Analysis, 41*, 417–422.

Crockett, J. L., Fleming, R. K., Doepke, K. J., & Stevens, J. S. (2007). Parent training: Acquisition and generalization of discrete trials teaching skills with parents of children with autism. *Research in Developmental Disabilities, 28*, 23–36.

Cuvo, A. J., & Vallelunga, L. R. (2007). A transactional systems model of autism services. *The Behavior Analyst, 30*, 161–180.

Demchak, M. A. (1987). A review of behavioral staff training in special education settings. *Education and Training in Mental Retardation, 22*, 205–217.

Demchak, M. A., & Browder, D. M. (1990). An evaluation of the pyramid model of staff training in group homes for adults with severe handicaps. *Education and Training in Mental Retardation, 25*, 150–163.

Detrich, R., Keyworth, R., & States, J. (2008). A roadmap to evidence-based education: Building an evidence-based culture. In R. Detrich, R. Keyworth, J. States (Eds.), *Advances in evidence-based education, Volume 1: A roadmap to evidence-based education* (pp. 3–25). Oakland, CA: The Wing Institute.

DiGennaro, F. D., Martens, B. K., & Kleinmann, A. E. (2007). A comparison of performance feedback procedures on teachers' treatment implementation integrity and students' inappropriate behavior in special education classrooms. *Journal of Applied Behavior Analysis, 40*, 447–461.

Dyer, K., Martino, G. M., & Parvenski, T. (2006). The River Street Autism Program: A case study of a regional service center behavioral intervention program. *Behavior Modification, 30*, 1–19.

Fisk, K. E. (2008). Treatment integrity of school-based behavior analytic interventions: A review of the research. *Behavior Analysis in Practice, 1*(2), 19–25.

Gardner, J. M. (1972). Teaching behavior modification to nonprofessionals. *Journal of Applied Behavior Analysis, 5*, 517–521.

Green, C. W., & Reid, D. H. (1994). A comprehensive evaluation of a train-the-trainers model for training education staff to assemble adaptive switches. *Journal of Developmental and Physical Disabilities, 6*, 219–237.

Greene, B. F., Willis, B. S., Levy, R., & Bailey, J. S. (1978). Measuring client gains from staff-implemented programs. *Journal of Applied Behavior Analysis, 11*, 395–412.

Harchik, A. E., & Campbell, A. R. (1998). Supporting people with developmental disabilities in their homes in the community: The role of organizational behavior management. *Journal of Organizational Behavior Management, 18*(2/3), 83–101.

Ingersoll, B., & Dvortcsak, A. (2009). Including parent training in the early childhood special education curriculum for children with Autism Spectrum Disorders. *Journal of Positive Behavior Interventions, 8*, 79–87.

Jahr, E. (1998). Current issues in staff training. *Research in Developmental Disabilities, 19*, 73–87.

Jones, F. H., Fremouw, W., & Carples, S. (1977). Pyramid training of elementary school teachers to use a classroom management "skills package". *Journal of Applied Behavior Analysis, 10*, 239–253.

Koegel, R. L., & Koegel, L. K. (2006). *Pivotal response treatments for autism: Communication, social, & academic development*. Baltimore, MD: Paul H. Brookes.

Koegel, L. K., Nefdt, N., Koegel, R. L., Bruinsma, Y. E. M., & Fredeen, R. M. (2006). A screening, training, and education program: First S.T.E.P. In R. L. Koegel, L. K. Koegel (Eds.), *Pivotal response treatments for autism: Communication, social, & academic development* (pp. 31–52). Baltimore, MD: Paul H. Brookes.

Lerman, D. C., Tetreault, A., Hovanetz, A., Strobel, M., & Garro, J. (2008). Further evaluation of a brief, intensive teacher-training model. *Journal of Applied Behavior Analysis, 41*, 243–248.

Macurik, K. M., O'Kane, N. P., Malanga, P., & Reid, D. H. (2008). Video training of support staff in intervention plans for challenging behavior: Comparison with live training. *Behavioral Interventions, 23*, 143–163.

Matson, M. L., Mahan, S., & Matson, J. L. (2009). Parent training: A review of methods for children with autism spectrum disorders. *Research in Autism Spectrum Disorders, 3*, 868–875.

McGimsey, J. F., Greene, B. F., & Lutzker, J. R. (1995). Competence in aspects of behavioral treatment and consultation: Implications for service delivery and graduate training. *Journal of Applied Behavior Analysis, 28*, 301–315.

Miles, N. I., & Wilder, D. A. (2009). The effects of behavioral skills training on caregiver implementation of guided compliance. *Journal of Applied Behavior Analysis, 42*, 405–410.

Montegar, C. A., Reid, D. H., Madsen, C. H., & Ewell, M. D. (1977). Increasing institutional staff to resident interactions through in-service training and supervisor approval. *Behavior Therapy, 8*, 533–540.

Moore, J., & Shook, G. L. (2001). Certification, accreditation, and quality control in behavior analysis. *The Behavior Analyst, 24*, 45–55.

Moore, J. W., & Fisher, W. W. (2007). The effects of videotape modeling on staff acquisition of functional analysis methodology. *Journal of Applied Behavior Analysis, 40*, 197–202.

Neef, N. A. (1995). Pyramidal parent training by peers. *Journal of Applied Behavior Analysis, 28*, 333–337.

Neef, N. A., Trachtenberg, S., Loeb, J., & Sterner, K. (1991). Video-based training of respite care providers: An interactional analysis of presentation format. *Journal of Applied Behavior Analysis, 24*, 473–486.

Nielsen, D., Sigurdsson, S. O., & Austin, J. (2009). Preventing back injuries in hospital settings: The effects of video modeling on safe patient lifting by nurses. *Journal of Applied Behavior Analysis, 42*, 551–561.

Page, T. J., Iwata, B. A., & Reid, D. H. (1982). Pyramidal training: A large-scale application with institutional staff. *Journal of Applied Behavior Analysis, 15*, 335–351.

Parsons, M. B. (1998). A review of procedural acceptability in Organizational Behavior Management. *Journal of Organizational Behavior Management, 18*, 173–190.

Parsons, M. B., & Reid, D. H. (1995). Training residential supervisors to provide feedback for maintaining staff teaching skills with people who have severe disabilities. *Journal of Applied Behavior Analysis, 28*, 317–32.

Parsons, M. B., Reid, D. H., & Green, C. W. (1996). Training basic teaching skills to community and institutional support staff for people with severe disabilities: A one-day program. *Research in Developmental Disabilities, 17*, 467–485.

Parsons, M. B., Reid, D. H., & Lattimore, L. P. (2009). Increasing independence of adults with autism in community activities: A brief, embedded teaching strategy. *Behavior Analysis in Practice, 2*, 40–48.

Pelios, L. V., & Lund, S. K. (2001). A selective overview of issues on classification, causation, and early intensive behavioral intervention for autism. *Behavior Modification, 25*, 678–697.

Petscher, E. S., & Bailey, J. S. (2006). Effects of training, prompting, and self-monitoring on staff behavior in a classroom for students with disabilities. *Journal of Applied Behavior Analysis, 39*, 215–226.

Phillips, J. F. (1998). Applications and contributions of organizational behavior management in schools and day treatment settings. *Journal of Organizational Behavior Management, 18*, 103–129.

Powers, M. D. (2000). *Children with Autism: A parents' guide* (2nd ed.). Bethesda, MD: Woodbine House.

Reid, D. H. (2004). Training and supervising direct support personnel to carry out behavioral procedures. In J. L. Matson, R. B. Laud, M. L. Matson (Eds.), *Behavior modification for persons with developmental disabilities: Treatments and supports* (pp. 73–99). Kingston, NY: NADD Press.

Reid, D. H., O'Kane, N. P., & Macurik, K. M. (in press). Staff training and management. In W. Fisher, C. Piazza, H. Roane (Eds.), *Handbook of applied behavior analysis*. New York: Guilford Publications.

Reid, D. H., & Parsons, M. B. (1995). Comparing choice and questionnaire measures of the acceptability of a staff training procedure. *Journal of Applied Behavior Analysis, 28*, 95–96.

Reid, D. H., & Parsons, M. B. (1996). A comparison of staff acceptability of immediate versus delayed feedback in staff training. *Journal of Organizational Behavior Management, 16*, 35–47.

Reid, D. H., & Parsons, M. B. (2000). Organizational behavior management in human service settings. In J. Austin, J. E. Carr (Eds.), *Handbook of applied behavior analysis* (pp. 275–294). Reno, NV: Context Press.

Reid, D. H., & Parsons, M. B. (2002). *Working with staff to overcome challenging behavior among people who have severe disabilities:*

A guide for getting support plans carried out. Morganton, NC: Habilitative Management Consultants.

Reid, D. H., & Parsons, M. B. (2006). *Motivating human service staff: Supervisory strategies for maximizing work effort and work enjoyment, 2nd Edition*. Morganton, NC: Habilitative Management Consultants.

Reid, D. H., Parsons, M. B., & Green, C. W. (2011). *The supervisor training curriculum: Evidence-based ways to promote work quality and enjoyment among support staff*. Washington, DC: American Association on Intellectual and Developmental Disabilities.

Reid, D. H., Parsons, M. B., Lattimore, L. P., Towery, D. L., & Reade, K. K. (2005). Improving staff performance through clinician application of outcome management. *Research in Developmental Disabilities, 26*, 101–116.

Reid, D. H., Rotholz, D. A., Parsons, M. B., Morris, L., Braswell, B. A., Green, C. W., et al. (2003). Training human service supervisors in aspects of positive behavior support: Evaluation of a statewide, performance-based program. *Journal of Positive Behavior Interventions, 5*, 35–46.

Rosenwasser, B., & Axelrod, S. (2001). The contributions of applied behavior analysis to the education of people with autism. *Behavior Modification, 25*, 671–677.

Sarokoff, R. A., & Sturmey, P. (2004). The effects of behavioral skills training on staff implementation of discrete-trial teaching. *Journal of Applied Behavior Analysis, 37*, 535–538.

Schell, R. M. (1998). Organizational behavior management: Applications with professional staff. *Journal of Organizational Behavior Management, 18*, 157–171.

Schepis, M. M., Reid, D. H., Ownbey, J., & Parsons, M. B. (2001). Training support staff to embed teaching within natural routines of young children with disabilities in an inclusive preschool. *Journal of Applied Behavior Analysis, 34*, 313–327.

Shore, B. A., Iwata, B. A., Vollmer, T. R., Lerman, D. C., & Zarcone, J. R. (1995). Pyramidal staff training in the extension of treatment for severe behavior disorders. *Journal of Applied Behavior Analysis, 28*, 323–332.

Shriver, M. D., & Allen, K. D. (2008). *Working with parents of noncompliant children: A guide to evidence-based parent training for practitioners and students*. Washington, DC: American Psychological Association.

Smith, T., Parker, T., Taubman, M., & Lovaas, O. I. (1992). Transfer of staff training from workshops to group homes: A failure to generalize across settings. *Research in Developmental Disabilities, 13*, 57–71.

Steege, M. W., Mace, F. C., Perry, L., & Longenecker, H. (2007). Applied behavior analysis: Beyond discrete trial teaching. *Psychology in the Schools, 44*, 91–99.

Sturmey, P. (1998). History and contribution of Organizational Behavior Management to services for persons with developmental disabilities. *Journal of Organizational Behavior Management, 18*(2/3), 7–32.

Sturmey, P., & Stiles, L. A. (1996). Training needs of shift supervisors in a residential facility for persons with developmental disabilities: Shift supervisor's and middle manager's perceptions. *Behavioral Interventions, 11*, 141–146.

Symon, J. B. (2001). Parent education for autism: Issues in providing services at a distance. *Journal of Positive Behavior Interventions, 3*, 160–174.

Symon, J. B. (2005). Expanding interventions for children with autism: Parents as trainers. *Journal of Positive Behavior Interventions, 7*, 159–173.

Symon, J. B., Koegel, R. L., & Singer, G. H. S. (2006). Parent perspectives of parent education programs. In R. L. Koegel, L. K. Koegel (Eds.), *Pivotal response treatments for autism: Communication, social, & academic development* (pp. 93–115). Baltimore, MD: Paul H. Brookes.

Vollmer, T. R., Sloman, K. N., & Peter Pipkin, C., St. (2008). Practical implications of data reliability and treatment integrity monitoring. *Behavior Analysis in Practice, 1*, 4–11.

van den Pol, R. A., Reid, D. H., & Fuqua, R. W. (1983). Peer training of safety-related skills to institutional staff: Benefits for trainers and trainees. *Journal of Applied Behavior Analysis, 16*, 139–156.

Weiss, M. J. (2005). Comprehensive ABA programs: Integrating and evaluating the implementation of varied instructional approaches. *The Behavior Analyst Today, 6*, 214–221.

Wilder, D. A., Atwell, J., & Wine, B. (2006). The effects of varying levels of treatment integrity on child compliance during treatment with a three-step prompting procedure. *Journal of Applied Behavior Analysis, 39*, 369–373.

Adults with Autism Spectrum Disorders

33

Sara Mahan and Alison M. Kozlowski

Introduction

Autism spectrum disorders (ASD), otherwise referred to as pervasive developmental disorders, first appeared in the *Diagnostic and Statistical Manual, Third Edition* (American Psychiatric Association, 1980). Since the debut of this spectrum of disorders 29 years ago, changes in diagnostic criteria as well as increased recognition and available assessments have been thought to increase the prevalence of ASD over time (Rutter, 2005; Wing & Potter, 2002). With the development of instruments to assess for ASD among those with Intellectual Disability (ID) and the increased knowledge of ASD, adults with ID living in a variety of settings began to be assessed and given a comorbid ASD diagnosis. Currently, up to 70% of individuals with ASD also have a diagnosis of ID (Fombonne, 2005; La Malfa, Lassi, Bertelli, Salvini, & Placidi, 2004; Matson & Shoemaker, 2009).

As these children and adolescents with ASD mature, they become adults with ASD. The time span of adulthood is greater than that of childhood and adolescence combined. Childhood and adolescence span 18 years whereas adulthood has the potential to span more than 50 years. As such, the adult ASD population comprises and will continue to comprise the majority of the ASD population. Since the symptoms of ASD persist into adulthood (Seltzer, Shattuck, Abbeduto, & Greenburg, 2004), the disorder will affect an individual's ability to live independently as well as gain and maintain employment. Despite this, the focus of research and public attention is on children with ASD. Although early intervention is important, research focusing on specific interventions, training programs, and various supports for adults with ASD is also imperative. In an effort to highlight the needs and service provision for adults with ASD, this chapter

will provide an overview of treatment techniques used among adults with ASD, prognosis, living placements, transition from high school, employment options and supports, specific models providing multiple services, and training programs focusing on relationships and sexuality.

Treatment

Within the adult ASD population, deficits in communication and socialization skills, restricted and repetitive interests, and associated behaviors (e.g., challenging behaviors) are targeted in the same manner as in children and adolescents with ASD. Interventions for the treatment of core symptoms of ASD in adults include a variety of methods based on the behavioral model (Rosenwasser & Axelrod, 2002) to increase communication and social skills, to improve restricted and repetitive patterns of behavior, and to decrease challenging behaviors. However, despite the widespread use of behavioral interventions and the plethora of research supporting their effectiveness among children with ASD, there is a paucity of research in this area within the adult population. The limited research consists mostly of case studies and primarily focuses on adults with comorbid ID and ASD. Research focuses on skills training and operant conditioning utilizing such techniques as modeling, fading, and differential reinforcement.

One of the overarching theories in the development of ASD is theory of mind. This theory posits that individuals with ASD lack the ability to take others' perspectives and that this primary deficit leads to problems in a variety of areas, including social skills (Schreibman, 2005). In conjunction with this theory, one study has used an adapted version of the Social Cognition and Interaction Training for Adults (SCIT-A) (Turner-Brown, Perry, Dichter, Bodfish, & Penn, 2008), which was originally designed for use with adults with psychotic disorders, to examine whether a specific intervention could increase theory of mind abilities, as

S. Mahan (✉)
Department of Psychology, Louisiana State University, Baton Rouge, LA 70803, USA
e-mail: srm101010@gmail.com

J.L. Matson, P. Sturmey (eds.), *International Handbook of Autism and Pervasive Developmental Disorders*, Autism and Child Psychopathology Series, DOI 10.1007/978-1-4419-8065-6_33, © Springer Science+Business Media, LLC 2011

521

well as emotional identification, among adults with high-functioning autism (HFA). The adapted SCIT-A consisted of three phases which taught adults to identify emotions, understand situations, and integrate skills while generalizing them to real-life situations over the course of 18 weeks. The authors concluded that this paradigm significantly increased the performance on a theory of mind task and an emotional identification task, which are issues considered to be related to core features of ASD.

Other researchers focusing on the core symptoms of ASD have successfully improved communication deficits using behavioral interventions. Farmer-Dougan (1994) increased appropriate verbal communication skills in six adults with ID, one who was also diagnosed with an ASD, in a natural setting (i.e., mealtimes) by providing food contingent on appropriate verbalizations. When the intervention was removed, these increases in appropriate verbal communication remained and the skills generalized across other mealtimes and individuals. Additionally, other behavioral interventions used to improve communication deficits in the child and adolescent population, such as picture exchange communication systems and mand training (Charlop-Christy, Carpenter, Le, LeBlanc, & Kellet, 2002; Ganz & Simpson, 2004; Matson, Sevin, Fridley, & Love, 1990), are consistently applied to adults with ASD.

Although there is limited research examining the effectiveness of behavioral techniques in increasing social skills in adults with ASD, these techniques have been well studied and frequently applied to younger populations (Matson & Minshawi, 2006; Schreibman, 2000; Zachor, Ben-Itzchak, Rabinovich, & Lahat, 2007). Social skills interventions primarily include skills training combined with reinforcement for appropriate use of these learned skills. In regard to repetitive and restricted interests or behaviors, a mixture of differential reinforcement and non-exclusionary time-out was effective in greatly decreasing the frequency of stereotyped behavior (i.e., hand slapping on objects) in an adult male diagnosed with comorbid ID and ASD (McKeegan, Estill, & Campbell, 1984). Hand slapping on objects decreased from an average of 57.5 to 0.25 times per hour after 1-month follow-up. Other strategies for decreasing stereotyped behavior include replacing it with functionally equivalent behaviors coupled with a schedule of reinforcement. For insistence on sameness in routines, interventions primarily focus on using schedules, pictures, and/or written material, so the individuals will better understand their activities for the day. For more in-depth information regarding specific intervention techniques, the reader is referred to previous chapters of this book.

With respect to challenging behaviors, the most effective forms of treatment across populations are also based on behavioral strategies (Matson, 2007a, 2007b; Matson, Wilkins, & Gonzalez, 2008; Schreibman, 2005) utilizing reinforcement and punishment. The use of punishment, often referred to as aversive strategies, consists of time-out, over-correction, response cost, or verbal reprimand, among other methods. Aversive strategies are often considered to be more restrictive in nature and are often employed when less restrictive methods have proven ineffective. Due to this more restrictive nature, there has been a recent emphasis on the use of positive behavioral supports. These strategies are based on assessment with the goal being to decrease challenging behaviors by increasing pro-social behaviors, such as through improving communication and social skills. To help increase appropriate behavior, desired behavior is rewarded using various schedules of reinforcement and forms of differential reinforcement.

Smith (1986) utilized competing appropriate stimuli to successfully decrease the frequency of rectal digging in a young woman with comorbid ASD and ID. Similarly, researchers who conducted separate case studies found that differential reinforcement methods were successful in decreasing a variety of challenging behaviors (i.e., pica-like behavior, throwing items, pushing items, screaming, and finger picking) in adults with comorbid ID and ASD (Richman, Wacker, Asmus, & Casey, 1998; Smith, 1987). Using an ABAB design, Smith (1987) found that differential reinforcement of incompatible behavior was successful in reducing the daily frequency of pica-like behavior from a mean of 21.3 to 4.6. These effects continued at 1-year follow-up with a daily mean of 0.5 occurrences of pica-like behavior. Likewise, Richman and associates (1998) utilized extinction and differential reinforcement of appropriate behavior to decrease several challenging behaviors, including finger picking. During the baseline extinction condition, finger picking did not decrease. However, when differential reinforcement of appropriate behavior was added to the extinction procedure, finger picking decreased to near-zero frequencies.

Although there is a focus on the use of positive behavioral supports to the exclusion of incorporating aversive techniques, the use of positive behavioral supports alone has not been supported by the research (Matson & Minshawi, 2006). Rather, for severe challenging behaviors it appears that the use of aversive techniques along with positive behavioral supports may be the most effective (Foxx, 2005). Reese, Sherman, and Sheldon (1998) found that a mixture of differential reinforcement, response cost, and relaxation training was helpful in decreasing the frequency of a variety of challenging behaviors (i.e., verbal aggression, physical aggression, and property destruction) in a 26-year-old male with comorbid ID and ASD. Another case study found that non-contingent reinforcement (NCR) combined with response cost was more effective than NCR alone in reducing the frequency of inappropriate vocalizations in an 18-year-old male diagnosed with autism (Falcomata, Roane,

Hovanetz, & Kettering, 2004). From baseline, the percentage of inappropriate vocalizations decreased from 99.1 to 55.6% for the NCR condition alone. When response cost was added to NCR, the percentage of inappropriate vocalizations decreased by an additional 54.4% (from 55.6 to 1.2%). During reversal to baseline, this behavior increased to 98.9% but subsequently decreased to 0.3% during the NCR plus response cost condition. Further supporting that response cost is effective above and beyond NCR alone, during reversal to the NCR alone condition, the frequency of inappropriate vocalizations increased to 60.9%. Yet, when the NCR plus response cost condition was employed once again, the frequency reduced to 1.6%. For further discussion on the topic of positive behavioral supports and aversive techniques the reader is referred to Matson and Minshawi (2006) as well as Foxx (2005). It is important to note that effective interventions utilizing the least aversive strategies are optimal.

Although there is limited research specific to the adult ASD population on the efficacy of behavioral techniques to improve core symptoms of ASD and associated features, these strategies are consistently applied to this population. There is a call for more research using larger sample sizes to examine the effectiveness of behavioral strategies in general and to compare various behavioral strategies against each other for different target behaviors. As the number of adults with ASD grows, this will provide valuable information for their treatment and improving their quality of life.

Prognosis

An area of increased interest within ASD is outcome of these individuals in adulthood in the domains of intellectual functioning, language ability, self-help skills, employment, and social skills. This information is critical in establishing the prognosis of these individuals at younger ages so that appropriate supports can be implemented earlier to increase adulthood independence. Many studies classify the outcome of these adults as "very good," "good," "fair," "poor," and "very poor." Yet, the meanings of the terms within this classification system (i.e., ranging from "very good" to "very poor") are not always identical between studies, which can lead to confusion when comparing studies describing outcomes. However, it should be assumed that those with "very good" and "good" outcomes achieve an adequate level of independence, including employment, and sufficient social skills while those with "poor" and "very poor" outcomes require ongoing enhanced supports and demonstrate a lack of independence.

The overall outcome of adults with ASD varies depending on many factors. Unfortunately, prognostic indicators are considered to be either static in the individual or very resistant to change. Quite possibly the best predictor of later outcome in those with ASD is that of IQ (Howlin, Goode, Hutton, & Rutter, 2004; Seltzer et al., 2004). It has been well established that comorbidity of ASD with ID is common, with comorbidity rates reaching up to 70% (Fombonne, 2005; La Malfa et al., 2004; Matson & Shoemaker, 2009). Therefore, most studies of predictors of later outcome in ASD focus on IQ (LeBlanc, Riley, & Goldsmith, 2008). However, it should be noted that IQ is not the sole predictor of later outcome and that results are not linear (i.e., an IQ of 90 does not necessarily mean a better outcome than an IQ of 80) (Howlin et al., 2004). The relative cutoff IQ score to differentiate "good" from "poor" outcome is not agreed upon, but most studies tend to view individuals with mild ID to average intelligence as possessing better outcomes than those with moderate ID and below (Howlin, 2005; Seltzer et al., 2004). Based on findings that individuals with greater deficits in intellectual functioning in the absence of ASD also have poorer prognoses (Nordin & Gillberg, 1998), it is unclear if intellectual functioning as measured by standardized tests or if comorbid ID guides the outcome of such individuals. Therefore, more research needs to be conducted with individuals diagnosed with an ASD in the absence of ID while focusing on IQ as a predictor.

Another useful predictor of later outcome in those with ASD is language ability (Howlin et al., 2004; Mawhood, Howlin, & Rutter, 2000; Nordin & Gillberg, 1998). In general, those who do not develop communicative speech by 5–6 years of age have a poorer prognosis. However, with the implementation of educational lessons to teach language to nonverbal children with ASD, it is possible for these individuals to attain later language abilities (Howlin, 2005). As these strategies have been employed more frequently in recent years, it is possible that the cutoff age for achievement of communicative speech, which influences prognosis, has been increasing. As a result, further research is warranted to investigate the prognosis for individuals who begin displaying language abilities at later ages in childhood.

Although specific self-help skills, also known as activities of daily living (ADLs), are not expressly included in outcomes studies, these affect an individual's ability to achieve full independence. ADLs vary widely in the adult ASD population with comorbidity of ID also playing a major role. When comparing the ADLs of adults with ASD versus those with a developmental receptive language disorder, adults with ASD presented with significantly lower scores despite the groups being matched on nonverbal IQ (Howlin, Mahwood, & Rutter, 2000). Overall, ADLs dealing with hygiene, dressing, and eating were found to be significantly poorer in the ASD group relative to the language disorder group. In fact, only 38.9% of adults in the ASD group achieved at least adequate overall functioning with ADLs. Furthermore, only 27.8% of the ASD group demonstrated full independence when money management and transportation were also taken into consideration. The remaining 72.2% did not achieve full independence. Likewise, Matson, Dempsey, and Fodstad (2009) found that adults with comorbid ASD and ID displayed significantly greater deficits in dressing, grooming, and hygiene than did adults with ID alone. Only in grooming were there significant differences between adults with autistic disorder and pervasive developmental disorder, not otherwise specified, with the autistic disorder group presenting with greater deficits. Although bathing, housekeeping, and meal preparation did not significantly differ among groups, all of the groups demonstrated impairment in each domain.

Many researchers have investigated the adolescent and adulthood outcomes of individuals with ASD (Ballaban-Gil, Rapin, Tuchman, & Shinnar, 1996; Gillberg & Steffenburg, 1987; Kobayashi, Murata, & Yashinaga, 1992; Szatmari, Bartolucci, Bremner, Bond, & Rich, 1989). Overall, these studies have concluded that outcomes for adults with ASD are generally "very poor" to "fair." One of the largest longitudinal studies following individuals with ASD from childhood through adulthood, with 120 participants, found that 78% of the individuals had either "very poor" or "poor" outcomes (Billstedt, Gillberg, & Gillberg, 2005). The remainder of the participants were considered to have "fair" outcomes with no participants achieving a "good" outcome status. Consistent with previously discussed predictive variables, individuals' prognoses were highly correlated with their IQ scores as well as the presence of communicative speech by 6 years of age.

Another longitudinal study assessed 48 individuals with ASD, from 19 through 31 years of age, with a mean age of 24, via telephone interviews with caregivers (Eaves & Ho, 2008). In this sample, approximately half of the young adults had a "fair" or "good" outcome while the remaining half were labeled as having "poor" outcomes. These outcomes were based on employment, social relationships, and independence and were each rated on a 0 (*very good*) to 3 (*very poor*) scale. A global outcome rating, from 0 (*very good*) to 11 (*very poor*), was then computed from these scores. Once again, IQ scores, both verbal and performance, correlated with overall better outcome later in life. It is important to note that this study looked at the relationship between outcomes and IQ and ASD severity for children and adolescents (ages ranging from 8 to 17 years of age), but not young adults. Despite this limitation, this study still provides useful information in terms of prognosis. Moderate negative correlations of −0.58 and −0.56 were found between verbal and performance IQ, respectively, and overall outcome. It should also be noted that ASD severity ratings combined with those of IQ did not indicate a statistically significant relationship. Therefore, it does not appear that the severity of ASD directly influences later outcome above and beyond IQ.

As it is accepted that individuals with ASD with low IQ scores generally have poor outcomes, another study looked specifically at individuals with IQ scores above 50 (Howlin et al., 2004). Out of this sample, 22% had "very good" or "good" outcomes, 19% had "fair" outcomes, and the remaining 58% had "poor" or "very poor" outcomes. Once again, outcomes were based on employment status, social relationships, and overall independence. Correlations between adult outcome and verbal and performance IQ were 0.81 and 0.66, respectively. Thus, these findings demonstrated that as verbal and performance IQ increased, so did adult outcomes. Additionally, the authors noted that individuals with an IQ score representing no ID (i.e., > 70), were the group most likely to have good outcomes. This finding appears to coincide with previous research stating that individuals with ID, with or without an ASD, are more likely to have poor outcomes as adults (Nordin & Gillberg, 1998).

The aforementioned findings describe outcomes mainly based on achievement of independence as well as the attainment of social relationships. Based on these criteria, the overall outcome for individuals with ASD is fair at best (Ruble & Dalrymple, 1996). The majority of adults with ASD will continue to require structured support networks and repeated instruction with socialization and communication skills. Yet, knowledge of this information still leaves many questions about adulthood unanswered. Therefore, Ruble and Dalrymple (1996) suggest assessing outcome from a different point of view. They posit that predictive variables should include the individual's strengths and weaknesses, advocates and support networks, others' perceptions of competence, the individual's perception of his or her quality of life, and stressors. When these predictive variables are used, with related constructs being the determinants of outcome, the outcome for individuals increases and can more likely be labeled as "good."

Living Arrangements

As individuals with ASD approach adulthood, a time at which most individuals gain their full independence and begin the transition from living at home with their family to living on their own, many lifestyle choices need to be made. Unfortunately, very little is reported about the residential opportunities for adults with ASD, much less the advantages and disadvantages of alternative placements. Therefore, much of the current information regarding residential options for adults with ASD is derived from literature discussing the variety of placements available for those with ID. Given the high comorbidity of these two disorders and the overall impact ID has on the outcome of adults with ASD, as was reviewed previously, it appears appropriate to employ these resources initially developed for individuals with ID when attempting to find a suitable placement for adults with ASD.

In most cases, the preferred option for living arrangements is complete independence (e.g., living in an apartment without assistance). However, based on prognosis, this is not usually a viable option. Only about 10% of individuals with ASD are able to achieve such a residential status in adulthood (Billstedt et al., 2005; Eaves & Ho, 2008; Howlin et al., 2004; Larkin, 1997). Most individuals with ASD who achieve independent living are higher functioning (i.e., those with Asperger's disorder or HFA). When looking at adults with HFA ranging from 17 to 31 years of age, approximately 33% were able to live independently (Szatmari et al., 1989).

When independent living is not possible, another common living arrangement is for the adult to continue living with his or her family. Researchers have found that this co-residential living arrangement supports a third to more than half of adults with ASD (Eaves & Ho, 2008; Howlin et al., 2004; Krauss, Seltzer, & Jacobson, 2005; Szatmari et al., 1989). Although this option may not appear optimal, mothers of adults with ASD who co-reside with their son or daughter reported many positive factors, including the ability to spend time with their child, certainty of good care, and a general "peace of mind" (Krauss et al., 2005). However, mothers also reported negative factors, such as having to frequently manage challenging behaviors and provide constant support.

Furthermore, this co-residency arrangement cannot be considered permanent. Although mortality rates are doubled within the ASD population (Shavelle, Strauss, & Pickett, 2001), many individuals outlive their parents. Therefore, parents will generally be unable to support their son or daughter throughout adulthood. Given this information, the family needs to plan for alternative placements early on, so that when they are no longer able to care for their child there can be a more seamless transition. Even when future alternative placements are arranged through early planning, this future transition may still be difficult for the individual due to the core symptoms of ASD severely impeding the ability for these individuals to make smooth transitions.

Although institutions, including psychiatric hospitals and developmental centers, are among the less preferred options of living for adults with ASD, these facilities are frequently found to support such individuals and are often necessary for more medically fragile adults. Within the institutions category, there are different levels of restriction. For example, developmental centers would be considered a less restrictive environment than psychiatric hospitals. However, as a collective group, these facilities are regarded as the most restrictive environments. Individuals living within these settings generally require more extensive supports than those living within the community. Although deinstitutionalization efforts and promotion of increased independent living have now been in effect for several decades (Wilson, Reid, & Green, 2006), up to 70% of adults with ASD are institutionalized at some point in their lives (Howlin et al., 2004; Larkin, 1997). In fact, although there has been an emphasis on deinstitutionalization within Western countries, Taiwan has actually experienced an increase in the number of individuals with disabilities residing in institutions (Yen, Lin, Wu, & Kang, 2009).

When out-of-home living is required, but an institution is not necessary or preferred, a somewhat less restrictive and more community-based lifestyle exists. Overall, it is estimated that 25% of individuals with ASD may demonstrate improvements in skills required for independent living over time, but still require supervision as adults (Larkin, 1997). As such, group homes may be more appropriate for these individuals. In general, group homes support several adults within one home where individuals typically either have their own bedroom or one roommate while family areas such as living rooms, dining rooms, bathrooms, and kitchens are shared. Residential staff assist the individuals throughout the day and night in completing ADLs, housekeeping duties, transportation services, and meaningful activities, among other essential and preferred activities. Although many of the services provided within group homes are similar to those provided within institutional settings, the individuals are generally more immersed within the community, and residents share the living quarters with fewer peers.

Given the popularity of research reviewing deinstitutionalization among those with developmental disabilities (Matson & Boisjoli, 2009), the majority of research comparing the advantages and limitations of different residential placements focuses on the differences between institutions and community placements, namely group homes. In general, group homes are frequently reported to have more advantages than institutional living arrangements. Group homes tend to have higher staff to resident ratios than institution settings, thus increasing the availability of one on one attention for residents (Hundert, Walton-Allen, Vasdev, Cope, & Summers, 2003). Additionally, findings within the developmental disabilities population suggest that group home residents appear to posses greater adaptive behavior functioning (Spreat, Conroy, & Rice, 1998) and increased family contact (Spreat & Conroy, 2002). Although a better quality of life may be observed in group home residents compared to institution residents, a change in environment does not necessarily improve all aspects of life. For example, the presence of challenging behaviors, such as physical aggression and self-injury, was not significantly different among 17 adult individuals with developmental disabilities who transitioned from an institution to group homes (Hundert et al., 2003).

Additionally, individuals residing in institutions compared to group homes in Israel appeared to have a lower rate of certain diseases, including cardiovascular difficulties and diabetes (Lifshitz, Merrick, & Morad, 2008). The authors attributed this finding to differences in lifestyles and the availability of medical resources within such settings. However, it should be noted that these authors also found other pertinent issues (e.g., psychiatric and digestive) to occur more frequently within institutional settings. Since institutions are more equipped to manage severe medical and behavioral problems, this difference may be due to placements being predetermined based on the prevalence of such issues.

When residential and group home options are deemed too restrictive and independent living and co-residency are not feasible, another more recent choice is supported independent living (SIL). In SIL the individuals live in their own apartment or house and receive supports (e.g., skills training, transportation) from staff who work with them for specified periods of time. Individuals may have roommates in SIL, but unlike group homes, staff are generally not available throughout the entire day and night. The number of hours of support received varies depending on an individual's needs and level of independence. Researchers have demonstrated that individuals in SIL placements are presented with a larger variety of community activities and more frequent opportunities to participate in such activities compared to residential facilities (e.g., institutions or group homes) (Howe, Horner, & Newton, 1998). With this larger emphasis on community participation, a wider social network is created. However, other researchers have suggested that severely developmentally disabled individuals in SIL may not receive sufficient opportunities to engage in leisure activities while at home (Wilson et al., 2006). During baseline observations of three individuals residing in SIL, no resident was found to be actively engaged with preferred activities while at home. However, following implementation of an intervention requiring staff to present potentially preferred activities in pairs to the resident, residents were observed engaging in leisure activities while at home more than 50% of the observed time. This suggests that SIL placements may only be an improvement over other placements if residential staff are accurately trained and supervised. However, given the typical supervisory environment of SIL and other less restrictive environments (e.g., group homes), frequent observations and feedback are not always possible (Harchik & Campbell, 1998).

Although residential options may seem limited at first glance, there are actually a variety of available options. However, eligibility requirements vary depending on regions, as do financial costs. This information needs to be coupled with a weighing of the potential benefits of each living arrangement so that an appropriate placement can be made. No single residential status can be considered best for all adults with ASD as individual characteristics and needed supports vary widely. As such, it is recommended that families of adults with ASD research their options and decide what type of residential status would be best for their child as an individual and not simply base placement decisions on which residential status appears the most attractive.

Transition from High School to College

Prior to beginning employment, many young adults attend college to determine what their future career goals are and to enhance their knowledge in that selected area. Adults with ASD are frequently unable to attain post-secondary education, which is often a result of the high rate of ID comorbidity discussed earlier. However, in cases of HFA and Asperger's disorder, individuals tend to function within the normal limits of intellectual functioning or above. As more recent laws require that children with ASD receive appropriate education (i.e., Individuals with Disabilities Education Act, PL 108-446), there has been an increase in high school attendance in this population. This increase in secondary education may help these young adults be more eligible to attend institutions of higher education than in the past (MacLeod & Green, 2009; VanBergeijk, Klin, & Volkmar, 2008). Not only has their ability to attend college increased, but also many individuals with ASD express an interest in doing so (VanBergeijk et al., 2008). As such, an increased interest in post-secondary education within this population has emerged. Thus, the service provisions required to assist this population in successfully completing college degrees need to be considered.

Individuals with ASD present with unique academic difficulties, such as issues arising from impairment in executive functioning (Holmes & Chaffee, 2007; MacLeod & Green, 2009; VanBergeijk et al., 2008). Individuals may struggle with organizational skills, time management, problem solving, and the ability to complete large, complex tasks. In high school settings, adolescents with ASD typically receive specialized services and teachers are available to identify and assist students in managing these difficulties. However, college requires more independence in a less individualized atmosphere. For instance, while high school education typically consists of small classrooms where individualized attention is readily available when needed, college courses are often composed of up to several hundred students per lecture or seminar. In these cases, students are expected to identify problems that may arise and seek out assistance from the professor, which may be difficult for individuals with ASD (MacLeod & Green, 2009). Additionally, professors do not often collaborate with each other like high school teachers do, so as to avoid conflicting deadlines for assignments and to share effective teaching strategies.

Therefore, it is critical to address these executive functioning issues to promote success in the individual. Utilization of colors and sub-dividers can be encouraged in order to increase organizational skills (VanBergeijk et al., 2008). Time management can be taught by providing individuals with planners, calendars, or electronic devices, so that deadlines are known and can be visualized (Holmes & Chaffee, 2007; VanBergeijk et al., 2008). In more severe cases, it may be necessary for the college to accommodate the student by providing a specialist to meet with the student regularly in order to assist in organizational and time management tasks (Holmes & Chaffee, 2007; MacLeod & Green, 2009). When this occurs, the specialist can also serve as a liaison between the student and his or her professors. The student should also be taught skills to break large, complex tasks into small, more manageable units (MacLeod & Green, 2009; VanBergeijk et al., 2008).

In addition to difficulties related to executive functioning, socialization deficits and insistence on routines that are characteristic of ASD continue to persist throughout adulthood. These problems have the potential to hinder a successful college transition as well as impede the ability to build new support networks. College life lacks the individual support high school provides for a variety of skills, including socialization skills. Also, if the individual lives away from home, the previously available family support network will no longer be readily accessible (Glennon, 2001; MacLeod & Green, 2009). Therefore, socialization impairments that were previously mediated by family support may become more prominent. As such, it is critical that the individual learns how to socialize appropriately in order to form new relationships that may be necessary in navigating through the college social network.

Situations in which appropriate social skills can be pivotal include group projects, mealtimes, and dormitory living (Glennon, 2001). In these situations, social stories may be extremely effective in improving socialization skills of those with adequate cognitive functioning and language skills (Gray & Garand, 1993). Social skills may become even more important if the student chooses to live on campus as he or she will most likely acquire a roommate. This may be a relationship that the individual has not previously experienced. Therefore, prior to attending post-secondary education, the individual should begin correspondence with his or her future roommate (Glennon, 2001). By beginning this relationship early, the individual may have a more successful transition into dormitory life. However, it should be recognized that some adults with ASD have been able to form friendships more easily at college, which has been attributed to the increase in diversity of many college campuses (Holmes & Chaffee, 2007).

In order to help prevent some of the aforementioned possible causes for setbacks, the transition process from high school to college should be addressed early on with accommodations being put in place as needed. It may be ideal for the individual to be exposed to college while still attending high school (VanBergeijk et al., 2008). For example, some school districts in New York have included an extra year in the individual's Individualized Education Plan, referred to as the 13th grade. During this year, students enroll in one to two college courses at a nearby community college while remaining in high school for part of the day. This is done to make the transition from high school to college a more gradual process while providing necessary supports.

Once enrolled in college, further supports should be offered and implemented if needed. This can be accomplished through service provisions offered by an institution's disability team (MacLeod & Green, 2009). Unfortunately, many individuals with Asperger's disorder and HFA may not readily disclose their disability, which limits the potential effectiveness of these service provisions. If an individual's disability is not initially disclosed, services can still be provided in the future; however, these services may not be immediately available once requested. Therefore, it is recommended that young adults with ASD who wish to acquire further education disclose their disability to the appropriate departments so that they can obtain provided supports which help increase their success. In cases in which post-secondary education is neither required nor feasible due to current levels of functioning, individuals may benefit more from vocational training which aids in attainment of specific employment.

Employment

Employment is an important aspect of life. It not only provides monetary compensation to support living expenses but also offers a social network and a sense of accomplishment. It has long been recognized that adults with a variety of developmental disabilities, including ASD, can acquire new skills that can be utilized in the work force. Although everyone has the potential to contribute in the work environment, individuals with ASD often require additional supports due to hindrances caused by the core symptoms of the disorder and associated features (e.g., challenging behaviors, sensory concerns). Individuals with ASD often present with impairments in understanding social situations, communication deficits, a restricted range of activities or interests, and insistence on sameness (APA, 2000). These influence an individual's ability to successfully interact with co-workers and clients, facilitate successful work experiences, as well as impact an individual's ability to cope with change in the workplace. Further impairing work performance and abilities, up to 70% of individuals with an ASD also present with ID (La Malfa et al., 2004; Matson & Shoemaker, 2009). Just as individuals with an ASD diagnosis are heterogeneous, the type and level of supports required are also varied.

In the United States there are several government acts which provide individuals with disabilities, including

ASD, equal access to education, employment, transportation, and other services necessary for living in today's world. These acts include the Americans with Disabilities Amendments Act of 2008 (PL 110-325), the Individuals with Disabilities Education Act of 2004 (PL 108-446), and the Rehabilitation Act Amendments of 1998 (PL 105-220). The Americans with Disabilities Amendments Act of 2008 and the Rehabilitation Act Amendments of 1998 relate more specifically to adults with ASD as these acts provide for the appropriate service provision and anti-discrimination laws that allow this population access to equal employment opportunities. For adults with ASD, these laws provide vocational training services, such as supported employment, through a government office of vocational rehabilitation. Adults with ASD receive eligibility for services through vocational rehabilitation if they require extra supports to obtain or retain employment, if their symptoms of ASD hinder employment in any manner, or if they are eligible for Social Security Disability Insurance (Quirk, Zeph, & Uchida, 2007). Australia and European countries have similar legislation providing employment supports to those with disabilities (O'Brien & Dempsey, 2004).

Currently, the preferred employment model is supported employment. Supported employment provides supports to individuals with disabilities in an integrated work setting where the main goal is independent competitive employment (Office of Disability Employment Policy, n.d.; Uchida, 2007). It is important to understand that competitive employment is not guaranteed employment. Rather it is employment in an integrated environment where a person has to compete with others to obtain a position. Unlike the various types of supported employment, no additional supports are provided in the workplace with competitive employment.

There are various types of supported employment which differ in the level of supports provided (i.e., individual placement, clustered/enclave, mobile crew, or entrepreneurial). The different levels of support allow this form of employment to be feasible for all adults with ASD. Some adults with ASD require more constant supports due to severe challenging behaviors, comorbid psychiatric disorders, and more severe intellectual impairment. In order to be considered supported employment, the job must occur in an integrated setting with individuals without disabilities where natural and/or artificial support is provided to help the individual maintain his or her job, and salary as well as vacation time are similar to that of individuals without disabilities holding similar jobs (Office of Disability Employment Policy, n.d.). Natural supports, or workplace supports, are supports that naturally occur at the job site (Brooke, Inge, Armstrong, & Wehman, 1997). Natural supports include such elements as co-worker support, supportive family members, and volunteers from the community (West, Kregel, Hernandez, & Hock, 1997), whereas artificial supports include training

from a job coach. Use of natural supports was reported by 85% of supported employment programs who indicated that these supports were not only effective in the majority of cases (81.8%), but also helped decrease costs (West et al., 1997). Training stemming from artificial supports focuses on building skills, often with the use of task analysis to determine which skills the individual already possesses and which skills the individual needs to improve upon to complete his or her job successfully (Brooke et al., 1997).

Task analysis informs job coaches about an individual's ability to complete distinct actions that comprise an overall skill. In conducting a task analysis, the whole task is deconstructed into more manageable discrete tasks. Then the individual is observed performing each discrete task. For example, a task of stocking shelves can be broken down into many smaller steps: wheeling the cart with supplies, identifying and going to the correct isle, identifying the correct location in the isle, picking up the item using correct form, putting the item on the shelf in the correct manner, repeating the necessary steps until the specified shelves are full, returning the cart to the stockroom, and contacting the job supervisor. In an effort to promote independent completion of the overall task, the individual would then receive further training for specific steps he or she was unable to complete independently.

Task analysis helps inform not only skills training but also what supports the individual will benefit from in the workplace. When teaching skills to complete workplace duties, behavioral techniques, similar to those discussed previously, are recommended. Recently, video modeling has been used in conjunction with behavioral techniques to enhance training. Video modeling has proven effective in increasing a variety of skills among those with ASD (Delano, 2007; Weiss, LaRue, & Newcomer, 2009), including skills that are beneficial to the workplace. Traditional video modeling entails having an individual watch a video of another individual demonstrating how to perform a skill or part of a skill. Then the individual is prompted to do the same task as the video demonstrated. Another form of video modeling is video self-modeling, where the individual watches himself or herself perform a task. This type of video modeling has proven effective in increasing functional skills and behavior among a variety of children (Hitchcock, Dowrick, & Prater, 2003); however, studies have not found it more effective than traditional video modeling (Sherer et al., 2001). Further research is necessary to determine the usefulness of video self-modeling in increasing work-related tasks among adults with ASD. Overall, task analysis, behavioral methods, and the use of technology to increase skills are useful in increasing skills for individuals in all forms of supported employment.

The most independent model of supported employment is individual placement. Individual placement is for the most independent individuals with ASD and entails working in an integrated setting and performing job tasks with the help of a job coach (Gerhardt & Holmes, 2005; Keel, Mesibov, & Woods, 1997). Although more adults with ASD are increasing their wages through supported employment, many of these individuals tend to work and take breaks alone (Rogan, Banks, & Howard, 1999). A job coach not only helps facilitate interactions with co-workers but also assists in skills training, locating and obtaining the job, and training co-workers on how to best interact with the individual. Through teaching co-workers about ASD and training them on how to best interact with individuals with ASD, job coaches increase the availability of natural supports. Although a job coach may initially provide intensive on-the-job training, this training is faded over time as skills improve.

Wehman and Kregel (1985) discuss four components of supported employment that should be provided in individual placement: (1) job placement, (2) advocacy and training, (3) monitoring, and (4) job retention. Job placement consists of finding a match between a job and the individual's abilities and interests, as well as organizing transportation. In determining job match, it is important to take into consideration not only the individual's skills but also their preferences. Researchers have demonstrated that when jobs are allocated based on an individual's preferences, there is greater on-task behavior and accuracy (Kern et al., 1998). Preference assessments have been able to predict future engagement in job tasks (Lattimore, Parsons, & Reid, 2003; Reid, Parsons, & Green, 1998). Yet, they have been better able to predict choice in job tasks among individuals who consistently choose a task throughout preference assessments than among adults with weaker preferences (Lattimore et al., 2003). Choice in work schedule and the order of task completion have also increased on-task behavior and accuracy (Kern et al., 1998; Watanabe & Sturmey, 2003).

The types of jobs adults with ID have obtained include employment in the food services, janitorial, clerical, retail, warehouse, manufacturing, grounds keeping, sorting, and childcare (Mank, Cioffi, & Yovanoff, 2003). Researchers have found that adults with ASD have found jobs working with computers, in the food services (e.g., cleaning dining areas, serving food, setting tables), in clerical settings (e.g., copying, labeling, checking documents), stocking shelves at community stores, as custodial staff in a variety of settings, as lab technicians cleaning and preparing research materials, and in manufacturing (e.g., assembly line type job), among other jobs (Howlin, Alcock, & Burkin, 2005; Keel et al., 1997; Mawhood & Howlin, 1999).

The second concern after job placement is job site advocacy and training of the individual, which entails behavioral-based methods to increase an individual's skills and performance specific to a job, as well as training co-workers on how to best help the supported individual (Wehman & Kregel,

1985). The third component consists of ongoing monitoring of an individual's performance at work and the individual's job satisfaction. Behavioral data as well as feedback from the employer should be utilized. The final component relates to job retention and follow-up. In this final component, the focus is on fading staff intervention at the job site. However, information regarding the individual's work performance should continue to be obtained through communication with the employer and through periodic observations at the job site. Helping the individual find new employment also falls under this final component (Wehman & Kregel, 1985).

The next type of supported employment is single or dispersed clustered/enclave placement. In this placement a job coach works with a small group of individuals, approximately two to six individuals per group, who all work at the same job site (single model) or at different sites within the same company (dispersed model). This type of placement is best suited for individuals who require daily, but not constant, supports to function appropriately at work (Keel et al., 1997) since the job coach provides daily training and additional supports. For individuals who require even more supports to be successful in the work place, a mobile crew model of supported employment may be utilized. In this model of supported employment, a job coach provides constant supervision to a small number of individuals, approximately three to four. Although jobs are in an integrated setting, social interaction with other non-disabled co-workers is minimal. Mobile crew jobs are typically contracted jobs from the private sector, such as janitorial work (Gerhardt & Holmes, 2005).

Another type of supported employment is entrepreneurial (Gerhardt & Holmes, 2005). In the entrepreneurial model a for-profit organization is developed based on the interests and skills of a small group of individuals with disabilities, up to approximately six individuals (Office of Disability Employment Policy, n.d.). For this small business model to be considered supported employment, the business needs to employ an equal or greater number of employees without disabilities (Office of Disability Employment Policy, n.d.). A limitation is that start-up costs are high and there is no guarantee of a profit to pay the individuals and for the individuals that support them in this job (Gerhardt & Holmes, 2005).

In the United States the number of supported employment agencies increased from 324 to 3,739 during 1986–1993 (Wehman & Revell, 1996). With the increase in the number of supported employment programs, the number of individuals served across all of the states and territories of the United States increased from 10,000 to 105,000 during 1986–1993. Reports from 1993 indicated that the majority of supported employment programs utilized the individual placement model (79%). Only 21% used a group model (e.g., clustered/enclave or mobile crew). From 1986 to 1993, programs focusing on individual placement increased from 52.1

to 79%. This increase is likely due to the fact that this form of supported employment costs less to implement and allows greater financial gain for the individual and society compared to other forms of supported employment (Wehman & Revell, 1996).

Although many adults with disabilities, including ASD, are being served through supported employment programs, in 2005 the rates of unsuccessful employment closure (i.e., they did not obtain a job) were one and a half times higher than successful employment closure for adults with autistic disorder being served through vocational rehabilitation government programs (Uchida, 2007). In 2003, only 719 (61%) adults with autistic disorder successfully found employment through the vocational rehabilitation system (Uchida, 2007). Unfortunately, research conducted by the Rehabilitation Services Administration only focused on one subtype of ASD, autistic disorder, rather than on the various subtypes or ASD as a whole. Using a specialized supported employment for adults with HFA or Asperger's disorder in the United Kingdom, these adults were more apt to obtain paid employment (63.3%) than a matched control group (25%) who only had access to "generic" employment services (Mawhood & Howlin, 1999). An 8-year follow-up of these same individuals found that 68% in the specialized supported employment program had paid employment, mostly in technical, computing, and administrative-type jobs (Howlin et al., 2005). This indicates that to provide more successful work situations, more specialized supported employment programs should be used for adults with ASD.

Despite the notion that supported employment is considered more financially viable in the long run for the individual and society (McCaughrin, Ellis, Rusch, & Heal, 1993; Wehman & Revell, 1996), other forms of employment, such as secure or sheltered employment, are frequently used. Other interchangeably used terms for sheltered employment include sheltered workshops, affirmative industries, vocational workshops, rehabilitation workshops, training workshops, and workshops (Migliori, Mank, Grossi, & Rogan, 2007). Jobs in sheltered workshops are guaranteed, non-integrated with typically developing employees, and located in facility-like settings. Job tasks are generally simple and repetitive, and work productivity is typically not emphasized by staff (Levy, 1983). Job tasks are generally contracted from private corporations or the government and include such duties as packaging products (e.g., bird seed, bandages), labeling, and paper shredding.

Sheltered employment work environments were first developed in the 1840s under the notion of providing vocational training in the absence of the frustrations of a typical work environment (Gill, 2005). This was thought to allow for skill development and aid in transition to more integrated employment. However, individuals with disabilities rarely transitioned to other more independent forms of employment. In some studies only 3.5% of individuals working in sheltered workshops transitioned to more community-integrated work environments (Taylor, 2002). Furthermore, adults working in sheltered workshops consistently produce lower wages (Inge, Banks, Wehman, Hill, & Shafer, 1988; Kregel & Dean, 2002; Krupa, Lagarde, & Carmichael, 2003). For example, Krupa and colleagues (2003) found that adults working in sheltered workshops earned no more than $1.00 an hour whereas adults within supported employment earned an average of $6.84 an hour. Other researchers reported that individuals in supported employment earn 250% more than individuals working in sheltered workshops (Kregel & Dean, 2002). Adults in sheltered workshops also tend to receive less training compared to adults in supported employment (Gerhardt & Holmes, 2005), thereby affecting their ability to gain other employment. In conjunction with these findings, adults diagnosed with ID working in more integrated work environments, as compared to sheltered workshops, had greater improvements in social skills, work skills, and money management skills (Inge et al., 1988).

Transitioning from sheltered workshops to supported employment models benefits not only the individual financially and their quality of life but also the society financially (Cimera, 2008; Hill & Wehman, 1983; McCaughrin et al., 1993; Wehman & Revell, 1996). For example, Cimera (2008) found that individuals diagnosed with ID in supported employment required significantly less funding, across 12 fiscal quarters ($6,618.76) than did individuals in sheltered employment ($19,388.04). Therefore, the cost of funding one individual in sheltered employment would support three individuals partaking in supported employment. Although supported employment is beneficial for all individuals with disabilities, research indicates that it is more cost-effective for individuals with mild ID as opposed to severe ID (Cimera, 2000). Also, out of all forms of supported employment, individual placement appears to be the most cost-effective (Cimera, 2000).

Although there has been an increase in supported employment, the majority of individuals with disabilities throughout the United States, up to 76%, are being served in facility-based employment (Migliori et al., 2007). This high percentage of adults with disabilities still being served by secured employment does not appear to be due to preference. Rather, 74% of individuals working in a sheltered workshop reported a desire to work in a community-based job (Migliori et al., 2007). A significantly greater number of adults with ASD utilizing supported employment services found employment (75.3%) compared to controls attempting to gain employment without these services (58.4%; Schaller & Yang, 2005).

The success of supported employment appears to be owed to this process' focus on training of the individual and co-workers; availability of job supports for skills building in communication, socialization, appropriate behavior, and completion of job tasks, as well as inclusion of multiple agencies and family members in the employment process. Duffy, Oppermann, Smith, and Shore (2007) discuss five strategies to enhance supported employment. The first strategy relates to employer relationship and understanding of the individual with ASD. The authors highlight the importance of teaching co-workers about ASD and how to interact and work effectively with these individuals. The second strategy discusses the importance of communication in gaining and retaining employment. Not only is communication training for the adult with ASD necessary, but so are open lines of communication between the individual, employer, job coach, individual's family, and other services providers (e.g., transportation). In fact, other service provision can impact an individual's ability to gain and maintain employment. For instance, many adults with ASD view inadequate transportation as hindering their ability to find employment (State of New Jersey, Adults with Autism Task Force, & Department of Human Services, 2009).

Providing workplace accommodations is the third strategy discussed by Duffy and colleagues (2007). These accommodations include having a job coach and mentor, providing structure for the individual, and altering environmental aspects to enhance job performance (e.g., noise level, lighting). Providing structure for the individual entails allowing for a predictable routine as well as providing supports to aid the individual in remembering his or her job schedule and how to successfully complete job tasks. A fourth strategy is teaching adults with ASD self-advocacy skills so that they can communicate their needs in an appropriate manner. These skills relate to social skills training. Although individuals with ASD are able to learn the skills to complete various types of jobs, they also have difficulty navigating the social aspects of the workplace. To help an adult with ASD become more successful at work, it is important to explain unwritten rules of conduct and expectations. Lastly, the fifth strategy is ensuring that staff providing supports to those with ASD have supports themselves. These supports include continuous education and training so that these agencies and employees can better provide enhanced services to individuals with ASD (Duffy et al., 2007).

Despite the optimism with the implementation of supported employment, there is limited research regarding the best practice of employment among adults with ASD. Future research is required to determine the best way to ensure a job match, develop natural supports, and use video modeling effectively in teaching skills (Hundley & Sullivan, 2007). Future research should also examine the long-term effects of supported employment on adults with ASD. Although individual-supported employment appears to be the most attractive supported employment type, it is not ideal for all individuals with ASD. An individual's specific skills, limitations, and preferences need to be taken into account when determining employment so that the individual is more likely to have success and enjoy his or her job.

Specific Models of Living

As previously discussed, most adults with ASD require living and employment supports. These supports do not exist independently. Rather, agencies support an individual in many aspects of life, including home, work, and transportation. The National Association of Residential Providers for Adults with Autism (NARPAA) lists 26 member agencies across 20 states of the United States (National Association of Residential Providers for Adults with Autism, n.d.) which provide living and employment supports, among other supports. Like many similar agencies and government funded and run residential or developmental centers, these agencies have the philosophy that individuals of any age with ASD can learn and they focus on positive programming. Overall, these agencies take a person-centered approach where employment, living environment, increased skills training, and interventions for challenging behaviors, specific to each individual, are addressed. Despite the recently growing number of agencies providing a variety of services to adults with ASD, this section will focus on farmstead models of living and the Treatment and Education of Autistic Children and related Communication-handicapped CHildren (TEACCH) model.

The first farmstead model for adults with ASD (i.e., Somerset Court) was developed in England by Sybil Elgar in 1974 (Bittersweet Inc., n.d.). Farmstead models provide residential and vocational supports, skills building, and behavioral intervention to adults with ASD. With the establishment of Bittersweet Farms in 1975 in Ohio, the farmstead approach for adults with ASD was transported to the United States (Giddan & Obee, 1996). In 1982, the first homes of Bittersweet Farms were built on an 80-acre farm in Toledo, Ohio (Kay, 1990). Today, Bittersweet Inc. has expanded to three properties: Bittersweet Farms and Bittersweet Pemberville, which provide residential, vocational, and skills-building services, and Betty's Farm which provides transition services, social skills training, and recreational activities (Bittersweet Inc., n.d.). Bittersweet Inc. also provides services for supported living and other specialized services (e.g., community training, advocacy, respite care) (Bittersweet Inc., n.d.). Bittersweet Farms, like all farmstead models, were developed with the notion of providing all the services needed to promote skill acquisition and appropriate behavior in one location with the spirit of collaboration between individuals and staff (Kay, 1990).

The key element making the farmstead model different from others is the central element of the farm lifestyle, with vocational activities revolving around the farm and home life. The notion is that the farm setting provides a variety of activities for individuals with diverse skills and preferences and that the farm's activities are considered meaningful to the individuals because they can see the end results (Bittersweet Inc., n.d.). Furthermore, the farm model is inherent to promoting collaboration. Individuals working at Bittersweet Farms have the opportunity to engage in a variety of work tasks, such as horticulture, animal care, carpentry and woodworking, maintenance, housekeeping, and food preparation (Kay, 1990). Additionally, Bittersweet Farms utilizes a variety of methods to increase the individuals' independence and success, such as environmental organization, meaningful activities, structured programming, behavioral strategies to decrease repetitive behaviors, and activities to enhance interaction (Giddan & Obee, 1996). Since the establishment of Bittersweet Farms, many other farmsteads have emerged throughout the United States. Also, other agencies or models, such as TEACCH which is discussed next, have incorporated elements of the farmstead into their programming.

TEACCH evolved from a research project funded by the National Institute of Mental Health (NIMH), United States Office of Education in 1966 (Mesibov, Schopler, & Sloan, 1983). In 1972, it became the first legally mandated statewide program for children with ASD. TEACCH focuses on the lifelong nature of ASD and provides a continuum of services for children, adolescents, and adults. Adult services currently include residential placement, training on life skills, vocational training and placement, and respite care (Mesibov et al., 1983; Mesibov, Shea, & Schopler, 2006). TEACCH was founded on five principles that were necessary when developing residential and day programs for adolescents and adults with an ASD. These five principles focused on (1) individualized skills training and behavioral intervention programs, (2) utilizing diagnostic evaluation and other assessments according to an individual's development, (3) collaboration between parents and professionals, (4) the use of small, structured classrooms, and (5) specialized services, such as living supports, vocational placement and supports, as well as respite care (Mesibov et al., 1983). Ongoing assessment, similar to other placements, is also an important aspect of TEACCH.

In the late 1970s, as children with ASD became adults with ASD, TEACCH expanded their services to provide for this aging population (Mesibov et al., 2006). Although TEACCH began providing living supports for adults with ASD in 1977, Carolina Living and Learning Center (CLLC), which is a residential program for adults with ASD in North Carolina, was not opened until 1990. The foundation of CLLC was built on (1) continuing services with integration between vocational and residential services at the same location, (2) instilling collaboration between agency, parents, and individuals, and (3) conducting research on the adaptation of techniques used with children with ASD to adults with ASD (Mesibov et al., 2006).

Similar to Bittersweet Farms, CLLC is also located on a farm where aspects of the farmstead model are applied, such as collaborative work between staff and individuals to complete home and farm activities. During the day, individuals who reside at CLLC and who attend day service programs facilitated at the center complete various tasks, including planting, harvesting, cooking, baking, and landscaping (Mesibov et al., 2006). In completing these tasks, a skills-building approach is taken. Tasks that an individual is unable to complete independently are taught to him/her using behavioral methods coupled with structured teaching. Structured teaching utilizes environmental organization, visual cues and schedules to provide structure for activities, routines incorporating flexibility so as to reflect real-life activities, and a predictable sequence of events (Mesibov et al., 2006). These structured teaching techniques are utilized to help enable the individual to gain more skills (Mesibov et al., 2006). As of 2006, only 15 adults lived at CLLC, with an additional five individuals attending its day service program while residing elsewhere (Mesibov et al., 2006).

To assess the success of this model, Persson (2000) examined the long-term gains for individuals in independence, skills, and quality of life. Adults living in homes implementing the TEACCH model had increases in all skill areas, including vocational skills, self-help skills, and interpersonal behavior. Although this study found increases in skills, there was no comparison group. As such, it is unknown whether the supported living environment overall or the specific TEACCH model was the catalyst for the skill increases observed in these individuals. To examine whether individuals living in group homes based on the TEACCH model as compared to other living situations had greater quality of treatment program, parent satisfaction, skills, and behaviors, Van Bourgondien, Reichle, and Schopler (2003) compared individuals living in CLLC, group homes, individual homes, and institutions. Although there were no differences in regard to skill acquisition or challenging behaviors, parents of individuals living at CLLC reported significantly greater satisfaction than parents of individuals living in group homes. Furthermore, CLLC utilized a significantly greater quality of treatment program, in that they used significantly greater amounts of visual structure, assessment and program development focusing on developmental level, behavior management strategies, as well as socialization and communication programming, than all other living placements.

TEACCH also offers a supported employment program, which supports a greater number of adults with ASD than does CLLC. This employment program was initiated in 1989 in conjunction with the North Carolina Vocational Rehabilitation Services and Autism Society of North Carolina (Mesibov et al., 2006) and has served over 300 individuals in gaining employment (Division TEACCH, n.d.). The TEACCH Supported Employment Program, like other employment programs for individuals with disabilities, utilizes several of the employment models previously discussed, including individual placement, enclave, and mobile crews. Placement into a specific model is determined, in part, by the level of supports required by the individual. Additionally, placement is also determined by the predictability of the job and whether the job can be adapted for the individual (Keel et al., 1997).

Although the farmstead and TEACCH models are appealing due to their founding philosophies and focus on assessment, behavioral interventions, skills building, collaboration, training, and continuum of services throughout the lifespan, there is a lack of empirical research to suggest that these models are more beneficial than other currently available placements. This is partially due to the limited research comparing TEACCH and farmstead agency outcomes to outcomes of individuals living in more generic settings. However, this may also be due to the increased focus of all agencies to use empirically supported interventions and person-centered planning. Regardless, these models were innovative at the time of their conception, have inspired service provision around the globe (Carminati, Gerber, Baud, & Baud, 2007), and have affected how we view and implement adult services today.

Relationships and Sexuality

It is often proclaimed that individuals with disabilities, including ASD, possess the same human rights as all other individuals. Although this statement is true, attention is seldom given to rights involving sexuality, love, marriage, romance, and the like. As individuals with ASD approach adolescence and adulthood, these specific human rights need to be addressed while taking into consideration many of the deficits associated with these disorders (e.g., socialization skills and challenging behaviors).

First, it is important to understand that individuals with ASD physically develop in the same manner as those individuals without an ASD, including experiencing puberty (Sullivan & Caterino, 2008). Despite this, it has previously been assumed that adolescents and adults with ASD were sexually unaware, therefore lacking an interest in sex and intimacy. These individuals came to be categorized as being asexual, or worse, sexual deviants (Ailey, Marks, Crisp, & Hahn, 2003). Fortunately, current research has proven that this is no longer considered to be the case.

It is now being found that the majority of adolescents and adults with ASD do show interest in sexuality and do engage in some form of sexual behavior (Hellemans, Colson, Verbraeken, Vermeiren, & Deboutte, 2007; Konstantareas & Lunsky, 1997; Ousley & Mesibov, 1991; Shea & Mesibov, 2005; Van Bourgondien, Reichle, & Palmer, 1997). Based

on interviews with adolescents and adults with HFA compared to those with ID alone, it has been found that although those with ID alone appear to have more experience with sexuality, there are no differences in the individuals' interest in sexuality and both groups are interested in and knowledgeable about this topic (Ousley & Mesibov, 1991). Furthermore, though experience is limited, many individuals with autism do engage in sexual behavior. Most commonly, instances of sexual behavior are expressed through masturbation (Hellemans et al., 2007; Konstantareas & Lunsky, 1997; Ousley & Mesibov, 1991; Van Bourgondien et al., 1997). Through interviews, Ousley and Mesibov (1991) found that 55% of adolescent and adult males with HFA engaged in masturbation at one point in their lifetime, compared to 20% of females. A more recent study found that 42% of males diagnosed with HFA engaged in masturbation (Hellemans et al., 2007). In regard to adults with autistic disorder, 77.8% of men and 33.3% of females engaged in masturbation (Konstantareas & Lunsky, 1997). Other researchers found similar results for all levels of ASD and ID, with findings that 75% of males and 24% of females engaged in masturbation (Van Bourgondien et al., 1997).

Although masturbation is the most common sexual behavior that individuals with ASD engage in, it is not the only sign of their interest in sexuality. Many of the previously discussed studies have also noted that individuals with ASD hold hands, hug, kiss, touch others or have others touch them, and have sexual intercourse (Hellemans et al., 2007; Konstantareas & Lunsky, 1997; Ousley & Mesibov, 1991; Van Bourgondien et al., 1997). Within this population, kissing occurs in 10–86.7% of individuals (Hellemans et al., 2007; Konstantareas & Lunsky, 1997; Ousley & Mesibov, 1991; Van Bourgondien et al., 1997), touching others in 17–46.7% of individuals (Hellemans et al., 2007; Konstantareas & Lunsky, 1997; Van Bourgondien et al., 1997), and attempted or successful sexual intercourse in 4–26.7% of individuals (Hellemans et al., 2007; Konstantareas & Lunsky, 1997; Van Bourgondien et al., 1997). Clearly, these rates are not consistent across studies, indicating that more research is needed to determine more accurate rates. Nevertheless, it is increasingly evident that sexual behaviors involving others, not just masturbation, are expressed by individuals with ASD.

Individuals with ASD also show interest in intimacy and relationships. Although it is not a common finding, researchers demonstrate that some individuals with ASD date, marry, and even have children. In fact, a longitudinal sample looking at 16 adults with HFA found that, in their lifetime, nearly 50% had participated in dating, 25% had dated regularly and had even initiated doing so, and one individual had married (Szatmari et al., 1989). Another study focusing on adults with Asperger's disorder and autistic disorder found that a third of the individuals with Asperger's disorder married and had children while no individuals in the autistic disorder group had done so (Larsen & Mouridsen, 1997). In the Asperger's disorder group, two of the three marriages resulted in divorce after several years of marriage. It is also noteworthy to mention that the individuals who married possessed IQ scores of average intelligence or slightly below. Another outcome study discovered that in a sample of 68 individuals with ASD, all with IQ scores of 50 or above, three had married with one of the marriages ending in divorce (Howlin et al., 2004). Based on these studies, it is evident that although marriage is not frequently seen among individuals with ASD, it does occur and IQ may be a good predictor of this possibility.

Given this current knowledge demonstrating that individuals with ASD have interest in sexuality and intimate relationships, it is necessary that sexual education be offered to this population. Without the implementation of such programs and workshops, sexuality may continue to be deemed taboo with those engaging in such behaviors receiving negative attention. Until recently, adapted sexual education programs existed for those with developmental delay in general and ID. However, these programs are not always sufficient for use with the ASD population as many aspects of ASD, such as socialization deficits, are not taken into account (Sullivan & Caterino, 2008). Yet many of the lesson topics ascribed for intellectually disabled and developmentally disabled adults should be taught in sexual education programs for adults with ASD. These topics may include, but are not limited to, sex and sexuality, body part identification, body changes, menstruation, self-esteem, relationships, dating, marriage, intimacy, sexual abuse, masturbation, childbirth, sexually transmitted diseases, contraceptives, and pregnancy (Ailey et al., 2003).

Perhaps what is at the forefront in programs for sexual education for those with ASD is the one operated by Division TEACCH run by the University of North Carolina at Chapel Hill (Sullivan & Caterino, 2008). The population TEACCH serves includes individuals with an ASD of nearly all ages (i.e., approximately 1–60 years of age) as well as those with a variety of levels of intellectual functioning. Specifically, TEACCH's sexual education program is comprised of four levels (Mesibov, 1982). It should be noted that cognitively lower functioning individuals, such as those with profound or severe ID, are only taught the first two levels. The first level is discrimination learning during which individuals are taught when and where to engage in sexual behaviors (e.g., masturbation). Reinforcement and punishment are used to increase appropriate sexual behaviors while decreasing inappropriate ones. The next level focuses on personal hygiene and includes lessons related to menstrual periods, the wearing of deodorant, and proper bathing. Following these two levels, higher functioning individuals (i.e., those functioning with moderate ID or above) learn about body parts and

their functions and then participate in a sexual education program in which heterosexual relationships and sexuality are discussed.

Another sexual education program that has received much attention in the literature is that of Benhaven, located in New Haven, Connecticut (Melone & Lettick, 1983). Benhaven takes a different approach to the topic of sexual education than TEACCH. At Benhaven, individuals are viewed as not possessing an invested interest in sexuality or romantic relationships with others. Rather, this program was designed to educate individuals on appropriate social behavior related to sexuality, such as appropriate touching and environments to engage in masturbation. A sexuality program designed for adults with ID was adapted to better meet the needs of adults with ASD. Sections that were adapted were those relating to communication and socialization skills, which are impaired in the ASD population. To make this sexuality program more appropriate for individuals with ASD, a pilot program was constructed involving six units: (1) identification of body parts, (2) menstruation, (3) masturbation, (4) physical examinations, (5) personal hygiene, and (6) social behavior. Melone and Lettick (1983) reported a good outcome with this program as its participants demonstrated gains in knowledge related to sexuality, such as understanding that it is acceptable to masturbate as long as it is done in private.

Overall, it has come to the attention of researchers, clinicians, and teachers alike that individuals with ASD do engage in sexual behavior and express interest in sexuality. Data continue to support these conclusions; however, more research in the area is needed. As of yet, few specific sexual education programs have been designed, and additional techniques to teach these lessons should be explored. One possible technique that may be useful is the use of social stories (Tarnai & Wolfe, 2008); however, data regarding its effectiveness in these situations is lacking. With the implementation of such programs, individuals with ASD may be better able to understand how their bodies work and what behaviors are appropriate to engage in with and without others.

Concluding Comments

Although the majority of individuals diagnosed with ASD are adults, current literature and services primarily concentrate on children with ASD. Early intervention is imperative; however, since ASD is a life-long disorder that continues to impact individuals into adulthood, it is critical to widen the field's focus to include adults as well. Currently, the preponderance of adults with ASD are suspected to only have a fair prognosis (Ruble & Dalrymple, 1996). This, along with the ever growing adult ASD population, makes it important to examine the current state of adult service provision as well as the multitude of factors affecting adulthood outcome.

Presently, there is an assortment of living and employment options available for adults with ASD which provide these individuals with the skills necessary to increase independence and function in today's society. A variety of services and levels of support are vital since the services required for adults with ASD vary drastically depending on individual skills and preferences. Despite the variety of service options providing a range of supports, from living to vocational, there is a paucity of research on which types of service provision are best for ASD overall and which are best for different sub-types of ASD. To better serve adults with ASD, there is a need for more research to compare the outcomes (e.g., increases in self-help or vocational skills, increases in number of individuals employed, increases in work attendance, and increases in the ability to communicate wants and needs appropriately) of different models of service provision.

It is also important to recognize that although many individuals with ASD function below age level intellectually and adaptively, they do mature into adults and deserve the same rights as everyone else. Therefore, they should be treated with respect and dignity, as well as given as much independence as possible. Additionally, future research should focus on specific interventions and trainings (e.g., sexuality, postsecondary education) to increase appropriate behaviors and quality of life as well as to give these individuals greater opportunities to partake in everyday adult life. Overall, such planning for service provision in adulthood should begin early and take into account an individual's abilities and preferences. By focusing on an individual's overall skill development early in life, one can better help the individual be more independent.

References

Ailey, S. H., Marks, B. A., Crisp, C., & Hahn, J. E. (2003). Promoting sexuality across the life span for individuals with intellectual and developmental disabilities. *The Nursing Clinics of North America, 38*, 229–252.

American Psychiatric Association. (1980). *Diagnostic and statistical manual of mental disorders* (3rd ed.). Washington, DC: Author.

American Psychiatric Association. (2000). *Diagnostic and statistical manual of mental disorders* (4th ed., text revision). Washington, DC: Author.

Americans with Disabilities Amendments Act of 2008 (Pub. L. No. 110-325, 122 Stat. 3553). (2008).

Ballaban-Gil, K., Rapin, I., Tuchman, R., & Shinnar, S. (1996). Longitudinal examination of the behavioral, language, and social changes in a population of adolescents and young adults with autistic disorder. *Pediatric Neurology, 15*, 217–223.

Billstedt, E., Gillberg, C., & Gillberg, C. (2005). Autism after adolescence: Population-based 13- to 22-year follow-up study of 120 individuals with autism diagnosed in childhood. *Journal of Autism and Developmental Disorders, 35*, 351–360.

Bittersweet Inc. (n.d.). *Bittersweet: Serving people with autism.* Retrieved November 4, 2009, from http://home.tbbs.net/semisweet/index.html

Brooke, V., Inge, K., Armstrong, A., & Wehman, P. (1997). *Supported employment handbook: A customer-driven approach for persons with significant disabilities.* Richmond, VA: Rehabilitation Research and Training Center on Workplace Supports.

Carminati, G. G., Gerber, F., Baud, M. A., & Baud, O. (2007). Evaluating the effects of a structured program for adults with autism spectrum disorders and intellectual disabilities. *Research in Autism Spectrum Disorders, 1*, 256–265.

Charlop-Christy, M. H., Carpenter, M., Le, L., LeBlanc, L. A., & Kellet, K. (2002). Using the picture exchange communication system (PECS) with children with autism: Assessment of PECS acquisition, speech, social communicative behavior, and problem behavior. *Journal of Applied Behavior Analysis, 35*, 213–231.

Cimera, R. E. (2000). The cost-efficiency of supported employment programs: A literature review. *Journal of Vocational Rehabilitation, 14*, 51–61.

Cimera, R. E. (2008). The cost-trends of supported employment versus sheltered employment. *Journal of Vocational Rehabilitation, 28*, 15–20.

Delano, M. E. (2007). Video modeling interventions for individuals with autism. *Remedial and Special Education, 28*, 33–42.

Division TEACCH, University of North Carolina School of Medicine (n.d.). *TEACCH autism program.* Retrieved November 10, 2009, from http://www.teacch.com/supportedemployment.html

Duffy, T., Oppermann, R., Smith, M. R., & Shore, S. (2007). Supporting successful employment. In D. W. Dew & G. M. Alan (Eds.), *Rehabilitation of individuals with autism spectrum disorders* (Institute on Rehabilitation Issues Monograph No. 32) (pp. 89–118). Washington, DC: The George Washington University, Center for Rehabilitation Counseling Research and Education.

Eaves, L. C., & Ho, H. H. (2008). Young adult outcome of autism spectrum disorders. *Journal of Autism and Developmental Disorders, 38*, 739–747.

Falcomata, T. S., Roane, H. S., Hovanetz, A. N., & Kettering, T. L. (2004). An evaluation of response cost in the treatment of inappropriate vocalizations maintained by automatic reinforcement. *Journal of Applied Behavior Analysis, 37*, 83–87.

Farmer-Dougan, V. (1994). Increasing requests by adults with developmental disabilities using incidental teaching by peers. *Journal of Applied Behavior Analysis, 27*, 533–544.

Fombonne, E. (2005). The changing epidemiology of autism. *Journal of Applied Research in Intellectual Disabilities, 18*, 281–294.

Foxx, R. M. (2005). Severe aggressive and self-destructive behavior: The myth of the nonaversive treatment of severe behavior. In J. W. Jacobson, R. M. Foxx, & J. A. Mulick (Eds.), *Controversial therapies for developmental disabilities* (pp. 295–310). Mahwah, NJ: Lawrence Erlbaum Associates.

Ganz, J. B., & Simpson, R. L. (2004). Effects on communicative requesting and speech development of the Picture Exchange Communication System in children with characteristics of autism. *Journal of Autism and Developmental Disorders, 34*, 395–409.

Gerhardt, P. F., & Holmes, D. L. (2005). Employment: Options and issues for adolescents and adults with autism spectrum disorders. In F. R. Volkmar, R. Paul., A. Klin., & D. J. Cohen (Eds.), *Handbook of autism and pervasive developmental disorder: Vol. 2. Assessments, interventions, and policy* (3rd ed., pp. 1087–1101). Hoboken, NJ: John Wiley & Sons.

Giddan, J. J., & Obee, V. L. (1996). Adults with autism: Habilitation challenges and practices. *Journal of Rehabilitation, 62*, 72–76.

Gill, M. (2005). The myth of transition: Contractualizing disability in the sheltered workshop. *Disability and Society, 20*, 613–623.

Gillberg, C., & Steffenburg, S. (1987). Outcome and prognostic factors in infantile autism and similar conditions: A population-based study of 46 cases following through puberty. *Journal of Autism and Developmental Disorders, 17*, 272–288.

Glennon, T. J. (2001). The stress of the university experience for students with Asperger syndrome. *Work, 17*, 183–190.

Gray, C. A., & Garand, J. D. (1993). Social stories: Improving responses of students with autism with accurate social information. *Focus on Autism and Other Developmental Disabilities, 8*, 1–10.

Harchik, A. E., & Campbell, A. R. (1998). Supporting people with developmental disabilities in their homes in the community: The role of organizational behavior management. *Journal of Organizational Behavior Management, 18*, 83–101.

Hellemans, H., Colson, K., Verbraeken, C., Vermeiren, R., & Deboutte, D. (2007). Sexual behavior in high-functioning male adolescents and young adults with autism spectrum disorder. *Journal of Autism and Developmental Disorders, 37*, 260–269.

Hill, M., & Wehman, P. (1983). Cost benefit analysis of placing moderately severely handicapped individuals in competitive employment. *Journal of the Association for the Severely Handicapped, 8*, 30–38.

Hitchcock, C. H., Dowrick, P. W., & Prater, M. A. (2003). Video self-modeling intervention in school-based settings. *Remedial and Special Education, 24*, 36–45.

Holmes, D. L., & Chaffee, K. (2007). Transition planning for individuals with autism spectrum disorders. In D. W. Dew & G. M. Alan (Eds.), *Rehabilitation of individuals with autism spectrum disorders* (Institute on Rehabilitation Issues Monograph No. 32) (pp. 15–34). Washington, DC: The George Washington University, Center for Rehabilitation Counseling Research and Education.

Howe, J., Horner, R. H., & Newton, J. S. (1998). Comparison of supported living and traditional residential services in the state of Oregon. *Mental Retardation, 36*, 1–11.

Howlin, P. (2005). Outcomes in autism spectrum disorders. In F. R. Volkmar, R. Paul, A. Klin, & D. Cohen (Eds.), *Handbook of autism and pervasive developmental disorders* (3rd ed., pp. 201–220). New York: John Wiley & Sons.

Howlin, P., Alcock, J., & Burkin, C. (2005). An 8 year follow-up of a specialist supported employment for high-ability adults with autism or Asperger syndrome. *Autism, 9*, 533–549.

Howlin, P., Goode, S., Hutton, J., & Rutter, M. (2004). Adult outcomes for children with autism. *Journal of Child Psychology and Psychiatry, 45*, 212–229.

Howlin, P., Mahwood, L., & Rutter, M. (2000). Autism and developmental receptive language disorder – A follow-up comparison in early adult life II: Social, behavioral, and psychiatric outcomes. *Journal of Child Psychology and Psychiatry, 41*, 561–578.

Hundert, J., Walton-Allen, N., Vasdev, S., Cope, K., & Summers, J. (2003). A comparison of staff-resident interactions with adults with developmental disabilities moving from institutional to community living. *Journal on Developmental Disabilities, 10*, 93–112.

Hundley, A. P., & Sullivan, R. C. (2007). Challenges and recommendations. In D. W. Dew & G. M. Alan (Eds.), *Rehabilitation of individuals with autism spectrum disorders* (Institute on Rehabilitation Issues Monograph No. 32) (pp. 119–134). Washington, DC: The George Washington University, Center for Rehabilitation Counseling Research and Education.

Individuals with Disabilities Education Act of 2004 (Pub. L. No. 108-446, 118 Stat. 2647). (2004).

Inge, K. J., Banks, P. D., Wehman, P., Hill, J. W., & Shafer, M. S. (1988). Quality of life for individuals who are labeled mentally retarded: Evaluating competitive employment versus sheltered workshop employment. *Education and Training in Mental Retardation, 23*, 97–104.

Kay, B. R. (1990). Bittersweet Farms. *Journal of Autism and Developmental Disorders, 20*, 309–321.

Keel, J. H., Mesibov, G. B., & Woods, A. V. (1997). TEACCH-supported employment program. *Journal of Autism and Developmental Disorders, 27*, 3–9.

Kern, L., Vorndran, C. M., Hilt, A., Ringdahl, J. E., Adelman, B. E., & Dunlap, G. (1998). Choice as an intervention to improve behavior: A review of the literature. *Journal of Behavioral Education, 8*, 151–169.

Kobayashi, R., Murata, T., & Yashinaga, K. (1992). A follow-up study of 201 children with autism in Kyushu and Yamaguchi, Japan. *Journal of Autism and Developmental Disorders, 22*, 395–411.

Konstantareas, M. M., & Lunsky, Y. J. (1997). Sociosexual knowledge, experience, attitudes, and interests of individuals with autistic disorder and developmental delay. *Journal of Autism and Developmental Disorders, 27*, 397–413.

Krauss, M. W., Seltzer, M. M., & Jacobson, H. T. (2005). Adults with autism living at home or in non-family settings: Positive and negative aspects of residential status. *Journal of Intellectual Disability Research, 49*, 111–124.

Kregel, J., & Dean, D. (2002). Sheltered vs. supported employment: A direct comparison of long-term earnings outcomes for individuals with cognitive disabilities. In J. Kregel, D. Dean, & P. Wehman (Eds.), *Achievements and challenges in employment services for people with disabilities: The longitudinal impact of workplace supports* (pp. 63–84). Richmond, VA: Virginia Commonwealth University, Rehabilitation Research and Training Center on Workplace Supports.

Krupa, T., Lagarde, M., & Carmichael, K. (2003). Transforming sheltered workshops into affirmative business: An outcome evaluation. *Psychiatric Rehabilitation Journal, 26*, 359–367.

La Malfa, G., Lassi, M., Bertelli, R., Salvini, R., & Placidi, G. F. (2004). Autism and intellectual disability: A study of prevalence on a sample of the Italian population. *Journal of Intellectual Disability Research, 48*, 262–267.

Larkin, M. (1997). Approaches to amelioration of autism in adulthood. *The Lancet, 349*, 186.

Larsen, F. W., & Mouridsen, S. E. (1997). The outcome in children with childhood autism and Asperger syndrome originally diagnosed as psychotic: A 30-year follow-up study of subjects hospitalized as children. *European Child and Adolescent Psychiatry, 6*, 181–190.

Lattimore, L. P., Parsons, M. B., & Reid, D. H. (2003). Assessing preferred work among adults with autism beginning supported jobs: Identification of constant and alternating task preferences. *Behavioral Interventions, 18*, 161–177.

LeBlanc, L. A., Riley, A. R., & Goldsmith, T. R. (2008). Autism spectrum disorders: A lifespan perspective. In J. L. Matson (Ed.), *Clinical assessment and intervention for autism spectrum disorders* (pp. 65–87). Burlington, MA: Academic Press.

Levy, S. M. (1983). School doesn't last forever; then what? Some vocational alternatives. In E. Schopler & G. B. Mesibov (Eds.), *Autism in adolescents and adults* (pp. 133–148). New York: Plenum Press.

Lifshitz, H., Merrick, J., & Morad, M. (2008). Health status and ADL functioning of older persons with intellectual disability: Community residence versus residential care centers. *Research in Developmental Disabilities, 29*, 301–315.

MacLeod, A., & Green, S. (2009). Beyond the books: Case study of a collaborative and holistic support model for university students with Asperger syndrome. *Studies in Higher Education, 34*, 631–646.

Mank, D., Cioffi, A., & Yovanoff, P. (2003). Supported employment outcomes across a decade: Is there evidence of improvement in the quality of implementation? *Mental Retardation, 41*, 188–197.

Matson, J. L. (2007a). Current status of differential diagnosis for children with autism spectrum disorders. *Research in Developmental Disabilities, 28*, 109–118.

Matson, J. L. (2007b). Determining treatment outcome in early intervention programs for autism spectrum disorders: A critical analysis of measurement issues in learning based interventions. *Research in Developmental Disabilities, 28,* 207–218.

Matson, J. L., & Boisjoli, J. A. (2009). An overview of developments in research on persons with intellectual disabilities. *Research in Developmental Disabilities, 30,* 587–591.

Matson, J. L., Dempsey, T., & Fodstad, J. C. (2009). The effect of autism spectrum disorders on adaptive independent living skills in adults with severe intellectual disability. *Research in Developmental Disabilities, 30,* 1203–1211.

Matson, J. L., & Minshawi, N. F. (2006). *Early intervention for autism spectrum disorders: A critical analysis.* Oxford, England: Elsevier Science, Inc.

Matson, J. L., Sevin, J. A., Fridley, D., & Love, S. R. (1990). Increasing spontaneous language in three autistic children. *Journal of Applied Behavior Analysis, 23,* 227–233.

Matson, J. L., & Shoemaker, M. (2009). Intellectual disability and its relationship to autism spectrum disorders. *Research in Developmental Disabilities, 30,* 1107–1114.

Matson, J. L., Wilkins, J., & Gonzalez, M. (2008). Early identification and diagnosis in autism spectrum disorders in young children and infants: How early is too early? *Research in Autism Spectrum Disorders, 2,* 75–84.

Mawhood, L., & Howlin, P. (1999). The outcome of a supported employment scheme for high-functioning adults with autism or Asperger's syndrome. *Autism, 3,* 229–254.

Mawhood, L., Howlin, P., & Rutter, M. (2000). Autism and developmental receptive language disorder – A comparative follow-up in early adult life I: Cognitive and language outcomes. *Journal of Child Psychology and Psychiatry, 41,* 547–559.

McCaughrin, W. B., Ellis, W. K., Rusch, F. R., & Heal, L. W. (1993). Cost-effectiveness of supported employment. *Mental Retardation, 31,* 41–48.

McKeegan, G. F., Estill, K., & Campbell, B. M. (1984). Brief report: Use of nonexclusionary timeout for the elimination of a stereotyped behavior. *Journal of Behavior Therapy and Experimental Psychiatry, 15,* 261–264.

Melone, M. B., & Lettick, A. L. (1983). Sex education at Benhaven. In E. Schopler & G. B. Mesibov (Eds.), *Autism in adolescents and adults* (pp. 169–186). New York: Plenum Press.

Mesibov, G. B. (1982, July). *Sex education for people with autism: Matching programs to level of functioning.* Paper presented at the meeting of the National Society for Children and Adults with Autism, Omaha, NE.

Mesibov, G. B., Schopler, E., & Sloan, J. L. (1983). Service development for adolescents and adults in North Carolina's TEACCH program. In E. Schopler & G. B. Mesibov (Eds.), *Autism in adolescents and adults* (pp. 411–432). New York: Plenum Press.

Mesibov, G. B., Shea, V., & Schopler, E. (2006). *The TEACCH approach to autism spectrum disorders.* New York: Springer.

Migliori, A., Mank, D., Grossi, T., & Rogan, R. (2007). Integrated employment or sheltered workshops: Preferences of adults with intellectual disabilities, their families, and staff. *Journal of Vocational Rehabilitation, 26,* 5–19.

National Association of Residential Providers for Adults with Autism. (n.d.). *Member agencies.* Retrieved November 22, 2009, from http://www.narpaa.org/agencies.asp

Nordin, V., & Gillberg, C. (1998). The long-term course of autistic disorders: Update on follow-up studies. *Acta Psychiatrica Scandinavica, 97,* 99–108.

O'Brien, J., & Dempsey, I. (2004). Comparative analysis of employment services for people with disabilities in Australia, Finland, and Sweden. *Journal of Policy and Practice in Intellectual Disabilities, 1,* 126–135.

Office of Disability Employment Policy. (n.d.). *A world in which people with disabilities have unlimited employment opportunities.* Retrieved November 2, 2009, from http://www.dol.gov/odep/archives/fact/supportd.htm

Ousley, O. Y., & Mesibov, G. B. (1991). Sexual attitudes and knowledge of high-functioning adolescents and adults with autism. *Journal of Autism and Developmental Disorders, 21,* 471–481.

Persson, B. (2000). Brief report: A longitudinal study of quality of life and independence among adult men with autism. *Journal of Autism and Developmental Disorders, 30,* 61–66.

Quirk, C., Zeph, L., & Uchida, D. (2007). Accessing the vocational rehabilitation system. In D. W. Dew & G. M. Alan (Eds.), *Rehabilitation of individuals with autism spectrum disorders* (Institute on Rehabilitation Issues Monograph No. 32) (pp. 55–88). Washington, DC: The George Washington University, Center for Rehabilitation Counseling Research and Education.

Reese, R. M., Sherman, J. A., & Sheldon, J. B. (1998). Reducing disruptive behavior of a group home resident with autism and mental retardation. *Journal of Autism and Developmental Disorders, 28,* 159–165.

Rehabilitation Act Amendments of 1998 (Pub. L. No. 105–220, 112 Stat. 936). (1998).

Reid, D. H., Parsons, M. B., & Green, C. W. (1998). Identifying work preferences among individuals with severe multiple disabilities prior to beginning supported work. *Journal of Applied Behavior Analysis, 31,* 281–285.

Richman, D. M., Wacker, D. P., Asmus, J. M., & Casey, S. D. (1998). Functional analysis and extinction of different behavior problems exhibited by the same individual. *Journal of Applied Behavioral Analysis, 31,* 475–478.

Rogan, P., Banks, B., & Howard, M. (1999). Workplace supports in practice: As little as possible, as much as necessary. *Focus on Autism and Other Developmental Disabilities, 15,* 2–11.

Rosenwasser, B., & Axelrod, S. (2002). More contributions of applied behavior analysis to the education of people with autism. *Behavior Modification, 26,* 3–8.

Ruble, L. A., & Dalrymple, N. J. (1996). An alternative view of outcome in autism. *Focus on Autism and Other Developmental Disabilities, 11,* 3–14.

Rutter, M. (2005). Etiology of autism: Findings and questions. *Journal of Intellectual Disability Research, 49,* 231–238.

Schaller, J., & Yang, N. K. (2005). Competitive employment for people with autism: Correlates of successful closure in competitive and supported employment. *Rehabilitation Counseling Bulletin, 49,* 4–16.

Schreibman, L. (2000). Intensive behavioral/psycho educational treatments for autism: Research needs and future directions. *Journal of Autism and Developmental Disorders, 30,* 373–378.

Schreibman, L. (2005). *The science and fiction of autism.* Cambridge, MA: Harvard University Press.

Seltzer, M. M., Shattuck., P., Abbeduto, L., & Greenburg, J. A. (2004). Trajectory of development in adolescents and adults with autism. *Mental Retardation and Developmental Disabilities, 10,* 234–247.

Shavelle, R. M., Strauss, D. J., & Pickett, J. (2001). Causes of death in autism. *Journal of Autism and Developmental Disorders, 31,* 569–576.

Shea, V., & Mesibov, G. B. (2005). Adolescents and adults with autism. In F. R. Volkmar, R. Paul, A. Klin, & D. Cohen (Eds.), *Handbook of autism and pervasive developmental disorder: Vol. 1. Diagnosis, development, neurobiology, and behavior* (3rd ed., pp. 288–311). New York: John Wiley & Sons.

Sherer, M., Pierce, K. L., Paredes, S., Kisacky, K. L., Ingersoll, B., & Schreibman, L. (2001). Enhancing conversation skills in children with autism via video technology. *Behavior Modification, 25,* 140–158.

Smith, M. D. (1986). Use of similar sensory stimuli in the community-based treatment of self-stimulatory behavior in an adult disabled by autism. *Journal of Behavioral Therapy and Experimental Psychiatry, 17,* 121–125.

Smith, M. D. (1987). Treatment of pica in an adult disabled by autism by differential reinforcement of incompatible behavior. *Journal of Behavioral Therapy and Experimental Psychiatry, 18,* 285–288.

Spreat, S., & Conroy, J. W. (2002). The impact of deinstitutionalization on family contact. *Research in Developmental Disabilities, 23,* 202–210.

Spreat, S., Conroy, J. W., & Rice, D. M. (1998). Improve quality in nursing homes or institute community placement? Implementation of OBRA for individuals with mental retardation. *Research in Developmental Disabilities, 19,* 507–518.

State of New Jersey, Adults with Autism Task Force, Department of Human Services. (2009, October). *Addressing the needs of adults with autism spectrum disorder: Recommendations for a plan of action for the state of New Jersey.* Retrieved December 15, 2009, from http://www.state.nj.us/humanservices/ddd/boards/AATFrpt.pdf

Sullivan, A., & Caterino, L. C. (2008). Addressing the sexuality and sex education of individuals with autism spectrum disorders. *Education and Treatment of Children, 31,* 381–394.

Szatmari, P., Bartolucci, G., Bremner, R., Bond, S., & Rich, S. (1989). A follow-up study of high-functioning autistic children. *Journal of Autism and Developmental Disorders, 19,* 213–225.

Tarnai, B., & Wolfe, P. S. (2008). Social stories for sexuality education for persons with autism/pervasive developmental disorder. *Sexuality and Disability, 26,* 29–36.

Taylor, S. J. (2002, September 2). *Disabled workers deserve real choices, real jobs.* Retrieved December 15, 2009, from http://www.accessiblesociety.org/topics/ecomomics-employment/shelteredwksps.html

Turner-Brown, L. M., Perry, T. D., Dichter, G. S., Bodfish, J. W., & Penn, D. L. (2008). Brief report: Feasibility of social cognition and interaction training for adults with high functioning autism. *Journal of Autism and Developmental Disorders, 38,* 1777–1784.

Uchida, D. R. (2007). Preamble. In D. W. Dew & G. M. Alan (Eds.), *Rehabilitation of individuals with autism spectrum disorders* (Institute on Rehabilitation Issues Monograph No. 32) (pp. vii–xii). Washington, DC: The George Washington University, Center for Rehabilitation Counseling Research and Education.

VanBergeijk, E., Klin, A., & Volkmar, F. (2008). Supporting more able students on the autism spectrum: College and beyond. *Journal of Autism and Developmental Disorders, 38,* 1359–1370.

Van Bourgondien, M. E., Reichle, N. C., & Palmer, A. (1997). Sexual behavior in adults with autism. *Journal of Autism and Developmental Disorders, 27,* 113–125.

Van Bourgondien, M. E., Reichle, N. C., & Schopler, E. (2003). Effects of a model treatment approach on adults with autism. *Journal of Autism and Developmental Disorders, 33,* 131–140.

Watanabe, M., & Sturmey, P. (2003). The effect of choice-making opportunities during activity schedules on task engagement of adults with autism. *Journal of Autism and Developmental Disorders, 33,* 535–538.

Wehman, P., & Kregel, J. A. (1985). A supported work approach to competitive employment of individuals with moderate and severe handicaps. *The Journal for the Association for Persons with Severe Handicaps, 10,* 3–11.

Wehman, P., & Revell, G. W. (1996). Supported employment from 1986 to 1993: A national program that works. *Focus on Autism and Other Developmental Disabilities, 11,* 235–244.

Weiss, M. J., LaRue, R. H., & Newcomer, A. (2009). Social skills and autism: Understanding and addressing the deficits. In J. L. Matson (Ed.), *Applied behavior analysis for children with autism spectrum disorders.* New York: Springer.

West, M. D., Kregel, J., Hernandez, A., & Hock, T. (1997). Everybody's doing it: A national study of the use of natural supports in supported employment. *Focus on Autism and Other Developmental Disabilities, 12,* 175–181.

Wilson, P. G., Reid, D. H., & Green, C. W. (2006). Evaluating and increasing in-home leisure activity among adults with severe disabilities in supported independent living. *Research in Developmental Disabilities, 27,* 93–107.

Wing, L., & Potter, D. (2002). The epidemiology of autism spectrum disorders: Is the prevalence rising? *Mental Retardation and Developmental Disabilities Research Reviews, 8,* 151–161.

Yen, C. F., Lin, J. D., Wu, J. L., & Kang, S. W. (2009). Institutional care for people with disabilities in Taiwan: A national report between 2002 and 2007. *Research in Developmental Disabilities, 30,* 323–329.

Zachor, D. A., Ben-Itzchak, E., Rabinovich, A., & Lahat, E. (2007). Change in autism core symptoms with intervention. *Research in Autism Spectrum Disorders, 1,* 304–317.

Subject Index

A

Aberrant Behavior Checklist (ABC)
  4-point rating scale, 241
Achenbach System of Empirically Based Assessment (ASEBA), 17
Active living with ASD
  ABA, 401
  antecedent physical activity
    closed/discrete movement skills, 403
    exercise, role of, 402–403
    open movement task, 403
    repetitive/stereotypical behaviors, 402
  education-based
    characteristics, 400
    intervention treatments, 400–401
  individualized instruction, 400
  key attitudes, 400
  physical activity skills
    evaluation, 402
    fading, 401
    prompt fading, 402
    recreational activities, 401
  in PRT
    goal of, 406
    language training, 406
    peer-mediated intervention interactions, 407
    physical activity participation, 408
    principles of, 406
    reinforcement use of, 407
    self-monitor performance, 408
    symbolic play, 407
    task variation, 407
  TEACCH program, 403–406
Activities of daily living (ADLs), 523–524
Adaptive and maladaptive behavior scales for CB
  AAIDD, 256
  CBCL, 256
  PDD Behavior Inventory (PDDBI)
    age-standardized scoring, 255
    behavioral dimensions, 255
    domains, related to, 255–256
  SIB-R, 256
  VABS-II, 256
Adaptive Behavior Task Analysis Checklist (ABTAC), 47
Adaptive skills interventions for ASD
  community
    helping others, 344–345
    shopping, 344
  domestic
    picture prompting, 340
    video, 340–341
  inclusion criteria, 339–340
  safety, 345–346

  self-care
    dressing, 342
    eating, 342
    grooming, 341–342
    toilet training, 343–344
Adjustment problems in ASD
  communication and interpretation difficulties, 56
  developmental risk factor, 56
  frequency of, 56–57
  pervasive developmental disorder, 56
  rituals and compulsive behavior, 57
  screening study, 56
  situational stressors, 56
  social interaction, 56
  social rules and conventions, 56
  stressors, 56
  unusual interests, 56
ADLs, *see* Activities of daily living (ADLs)
Adolescents and adults with ASD
  symptom patterns, 167
    comparative studies, 169
    Down syndrome (DS), 168
    identification, 168
    measurement problems, 168
    methodological limitations of studies, 170
Adults with autism
  adulthood, time span, 521
  diagnostic criteria, 521
  employment
    advocacy and training, 529
    Americans with Disabilities Amendments Act, 528
    artificial supports, 528
    communication training, 531
    employer relationship, 531
    enclave placement, 529
    entrepreneurial model, 529
    facility based, 530
    individual placement, 528–529
    Individuals with Disabilities Education Act, 526–528
    jobs, 528–529
    long-term effects, 531
    mobile crew model, 529
    natural supports, 528
    performance monitoring, 529
    Rehabilitation Act Amendments, 528
    secure and sheltered, 530
    self-advocacy skills, teaching, 531
    service provision and anti-discrimination laws, 528
    small business model, 529
    social network and sense of, 527
    Social Security Disability Insurance, 528
    staff supports, 531

Diagnostic instruments for ASD (*cont.*)
- core impairments, 215
- measures
  - ASD-DA, 224–225
  - ASD-DC, 225
  - BFI, 226
  - BISCUIT-Part 1, 225–226
  - PDDBI, 226–227

Diagnostic Interview for Social and Communication Disorders (DISCO)
- items in, 221–222
- psychometric analyses, 222

Differential reinforcement of alternative behavior (DRA), 357–358, 441, 484–485

Differential reinforcement of incompatible behavior (DRI), 356–357, 441

Differential reinforcement of other behavior (DRO), 356, 391, 418–419, 441

Direct observational methods for CB
- antecedent-behavior-consequence, 251
- continuous recording, 251
- interval recording, 251
- latency recording, 251
- momentary time sample recording, 252
- operational definition, 250–251
- partial interval recording, 251–252
- time length observation, 251
- visual product recording, 252
- whole interval recording, 252

Disability, 56

Discrete trial teaching (DTT), 10, 302

DNA replication
- deletion, 78
- duplication, 78
- frameshift mutation, 78
- genes, 78
- insertion, 78
- inversion, 78
- missense mutations, 78
- nonsense mutation, 78
- point mutations, 78
- RNA splicing mutation, 78
- silent mutation, 78

DRA, *see* Differential reinforcement of alternative behavior (DRA)
DRI, *see* Differential reinforcement of incompatible behavior (DRI)
DRO, *see* Differential reinforcement of other behavior (DRO)
Dyskinesia, 239

E

Early and intensive behavioral intervention (EIBI)
- changes in
  - NNT, 334
  - RCI, 333
- children with other diagnosis
  - intellectual disabilities, 334
- curriculum
  - advanced, 325
  - beginning, 325
  - intermediate, 325
- meta-analysis and effect size, 332–333
- moderators and mediators of treatment outcome, 334–335
  - pre-intervention variables and, 335
- multi-site young autism project, 328–330
- outcome study, 328, 330–332
  - LEAP, 327
  - treatment, 326

- principles
  - hand flapping and gazing, 324
  - motivational operations, 324–325
  - reinforcement, 324
- records, 326
- school-aged children, 334
- school integration, 325–326
- teaching methods
  - discrete trial teaching, 325
  - natural environment teaching, 325
  - task analyses and chaining, 325
- treatment, 324

Early detection of ASD
- communication
  - gestural, 200
  - pre-verbal, 200
  - vocal, 200
- diagnoses, 197–198
- EIBI, 197
- joint attention (JA)
  - echoics, 200
  - IJA, 199
  - intraverbals, 200
  - RJA, 199
  - social behavior, 199
  - tacting, 200
- motor and sensory
  - unusual posturing, 200
- response to name, 199
- siblings, risk, 198–199
- signs, early
  - behaviors, categories, 198
  - home videos, investigation of, 198
  - skill regression, 198
  - symptoms, 198

Early diagnosis of ASD
- AAP, recommendations
  - two-level system, 200–201
- awareness, 200

Early infantile autism, 30

Early intensive behavioral intervention (EIBI), 197, 201, 211

Early intervention for ASD, 322
- core deficits, 321
- evidence-based
  - requirements, 323
  - well-established, 323
- programs
  - ABA based, 323–324
  - ESDM, 322–323
  - treatment and education of children, 322

Early Screening of Autistic Traits Questionnaire (ESAT)
- 4 and 14-item, 208
- psychometric properties, 208
- sensitivity and specificity, 209
- studies, 208
- two-stage early screening program
  - diagnostic evaluation, 209
  - training, 209

Early start Denver model (ESDM), 322–323

Education of All Handicapped Children Act, 32

Edward's syndrome, 77

EFAs, *see* Experimental functional analyses (EFAs)

EIBI, *see* Early intensive behavioral intervention (EIBI)

"Emotional refrigeration," 4

Emotions
- recognition in people with ASD

CPSIA information can be obtained
at www.ICGtesting.com
Printed in the USA
LVOW06*1150180917

549085LV00009BA/98/P

9 781441 980649